Disease Control Priorities
in Developing Countries

A WORLD BANK BOOK

Disease Control Priorities in Developing Countries

EDITORS
Dean T. Jamison
W. Henry Mosley
Anthony R. Measham
José Luis Bobadilla

Published for the World Bank
Oxford University Press

Oxford University Press

OXFORD NEW YORK TORONTO
DELHI BOMBAY CALCUTTA MADRAS KARACHI
KUALA LUMPUR SINGAPORE HONG KONG TOKYO
NAIROBI DAR ES SALAAM CAPE TOWN
MELBOURNE AUCKLAND

and associated companies in

BERLIN IBADAN

Published by Oxford University Press, Inc.
200 Madison Avenue, New York, N.Y. 10016
Oxford is a registered trademark of Oxford University Press.

Manufactured in the United States of America
First printing October 1993

The findings, interpretations, and conclusions expressed in this
study are entirely those of the authors and should not be attributed in any manner to the World Bank, to its affiliated
organizations, or to members of its Board of Executive
Directors or the countries they represent.

The maps that accompany the text have been prepared solely for
the convenience of the reader; the designations and presentation of material in them do not imply the expression of any
opinion whatsoever on the part of the World Bank, its
affiliates, or its Board or member countries concerning the
legal status of any country, territory, city, or area, or of the
authorities thereof, or concerning the delimitation
of its boundaries or its national affiliation.

Library of Congress Cataloging-in-Publication Data

Disease control priorities in developing countries / editors, Dean T.
Jamison ... [et al.].
   p.   cm.
   Includes bibliographical references.
   ISBN 0-19-520990-7
   1. Public health—Developing countries. 2. Medicine, Preventive—
Developing countries. 3. Health planning—Developing countries.
I. Jamison, Dean T.   II. International Bank for Reconstruction and
Development.
   [DNLM: 1. Communicable Disease Control—economics. 2. Developing
Countries—economics. 3. Health Policy—economics. 4. Health
Priorities—economics.   WA 110 D611]
RA441.5.D57   1993
614'.42272'4—dc20
DNLM/DLC
for Library of Congress   92-48723
                                                                CIP

DEDICATION

This volume is dedicated to the men and women who, under the leadership of Dr. D. A. Henderson, participated in the World Health Organization's Intensified Smallpox Eradication Programme. The successful completion of that effort in 1977 obviated the need for a chapter on smallpox in this collection.

Contents

All dollar amounts are current U.S. dollars unless otherwise stated.

Preface

Between 1950 and 1990, life expectancy in developing countries increased from forty to sixty-three years with a concomitant rise in the incidence of the noncommunicable diseases of adults and the elderly (Feachem and others 1992). Yet there remains a huge unfinished agenda for dealing with undernutrition and the communicable childhood diseases. These trends lead to increasingly diverse and complicated epidemiological profiles in developing countries. At the same time, new epidemic diseases like AIDS are emerging; and the health of the poor during economic crisis is a source of growing concern. These developments have intensified the need for better information on the effectiveness and cost of health interventions. To assist countries to define essential health service packages, this book provides information on disease control interventions for the commonest diseases and injuries in developing countries.

The decision to undertake this review did not come easily. Several objections were immediately obvious. A review of disease control priorities in developing countries, given the magnitude of that topic, could not simultaneously do justice to the equally critical questions of implementation capacity and of financing. Nor could it cover the full range of tropical endemic diseases in any depth, given the likely resources. The decision was made to go ahead for two reasons. First, because the combined insights of economists, epidemiologists, and clinicians could give valuable guidance in the difficult choices facing decisionmakers in developing countries, aid agencies, and the World Bank. Second, because, for the most part, other reviews did not systematically assess the cost-effectiveness of available interventions. In the one major review that did provide information on cost-effectiveness (Walsh and Warren 1986), the range of diseases covered was restricted predominantly to the important diseases of childhood.

This collection is intended for health practitioners at every level. For health care providers, individual chapters offer preventive and case management guidelines critical to improving the quality of care; health program managers will find sets of chapters on such subjects as maternal and child health related conditions to help them set priorities more objectively. Planners at the district, regional, and national level will find information on how to improve the allocation of resources.

The need for health sector reform is virtually global. Developed and developing countries, centrally planned and market-oriented health systems, successful and flawed health institutions all seem to share two basic attitudes: a profound dissatisfaction with the present organization and financing mechanisms of health care delivery, and a conviction that there are ways to obtain better results with the available resources. To be effective, health-sector reformers will need to review existing services and adapt them to provide the most cost-effective interventions available. This book will meet its purpose if it contributes to this exercise.

The contents of this volume served as a major source of background information for the World Bank's *World Development Report 1993* on health. It is timely that this collection, which serves as a companion and a reference to the Report, should appear so soon after it.

References

Feachem, Richard G. A., Tord Kjellstrom, Christopher J. L. Murray, Mead Over, and Margaret Phillips, eds. 1992. *Health of Adults in the Developing World*. New York: Oxford University Press.

Walsh, Julia, and Kenneth S. Warren, eds. 1986. *Strategies for Primary Health Care: Technologies Appropriate for the Developing World*. Chicago and London: University of Chicago Press.

World Bank. 1993. *World Development Report 1993: Investing in Health*. New York: Oxford University Press.

Acknowledgments

We wish to acknowledge the high degree of support and encouragement we have received from many quarters following the decision to proceed with this review. The World Bank provided the bulk of the resources and the review was a principal activity of the Population and Human Resources Department under Ann Hamilton for four years. The World Health Organization provided invaluable support, mainly through the contributions of a large number of staff members, who either coauthored or reviewed chapters. We are indebted to the Rockefeller Foundation for critical financial support, which enabled us to hold review meetings in Woods Hole in 1990 and at the Bellagio Study and Conference Center on Lake Como in 1992. In 1991, the Centers for Disease Control and Prevention (CDC) hosted a major review meeting for selected chapters in Atlanta; the All-India Institute of Medical Sciences hosted a similar review meeting in New Delhi, early in 1992; and the International Clinical Epidemiology Network (INCLEN) arranged for critical discussion of many chapters at its 1992 annual meeting in Indonesia. This extensive series of reviews contributed greatly to the quality of this collection, and we are much indebted to the sponsoring institutions.

We are also deeply grateful to the many chapter authors and reviewers who worked extremely hard, throughout the long and difficult revision process, with virtually no compensation for their efforts. We wish particularly to acknowledge David Bell, Richard Feachem, and William Foege, who provided extensive and valuable comments. At the risk of omitting others whose contributions were extensive, we also wish to acknowledge major contributions from Jacques Baudouy, Alan Berg, Robert Black, John Briscoe, Guy Carrin, E. Chigan, Joseph Davis, Nicholas Drager, Davidson Gwatkin, Alaya Hammad, Ralph Henderson, Kenneth Hill, Jeffrey Koplan, Jean-Louis Lamboray, Joanne Leslie, Richard Morrow, Philip Musgrove, Richard Peto, Nancy Pielemeier, Barry Popkin, William Reinke, Julia Rushby, Ismail Sirageldin, Eleuther Tarimo, Anne Tinker, and David Werner. Finally, we thank the anonymous peer reviewers at the World Bank for their helpful evaluations of the text; Coni Benedicto and Christopher Wilson for tactical skills in keeping work on track; Joanne Ainsworth for splendid and tactful editing; and Jenepher Moseley for coordinating timely publication.

Contributors

EDITORS

Dean T. Jamison *is a professor of public health and of education at the University of California, Los Angeles. He serves as part-time adviser on population, health, and nutrition to the Latin America and the Caribbean Regional Office at the World Bank.*

W. Henry Mosley *is chairman of the Department of Population Dynamics at the Johns Hopkins School of Hygiene and Public Health.*

Anthony R. Measham *is adviser for population, health, and nutrition in the New Delhi resident mission of the World Bank.*

José Luis Bobadilla *is a senior health policy specialist in the Population, Health, and Nutrition Department at the World Bank.*

AUTHORS

Roy M. Anderson
Center for Infectious Disease Epidemiology
  Department of Zoology, University of Oxford

Howard Barnum
The World Bank

David E. Barmes
World Health Organization

Jeanne Bertolli
University of California, Los Angeles

Douglas Bratthall
World Health Collaborating Center, Malmö, Sweden

Logan Brenzel
REACH, *Arlington, Virginia*

J. Richard Bumgarner
World Health Organization

D. A. P. Bundy
Imperial College, London

Susan Burger
Emory University, Atlanta, Georgia

Lincoln C. Chen
Harvard School of Public Health

John Clements
World Health Organization

Susan Cochrane
The World Bank

Peter Cowley
The World Bank

Andrew Creese
World Health Organization

Carlos Cruz
Instituto Nacional de Salud Pública,
  Cuernavaca, Mexico

A. R. Davis
World Health Organization

Richard G. Feachem
London School of Hygiene and Tropical Medicine

Chris N. Feifer
The Rand Corporation, California

Stanley O. Foster
Centers for Disease Control and Prevention, Atlanta, Georgia

Tomas Frejka
*The Population Council, Regional Office
  for Latin America, Mexico City*

Julio Frenk
Instituto Nacional de Salud Pública, Cuernavaca, Mexico

Rae Galloway
The World Bank

Paul J. Gertler
The Rand Corporation, California

Lucy Gilson
London School of Hygiene and Tropical Medicine

E. Robert Greenberg
Dartmouth Medical School, Hanover, New Hampshire

Jean-Pierre Habicht
Cornell University

Scott B. Halstead
The Rockefeller Foundation

Jeffrey Hammer
The World Bank

Donald A. Henderson
United States Department of Health and Human Services

Myo Thet Htoon
Myanmar Ministry of Health

Dale Hu
Centers for Disease Control and Prevention, Atlanta, Georgia

Michel Jancloes
World Health Organization

Jonathan C. Javitt
Georgetown University Medical Center

A. Meredith John
Princeton University

Mark Kane
World Health Organization

Lies D. Kosasih
Jakarta

Henry M. Levin
Stanford University

Bernhard H. Liese
The World Bank

Alan D. Lopez
World Health Organization

Rafael Lozano
Instituto Nacional de Salud Pública, Cuernavaca, Mexico

José Martines
World Health Organization

Deborah A. McFarland
*Emory University and Centers for Disease Control
  and Prevention, Atlanta, Georgia*

William P. McGreevey
The World Bank

Judith McGuire
The World Bank

Joseph L. Melnick
Baylor College of Medicine, Houston

Catherine Michaud
Harvard School of Public Health

Anne Mills
London School of Hygiene and Tropical Medicine

Gavin Mooney
University of Aberdeen, Sydney, and Tromsø

Christopher Murray
Harvard School of Public Health

José A. Nájera
World Health Organization

Mead Over
The World Bank

Thomas A. Pearson
*Imogene Bassett Research Institute and Columbia
  University*

Allison Percy
REACH, *Arlington, Virginia*

Karen Peterson
Harvard School of Public Health

Margaret Phillips
Mexico City

Per Pinstrup-Andersen
*International Food Policy Research Institute (IFPRI),
  Washington, D.C.*

Peter Piot
World Health Organization

Ernesto Pollitt
University of California, Davis

Nicholas Prescott
The World Bank

André Prost
World Health Organization

Vulmiri Ramalingaswami
All India Institute of Medical Sciences, New Delhi

Annik Rouillon
International Union Against Tuberculosis, Paris

Frederick Sai
International Planned Parenthood Federation, London

Alfred Senft
Brown University

Donald S. Shepard
Brandeis University, Waltham, Massachusetts

Gordon Smith
*The Johns Hopkins University School of Hygiene
and Public Health*

Frank E. Speizer
*Harvard Medical School and Harvard School
of Public Health*

Kenneth Stanley
Harvard School of Public Health

Sally K. Stansfield
McGill-Ethiopia Project, Addis Ababa

Robert Steinglass
REACH, Arlington, Virginia

Claudio Stern
El Colegio de México, Mexico City

Karel Styblo
International Union Against Tuberculosis, Paris

Carl E. Taylor
*The Johns Hopkins University School of Hygiene
and Public Health, and* UNICEF

Alberto M. Torres
World Health Organization

Jorge Trejo-Gutierrez
The Regional Hospital, Guadalajara, Mexico

J. Patrick Vaughan
London School of Hygiene and Tropical Medicine

Julia A. Walsh
Harvard School of Public Health

Kenneth S. Warren
Biofield, New York

Richard Jed Wyatt
*National Institute of Mental Health Neurosciences
Center at St. Elizabeth's, Washington, D.C.*

PART ONE

Introduction

1

Disease Control Priorities in Developing Countries: An Overview

Dean T. Jamison

International health policy is at a time of transition. A pretransition environment dominated by high fertility, high mortality, infectious disease, and malnutrition is giving way to a low-mortality, low-fertility environment. For the past two decades much of the international public health community has focused attention on the communicable childhood diseases (CCDs). Although there are exceptions to this generalization—continued concern about the tropical diseases, for example—much of the debate and analysis has concentrated on whether CCD problems would be best addressed by broad-reaching strategies or by selective ones. Significant technical and programmatic progress has been made in this period, and the focus of concern on CCD has clearly been appropriate: the problems are great; the technological and epidemiological tools have become powerful; and the payoff for adapting and applying what is known is very high. The success of CCD control efforts combined with large and sustained fertility reductions in many developing countries has led, however, to the "health transition," that is, the change from a pretransition environment dominated by high fertility, high mortality, infectious disease, and malnutrition to a low-mortality, low-fertility environment with a disease profile that increasingly emphasizes noncommunicable conditions of adults and the elderly.[1] Figure 1-1 illustrates the progress of the health transition through demographic to epidemiologic change.

This collection reports the findings of the Health Sector Priorities Review, a review conducted by the World Bank of the implications for disease control priorities of the health transition. The core of this collection consists of analyses undertaken for the Health Sector Priorities Review that assess the significance to public health of individual diseases (or related clusters of diseases) and of what is now known about the cost and effectiveness of relevant interventions for their control.[2] To the extent possible, the cost-effectiveness of intervention has been summarized by estimates of marginal cost per disability-adjusted life-year (DALY) gained; although this measure is imperfect, and often varies with the scale of the control effort and across environments, its estimation, for each of a large number of interventions, does indicate priorities for

the allocation of resources to disease control. By addressing a broad range of conditions, the World Bank Health Sector Priorities Review was able both to estimate the cost-effectiveness of CCD interventions and to place them into the context of interventions for noncommunicable diseases and for communicable diseases of adults.[3]

This chapter has three purposes: to set the context for the collection as a whole by describing the Health Sector Priorities Review and outlining the methods of cost-effectiveness analysis used; to summarize the findings of the condition-specific analyses, which are reported in parts 2, 3, and 4 of this collection; and to draw a few broad conclusions. In chapter 29, Mosley, Bobadilla, and Jamison describe the health transition more fully and provide an amplified set of implications for policy.

Before proceeding with the substance of the chapter, I will put forth four caveats. First, any general discussion of conditions and priorities for so vast and diverse a set of countries as those that make up the developing world naturally runs the risks of overstating generalities and understating differences. The authors represented in this collection assume the reader to be already familiar with this diversity, and, therefore, we avoid continually repeating caveats about the limits to generalization. Nevertheless, our concern is with generalization—with addressing trends and findings that are important for a sufficiently large number of countries that they assume significance for the developing world as a whole. That said, the conclusions of this chapter, and of the collection as a whole, can best be viewed as a useful starting point for country-specific analyses and certainly not as a substitute for them.

A second caveat concerns limits to the coverage of the World Bank Health Sector Priorities Review. One shortcoming is the lack of attention to most mental and neurological illness; analyses structured like those in this collection for a broader range of neuropsychiatric conditions may be initiated soon, but results are currently unavailable.[4] Many other conditions—some minor, some more important—were omitted in order to keep the scope of the review manageable. Likewise, interventions associated with the very diverse range of tradi-

Figure 1-1. *Relationships between Demographic, Epidemiologic, and Health Transitions*

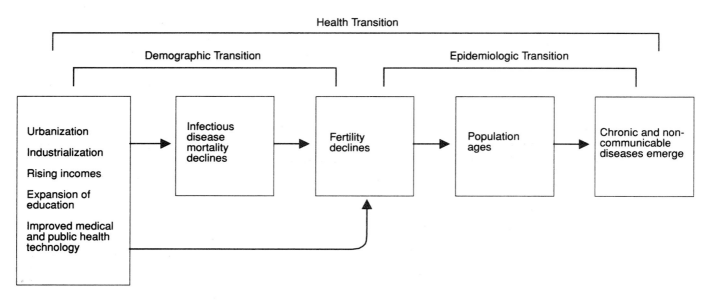

Source: Chapter 28.

tional medical practices were not included. These gaps in coverage genuinely limit the scope of the review. But I feel they do not significantly alter conclusions concerning the very broad range of conditions and interventions that were included.

A third caveat concerns the perspective of this document, which is that of governments or of development assistance agencies working with governments. Other perspectives—those of clinicians or of patients or of nongovernmental organizations, for example—are also important, and this review's findings concerning intervention cost-effectiveness have some relevance from those perspectives. But the review's main purpose is to identify those interventions that, on the basis of their cost-effectiveness, governmental policy should seek to encourage or discourage.

Fourth, we assume throughout this collection that the analysis of health policy can usefully be divided into three tasks: to choose attractive interventions; to design delivery systems for such interventions; and to choose appropriate governmental instruments to encourage these interventions. Because of the changing pattern of disease, delineated in chapters 3 and 29, this collection readdresses the first task of health planning, that of choosing interventions. For this reason I take the time here to consider the three tasks together. The first task, choosing interventions, assesses the cost-effectiveness of potential disease control technologies by combining technical analysis (epidemiological and clinical) with economic considerations; it will also, occasionally, extend to the task of assessing the benefits of intervention in relation to cost broadly defined.[5] The second task, designing delivery systems, has dominated thinking about health policy. Economically sensible delivery systems, however, must follow choice of what interventions are

to be implemented. In either the public or private sector the three key design elements for delivery systems—planning development of human and physical infrastructure, planning the logistical system for drugs and supplies, and planning appropriate information and incentive structures and financial instruments—all depend in important ways on the intervention mix. At the same time, the cost-effectiveness of interventions will vary with the capacity of local infrastructure to deliver them (Over 1988), as is well illustrated in chapter 14, "Dengue," by Halstead and Shepard. Ideally, then, the first two tasks of health policy analysis should be addressed iteratively rather than sequentially. The third task of policy, choice of the appropriate mix of governmental instruments, deals with what governments can do through provision of information, taxation, regulation, direct investment, and research.[6] The brief discussion of these instruments in this chapter points to their importance; it does not assess them in any depth.

If the familiar pattern of problems in developing countries—communicable childhood disease, undernutrition, and excess fertility—could be expected to continue their dominance of the epidemiological profile, then there would be little need for the broad reassessment of objectives attempted in this collection. Analyses aimed at improving the infrastructure, logistics, and financial aspects of the delivery systems so they are able to deal with the pretransition conditions could simply proceed. But massive epidemiological change is already deeply penetrating the developing world, and response to this change has typically been to import the high-cost approaches of the industrialized nations to the (very limited) extent that resources permit—hence the timeliness of broad assessment of the cost-effectiveness of intervention options. Reassessment of the design of delivery systems and the appropriate role for government also claims priority; but that reassessment must follow identification of the interventions to be delivered (or encouraged) and those to be discouraged.

The World Bank's 1980 policy paper on the health sector (World Bank 1980) focused on communicable diseases of childhood, but shortly after that paper was published another widely cited paper prepared at the World Bank (Evans, Hall, and Warford 1981) was drawing attention to the emergence of behavioral disorders and noncommunicable disease as significant problems in many developing countries. Although Evans, Hall, and Warford were explicitly pessimistic about prospects for cost-effective intervention to address these emerging problems, World Bank staff members were encouraged to begin addressing the issue in their work with individual governments, and analyses for China (Jamison and others 1984; Bumgarner and others 1990) and Brazil (Briscoe and others 1989) attempted to develop relevant policy responses in epidemiological environments characterized both by lingering problems of childhood disease and malnutrition and by rapid emergence of noncommunicable disease (NCD).[7] During the progress of these country studies it became clear that very little analysis indeed had gone into the task of selecting from and adapting the broad range of NCD interventions available in the industrialized countries to generate options relevant to the extremely cost-constrained environments of developing countries.

This lack of analysis of appropriate approaches for developing countries to take in dealing with NCDs provided the impetus, then, for the World Bank Health Sector Priorities Review. At the same time it seemed appropriate to reassess the cost-effectiveness of interventions addressing communicable conditions, malnutrition, and excess fertility; such a reassessment would both provide the context for judging the relative cost-effectiveness of interventions for NCDs and allow judgments to be made on intervention priority for child survival.

The World Bank Health Sector Priorities Review

The most important part of the review is a series of analyses on diseases and conditions of great importance in part or all of the developing world.[8] The first part of table 1-1 lists the included topics and indicates which chapter of the collection covers them; the second part lists potentially important conditions that were not included but that, ideally, should be addressed in further work. The authors of each chapter were asked to undertake three tasks: to assess the current and probable future public health significance of the conditions in developing countries; to judge the cost and effectiveness of alternative approaches to preventing the condition in different contexts; and to judge the cost and effectiveness of alternative approaches to case management for the conditions in various contexts. Ideally each chapter would have been written by an economist, an epidemiologist, and a clinician or biomedical scientist. Although each of these categories is well represented among the chapter authors, relatively few of the individual chapters ended up with all three.

Table 1-2 provides definitions of terms that are frequently used in this chapter and throughout the collection. After reviewing drafts of all the chapters, I concluded that dividing interventions between those that are public health oriented and those that are clinically oriented was more useful than distinguishing between preventive and case management interventions, a distinction that the chapter authors had originally been asked to make. In table 1-2 I define how we use these terms, and later in this chapter I divide the summaries of the findings of the condition-specific chapters into two sections, one on public health intervention and the other on clinical intervention.

In table 1-2 I also define the objectives of intervention, which, as we categorize them, include primary prevention, secondary prevention, cure, rehabilitation, and palliation. Although there is some tendency for public health interventions to have primary prevention as their main objective, this is far from universally true; by the same token, some clinical interventions also seek primary prevention. Hence the importance of clarity about objectives in discussing individual interventions. Table 1-2 also defines the instruments of government policy that can be used to encourage or discourage use of specific interventions.

The cost-effectiveness of any given intervention varies according to circumstances, and the main sources of such variation are discussed in the next section. A particularly important source of variation, however, results from the general mortality level of the environment, and each set of chapter authors was asked to consider two environments (if relevant to their conditions). One of these was a high-mortality, high-fertility environment with low gross national product (GNP) per capita and extremely limited resources available for the health sector; Nigeria might be an example. The other was an environment with relatively low fertility and mortality, a middle-income GNP, and more substantial resources for the health sector; Thailand would be typical here. Many of the authors of the disease-specific analyses used both these paradigms, whereas others used only one or found neither appropriate. What is important to note here, though, is that conclusions concerning intervention attractiveness can vary quite substantially depending on a country's progress through the health transition and that this point was very much a starting point for the analyses in the World Bank review.

Assessing the Cost-effectiveness of Intervention

This section contains a discussion of general issues associated with choosing interventions, that is, with criteria for cost-effective choice. The nature of the instruments open to government to promote cost-effective intervention is discussed in chapter 29. The purpose in both chapters is not to provide an account of methodological issues associated with economic assessment of intervention options; rather we wish simply to describe the basic concepts being applied and refer the reader to the relevant literature (for example, Drummond, Stoddart, and Torrance 1987).

Table 1-1. *Selected Clusters of Diseases and Conditions*

Status	Unfinished agenda	Emerging problems
Included	*Infections principally affecting children* Acute respiratory infections (chap. 4) Diarrheal diseases (chap. 5) Poliomyelitis (chap. 6) Helminthic infections (chap. 7) Measles (chap. 8) Tetanus (chap. 9)	Human immunodeficiency virus infection and sexually transmitted diseases (chap. 20) Cancers (chap. 21) Diabetes (chap. 22) Cardiovascular disease (chap. 23) Chronic obstructive pulmonary disease (chap. 24) Injury (chap. 25) Cataract (chap. 26) Oral health (chap. 27) Schizophrenia and manic-depressive illness (chap. 28)
	Other infections Rheumatic heart disease (chap. 10) Tuberculosis (chap. 11) Leprosy (chap. 12) Malaria (chap. 13) Dengue and yellow fever (chap. 14) Hepatitis B (chap. 15)	
	Reproductive health and malnutrition Excess fertility (chap. 16) Maternal and perinatal health (chap. 17) Protein-energy malnutrition (chap. 18) Micronutrient deficiency disorders (chap. 19),	
Omitted	Lymphatic filariasis African trypanosomiasis Chagas' disease Leishmaniasis Skin diseases	Epilepsy Affective disorders Alcohol and other drug abuse Arthritis Influenza Appendicitis Hernia

Source: Author.

The methods of assessing the cost and effectiveness of intervention vary from chapter to chapter, complicating the task of cross-chapter comparisons of the cost-effectiveness of intervention. Because of wide variation in the nature of the conditions and the adequacy of the literature, the chapters vary in the extent to which they provide quantitative estimates of cost-effectiveness; hence the results are sometimes difficult to compare. Nevertheless, the authors proceeded with similar objectives and methods, and, if one accepts the results as reasonable first approximations, the collection does generate the raw materials for comparative assessment of the cost-effectiveness of intervention. Often these first approximations rely on epidemiological or clinical judgments combined with the results of published studies, or, in those cases where published data were unavailable, judgments were made on the basis of discussion with experienced observers. Some reviewers of this effort have been uncomfortable with the explicit use of judgmental assessments; we have consistently encouraged them to let us know of any cases where current clinical or public health decisions are being made on the basis of better information on efficacy or cost than we use.

A critical choice in applications of economic analysis to resource allocation is that of whether to value outcomes be-

cause of their economic benefits or because of some more proximal effectiveness measure. Ideally, economic benefits would be the criterion; the results of the analysis—phrased in dollars of output value given the dollar value of inputs—provide standards for assessment of interventions across sectors: immunization as against irrigation as against smaller class sizes, say. When there are good markets for products, benefits can be assessed in monetary terms by using market prices (that is, willingness of consumers to pay) to value benefits. Even when willingness-to-pay valuation cannot be assessed directly because of lack of market prices, as is typically true in the health sector, questions in surveys are increasingly being used to elicit information about hypothetical willingness-to-pay. Briscoe and de Ferranti (1988) indicate the potential for this approach in valuation of water projects, but applicability in the health sector remains to be assessed. Nonetheless, pervasive problems of consumer ignorance of effectiveness of intervention (previously discussed) and a widespread tendency for individuals systematically to underestimate risks (Weinstein 1989) suggest that willingness-to-pay assessments will probably have limited application to health. An alternative approach—sometimes called the human capital approach—is to view health investments as instrumental to improving economic productivity;

Table 1-2. Definition of Terms

1. *Interventions.* The term "intervention" is used in this chapter to denote actions taken by or for individuals to reduce the risk, duration, or severity of an adverse health condition. Interventions are the *proximal* cause of deliberate changes in risks, duration, or severity; instruments of policy (see below) encourage, discourage, or undertake interventions. Stopping smoking, for example, is an intervention that an individual can take to reduce risk from a range of diseases; taxing tobacco products is a potential instrument of government policy to encourage this intervention. I divide interventions into those that are "public health" and those that are "clinical."

   1.1 *Public health interventions.* These are interventions sought of or directed toward entire populations or population subgroups; this chapter divides public health interventions into five broad categories—change of personal behavior, control of environmental hazards, immunization, mass chemoprophylaxis, and screening and referral. (Table 1-5 provides a broad range of examples of each of these strategies for population-based intervention.)

   1.2 *Clinical interventions.* These are interventions provided at facilities, usually to individuals. This chapter divides clinical interventions into those that can be provided at the clinic (community, private, work-based, or school-based), at a district hospital, or at a referral hospital.

2. *Objectives of Intervention.* The objectives of intervention are structured, in this chapter, into five categories:[a]

   2.1 *Primary prevention* aims to reduce the risk of a condition occurring by lowering the level of risk factors or instituting policies to forestall their emergence. (This latter is sometimes referred to as "primordial prevention.")

   2.2 *Secondary prevention* aims to reduce the duration or severity of a condition or physiological risk factor in order to forestall its leading to more adverse consequences.

   2.3 *Cure* of a condition aims to remove its cause and restore function to the status quo ante.

   2.4 *Rehabilitation* aims to restore (or partially restore) physical, psychological, or social function resulting from a previous or chronic condition.

   2.5 *Palliation* aims to reduce pain and suffering from a condition for which no means of cure or rehabilitation is currently available. (This may range from the use of aspirin for headaches to use of opiates to control terminal cancer pain.)

3. *Instruments of Policy.* These are the activities that can (potentially) be undertaken by governments or other entities that wish to encourage or discourage interventions, or, importantly, to expand the menu of potential intervention. I distinguish five major instruments or policy:

   3.1 Use of *information, education, and communication* (IEC) seeks to improve the knowledge of individuals (and service providers) about the consequences of their choices.

   3.2 Use of *taxes and subsidies* on commodities, services, and pollutants seeks to effect appropriate behavioral responses.

   3.3 Use of *regulation and legislation* seeks to limit availability of certain commodities, to curtail certain practices, and to define the rules governing finance and provision of health services.

   3.4 Use of *direct expenditures* seeks to provide (or finance provision of) selected interventions (e.g., immunizations) or to provide infrastructure (e.g., medical schools) that facilitates provision of a range of interventions.

   3.5 Undertaking *research and development* (or encouraging them through subsidies) is an instrument central to the goal of expanding the range of interventions available and reducing their cost.

a. The International Epidemiology Association's *Dictionary of Epidemiology* (Last 1988) provides a helpful discussion of different types of prevention but, interestingly, has no entries for "cure" or "rehabilitation." Their term "tertiary prevention," which is not used here, seems to encompass both "rehabilitation" and "palliation," as we define those terms.

Source: Author.

estimates of the effect of a health intervention on productivity thus provide a lower bound to total benefits. One example comes from assessing the effect on the productivity of rubber plantation workers of correcting iron deficiencies (Basta, Soekirman, and Scrimshaw 1979; Levin and others, chapter 19, this collection); other examples come from assessment of the effect on productivity of malaria control efforts (Najera and others, chapter 13, this collection). It is worth noting that willingness-to-pay and human capital approaches tend to imply different values to be attached to the life of different individuals of the same age in the same country. Phelps and Mushlin (1991) discuss relations between cost-effectiveness and cost-benefit analyses of health projects; they conclude that willingness to set a cutoff level of acceptable cost-effectiveness results in equivalence between cost-effectiveness and cost-benefit approaches.

More typically, however, outcomes will be assessed in deaths or disability averted, and the task is to come up with some measure for making such an assessment that allows comparisons across the health sector, even if intersectoral comparisons (cost-benefit analyses) remain infeasible.[9] There is now a valuable literature on how effectiveness measures to aggregate the disability-, morbidity-, and premature mortality-averting effects of interventions across the health sector might be constructed and applied (Barnum 1987; Zeckhauser and Shepard 1976; Over 1988; and Feachem, Graham, and Timaeus 1989). Such measures, in addition to providing the effectiveness measures for cost-effectiveness analyses, can be used with epidemiological information to assess the burden of disease in a population, as has recently been done for the major regions of the world (World Bank, 1993). Nonetheless, inherent difficulties remain, and these are usefully discussed in Murray (1990). Table 1-3 sets forth the characteristics of the main approaches to effectiveness measurement in the literature; from a practical perspective, the use of ratings based on expert judgment is probably the best that can now be done if the purpose of the analysis is to compare interventions across the sector, although, as Preston (1991) has noted, these measures must be used with care. This has been the approach adopted in the World Bank Health Sector Priorities Review.

I conclude that a workable measure for effectiveness for most of the analysis will be disability-adjusted life-years gained (or DALYs). The DALY gain associated with averting a death is, simply, the number of years between the age at which the death would have occurred and the individual's expected age at death, given survival to the given age, with years gained in future years discounted back to the present at a discount rate of 3 percent per annum in all chapters in this collection. Unhealthy life-years are given lower weights than healthy ones, depending on degree of disability (by the rating procedure described in the preceding paragraph) so that the effectiveness of interventions to address morbidity or disability can be measured in terms that permit comparison with interventions that avert mortality. The DALY measure used in this

collection is a particular form of the more general concept of "quality-adjusted life-year" (QALY) introduced by Zeckhauser and Shepard (1976).

Garber and Phelps (1992) provide the basic theoretical underpinnings for cost-effectiveness analyses in health that adjust life-years for quality. (See Johannesson [1992] for a general discussion of discounting healthy life-years, and see Cropper, Aydede, and Portney [1992] for empirical assessments of time preference for saving lives.) Authors of individual chapters assess the losses due to disability or morbidity in ways judged suitable to the conditions with which they are dealing. Thus, reduction in morbidity and disability can be explicitly considered in the analysis, and most chapters do so, if the conditions they deal with have significant consequences other than death. The approach used here explicitly values years of healthy life at all ages equally; this assumption can be readily relaxed, however, to give greater weight to those age groups likely, say, to have more dependents (Musgrove 1991).

Table 1-3. *Alternative Approaches to Measuring Effectiveness of Intervention*

Approach to measurement	Cost	Possible bias	Applicability[a]	Example
Mortality				
Deaths averted	Very low	Highly biased conditions involving disability	Medium	Assessment of priorities in child survival (Walsh and Warren 1979)
Years of potential life lost	Very low	Highly biased against conditions involving disability	Medium	Regularly used by Centers for Disease Control to assess burden of disease in the United States, (MMWR 1992)
Quality-of-life adjusted life-years[b]				
Expert ratings assessment	Low	Unrepresentative experts	High	Ghana Health Assessment Project Team (1981); this collection
Survey-based	Medium	n.a.	Low (in practice)	Rosser scale (Rosser and Kind 1978); European quality-of-life assessments (EuroQol Group 1990)
Risk tradeoffs	High	Questionable relevance of artificial gambles	Low (in practice)	Various quality-of-life assessments (Tan-Torres 1990)
Quantity-of-life high tradeoffs: Individual length vs quality of life	Medium/high	Probably low for patient-level decisionmaking	Medium	Various quality-of-life assessments (Tan-Torres 1990)
Quantity-of-life tradeoff: Across individuals	Medium	Probably low for social decisionmaking	Medium/high	Vaccine development study (Institute of Medicine 1986; Nord 1991)
Calibration of preexisting condition-specific studies	Medium	Probably low	Low	Cairns and Johnston 1991

n.a. Not applicable.

Note: This table does not review approaches to measuring the economic benefits of changes in health status. Such measures—based, for example, on willingness to pay for reductions in the probability of adverse outcomes or on assessment of health-related determinants of labor productivity (human capital)—allow conclusions to be drawn about the attractiveness of particular health interventions relative to their cost, not simply by comparison with other interventions (for examples, see chapter 19). No usable set of benefit measures is available across conditions.

a. Availability for application in health-sector-wide cost-effectiveness studies.

b. Each of the methods for quality of life measurement—ratings, risk tradeoffs, quantity-of-life tradeoffs, calibrations—can be undertaken by different groups, possibly with different results. The groups can be of "experts," respondents to a survey, or, in a clinical setting, potential patients. For the ratings method, this table comments on both expert and survey approaches: a similar breakdown could be provided for each method. See Fallowfield (1990) for a general discussion of these matters.

Source: See references in final column of table.

Costs are generally assessed at market prices. In some cases, however, for some inputs into health care, costs may be lower in developing countries (for example, for semiskilled labor). These costs are typically for inputs that cannot be traded internationally, and their existence undermines attempts to estimate costs that are not simply country-specific. Squire (1989) provides a general discussion of approaches to dealing with nontradables in project analysis; his results, though, are more relevant to country-specific assessments than to cross-national comparisons.

The working conclusion of this chapter is that for drugs, for most equipment, and for high-level manpower, considerations of cost variability between high- and low-income countries are essentially irrelevant. For facilities and lower-level manpower they are likely to change some numbers, but in most cases costs can more reasonably be expressed in constant dollars than, say, as fractions of local per capita income—a method that assumes essentially no health sector inputs to be internationally tradable. The chapters "Cancer," by Barnum and Greenberg (chapter 21, this collection), and "Tuberculosis," by Murray, Styblo, and Rouillon (chapter 11, this collection), attempt to divide costs into those for traded goods and those for nontradables. Their assessments do suggest that local costs will often be important and that those who attempt to assess the cost-effectiveness of intervention in a country-specific context should pay close attention to this issue unless there is a completely free market for foreign exchange and the costs of nontradables are similar to those of the comparator country.

Another important issue in cost analysis concerns assessment of the amount and value of time required of patients or caretakers; the importance of mothers' time, in particular, for compliance with child survival interventions has been stressed by Leslie (1989). These time costs are potentially difficult to value (Briscoe and de Ferranti 1988) and have been neglected in this collection. It is hoped that subsequent work will redress this omission. A related issue concerns treatment of costs that will ensue from intervention success; Levin and others (chapter 19, this collection) point out that substantial food costs can result from micronutrient supplementation or parasite control. The existence of such costs suggests the importance, in these cases, of broadening the definition of the intervention.

A final issue concerning cost analysis is that of joint costs, that is, the situation where several interventions are essentially made available with a (partially) common set of inputs. The chapters in this collection handle this in part by defining interventions in terms of natural packages; the chapter "Poliomyelitis," by Jamison and others (chapter 6, this collection), considers the preventive intervention for polio to be diphtheria-pertussis-tetanus vaccine plus polio immunization, and assesses the cost-effectiveness of that package, because polio immunization would (almost always) be given with the vaccine. In many cases, however, such packaging would get too

Table 1-4. Factors Influencing Variation in Cost-Effectiveness

Influencing factor	Examples
Epidemiological environment	
Prevalence of condition	Screening and referral programs for leprosy; for cervical and breast cancer
Incidence of condition	BCG immunization for tuberculosis; preventive measures for many injuries
Case-fatality rate	Measles immunization; oral rehydration therapy for diarrhea
Transmission dynamics of infectious conditions	Treatment of sexually transmitted diseases in core vs noncore groups; vector control for malaria, dengue
Existence of competing risks of synergisms	Measles vaccination: amplification of cost-effectiveness by strengthening individuals in a general way. Among the very young or elderly, competing risks reduce the cost-effectiveness of some targeted interventions.
Individual characteristics	
Age	Cancer treatment: more cost-effective for younger patients
Tendency to compliance	Tuberculosis chemotherapy; antihypertensive medication
Tendency to self-refer	Sexually transmitted diseases control
Levels of risk factors	Hypertension and hyperlipidemia
Individual variation in values	Attitude toward disability relative to risk of death; can lead to individual differences in intervention effectiveness
System characteristics	
Local costs of non-traded inputs to health care system	Real costs of care-intensive interventions (such as hospitalization to ensure compliance with tuberculosis chemotherapy) are low where wages are low, because most health care personnel are relatively immobile
Generalized systemic competence	Case management of dengue hemorrhagic fever: high cost and low effectiveness in unsophisticated systems. Cost-effectiveness, at the margin, of some interventions in a system with high level of professionalism and capacity may be much less than in less well developed systems
Discount rate	Hepatitis B immunization: where discount rates are high, interventions with payoffs well into the future become relatively less attractive, and age of the patient becomes a less significant determinant of cost-effectiveness

Source: Author.

Figure 1-2. *Increasing Costs per Disability-Adjusted Life-Year Associated with More Complete Control of Dengue*

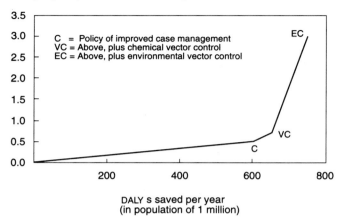

Cost per year (millions of U.S. dollars)

C = Policy of improved case management
VC = Above, plus chemical vector control
EC = Above, plus environmental vector control

DALY s saved per year
(in population of 1 million)

Source: Chapter 14.

bulky and the chapter authors have simply been asked to do the best they could while noting where joint costs would need to be considered in country-specific applications.

In this collection, then, for comparison across interventions we use the common denominator of dollar cost per DALY gained, with the understanding that intervention costs and cost-effectiveness will likely vary across locales (even after controlling for intervention quality) because of differences in individuals, in epidemiological conditions, in delivery system characteristics, and in the degree of penetration of the intervention into the population. Table 1-4 lists many important factors that lead to variation in cost-effectiveness, and, to the extent that interventions are first applied where their cost-effectiveness is highest, these factors collectively will lead to rising costs per DALY with increased application of an intervention.[10] Figure 1-2 illustrates this for control of dengue; up to a point, improved case management is most cost-effective, but beyond that point, if a higher level of control for dengue is to be sought, chemical and then environmental strategies of vector control must be introduced.

This phenomenon of rising costs per DALY comes up implicitly in many of the chapters; the cause of the phenomenon is, frequently, the lack of intervention specificity and, also frequently, costly targeting and compliance problems. *Intervention specificity* refers to what fraction of intervention recipients would benefit assuming that the intervention is applied exactly to the individuals to whom it should be applied (the factors "Prevalence of condition," "Incidence of condition," and "Levels of risk factors" in table 1-4). Take BCG (bacille Calmette-Guérin) vaccination as an example; it should be applied to all newborns, but it is a benefit, ex post, only to that tiny fraction of children who would have died in childhood from miliary tuberculosis (TB) without it. Tuberculosis chemo-

therapy for sputum positives, by contrast, although costly, will virtually never be applied when unneeded; it is highly specific. Targeting BCG or other interventions to populations at highest risk, at least until full coverage can be afforded, will maximize cost-effectiveness while simultaneously advancing equity objectives (Mosley and Jolly 1987). As an illustration, figure 1-3 (from Murray, Styblo, and Rouillon, chapter 11, this collection) shows how BCG cost-effectiveness improves with rising risk of infection (and, hence, rising intervention specificity), whereas chemotherapy remains of essentially constant attractiveness.

In addition, targeting costs and compliance costs can dilute cost-effectiveness. Treatment can be very cost-effective for self-referred compliant patients ("Tendency to compliance" and "Tendency to self-refer" in table 1-4); as compliance becomes more problematic, or targeting more costly, cost-effectiveness decreases. For example, oral rehydration therapy (ORT) in the hospital or clinic setting is highly cost-effective; it will only be used for severe cases of diarrhea, and it is likely to be applied effectively by qualified medical personnel. When ORT is taken to the community, however, cost-effectiveness declines substantially, both because of a decrease in intervention specificity (mild cases will be treated unnecessarily) and because home treatment will be applied less effectively than hospital treatment in severe cases. Similarly, targeting costs can be decreased if an immunization program to prevent neonatal tetanus shifts from trying to reach pregnant women to immunizing all childbearing women, although there will be a loss of specificity (at least with respect to preventing neonatal tetanus but not, presumably, with respect to adult tetanus).

Figure 1-3. *Cost-Effectiveness of BCG Immunization and Tuberculosis Case Treatment as Function of Annual Risk of Infection*

Cost per death averted (U.S. dollars)

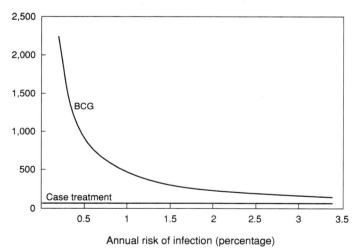

Annual risk of infection (percentage)

Source: Chapter 11.

When an intervention requires large fixed costs, total program costs need to be weighed against total effects; simple assessment of marginal cost and effectiveness fails to suffice. The fixed costs involved in, to take several examples, investing in major facilities, mounting a media-based health education program, or devising regulations and procedures can be substantial. Fixed costs need not be financial; managerial or political attention to a problem may have an important fixed cost element. When fixed cost may be important, understanding the total burden of disease is necessary for estimating potential total intervention effects (Mooney and Creese, appendix C, this collection).

These points are relatively obvious, but there is often an optimistic bias toward assessing cost-effectiveness under assumptions of favorable targeting and compliance costs and of favorable intervention specificity. One might expect, as previously noted, rising marginal costs and decreasing marginal effectiveness as interventions are extended through populations; these combine to dilute cost-effectiveness. Thus favorable case cost-effectiveness estimates can be real, but their margin of applicability may be limited. In principle, it is desirable to acquire some sense of the responsiveness of intervention cost-effectiveness to a range of parameters, particularly the extent of application of the intervention. In practice, sensitivity analysis is sometimes possible but often difficult—and comparisons are then made for "representative" estimates of marginal cost-effectiveness to provide general guidance to decisionmakers. When there are great differences in the marginal cost-effectiveness of different interventions—as this chapter concludes there to be—this "general guidance" can suggest important redirections of policy.[11] Figure 1-4 illustrates how differences in marginal costs per DALY across interventions can lead to inefficiency. In that example, intervention B is assumed to have a constant cost per DALY of $60 for the range of expenditure levels considered (up to $4,000); intervention A starts with a lower cost per DALY ($20) but one that is rising to $100 per DALY at an expenditure of $4,000. The point here is that when, at prevailing levels of expenditure on each intervention, cost per DALY is lower for one of them (as it would be for A at an expenditure of $1,000 on each of them), reallocation of money will increase output without increasing cost. Hence, the previous allocation would have been inefficient.

Finally, it is worth reiterating that the assessments to be summarized in this chapter provide only an ordering of interventions based on estimates of current marginal cost-effectiveness; epidemiological information is required to assess how much of each intervention needs to be acquired in light of rising costs per DALY gained (Prost and Jancloes, appendix D, this collection). For example, one of the most cost-effective interventions (for adults) is screening hospital blood supplies for human immunodeficiency virus (HIV) seropositivity; as cost-effective as this may be, relatively few deaths can be averted by it. Chemotherapy for patients with tuberculosis, conversely, although somewhat less cost-effective, could be expected to save hundreds of times more lives. Resource allo-

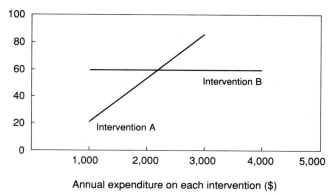

Figure 1-4. *Reaching Optimum Intervention Levels*

Cost per DHLY (U.S. Dollars)

Annual expenditure on each intervention ($)

Source: Author.

cation, then, for interventions, depends on both economic and epidemiological information because of the strong effect of epidemiology on the rate of increase in marginal costs. (Resource allocation to research, by contrast, should be driven much more by the epidemiological significance of diseases and researchers instincts about where advances might be realized.)

The Findings: Public Health Interventions

In this section I summarize the findings of the twenty-five condition-specific chapters of this collection. In the first section I noted our conclusion that dividing interventions into two broad categories—public health and clinical—was most conducive to discussing policy tradeoffs, and these summarizing remarks are so divided. (Table 1-2 defined what is included in each of these categories.) This section deals with public health interventions, and the following section deals with clinical ones.

Five Strategies of Public Health Intervention

Public health interventions are organized into five separate strategies in this collection—those designed to change personal behavior, to control environmental hazards, to immunize, to provide mass chemoprophylaxis, and to establish mechanisms for screening and referral. Appendix table 1A-1 lists various components of each of these strategies and provides examples of the condition(s) they might effectively address; this summary of the review's findings on public health intervention will, then, explicitly indicate which of these strategies is being assessed. I feel that in reviewing health policies, or intervention alternatives, it will often be useful to do so within each of these five broad strategies because of commonalities of logistics, policy instruments, and approaches within each. (This is true despite the frequently great diversity of conditions to be addressed within any one intervention strategy.)

Before turning to the condition-by-condition summary of findings, I should touch on the issue of joint costs (and multiple outcomes) of interventions in light of conclusions from the individual chapters. The analysis upon which this collection is based is structured by diseases (or adverse health conditions more generally), and the issues addressed in the individual chapters thus concern the nature, cost, and effectiveness of the interventions available for dealing with each condition. In many cases, of course, any given intervention will address multiple conditions and, indeed, may well have important effects outside the health sector altogether. Perhaps the clearest examples are control of smoking, breastfeeding, and environmental improvements. Limitation of smoking markedly reduces risk for lung cancer, ischemic heart disease, and chronic obstructive pulmonary disease; outside the health sector it reduces (at least to some extent) property damage from fire and frees productive resources for alternative use. Breastfeeding, likewise, has multiple health effects; it enhances child immunity, reduces exposure to infection, provides balanced nutrition and, by suppressing ovulation, postpones the next pregnancy (Anderson 1990). The cost of breastfeeding, however, includes, as do many health-promoting interventions, substantial amounts of mothers' time—which is not easily valued in terms, say, of wages forgone (Leslie 1992). Finally, whereas environmental interventions have beneficial health consequences, their main objectives often lie outside the health sector; World Bank (1992) provides a recent comprehensive discussion.

Appendix table 1A-2 lists a number of public health interventions that have a range of outcomes; in country-specific applications, assessment of the cost-effectiveness of these interventions should, ideally, quantitatively aggregate intervention effects along these multiple dimensions of outcome. Likewise for clinical intervention there will frequently be joint costs (associated, for one example, with the availability of diagnostic facilities in a district hospital); again, in country-specific application, these matters need to be assessed more quantitatively than they can be in a general overview.

Authors of the disease-specific chapters of this collection have generally noted where interventions for the condition they were addressing had multiple outcomes, and in this chapter, I too note the most important cases. It is clear, looking across findings of the individual chapters in this collection, that multiple effect and joint cost problems do complicate the task of assessing cost-effectiveness in many important instances; that said, it is more generally true that these problems are relatively minor or can be dealt with by reasonable approximations and simplifications in the analysis.

Findings

Appendix table 1A-3 presents, in very summary form, the findings from the chapters in this collection concerning public health interventions. For each disease category the first column of appendix table 1A-3 indicates relevant intervention strategies, and the second indicates, to be explicit, the objective of intervention—primary prevention, secondary prevention, cure, rehabilitation, or palliation (as defined in table 1-2). The first column states findings on cost-effectiveness and, where applicable, notes the most important factors (from table 1-4) likely to lead to variability in cost-effectiveness across circumstances.

Although the entries in appendix table 1A-3 are self-explanatory, a few general observations on each primary category of intervention may be worth making.

PERSONAL BEHAVIOR CHANGE. Some personal behavior changes that are favorable for health outcomes tend to occur naturally as incomes rise; these include, at least for many cultures, improved hygienic behaviors, increased energy intake and quality in the diet, and decreased crowding. Improvements in these behaviors are typically important for the pre-epidemiological transition diseases and, as entries in appendix table 1A-3 indicate, can often be affected by educational interventions even though the main force driving improvements—income increases—is beyond the domain of health policy.

Other behaviors are likely either to be less dependent on income levels (for example, breastfeeding behavior, sexual practices) or to be adversely influenced by income increases, at least for a period of time (for example, dietary excess, sedentary lifestyles, smoking, alcohol consumption). Most of these are risk behaviors for posttransition conditions. Although the natural course of development is unlikely to improve these behaviors, there is more of a scope for affordable government policy to influence them. Regulatory policies and, particularly, taxation policies for tobacco, alcohol, and fatty meats show great promise for inducing behavioral change and, currently, are very much underused. Education of elites and the public are complementary instruments, not least because they generate the political will and popular support for regulation and taxation. The extremely high cost-effectiveness of smoking control makes it, perhaps, the top priority for governmental action (Stanley, appendix A, this collection); although less well documented, the probably high cost-effectiveness of alcohol control makes it another priority.

ENVIRONMENTAL HAZARDS CONTROL. Rising incomes help with improving water supply and sanitation and that is likely to be important in prevention of a broad range of infectious and parasitic diseases. Vector control is at least marginally cost-effective for a number of conditions (malaria, onchocerciasis, dengue) in some environments. Industrialization introduces new hazards into the environment (lead, mercury, and the like) that can produce severe lifetime disability if not effectively controlled. Improvements in household ventilation, indoor fireplaces, and cookstoves can substantially reduce risks for chronic obstructive pulmonary disease (COPD); and occupational and transport safety measures are important in many specific instances. In principle, protective measures can be delivered through environmental intervention, and water fluoridation for prevention of caries is one example. Not explicitly mentioned in appendix table 1A-3 is the problem of lead toxicity resulting from excess use of lead-based paints and combustion of gasoline with high lead content. Recent research—reviewed in Pollitt (1990)—indicates that lead toxicity may be far more important than previously thought as a determinant of slow development and impaired mental functioning.

IMMUNIZATION, MASS CHEMOPROPHYLAXIS, AND SCREENING. The interventions listed on appendix table 1A-3 under the headings Immunization, Mass Chemoprophylaxis, and Screening all share certain common characteristics: (a) they involve the direct administration or application of a specific technical intervention to individuals on a one-by-one basis, (b) they are directed to certain target populations, and (c) the coverage of the target population is important to produce the desired effect. Technically, each of these intervention strategies is highly efficacious when correctly applied to a compliant subject, but their actual effectiveness in developing-country settings is strongly conditioned by the local administrative, managerial, and logistical capabilities, as well as by traditional cultural constraints.

Although it is no surprise, the all-pervasive potential of immunization programs is dramatically underlined in the findings set forth in appendix table 1A-3. Most immunization interventions are highly cost-effective; and many of them address highly prevalent conditions. Measles and tetanus vaccination appear particularly cost-effective and worthy of relatively greater attention within immunization programs. Far more could be efficiently spent on immunization than is now being spent; and, even though costs of delivery tend to rise as more marginal populations are reached, extending immunization programs to virtually universal coverage is likely to prove both cost-effective and a practical way of significantly improving the health of the poor.

One particularly promising application of mass chemoprophylaxis lies in the administration of anthelmintic medication and micronutrient supplements to school-age children. Here cost-effectiveness appears quite high for conditions that, although of extremely high prevalence, have only recently been seen to be of substantial importance for intellectual and physical development. A program of chemoprophylaxis for school-age children could, like the Expanded Programme on Immunization (EPI) for younger children, be expected to serve as the starting point for an ultimately much expanded capacity to deal with the health needs of this age group; the Rockefeller Foundation and the UNDP are jointly initiating such a program.

Perhaps the only significant cancers for which treatment is cost-effective (breast, cervical) are ones for which early screening and referral are important; so, as NCDs begin to emerge, this strategy will become increasingly relevant. The emerging strategies for treatment of acute respiratory infections in children all rely heavily on community-based programs for early detection and quick referral; with increased experience, improvements in capacity for cost-effective screening and referral programs can be expected to develop.

These comments only touch on some of the findings summarized in appendix table 1A-3 to give a sense of their range and diversity. Next is a discussion of clinical interventions.

The Findings: Clinical Interventions

Facilities to provide clinical intervention vary continuously in size, in the degree of complexity (and range) of the conditions that they address, in the sophistication of their facilities and equipment, and in the training and skill of their staff.[12] The authors have found it useful, nonetheless, to use generally accepted terminology in categorizing facilities into three groups—clinic-level, district hospitals, and referral hospitals— while recognizing that that categorization involves much simplification and that the appropriate classification structure will vary substantially from country to country. Appendix table 1A-4 indicates (in a very general way), for each of these three levels of facility, examples of the kinds of interventions they might address and what capacity such a facility might have for primary modes of diagnostic and therapeutic intervention.

Each chapter of this collection addresses the desirability not only of public health intervention but also of clinical interventions that might be mounted at various levels of the referral system. One lesson that emerges from these chapters is that currently such analyses are severely constrained by the paucity of data relating to the effect and cost of clinical interventions. In the absence of such analyses, it is perhaps natural for developing countries to import, to the extent that resources permit, the methods of case management used or being developed in high-income countries. The key phrase here is, of course, "to the extent that resources permit." Available resources permit importation of high-cost interventions for only a tiny proportion of a developing country's population.[13] In order to extend access to services for the rapidly emerging epidemic of acquired immunodeficiency syndrome (AIDS) as well as for the impending epidemic of noncommunicable disease, radically lower cost methods of case management will need to be developed from the rich range of technologies and procedures that now exist, or that are coming into being.

Appendix table 1A-5 summarizes data from the individual chapters on the cost-effectiveness of clinical intervention, by disease, subject to the caveat that potentially remediable data deficiencies have frequently left a high margin of uncertainty. The table includes discussion, for each condition, of the strategy (level of facility and mode of intervention) for treating it, indicates the objective of intervention, and summarizes findings on cost-effectiveness.

Several observations stand out from appendix table 1A-5:

• Curative care for tuberculosis and sexually transmitted diseases appears extremely cost-effective; further, such care is not now being provided to anything like the extent it should be, given the high burden of morbidity and mortality resulting from these conditions. Surgical treatment of cataract is also highly cost-effective.

- The extremely diverse range of clinical interventions of moderate cost-effectiveness (medical management of angina or diabetes are examples as is surgical management of cervical cancer) suggests that country-specific analyses of these conditions are required and that facilities capable of competently handling diverse conditions will need to be developed.
- The cost is sufficiently high for some clinical interventions to imply that even if they are effective (as is the case with coronary artery bypass grafting to deal with angina), their cost-effectiveness is so poor that their use should be actively discouraged until other, more cost-effective interventions can be delivered to their appropriate potential.
- Control of pain from terminal cancer could benefit perhaps 1.5 million individuals annually at acceptable costs; current legislation and standard practices greatly limit what is done in relation to what potentially could be done.
- Rehabilitation (in particular from leprosy, poliomyelitis, and injury) shows promise of being extremely cost-effective; but very little attention has been accorded rehabilitation, and little is known about how best to provide services on a population basis or what might be expected in terms of effectiveness and cost.

Again, as with the discussion of public health interventions, one theme that emerges from this review of clinical cost-effectiveness is that of complexity and diversity. Many interventions are clearly not cost-effective, and public policy should make every effort to discourage their use. But the available evidence does suggest that a broad range of interventions, addressing a similarly broad range of conditions, will prove cost-effective. Many of these interventions are not now being used to anything like the extent that they should be. Likewise, much of what is currently undertaken by the clinical system is misdirected (toward interventions of low cost-effectiveness) or simply inefficiently used. Redirection of substantial resources from interventions of low cost-effectiveness toward those with very high cost-effectiveness is clearly possible; a central task of health policy must be to design implementation strategies and government policy instruments that can promote these potential efficiency gains.

Conclusions

I draw five very broad conclusions—one methodological and the other four substantive—from this collection reporting on the World Bank's Health Sector Priorities Review. The methodological conclusion is that it is feasible, on a broad scale, systematically to assess intervention cost-effectiveness in the health sector. The effort required is substantial, but results that allow broad intrasectoral assessment of intervention priorities can be obtained.

One substantive conclusion is that the available evidence points to great variation, across interventions, in marginal cost-effectiveness.[14] Appendix table 1A-6 summarizes this evidence by grouping interventions into ranges of marginal cost per DALY in hypothetical (but realistic) environments. The challenge ahead is that of designing and implementing instruments of government policy that will greatly expand use of the interventions in the first two sections of appendix table 1A-6 while decreasing use of interventions, like those in the last section of the table, that provide very little value for money.

Garber and Phelps (1992) observe, though, that under a reasonable range of assumptions it will make economic sense to pay for DALYs up to a cost of about twice the level of income; this leads to a second substantive conclusion from appendix table 1A-6, which is that, in many countries, quite a broad array of interventions is likely to prove attractive by any reasonable economic standard.

My third substantive conclusion concerns the extent to which public health as opposed to clinical strategies tend to be more cost-effective and the extent to which seeking primary preventive objectives will tend to be more cost-effective than seeking other objectives. Appendix tables 1A-7 and 1A-8 summarize the material from appendix table 1A-6 in ways that allow these questions to be addressed. Although there are some patterns (in particular, primary prevention by way of immunization accounts for many highly cost-effective interventions), in general I conclude that there is no especially strong general tendency for primary prevention or public health interventions to have superior cost-effectiveness.

The fourth substantive conclusion is that virtually no cost-effective interventions require more specialized facilities than those available at district hospitals. Thus, even though one cannot argue in general in favor of prevention over cure or public health over clinical intervention, one *can* conclude that district hospitals and lower level facilities potentially offer almost all attractive interventions.

Appendix 1A: Clinical and Public Health Interventions

The eight tables in this appendix examine clinical and public health interventions and relate the characteristics of the different interventions to their cost-effectiveness.

Table 1A-1. Public Health Interventions

Intervention strategy	Adverse health outcomes avoided or treated
Promoting healthy behavior	
Dietary practices	
Maternal	Low birth weight
Infant/child	Growth-stunting infection, micronutrient deficiency
Adult	Obesity, diabetes, cancer, ischemic heart disease, hypertensive disease
Prevention against infection	
Personal hygiene	Diarrheal diseases, intestinal parasites, skin infections
Use of soap	
Food handling	
Defecation practices	
Household ventilation/crowding	Respiratory diseases
Sexual behaviors	Sexually transmitted diseases, premature fertility
Personal health practices	
Exercise	Obesity, heart disease
Stress control	Mental disease
Carelessness	Injuries, poisoning
Tobacco use	Cancer, heart disease, chronic obstructive pulmonary disease
Controlling substance abuse	
Alcohol	Hypertensive disease, cirrhosis, injuries
Drugs	Addiction, injuries, mental disease
Preventing intentional mutilation	Injuries
Reproductive practices	
Contraceptive practice	Unwanted pregnancy
Pregnancy care	Pregnancy outcome
Childbirth practice	Perinatal/maternal mortality
Breastfeeding practice	Malnutrition, diarrhea
Abortion	Maternal mortality, unwanted pregnancy
Home care	
Use of first aid	Injury
Use of oral rehydration therapy	Diarrheal disease, acute diabetic conditions
Clinic use	
Treatment of simple conditions	Entry into referral structure
Control of environmental hazards	
Household	
Water availability/quality	Water-related diseases
Waste disposal	Infectious diseases, toxic exposures
Food hygiene	Diarrhea, parasites
Air quality	Respiratory disease
Vector control	Malaria, yellow fever, river blindness
Community	
Housing quality	Injury, poisoning
Motor vehicle/road safety	Accidents, injuries
Occupational hazard control	Injury, toxic exposure
Public health services	
Immunization	
At birth	Hepatitis B, tuberculosis
First year of life	Polio, measles, diphtheria, tetanus, pertussis
School age	Tetanus
Adulthood	Tetanus, yellow fever, influenza
Mass chemoprophylaxis	
Food fortification	Iodine and other deficiencies
Micronutrient supplementation	Vitamin A and other deficiencies
Water fluoridation	Caries
School-based provision of anthelmintics	Schistosomiasis, intestinal helminths
Mass administration of antibiotics	Sexually transmitted diseases
Screening and referral	
Screening programs in clinics, schools, work sites, and so on	Selected infectious diseases (such as tuberculosis); cancers (such as cervix, breast); cardiovascular disease risk factors (such as hypertension, hyperlipidemia); high-risk pregnancy

Source: Author.

Table 1A-2. Selected Interventions with Multiple Outcomes

Intervention	Outcome		
	Main health outcome	Secondary health outcome	Nonhealth outcomes
Provision of water supplies and sanitation	Control of diarrheal diseases	Control of skin, respiratory, and helminthic infections	Saving of household time; welfare improvements
Provision of soap	Control of diarrheal diseases	Control of skin, respiratory, and helminthic infections	
Reduction of vehicle speed limits	Reduced severity and incidence of crash-related injuries		Reduction in property damage from vehicle crashes; energy conservation; time costs
Control of smoking	Reduced incidence of lung cancer, heart disease, and chronic obstructive pulmonary disease	Reduced incidence of minor cancers; reduction in burn injuries	Welfare loss for current addicts, welfare gain for nonsmokers; freeing of land and labor for uses other than tobacco production
Vector control	Reduced incidence of vector-borne diseases		Improved welfare when vectors, such as mosquitoes, are nuisances
Female education	Reduced child mortality rates	Improved child growth; reduced adult health	Higher levels of female productivity and earnings; improved congruence between actual and desired fertility levels
Breastfeeding	Improved child growth through improved nutrient availability and protection against diarrhea	Protection of child against infectious disease; postponement of next pregnancy; possible long-term cognitive benefits to child	Savings in costs of infant formula and bottles; time costs for mother
Family planning services	Reduced child mortality	Reduced maternal morbidity and mortality	Economic and welfare gains from improved control of level and timing of fertility

Source: Author.

Table 1A-3. Public Health Interventions: Cost and Effectiveness

Condition	Intervention strategy	Objective	Cost and effectiveness	Comments
Acute respiratory infections (ARI) (see chap. 4)	Screening and referral: households need to be educated to identify signs of pneumonia in children and bring them to clinics for treatment	Cure	Costs per disability-adjusted life-year (DALY) $20 in high-mortality environments to $50 in low-mortality environments	Has variable efficacy in all age groups. See ARI case management chapter for details of program
	Behavior change: breastfeeding promotion via education programs	Secondary prevention (via strengthening of child to reduce effects of infection)	Approximately $50 per DALY (for ARI consequences of breastfeeding only)	Multiple benefits, including averted infant mortality
	Reduced protein-energy malnutrition via supplementation programs	Secondary prevention (via strengthening of child to reduce effects of infection)	Estimated cost per DALY about $65	Depending upon food availability
	Immunization: for pertussis, see discussion of poliomyelitis; Pneumococcal vaccine For measles, see that entry	Primary prevention	For appropriate age groups (> 18 mo.), cost per DALY saved about $70	Has variable efficacy for all age groups
	Hemophilus influenzae vaccine	Primary prevention	No estimates available for cost-effectiveness; vaccine costs high, $2 to $14 per dose. Moderate efficacy in children over two years	Efficacy trials in early stages
Diarrheal diseases (see chap. 5)	Possible immunizations: using effective rotavirus vaccine	Primary prevention	Approximately $10 per DALY, assuming 80 percent vaccine efficacy	Effective vaccine still not available
	Using effective cholera vaccine	Primary prevention	Approximately $75 per DALY, assuming 70 percent vaccine efficacy	Current vaccines have low efficacies
	Immunization: measles vaccine	Primary prevention	Approximately $10 per DALY, assuming 85 percent vaccine efficacy	Rotavirus and measles-associated diarrhea is much more common than cholera, explaining much of the cost-effectiveness differences
	Control of environment: improving water supply and sanitation by upgrading of infrastructure	Primary prevention	Cost-effectiveness of diarrhea averted is unknown, but there are additional benefits	Estimated to reduce diarrhea morbidity and mortality by about 30 percent
	Behavior change: improved domestic and personal hygiene via education	Primary prevention	Approximately $170 per DALY, depending on case-fatality reductions, incidence rates, and wage levels	
	Breastfeeding promotion by various methods, including changes in hospital routine and mass-media education	Primary prevention	Approximately $30 per DALY, assuming a reduction in non-breastfeeding of 40 percent (< 2 months), 30 percent (3–5 months) and 10 percent (6–11 months) and assuming a judicious selection of interventions used	See above
	Improving weaning practices by education	Secondary prevention	Approximately $30 per DALY, in children < 75 percent weight-for-age, age six months to five years	See above

(Table continues on the following page.)

Table 1A-3 (continued)

Condition	Intervention strategy	Objective	Cost and effectiveness	Comments
Poliomyelitis (see chap. 6)	*Immunization:* oral or injectable polio vaccine in three or more doses to children under one year of age; given simultaneously with diphtheria, pertussis, and tetanus DPT immunization	Primary prevention; established a global objective: eradication of disease from wild polio virus by the year 2000	For polio plus DPT, cost per DALY approximately $20 in high-mortality environments and $40 in low-mortality environments; cost per DALY of DPT without polio vaccine somewhat higher and cost of polio without DPT immunization many times higher	If injectable used, there could be a reduced number of needed contact raising immunization rates and costs per fully vaccinated child in some environments
Helminthic infection (see chap. 7)	*Targeted mass chemotherapy:* school-based delivery of anthelmintics (praziquantel for schistosomes and albendazole for intestinal helmintics in high-endemicity areas without individual screening)	Secondary prevention	Ranging from $6 to $33 per DALY; low estimate assumes either 0.02 or 0.2 DALYs saved yearly and high estimate assumes either 0.05 or 0.5 DALYs saved yearly. Approximately 80 percent effectiveness and heavily reliant on intensity of infection	Cost-effectiveness figures are hypothetical, using range of program costs and empirical estimates of efficacy
	Targeted screening and treatment: praziquantel and albendazole given after screening in targeted groups	Secondary prevention	Depending upon intensity of infection	Generally two-thirds as effective at same cost as mass or targeted chemoprophylaxis
	Control of environment: onchocerciasis vector control with chemical pesticides	Primary prevention	$100–$200 per DALY saved, and closely tied with breeding patterns of vector	Variable efficacy in trials
	Cloth filters for crustacean intermediate of Dracunculus (guinea worm)	Primary prevention	Probable low cost	Only enclosed water supplies will eradicate disease
Measles (see chap. 8)	*Immunization:* four possible scenarios: • the current antigen at nine months of age • the above plus coverage at all "opportunities" • the E-Z antigen at six months • the E-Z antigen at six months and nine months	Primary prevention via individual protection; with high vaccination coverage rates, some protection resulting from interruption of transmission	With use of the current measles antigen at the recommended nine months of age, base cost per DALY gained $2 to $15, depending on case-fatality rates and cost of the measles portion of the program. Epidemiologic model to assess effectiveness of alternative antigens and two-dose schedules demonstrates that significantly more deaths could be averted over the base cost at costs per incremental DALY of twice the cost per DALY of the base case—still relatively attractive	Vaccination should begin earlier in life in areas with high measles mortality. This change in vaccination schedule would alter cost-effective figures
Tetanus (see chap. 9)	*Immunization:* routine vaccination targeting women of childbearing age, and pregnant women, schoolgirls, infants, and males	Primary prevention	Approximately $2–10 per DALY gained, predominantly from averted neonatal tetanus mortality. Depends on incidence rates, which in turn are tied with health infrastructure, especially birth practices	Choice of strategy and target group varies according to incidence, available resources, health service organization, channels for contact, immediacy of desired impact, and so on
	Behavior change: training birth attendants	Primary prevention	Suspected to be higher than costs for routine vaccination of pregnant women	Training, supervision, and support costs may be too high for much of the developing world

18

Disease	Type	Intervention	Cost	Comments
Rheumatic heart disease (see chap. 10)	Primary prevention	*Immunization:* to prevent incidence of rheumatic fever/rheumatic heart disease (RF/RHD) precursor, group A streptococcus	Possible low cost	Vaccine under development; unlikely to be available for many years
	Primary prevention of RF	*Screening and referral:* for children with pharyngitis refer to clinic for antibiotic prophylaxis against RF	Cost about $300 per DALY; high because proportion of pharyngitis cases that develop into RF is low	May encounter resistant strains, necessitating expensive antibiotics
Tuberculosis (see chap. 11)	Primary prevention	*Immunization:* BCG added to DPT program	$7 per DALY; cost-effectiveness drops substantially when annual risk of infection < 1 percent	Reported effectiveness of vaccine is widely variable. Costs of BCG program alone are four times those of adding it to preexisting EPI
	Primary and secondary prevention	*Targeted chemoprophylaxis:* selective screening in high-risk populations (AIDS patients and family members of tuberculosis patients) and treatment of smear-positive patients	Suspected to be reasonable	Mass prophylaxis has high costs with limited effectiveness
Leprosy (see chap. 12)	Primary prevention	*Immunization:* use of BCG vaccine to prevent leprosy	Probably reasonable, as costs be shared with tuberculosis immunization program. Will depend on incidence rates	Vaccine reported to be 30–80 percent effective against leprosy, depending on age at vaccination and regions studied
	Primary prevention	*Targeted screening:* passive screening via clinical exam	$0.50 per DALY, sensitive to percentage of cases which are multibacillary or paucibacillary (harder to diagnose clinically) and incidence rates	Does not include treatment costs (see appendix table 1A-5)
Malaria (see chap. 13)	Primary prevention	*Control of environment:* chemical vector control via intradomicillary spraying of insecticide to kill adult mosquitoes	$5–$250 per DALY, depending on type of mosquito which is the primary determinant of case fatality. Also linked with incidence rates and geographical distribution of the human and mosquito population	If population widespread, the marginal costs of eradication are high. Cost-effectiveness will decrease if spraying is carried out in nonuniform manner
	Primary prevention	Environmental vector control via drainage and land management techniques	Suspected to be high	Role limited to urban areas. Chemically impregnated bed netting with promising results
Dengue (see chap. 14)	Primary prevention	*Control of environment:* spraying of chemical insecticide for Aedes mosquito	$2,200 per DALY tied to how quickly Aedes replaces itself	Has to be repeated several times per year
	Primary prevention	Direct expenditures and education for eliminating breeding sites of Aedes mosquito	$3,500 per DALY needs integrated program to be effective	Closely related to labor costs. Has potential of sustained long-term control or eradication
	Primary prevention	*Possible immunization:* two-dose vaccination will probably be needed	$1,600 per DALY heavily dependent on incidence rates	Vaccine in planning stages

(Table continues on the following page.)

Table 1A-3 *(continued)*

Condition	Intervention strategy	Objective	Cost and effectiveness	Comments
Hepatitis B (see chap. 15)	*Immunization*: adding three dose vaccine to preexisting immunization program	Primary prevention	$25–$50 per DALY depending on prevalence of carrier state and ability of immunization program to provide adequate coverage using a three-dose schedule	Discounting of benefits is important, since vaccine is given at birth and averted mortality occurs late in life. Cost of treating significant morbidity important (especially cirrhosis). Vaccine costs are variable but have declined significantly for public sector programs. Maximum cost-effectiveness may be achieved only through integration into routine infant immunization programs
Excess fertility (see chap. 16)	*Behavior change*: increasing the use of condoms via education and subsidization	Primary prevention	$15–$75 per DALY will vary depending on number of births which exceed the resources of a family or society and the mortality associated with this excess. The effectiveness of the program is an essential component which will rely on personal acceptance of condoms	Only includes benefits derived from averted mortality by increasing birth interval and limiting teenage pregnancies. Assumes theoretical 100 percent effectiveness
	Use of information, education, and communication model to lengthen birth intervals by encouraging breastfeeding	Primary prevention	Suspected to be of low to moderate cost and is dependent upon cultural biases	Benefits from averted ARI and diarrhea cases in breastfed child are significant
Maternal and perinatal health (see chap. 17)	See entry in appendix table 1A-5			
Protein-energy malnutrition (see chap. 18)	*Targeted mass chemoprophylaxis*: food supplementation for preschool children resulting in a 100,000-calorie transfer and 0.5-kg average weight gain	Secondary prevention	$70 per DALY, based on relationship between food supplementation and child growth for particular weight-for-age child	Depends on percentage of target population that are severely or moderately malnourished, since standard food transfer will affect these groups differently
	Food supplementation for pregnant women resulting in a 100,000-calorie transfer and a 300-gram increase in birth weight	Secondary prevention	$25 DALY, based on relationship between food supplementation and fetal growth as it affects infant mortality	See above
Micronutrient deficiency disorders (see chap. 19)	*Targeted mass chemoprophylaxis*: daily self-administered oral iron supplementation for duration of pregnancy	Secondary prevention	$13 per DALY, depending on prevalence rates and severity of iron deficiency anemia	In regions of severe iron deficiency anemia
	Use of injected or oral iodinated oil once every two to five years in women of reproductive age	Secondary prevention	$20 per DALY varies with prevalence rates and severity of iodine deficiency	Clean syringes need to be used
	Semiannual mass dose of vitamin A for children age zero to five	Secondary prevention	$9 per DALY varies with prevalence rates and severity of vitamin A deficiency	Benefits include averted measles, respiratory and diarrheal mortality

	Type of prevention	Cost-effectiveness	Comments
Mass chemoprophylaxis: fortification of salt or sugar supplies with iron-containing compounds	Secondary prevention	$5 per DALY varies with prevalence rates and severity of iron-deficiency anemia	As with all food fortification programs, the carrier must be available and accepted by the groups at risk
Iodization of salt or water	Secondary prevention	$8 per DALY, depending on prevalence rates and severity of iodine deficiency	See above
Fortification of sugar with vitamin A compounds	Secondary prevention	$5 per DALY, depending on prevalence rates and severity of vitamin A deficiency	See above
HIV infection and other sexually transmitted diseases (see chap. 20)			
Screening and referral: blood screening for HIV among blood donors using rapid lab tests	Primary prevention	$1–$250 per DALY linked to the prevalence rate of HIV infection among blood donors and sexual activity group of proposed blood recipient	Cost of blood test relies on sophistication of health care system
Behavior change: information, education, and communication program to: (a) decrease frequency of sexual partner change, and (b) increase proportion of sex acts protected by condoms	Primary prevention	$1–$150 per DALY depends on sexual activity and prevalence of each type of sexually transmitted disease in target population (i.e., HIV transmission rates in population with syphilis greater than in population with chancroid)	Social barriers to condom usage are often important. Practical problems include the identification of the "access group" by which high-risk groups can be identified
Female education and employment: reduce supply of female sex workers by raising their opportunity cost and reduce demand for their services by attracting more women to urban areas	Primary prevention	Likely to be highly effective in the long run and may yield many benefits other than disease control	Cost-effectiveness difficult to compute
Cancers (see chap. 21)			
Screening and referral: use of PAP smear at five-year intervals to screen for cervical cancer	Secondary prevention	$100 per DALY, based on prevalence rates and health care setting in which program is carried out	Assumes that there will be an appropriate referral system for further treatment if indicated by PAP smear
Annual breast examinations to screen for breast cancer	Secondary prevention	$50 per DALY based on prevalence rates and health care setting in which program is carried out	Same as above and use of annual mammography at one-year intervals for women fifty-nine and above reduces cost-effectiveness tenfold
Behavior change: smoking cessation classes	Primary prevention	$20 per DALY tied to percentage of antismoking effort aimed at preventing "new starters" or those already smoking	Less expensive to prevent onset of smoking than to have smokers quit
Smoking reduction via tobacco tax	Primary prevention	See COPD entry in this table	See COPD entry in this table
Diabetes (see chap. 22)			
Behavior change: health education to improve dietary and exercise habits may hold potential for prevention of non-insulin-dependent diabetes (NIDDM)	Primary prevention of NIDDM	Costs might be $0.02 to $0.50 per capita per year; effectiveness unknown but probably low. Cost-effectiveness enhanced by similarity of the behavior changes for reducing cardiovascular and some cancer risks	NIDDM patients often have limited modification program rates
Screening and referral: screening for glucose intolerance in high-risk groups (such as obese, pregnant women) may allow for more precise targeting of health education and perhaps medication	Primary and secondary prevention of NIDDM	Unknown; cost-effectiveness depends on prevalence in the screened group and cost-effectiveness of referred interventions	High costs associated with complication (stroke, coronary artery disease, ketoacidosis, and coma)

(Table continues on the following page.)

Table 1A-3 (continued)

Condition	Intervention strategy	Objective	Cost and effectiveness	Comments
Cardiovascular disease (see chap. 23)	*Behavior change:* through a public prevention package (mass education and individual counseling); screening and referral services to those at high risk	Primary and secondary prevention	Costs perhaps less than $1 per capita per year in targeted population, about $150 per DALY	Effectiveness will depend on depth of impact.
Chronic obstructive pulmonary disease (see chap. 24)	*Behavior change:* smoking reduction via tobacco tax and education/cessation programs	Primary prevention	20 percent tax on tobacco might reduce overall tobacco consumption by about 20 percent and avert perhaps 40 deaths per year in a typical population of 200,000 smokers. Adding educational programs, $20 per DALY can be achieved	Heavy smokers (those with greatest risk) may be unresponsive to program
Injury (see chap. 25)	Alcohol taxation to discourage use resulting in 30 percent decrease in fall, transportation, and burn injuries	Primary prevention	Low to moderate cost per DALY depends on case-fatality rates and percentage of injuries that are alcohol attributable	If public is strongly against an alcohol tax, illicitly produced alcohol use may increase, resulting in excess mortality
	Education programs to reduce transportation, burn, and poisoning injuries by 40–50 percent	Primary prevention	Moderate cost per DALY depends on depth of impact and case-fatality rates	Injury education programs have limited effectiveness without safety laws. Alcohol awareness component often essential
	Control of environment: manufacture, modification, and use of products such as seat belts, safer stoves, and childproof caps to cause a 50 percent reduction in transportation, fall, burn, and poisoning injuries	Primary prevention	High cost per DALY depends on case-fatality rates and percentage of injuries which are preventable by environmental improvements	Safer product will still have to be inexpensive and some improvements will require enormous fixed costs
Cataract (see chap. 26)	*Behavior change:* ocular protection from solar radiation (e.g., hats and sunglasses)	Primary prevention	Inexpensive depending upon extent to which cataract progression is retarded by eye protection	Probably beneficial, but to what extent is unknown
Oral health (see chap. 27)	See appendix table 1A-5			
Schizophrenia and manic-depressive illness (see chap. 28)	See appendix table 1A-5			

Source: See chapters on individual diseases in this collection.

Table 1A-4. Clinical Intervention: Level of Facility and Mode of Intervention

Level of clinical facility	Typical conditions addressed	Intervention mode			
			Therapeutic		
		Diagnostic	Medical	Surgical	Physical or psychological therapy
Clinic (private, community, and school- and work-based)	Minor trauma; simple injections; support of population-based interventions; uncomplicated childbirth; family planning	Clinical	Short list of essential drugs (about 20)	Sutures	Important potential role for supervisng physical therapy
District hospital	Complicated childbirth fractures and burns; complicated infections; cataract; hernia; appendectomy; diabetes, hypertension, and similarly complex condition	Clinical; basic laboratory; basic radiologic facilities	Long list of essential drugs (about 200)	Capacity for dealing with abdominal surgery, many fractures, cesarean sections, some rehabilitative surgery	Design and management of more complex regimens of physical and psychological therapy
Referral hospital	More complicated medical and surgical conditions	More advanced laboratory and radiologic facilities	As above, but also specialized drugs, chemo-therapy, and radiotherapy	As above but also capacity for more complicated surgery of head and chest	Support capacity for district hospitals

Source: Author.

Table 1A-5. Clinical Interventions: Cost and Effectiveness

Condition	Intervention strategy	Objective	Cost and effectiveness	Comments
Acute respiratory infections (see chap. 4)	Clinic level: antibiotic treatment of pneumonia in young children (for whom case-fatality rates high). To succeed, control programs must educate families to bring children with cough or difficulty breathing to a facility quickly	Cure	Costs per disability-adjusted life-year (DALY) saved is $20 in high-mortality to $50 in low-mortality environments	Resistance to "first line" antibiotics will necessitate use of expensive antibiotics. Costs of allergic reaction to medication could be substantial.
Diarrheal diseases (see chap. 5)	Clinic level: education and distribution of ORT sugar-salt solution	Secondary prevention	Ranging from $35–$350 per DALY, depending on the case-fatality rate of target population and the cost of labor	Assuming cost per diarrhea of $1.00–$5.00 and 0.05%–0.5% of deaths prevented per case treated
	Use of antibiotics and antimotility agents	Curative	Very poor cost-effectiveness for most diarrhea cases for which they are either harmful or useless	May be indicated for dysentery or cholera
Poliomyelitis (see chap. 6)	Clinic level: physiotherapy, psychotherapy, provision of simple prostheses to enhance physical function and promote social integration	Rehabilitation	Potential high cost per DALY	Needs constant source of skilled labor
	District and referral hospital levels: surgery of varying degrees of complexity	Rehabilitation	Probable moderate to low cost per DALY	Developed health care system and expensive specialists when needed
Helminthic infection (see chap. 7)	See entry in appendix table 1A-3			
Measles	Clinic level: therapeutic doses of vitamin A for children with severe measles; other therapy (including use of antibiotics) to further reduce adverse consequences	Secondary prevention	Limited evidence that case-fatality rates can be reduced by 50 percent or more from their initial levels of 0.01–0.05. If such therapy costs $10, cost per DALY of therapy would be $20–$80	Proportion of measles morbidity and mortality which is preventable via supplementation is still being investigated
Tetanus (see chap. 9)	Referral hospital level: case management care including neurorespiratory resuscitation; antispasmodic therapy; antitoxin drugs, wound care, and intensive nursing	Cure	$100 per DALY and is tied to case-fatality reduction	Needs moderately sophisticated health care system, wide range in protocol costs. Few neonatal tetanus patients are brought for medical care.
Rheumatic heart disease (see chap. 10)	Clinical level: regular administration of antibiotics at three- to four-week intervals prevents recurrence in patients who have had rheumatic fever (RF), later bouts of RF, hence emergence of rheumatic heart disease	Secondary prevention	$100–$200 per DALY in compliant patients	Compliance is an issue
	Referral hospital level: open-heart surgery in higher-level referral hospitals to permit restoration of function in mitral or other valves (valvuloplasty)	Secondary prevention and rehabilitation	$1,000–$2,000 per DALY, depending on age of patient and local surgical costs	Needs advanced health care system

Disease (chapter)	Intervention	Type	Cost per DALY	Notes
Tuberculosis (see chap. 11)	*Clinic level:* short-course chemotherapy with two-month hospitalization	Cure Primary prevention	$3 per DALY linked to hospitalization costs. Standard chemotherapy has lower drug costs, but a lesser cure rate compared with short-course chemotherapy (with similar hospitalization periods)	Resistant strains could become a significant problem (especially among AIDS patients) causing an increase in costs
Leprosy (see chap. 12)	*Clinic level:* multidrug therapy with monthly visits to health center and daily oral medication	Cure	$7 per DALY will depend on percentage of cases which are multi- or paucibacillary since the latter has much higher treatment costs. Does not include benefits of decreased transmission	Compliance with daily oral medication and drug resistance needs to be considered in detail (see appendix table 1A-3) or capital costs ($3 per DALY)
	District hospital level: treatment of complications, including reconstructive surgery, ulcer therapy, and alternate medication	Rehabilitation	$190 per DALY, depending on level of services provided	Sensitive to labor and hospital costs
Malaria (see chap. 13)	*District level:* treatment of passively detected malarial patients in regions of moderate-to-high endemicity and chemical vector control	Cure Primary prevention	$200–$500 per DALY tied to case-fatality rates and levels of endemicity	See appendix table 1A-3 for chemical vector control data. Active case searches are expensive and drug resistance may be a problem if antimalarials are used haphazardly
Dengue (see chap. 14)	*District or referred hospital levels:* Improved case management with better education of physicians, lab facilities, and pharmacies	Cure Palliation	$630 per DALY, tied to status of health care system	Difficult to define shared costs. Possible only in countries with system as defined
	Improved case management and possible immunization	Cure Palliation Primary prevention	$1,250 per DALY saved	See appendix table 1A-3
	Improved case management and chemical vector control	Cure Palliation Primary prevention	$1,200 per DALY saved	See appendix table 1A-3 for chemical vector control data
	Improved case management and environmental vector control	Cure Palliation Primary prevention	$3,400 per DALY saved	See appendix table 1A-3 for environmental vector control
Hepatitis B (see chap. 15)	See cancer entry in this table			
Excess fertility (see chap. 16)	*Clinic level:* insertion of intra-uterine (IUDs) and oral contraceptives (OCPs) disbursement	Primary prevention	$30–$150 per DALY saved	While the initial cost of an IUD will be greater than the initial OCP outlay, the amortized IUD cost (over its lifetime) is lower
Maternal and perinatal health (see chap. 17)	*Clinic and district hospital level:* improving the community-based outreach system which provides prenatal and birth attendant care. Upgrading building facilities to ensure safe deliveries (including surgical capabilities)	Primary prevention	Approximately $30–$250 per DALY linked to level of services provided, reductions in maternal/perinatal death rates and number of low-birth-weight babies prevented via the intervention	Calculations are theoretical. Family planning may be added in areas of low contraceptive prevalence

(*Table continues on the following page.*)

Table 1A-5 (continued)

Condition	Intervention strategy	Objective	Cost and Effectiveness	Comments
Protein-energy malnutrition (see chap. 18)	*District and hospital level:* treatment with feeding for child, education of mothers, and medication for infections	Rehabilitation	Approximately $150–$250 per DALY tied to case-fatality reduction and level of services provided	Cost-effectiveness figures are still theoretical
Micronutrient deficiency disorders (see chap. 19)	*Clinic level:* blood transfusion of severely anemic patients (especially pregnant women prior to delivery)	Cure	Moderate-to-high cost per DALY, depending on case-fatality reduction from transfusion	All blood has to be tested for HIV and hepatitis, which will raise costs
HIV infection and other sexually transmitted diseases (see chap. 20)	*Clinic level:* use of ophthalmic antibiotic ointment at birth to prevent gonococcal ophthalmia neonatorum	Primary prevention	$5–$125 per DALY with lower values at higher prevalence rates	Ointment easily applied and usually requires one dose
	Treatment of sexually transmitted diseases with antibiotics	Cure Primary prevention	$1–$55 per DALY. Most cost-effective interventions are those targeted at most sexually active group in an HIV epidemic	Cost-effectiveness linked to health care setting
	Clinic and district hospital level: treatment of AIDS with medical and surgical interventions	Palliation	$80–$1,250 per DALY, depending on level of services provided, with lower costs for home care and higher costs for antivirals	Unreliable decreases in morbidity with use of antivirals
Cancers (see chap. 21)	*Referral hospital level:* case management treatment of various cancers via surgery, supportive care, and chemotherapy	Cure Palliation	Cost per DALY as follows: leukemia—$10,000; cervix—$2,600; breast—$3,100; lung—$12,000; liver—$11,000; colon and rectum—$5,000; stomach—$10,500; esophagus—$10,600; mouth and pharynx—$3,700; depends on improvements in case-fatality rates	$150 per DALY when program is confined to pain relief. With the exceptions of early stage oral, cervix, breast, and rectum, technically advanced treatment with high foreign exchange content is needed for most cures
Diabetes (see chap. 22)	*Clinic level:* oral hypoglycemics to stabilize non-insulin-dependent diabetes mellitus (NIDDM); concomitant health education	Secondary prevention	Cost of outpatient provision of oral hypoglycemics about $25 per patient per year; can be quite effective in forestalling complications, including insulin-dependent diabetes (IDDM)	Limited compliance rates reported with long-term use of daily medication
	Injected insulin and health education for IDDM	Secondary prevention	Cost of insulin therapy (life-saving) about $210 per year; estimated cost per DALY about $240	The misuse of insulin could lead to excessive morbidity and mortality
Cardiovascular disease (see chap. 23)	*Primary care level:* medical management of hypertension	Secondary prevention	Cost per DALY gained about $2,000 for typical case, linked to mortality reduction	Medication costs often expensive
	Medical management of hypercholesterolemia	Secondary prevention	Cost per DALY gained about $4,000 in typical case, linked to mortality	See above

Intervention	Type	Cost per DALY	Comments
Medical management of stable angina	Secondary prevention / Rehabilitation	Cost per DALY gained $100–$200	Depends on level of service provided and costs of medication
Management after stroke or myocardial infarction (MI) by behavioral change and appropriate medication	Secondary prevention	Cost per DALY gained $150–$200, tied to disability and mortality reductions	With all cardiovascular interventions
District hospital level: low-cost management of unstable angina acute MI	Secondary prevention / Rehabilitation	Cost per DALY gained approximately $150–$350	Needs advanced health care system
High-cost management of unstable angina or acute MI	Secondary prevention / Rehabilitation	Perhaps $30,000 per DALY saved	
Referral hospital level: angioplasty or bypass graft surgery	Secondary prevention / Rehabilitation	Over $5,000 per DALY gained	See above
Chronic obstructive pulmonary disease (see chap. 24) *District hospital level:* treatment of exacerbation, including mechanical ventilatory assistance, steroids, and fluids	Palliation	Approximately $200–$300 per day for treatment in hospital with a minimal effect on mortality rates	Needs advanced health care system
Injury (see chap. 25) *District or referral hospital level:* treatment of injuries including medical and surgical interventions	Cure / Rehabilitation	Probably expensive, since based on types of injuries treated	Very difficult to estimate cost-effectiveness, as it depends on levels of treatment
Cataract (see chap. 26) *Clinic level:* use of fixed surgical facilities, mobile surgical teams, or eye camps to provide unilateral or bilateral cataract extraction	Cure	$20–$40 per DALY. Some variation expected, depending on societal and personal perception of disability from blindness	Includes costs for glasses every five years
Oral health (see chap. 27) *Clinic level:* plaque and calculus removal, fissure sealants, and topical fluoride. Extraction of teeth with advanced caries	Secondary prevention / Cure	Cost per treatment episode could range between $5 and $20. Cost per DALY saved will depend on number of cases treated to prevent one advanced case of caries and is suspected to be moderately high, since there is no mortality burden. Costs also very sensitive to who is performing intervention; preventive care may also be done with lower costs	Pain and inability to chew as a result of advanced untreated caries causes significant disability. Societal demand for dental procedures often high. Fluoridation of water supply requires advanced supply system. Identification of high-risk groups may be effective in reducing costs
Schizophrenia and manic-depressive illness (see chap. 28) *Clinic level:* use of antipsychotic medication to treat schizophrenic patients with additional use of lithium to treat manic-depressive patients.	Rehabilitation	Cost per DALY gained is $250–$300 for either the schizophrenia or manic-depressive treatment program. Highly sensitive to clinical/societal perception of disability	Clinical training of health center staff, outreach, and compliance components of case are important.

Source: See chapters on individual diseases in this collection.

Table 1A-6. Intervention Characteristics and Cost-Effectiveness

Potential intervention	Strategy	Objective application	Potential group[a]	Age
$25 per DALY[b]				
Breastfeeding promotion	Public health: Behavior change	Secondary prevention	Moderate	Childhood
Diphtheria-pertussis-tetanus plus polio immunization	Public health: Immunization	Primary prevention	Substantial	Childhood
Measles immunization	Public health: Immunization	Primary prevention	Substantial	Childhood
Tuberculosis immunization	Public health: Immunization	Primary prevention	Moderate	Childhood
Iodization of salt	Public health: Mass chemoprophylaxis	Secondary prevention	Substantial	All ages
Fortification of sugar with vitamin A	Public health: Mass chemoprophylaxis	Secondary prevention	Substantial	Childhood
Semiannual mass dose of vitamin A	Public health: Mass chemoprophylaxis	Secondary prevention	Substantial	Childhood
Rotavirus immunization	Public health: Immunization	Primary prevention	Limited	Childhood
Hepatitis B immunization	Public health: Immunization	Primary prevention	Substantial	Childhood
Medical treatment of measles with vitamin A	Clinical: Primary care	Cure	Limited	Childhood
Medical treatment of acute respiratory infections with antibiotics	Clinical: Primary care	Cure	Moderate	Childhood
Use of ophthalmic ointment at birth to prevent gonococcal infection	Clinical: Primary care	Primary prevention	Substantial	Childhood
Targeted mass anthelmintics	Public health: Mass chemoprophylaxis	Secondary prevention	Substantial	School age
Antituberculosis chemotherapy with short-course hospitalization	Clinical: District hospital	Cure	Substantial	All ages
Smoking prevention or cessation programs	Public health: Behavior change	Primary prevention plus secondary prevention	Substantial	Adults
Use of condoms to prevent excess births and sexually transmitted diseases	Public health: Behavior change	Primary prevention	Moderate	Adults
Blood screening for HIV	Clinical: District hospital, Referral hospital	Primary prevention	Limited	Adults
Iodine injections for pregnant women	Public health: Mass chemoprophylaxis	Secondary prevention	Substantial	Adults
Daily oral iron for pregnant women	Public health: Mass chemoprophylaxis	Secondary prevention	Limited	Adults
Cataract removal	Clinical: District hospital	Cure	Substantial	Elderly
Medical treatment of leprosy	Clinical: Primary care	Cure	Moderate	Adults
Malaria control with chemical pesticides	Public health: Environmental	Primary prevention	Moderate	All ages
$25–$75 per DALY				
Pneumococcal immunization	Public health: Immunization	Primary prevention	Moderate	All ages
Use of oral rehydration solutions	Public health: Behavior change	Secondary prevention	Substantial	School age
Improved weaning practices	Public health: Behavior change	Secondary prevention	Moderate	Childhood
Food supplements for children	Public health: Mass chemoprophylaxis	Secondary prevention	Limited	School age
Food supplements for pregnant women	Public health: Mass chemoprophylaxis	Secondary prevention	Limited	Adults
Improved antenatal care by upgrading facilities and providing family planning	Clinical: Primary care, District hospital, Referral hospital	Primary prevention	Limited	Adults
$75–$250 per DALY				
Medical treatment of tetanus	Clinical: District hospital	Cure	Limited	Childhood
Cholera immunization	Public health: Immunization	Primary prevention	Limited	Childhood
Malaria control with passive case finding and chemical pesticides with treatment	Clinical: Primary care, Public health, Environmental	Primary prevention plus cure	Moderate	All ages

Intervention	Delivery	Type	Level	Age group
Medical and surgical treatment of leprosy complications	Clinical: Primary care, District hospital	Rehabilitation plus palliation	Limited	All ages
Antibiotic prophylaxis for children with history of rheumatic fever	Clinical: Primary care	Secondary prevention	Limited	Childhood
Public preventive package for most cardiovascular risk factors	Public health: Behavior change	Primary prevention plus secondary prevention	Moderate	Adults
Insulin therapy for non-insulin-dependent diabetic individuals	Clinical: Primary care	Secondary prevention	Limited	Adults, elderly
Management of stable angina with medication	Clinical: Primary care	Rehabilitation plus secondary prevention	Limited	Adults, Elderly
Management of post-myocardial infarction or post-stroke patients	Clinical: Primary care, Public health, Behavior change	Secondary prevention	Moderate	Adults, Elderly
Low-cost medical management of unstable or myocardial infarction	Clinical: District hospital	Rehabilitation plus secondary prevention	Limited	Adults, Elderly
Cancer pain management	Clinical: Primary care	Palliation	Substantial	All ages
Onchocerciasis control with chemical pesticides	Public health: Environmental	Primary prevention	Moderate	All ages
Schizophrenia or manic-depressive illness treatment with medication	Clinical: Primary care	Rehabilitation	Moderate	Adults
$250–$1,000 per DALY				
Referral of pharyngitis cases for antibiotic prophylaxis to prevent rheumatic fever and rheumatic heart disease	Public health: Screening and referral	Primary prevention	Limited	Childhood
Improved dengue case management via education of health care providers	Clinical: Behavior change	Primary prevention	Limited	All ages
> $1,000 per DALY				
Medical and surgical management of chronic obstructive pulmonary disease	Clinical: Referral hospital	Rehabilitation plus palliation	Limited	Adults, Elderly
Surgery for rheumatic heart disease	Clinical: Referral hospital	Rehabilitation plus secondary prevention	Limited	Adults
Management of moderate hypertension with medication	Clinical: Primary care	Secondary prevention	Moderate	Adults, Elderly
Management of hypercholesterolemia with medication	Clinical: Primary care	Secondary prevention	Limited	Adults, Elderly
High-cost management of MI or unstable angina	Clinical: District hospital	Secondary prevention	Limited	Adults, Elderly
Management of coronary artery disease with surgery	Clinical: Referral hospital	Rehabilitation plus secondary prevention	Limited	Adults, Elderly
Medical and surgical management of cancers	Clinical: Referral hospital	Cure plus palliation	Limited	All ages
Dengue control with chemical pesticides with or without improved case management	Public health: Environmental	Primary prevention	Moderate	All ages
Dengue control via drainage and land management with or without improved case management	Public health: Environmental	Primary prevention	Limited	All ages

a. Age groups are defined as follows: Childhood = age 0 to 4; School age = age 5 to 14; Adults = age 15 to 59; Elderly = age 60 plus. Most interventions will be useful for a range of age groups; the principal age group to whom the intervention would be addressed is indicated.

b. DALY = disability-adjusted life-years.

Source: Tables 1A-3 and 1A-5.

Table 1A-7. Intervention Cost-Effectiveness by Objective

Cost per DALY	Number[a]	Primary prevention	Secondary prevention	Cure	Rehabilitation	Palliation
< $25	22	10	8	5	0	0
$25–$75	6	2	4	0	0	0
$75–$250	13	4	6	0	2	1
$250–$1,000	2	2	0	0	0	0
> $1000	9	2	5	1	3	2
Total	52	20	23	6	5	3

a. The total number of interventions does not equal the number of objectives, as some interventions have multiple objectives.
Source: Appendix table 1A-6.

Table 1A-8. Intervention Cost-Effectiveness by Public Health and Clinical Strategy

Cost per DALY	Public health					Clinical		
	Environ-mental	Mass chemo-prophylaxis	Immunization	Screening and referral	Behavior change	Primary care	District hospital	Referral hospital
< $25	1	6	5	0	3	4	3	1
$25–$75	0	1	1	0	2	1	1	1
$75–$250	2	0	1	0	2	8	3	0
$250–$1,000	0	0	0	1	1	0	0	0
> $1,000	0	0	0	0	0	2	1	4
Total	3	7	7	1	8	15	8	6

Source: Appendix table 1A-6.

Appendix 1B: Countries and Territories as Grouped in this Collection

The table on the facing page lists the country and territorial groupings used for aggregating country into regional data throughout this collection. The *Industrialized transition econo-* mies grouping was previously labeled *Industrialized nonmarket economies.*

Analyses in the collection sometimes further aggregate countries into *industrialized economies* included in the first and second groups in this table and *developing economies* as shown in the third, fourth, fifth, and sixth groups.

Table 1B-1. Regional Groupings of Countries and Territories

Industrial market economies	Industrialized transition economies	Latin America and the Caribbean	Sub-Saharan Africa	Middle East and North Africa	Asia and the Pacific
Austrialia	Albania	Antigua and Barbuda	Angola	Afghanistan	Bangladesh
Austria	Bulgaria	Argentina	Benin	Algeria	Bhutan
Belgium	Czechoslovakia	Bahamas	Botswana	Bahrain	Brunei
Canada	Former German Dem. Rep.	Barbados	Burkina Faso	Egypt, Arab Rep. of	Cambodia
Channel Islands	Hungary	Belize	Burundi	Gaza Strip	China (excluding Taiwan)
Cyprus	Poland	Bolivia	Cameroon	Iran, Islamic Rep. of	Fiji
Finland	Romania	Brazil	Cape Verde	Iraq	French Polynesia
France	U.S.S.R.	Chile	Central African Republic	Israel	Guam
Germany, Fed. Rep. of	Yugoslavia	Colombia	Chad	Jordan	Hong Kong
Greece		Costa Rica	Comoros	Kuwait	India
Iceland		Cuba	Congo, People's Rep. of the	Lebanon	Indonesia
Ireland		Dominica	Côte d'Ivoire	Libya	Kiribati
Italy		Dominican Republic	Djibouti	Morocco	Korea, Dem. People's Rep. of
Japan		Ecuador	Equatorial Guinea	Oman	Korea, Republic of
Luxembourg		El Salvador	Ethiopia	Pakistan	Lao People's Dem. Rep.
Malta		Grenada	Gabon	Qatar	Macao
Netherlands		Guadeloupe	Gambia, The	Saudi Arabia	Malaysia
New Zealand		Guatemala	Ghana	Syrian Arab Republic	Maldives
Norway		Guyana	Guinea	Tunisia	Mongolia
Portugal		Haiti	Guinea-Bissau	Turkey	Myanmar
Spain		Honduras	Kenya	United Arab Emirates	Nepal
Sweden		Jamaica	Lesotho	West Bank	New Calednoia
Switzerland		Martinique	Liberia	Yemen, People's Dem. Rep. of	Pacific Islands
United Kingdom		Mexico	Madagascar	Yemen Arab Republic	Papua New Guinea
United States		Montserrat	Malawi	Other North Africa	Philippines
Other Europe		Netherlands Antilles	Mali		Singapore
Other North America		Nicaragua	Mauritania		Solomon Islands
		Panama	Mauritius		Sri Lanka
		Paraguay	Mozambique		Taiwan
		Peru	Namibia		Thailand
		Puerto Rico	Niger		Tonga
		St. Kitts and Nevis	Nigeria		Vanuatu
		St. Lucia	Réunion		Viet Nam
		St. Vincent and the Grenadines	Rwanda		Western Samoa
		Suriname	Saô Tomé and Principe		Other Micronesia
		Trinidad and Tobago	Senegal		Other Polynesia
		Uruguay	Seychelles		
		Venezuela	Sierra Leone		
		Virgin Islands (U.S.)	Somalia		
		Other Latin America	South Africa		
			Sudan		
			Swaziland		
			Tanzania		
			Togo		
			Uganda		
			Zaire		
			Zambia		
			Zimbabwe		
			Other West Africa		

Notes

I am deeply indebted to many of my colleagues for comments and discussions concerning earlier drafts of parts of this material; they include Jacques Baudouy, Robert Black, John Briscoe, J. Richard Bumgarner, Donald Bundy, Guy Carrin, Lincoln Chen, E. Chigan, Andrew Creese, Joseph Davis, Nicholas Drager, William Foege, Davidson Gwatkin, Jean-Pierre Habicht, Ann Hamilton, Alaya Hammad, Jeffrey Hammer, D. A. Henderson, Ralph Henderson, Kenneth Hill, Michel Jancloes, Jeffrey Koplan, Jean-Louis Lamboray, Joanne Leslie, Bernhard Liese, Judith McGuire, Richard Morrow, Christopher Murray, Philip Musgrove, Mead Over, Thomas Pearson, Richard Peto, Margaret Phillips, Nancy Pielemeier, André Prost, William Reinke, Julia Rushby, Robert Steinglass, Eleuther Tarimo, Carl Taylor, Anne Tinker, Kenneth Warren, and David Werner.

David Bell, José-Luis Bobadilla, Richard Feachem, Anthony Measham, and W. Henry Mosley provided me with particularly useful insights and comments. Peter Cowley provided valuable assistance with preparation of the tables in the chapter and helpful comments on the chapter as a whole.

The opportunity to give the Heath Clark Lecture for 1989–90 at the London School of Hygiene and Tropical Medicine provided me both with valuable feedback on portions of this chapter and with the chance to work on it for several months in a highly stimulating environment. Much of this work was done while I was at the University of California, Los Angeles, which has been in every way supportive of this effort.

1. Issues associated with the health transition and its implications for policy are increasingly widely discussed; for example, see Bell 1992; Bicknell and Parks 1989; Bobadilla and others, chapter 3, this collection; Chen and others 1992; Chesnais 1990; Evans, Hall, and Warford 1981; Foege and Henderson 1986; Harlan, Harlan, and Oii 1984; Jamison and Mosley 1991; and Mosley and Cowley 1991. The work of Julio Frenk and his colleagues in Mexico—for example, Frenk and others 1989—has provided a particularly influential impetus for work in this area.

2. General economic conditions and behavioral patterns in society influence health outcomes (Bell and Reich 1988; Behrman 1990; Berman, Kendall, and Bhattacharyya 1989; Cochrane, Leslie, and O'Hara 1982; DaVanzo and Gertler 1990). This collection deals with these wider issues, for both adults and children, only insofar as they can be addressed by health-related intervention.

3. A comprehensive analysis of health problems of adults in the developing world that calls for more explicit policy and programmatic attention in addressing those problems has recently been completed for the World Bank (Feachem and others 1992).

4. A recent assessment of intervention options for mental disorders by the World Health Organization concludes—although treatment costs are not explicitly considered—that relatively simple interventions could be much more widely used to address widespread mental disorders (World Health Organization 1991).

5. The very different character of health interventions from other "goods" typically "chosen" by market forces—in particular consumer (and provider) ignorance about links between interventions and health improvement—generates a need for specialist assessment of intervention choice and for serious consideration of mechanisms that deal with market failure to decide on the level and composition of interventions to be provided. For a valuable review, see Barr 1992. A comprehensive approach to dealing with market failure through "managed competition" is provided by Enthoven 1988. Implications of this literature from the perspective of developing countries have been drawn in a major recent publication of the World Bank (World Bank 1993).

6. These elements need consideration, obviously, independently of whether the government, the private sector, or nongovernmental organizations are responsible for delivering the relevant service. Akin, Birdsall, and de Ferranti (1987) discuss these issues from the perspective of financing health systems; Birdsall (1989) further discusses the government role in the health sector; and Stiglitz (1989) provides a valuable general overview of the economic role of the state.

7. At about the same time, the World Health Organization was also beginning to address these issues; Dr. Hiroshi Nakajima, the current director-general, observed: "Even before we win our battle against the communicable diseases, which has engaged us since our earliest days, many developing countries must now, in addition, face the burden of ageing and chronic and degenerative diseases" (World Health Organization 1988, p. 102).

8. In many ways this review is very much in the spirit of Walsh and Warren's (1979, 1986) assessment of priorities for control of communicable childhood diseases in developing countries; the current effort involves more extensive use of economic analysis and covers a much broader range of conditions. In subsequent work for the United Nations Development Programme (UNDP), Walsh (1988) has extended her earlier work with Warren. Amler and Dull (1987) and the Department of Health and Human Services (1991) have reviewed a broad range of preventive intervention policies for the United States, and, more for clinical preventive services, the U.S. Preventive Services Task Force (1989) has reviewed the effectiveness of 169 interventions. The state of Oregon in the United States has ordered over 700 interventions, using cost-effectiveness and other criteria, for the purpose of rationing limited public resources to provide health care for the poor; a recent edited collection (Strosberg and others 1992) discusses many facets of the Oregon plan. Patel (1989) has reviewed estimates of cost and effectiveness of a range of health interventions for UNICEF, and Udvarhelyi and others (1992) provide a comprehensive review of medical cost-effectiveness and cost-benefit studies from the perspective of their methodological adequacy. All these approaches to the analytic evaluation of health practices fall within the general area of what is increasingly known as "health technology assessment"; Garber and Fuchs (1991) provide a valuable general overview of the field.

9. If one is simply assessing the relative attractiveness of alternative means for achieving a single, specific health objective—for example, reducing infant mortality—this measurement problem disappears, and one can judge intervention cost-effectiveness simply in terms of, say, cost per infant death averted.

10. There is at least anecdotal evidence to suggest that in immunization programs immunizations are often first provided where the cost per child contact is lowest; if, as is likely, these children have relatively low incidence rates (for example, of tuberculosis) or case-fatality rates (for example, of measles), then the Expanded Programme on Immunization may not be starting with the most cost-effective population subgroups.

11. In an early application of cost-effectiveness analysis within the health sector, Barnum and others (1980) go beyond comparing marginal cost-effectiveness to attempting an analysis of maximization of total outcome for different levels of expenditure on child survival; Forgy (1991) uses data from this collection on child survival to undertake a similar analysis.

12. It is important to recognize that some facilities address only a narrow range of conditions—for example, there are cancer and TB hospitals. Over and Piot (chapter 20) discuss the usefulness of clinics for sexually transmitted diseases, and Javitt (chapter 26) discusses use of mobile surgical camps (district-hospital level, in some sense) to deal with cataract.

13. Health care expenditures of approximately $460 billion in 1986 for the 242 million people of the United States well exceeded the GNP of China ($320 billion), with a population of 1.05 billion; it was close to triple the combined GNPs of all the World Bank member countries of Sub-Saharan Africa, which had a total population of about 425 million and a combined GNP of about $175 billion.

14. A separate line of evidence, albeit only suggestive, for inefficiency resulting from variation in marginal cost-effectiveness is the very high degree of observed variation in procedure frequence in somewhat similar environments (Sanders, Coulter, and McPherson 1989).

References

Akin, J., Nancy Birdsall, and D. de Ferranti. 1987. *Financing Health Services in Developing Countries*. Washington, D.C.: World Bank.

Amler, R. W., and H. B. Dull, eds. 1987. *Closing the Gap: The Burden of Unnecessary Illness*. New York: Oxford University Press.

Anderson, M. A. 1990. "Nature and Magnitude of the Problem of Suboptimal Breastfeeding Practices." Paper presented at the International Policymakers Conference on Breastfeeding, Florence, Italy, July 30–August 1.

Barnum, Howard. 1987. "Evaluating Healthy Days of Life Gained from Health Projects." *Social Science and Medicine* 24(10):833–41.

Barnum, Howard, R. Barlow, L. Fajardo, and A. Pradilla. 1980. *A Resource Allocation Model for Child Survival*. Cambridge, Mass.: Oeldeschlager, Gunn and Hain.

Barr, Nicholas. 1992. "Economic Theory and the Welfare State: A Survey and Interpretation." *Journal of Economic Literature* 30:741-803.

Basta, S. S., D. K. Soekirman, and N. S. Scrimshaw. 1979. "Iron Deficiency Anemia and the Productivity of Adult Males in Indonesia." *American Journal of Clinical Nutrition* 32:916–25.

Behrman, J. R. 1990. "A Survey on Socioeconomic Development, Structural Adjustment and Child Health and Mortality in Developing Countries." In K. Hill, ed., *Child Survival Programs: Issues for the 1990s*. Baltimore: Johns Hopkins University School of Hygiene and Public Health, Institute for International Programs.

Bell, D. E. 1992. "Some Implications of the Health Transition for Policy and Research." In L. Chen, A. Kleinman, J. C. Caldwell, J. E. Potter, and N. Ware, eds., *Health and Social Change*. Westport, Conn.: Auburn House.

Bell, D. E., and M. R. Reich, eds. 1988. *Health, Nutrition, and Economic Crisis*. Dover, Mass.: Auburn House for the Harvard School of Public Health.

Berman, P., C. Kendall, and K. Bhattacharyya. 1989. "The Household Production of Health: Putting People at the Center of Health Improvement." In *Towards More Efficacy in Child Survival Strategies: Understanding the Social and Private Constraints and Responsibilities*. Baltimore: Johns Hopkins University School of Hygiene and Public Health.

Bicknell, W. J., and C. L. Parks. 1989. "As Children Survive: Dilemmas of Aging in the Developing World." *Social Science and Medicine* 28(1):59–67.

Birdsall, Nancy. 1989. "Thoughts on Good Health and Good Government. *Daedalus* 118:23.

Briscoe, J. 1989. "Adult Health in Brazil: Adjusting to New Challenges." Report 7807-BR, World Bank, Washington, D.C.

Briscoe, J., and D. de Ferranti. 1988. *Water for Rural Communities*. Washington, D.C.

Bumgarner, J. R. 1992. *China: Long-term Issues and Options in the Health Transition*. A World Bank Country Study. Washington, D.C. World Bank.

Cairns, J., and K. Johnston. 1991. "Condition-Specific Outcome Measures as an Alternative to Across-Programme QALYs." Health Economics Unit, University of Aberdeen.

Chen, L., A. Kleinman, J. C. Caldwell, J. E. Potter, and N. Ware, eds. 1992. *Health and Social Change*. Westport, Conn.: Auburn House.

Chesnais, J-C. 1990. "Demographic Transition Patterns and Their Impact on the Age Structure." *Population and Development Review* 16(2):327–36.

Cochrane, S., J. Leslie, and D. O'Hara. 1982. "Parental Education and Child Health: Intracountry Evidence." *Health Policy and Education* 2:213–50.

Cropper, Maureen L., Sema K. Aydede, and Paul R. Portney. 1992. "Rates of Time Preference for Saving Lives." *American Economic Review* 82:469–72.

DaVanzo, J., and P. Gertler. 1990. "Household Production of Health: A Microeconomic Perspective on Health Transitions." Rand N-3014-RC. Rand Corporation, Santa Monica, Calif.

Drummond, M. F., G. L. Stoddart, and G. W. Torrance. 1987. *Methods for the Economic Evaluation of Health Care Programs*. Oxford: Oxford University Press.

Enthoven, Alain C. 1988. *Theory and Practice of Managed Competition in Health Care Finance*. Amsterdam: North Holland.

EuroQol Group. 1990. "EuroQol—A New Facility for the Measurement of Health-Related Quality of Life." *Health Policy* 16:199–208.

Evans, J. R., K. L. Hall, and J. Warford. 1981. "Health Care in the Developing World: Problems of Scarcity and Choice." *New England Journal of Medicine* 305:1117–27.

Fallowfield, Leslie. 1990. *The Quality of Life*. London: Souvenir Press.

Feachem, R. G. A., W. J. Graham, and I. M. Timaeus. 1989. "Identifying Health Problems and Health Research Priorities in Developing Countries." *Journal of Tropical Medicine and Hygiene* 92(3):133–91.

Feachem, R. G. A., T. Kjellstrom, C. J. L. Murray, Mead Over, and M. A. Phillips. 1992. *The Health of Adults in the Developing World*. New York: Oxford University Press.

Foege, W. H., and D. A. Henderson. 1986. "Management Priorities in Primary Health Care." In J. A. Walsh and K. S. Warren, eds., *Strategies for Primary Health Care*. Chicago: University of Chicago Press.

Forgy, Lawrence. 1991. "Cost-Effectiveness in Child Health: A Minimum Information Approach to Planning and Forecasting." Paper presented at the seminar on Child Survival Interventions: Effectiveness and Efficacy, at the Johns Hopkins University School of Hygiene and Public Health, Baltimore, June 20–22.

Frenk, J., J.-L. Bobadilla, Jaime Sepúlveda, and M. Lopez Cervantes. 1989. "Health Transition in Middle-Income Countries: New Challenges for Health Care." *Health Policy and Planning* 4:29–39.

Garber, Alan M. and Victor R. Fuchs. 1991. "The Expanding Role of Technology Assessment in Health Policy." *Stanford Law and Policy Review* 3:203–9.

Garber, Alan M., and Phelps, Charles E. 1992. "Economic Foundations of Cost-Effectiveness Analysis." Working Paper 4164. National Bureau of Economic Research, Cambridge, Mass.

Ghana Health Assessment Project Team. 1981. "Quantitative Method of Assessing the Health Impact of Different Diseases in Less Developed Countries." *International Journal of Epidemiology* 10(1):73–80.

Harlan, W. R., L. C. Harlan, and W. L. Oii. 1984. "Changing Disease Patterns in Developing Countries: The Case of Malaysia." In P. Leverton and L. Massi, eds., *Health Information Systems*. New York: Praeger Scientific.

Institute of Medicine. 1986. *New Vaccine Development: Establishing Priorities*. Vols. 1 and 2. Washington, D.C.: National Academy Press.

Jamison, D. T., J. R. Evans, T. King, I. Porter, N. Prescott, and A. Prost. 1984. *China: The Health Sector*. A World Bank Country Study. Washington, D.C.

Jamison, D. T., and W. H. Mosley. 1991. "Selecting Disease Control Priorities in Developing Countries: Health Policy Responses to Epidemiological Change." *American Journal of Public Health* 81:15–22.

Johannesson, Magnus. 1992. "On the Discounting of Gained Life-Years in Cost-Effectiveness Analysis." *International Journal of Technology Assessment in Health Care* 8:359–64.

Last, J. M., ed. 1988. *A Dictionary of Epidemiology*. 2d ed. New York: Oxford University Press for the International Epidemiological Association.

Leslie, Joanne. 1989. "Women's Time: A Factor in the Use of Child Survival Technologies?" *Health Policy and Planning* 4(1):1–16.

———. 1992. "Women's Time and the Use of Health Services." *IDS Bulletin* 23:4–7.

MMWR (*Morbidity and Mortality Weekly Report*). 1992. "Years of Potential Life Lost before Ages 65 and 85—United States, 1989–1990." MMWR 41(18):313–15.

Mosley, W. H., and P. Cowley. 1991. "The Challenge of World Health." *Population Bulletin* 46(4):1–39.

Mosley, W. H., and R. Jolly. 1987. "Health Policy and Program Options: Compensating for the Negative Effects of Economic Adjustment." In G. A. Cornia, R. Jolly, and F. Stewart, eds., *Adjustment with a Human Face*. Oxford: Clarendon Press.

Murray, C. J. 1990. "Rational Approaches to Priority Setting in International Health." *Journal of Tropical Medicine and Hygiene* 93(5):303–11.

Musgrove, Philip. 1991. "The Burden of Death at Different Ages: Assumptions, Parameters and Values." Occasional Paper 12. Latin America and the Caribbean Regional Office, Human Resources Division, Technical Department, World Bank, Washington, D.C.

Nord, Erik. 1991. "The Relevance of QALYs in Prioritizing between Different Patients." Paper presented at the 12th Nordic HESG meeting, Copenhagen, August.

Over, Mead. 1988. "Cost-Effective Integration of Immunization and Basic Health Services in Developing Countries: The Problem of Joint Costs." Working Paper 23. World Bank, Washington, D.C.

Patel, Mahesh S. 1989. "Eliminating Social Distance between North and South: Cost-Effective Goals for the 1990s." Staff Working Paper 5. UNICEF, New York.

Phelps, Charles E., and Alvin I. Mushlin. 1991. "On the (Near) Equivalence of Cost-Effectiveness and Cost-Benefit Analysis." *International Journal of Technology Assessment in Health Care* 7:12–21.

Pollitt, E. 1990. *Malnutrition and Infection in the Classroom.* Paris: UNESCO.

Preston, S. H. 1991. "Health Indexes and Health Sector Planning." Paper presented at the Workshop on the Policy and Planning Implications of the Epidemiological Transition in Developing Countries, at the National Research Council, Washington, D.C., November 20–22.

Rosser, R. M., and P. Kind. 1978. "A Scale of Valuations of States of Illness: Is There a Social Consensus?" *International Journal of Epidemiology* 7(4): 347–58.

Sanders, D., A. Coulter, and K. McPherson. 1989. "Variation in Hospital Admission Rates: A Review of the Literature." King's College Fund, Paper 79. London.

Squire, Lyn. 1989. "Project Evaluation in Theory and Practice." In B. Hollis Chenery and T. N. Srinivasan, eds., *Handbook of Development Economics*, Vol. 2. Amsterdam: North Holland.

Stiglitz, J. 1989. "On the Economic Role of the State." In A. Heertje, ed., *The Economic Role of the State*. Cambridge, Mass.: Basil Blackwell in association with Bank Insinger de Beauford NV.

Strosberg, Martin A., Joshua M. Weiner, and Robert Baker, with I. Alan Fein, (ed.) 1992. *Rationing America's Medical Care: The Oregon Plan and Beyond.* Washington, D.C.: The Brookings Institution.

Tan-Torres, Teresa. 1990. "Comparison of Different Methods of Eliciting Utilities for Outcome States in Leprosy." University of the Philippines, Department of Medicine, Clinical Epidemiology Unit.

Udvarhelyi, I. Steven, Graham A. Colvitz, Arti Rai, and Arnold M. Epstein. 1992. "Cost-Effectiveness and Cost-Benefit Analyses in the Medical Literature." *Annals of Internal Medicine* 116:238–44.

USDHHS (U.S. Department of Health and Human Services). 1991. *Healthy People 2000: National Health Promotion and Disease Prevention Objectives.* Washington, D.C.: U.S. Government Printing Office.

U.S. Preventive Services Task Force (R. S. Lawrence, Chairman). 1989. *Guide to Clinical Preventive Services.* Baltimore: Williams and Wilkins.

Walsh, J. A. 1988. *Establishing Health Priorities in the Developing World.* Boston: Adams Publishing Group for the United Nations Development Programme.

Walsh, J. A., and K. S. Warren. 1979. "Selective Primary Health Care—An Interim Strategy for Disease Control in Developing Countries." *New England Journal of Medicine* 301:967–74.

———, eds. 1986. *Strategies for Primary Health Care: Technologies Appropriate for the Control of Disease in the Developing World.* Chicago: University of Chicago Press.

Weinstein, N. D. 1989. "Optimistic Biases about Personal Risks." *Science* 246:1232–33.

WHO (World Health Organization). 1988. *From Alma-Ata to the Year 2000: Reflections at the Midpoint.* Geneva.

———. 1991. *Evaluation of Methods for the Treatment of Mental Disorders.* WHO Technical Report 812, Geneva.

World Bank. 1980. *Health Sector Policy Paper.* Washington, D.C.

———. 1992. *World Development Report 1992: Development and the Environment.* Washington, D.C.

———. 1993. *World Development Report 1993. Investing in Health.* Washington, D.C.

Zeckhauser, R., and D. Shepard. 1976. "Where Now for Saving Lives?" *Law and Contemporary Problems* 40:5–45.

2

Causes of Death in Industrial and Developing Countries: Estimates for 1985–1990

Alan D. Lopez

Information about the cause structure of mortality has for many years served as the cornerstone for monitoring health progress and for the determination of health priorities. Over the years, information systems on routine causes of death have been established in many countries and, throughout the industrial world at least, these have evolved to the point at which there is now virtually complete coverage of deaths and medical certification. A handful of developing countries, primarily in Latin America and East Asia have achieved comparable standards of reliability of their cause-of-death statistics. In several other countries, considerable progress has been achieved toward obtaining reasonably reliable mortality information for at least the urban populations, although calculation of mortality rates is often impeded by lack of information about the population at risk. For the majority of developing countries, however, the reliability of cause-of-death data emanating from vital registration systems—where they exist—is sufficiently poor essentially to preclude their use for assessment of the national health situation.

In the absence of reliable information on medically certified causes of death, countries are increasingly adopting lay reporting schemes to obtain at least a broad overview of health conditions in populations in which deaths are not routinely recorded or medically certified. This technique has undoubtedly generated useful information for several populations, but it has not been nearly as widely exploited as, for example, the indirect techniques for assessing levels of mortality on the basis of information from women about children ever born and children surviving. As a result, global and regional patterns of mortality by age and sex can be, and have been, established with some confidence, whereas the cause structure of mortality, for at least half of the world's population, is, at best, uncertain.

One method of estimating causes of death in countries without reliable information is to develop a model of the epidemiological transition based on the experience of the industrial countries. Hakulinen and others (1986), for example, estimated a series of cause-specific regression equations to predict the level of mortality for a given cause (among twelve broad cause-of-death groups) from information about the crude death rate. Perhaps the greatest limitation of this method is that it implicitly assumes that the cause-level relationship is invariant over time. This is unlikely to be the case in contemporary developing countries, where modernization, social and economic change, and the infusion of medical technology have undoubtedly altered the nature and severity of disease epidemics. Adjustment of the estimates generated by the model on the basis of a critical appraisal of available epidemiological information, as has been done in Indonesia, for example (see Hull, Rohde, and Lopez 1981), increases the reliability of the estimates. This type of complementary analysis is clearly quite complicated at a global, or even regional, level, however, and hence the indirect estimates of cause-of-death patterns should be viewed only as a first approximation to the underlying epidemiological environment. The method followed in this chapter of estimating the global and regional mortality situation in 1985 is one of progressively assembling nationally representative mortality patterns according to the degree of confidence in their reliability.[1] Thus the first section of the chapter deals exclusively with the industrialized market and nonmarket countries. The market economies include the following:

Australia	Greece	New Zealand
Austria	Iceland	Norway
Belgium	Ireland	Portugal
Canada	Italy	Spain
Denmark	Japan	Sweden
Finland	Luxembourg	Switzerland
France	Malta	United Kingdom
Germany, Fed. Rep.	Netherlands	United States

The countries listed below are considered industrial nonmarket economies:

Albania	German Dem. Rep.	Romania
Bulgaria	Hungary	U.S.S.R.
Czechoslovakia	Poland	Yugoslavia

These thirty-three countries in 1985 accounted for a population of about 1.2 billion people (that is, 1,200,000,000) or approximately 25 percent of the world total.[2] Some 11 million deaths occur each year in these countries (out of a global total of roughly 50 million), virtually all of which are medically certified.[3] There remain, however, important differences in diagnostic and coding practices among these countries due to differences in medical training, availability of diagnostic aids, and the like. Percy and Muir (1989), for example, in their study of the international comparability of cancer mortality data in seven industrialized countries, found that cancer deaths were typically overreported by 3 to 4 percent compared with the United States. The largest difference was estimated for France, where coding procedures resulted in a 10 percent higher death rate for cancer than would have been the case if the procedures in use in the United States had applied. The implications of artifacts such as these for comparative mortality analyses could be quite substantial. For example, the age-adjusted cancer death rate for France in 1984 was 139.5 per 100,000, or about 5 percent more than what was observed in the United States (132.4 per 100,000). After allowing for coding differences, the French cancer death rate was recalculated by Percy and Muir at 127.5 per 100,000, almost 5 percent less than the rate for the United States. Although these artifacts are likely to be less of a problem for aggregate analyses, such as those reported in this study, it must be kept in mind that the resulting cause-of-death pattern, even for industrial countries, is not exact. Nonetheless, for broad cause-of-death groups at least, the structure of mortality can be reasonably well established from the data available.

The estimation of cause-specific mortality for the developing regions of the world is even less precise. Global estimates of disease-specific morbidity and mortality have been prepared by several technical programs in the World Health Organization. These estimates are frequently based on studies carried out at the community level in various developing countries and then extrapolated to yield regional and global figures. This is clearly a very imprecise method, but in the absence of vital registration there is little alternative but to "evaluate and extrapolate." In addition, cause-of-death data are available for a number of developing countries, particularly in Latin America, and provided the coverage and reliability of the information is known, even approximately, these data can be exploited to estimate national cause-of-death patterns. Regional and global estimates can then be obtained, although this aggregation introduces an additional degree of uncertainty into the estimates because of missing data for some countries. For some large populations in the developing world, cause-of-death information is now becoming available which is of sufficient quality and representativeness to permit reasonable estimates of the epidemiological situation for the country as a whole. China now has routine mortality data, almost all of which is medically certified for over 100 million people in rural and urban areas in the eastern half of the country, where the bulk of the population resides. India also has implemented a rural survey of causes of death. It is based on lay reporting of the cause of death, with verification on a sample basis by physi-

Table 2-1. Population of the Developing World

Region	Population (millions)	Percentage of total population
Sub-Saharan Africa	456	12.4
Middle East/North Africa	376	10.2
Latin America/Caribbean	402	11.0
India	765	20.9
China	1,065	29.0
Other Asia/Pacific	604	16.5
Total	3,668	100.00

Source: Author.

cians at district primary health care centers. Obviously, reliable information about the mortality pattern for these two countries will have a significant effect on the estimation procedure for all developing countries. Indeed, in 1985, one-half of the population of the developing world were living in China and India as shown in table 2-1.

Causes of Death

The causes of death selected for mortality estimation are shown in table 2-2, along with the corresponding codes of the International Classification of Diseases (ICD). For the ninth revision of the ICD (ICD-9), the codes refer to items in the Basic Tabulation List, whereas for ICD-8, the numbers refer to diseases and injuries included in list "A." Both of these are summary or "short" lists and are used by WHO to collect and store mortality information. In some cases, the items available in the summary lists do not correspond exactly to the composition of cause-of-death categories defined on the basis of the detailed rubrics of the ICD. The discrepancies are generally minor, however, and in any case will have much less effect on the estimates than the artifacts and uncertainties mentioned above.

Eight broad categories of causes of death are considered:

- Infectious and parasitic diseases
- Neoplasms
- Diseases of the circulatory system and other selected degenerative diseases[4]
- Chronic obstructive lung diseases (principally chronic bronchitis and emphysema)
- Complications of pregnancy
- Perinatal conditions
- Injury and poisoning (all external causes)
- All other causes

For the industrial countries at least, the remainder category has been further disaggregated into "other specific causes" and "symptoms and ill-defined conditions." For some categories, namely, infectious and parasitic diseases, diseases of the circulatory system, and the remainder category, estimates of mortality from more specific conditions listed in table 2-2 have also been attempted. This was done because disease-specific esti-

Table 2-2. Causes of Death and Corresponding Categories in the International Classification of Diseases, Injuries, and Causes of Death (ICD)

Cause of death	ICD-8 List A	ICD-9 Basic Tabulation List
Main Categories		
Infectious and parasitic diseases	A1–44, A90–92, A99	01–07, 320–322
Neoplasms	A45–61	08–17
Circulatory system and certain degenerative diseases	A64, A80–88, A98, A102, A105–106	25–30, 181, 341, 347, 350
Chronic obstructive pulmonary (lung) disease	A93, A96	323–326
Complications of pregnancy	A112–118	38–41
Perinatal conditions	A131–135	45
Injury and poisoning	A138–150	E47–E56
Ill-defined causes	A136, A137	46
Other causes	Other codes	All other codes
Infectious diseases		
Diarrhea	A1–5, A99	01
Tuberculosis	A6–10	02
Acute respiratory infection	A15–17, A89–92	033–035, 320–322
Measles	A25	042
Polio	A22–23	040, 078
Yellow fever, dengue, and encephalitis	A26–27	044–045
Malaria	A31	052
Schistosomiasis and filariasis	A39, A41	072, 074
Intestinal parasites	A42–43	075–076
Circulatory and degenerative diseases		
Ischemic heart disease	A83	27
Cerebrovascular disease	A85	29
Other cardiovascular diseases	A80–82, A84, A86–88	25, 26, 28, 30
Diabetes	A64	181
Certain degenerative diseases (nephritis, cirrhosis, ulcers)	A98, A102, A105, A106	341, 347, 350
Other disorders		
Mental disorders	A69	210–212
Oral health diseases	A97	330
Micronutrient deficiency	A62–63, A67	180, 193, 200
Malnutrition	A65	190–192

Source: International Classification of Diseases, Injuries, and Causes of Death.

mates are undoubtedly of much greater relevance for determining health priorities than an aggregate of conditions which may require substantially different strategies for prevention and control.

Causes of Death in Industrial Countries in 1985

Tables 2-3, 2-4, and 2-5 summarize the cause-of-death structure for the industrialized world as a whole (table 2-3) as well as for the groups of industrial market economies (table 2-4) and the industrial nonmarket economies (table 2-5) separately.

All Industrial Countries

The structure of mortality shown in table 2-3 for the industrialized countries as a whole is very much what one would expect for a population with an average life expectancy of seventy-four years. Of the 11.05 million deaths reported for these countries during 1985, 7.63 million, or approximately 70 percent, occurred at age sixty-five and over. Another 2.3 million were at age forty-five through sixty-four. That is, almost 10

million (90 percent) of the 11 million deaths were at age forty-five and over. In contrast, there were 355,000 infant and child deaths below age five (3.2 percent of the total), 275,000 of which occurred among infants. The vast majority of these infant deaths in turn occurred very early in life (typically within the first week) and were due to various perinatal and congenital conditions which are difficult to eliminate. Nonetheless, further progress in reducing this toll of over 350,000 young-child deaths each year can be expected through the reduction of inequalities in access to, and use of, prenatal care and infant and child health services among different sectors of the population. Indeed, reduction of such inequalities is central to the health-for-all-strategies in these countries and applies not only during infancy and childhood but at later ages as well.

Infectious and parasitic diseases (including acute respiratory diseases) claimed just over half a million deaths in the industrialized countries about 1985, two-thirds of which were among the elderly (sixty-five years and over). Even so, 110,000 of these deaths were among children below the age of five, with all but about 6,000 of these occurring in the nonmarket coun-

Table 2-3. Causes of Death in Industrial Countries, 1985

Cause of death	Number (thousands)			Percentage		
	Males	Females	Total	Males	Females	Total
Infectious and parasitic diseases	266	240	506	4.7	4.4	4.6
Acute respiratory infections	184	184	368	3.3	3.4	3.3
Tuberculosis	30	10	40	0.5	0.2	0.4
Neoplasms	1,263	1,030	2,293	22.5	18.9	20.8
Circulatory and certain degenerative diseases	2,720	3,210	5,930	48.6	59.0	53.7
Ischemic heart disease	1,199	1,193	2,392	21.4	21.9	21.7
Cerebrovascular disease	590	914	1,504	10.5	16.8	13.6
Diabetes	59	94	153	1.1	1.7	1.4
Complications of pregnancy	0	4	4[a]	0.0	0.1	0.0
Perinatal conditions	60	40	100	1.1	0.7	0.9
Chronic obstructive lung diseases	245	140	385	4.4	2.6	3.5
Injury and poisoning	536	236	772	9.6	4.3	7.0
Ill-defined causes	115	132	247	2.1	2.4	2.2
All other causes	397	410	807	7.1	7.5	7.3
Total	5,601	5,444	11,045	100.0	100.0	100.0

a. Estimated at 6,000 due to under-reporting.
Source: Calculated from WHO mortality database.

tries. It should be emphasized here that this category does not include deaths coded to acquired immunodeficiency disease (AIDS) because it was not possible to distinguish these deaths from other causes in the mortality data reported to WHO. Still, the number of new AIDS cases reported for the industrialized countries about 1985 was less than 30,000, and hence the mortality from AIDS would not have altered dramatically the overall total of deaths from infectious and parasitic diseases. Rather, acute respiratory infections, primarily pneumonia among the elderly, account for about two-thirds of the deaths from infections in industrial countries. Another 40,000 deaths are attributable to tuberculosis, primarily at age forty-five and over. Acute respiratory infections and tuberculosis are thus the

principal causes of death from infectious diseases in industrial countries, accounting for four-fifths of the half-million deaths still due to infections in the industrialized world.

In these countries, cancer, primarily malignant neoplasms, claims the lives of 2.3 million persons each year, 55 percent of which are males. Cancer too has a relatively high average age at death, with 1.4 of the 2.3 million deaths occurring beyond age sixty-five. Nonetheless, there is still very substantial scope for preventing premature death from neoplastic diseases. Of the remaining 900,000 cancer deaths, all but a handful (15,000) occurred between the ages of fifteen and sixty-four.

The causes of cancer are still very much a matter of investigation, but in countries such as the United States, where

Table 2-4. Causes of Death in Industrialized Market Countries, 1985

Cause of death	Number (thousands)			Percentage		
	Males	Females	Total	Males	Females	Total
Infectious and parasitic diseases	152	156	308	4.3	4.8	4.5
Acute respiratory infections	115	126	241	3.3	3.8	3.5
Tuberculosis	9	4	13	0.3	0.1	0.2
Neoplasms	888	719	1,607	25.1	21.9	23.6
Circulatory and certain degenerative diseases	1,682	1,773	3,455	47.6	54.1	50.7
Ischemic heart disease	730	595	1,325	20.6	18.1	19.4
Cerebrovascular disease	334	467	801	9.5	14.2	11.8
Diabetes	48	73	121	1.3	2.2	1.8
Complications of pregnancy	0	1	1	0.0	0.0	0.0
Perinatal conditions	24	18	42	0.7	0.5	0.6
Chronic obstructive lung diseases	168	86	254	4.7	2.6	3.7
Injury and poisoning	288	143	431	8.1	4.4	6.3
Ill-defined causes	83	99	182	2.3	3.0	2.7
All other causes	251	284	535	7.2	8.7	7.9
Total	3,536	3,279	6,815	100.0	100.0	100.0

Source: Calculated from WHO mortality database.

Table 2-5. Causes of Death in Industrialized Nonmarket Countries, 1985

Cause of death	Number (thousands)			Percentage		
	Males	Females	Total	Males	Females	Total
Infectious and parasitic diseases	114	84	198	5.5	3.9	4.7
Acute respiratory infections	68	58	126	3.3	2.7	3.0
Tuberculosis	21	6	27	1.0	0.3	0.6
Neoplasms	375	312	687	18.2	14.4	16.2
Circulatory and certain						
degenerative diseases	1,038	1,437	2,475	50.3	66.4	58.5
Ischemic heart disease	469	598	1,067	22.7	27.5	25.2
Cerebrovascular disease	255	448	703	12.4	20.7	16.6
Diabetes	12	21	33	0.6	1.0	0.8
Complications of pregnancy	0	3	3	0.0	0.2	0.1
Perinatal conditions	35	23	58	1.7	1.1	1.4
Chronic obstructive lung diseases	77	54	131	3.7	2.5	3.1
Injury and poisoning	248	93	341	12.0	4.3	8.1
Ill-defined causes	32	33	65	1.6	1.5	1.5
All other causes	146	126	272	7.1	5.8	6.4
Total	2,065	2,165	4,230	100.0	100.0	100.0

Source: Calculated from WHO mortality database.

cigarette smoking has been prevalent for several decades, it has been estimated that roughly one-third of cancer deaths can be directly attributed to cigarette smoking (Doll and Peto 1981). Recent estimates (WHO 1991a) have attributed 42 percent of all male cancer deaths and 8 percent of female cancer deaths in the industrial countries to cigarette smoking. Dietary factors are also thought to account for a similar proportion (one-third) of cancer deaths. Other behavioral factors have been causally associated with certain sites of the disease, including excessive alcohol consumption (esophagus, pharynx), reproductive and sexual behavior, occupation, and pollution.

By far the leading type of cancer causing death in the industrialized world today is lung cancer. Almost 500,000 lung cancer deaths were diagnosed in industrial countries in 1985, three-quarters of them among males. Other leading types of cancer include stomach cancer (380,000 deaths), breast cancer (165,000 female deaths), and prostatic cancer (95,000 male deaths). Overall, since 1950, there has been relatively little change in nonlung cancer mortality—death rates have risen slightly for males and declined slightly for women. Lung cancer mortality, almost all of which can be attributed to cigarette smoking (USDHHS 1989), has risen dramatically in industrial countries during the last forty years or so (see figure 2-1), although there are signs that the epidemic, at least among males, has stabilized in several countries, including the United States, Australia, Switzerland, and the former Federal Republic of Germany (Lopez 1989). Male lung cancer death rates in these countries may soon begin to decline, as they have already begun to do in England, Wales, and Finland. Among women, by contrast, death rates from lung cancer are rising virtually throughout the industrialized world as a result of the widespread adoption of cigarette smoking among women during the 1950s and 1960s.

More than one-half of all deaths in industrial countries (5.93 million, or 54 percent) are attributed each year to the circula-

tory diseases and to certain degenerative diseases. Circulatory diseases alone claim 5.45 million lives each year, or almost exactly 50 percent of the total. More females than males die from circulatory and certain degenerative diseases (3.21 million, compared with 2.72 million), although among what might be termed "premature deaths," males predominate, with roughly 785,000 males succumbing each year to these diseases before the age of sixty-five, compared with 390,000 females.

Of the circulatory diseases, the principal cause of death is ischemic heart disease, which each year claims 2.4 million lives, 1.9 million (or roughly 80 percent) of which occur among those age sixty-five and over. The numbers of deaths are roughly evenly divided between males and females, although premature death from the disease (that is, before age sixty-five) is much (in fact, three times) more common among males. There has been considerable research into the causes of ischemic heart disease and a number of risk factors have been identified, the principal ones being hypertension, cigarette smoking, and elevated serum cholesterol. In countries such as the United States, Australia, and Canada, where health promotion campaigns to reduce the prevalence and severity of risk factors in the population have been in operation for several years, marked declines in death rates, of the order of 30 to 50 percent, have been observed since the late 1960s.

Another leading cause of death from circulatory disease is stroke (cerebrovascular disease), which each year claims the lives of 1.5 million persons in industrial countries, 60 percent of whom are women. Most of these deaths occur at the advanced ages with slightly less than 240,000 deaths occurring before age sixty-five. The sex differential in premature mortality from stroke is less marked than for ischemic heart disease, the proportion of male deaths being only marginally higher than female deaths (55 percent compared with 45 percent).

The principal other cardiovascular disease causing death is nonischemic heart disease, including pulmonary and hyper-

Figure 2-1. Relative Mortality Trends from Selected Causes of Death, by Gender, in Industrial Countries, 1950–86

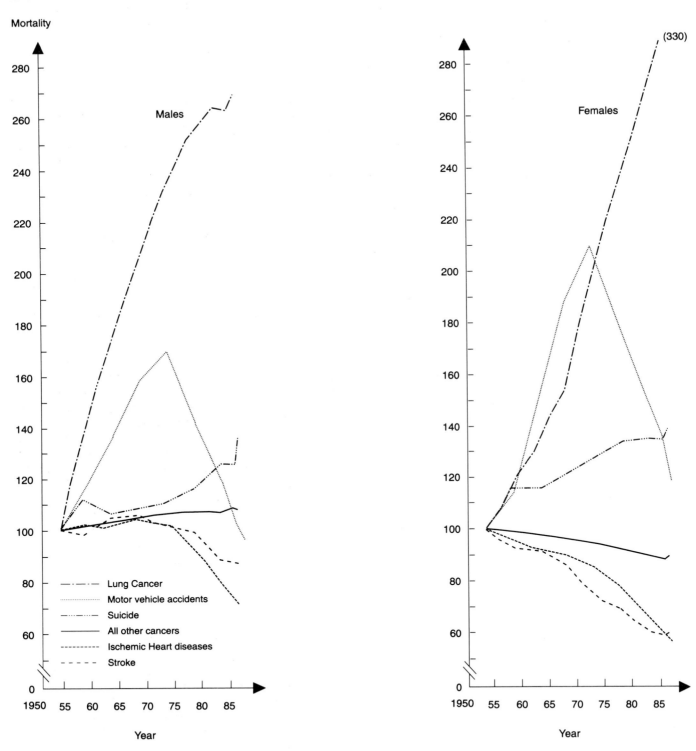

Note: Mortality in the base period, 1950–54, is set at 100, and mortality in other years is determined in relation to this base.
Source: Lopez 1990b.

tensive heart disease. This category of causes accounted for the death of an additional 1.5 million persons in 1985, almost 900,000 of whom were females. These diseases were also characterized by a high average age at death—1.3 million (87 percent) of the deaths assigned to this category occurred beyond age sixty-five.

The remainder of this broad category of circulatory and degenerative diseases consists of four specific conditions; cirrhosis of the liver, diabetes mellitus, ulcer of the stomach and duodenum, and nephritis and nephrosis. Roughly 480,000 deaths are coded each year to these conditions, of which diabetes and cirrhosis of the liver each claim about 150,000. Interestingly, the sex ratio of mortality is reversed for the two diseases. Twice as many females die of diabetes than males, whereas twice as many males die of cirrhosis of the liver. This outcome is certainly consistent with observations on the alcohol consumption patterns of men and women (Capocaccia and Farchi 1988).

The substantial improvements in public health in industrial countries during the course of the twentieth century have virtually eliminated pregnancy-related deaths among women. In 1985 only about 4,500 such deaths were reported in the industrial countries, the vast majority (80 percent) in the nonmarket group. Still, misdiagnosis of maternal deaths is estimated to be of the order of 50 percent in industrial countries (Royston and Lopez 1987), and thus the true mortality from maternal causes is probably closer to 6,000 deaths per year. Virtually all these deaths occur between the ages of fifteen and forty-four and are largely preventable.

Perinatal conditions claimed the lives of 100,000 babies in the industrialized world in 1985, 60 percent of whom were boys. In almost all cases these deaths occur during the neonatal period (up to twenty-eight days after birth) and to a large extent are due to congenital anomalies, birth trauma, and other circumstances of birth. Given the constitutional (rather than environmental) nature of these deaths, it is difficult to see how this mortality can be reduced much further, although the much more common occurrence of such deaths in the nonmarket countries suggests that there is still scope for a reduction in death rates in this group.

A further 1.17 million deaths in 1985 were ascribed to other specific diseases, of which the chronic obstructive pulmonary diseases (primarily chronic bronchitis and emphysema) accounted for almost 400,000. Of these, roughly 250,000 were male deaths. This group of conditions, for which the principal risk factor is cigarette smoking (USDHHS 1989), also tends to claim most lives at the higher ages, with 80 percent of deaths occurring among people age sixty-five and over.

The other remaining broad category of causes of deaths, namely, injury and poisoning (external causes), accounted for about 770,000 deaths in the industrialized world in 1985. Male deaths from violent causes (536,000) were more than twice as common as female deaths from such causes (236,000). Moreover, roughly one-half (260,000) of the male deaths occurred between the ages of fifteen and forty-four, and roughly half that number again (147,000) between forty-five and sixty-four. Only about 17 percent (92,000) of all male deaths due to violence occurred at age sixty-five and over. There is thus considerable scope for additional preventive measures to counter premature male mortality from violence (principally motor vehicle accidents) which each year accounts for almost 10 percent of all male deaths in industrial countries. Mortality from violent deaths among females is much lower (4.3 percent), with almost 50 percent of these deaths occurring among women age sixty-five and over. Accidental falls are a leading cause of death from violence among elderly women.

The quality of cause-of-death statistics for industrial countries as a whole is reflected in the relatively low proportion of deaths for which a specific diagnosis could not be offered.[5] In 1985, the number of deaths coded to the category of signs, symptoms, and ill-defined conditions was approximately 250,000, of which 180,000 were deaths among the elderly. Certainly the ascertainment of a single underlying cause of death in the presence of multiple pathologies, as is often the case for death at advanced ages, is difficult, and the verdict of senility is sometimes applied. Ill-defined conditions account for only about 2.3 percent of deaths overall in the industrial world, and even among the elderly, where they are most common, the percentage is essentially the same. Slightly more female than male deaths are coded to ill-defined conditions, primarily because of the higher average age at death for women.

Industrial Market and Nonmarket Mortality Compared

Tables 2-3 through 2-5 are obviously not appropriate for making mortality comparisons between the industrialized market and nonmarket countries in view of differences in population size and structure between the two groups. Of the 1.17 billion population living in industrial countries, roughly two-thirds (760 million) live in the market economies and the remaining one-third in the nonmarket countries. In order to control for differences in population size and composition, age-standardized death rates have been computed for various causes of death, using the "European" population age structure as the standard. The results are shown in table 2-6.

For both males and females, total mortality rates are about 40 percent higher in the nonmarket countries than in the market economies. Death rates from infectious and parasitic diseases are low (of the order of 30 to 60 per 100,000 population) in both groups of industrial countries but are nonetheless still higher in nonmarket countries, especially for males. These higher rates are largely due to the higher tuberculosis mortality among the elderly in the nonmarket group. Interestingly, overall death rates from neoplasms are virtually identical for males in the two country groups but are higher for females in the market economies. This no doubt reflects the rapid rise in female lung cancer mortality in several countries such as the United States, Australia, Denmark, and the United Kingdom, a phenomenon which is much less apparent in Eastern Europe.

Circulatory and certain degenerative diseases contribute most to the higher overall death rates observed in the nonmarket countries. The age-standardized death rate for males in these countries is almost 850 per 100,000, about 65 percent higher than the level observed in the market economies. Among women, the differential is even greater, with death rates from these diseases in Eastern Europe being 80 percent higher overall than in other industrial countries. Moreover, mortality rates in the nonmarket countries are uniformly higher for all major component diseases of the circulatory system, in particular ischemic heart disease and stroke, and for chronic obstructive lung diseases. By contrast, diabetes death rates are higher in the market economies, although the net effect of this differential on comparative mortality for the

Table 2-6. Age-Standardized Death Rates (per 100,000) for Selected Causes, Industrial Country Groups, 1985

Cause of death	Market economies		Nonmarket economies		Total	
	Males	Females	Males	Females	Males	Females
Infectious and parasitic diseases	48.3	28.5	62.0	36.1	57.5	33.9
Tuberculosis	2.7	0.8	12.7	2.6	6.1	1.5
Acute respiratory infections	37.3	22.2	37.6	24.8	41.0	25.2
Neoplasms	264.6	154.4	266.3	136.1	268.7	149.2
Circulatory and certain degenerative diseases	516.7	323.3	847.5	582.2	605.6	405.3
Ischemic heart disease	222.4	108.8	382.1	241.0	265.1	149.5
Cerebrovascular disease	102.7	83.1	210.7	180.0	131.9	114.4
Other cardiovascular diseases	138.1	98.7	203.4	134.5	155.1	110.4
Diabetes	14.2	14.0	8.5	8.6	12.8	12.3
Other degenerative diseases	39.2	18.6	42.8	18.1	40.7	18.7
Complications of pregnancy	n.a.	0.2	n.a.	1.6	n.a.	0.7
Perinatal conditions	7.5	5.8	14.3	9.7	10.5	7.5
Injury and poisoning	79.5	31.8	137.0	41.9	99.2	35.7
Ill-defined causes	26.8	18.7	26.2	14.2	26.5	17.3
All other causes	127.5	72.7	153.4	71.9	136.6	73.6
Total	1,070.9	635.3	1513.6	897.2	1,206.5	724.3

n.a. Not applicable
Note: Data are standardized onto the WHO "European" population structure.
Source: Calculated from WHO mortality database.

category as a whole is negligible in view of the relatively low mortality from diabetes. The remaining degenerative diseases (which include cirrhosis of the liver) exhibit virtually identical mortality levels in the two groups of countries.

The only other significant category of causes of death for which the mortality differential is quite substantial is injuries and poisonings, especially among males. In the nonmarket countries, the male death rate from violence of 137 per 100,000 is more than 70 percent higher than the average in the other industrial countries. Among females, mortality from violence has traditionally been much lower than for males, and hence the relatively large differential in favor of women in the market economies (approximately 25 percent) has comparatively little effect on the overall mortality differential among females in the two groups of countries.

Certainly, a more detailed investigation of specific causes of death would help to shed more light on the underlying factors which contribute to the mortality differentials observed between the market and nonmarket countries. Differences in individual lifestyle, including cigarette consumption, diet, and general health consciousness, no doubt account for a substantial proportion of the differences in mortality. The mortality rates are aggravated by more pervasive environmental factors, such as pollution and occupational hazards for certain cancers and respiratory diseases. Yet any interpretation of aggregate-level mortality differences such as those outlined above must take into account the substantial heterogeneity of the populations being compared. This is particularly true for the nonmarket countries. The former U.S.S.R., which alone accounted for two-thirds of the population of the industrialized nonmarket economies, was itself a very heterogeneous country with mortality profiles for subpopulations which vary from the Central–Eastern European pattern to a structure more typical of Asian countries. At best, therefore, the broad mortality comparisons presented here provide a *summary* perspective on health conditions for roughly one-quarter of the world's population.

Mortality in Industrial Countries: Update for 1990

More recent data for the late 1980s and, for several countries, 1990, are now available at WHO. Not surprisingly, the cause pattern of mortality in 1990 is much the same as for 1985, given the relative inertia of a mortality structure dominated by the chronic diseases.

CANCER. In 1990 there were 2.42 million deaths—1.35 million males, 1.07 million females. The leading type was lung cancer (400,000 males deaths, 120,000 female deaths), followed by colon-rectum cancer (276,000 deaths, both sexes combined), stomach cancer (244,000), breast cancer (175,000 women), and prostatic cancer (105,000 men).

CARDIOVASCULAR DISEASES. During 1990, 5.43 million deaths were coded to this category—2.46 million males and 2.97 million females. By far the largest category was ischemic heart disease (2.33 million), followed by cerebrovascular diseases (stroke) (1.48 million). Other (nonischemic) heart diseases claimed 1.06 million lives in 1990.

CERTAIN DEGENERATIVE DISEASES. Diabetes mellitus caused 170,000 deaths in 1990; ulcer of stomach and duodenum, 50,000; cirrhosis of the liver, 175,000; nephritis, nephrotic syndrome, and nephrosis, 125,000.

CHRONIC OBSTRUCTIVE PULMONARY DISEASES. In 1990 there were 388,000 deaths, 240,000 among men.

INJURIES AND POISONINGS. During 1990, some 865,000 deaths occurred in industrial countries from external causes, the majority (615,000) among males. Motor vehicle accidents claimed the lives of 215,000 persons, of whom 160,000 were males. The other leading cause of violent death was suicide, with 140,000 male deaths and 50,000 female deaths in 1990.

Estimated Cause-of-Death Patterns in 1985

The estimates for specific causes of death in developing countries are summarized in table 2-7 for children and adults separately and are discussed in more detail in this section according to their etiology. Table 2-8 provides an estimated distribution of mortality by broad cause groups within each of four geographic regions, which together encompass the entire developing world. The method of estimation and the sources used are also given in this section. It is immediately apparent that there is a substantial degree of uncertainty in the mortality estimates for specific causes, and hence the estimates must be viewed with considerable caution, particularly for individual diseases.

Quite apart from these more methodological considerations, the vast majority of childhood deaths in developing countries

occur within a complex epidemiological environment. Children are often afflicted with multiple infections, which in turn are aggravated by malnutrition and poverty. The estimation of mortality attributable to a single underlying cause is thus extremely difficult in developing countries, where infectious diseases are still common. One must be prepared to accept a considerable degree of overlap between estimates for specific diseases (there is a parallel in the industrial countries but at the other extreme of life, that is, at the advanced ages, when there are often several pathologies present at or about the time of death).

As a consequence, the estimates of mortality from leading causes of death in developing countries are presented here along with these disease interactions. This is clearly a departure from the convention of specifying a *single* underlying cause of death, but it is no doubt much closer to the reality which prevails in many parts of the developing world. Measles is a case in point. The most common complications of measles include pneumonia, diarrhea, and malnutrition. Studies in Latin America (Puffer and Serrano 1973) and Africa (Ofosu-Amaah 1983) have shown that many measles deaths were in fact attributed to complications of the disease, resulting in considerable underascertainment. The quantification of measles mortality shown in table 2-7 explicitly recognizes these relationships between underlying, immediate, and associated causes of death—the global estimate of 2 million measles

Table 2-7. Estimated Causes of Death in Developing Countries, by Age, 1985
(thousands)

Cause of death	Age		
	Under five	Five and over	All ages
Infectious and parasitic diseases	10,500	6,500	17,000
Diarrheal diseases	4,000	1,000	5,000
Tuberculosis	300	2,700	3,000
Acute respiratory diseases	4,300	2,000	6,300
Measles, whooping cough, and diphtheria	1,500	—	1,500
Other acute respiratory diseases	2,800	2,000	4,800
Other measles and whooping cough[a]	700	—	700
Malaria	750	250	1,000
Schistosomiasis	—	200	200
Other Infectious and parasitic diseases	450	350	800[b]
Complications of pregnancy	—	500	500
Perinatal conditions	3,200[c]	—	3,200
Neoplasms	—	2,500	2,500
Chronic obstructive lung diseases	—	2,300	2,300
Circulatory diseases and certain degenerative diseases	—	6,500	6,500
External causes	200	2,200	2,400
Other and unknown causes	700	2,800	3,500[b]
Total	14,600	23,300[d]	37,900

— Negligible

a. Does not include 400,000 measles-related deaths included under diarrheal diseases.

b. Some of these deaths actually may be attributable to malaria. The global estimate of mortality from the disease is between 1 and 2 million annually.

c. Includes an estimated 775,000 deaths from neonatal tetanus.

d. Of these, an estimated 1.6 million deaths occur at ages 5 to 14 years. Diarrheal diseases and acute respiratory disease are each estimated to account for about 300,000 deaths at these ages; another 150,000 or so are due to malaria and tuberculosis. Accidents and violence are a leading cause od death at these ages and may well claim 200,000 to 300,000 lives each year in this age group in developing countries.

Source: Author's estimates.

Table 2-8. Estimated Causes of Death in Developing Countries, by Region, 1985
(thousands)

Cause of death	Latin America and the Caribbean	Sub-Saharan Africa	Middle East/ North Africa	Asia	Total
Infectious and parasitic diseases	900	4,500	2,400	9,200	1,700
Neoplasms	300	250	200	1,750	2,500
Circulatory diseases and certain degenerative diseases	900	650	550	4,400	6,500
Complications of pregnancy	35	125	80	260	500
Perinatal conditions	300	680	420	1,800	3,200
Chronic obstructive pulmonary diseases	90	60	50	2,100	2,300
External causes	250	350	200	1,600	2,400
Other and unknown causes	425	585	400	2,090	3,500
Total	3,200	7,200	4,300	23,200	37,900

Source: Author's estimates.

deaths in 1985 has been disaggregated into estimates of the components of the disease-complication interaction. Many of these deaths would in turn be associated with malnutrition.

Several other examples could be cited, including the complexity of malarial infection. Severe anemia is often a consequence of repeated attacks of malaria but can also result from hookworm infection and nutritional deficiencies. Although this epidemiological complexity makes the estimation of mortality from specific diseases uncertain, there are clear implications for health interventions. Health care programs primarily designed to control the spread of infection from a single disease can be expected to exert a disproportionate effect on child survival by simultaneously reducing mortality from associated causes.

Infectious and Parasitic Diseases

The basis for the estimates of mortality from specific infectious diseases is given below. Although joint estimates are provided, the very poor quality of the data and information available to make them suggests that they be viewed extremely cautiously. Confidence intervals of the order of 50 percent around each estimate would seem reasonable.

DIARRHEAL DISEASES. In their review of morbidity and mortality from diarrheal diseases based on twenty-four studies in the developing world, Snyder and Merson (1982) estimated that there were roughly 4.6 million childhood deaths (below age five) each year associated with these diseases. Allowing for the effect of oral rehydration treatment in the meantime, and for population growth, the annual number of deaths is currently thought to be about 4.4 million. However, evidence on the case-fatality rate from the disease and the number of episodes (1,300 million per year) suggests just under 4 million childhood deaths.

The distinction between "association" and "cause" is emphasized by the authors. Acute diarrheal diseases are thus estimated to be associated with approximately 4 million child-

hood deaths, although the actual underlying cause of death may have been some other condition. Childhood mortality in many cases is the result of multiple infections, often aggravated by malnutrition, and the attribution of death to a single underlying cause is often extremely difficult in these circumstances. In the absence of more precise diagnostic information about the underlying cause of death, however, the estimate of 4 million childhood deaths will be taken as indicative of the volume of mortality due to diarrheal diseases, with about 10 percent of these (that is, 400,000) arising as a complication of measles.

Snyder and Merson do not provide estimates of diarrheal disease mortality in the population age five and over. Still, the studies which they reviewed suggest an annual death rate from diarrheal diseases in the adult population of about 1.4 per 1,000 in 1980. Applying this estimate to the estimated adult population in developing countries (excluding China) yields a total of about 3.1 million adult deaths. By contrast, age-specific data on morbidity from diarrheal diseases reported by Snyder and Merson suggest about 0.2 episodes per adult per year. Assuming the same case-fatality ratio as estimated for children (0.3 percent), this yields an estimate of about 1.3 million adult deaths. A third way to estimate diarrheal disease mortality is to use figures on the age-specific death rates from these diseases observed for the industrial countries at levels of life expectancy comparable to that of contemporary developing countries, excluding China (Preston 1976, p. 93). This method suggests a total of about 700,000 adult deaths and, interestingly, a total of about 3.9 million deaths below age five, or roughly the same estimate obtained earlier. In view of this proportionality between child and adult deaths, and the more recent evidence used in the method of case-fatality rate per episode, a figure of about 1 million adult deaths from diarrheal diseases would seem plausible, with about 300,000 of these occurring at age five through fourteen, based on age-specific fatality rates reported in community studies (Kirkwood 1990a).

These estimates are unlikely to be drastically altered by the addition of mortality in China. On the basis of the information for reporting areas, the number of diarrheal disease deaths among adults is unlikely to exceed 50,000 per year, which is well within the margin of uncertainty of the global estimates derived above.

TUBERCULOSIS. The experience of the WHO Tuberculosis Control Programme suggests that the most reliable estimates of mortality in developing countries are obtained from the case-fatality ratio among detected cases. This is predicated on the knowledge that without appropriate chemotherapy, tuberculosis infection is highly fatal. A review of studies on the proportion of cases detected that are also treated suggests that, overall, the case-fatality rate of the disease in developing countries is probably on the order of 15 percent (Murray, Styblo, and Rouillon, chapter 11, this collection). Applying this to incidence data yields an estimate of about 3 million tuberculosis deaths each year in developing countries. Approximately 200,000 of these deaths occur in China, leaving a total for other developing countries of 2.6 million deaths. Murray, Styblo, and Rouillon (1989) estimate that about 15 percent of these deaths (or 450,000) occur below age fifteen and of these, about two-thirds (or 10 percent of the total) are deaths of children under five. Thus roughly 300,000 childhood deaths (birth through age four) which occur each year in developing countries are estimated to be due to tuberculosis.

ACUTE RESPIRATORY INFECTIONS (ARI). A review of information available to WHO on causes of mortality in young children suggests that between 25 and 30 percent of deaths among the under-fives are attributable to these diseases (Leowski 1986). This estimate is supported by results obtained from longitudinal mortality surveys of communities conducted in Nepal, Pakistan, the Philippines, and Tanzania, using verbal autopsies. Despite the caveats associated with this type of estimation procedure, it is probable that acute respiratory infections account for about 4.3 million child deaths (that is, from birth through age four) each year in developing countries. The rationale underlying this estimate is outlined below.

Essentially, the group of acute respiratory infections can be classified into two broad subcategories, namely, certain vaccine-preventable diseases (measles, tuberculosis, whooping cough, and diphtheria) and other respiratory diseases (primarily pneumonia, influenza, acute bronchitis, and bronchiolitis). Separate estimates of mortality are available for the component diseases of the first category. According to estimates prepared by the WHO Expanded Programme on Immunization, there were approximately 2 million measles deaths and some 600,000 deaths from whooping cough in 1985 among children in developing countries. These estimates were prepared on the basis of assumptions about vaccine effectiveness (95 percent for measles, 80 percent for whooping cough), susceptibility of the unexposed population (100 percent for measles, 80 percent for whooping cough), estimated coverage by immunization, and case-fatality rates.

Information from community-level studies available to WHO indicates that about 1.1 million, or slightly more that half of the 2 million measles deaths, are due to ARI. Similarly, about two-thirds (or 400,000) of the pertussis deaths in 1985 were also attributable to ARI. Evidence from the industrial countries at an earlier stage of the epidemiological transition suggests a mortality ratio of about 0.7 between acute respiratory diseases (influenza, pneumonia, bronchitis) and diarrheal diseases. On this basis, the volume of mortality from the remaining respiratory diseases should be about 2.8 million deaths of children under age five. This yields a total of about 4.3 million for ARI-related deaths under age five.

Acute respiratory infections, particularly pneumonia, also claim a substantial number of lives at older ages. A comparison of age-specific death rates among adults from influenza, pneumonia, and bronchitis with those from diarrheal diseases (Preston 1976) suggests that death rates from the respiratory category are roughly two to four times higher. This would imply an annual toll of between 2 million and 4 million adult deaths from acute respiratory diseases in developing countries each year.[6] Data from China, India, and Latin America, however, suggest that the lower limit of this range is more reasonable, and hence an estimate of 2 million deaths beyond age five from these diseases is proposed. According to survey data for Sub-Saharan Africa reported by Kirkwood (1990b), about 300,000 of these deaths occur from age five through age fourteen.

VACCINE-PREVENTABLE DISEASES. Separate estimates for three of these diseases (poliomyelitis, tuberculosis, and neonatal tetanus) are presented elsewhere in this section. The overwhelming majority of deaths from the remainder are from measles and whooping cough. As mentioned earlier, measles probably claimed about 2 million lives below the age of five in 1985. Of these deaths, 1.1 million were also associated with ARI and another 400,000 with diarrhea. Whooping cough is estimated to have killed about 600,000 children in 1985, and 400,000 of these deaths were likewise associated with ARI. Taken together, the vaccine-preventable diseases either were the cause of, or were closely associated with, 3.7 million deaths of young children in 1985, of which 2 million were from measles, 600,000 from whooping cough, 300,000 from tuberculosis, about 800,000 from neonatal tetanus, and 25,000 from poliomyelitis.

POLIOMYELITIS. The immunization coverage rate for this disease is about 70 percent globally (WHO 1989). It is estimated by WHO that about 70 percent of the world's population lives in polio-endemic areas and that the annual incidence of the disease is about 250,000 cases. Overall, 25,000 deaths per year are estimated to occur from the disease.

YELLOW FEVER, DENGUE, AND ENCEPHALITIS. The estimation of annual mortality from these diseases is particularly difficult because of their epidemic nature, which results in considerable fluctuations from year to year. The estimated total mortality from these diseases in 1985 was about 15,000, but it should be noted that yellow fever in Nigeria was comparatively low in that year. Since the number of yellow-fever deaths in Nigeria during epidemic years can easily reach 10,000, the figure of 15,000 annual deaths from these diseases has been increased to 20,000 in an attempt to allow for epidemic variations.

MALARIA. Estimates of malaria mortality in Africa made some thirty years ago suggested that there were about 1 million deaths each year from the disease. Recent studies, based on active surveillance and intervention projects in Africa, suggest that the global total number of deaths is probably in the range of 1 to 2 million deaths per year. There is much more confidence in this range than in a point estimate, but for the purposes of this study, and without any additional guidance as to what part of the range is more probable, the lower limit has been chosen, yielding an estimate of 1 million deaths per year. Of these, about 500,000 are estimated to occur among children in Africa. The widespread and relatively indiscriminate use of chloroquine as practiced in Africa, keeps mortality down but also favors the selection of chloroquine-resistant parasites. As chloroquine resistance increases in geographic extension, frequency, and intensity, there is a serious threat of rising mortality, because there is no alternative drug that is equally safe and cheap.

Data from lay reporting of causes of death in rural India suggest that about 1 percent of deaths in India, or about 150,000, are due to malaria. Half of these deaths occur among infants and young children. On the basis of age-specific mortality data for certain endemic countries, malaria is also estimated to account for about 150,000 of the 1.6 million childhood deaths each year at age five through fourteen.

SCHISTOSOMIASIS. The prevalence of schistosomiasis is estimated at about 200 million people and is endemic in seventy-six countries. Information about the severity and age-specific prevalence of the disease, however, indicates that the upper limit of the estimated number of persons with severe infection is of the order of 13 million. Assuming a 0.1 percent case-fatality rate (limited to cases of severe infection), this implies a global total of about 13,000 deaths per year. Walsh (1988, p. 15) has estimated an annual mortality of between 250,000 and 500,000, apparently based on the assumption of a case-fatality rate for all cases (not only severe manifestations) of between 0.1 and 0.25 percent. Thus the range of mortality estimates varies from 13,000 to 500,000. An approximate mid-point of the range (200,000 deaths) may be taken as a rough guide to the annual toll of mortality but, as with many other of the diseases under consideration here, the degree of uncertainty is substantial. Information on the likely range of estimates is probably of greater relevance for establishing health priorities than these attempts at providing more precise figures.

SUMMARY FOR INFECTIOUS AND PARASITIC DISEASES. Summing up the estimates for the diseases listed above yields an annual mortality of about 17 million deaths (see table 2-6), about 10.5 million of which are estimated to occur among infants and children less than five years of age. These are undoubtedly the most significant communicable diseases, but other infectious and parasitic diseases, including amebiasis, hookworm, AIDS, and hepatitis B, undoubtedly claim several hundred thousand lives each year (neonatal tetanus is considered with the group of perinatal conditions). It is estimated on the basis of regional estimates for the major component diseases of this category that of these 17 million, slightly more than one-half occur in Asia and about one-quarter in Sub-Saharan Africa. The lowest mortality is estimated for Latin America, where about 900,000 deaths are estimated to have occurred in 1985 from infectious and parasitic diseases.

Complications of Pregnancy, Childbirth and the Puerperium, and Perinatal Conditions

In this section, separate estimates have been provided for two broad categories of cause of death since they are restricted to specific population groups, namely pregnant women (maternal causes) and newborn infants (perinatal conditions).

MATERNAL MORTALITY. It is well known that registered data on maternal deaths generally underestimate the extent of maternal mortality, even in industrial countries (see Ziskin and others 1979; Smith and others 1984; Rubin and others 1981). Mortality models based on these data, such as models of the epidemiological transition, will therefore tend systematically to underestimate deaths due to complications during pregnancy or the birth process, irrespective of the overall level of female mortality. Typically, the higher the level of female mortality, the greater the underestimation of deaths from such causes. As an alternative procedure, selected community-wide studies have been evaluated (see, for example, Fortney and others 1986; Royston and Lopez 1987) in order to estimate the relation between the overall level of female mortality and mortality from pregnancy complications or the birth process in various sociocultural settings. Applying these community-based estimates to estimates of the number of births in major regions leads to an overall estimate of approximately 500,000 maternal deaths in developing countries in 1985. Of these, an estimated 35,000 occurred in Latin America and the Caribbean, 125,000 in Sub-Saharan Africa, 80,000 in the Middle East and North Africa, and about 260,000 in Asia and Oceania.

PERINATAL CONDITIONS. On the basis of community-level data, WHO has estimated the annual number of perinatal deaths each year to be approximately 7.3 million, of which only about 300,000 occur in industrial countries (WHO 1989). Of the remaining 7 million perinatal deaths, the proportion which are early neonatal deaths (birth to six days) appears to vary between 40 and 50 percent in developing countries, according to statistics published in the United Nations Demographic Yearbook. This percentage implies an estimate of about 3.2 million early neonatal deaths, almost all of which can probably be attributed to one of the perinatal conditions. Neonatal tetanus alone would account for about one-quarter (or roughly 800,000) of these deaths. Out of a total of 3.2 million deaths, almost 60 percent (1.8 million) are estimated to have occurred in Asia, 680,000 in Sub-Saharan Africa, 300,000 in Latin America and the Caribbean, and about 420,000 in the Middle East–North Africa region (see table 2-8).

Chronic Diseases and Violent Death

Specific mortality estimates for the major non-communicable diseases and violence are discussed below. Although the etiology of the constituent diseases (e.g. different types of cancer) can vary considerably, arguing for more specific estimates, only broad categories of causes are discussed here in view of the uncertain diagnostic accuracy of the cause of death information upon which they are based.

NEOPLASMS. On the basis of incidence data reported to the International Agency for Research on Cancer, Parkin, Läärä, and Muir (1988) have estimated that there were a little over 3.2 million new cases of cancer in the developing world in 1980. This corresponds to an incidence rate of 94.5 per 100,000. Applying this figure to the estimated 1985 population yields a total of about 3.6 million new cases in 1985. This may well be an underestimate, however, as population aging in the developing world will certainly imply an increased burden of illness from cancer, even if the relative levels of prevalence of risk factors were to remain unchanged. This is certainly not the case, as is evident from the dramatic increase in cigarette consumption in developing countries in recent years (WHO 1985). Nonetheless, the figure of 3.6 million new cases in 1985 provides a reasonable, if conservative, benchmark from which to derive estimates of mortality. .

A very crude first approximation can be obtained from the observed relation between incidence and mortality in the industrial countries. In 1985 there were an estimated 3.25 million new cases of cancer in the industrialized world and 2.3 million deaths, yielding a mortality-to-incidence ratio of 0.7. If this ratio were to apply in developing countries, the estimated number of deaths would be on the order of 2.5 million. Still, health services for cancer patients are undoubtedly more widely available in industrial countries and are probably more effective in treating the disease. One would therefore expect that not only is the average age at death from cancer lower in developing countries but also the mortality-to-incidence ratio is probably higher than in industrial countries. Thus the annual toll of cancer deaths is no doubt higher than the 2.5 million suggested by this method of estimation, but how much higher is rather uncertain.

In China alone, there are about 1 million cancer deaths each year, according to the mortality data from reporting areas. Lay reporting of the cause of death in rural India suggests that about 4 percent of all deaths in India are due to cancer, and this proportion is confirmed by studies carried out in communities in Andhra Pradesh; Goa, Daman, and Diu; and Maharashtra states. This would suggest an annual mortality from cancer in India of about 400,000 deaths, or 50 per 100,000 population. National data for Latin America and the Caribbean, although

incomplete, yield an estimate of about 300,000 deaths per year, which is just under 10 percent of all deaths. The information on overall life expectancy in Sub-Saharan Africa and the Middle East–North Africa region, and the regional incidence estimates reported by Parkin, Läärä, and Muir (1988), suggest levels of cancer mortality comparable to what was observed for India. Such levels yield another 450,000 cancer deaths (neoplasms) in these two regions (table 2-8).

On the basis of the incidence levels for cancer reported by Parkin, Läärä, and Muir (1988), it may be estimated that there were some 300,000 to 400,000 deaths from cancer for the remainder of Asia in 1985. The addition of these deaths yields an overall total of 2.5 million cancer deaths each year in the developing world. This process of aggregation thus leads to an estimate of cancer mortality which is identical to that estimated from the mortality-to-incidence ratio method. The fact that the two estimates do not differ should not be seen as necessarily a verification of either method. The evidence, however, would seem to suggest that the annual number of cancer deaths in the developing world is at least 2.5 million. On the basis of incidence data, the principal sites of cancer mortality in the developing world are stomach, mouth-pharynx, esophagus, and lung among males, and cervix, breast, stomach, and mouth-pharynx (particularly in India) among females.

CHRONIC OBSTRUCTIVE LUNG DISEASE (COLD). Global and regional estimates for this category of diseases are particularly difficult because of the lack of reliable data for the majority of developing countries. The mortality information available from China suggests that as much as 15 percent of all deaths are due to these diseases, which would imply about 1 million deaths. In China, at least, there is some basis for expecting high COLD mortality in view of past smoking patterns, particularly among males, and the very high levels of indoor air pollution emanating from the cooking and heating fuels used (World Bank 1989). In India, data from the lay reporting system in rural areas suggest a COLD mortality figure of about 6 to 8 percent, a proportion which is at least consistent with prevalence studies in specific communities (see, for example, Malik and Wahi 1978). This would imply an additional 700,000 to 800,000 deaths in India alone. Death rates of the order of 40 to 60 per 100,000 have been reported to WHO for other parts of Asia. From these estimates, an additional 350,000 deaths from COLD in the remainder of Asia and the Pacific are estimated for 1985. Data for Latin America suggest that at least 90,000 adults succumbed to these diseases in 1985. On the basis of comparative life expectancy, the annual mortality in Sub-Saharan Africa and the Middle East–North Africa region is estimated at 60,000 and 50,000, respectively, yielding a total for all developing countries of 2.3 million deaths. There is, however, considerable uncertainty associated with this estimate.

CIRCULATORY DISEASES AND SELECTED DEGENERATIVE DISEASES. As for the chronic obstructive lung diseases, perhaps the best way to proceed in estimating global mortality for this group of diseases is by considering the situation in major regions separately. In China, available data suggested that there are at least 1 million deaths from stroke alone each year and another million deaths from all forms of heart disease. The estimated total for the four specific degenerative diseases is about 400,000, suggesting an overall total for this category of diseases in China of about 2.5 million deaths per year. In rural areas of India, on the basis of data from the Rural Cause of Death Survey (Indian Office of the Registrar General 1989), diseases of the circulatory system (primarily heart diseases and stroke) account for about 10 percent of deaths. The remaining degenerative diseases make up an additional 2 percent or so of all deaths, suggesting an annual mortality from this category of about 1.1 million.

The group of countries that make up the remainder of Asia (excluding India, China, and western Asia) has an average life expectancy of about fifty-seven years, which, if one uses the indirect mortality estimation techniques described by Hakulinen and others (1986), would imply a relative mortality of about 12 percent due to the cardiovascular and other chronic degenerative diseases. This estimate yields a further 800,000 deaths in the remainder of Asia and the Pacific, or a grand total for Asia of 4.4 million deaths each year.

Data from countries of Latin America, when aggregated and adjusted for underreporting, yield another 800,000 to 900,000 deaths from these causes. Very little information on the extent of mortality from cardiovascular disease is available for the African and Middle East regions, but with life expectancy in these areas typically on the order of fifty to fifty-five years, it is difficult to see how less than 10 percent or so of deaths could be ascribed to these diseases. As a very rough estimate, accompanied by a substantial degree of uncertainty, an additional 1.2 million deaths have been attributed to these causes in the two regions combined as shown in table 2-8. The global total for this category is thus estimated at about 6.5 million deaths per year, of which the four specific degenerative diseases probably claim between 600,000 and 1 million lives each year.

INJURY AND POISONING. In almost all cases, the attribution of death to a violent cause as opposed to a disease is relatively straightforward. This is not to deny that the disaggregation of violent deaths into accidents, suicides, homicides, and other violence is often quite complicated and may well be influenced by sociocultural or legal factors, for example, mitigating against a verdict of suicide in some cultures. In this review attention will be confined to the broad category of violent deaths, and hence for the most part, these considerations would not apply. Moreover, because of the relative ease of distinguishing a violent death from other causes, one can have greater confidence in the data generated by alternative collection schemes, such as lay reporting.

In China, roughly 700,000 deaths from external causes are estimated to occur each year, or about 10 percent of the total. In India, the proportion is less, about 6 percent, or 550,000 deaths, from accidents and violence. Data for Latin America, after adjusting for incomplete coverage, indicate that there

were about 250,000 violent deaths in the region in 1985, this being about 8 percent of all deaths. Evidence from other developing regions suggests that violence is less important as a cause of death and a proportionate mortality of about 5 percent is probably not unreasonable. This assumption yields an estimate of 350,000 deaths in Sub-Saharan Africa, 200,000 in the Middle East–North Africa region, and 350,000 in the remainder of Asia. The estimated total number of violent deaths is thus 2.4 million deaths per year for the developing world, of which about 8 to 9 percent (that is, 200,000) are estimated to occur before age five.

Maternal and Childhood Mortality: Update for 1990

The number and relative importance of deaths from chronic diseases among adults in developing countries are likely to have altered very little between 1985 and 1990. But given the natural history of these diseases, one might reasonably expect to see a significant change brought about by child health interventions in this short period of time. According to WHO (1992), this has indeed been the case. The number of infant and child deaths declined to about 12.9 million in 1990. In large part, this decline has been attributed to the rapid improvement in immunization coverage since the mid-1980s (WHO 1992). In 1990, measles was estimated to have caused 880,000 deaths of children under age five in developing countries, down from 2 million in 1985. Relatively few of these deaths were attributable to measles alone (220,000), the majority arising from interactions with acute respiratory infections (480,000) and diarrhea (180,000). Similarly, whooping cough in 1990 was estimated to have caused 360,000 child deaths, 260,000 of which were estimated to have occurred in conjunction with acute respiratory infections. There has also been a dramatic decline in neonatal tetanus deaths, from 800,000 in 1985 to 560,000 in 1990.

By contrast, relatively little change has occurred in the other principal causes of child death. Allowing for the association with measles, diarrheal diseases are estimated to have claimed about 3.2 million children in 1990. Acute respiratory infections, primarily pneumonia, were the cause of 3.5 to 3.6 million child deaths in 1990; if one includes the deaths associated with measles and whooping cough mentioned above, this toll rises to about 4.3 million deaths a year. Mortality from other traditional diseases of childhood, such as malaria, has remained essentially unchanged, as has the category of perinatal conditions (including neonatal tetanus), which, in 1990, are estimated to have caused about 3 million early infant deaths.

Finally, a recent update of the annual number of maternal deaths in developing countries shows relatively little change compared with 1983–85 (WHO 1991b). In 1988–90 the annual number of maternal deaths in developing countries was estimated at just over half a million (505,000), with an approximate 5 percent decline in risk being more than compensated for by a 7 percent rise in the number of women exposed to risk. Maternal mortality appears to have increased by about 10 percent in Africa (170,000 deaths in 1988–90), declined slightly in Latin America (25,000 deaths), and remained unchanged in Asia.

Summary and Conclusions

The estimation of mortality levels, structure, and trends is fundamental to any assessment of the health situation. For several countries, including virtually all the industrialized world as well as a number of countries in Latin America and eastern Asia, reasonably reliable and comparable mortality statistics are available to determine the age, sex, and cause of mortality. In the group of industrial countries, which together made up about one-quarter of the world's population in 1985, the leading causes of death are those conditions for which prevention is largely a matter of personal lifestyle. Diseases such as ischemic heart disease, stroke, cancer, and, in particular, lung cancer, the chronic obstructive lung diseases, diabetes, and cirrhosis of the liver, which dominate the mortality pattern in industrial countries, all have a significant behavioral component. Cigarette smoking, for example, is by far the principal risk factor for lung cancer, chronic bronchitis, and emphysema and is also causally associated to varying degrees with ischemic heart disease, stroke, and several other types of cancer. Indeed, cigarette smoking is probably the leading cause of mortality in the industrial countries, claiming an estimated 2.1 million lives each year (or 20 percent of the total) in these countries. This number can be expected to rise to at least 3 million by the 2020s as the full effect of the smoking epidemic among women is felt (Peto and others 1992).

By and large, the industrial countries, particularly those with market economies, have been very successful in deferring death to higher and higher ages. In these countries, the challenge will be to ensure a comparable delay in the onset of chronic disease, thus minimizing the proportion of the years of life gained which are spent in a state of chronic morbidity or disability. Further reductions in inequalities in health status within national populations will also bring rewards in terms of gains in life expectancy, particularly for adults. Accidental deaths, suicide, and other violence continue to claim a significant proportion (7 to 8 percent) of lives in industrial countries and constitute a very substantial cost to society in terms of potential years of life lost. Behavioral factors—in particular, alcohol abuse—similarly underlie many of these deaths.

Mortality rates from most leading causes of death are significantly higher in nonmarket industrial countries. Indeed, in some cases, most notably Hungary, death rates from major chronic diseases among men have been rising for several years. Information on the prevalence and distribution of risk factors is clearly an essential component of health strategies designed to counter these trends.

Although the health situation in developing countries has been assessed collectively, it is absolutely imperative to keep in mind the heterogeneity of this group when interpreting the estimates of the cause-of-death structure. Mortality levels within the group vary from high-mortality countries in Africa and Asia, where infant mortality rates exceed 200 per 1,000 live births, to countries such as China, Cuba, Argentina, Chile, and Uruguay, where life expectancy is comparable to that observed in many industrial countries. Not surprisingly, the cause-of-death structure in the former category is dominated by the communicable diseases, whereas in the latter group the chronic diseases are of most concern. Other developing countries, with life expectancy in the range of about fifty-five to sixty-five years, are intermediate in their progression through the epidemiological transition. Clearly, in these countries, as with very high-mortality populations where infant and child deaths continue to claim up to 50 to 60 percent of the total, health strategies must continue to focus on the prevention and control of infectious diseases, particularly the diarrheal diseases, respiratory infections, and the vaccine-preventable diseases. Malaria, too, is a leading cause of child death in some areas. Effective primary health care delivery undoubtedly offers the greatest hope for success in rapidly bringing down mortality levels for these diseases.

But what is also clear is that the chronic diseases have already emerged as a significant, if not the significant, health problem in a sufficient number of developing countries to warrant increasing attention. There are now at least as many cancer deaths in developing countries as in the industrialized world and at least another 9 million deaths each year in developing countries from other chronic diseases. To some extent, this is an inevitable consequence of progress toward the conquest of infectious diseases. Still, the widespread adoption of cigarette smoking in many parts of the developing world is rapidly eroding some of the gains in life expectancy which have been achieved as a result. Although the annual amount of tobacco-attributable mortality in the developing world is currently less than that of the industrial countries (about 1 million to 1.5 million deaths per year), this death toll is projected to rise rapidly during the next three to four decades to reach 6 million to 8 million in the 2020s (Peto and Lopez 1991). A substantial proportion of this premature mortality is expected to occur in China, where the dramatic increase in consumption of manufactured cigarettes during the last twenty years or so (China now consumes one-quarter of the world total) can be expected to result in 2 million to 3 million smoking-attributable deaths in the 2020s, almost a million of which will be from lung cancer (Peto and Lopez 1991).

The rapidly emerging epidemic of smoking-attributable mortality is one of the principal public health issues which developing countries will face during the next few decades, and in many cases it will be superimposed on a health system still preoccupied with the control of infectious diseases. The inevitability of death thus implies that, although this transition to chronic diseases is to be expected, what is important is that these deaths be postponed to as late in life as possible. As for the industrial countries, effective preventive strategies have a much greater likelihood of achieving this than costly attempts at cure.

Notes

This chapter was prepared while I was a staff member of WHO's Division of Global Epidemiological Surveillance and Health Situation and Trend Assessment. The views expressed here are mine and do not necessarily reflect the opinions or policies of the World Health Organization. Nonetheless, my research has benefited from the contribution and comments of many colleagues at WHO, particularly those in technical programs concerned with the health problems specifically discussed in the chapter. Their contribution is gratefully acknowledged. I should also like to express my sincere gratitude to Dean Jamison for his insistence that this type of assessment should and could be done, and for his very helpful remarks on several earlier versions of it. The paper has also benefited from a critical review by Timo Hakulinen and Althea Hill. In acknowledging the very considerable assistance which I received in the preparation of this chapter, I also accept that any errors and omissions are my responsibility.

1. The year 1985 has been chosen in order to present a mid-decade review. Whenever possible, estimates for 1990 have been included as well.

2. The populations of the former Yugoslavia, the former German Democratic Republic (GDR), and the former U.S.S.R. are shown in this chapter, since they were countries at the time the data were provided to the World Health Organization (WHO).

3. The only industrial country for which cause-of-death data about 1985 are not available to WHO is Albania. This is unlikely to affect the results for the group as a whole, since the total annual number of deaths in Albania is of the order of 17,000, which is less than 0.2 percent of the total for the industrialized world.

4. Namely, cirrhosis of the liver, ulcers of the stomach and duodenum, nephritis and nephrosis, and diabetes mellitus.

5. This diagnostic specificity does not, however, guarantee international comparability due to the reasons mentioned earlier.

6. Some adult deaths from the vaccine-preventable diseases would also be expected, but these are likely to be comparatively few compared with adult mortality from acute bronchitis and pneumonia.

References

Capocaccia, Riccardo, and Gino Farchi. 1988. "Mortality from Liver Cirrhosis in Italy: Proportion Associated with Consumption of Alcohol." *Journal of Clinical Epidemiology* 41(4):347–57.

Doll, Richard, and Richard Peto. 1981. *The Causes of Cancer.* Oxford: Oxford University Press.

Fortney, J. A., Irene Susanti, Saad Gadalla, Saneya Saleh, Susan Rogers, and Malcolm Potts. 1986. "Reproductive Mortality in Two Developing Countries." *American Journal of Public Health* 76(2):134–36.

Hakulinen, Timo, Harold Hansluwka, Alan Lopez, and Tadashi L. Nakada. 1986. "Global and Regional Mortality Patterns by Cause of Death in 1980." *International Journal of Epidemiology* 15(2):226–33.

Hull, T. H., J. E. Rohde, and A. D. Lopez. 1981. "A Framework for Estimating Causes of Death in Indonesia." *Majalaj Demografi Indonesia* 15:77–125.

Indian Office of the Registrar General. 1989. *Survey of Causes of Death (Rural).* Annual Report, 1987. Series 3, 20. Delhi.

Kirkwood, Betty R. 1991a. "Diarrhoea." In R. G. A. Feachem and D. T. Jamison, eds., *Disease and Mortality in Sub-Saharan Africa.* New York: Oxford University Press.

———. 1991b. "Acute Respiratory Infections." In R. G. A. Feachem and D. T. Jamison, eds., *Disease and Mortality in Sub-Saharan Africa.* New York: Oxford University Press.

Leowski, Jerzy. 1986. "Mortality from Acute Respiratory Infections in Children under 5 Years of Age: Global Estimates." *World Health Statistics Quarterly* 39:138–144.

Lopez, A. D. 1990a. "The Interrelationship between Lung Cancer and Tobacco Consumption: Evidence from National Statistics." In Matti Hakama, Valerie Beral, J. W. Cullen, and D. M. Parkin, eds., *Evaluating Effectiveness of Primary Prevention for Cancer.* Scientific Publication 103, IARC. Lyon: International Agency for Research on Cancer.

———. 1990b. "Competing Causes of Death: A Review of Recent Trends in Mortality in Industrialized Countries with Special Reference to Cancer." *Annals of the New York Academy of Science* 609 (November 2):58–76.

Malik, S. K., and P. L. Wahi. 1978. "Prevalence of Chronic Bronchitis in a Group of North Indian Adults." *Journal of the Indian Medical Association* 70(1):6–8.

Ofosu-Amaah, Samuel. 1983. "The Control of Measles in Tropical Africa: A Review of Past and Present Efforts." *Review of Infectious Diseases* 5(3):546–53.

Parkin, D. M., E. Läärä, and C. S. Muir. 1988. "Estimates of the Worldwide Frequency of Sixteen Major Cancers in 1980." *International Journal of Cancer* 41:184–97.

Percy, Constance, and Callum S. Muir. 1989. "The International Comparability of Cancer Mortality Data: Results of an International Death Certificate Study." *American Journal of Epidemiology* 129(5):934–46.

Peto, Richard, and A. D. Lopez. 1991. "Worldwide Mortality from Current Smoking Patterns." In Betty Durston and Konrad Jamrozik, eds., *Tobacco and Health 1990: The Global War.* Proceedings of the Seventh World Conference on Tobacco and Health, Perth, Australia, April 1–5, 1990. Health Department of Western Australia.

Peto, Richard, A. D. Lopez, Jillian Boreham, Michael Thun, and Clark Heath. 1992. "Mortality from Tobacco in Developed Countries: Indirect Estimation from National Vital Statistics." *Lancet* (23 May) 1268–78.

Preston, S. H. 1976. *Mortality Patterns in National Populations.* New York: Academic Press.

Puffer, R. R., and C. V. Serrano. 1973. *Patterns of Mortality in Childhood.* Scientific Publication 262, PAHO (Pan-American Health Organization). Washington, D.C.

Royston, Erica, and A. D. Lopez. 1987. "On the Assessment of Maternal Mortality." *World Health Statistics Quarterly* 40(3):214–24.

Rubin, George, Brian McCarthy, James Shelton, Roger Rochat, and Jules Terry. 1981. "The Risk of Childbearing Re-evaluated." *American Journal of Public Health* 71(7):712–16.

Smith, Jack C., J. M. Hughes, P. S. Pekow, and R. W. Rochat. 1984. "An Assessment of the Incidence of Maternal Mortality in the United States." *American Journal of Public Health* 74(8):780–83.

Snyder, J. D., and M. H. Merson. 1982. "The Magnitude of the Global Problem of Acute Diarrhoeal Disease: A Review of Active Surveillance Data." *Bulletin of the World Health Organization* 60(4):605–13.

USDHSS (United States Department of Health and Human Services). 1989. *Reducing the Health Consequences of Smoking: 25 Years of Progress. A Report of the Surgeon General.* Rockville, Md.: Centers for Disease Control, Office on Smoking and Health.

Walsh, J. A. 1988. *Establishing Health Priorities in the Developing World.* Boston: Adams Publishing Group for the United Nations Development Programme.

World Bank. 1989. "China: Long-term Issues in Options for the Health Sector."

WHO (World Health Organization). 1985. *World Health Statistics Annual 1985.* Geneva.

———. 1989. *Expanded Programme on Immunization: Update.* May. Geneva.

———. 1991a. "Smoking as a Cause of Cancer." *Tobacco Alert* October:2.

———. 1991b. "New Estimates of Maternal Mortality." *Weekly Epidemiological Record.* 66:345–48.

———. 1992. *Eighth Report on the World Health Situation.* Geneva.

Ziskin, Leah Z., Margaret Gregory, and Michael Kreitzer. 1979. "Improved Surveillance of Maternal Deaths." *International Journal of Gynaecology and Obstetrics* 16:282–86.

3

The Epidemiologic Transition and Health Priorities

José Luis Bobadilla, Julio Frenk, Rafael Lozano,
Tomas Frejka, and Claudio Stern

The world approaches the end of a century and a millennium having achieved, during the last century, the most intensive and extensive health changes in history. Advances in our knowledge of the causes and effects of diseases, progress in sanitation and nutrition, development of vaccines and drugs, expansion of a vast network of facilities and personnel, appearance of a whole sector of the economy devoted to health-related goods and services, predominance of medical over religious or legal considerations in the interpretation of human experience: these are but a few of the shifts that have radically transformed the health scene in most countries.

The results are well known: more people enjoy the benefits of good health than ever before. Yet, as with all true progress, improvement in health has created new problems and challenges. In a very real sense, it can be said that the health field has been a victim of its own successes. Thus, the dramatic reduction in the incidence and severity of infectious diseases has allowed the survival of a large number of individuals who, for that very reason, become increasingly exposed to the risk of chronic ailments and injuries. Similarly, control of fertility is modifying structure of the population, leading to an unprecedented proportion and quantity of elderly people, who pose enormous demands on the health care system.

In addition, the general process of industrialization, urbanization, and modernization—of which the expansion in health services has been both a consequence and a facilitator—has entailed high costs. The environment has been seriously and permanently damaged in many parts of the world. We have learned that mass consumption of tobacco is directly responsible for a large burden of premature deaths and disabilities. The shift in diet from vegetables and cereals to animal foodstuffs and some artificial products has been recognized as contributing to cardiovascular disease and some cancers of the digestive system.

The net result of these changes has been that the health field has achieved a level of complexity never seen before. Such complexity is compounded by the fact that the benefits of progress have been very unequally distributed both between and within nations. Together with the explosion in science and technology there has been a widening of the gap between

what is achievable by current knowledge and what is actually achieved. To the extent that controlling certain diseases becomes technically feasible, their continuing existence among deprived populations becomes morally compelling. The problem of equity has thus emerged as one of the central concerns of our times.

As part of the increasing complexity of the health field, most governments around the world have developed various forms of organized social response to the problems of their populations. Although the role of the state in providing health services has recently decreased in some countries, the overall trend after World War II has been oriented toward an incremental participation. Modern nations, on the whole, now consider health an essential element of development, requiring integration into national plans.

The simultaneous presence of more complex health conditions, on the one hand, and increased commitment to extending health services, on the other, has given a strategic character to the definition of priorities. This is compounded, in many countries, by a situation of stagnant and even shrinking resources. In such a context, it has become imperative to develop methods for long-term health planning that are solidly grounded on demographic and epidemiologic information. Needless to say, many economic and political variables outside the planning process affect the final allocation of resources. At the very least, health planning allows us to know the way in which those other variables make resource allocation deviate from the technically defined optimum. At its best, health planning can constitute a force for mobilizing social resources toward the satisfaction of health needs.

Indeed, our ability to identify new health changes and opportunely respond to them depends on a clear understanding of the determining factors and on the consequent design of innovative models for health promotion, and for disease prevention and treatment. In this chapter we attempt to apply the theory of the epidemiologic transition to explain the recent transformations and the future evolution of health needs in populations. We particularly refer to middle-income countries, where such transition adopts specific forms and where the gap between the changing character of health problems and the adequacy of the social response is of significant concern. Among the middle-income countries, Mexico is used to illustrate the basic information and methods required to incorporate demographic and epidemiologic criteria into the process of planning for health services and related programs.

The opening section of the chapter presents the conceptual basis for understanding the epidemiologic transition in middle-income countries and the main components of health planning. In it we define demographic variables as important measures of population health needs and therefore as fundamental elements for setting priorities. Next, we describe some of the important social and demographic changes which have occurred in Mexico during the past fifty years. An account of the main aspects of the epidemiologic transition in Mexico follows, in which we propose that it might be a new model not hitherto considered by the original theory. The following section presents projections of the most important demographic and epidemiologic variables from 1980 to 2010 and the general trends of social variables in that time period. The last section includes an analysis of the likely implications that the main described changes will have on the health system, and we suggest some reforms that should be introduced to deal with the complex health scenario of the next twenty years.

Conceptual Framework

Although some authors may consider it possible to identify a common pattern of epidemiologic transition for the industrial nations, for the so-called developing countries this is almost impossible without incurring significant mistakes or superficial generalizations. Actually, not all poor countries are continuously in the process of developing; at times of crisis they seem to be static or even underdeveloping. In many respects, the differences among poor countries are often greater than those between industrial and developing nations. The picture is even more complex in the areas of health and health care, since many relatively poor countries resemble industrial nations in these respects (as is true of Costa Rica, Cuba, and Sri Lanka). However, most countries rich and poor present serious inequalities among different social groups, leading to internal heterogeneity. Many rich nations are characterized by development with pockets of underdevelopment; conversely, most of the developing nations are composed in varying proportions of underdevelopment with pockets of development.

Attempting to describe the health transition for the developing countries as a whole is thus inappropriate. In the absence of an optimal classification of countries, we will adopt the one used by the World Bank, based on national income per capita. In particular we will refer to "middle-income" countries, which in 1990 had a median gross national product per capita between US$611 and US$7,619 (World Bank 1992).

The Health Transition

Our analysis of the dynamics of health in human populations begins with the differentiation of two basic elements. On the

one hand, there are the *health conditions* or needs of the population; these are represented mostly by negative deviations from physical and psychological function, although they also include nonmorbid conditions like pregnancy and, in the most comprehensive perspective, positive well-being. On the other hand, there is the *organized social response* to the health needs of the population; this entails any organized collective action aimed at promoting health, or at preventing and treating disease. In this context, the *health transition* refers to the changes over time of both the health conditions and the organized social response. In turn, the health transition comprises two sets of processes, corresponding to the foregoing differentiation. The first one is what Omran (1971) described as the *epidemiologic transition*, that is, changes in health conditions. The second is the *health care transition*, that is, changes in the organized social response (Frenk and others 1989b). Empirical evidence shows that these two transitions are dependent on each other. For example, universal coverage of effective health services has contributed to the decline of childhood mortality due to infectious diseases in countries like China, Costa Rica and Sri Lanka. What is less common is the anticipatory adaptation of the health system to ongoing changes in the health needs of the population. In any case, we have a more elaborate theory of the epidemiologic than of the health care transition.

The theory of the epidemiologic transition as developed to date refers to the changes in the population parameters and in the health and disease patterns, which occur over decades or centuries. The elements of this theory are: (a) the description of the strong links between demographic changes and health needs of populations, as measured by the mix of causes of death and the age structure of mortality; (b) the coherent classification of eras that allows for the identification of important socioeconomic changes that affect survival at different times; and (c) the potential for anticipating changes in disease patterns and the opportunities offered by such anticipation to strategic health planning.

In his original formulation, Omran (1971) proposed three eras of the epidemiologic transition that countries experience at different stages of their social and economic development:

The era of *pestilence and famine*, when life expectancy is low (20 to 39 years) and the major causes of death are associated with malnutrition, infection, and complications of reproduction.

The era of *receding pandemics*, when the disease pattern is still dominated by infectious diseases and malnutrition, but major mortality fluctuations, including peaks, are less common. Life expectancy rises to between 30 and 50 years, and there is a tendency for increasing control of the biological pollution of the environment, as a result of improved sanitation, with declining rates of infection.

The era of *degenerative and man-made diseases*, characterized by the rise of cardiovascular diseases, cancer, diabetes, and other degenerative diseases. Life expectancy is over 50 years and fertility becomes a crucial factor of population growth.

The original description of the theory and some of the later updates acknowledge the heterogeneity of social and economic development among countries. Accordingly, Omran (1971) suggested that at least three models can be recognized: the classical or Western model, the accelerated model (such as that followed by Japan), and the delayed or contemporary model, the main differences among them being the timing and the pace of change. The delayed (or contemporary) model described the incomplete transition of most developing countries. The important decline of mortality started after World War II and was mainly a result of the adoption of imported public health measures and some medical interventions, and not so much to improvements in economic and social factors, as was the case in the classical or Western model. Although the gains in child survival have been substantial in this model, the mortality rates are still relatively high.

More recently, Frenk and others (1989b) have proposed a new model, called the "protracted-polarized model" of the epidemiologic transition. Its formulation is largely based on observations from some large middle-income countries. Its main features are as follows:

- The decline of mortality takes place in very short periods of time, as compared with the classical model. Western European countries that followed the classical model took more than 130 years to reduce mortality from 35 deaths per 1000 population to 10, whereas many middle-income countries have achieved a similar decline in less than 70 years.

- The onset of the mortality decline starts in the twentieth century, reaching low levels near the end of the century.

- Despite significant reductions in mortality by infectious diseases, these diseases are not brought fully under control, and their incidence rates remain relatively high by the end of the century. This situation, together with the increase of noncommunicable diseases, produces an *overlap of eras*.

- The unequal distribution of wealth and the incomplete coverage of interventions gives place to a widening of the gap in health status among social classes and geographical regions. This process has been described as "epidemiologic polarization" (Frenk and others 1989a). Even though this process might have occurred under other transition models, in the protracted model polarization possibly goes on for longer periods.

- A review of morbidity data reveals the reemergence of epidemic diseases that had been controlled or eradicated, which produces a *countertransition*.

The first two characteristics of this model serve to differentiate it from others previously described. The other features have not been examined for countries presenting the classical or the delayed model. It is proposed that they also might differ between the protracted-polarized and the other models of epidemiologic transition.

There are two implicit assumptions in transition theory that need to be critically examined. One is that each era is more desirable than the previous ones because it reflects "progress." Yet, even when survivorship increases, morbidity and disability do not necessarily decline in the same proportion; and

actually the health conditions for a large proportion of adults might not improve or might even worsen (Wildavsky 1977). It could be that the third era represents an advanced stage of a longer transitional era, so that in a fourth era it might be possible to live in societies with low mortality and morbidity rates of both infectious and noncommunicable diseases and of accidents, violence, and mental diseases.

The second assumption refers to the sequence of the transition from one era to the other. It has been proposed that some modifications to the original theory might be introduced to accommodate experiences from some middle-income countries (Frenk and others 1989b). First, the eras are not necessarily sequential, since two or more may overlap at the same time. Second, the evolutionary changes in the pattern of morbidity and mortality are reversible, so that there can be backward movements, as we pointed out earlier.

In addition, the theory presents some limitations that need to be highlighted:

- It has limited potential to explain heterogeneity in disease patterns within countries. As we postulated previously, within a given country, it is possible to recognize social groups with common infectious diseases, coexisting with social groups affected by noncommunicable diseases.

- The implicit and operational concept of health is exclusively limited to health losses that can be documented through mortality. Several health problems that predominantly produce morbidity, let alone positive aspects of health, are by definition ignored. This is extremely important, since the advance in therapeutics often postpones or averts death but does not cure the disease.

- The capacity to relate social and economic changes to health improvements is relevant only to the general aspects of development. Unfortunately, the theory as it stands cannot explain how social and economic changes are related to health transformations; it also has a limited value to explain the role of different forms of social organization on the timing, pace, and modality of the epidemiologic transition.

Health Planning: Using the Transition to Set Priorities

As experience in the developing countries accumulates and as new analyses are elaborated, our knowledge will expand and the progression of epidemiologic transition theory may help us to understand current health dynamics in a variety of countries. Such understanding is essential not only to advance our theories about the nature of change in the health field but also to shape future reforms.

With respect to budgetary allocations, there are two main methods of planning for health services. The first one, which is the most commonly used, can be called the retrospective method, because it commonly starts out from a fixed budget and then moves to the allocation of those resources to different health programs, according to previously established priorities.

The alternative method, which can be called prospective, begins with a definition of population health needs. In this context, the term "needs" refers specifically to health conditions that require care but not to the care itself (Donabedian 1973). That is to say, needs can be defined as health and disease processes, such as death, disease, and disability, as well as nonpathological conditions that require care, such as pregnancy or the monitoring of childhood growth and development. The two most important demographic determinants of health needs in a population are the absolute number of individuals and the age composition (Jones 1975). Other important determinants include changes in the prevalence rates of disease, injury, and disability, as well as changes in the demand for health services, which are influenced by rising expectations and disposable income.

From these needs, the planning process moves on to determine the health services that would be required to meet them. Finally, service production targets are used to estimate the required resources, including human and material, as well as their financial expression in a budget. The translation of health needs into their service and resource equivalents is achieved through a series of mediating factors. Thus, the satisfaction of health needs by the use of services is mediated by the quality, technological content, and equity in the distribution of those services. In turn, the amount of services that are actually produced and used is determined by the availability, accessibility, and productivity of resources. The planning process makes use of both normatively and empirically derived standards that provide the quantitative elements required to translate needs into services and into resources (Donabedian 1973; Frenk and others 1988). The retrospective approach to health planning has the undeniable advantage of establishing, from the outset, the budgetary limitations that the planner unavoidably has to face. Its major disadvantage, especially for long-term planning, is that it tends to perpetuate existing conditions. Therefore, if the purpose of planning is to anticipate the future in order to transform it, it must adopt a prospective view that begins by estimating future health needs and derives from them the resource requirements. In this respect, the theory of the epidemiologic transition provides an invaluable framework for projecting likely scenarios of health needs. Such an anticipatory exercise is the only rational way to determine health priorities for the long run.

For these reasons, the present chapter adopts a prospective approach in illustrating the nature of the health transition in Mexico. We use the most straightforward measures of health needs, namely, population size and mortality. All our calculations and projections to the year 2010 are based on age- and cause-specific mortality rates, in combination with projections of population age groups. From this point of departure, we analyze the changes that must be introduced if the health care system is to respond in an effective manner to an increasingly complex set of population needs.

Mexico: Historic Trends

Mexico has experienced a significant process of social and economic change during the last fifty years, yielding considerable improvements in the living conditions of the population

(table 3-1). This process has been causally associated with the demographic and epidemiologic transitions. These are dealt with below in terms of Mexico's social, demographic, and health care variables.

Socioeconomic Factors

From a predominantly rural and agrarian country, Mexico has moved a long way toward becoming an urban and industrial nation. Although economic growth in Mexico during this period was substantial until the early 1980s (when the financial crisis and economic stagnation began), various factors have contributed to maintain a highly unequal social and economic structure.

Among the factors which have contributed to this high degree of social and economic inequality among the Mexican population, the following are important: mountainous land, populated since ancestral times by a large number of different ethnic groups; three centuries of colonial rule during which a racially based unequal social structure was institutionalized; a model of capital-intensive industrial development during the last fifty years (which is not easily compatible with greater social equality, since it benefits the urban upper- and middle-class groups to a much greater extent than the rural population and the urban working classes); a very fast rate of population growth since the 1940s, demanding large resources for basic social and economic infrastructure (also very unequally distributed, owing to the other reasons given); political centralization and uninterrupted management for the last seventy years by the same political party.

As a result of some of these factors, territorial, economic, and social "development" has taken place in a highly concentrated manner. Industrialization and urbanization are highly concentrated and coexist with rural dispersion and extended traditional agrarian forms of production and subsistence. Distribution of income is among the most unequal in the world. Differences in living standards are vast. A few have much more than they need (the top 10 percent of the population concentrate about 40 percent of national income), whereas a large proportion of the population subsists at substandard levels in every respect, including, of course, health (López-Gallardo 1984).

Thus, Mexico has undoubtedly experienced a process of economic growth, and important changes in its economic and social structure have been taking place. The labor force working in agriculture decreased from 65 to 23 percent between 1940 and 1990 (see table 3-1); the urban population increased from 20 to 57 percent between 1940 and 1990; the literate population increased from 43 to 88 percent between 1940 and 1990; houses with running water increased from 17 percent in 1950 to 79 percent in 1990; and so forth. But great inequalities not only persist; they have become aggravated as a result of the financial and economic crisis prevailing in the 1980s. Income and wealth have become even more unequally concentrated; unemployment and underemployment are on the rise, and there are fewer public resources to mitigate poverty and extend the economic infrastructure and social services to the whole

Table 3-1. **Indicators of Social and Economic Development in Mexico: 1940–90**

Indicators	1940	1950	1960	1970	1980	1990
Labor force in agriculture (percent of economically active population)	65.4	50.2	49.4[a]	39.2	25.8	22.6
Literate (percent of population aged 15 and over)	43.2	55.9	65.5	74.1	82.7	87.6
Percent of urban population[b]	20.0	28.0	36.5	44.9	51.8	57.4
Percent of rural population[c]	70.0	56.7	48.3	40.4	33.7	28.7
Percent of houses with running water	—	17.0	23.4	61.4	70.2	79.4
Percent of houses with sewer	—	—	29.7	41.0	51.2	63.6
Percent of houses with one room	—	60.4	57.8	39.8	29.8	—
Occupants per house (average number of persons)	—	4.9	5.5	5.8	5.5	5.0
Gross domestic product per capita (in 1980 U.S. dollars)[d]	—	1,408	1,547	2,180	3,096	2,708

— Data not available.
a. Estimated from Altimir, 1974.
b. Localities with more than 15,000 inhabitants.
c. Localities with less than 2,500 inhabitants.
d. Data from Gómez-de-Léon and Frenk, 1992.
Source: Generally, 1940–80: United Nations, 1989a; 1990: México, Instituto Nacional de Estadística, Geografía, e Informática (INEGI), 1992. Exceptions indicated above.

Historic Trends in Population and Health

During most of the twentieth century Mexico was a typical example of a country with high levels of fertility and declining mortality, a situation that resulted in one of the highest rates of population growth in the world. In the decades of the 1950s, 1960s, and 1970s, the annual population growth rate for Mexico was over 3 percent. Figure 3-1 depicts the trends of the birth and mortality rates during the twentieth century.

Until 1970 the rate of population growth was one of the most important determinants of health needs. Two out of the other three primary demographic indicators relevant for health planning remained fairly constant: the age structure of the population during the period 1950 to 1980 showed a pyramidal form, with 43 to 47 percent of the inhabitants under fifteen years of age, and the absolute number of deaths was similar in 1950 to that of 1980, about 450,000. The number of births was the exception: it increased by 74 percent from 1950 to 1970 (table 3-2).

During these three decades the rate of economic growth was higher than that of the population (Wilkie 1978). Similarly, health services expanded both in scope and coverage, at a rate faster than the population.

The intervention of the Mexican state in the provision of health services was institutionalized and strengthened as early as the 1940s. A social security system and the Ministry of Health were created (Frenk, Hernández-Llamas, and Alvarez-Klein 1980). Health was seen as an essential input to economic development. The social security system, which has become the dominant scheme for the provision of medical care, is limited to those who are formally employed, especially those in the industrial and service sectors. In 1990 it covered about 55 percent of the population of Mexico.

During the postwar period in Mexico, health indicators tended to improve. Infectious diseases were displaced as the

population (Consejo Consultivo del Programa Nacional de Solidaridad, 1990).

main causes of death, and the infant mortality rate in 1991 is estimated to have declined to less than a third of its level in 1950. The increase of deaths due to noncommunicable diseases was detected before 1950, but it was not until the late 1960s that substantial increments began (table 3-2). The sharp increase of noncommunicable diseases between 1970 and 1980 is overestimated. A large proportion can be explained by the improvement in the certification of cause of death during the decade of the 1970s, and the expansion of health facilities with more accurate diagnostic technologies.

In the decades of reference, 1950 to 1980, estimates of the population size and of the numbers of births were quite sufficient to anticipate the load of morbidity, injury, and disability to be carried by the health services in any subsequent ten or fifteen years. There was less need for strategic planning, for several reasons, than at present. The rate of economic growth

Figure 3-1. **Death and Birth Rates in Mexico, 1900–2010**

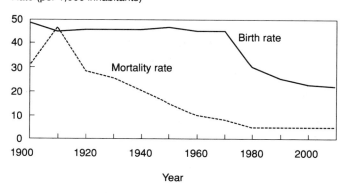

Note: Actual data 1900-80; estimates 1990-2010.
Source: 1900-1970: Alba 1971; 1980: México, INEGI 1984; 1990-2010; México, INEGI y CONAPO 1985; 1990-2010: Instituto Nacional de Estadistica 1986.

was faster than that of the population, so that maintaining at least a constant level of coverage and quality was taken for granted. Table 3-2 presents in the bottom row the growth rate in gross domestic product for three decades, showing a steep increase from the 1950s to the 1970s. In sharp contrast, the trend is reversed during the 1980s, when the same indicator yields an average of 1 per cent for the decade 1981–90. Although economic growth rates have recovered somewhat over the first two years of the 1990s, most projections anticipate lower growth rates for the period 1993–96, than those reached in the 1970s.

A significant demographic change of the 1970s was the onset of a rapid fertility decline. The total fertility rate declined from 6.7 (children per fertile age woman) in 1970 to 5.7 in 1975–76 and to 4.3 by 1981. For 1990 the total fertility rate was estimated at 3.3 children for every woman of child-bearing age. This fertility decline is expected to continue, although at a slower pace, for the foreseeable future. Figure 3-2 shows the age-specific fertility rates (per 1,000 fertile women) in three different periods between 1970 and 1986, when significant decline in fertility occurred.

The Epidemiologic Transition in Mexico

The changes in the patterns of morbidity and mortality, which are closely related to the demographic transition, constitute the main elements of the epidemiologic transition (Omran 1971). It is suggested that Mexico might be undergoing an

Figure 3-2. Age-Specific Fertility Rates in Mexico during Period of Fertility Decline

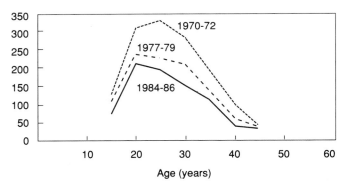

Source: Aparicio-Jiménez 1988.

epidemiologic transition under the protracted-polarized model (Frenk and others 1989b) described earlier, characterized by infectious diseases and malnutrition coexistent with noncommunicable diseases and injury.

Mortality in Mexico started to decline early in the twentieth century. At the beginning of the century, life expectancy at birth was estimated to be about twenty-five years. By 1950, life expectancy had almost doubled. For 1950, estimates of life expectancy range from 46.2 to 49.1 years for men and 49.0 to

Table 3-2. Selected Demographic, Epidemiologic, and Economic Measures for Mexico, 1950–2010

Measures	1950	1960	1970	1980	1990	2000	2010
Demographic							
Population (thousands)	27,376	37,073	51,176	69,655	81,250	103,996	123,158
Annual population growth rate (over previous ten years)	—	3.0	3.2	3.1	2.6	1.9	1.7
Age groups (percentage)							
0–14	43	46	47	44	38	31	29
15–64	54	51	50	53	57	64	65
65 and over	3	3	3	3	4	5	6
Deaths (thousands)	443	419	499	462	423	535	665
Births (thousands)	1.278	1.663	2.224	2.100	2.352	2.520	2.745
Epidemiologic: cause of death							
Infectious and parasitic diseases							
thousands	214	158	196	83	66	50	41
percentage	48.4	37.6	39.2	17.6	15.6	9.3	6.1
Cardiovascular diseases, cancer, diabetes, other selected chronic diseases, and violent deaths							
thousands	66	77	111	217	229	388	526
percentage	15.0	18.3	22.3	46.9	54.3	72.6	79.4
Economic							
GDP annual growth rate per capita (over previous ten years)	—	3.0	3.7	5.5	1.0	—	—

— Data not available.

Note: Projections for years 2000 and 2010.

Source: Demographic measures 1950–80: United Nations 1986; 1990: México, Instituto Nacional de Estadística, Geografía e Informática, 1992. Demographic projections: México, Instituto Nacional de Estadística, Geografía, e Informática y Consejo Nacional de Población 1985. Epidemiologic measures, 1950–90: México, Dirección General de Estadística, from vital statistics of the Civil Registrar for 1950, 1960, 1980, and 1990 (unpublished); 2000–2010: Expert opinion on linear trends 1950–80; 1960–80: Economic Commission for Latin America and the Caribbean 1986; 1990: World Bank 1992.

52.1 for women (Camposortega 1988). The mortality decline has continued since then, and by 1990, life expectancy was estimated at about seventy years (World Bank 1992).

According to the original theory proposed by Omran (1971), and judged solely by the time of onset and the rapid speed of the mortality decline, Mexico would fit in the accelerated model. The common denominator of the delayed model and its transitional variant (Omran 1983) is the starting point of the pronounced decline in death rates in the decade of the 1950s. Clearly the decline of mortality in Mexico started earlier, in the 1920s. For this reason Mexico does not fit the delayed model nor its transitional variant.

One of the universal characteristics of the epidemiologic transition is the shift of the age structure of mortality from the young ages to the old ages. Figure 3-3 presents the age distribution of deaths in Mexico for the period 1940–85. It is interesting that the greatest changes in the age structure of mortality occur between 1970 and 1985. Similar to what Omran (1983) described for the transitional variant of the delayed model, the reductions in infant and child mortality (birth through four years) in Mexico are substantial, but the levels slacken at relatively high rates. For the period 1981–86 the infant mortality rate was 43 deaths per 1,000 live births (Bobadilla and Langer 1990), representing about 20 percent of the total deaths (figure 3-3). It is likely that the low percentage of infant deaths in 1940 is affected by heavy underregistration. The percentage of total deaths which correspond to the elderly (over sixty years) increases from 18 percent in 1940 to almost 40 percent in 1985. The latest information on mortality shows that 50 percent of all registered deaths in 1990 occurred among the elderly.

As life expectancy at birth increases, the structure of mortality by causes of death changes (Omran 1971). The general

Figure 3-4. Deaths by Cause, According to Life Expectancy at Birth

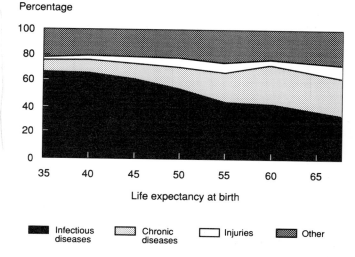

Source: México; INEGI 1986.

trend is as would be expected: as life expectancy rises, the proportion of infectious diseases declines and the proportion of noncommunicable diseases rises. Figure 3-4 depicts, at different levels of life expectancy, the relative distribution of deaths by cause of death. It is interesting that, due to the young age structure of the Mexican population, at the highest level of life expectancy shown (sixty-eight years) the proportion of infectious disease is still high (representing about 35 percent of the deaths).

Improvements in living conditions reduced the incidence rates of diarrheal and other infectious diseases. In addition, the antimalaria and the mass vaccination campaigns contributed significantly to the decline of infections. The introduction of more effective therapy reduced the fatality rates for many infectious diseases and also contributed to the decline in the death rate.

As pointed out earlier, the trends of morbidity are not considered in the original description of the epidemiologic transition. The study of morbidity is particularly important in countries where the greater survival rates have been obtained through reductions of lethality, sometimes in the absence of reductions of incidence rates. In Mexico many infectious diseases that have very low rates of mortality still present high rates of incidence or prevalence. Two groups can be distinguished according to their trends: first, the diseases preventable through vaccination—such as measles, poliomyelitis, and diphtheria—that are clearly declining; second, diseases that have been previously controlled, such as malaria, dengue fever, and cholera, but have recently shown a reemergence (Soberón and others 1988). Figure 3-5 shows the trends of the absolute number of newly diagnosed malaria cases in Mexico for the period 1942–87. In the early 1940s there were more than 140,000 cases per year. This figure declined to less thus 5,000 in the early 1960s, but then started to increase, so that by 1985

Figure 3-3. Deaths in Mexico by Age, 1940–85

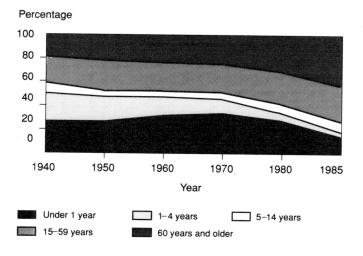

Source: México: Secretaría de Salud 1987.

Figure 3-5. Incidence of Malaria in Mexico, 1942–88

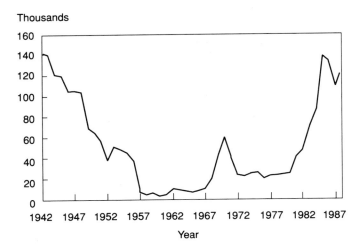

Source: México: Dirección General de Epidemiología 1989.

there were more than 130,000 cases. This is a typical example of the process called countertransition mentioned earlier.

The overlap of eras is closely related to the pace of the epidemiologic transition among different social groups. The universal social inequalities in health have been usually described in quantitative terms, because the burden of disease and death is greater among the poor. The mortality decline starts among the higher social classes, and eventually the lower classes catch up and close the gap. This is described as a general pattern of transition (Omran 1983) and is probably applicable to all countries regardless of the model of epidemiologic transition they pass through. Under the protracted model, however, the lower social classes show very small improvements, which raises questions about the time required to catch up with the upper classes. Thus the period of polarization seen in other models probably takes longer in the protracted model. Table 3-3 shows the gap between the infant mortality rate in the poorest states of Mexico, those of the southern region, and that of the wealthier states in the northern region of the Mexican territory. It is shown that the excess of mortality in the poorer

states rises from 1.6 to 3.3, as compared with the wealthier states.

The different patterns of epidemiologic change within the country provide further evidence of the epidemiologic polarization in Mexico. In table 3-4 we compare the cause-specific death rates for diarrheal diseases and acute respiratory infections with those for cardiovascular diseases and cancer. The death rate for diarrheal diseases and acute respiratory infections was 1.6 times higher in the southern region in 1940, whereas in 1985 it was almost four times higher in the southern region than in the northern. Both regions show an impressive absolute decline, but the greatest occurred in the northern region, where the corresponding death rate was reduced by 94 percent from 554 (deaths per 100,000 population) in 1940 to 31 in 1985. In the southern region the rate was reduced by 86 percent during the same period, from 878 to 122.

The trend of the death rates due to the selected chronic diseases shows very little change for the northern region, with an increase of 25 percent, whereas in the southern region the increase was about 85 percent. This discrepancy in the rate of increase of chronic diseases leads to a convergence of the corresponding rates in both regions (table 3-4). It can be concluded from table 3-4 that the inhabitants of the northern region have been able to control infectious disease and probably have entered into the third era of the epidemiologic transition. They have not, however, had the expected increase of cardiovascular diseases and cancer. The death rate for cardiovascular diseases in the United States in 1986 was 3.5 times as high as that in the northern region of Mexico.

The final outcome of this process of regional polarization is summarized in the last three rows of table 3-4. The ratio of the selected infectious to chronic diseases changes from 6.1 to 0.3 in the northern region, with the crossover occurring in the 1970s. In contrast, in the southern region the change is from 19.8 to 1.5, with no crossover by 1985. The difference in the ratios between the two regions increased from 3.2 to 5.0 in the period 1940–85.

Future Demographic, Epidemiologic, and Social Changes

In the next twenty years, many middle-income countries will continue to show substantial improvements in child health

Table 3-3. Infant Mortality Rate (IMR) in Southern and Northern Regions of Mexico, 1962–86

| Period | Southern region[a] | | Northern region[b] | | Southern/northern |
	Infant deaths	IMR [c]	Infant deaths	IMR [c]	
1962–66	39	147	26	92	1.60
1967–71	46	93	55	73	1.28
1972–76	73	112	74	69	1.62
1977–81	71	92	51	45	2.02
1982–86	66	92	32	28	3.26

a. Includes Tabasco, Yucatán, Campeche, Quintana Roo, Oaxaca, Chiapas, Puebla, and Tlaxcala.
b. Includes Baja California, Baja California Sur, Sonora, Sinaloa, Nayarit, Nuevo León, and Tamaulipas.
c. IMR (Infant mortality rate) refers to deaths of children under one year of age per 1,000 live births.
Source: México, Dirección General de Planificación Familiar 1989.

Table 3-4. Cause-Specific Death Rates for Selected Infectious and Chronic Diseases in Southern and Northern Regions of Mexico, 1940–85
(per 100,000 inhabitants)

Cause of death	Region[a]	1940	1950	1960	1970	1980	1985
Diarrhea and acute respiratory infections	Southern	878	507	403	403	178	122
	Northern	554	323	227	196	66	31
	Southern/northern	1.58	1.57	1.77	2.06	2.70	3.94
Cardiovascular diseases and cancer	Southern	44	57	56	54	64	81
	Northern	91	121	110	110	112	114
	Southern/northern	0.48	0.47	0.51	0.49	0.57	0.71
Ratio (infectious/chronic)	Southern	19.8	8.8	7.2	7.5	2.8	1.5
	Northern	6.1	2.7	2.0	1.8	0.6	0.3
	Southern/northern	3.2	3.3	3.6	4.2	4.7	5.0

a. Southern region includes Tabasco, Yucatán, Campeche, Quintana Roo, Oaxaca, Chiapas, Puebla, and Tlaxcala. Northern region includes Baja California, Baja California Sur, Sonora, Sinaloa, Nayarit, Nuevo León, and Tamaulipas.
Source: 1940: México, Secretaría de Salubridad y Asistencia 1946; 1950, 1960: México, Instituto Nacional de Estadística 1980; 1970, 1980, 1985: México, Dirección General de Estadística 1973, 1984, 1988.

and life expectancy. Most of them will also witness, paradoxically, a greater burden of disease. In this section we examine the projected trends of the main determining factor of health needs and demand for health care in Mexico.

Population Projections and Future Health Needs

In the early 1980s the Mexican government (Mexico, INEGI/CONAPO, 1985) anticipated that fertility would continue to decline rather rapidly, at least through the 1980s, and probably also into the 1990s. On the basis of this assumption, a "programmatic" projection aiming for replacement-level fertility by 2010 was calculated. The actual fertility reduction of the 1980s, however, was somewhat slower, corresponding more closely to the "alternative" projection of remaining at 28 percent above replacement fertility in 2010, the projection used in this chapter. According to this projection, the annual absolute additions of population will increase, although the population growth rate will decrease from 3.1 percent in the 1970s to 1.7 percent in the period 2000–10.

The transition from high to low fertility is leading to significant changes in the age structure. The percentage of children under fifteen will decline from 44 in 1980 to 29 in 2010, whereas the absolute number will more than only increase from 30 million to 35 million. The group of adults age fifteen through sixty-four will increase from 53 to 65 percent of the population, whereas the absolute number will rise from 37 million to 80 million, more than a twofold increase. The percentage of the population age sixty-five and above will double, from 3 to 6 percent, between 1980 and 2010, and the absolute number will more than triple from 2.3 million in 1980 to 7.1 million in 2010 (table 3-2).

The aging process will entail an increase in the number of deaths, larger than any other increase in this century. By the year 2010 the total number of deaths will be 665,000, about 44 percent more than in 1980.

Despite the continuous decline in the total fertility rate, the total number of births will not decrease. The slight downward trend of the 1970s will be reversed and, according to this projection, an increase of 31 percent is expected between 1980 and 2010 (table 3-2).

Projections of the Mortality Structure by Cause of Death

In order to estimate the effect of the aging of the population on the relative contribution of the different causes of death, the 1980 age-specific death rates for eleven groups of causes of death were applied to all the age groups projected for 2010, according to the alternative projection. The results are presented in the second column of table 3-5, which shows the distribution (per thousand) of the selected causes of death. Deaths due to malignant tumors would rise from 67 to 81 per thousand. An increase can be seen in the proportion of deaths due to heart and circulatory diseases, which would rise from 169 to 204 per thousand, a 21 percent increase. The total number of deaths due to these causes would increase from 74,000 in 1980 to 136,000 in 2010, an 84 percent increase. It is interesting to note that even though the proportion of deaths caused by diarrheal diseases and acute respiratory infections would decline from 169 per thousand in 1980 to 130 in 2010, the absolute number of deaths for these two groups would increase from about 78,000 to 86,000. Planning for health services in the next thirty years cannot be done without reliable estimates of future trends in incidence rates and possible changes in fatality rates of the main diseases and injury. Projections of the future incidence rates of diseases, accidents, and violence will probably follow trends of the past twenty-five years or so. Infectious diseases will continue to decline to a certain floor, and noncommunicable diseases will continue to increase, although the pace might be less pronounced. Saturation or competition among causes will modify the increase. The same can be said for deaths due to accidents and violence.

Table 3-5. Deaths in Mexico by Main Causes, 1980 and Projections for 2010

(per thousand)

Cause of death	ICD-9 codes	1980	2010 Using 1980 age-specific mortality rates	Projecting linear trend from 1965, 1970, 1981	Linear trends corrected by experts' opinions
Malignant tumors	140–165, 170–175, 179–208, 230–234	67	81	89	78
Accidents and violence	E800–E848, E850–E869, E880–E888, E890–E999	161	156	287	272
Heart and circulatory diseases	390–398, 401–405, 410–438, 440–459	169	204	409	332
Chronic bronchitis and other chronic respiratory diseases	466–490, 493	32	32	6	21
Acute respiratory infections	460–465, 470–478, 480–487	82	66	0	33
Diarrheal diseases	001–009, 120–129	87	64	5	24
Cirrhosis and other liver diseases	571	35	41	52	44
Other child infections	032–037, 045–055, 138	6	5	0	1
Diabetes	250	37	48	98	80
Perinatal problems	760–779	56	32	20	16
All other causes		268	271	34	99
Total		1,000	1,000	1,000	1,000

Source: 1980: México, Secretaría de Programación y Presupuesto y Secretaría de Salubridad y Asistencia 1984; 2010: Authors' calculations.

Two different procedures were applied in estimating the relative contribution of the eleven groups of causes of death for the year 2010. First, the distribution of deaths was estimated by applying the age-specific incidence rates that would result if past trends were to continue linearly. Three points in time were used to estimate the slope and intercept of the linear trend (age- and cause-specific death rates for the years 1965, 1970, and 1981). The results, shown in the third column of table 3-5, are not plausible, as can be concluded, for example, from the virtual disappearance of deaths due to diarrheal diseases and acute respiratory infections. For this reason, we followed a second procedure. The opinions of seven epidemiologists on the future trends (previously described) of each cause of death for all age groups were used to estimate more plausible figures. The aggregated results are presented in the fourth column of table 3-5. The effect of having introduced experts' opinions is the moderation of the linear trends and the modification of straight lines into curves. The contribution of deaths due to diarrhea and acute respiratory infections is quite plausible. The same can be said for the corresponding data on accidents and violence. Deaths due to heart and cardiovascular diseases more than double their contribution, rising from 169 to 352 per 1,000 deaths. This is most likely an overestimation.

Even though the methodology to estimate the future number of deaths by specific causes could be more sophisticated and yield more plausible results, the three alternative projections shown in table 3-5 provide a guide for strategic planning. The calculations obtained using static 1980 rates give an idea of the minimum number of expected deaths in the three main causes of death (malignant tumors, heart and circulatory diseases, accidents and violence). By contrast, the results obtained by applying the regression coefficients of the linear trend provide estimates of the maximum expected contribution for the same

causes of death. In other words, the first three causes of death will be responsible for 44 to 79 percent of all deaths in the year 2010. In any case, the point is made that the Mexican population in the twenty-first century will be dying from causes, most of which are preventable, that affect mainly adults and the elderly. The complexity and the costs of preventing, controlling, and treating many of the main diseases of the period 2000 to 2010 will be considerably larger than those prevailing at present. The implications of this situation for the health system will be discussed later.

Future Social Change and the Demand for Health Care

Up to this point plausible demographic and epidemiologic changes have been assumed in the estimates of health needs in the year 2010. Other economic and social changes, however, are taking place in Mexican society that will affect future health needs and that should be taken into account in health planning. In this section we briefly mention some of the trends in the areas of urbanization, education, employment, and social inequality and will speculate about their possible effects on future health needs and demands.

URBANIZATION. According to existing projections (Nuñez and Moreno 1986), by the year 2000 approximately 76 percent of the Mexican population will live in communities with 2,500 or more inhabitants. A significant part of urban growth will take place in middle-size cities (50,000 to 500,000 inhabitants), although the large metropolitan areas will also continue to grow significantly. At the same time, tens of thousands of rural localities will persist. A continued process of urbanization in a context of greater poverty will have repercussions on the incidence of diseases and disabilities related to these conditions, most notably injuries, mental disorders, alcoholism, and probably drug abuse.

EMPLOYMENT. According to estimates and projections made by Trejo (1988), it will be very difficult to create formal employment in the quantity and at the pace that will be required during the next years. As was shown before, the working-age population (fifteen through sixty-four years) will grow significantly faster than the total population during the rest of the century. The annual growth rate of this population has been estimated at 3.5 percent in 1985–90, 2.7 percent in 1990–95, and 2.3 percent in 1995–2000. An average of one million jobs would have to be created yearly during the next twelve years in order to satisfy the requirements of the new population entering the labor market. The rates of economic growth required to yield so many jobs, about 6 percent annually, seem to be difficult to attain in this period. Unemployment and informal employment are likely to increase, leading to a rapid growth of population not entitled to social security. In addition, women will continue to enter the labor market at a faster rate than the general population, imposing additional pressure on the demand for jobs.

The incorporation of large numbers of people into the informal labor market will generate a much greater demand on the health subsystem for the noninsured population (that is, services provided by the Ministry of Health, other public assistance institutions, and to some extent private institutions). This, in turn, could lead to more extreme health inequities between the poor and those with formal jobs, who are entitled to social security. The increasing participation of women in the labor market could have repercussions on their health and especially on the health of their children, given the scarcity of institutionalized child care. Studies undertaken in the fast-growing assembly plants along the Mexican border with the United States are showing that children born to working women in these industries tend to have lower birth weight than those of comparable women. Also, the demand for nurseries might increase considerably.

EDUCATION. If the trend in formal education that took place in the 1970s continues, it might be expected that by the end of the century almost the whole adult population will know how to read and write, and the vast majority will have finished primary school. The average number of years of education grew from 3.5 to 5.5 years between 1970 and 1980 and to 6.2 in 1990. The average might increase to more than 9 years by the year 2010. The improvement of education and heightened exposure to mass media is likely to increase the demand for health services and for a better quality of services. It can also lead to a greater participation of the population in taking care of its own health.

SOCIAL INEQUALITY. Mexico presents one of the highest levels of wealth concentration (Hernández-Laos 1984). The degree of social mobility (access of growing sectors of the population to better jobs, salaries, and living conditions), which was a permanent characteristic of Mexican society up

to the mid-1970s, will probably continue to diminish, as it did in the 1980s. As a result, it is possible to predict a greater polarization of Mexican society. The size of the middle class will be reduced, and the lower classes might again encompass 60 percent or more of the total population.

Implications for the Health Care System

From the foregoing analysis it is possible to conclude that early in the twenty-first century health needs will be governed in Mexico by an increase in the number of people who suffer from noncommunicable diseases, only moderate reductions in the absolute number of infectious diseases, and an increase in the number of births. Increasing amount and complexity in the health needs will have profound implications for the organization and delivery of health services.

Allocation of Resources for Competing Health Needs

So far, estimates of health needs have been derived only from basic information on mortality. The relation between mortality and causes of death, on the one hand, and morbidity and causes for medical care demand, on the other, is far from being straightforward. This is particularly true for countries that are in the midst of the epidemiologic transition. The discrepancy between mortality and morbidity indicators is particularly relevant for the estimation of health needs that are met through hospitalization. Often the causes for hospital admission are not represented in the main causes of death. About 65 percent of the budget for health care goes for hospital-related expenses. Thus, it is important to introduce a series of considerations into the estimates of health needs derived from mortality data.

First is the estimate of hospital use due to needs derived from reproduction and its regulation. According to hospital records, at least 40 percent of the persons hospitalized in Mexico in 1986 were women who were delivering children, either normal or with complications. This number excludes other related causes of hospital admission such as female surgical sterilization and neonatal admissions, which together might account for 3 to 6 percent of the total number of persons admitted to hospitals (Mexico, Instituto Mexicano del Seguro Social 1986).

Second is the fact that at the present time the provision of hospital services is insufficient to meet the needs of the population. Planning for future services should take into account resources required to close the gap between supply and needs. It is almost impossible to estimate the health needs to be met through hospital services using data from current information systems. The magnitude of unmet need is often a matter of speculation and debate. It is, however, possible to estimate the resource equivalents that would be required to meet the health needs derived from births, given the prevailing health care model. According to the 1987 National Health Survey (Mexico, Dirección General de Epidemiología 1988), about 30 percent of the births were not attended by a health professional, which in the Mexican context means an unmet need of about that magnitude. Considering that the absolute number of births will increase about 30 percent from 1980 to 2010, and that 30 percent of the present deliveries are not being cared for properly, the real increase in the requirement of beds for birth care is about 85 percent (in relation to the total available). The required budget to build the hospital beds to deliver annually more than a million additional babies in the first ten years of the next century is formidable.

Third, the coexistence of noncommunicable diseases and problems related to reproduction will most likely pose a dilemma in the allocation of beds, which might not be resolved rationally. This problem can be portrayed as a competition between patients: on the one hand, pregnant or delivering women, a large proportion of whom will come from the deprived socioeconomic groups and the rural areas; on the other hand, adult and elderly patients suffering from cardiovascular disorders, cancer, diabetes, and disabilities due to accidents. There is evidence that infectious diseases and problems linked to reproduction are more prevalent in the rural areas and among the least privileged socioeconomic groups. Past experience with the decisionmaking process suggests that the outcome in the allocation of resources between the two groups will be biased toward the needs of the wealthier. Reproductive and infectious problems might become neglected health needs in the period 2000–10 if the health care model and the decisionmaking process continue as now.

Changing Priorities in the Delivery of Health Services

Probably the top priority of countries like Mexico, which are undergoing a protracted-polarized transition, is to avoid the pernicious competition among types of pathology. Yet, important segments of the health planning community—both at the national and the international levels—have themselves become polarized in two bands: those who claim that the first order of business is to bring common infections and undernutrition under control, and those who see in the rising prevalence of chronic ailments and injuries the need for a shift in priorities. Still, the complex reality of many countries means that there is no alternative but to address the pretransitional and the posttransitional problems simultaneously. Basic notions of equity demand that the gap between knowledge and action be closed for all population groups, so that the "left-over ills" (Frenk and others 1989a) represented by common infections and malnutrition cease to affect the least privileged segments of society. Eliminating the epidemiologic polarization occupies, therefore, a top place in the list of priorities.

Furthermore, there are close links between the two groups of pathology. For instance, the most common reason for heart surgery in Mexico continues to be valve replacement to repair damage produced by rheumatic heart disease—a pretransitional condition. If the relatively inexpensive preventive measures against rheumatic fever were implemented, specialized resources could be freed for the treatment of other heart conditions for which prevention is not so effective. Similarly, a large proportion of resources in the complex fields of neurology and neurosurgery continue to be used to correct prevent-

able conditions, such as epilepsy due to birth trauma and brain cysticercosis. Addressing pretransitional pathology would reinforce the care of posttransitional diseases.

Recognizing the need to control the common infectious and reproductive problems should not lead to the conclusion that chronic diseases and injuries will have to wait their turn. Such a conclusion would most likely transform the posttransitional conditions from emerging to epidemic. To avoid this future scenario, the control of chronic diseases, especially cancer and ischemic heart disease, will require an emphasis and reliance on primary prevention programs, such as those aimed at reducing the number of individuals exposed to the risk factors or the causal agents of disease. Even wealthy countries with large investments in health care have to turn to primary prevention, as the costs of treatment and rehabilitation rapidly increase (Litvak and others 1987). Thus far, Mexico, as many other middle-income countries, has given a very low priority to such programs. The only way to reduce the demand for hospital and other specialized medical services by the year 2010 will be to implement vigorous campaigns in order to reduce the consumption of tobacco, alcohol, animal fats, sugar, and salt. The role of legislation and sanitary regulation as instruments to control the exposure to many noxious agents has not been fully exploited.

Reshaping the Health Care Model

The limitations of the health care model based on curative services in hospital settings have been clearly demonstrated in most industrial countries. No single country has been able to cope adequately with the rising costs of medical care. The health needs of the Mexican population in the foreseeable future suggest that its imported health care model could be exhausted soon. Aiming at delivering all births in hospitals is not only financially impossible but also medically unnecessary. In a similar way, performing all surgical operations in hospitals results in undue costs. The social needs of hospitalized patients will have to be met through means other than keeping them in hospitals. Many of these changes are being successfully implemented in developing countries, including Mexico, through demonstration projects. Still, changing entrenched practice patterns may take many years. Until now the health needs of the Mexican population have been growing faster than the ability to react and adapt to the new conditions. The transfer of care of some health problems from hospitals to health centers and to the homes of the affected would require a strong component of community participation. Of paramount importance is the strengthening of family and social networks to maintain the support for the disabled and the chronically ill.

Restructuring the health care model will undoubtedly require innovations. The social response to the complex health needs of the twenty-first century will have to be based on scientifically validated information. Research to design alternative modes of effectively meeting the needs of the population must be one of the key strategies of any health care system that aspires to shape the future.

Notes

We would like to acknowledge the valuable comments given to an earlier version of this chapter by Dean Jamison, Henry Mosley, Joseph Decosas, and Stephen Simons.

References

Alba, Francisco. 1971. *La Población de México: Evolución y Dilemas*. México, D. F.: El Colegio de México.

Altimir, Oscar. 1974. La medición de la población economicamente activa de México, 1950–1970. *Demografía y Economía* 8:50–83.

Aparicio-Jimenez, Ricardo. 1988. Niveles, tendencias e impacto demográfico de la anticoncepción. En: Dirección General de Planificación Familiar. *Memoria de la Reunion Sobre Avances y Perspectivas de la Investigación Social en Planificación Familiar en México*. México, D. F.: Secretaría de Salud.

Bobadilla, José Luis, and Ana Langer. 1990. "La mortalidad infantil en México: Un fenómeno en transición." *Revista Mexicana de Sociología* 1:111–32.

Camposortega, Sergio. 1988. "El nivel y la estructura de la mortalidad en México, 1940–1980." In Mario Bronfman and José Gómez de Léon, eds., *La mortalidad en México: Niveles, tendencias y determinantes*. México, D. F.: El Colegio de México.

Consejo Consultivo del Programa Nacional de Solidaridad. 1990. *El Combate a la Pobreza*. México, D. F.: El Nacional.

Donabedian, Avedis. 1973. *Aspects of Medical Care Administration*, Cambridge, Mass.: Harvard University Press.

Economic Commission for Latin America and the Caribbean. 1986. *Statistical Yearbook for Latin America and the Caribbean*. New York: United Nations.

Frenk, Julio, José Luis Bobadilla, Jaime Sepúlveda, and Malaquias López-Cervantes. 1989a. "Health Transition in Middle-Income Countries: New Challenges for Health Care." *Health Policy and Planning* 4:29–39.

Frenk, Julio, José Luis Bobadilla, Jaime Sepúlveda, Jorge Rosenthal, and Enrique Ruelas. 1988b. "A Conceptual Model for Public Health Research." PAHO *Bulletin* 22:60–71.

Frenk, Julio, Tomas Frejka, José Luis Bobadilla, Claudio Stern, Jaime Sepúlveda, and Marco José. 1989. "The Epidemiological Transition in Latin América." In IUSSP (International Union for the Scientific Study of Population), *International Population Conference*, New Delhi. Liège 1989.

Frenk, Julio, Hector Hernández-Llamas, and Lourdes Alvarez-Klein. 1980. "El mercado de trabajo médico: II. Evolución histórica en México." *Gaceta Médica de México* 116:20–21 and 57–60.

Gómez-de-Léon, José, Julio Frenk, 1992. *Population and Health Challenges in Mexico on the Eve of the 21st Century*. Unpublished.

Hernández-Laos, Enrique. 1984. "La desigualdad regional en México (1900–1980)." In Rolando Cordera and Carlos Tello, eds., *La desigualdad en México*. México, D.F.: Siglo Veintiuno.

Jones, G. W. 1975. "Population Growth and Health and Family Planning." In W. C. Robinson, ed., *Population and Development Planning*. New York: Population Council.

Litvak, Jorge, L. Ruiz, Helena E. Restrepo, and Alison McAlister. 1987. "El problema creciente de las enfermedades no transmisibles, un desafío para los países de las Américas." *Boletín de la Oficina Sanitaria Panamericana* 103:433–449.

López-Gallardo, Juan 1984. "La distribución del ingreso en México: Estructura y evolución." In R. Cordera and C. Tello, eds., *La desigualdad en México*. México, D.F.: Siglo Veintiuno.

México, Dirección General de Estadística. 1973. "Computer Data on Deaths for 1970." México, D. F.: Instituto Nacional de Estadística, Geografía e Informática.

———. 1984. "Computer Data on Deaths for 1980." México, D. F.: Instituto Nacional de Estadística, Geografía e Informática.

———. 1988. "Computer Data on Deaths for 1985." México, D. F.: Instituto Nacional de Estadística, Geografía e Informática.

México, Dirección General de Epidemiología. 1988. *Encuesta Nacional de Salud: Resultados nacionales*. México, D. F.: Secretaría de Salud.

———. 1989. *Paludismo y otras enfermedades transmitidas por vector*. México, D. F.: Secretaría de Salud.

México, Dirección General de Planificación Familiar. 1989. *Encuesta Nacional de Fecundidad y Salud 1987*. Computer tapes. México, D. F.

México, Instituto Mexicano del Seguro Social. 1986. "Computer data on hospital discharges by cause and age groups." México, D. F.

México, INEGI (Instituto Nacional de Estadística, Geografía e Informática). 1980. *Incidencia de la mortalidad en los Estados Unidos Mexicanos*. México, D. F.: Secretaría de Programación y Presupuesto.

———. 1984. *Agenda Estadística*. México, D. F.: Secretaría de Programación y Presupuesto.

———. 1986. *Estadisticas Históricas de México*. México, D. F.: Secretaría de Programación y Presupuesto.

———. 1992. *Perfil Sociodemografico. XI Censo General de Población y Vivienda*. México, D. F.: INEGI.

México, INEGI y CONAPO (Instituto Nacional de Estadística, Geografía e Informática y Consejo Nacional de Población). 1985. *Proyecciones de la población de México y de las Entidades Federatives: 1980–2010*. México, D. F.: Secretaría de Programación y Presupuesto.

México, Secretaría de Programación y Presupuesto y Secretaría de Salubridad y Asistencia. 1984. *Boletín de Información Estadística No. 1*. México, D. F.

México, Secretaría de Salubridad y Asistencia. 1946. *Anuario Estadística de Salubridad y Asistencia*. México, D. F.: Secretaría de Salubridad y Asistencia.

México, Secretaría de Salud. 1987. *Anuario Estadístico 1987*. México, D. F.: Secretaría de Salud.

Nuñez, Leopoldo, and Lorenzo Moreno. 1986. *Proyecciones de la población urbana y rural, 1980–2010*. México, D. F.: Asociación Mexicana de Demografía Médica.

Omran, Abdel. 1971. "The Epidemiologic Transition: A Theory of the Epidemiology of Population Change." *Milbank Memorial Fund Quarterly* 49:509–38.

Omran A. R. 1983. "The Epidemiologic Transition Theory: A Preliminary Update." *Journal of Tropical Pediatrics* 29:305–16.

Soberón, Guillermo, Jesus Kumate, and José Laguna. 1988. *La salud en México: Testimonio* Vol. 1, *Problemas y programas de salud*. México, D. F.: Fondo de Cultura Económica.

Trejo, Saúl. 1988. *Empleo para todos: El reto y los caminos*. México, D. F.: Fondo de Cultura Económica.

United Nations. 1986. *World Population Prospects*. Population Studies No. 98. New York: United Nations.

———. 1989a. *Case Study in Population Policy: Mexico*. New York.

———. 1989b. *World Population Prospects, 1988*. New York.

Wildavsky, Aaron. 1977. "Doing Better and Feeling Worse: The Political Pathology of Health Policy." In *Doing Better and Feeling Worse: Health in the United States*. Proceedings of the American Academy of Arts and Sciences, 106, no. 1. Boston, Mass.

Wilkie, James W. 1978. *La Revolución Mexicana: Gasto federal y cambio social*. México, D. F.: Fondo de Cultura Económica.

World Bank. 1992. *World Development Report 1992: Development and the Environment*. Washington, D.C.

PART TWO

The Unfinished Agenda, I
Infectious Disease

Acute Respiratory Infection
Diarrheal Diseases
Poliomyelitis
Helminth Infection
Measles
Tetanus
Rheumatic Heart Disease
Tuberculosis
Leprosy
Malaria
Dengue
Hepatitis B

4

Acute Respiratory Infection

Sally K. Stansfield and Donald S. Shepard

Acute respiratory infection (ARI) is the most frequent illness globally and a leading cause of death in the developing world. Among children under five alone, four million deaths annually are ascribed to ARI, most of which are due to pneumonia. That mortality due to pneumonia is ten to fifty times higher in developing countries suggests that there is ample room for improvement in addressing this important public health problem. The heterogeneity of the clinical presentations and causative organisms in ARI, however, has hampered efforts to design simple and effective interventions.

The classification and management of ARI in the industrialized world are founded on epidemiologic, radiologic, and microbiologic data, in addition to clinical history and physical examination. The syndromes of ARI, which are complex clinical conditions of varying etiology and severity, are most frequently categorized on the basis of anatomical location.

Common diagnostic categories for uncomplicated ARI with etiologic and clinical correlates are detailed in table 4-1. As suggested by this table, ARI includes the minor upper respiratory infections (URIS), such as colds and sore throats, in addition to the more serious (and potentially fatal) acute lower respiratory infections (ALRIs) of pneumonia and bronchiolitis.

Most of the studies of ARI from developing countries have been conducted among infants and children. Programs which have been developed to prevent or treat ARI have often focused exclusively on children, on the argument that the principal opportunities to reduce ARI mortality are among children under five. Although adults, particularly the elderly, may benefit from preventive and therapeutic interventions, the most significant reduction in years of life lost will be seen among infants and children. The data and strategies outlined in this chapter therefore focus primarily on children under five.

Table 4-1. *Clinical Summary of Acute Respiratory Infections in Infants and Young Children*

Type	Diagnosis	Most common etiology	Age at peak incidence (months)	Mortality
Upper respiratory infections	Nasopharyngitis (coryza, colds)	Viral (various)	—	No
	Otitis media (middle ear infection)	Bacterial (pneumococcus, *Hemophilus influenzae*)	6–7	No
	Pharyngo-tonsillitis	Viral (various) and bacterial (*Streptococcus pyogenes, Corynebacterium diphtheriae*)	—	No (except diphtheria)
	Epiglottitis	Bacterial (*Hemophilus influenzae*)	24–47	Yes
Lower respiratory infections	Laryngitis (croup)	Viral (especially parainfluenza and measles)	12–23	Rare
	Tracheobronchitis	Viral and bacterial (various)	Constant	No
	Bronchiolitis	Viral (RSV, parainfluenza 3)	0–11	Yes
	Pneumonia	Bacterial (pneumococcus, *Hemophilus influenzae*) and viral (RSV, influenza, parainfluenza, measles, adenovirus)	24–35	Yes

— Not available.
Source: Authors' data.

Risk Factors for ARI

Treatment of pneumonia clearly reduces ARI mortality, but the definitive solution to the problem of high numbers of ARI deaths in developing countries will ultimately be found in prevention of pneumonia. Although the epidemiologic data from the developing world are limited, a review of the available information suggests possible ways to reduce ARI mortality through reducing the risk of pneumonia. Table 4-2 summarizes the following discussion of some of the known and suspected risks for pneumonia incidence and mortality.

Age and Sex

The incidence of ARI (most of which is URI) is inversely related to age, peaking at four to nine infections in each of the first two years of life, dropping to three to four by school age, and remaining at two to three per year for adults (Datta Banik, Krishna, and Mane 1969; Kamath and others 1969; Monto and Ullman 1974; Friej and Wall 1977; Spika and others 1989). The frequency of pneumonia and the case-fatality ratio, however, are highest among both the very young and the very old (Bulla 1978; Berman and others 1983; Ngalikpima 1983). Studies in several developing countries have demonstrated that pneumonia occurred 1.5 to 1.8 times as frequently among infants as among children two to fours years of age (Berman and McIntosh 1985). There is a slightly increased incidence of both overall ARI and pneumonia among male children (Bulla 1978; Berman and others 1983; Narain and Sharma 1987; Selwyn 1990), although female children have been observed to have a higher case-fatality ratio in some countries, probably as a result of poorer access and quality of care during illness episodes (Tupasi and others 1990).

Socioeconomic Status and Child-Rearing Practice

Low socioeconomic status and crowding have been well documented as risk factors for mild respiratory infections in the industrialized world. Studies in developing countries (Verma and Menon 1981; Stansfield 1987; Tupasi and others 1988; Borrero and others 1990; Vathanophas and others 1990) have also demonstrated an increased frequency of pneumonia re-

quiring hospitalization among persons from lower socioeconomic groups and in more crowded households. Aaby (1988) has suggested that crowding is a predictor of an increased case-fatality ratio due to measles, in addition to an increased risk of infection.

Both poverty and crowding may, however, be proximate measures for other known or as yet unrecognized risk factors. For example, the frequent association of these factors with lower educational levels, poor nutrition, and certain child-care practices further confounds analysis of risks for pneumonia. Existing evidence suggests, however, that infants with restricted respiratory excursion of the chest wall due to obesity (Tracey, De, and Harper 1971) or swaddling (Yurdakok, Yavuz, and Taylor 1990) may have increased risk of pneumonia. Family stress also increases the risk of infections such as pneumonia among both children and adults (Foulke and others 1988; Graham and others 1990; Cohen, Tyrell and Smith 1991), probably because of interference with immune competence (Kiecolt-Glaser and Glaser 1986). Although chilling is frequently cited as a risk factor for URI or pneumonia, most studies have provided no evidence of this association (Jackson and others 1963; Douglas, Lindgram, and Cough 1968).

Nutritional Status and Practices

Poor nutrition lowers both systemic and local defenses against ARI, including reduction of the effectiveness of epithelial barriers, systemic immune responses, and cough reflexes. Nutritional status is inversely related to both the incidence and the case-fatality ratio for pneumonia (Kielmann and McCord 1978; Pio, Leowski, and Luelmo 1982; Berman 1983; Sommer 1983; Sommer, Katz, and Tarwotjo 1984; Berman and others 1991). Investigators have documented an incidence of pneumonia twelve to twenty times greater in undernourished children than in children of normal weight-for-age (James 1971; Berman and others 1983; Tupasi and others 1988). Mortality due to each of these already more frequent episodes of pneumonia increases two- to thirteenfold for each decile below 80 percent weight-for-age (Escobar, Dover, and Duenas 1976; Kielmann and McCord 1978; Tupasi 1985).

While nutritional deficiency diseases augment the chances of ARI episodes, so episodes of ARI contribute to nutritional

Table 4-2. Risk Factors for Pneumonia

Increased incidence	Increased case fatality
Age less than two years or more than sixty-five	Age less than two years or more than sixty-five
Male	Low socioeconomic status
Poor nutritional status	Poor nutritional status
Low birth weight	Low birth weight
Lack of breastfeeding (in infants)	Lack of breastfeeding (in infants)
Smoking, air pollution	Lack of maternal education
Crowding	Reduced access to health care
Incomplete immunization	Crowding
Swaddling	Underlying chronic disease
Vitamin A deficiency	

Source: Authors' data.

deficiency, thus further increasing the risk of subsequent infection and death. A prospective study in the Gambia (Rowland, Rowland, and Cole 1988) showed that pneumonia reduced weight gain in young children by 14.7 grams for each day of infection. Recurrent ARI episodes, as a principal cause of the weight shortfall during infancy, therefore progressively increase the risk of death due to other childhood diseases.

Low birth weight, seen in 20–40 percent of infants in many developing countries, also increases the risk and case-fatality ratio of pneumonia. Studies (Datta 1987; WHO 1988) have shown relative risks of mortality due to pneumonia which are 2.5- to 8-fold greater among infants of low birth weight. Other than malaria and tobacco chewing, the only factors associated with low birth weight for which cause-and-effect relationships have been established in developing countries (and which are modifiable over the short term) are low prepregnancy weight, low gestational weight gain, and low caloric intake (WHO/EPI 1987). Short birth intervals, teenage pregnancy, certain genital infections, and arduous work after mid-pregnancy are other potentially modifiable factors associated with low birth weight. Although reduction of the incidence of low birth weight would be expected to reduce ARI mortality, no prospective studies have demonstrated the feasibility and effectiveness of interventions to address this important problem.

The few well-conducted studies on infant feeding practices and the incidence of pneumonia demonstrate a protective effect of breastfeeding. The literature has suffered from wide variations in definitions, both of specific feeding practice and of ARI. Although several studies summarized in a review by Jason and others (1984) failed to document any protective effect of breastfeeding, others have found a two- to fivefold decreased incidence of pneumonia (Chandra 1979; Singhi and Singhi 1987) and decreased case-fatality ratio due to pneumonia (LePage, Munyakazi, and Hennart 1981). A more rigorous study in southern Brazil (Victors and others 1987) demonstrated that infants who were completely weaned had a risk of death due to pneumonia 3.6 times higher than breastfed infants.

Vitamin A deficiency, which often accompanies protein-calorie malnutrition, results in keratinization of the respiratory epithelium and depression of the immune response, thus presumably decreasing both local and systemic resistance to bacterial colonization and infection. Still, the literature on vitamin A deficiency and its association with ARI morbidity and mortality is sparse and controversial. Two studies (Sommer, Katz, and Tarwotjo 1984; Bloem and others 1990) have suggested a two- to fourfold increase in the relative risk of ARI associated with serologic or ophthalmic signs of vitamin A deficiency. In the Sommer study (1983), mortality in the clinically vitamin A-deficient group was 8.6 times that in non-xerophthalmic children.

Several prospective studies have noted a reduction in overall mortality among children whose diets were supplemented with vitamin A. Vitamin A supplements given to children with severe pneumonia or measles has improved clinical outcome and reduced mortality (Barclay, Foster, and Sommer 1987; Hussey and Klein 1990). Prospective studies of the effect of vitamin A supplementation in children from areas with endemic vitamin A deficiency (who are, therefore, presumed to be subclinically deficient) have not, however, demonstrated an effect on ARI-specific morbidity or mortality (Rahmathullah and others 1990; Vijayaraghavan and others 1990; Rahmathullah and others 1991). The effect of vitamin A supplementation on ARI-specific morbidity and mortality among children who are not clinically xerophthalmic remains speculative.

Smoking and Air Pollution

There is a large and expanding literature from industrialized countries on the increase in risk of pneumonia from active and passive smoking. Investigators in both industrialized and developing countries have demonstrated a 1.5- to 4-fold increased incidence of pneumonia among smokers and among children whose parents smoke (Harlap and Davies 1974; Leeder and others 1976; Ekwo, 1983; Weiss and others 1983; Ware and others 1984; Pedreira and others 1985; Chen, Wanxian, and Shunzhang 1986; Burchfiel and others 1986; Lipsky and others 1986; Samet, Marbury, and Spengler 1987; USDHHS 1989). Maternal smoking also predisposes to low birth weight (Martin and Bracken 1986; Ruben and others 1986), thus increasing the risk of pneumonia mortality for the infant after birth. There are no prospective data currently available from developing countries to establish that programs to reduce smoking will reduce ARI-specific mortality. The recent alarming increases in the numbers of persons who smoke in developing countries, however, argue for prompt intervention, particularly since successful reduction of smoking may be expected to yield health benefits beyond the reduction of ARI morbidity and mortality.

Exposure to both outdoor and indoor air pollution have been suspected to increase the risk of ARI in many developing countries (Kamat and others 1980; WHO/UNEP 1988; Chen and others 1990). There is growing concern regarding the health effects of the products of combustion (including carbon monoxide, particulates, and sulfur and nitrogen dioxides) from cooking and heating fires. It has been estimated that 300 million to 400 million people, mostly in the rural areas of developing countries, are adversely affected by these organic fuel emissions (de Koning, Smith, and Last 1985). Although there is a clear relation between exposure to such emissions and chronic obstructive pulmonary disease (WHO/EPP 1984; Chen and others 1990), the relation to pneumonia in the developing world is less well documented.

Indoor particulate concentrations, probably the best single indicator of toxic (noncarcinogenic) effects, are twenty times higher in the villages of developing countries than in households where two packs of cigarettes are smoked per day (Pandey, Boleij, Smith, and Wafula 1989). Several studies in developing countries have suggested that an increased incidence of pneumonia is associated with exposure to organic fuel emissions (Sofoluwe 1968; Kossove 1982; Honicky 1985; Campbell, Armstrong, and Byass 1989; Penna and Duchiade 1991), although several studies have had problems with confounding variables such as socioeconomic status and crowding. One study in Nepal (Pandey, Neupane, Gautam, and Shrestha 1989) has demonstrated that the number of episodes of life-threatening pneumonia among children under two is directly proportional to the reported hours per day spent near the stove. Studies in the Gambia suggest that carriage on the mother's back during cooking may predispose children to pneumonia (Armstrong and Campbell 1991). Prospective trials are required to assess the effectiveness of interventions such as improvements in stove design, improved ventilation, and behavioral change to reduce exposure.

Clinical Syndromes Causing ARI Mortality

The predominant known causes of ARI mortality are bacterial and viral pneumonia, measles, and pertussis. Additional epidemiologic data are needed to characterize the importance of other clinical syndromes and etiologic agents, including diphtheria, bacterial pharyngitis, and the "opportunistic" viral and bacterial infections which are likely important causes of pneumonia mortality among the very young, the very old, and those immunocompromised by acquired immunodeficiency syndrome (AIDS) or malnutrition.

Pneumonia

Pneumonia is an inflammatory process of the pulmonary interstitial space or alveoli which may be diffuse or confined to lung segments or lobes. Clinically, patients with pneumonia most frequently present with cough and tachypnea (rapid breathing);retractions (indrawing of the lower chest wall on inspiration) may also be present in more severe cases. Among neonates and younger infants, however, cough is often absent.

Available information from developing countries suggests that more than 75 percent of ARI deaths are caused by pneumonia, both bacterial and viral (Bulla and Hitze 1978; Berman 1991). Microbiologic data is difficult to obtain and of variable quality, yet most investigators agree that the bulk of ARI mortality among both children and adults is due to pneumonias caused by two bacteria, *Streptococcus pneumoniae* and *Hemophilus influenzae* (Berman and others 1983; Denny and Clyde 1983; Shann and others 1984; Selwyn 1990; WHO/ARI 1991b). Viral agents which cause fatal pneumonia include respiratory syncytial virus (RSV), measles, parainfluenza, influenza, and adenovirus. Mixed viral and bacterial infections are frequently documented (Berman 1991). Clinical malaria has also been found to coincide frequently with the clinical and radiologic diagnosis of pneumonia (Byass and others 1991).

Measles

Measles is a vaccine-preventable disease causing an acute febrile eruption which occurs naturally only in humans. The viral infection itself may result in any of several clinical syndromes, including croup (laryngotracheobronchitis), bronchitis, bronchiolitis, or even viral pneumonia, particularly in children immunocompromised by severe malnutrition. These manifestations may occur in the absence of the typical measles rash. Common complications of measles include growth faltering, chronic diarrhea, otitis media (middle ear infection), encephalitis, and pneumonia. Pneumonia, including primary measles pneumonia as well as superinfection by viruses and bacteria, is the most common complication of measles and often represents the principal proximal cause of death.

In unimmunized populations, epidemics occur in two-year cycles with secondary attack rates exceeding 90 percent among susceptible household contacts (Keja and others 1988). Although generally a disease of childhood, measles can occur at any age in susceptible populations. Infants in industrialized countries are not usually affected under the age of six to eight months, presumably because of placentally transmitted maternal antibodies. In parts of Africa, however, 20 to 45 percent of children are infected with measles before they attain the recommended age for immmunization at nine months.

Although improving immunization coverage progressively reduces infection rates, it was estimated in 1989 that there were 70 million annual cases of measles, and that 1.5 million to 2 million of those affected would die during the month following infection. Although generally a mild disease in temperate climates, an estimated 1 to 5 percent of all affected children in developing countries will die of measles or its complications. Children who survive the acute episode have an increased risk of mortality for weeks to months following infection. Most investigators, therefore, report deaths which occur within one month of the measles rash as "measles-associated."

Partly because of such variations in methods of ascertaining deaths due to or associated with measles, the reported case-fatality ratios vary widely. Williams and Hull (1983) documented a 5 percent case-fatality ratio during the acute phase of the disease, and a cumulative rate of 15 percent during the nine months following the rash. The case-fatality ratios obtained from prospective population-based studies range from 2 percent in Bangladesh to 34 percent in Guinea Bissau (WHO/EPI 1987). Rates of 50 percent or more have been described in severely undernourished populations. It has been suggested, however, that deaths prevented by measles immunization will be "replaced" by deaths from other causes, such that measles immunization may prevent fewer deaths than these mortality ratios would suggest.

Pertussis

The majority of cases of whooping cough, or the pertussis syndrome, are vaccine-preventable infections caused by *Bordetella pertussis*. The paroxysms of coughing, often associated with a characteristic inspiratory gasp (the whoop), may persist for four to ten weeks. Pertussis is often associated with dehydration and weight loss; and encephalitis is an occasional complication. Pneumonia, resulting either from the organism itself or from secondary bacterial infection, is the proximal cause of death in over 90 percent of cases.

Although pertussis occurs endemically, it tends to produce epidemics every three to four years, with up to 90 percent of exposed susceptibles developing the disease (Broome 1981;

Muller, Leeuwenburg, and Pratt 1986). Incidence is higher among girls than boys. Population-based studies have suggested an annual incidence of 1 to 5 percent among children under fifteen, although infants have a 16 percent chance of infection in Kenya (Voorhoeve and others 1977). The case-fatality ratio averages about 1 percent, although up to 15 percent of cases were fatal in studies in Uganda (Bwibo 1971) and Santa Maria Cauque (Mata 1978). The highest mortality is observed among females and children under two, with an estimated 500,000 to 1 million infant deaths annually due to pertussis (Muller, Leeuwenburg, and Pratt 1986; Keja and others 1988).

Diphtheria

The epidemiology of diphtheria in the developing world is poorly understood. Although the causative organism, *Corynebacterium diptheriae*, is widely present in Africa, and over 96 percent of unvaccinated adults are immune (Ikejani 1961; Muyembe and others 1972), there are few reported cases of this vaccine-preventable disease. It has been suggested that immunity may result from subclinical or misdiagnosed infections, an explanation supported by the finding of carriage of the organism in 4 to 9 percent of the population (Ikejani 1961; Muyembe and others 1972).

There are no community-based studies, but data from hospitals suggest diphtheria may be an important cause of pharyngitis and croup. Of 180 children hospitalized with respiratory infections in Colombia (Escobar, Dover, and Duenas 1976), seven of the nine cases of croup were caused by diphtheria. Investigators in the Gambia found evidence to suggest an annual incidence of 6 per 1,000 children under five. Salih and others (1985) have reported epidemic diphtheria and suggest that it is one of the most important diseases of childhood in the Sudan.

Pharyngitis

Pharyngitis is an upper respiratory tract infection that is most commonly viral and, therefore, self-limited. Bacterial pharyngitis, although less common, is of greater public health importance. Though acute bacterial pharyngitis (except when due to diphtheria) is not a significant primary cause of mortality, acute rheumatic fever (ARF) is an occasional late complication of untreated pharyngitis caused by group A betahemolytic streptococci (*Streptococcus pyogenes*). Acute rheumatic fever has been reported at rates of 27 to 100 cases per 100,000 per year (WHO 1988), although it is much less frequent in industrialized countries. Microscopic cardiac damage during ARF may progress over subsequent years, frequently causing incapacitation and, ultimately, death owing to changes in cardiac function.

Antibiotic therapy of bacterial pharyngitis is recommended in industrialized countries to prevent ARF and other sequelae of streptococcal pharyngitis. Management of streptococcal pharyngitis has been controversial, however, and even less is known of the epidemiology of streptococcal disease to guide its management in the developing world (Markowitz 1981). In view of additional concerns regarding the cost and insensitivity of the laboratory tests, and the lack of criteria to distinguish streptococcal pharyngitis on clinical grounds, it is currently difficult to establish in developing countries a strategy for management of pharyngitis which will effectively prevent poststreptococcal complications. Antibiotic prophylaxis for patients with a history of rheumatic fever has, therefore, been recommended as the most feasible strategy to prevent rheumatic heart disease in developing countries (WHO 1988).

Other Causes of ARI Mortality

Additional causes of ARI mortality include viral bronchiolitis and epiglottitis. Bronchiolitis, especially that resulting from RSV and parainfluenza 3, may be responsible for up to one-third of ALRI among children under five, most of which occurs in infants (Cherian and others 1990). The virology of these infections is apparently similar to that observed in industrialized countries (Selwyn 1990). The difficulty of the laboratory techniques and lack of cost-effective measures for prevention and treatment of these infections have hampered efforts to address these important causes of mortality.

Epiglottitis, which is usually caused by *Hemophilus influenzae* type b, is an occasional cause of death when the infected epiglottis obstructs respiration. Additional epidemiologic investigations are needed to define the role of other organisms as causes of mortality due to pneumonia, including group B streptococcus, *Chlamydia trachomatis* and *C. pneumoniae*, *Mycoplasma pneumoniae*, *Ureaplasma urealyticum*, and *Pneumocystis carinii*. These bacterial and parasitic pneumonias may be important causes of mortality, especially among neonates or persons immunocompromised, such as by malnutrition or AIDS. Tuberculosis and some helminthic infections may also present as pneumonia; these more chronic infections are often distinguished clinically by their failure to respond to the usual antibiotic therapy.

Public Health Significance

Comparison of results from investigations on the public health significance of ARI in different countries is all but prevented by wide variations in study design, case definitions, and culture techniques. Meaningful comparison of study results is difficult, for example, when some investigators have used sensitive case definitions which include all coughs and colds, whereas others focus only on the more severe ARI that comes to the attention of health care workers.

Current Levels and Trends in the Developing World

The few well-conducted community-based prospective studies performed suggest that overall incidence of ARI in the developing world is similar to that observed in the industrialized world.

MORBIDITY AND MORTALITY LEVELS, CIRCA 1985. Prevalence figures show that children spend from 22 to 40 percent of observed weeks with ARI, and from 1 to 14 percent of observed weeks with ALRI, such as pneumonia or bronchiolitis. Acute respiratory infections account for 20 to 40 percent of adult outpatient consultations and 20 to 60 percent among children. Of all pediatric admissions to hospitals, 12 to 45 percent are for ARI, whereas 20 to 30 percent of adult inpatients have been admitted for ARI treatment (Bulla and Hitze 1978; PAHO 1980; Leowski 1986).

The reported incidence of ALRI varies widely, from country to country as well as with age and nutritional status. Whereas the annual incidence of pneumonia is 3 to 4 percent in children under five in the industrialized countries, it ranges from 10 to 20 percent in most developing countries, reaching as high as 80 percent in populations with a high prevalence of malnutrition and low birth weight. In Papua New Guinea in 1973, for example, there were 72 episodes per 1,000 children of one to four years of age and 1,074 episodes per 1,000 infants (Riley and Douglas 1981). In Costa Rica an annual incidence of pneumonia of 37 per 1,000 children was observed among those of normal nutritional status, while the rate was 457.8 per 1,000 among malnourished children (Pio, Leowski, and ten Dam 1985). The overall incidence of ARI, most of which is coughs and colds, is comparable to that in the industrialized world. The greater public health importance of ARI in developing countries is manifest, however, in the increased frequency of lower respiratory tract infections and in the disease-specific mortality rates that are ten to fifty times higher than in industrialized countries (WHO 1984; Mohs 1985; Camargos, Guimaraes, and Drummond 1989). Most vulnerable to death due to pneumonia are the very young and the very old.

Of the estimated 15 million deaths occurring each year among children under five, 25 to 30 percent are due to ARI. As the cause of approximately 4 million deaths annually among this age group alone, ARI often surpasses diarrhea in importance as a cause of mortality (Bulla and Hitze 1978; Balint and Anand 1979; Shann and others 1984; Pio, Leowski, and ten Dam 1985; Spika and others 1989). Pneumonia causes from 2 to 8 percent of adult deaths in countries for which data are available (Hayes and others 1989), ranking from second to tenth as a cause of death among those age fifteen through sixty-four.

TRENDS IN THE PERIOD 1970 TO 1985. Although surveillance data for overall ARI morbidity in the developing world are limited, it is likely that these rates have remained unchanged in the past fifteen to twenty years, just as they have in the industrialized countries. Reductions in incidence of ARI as a result of improved immunization coverage (with measles, diphtheria, and pertussis vaccines) would have little effect on the overall incidence of ARI, because the frequency of viral upper respiratory infections would remain largely unchanged.

Pneumonia mortality, however, has been reduced significantly over the past fifteen to twenty years in the United States for all age groups except the elderly. Similar reductions in mortality would be expected in developing countries where the risk factors such as nutritional or socioeconomic status, immunization coverage, and access to health care have improved. In many countries, however, ARI has increased in relative importance, frequently emerging as the first cause of childhood death where diarrheal disease mortality rates have been successfully reduced (Chen, Rahman, and Sarder 1980; Zimicki 1988). Mortality from ARI has increased in relative importance even in settings where high coverage with measles immunization has been achieved (Greenwood and others 1988; Zimicki 1988).

Data from industrialized countries suggest that changes in immunization policy may increase the incidence of disease. With intensive control efforts, for example, the incidence of measles in the United States had fallen to the lowest level ever recorded in 1983. When expenditure for immunization was reduced in 1984, however, increased outbreaks were observed. A similar resurgence of pertussis has been noted in countries in which changes in public opinion or immunization policy have led to a reduction in immunization coverage.

Possible Morbidity and Mortality Patterns: 2000 and 2015

As viral upper respiratory infections, which account for the bulk of ARI morbidity, are unlikely to be eradicated in the foreseeable future, the overall incidence of ARI is likely to be substantially unchanged for the next twenty-five years. Considerable opportunity exists, however, to reduce the incidence of vaccine-preventable ARI and to reduce the case-fatality ratio for pneumonia, thereby reducing ARI mortality.

Changing demographic patterns, such as birth spacing and consequent improvements in nutritional status would be expected to substantially reduce mortality due to pneumonia during the next twenty-five years. Increased life expectancies may later create larger populations of the elderly, among whom pneumonia will likely remain a significant cause of mortality. Progress in improving the access to and quality of care will be instrumental in controlling mortality among both the young and the elderly.

Of potential future concern, however, is the evolution of antimicrobial resistance among the pathogens causing bacterial pneumonia, which may interfere with the effectiveness of interventions. Although the development of newer antimicrobials has, to date, kept pace with the evolution of resistance to them, the cost of later-generation antibiotics will not be so easily borne in developing countries. And there is evidence to suggest that inappropriate use of antimicrobials, so frequent throughout the world, speeds the evolution of resistance.

Coverage with the vaccines currently included in WHO's Expanded Programme on Immunization (EPI) may be expected to continue to increase, also leading to reduction in the number of deaths from ARI. In addition, improved vaccine technology will likely alter the currently observed patterns of mortality due to ARI during the next twenty-five years. New vaccines, too, increase hopes of reducing childhood ARI mortality due to measles and bacterial pneumonias caused by S. *pneumoniae* and H. *influenzae*.

Economic Costs of ARI

Acute respiratory infections account for an average of 35 percent of all outpatient visits globally (Bulla and Hitze 1978) and generally similar proportions of all hospitalizations among children.

DIRECT COSTS. The minimal direct cost of ALRI for children in the first two years of life in the United States has been estimated at $35.14 per child, 56 percent of which is attributable to hospitalization (McConnochie, Hall, and Barker 1988).[1]

In many developing countries, the economic burden of treatment of ARI already exceeds the expected cost of ARI case management with improved effectiveness and broader coverage. More appropriate use of existing health personnel and pharmaceutical resources might be expected, in many countries, to avert mortality with little or no additional expenditure. For example, the prevalence of the inappropriate use of pharmaceuticals for the management of ARI suggests that a net cost savings might be achieved by improving use patterns (Stansfield 1990; Foreit and others 1991). Frequently, more than half of antibiotic use is unnecessary (Hossain, Glass, and Khan 1982; Stein and others 1984; Quick and others 1988). A study in Peru (Foreit and Lesevic 1987) showed that approximately 50 percent of the expenditure for medications to treat ARI episodes was inappropriate, at an excess cost of $18.47 to $21.97 per child covered. The authors of the study estimated that an 89 percent reduction in treatment costs would be achieved through altering outpatient treatment of ARI to conform to WHO guidelines. Both inappropriate prescription of antibiotics and poor compliance probably also contribute to the development of antimicrobial resistance and will greatly increase the future direct costs of ARI treatment as the use of more expensive antimicrobial agents becomes necessary.

INDIRECT COSTS. Acute respiratory infections account for an average of one-third of all absences from work (Bulla 1978). In Britain, one to two weeks of schooling are lost per child per year due to ARI (Crofton and Douglas 1975). Data from Ghana (Ghana Health Project Assessment Team 1981) indicate that over 94 percent of the fifty-two days of life lost per case of ARI is due to mortality rather than disability. Particularly in the setting of developing countries, where case-fatality ratios are high and access to services limited, the bulk of costs attributable to ARI are indirect costs due to mortality. No such estimates are available for the developing world, but ARI also likely takes a relatively greater toll in these settings in the form of growth deficits, malnutrition, and resulting learning disabilities. Although these indirect costs of ARI are difficult to quantify, it is probable that they greatly reduce the potential productivity of those affected.

Lowering the Incidence of ARI

Possible preventive approaches to reduce ARI morbidity and mortality include immunization and alteration of other risk factors which predispose children and adults to pneumonia.

Elements of the Preventive Strategy

Although the data are adequate to support the use of immunization in the control of ARI, the limitations of current knowledge regarding the feasibility and effectiveness of other preventive strategies are, for the moment, a barrier to their use in programs to reduce ARI morbidity and mortality. It has been estimated that deaths due to the four vaccine-preventable respiratory diseases (measles, diphtheria, pertussis, and tuberculosis) may account for up to 25 percent of the total mortality among children under five in the developing world.

Although the immunization programs must be part of any strategy to prevent ARI, available data do not yet justify the design and implementation of programs to reduce environmental and nutritional risk factors for ARI control. The evidence does suggest, however, that such programs may be effective. Several potential preventive interventions that might be considered for inclusion in ARI control programs have been included in the following discussion. Those for which evidence of feasibility and effectiveness are strongest are included in a comparative model of cost-effectiveness, which is summarized in table 4-3. It is important to recognize, however, that the actual benefits from these interventions would be broader than those calculated, since each would reduce morbidity and mortality resulting from many health problems beyond ARI alone. Sources for the data used and the methods for calculating the cost-effectiveness estimates are specified in the appendix to this chapter.

MEASLES IMMUNIZATION. Operational problems in maintaining the necessary cool temperatures for handling the measles vaccine are a frequent barrier to maintaining vaccine viability and efficacy. The World Health Organization has estimated the efficacy of the vaccine to be 90 percent when maintained at appropriately cool temperatures (Keja and others 1988). Because of variability in study design and alterations in vaccine viability as a result of handling, the measured efficacy of the vaccine may vary broadly, although Hull, Pap, and Oldfield (1983) achieved an efficacy of 89 percent in the Gambia.

Considerable controversy surrounds the issue of immunization strategy for measles. Studies with the currently available (Schwartz) vaccine have demonstrated that residual levels of maternal antibody restrict the effectiveness of the vaccine in the first few months of life. Available data regarding age-specific seroconversion and measles incidence rates suggest that immunization at nine months of age will prevent the maximal number of cases (WHO/EPI 1982). These data were the basis for the WHO recommendation of one dose of measles vaccine to be given between nine and twelve months of age.

Yet, in many countries, 20 to 45 percent of measles cases occur among infants before nine months of age, when they are most vulnerable to measles mortality. It had been suggested that "herd immunity" achieved with adequate immunization coverage among older infants and children may serve to reduce the infection rate among younger infants (Black 1982; Heymann and others 1983). Recent evidence, however, suggests that in areas of high population density, there is no shift in the age distribution of cases or reduction in incidence greater than the level of vaccination coverage (Dabis and others 1988; Taylor and others 1988). Particularly in the urban areas of Africa, the increased transmission rates may lower the optimal age for immunization (McLean and Anderson 1988; Taylor and others 1988).

Table 4-3. Calculated Cost-Effectiveness of Interventions for ARI Control
(U.S. dollars)

Intervention	Expected disease-specific mortality reduction[a] (percent)	Proportion of ARI mortality addressed (percent)	Expected ARI-specific mortality reduction (percent)	Deaths averted in children under five (per million population)	Cost per person in target population	Total cost (per million population)	Cost per death averted	Cost per disability-adjusted life-year saved
Case management	60–90 (80)	38–52 (49)	23–47 (39)	351–676 (585)	$3.61	$220,000–$940,000 ($541,877)	$379–$1,610 ($926)	$37
Breastfeeding promotion	50–80 (72)	4	2–3.2 (2.8)	15–96 (42)	$5.00	$40.00	$417–$2,667 ($952)	$38
EPI vaccines	44–80 (65)	20–25 (22.5)	8.8–20 (14.6)	66–600 (219)	$9.08	$122,580–$245,160 ($217,920)	$409–$1,857 ($995)	$40
Reduction of malnutrition	50–95 (80)	70–90 (80)	35–85 (64)	263–2,550 (960)	$15.00 (malnourished) $11.85 (all children)	$810,000–$1,777,500 ($1,500,000)	$697–$3,080 ($1,563)	$63
Pneumococcal vaccine	0–30 (15)	30–50 (40)	0–15 (7)	0–450 (105)	$7.28	$98,280–$196,560 ($174,720)	$437 ($1,664)	$67

Note: Most likely values in parentheses.
a. Disease is pneumonia except for EPI vaccine, where disease is pertussis and measles; for pneumococcal vaccine, disease is pneumococcal pneumonia.
Source: Authors' data.

In 1989, the World Health Organization recommended the use of the higher titer Edmonsten-Zagreb vaccine at or before six months of age in areas where measles is a major cause of infant mortality (WHO/EPI 1990). Subsequent reports of increased late mortality among children immunized with such higher titer vaccines (Garenne, Leroy, and Sene 1991) has, however, prompted a suspension of that recommendation. Alternatives to the current measles vaccines must be developed which are effective in younger infants.

Ongoing studies of the effectiveness, optimal dose, nonparenteral routes of administration (in order to overcome residual maternal antibodies), and booster response to the new vaccines will help further to refine immunization policies in the near future. More studies are needed to explore the cost-effectiveness of a two-dose schedule, such as initial measles immunization with the third diphtheria-pertussis-tetanus vaccine (DPT) dose (followed by a second dose at six to twelve months of age). High drop-out rates, which are a major barrier to the success of immunization programs, also argue in favor of using earlier opportunities for immunization, even if children are less than the ideal age for achieving seroconversion or optimum protection. Some investigators, however, have raised the concern that earlier immunization may interfere with antibody response at the time of revaccination (Wilkins and Wehrle 1979; Linnemann and others 1982; Stetler and others 1986).

PERTUSSIS IMMUNIZATION. The vaccine for pertussis is delivered together with the diphtheria and tetanus vaccines. The efficacy of pertussis vaccine for the fully immunized child (three doses) has been recently questioned but is estimated at 70 to 90 percent in the industrialized world (Church 1979; Koplan and others 1979) and 50 to 90 percent in developing countries. As for measles, however, transmission rates in endemic areas are such that many children are infected and most deaths occur prior to the usual age of completed immunization.

Pertussis immunization coverage in some industrialized countries has fallen off in the last fifteen years, primarily because of concern about associated adverse neurological effects, most notably encephalopathy (Brahmans 1986), although there is also some controversy about the vaccine's effectiveness (Fine and Clarkson 1987). Outbreaks of pertussis have been observed in Great Britain, Japan, and Sweden, where policy changes or public opinion have led to a reduction of immunization coverage. Even with the current preparation, however, the benefit of the vaccine far outweighs the risk of adverse effects (Koplan and others 1979; Cherry 1984). Accelerated research has led to the development of acellular pertussis vaccines, which offer hope in the near future for both improved effectiveness and fewer adverse effects (Miller and others 1991).

PNEUMOCOCCAL IMMUNIZATION. The pneumococcal vaccine licensed for use in the United States is composed of the purified polysaccharide extracted from twenty-three of the eighty-four types of *Streptococcus pneumoniae*. These capsular subtypes are responsible for approximately 90 percent of invasive pneumococcal disease in the United States. Still, over 30 percent of blood culture isolates from patients with pneumonia in developing countries have been pneumococcal serotypes which are not included in the current vaccine (Ghafoor and others 1990; Mastro and others 1991). In addition, the vaccine induces little immunity in children under eighteen months of age, who are most vulnerable to mortality due to pneumococcal infections.

Studies in the United States have suggested that the currently available vaccine is 50 to 80 percent effective in preventing bacteremia and pneumonia in adults. Results of studies among the very elderly or chronically ill (Simberkoff and others 1986) and among children under eighteen months have been less encouraging. The vaccine has also been tested in Papua New Guinea, which reports that up to 50 percent of pneumonia is due to pneumococcal infection. Clinical trials there (Riley and others 1986) among children age six months through fifty-nine months have shown a 50 percent reduction in pneumonia-specific mortality rates during periods of one to five years after immunization. There appears to have been no reduction in pneumonia incidence, and there is little evidence to suggest that the vaccine was immunogenic in the younger age groups. The cause of the mortality reduction is, therefore, not clear, and the results need to be replicated in other developing countries. Also of potential interest was the finding that infants of mothers immunized during their last trimester had a 32 percent lower rate of pneumonia (Riley and Douglas 1981). Such "passive" protection of infants while they await completion of immunization series deserves further investigation.

H. INFLUENZAE VACCINE. Like pneumococcal vaccine, which is also a polysaccharide vaccine, the current *H. influenzae* vaccine has limited immunogenicity in infants and young children. The vaccine is made from *H. influenzae* type b polysaccharide, since this type accounts for virtually all invasive disease in the industrialized world. The effective protection (measured by the prevention of invasive disease, mainly meningitis and bacteremia) found in children over twenty-four months of age has ranged from 0 to 90 percent (Granoff and others 1986; Harrison and others 1987; Black and others 1988; Gilsdorf 1988). The effectiveness of the *H. influenzae* type b vaccine in reducing pneumonia morbidity and mortality cannot be estimated from U.S. data, since the frequency of pneumonia due to Hib is too low.

An increase in early cases after Hib immunization has been variously ascribed to unmasking of latent infection or shortening of the incubation period, perhaps because of transient postvaccination reductions in antibody levels (Black and others 1988). One study (Osterholm and others 1987) actually calculated an increased risk of *H. influenzae* infection of 45 percent, leaving the protective effect of Hib vaccine in some doubt.

The newer Hib conjugate vaccines, which link Hib antigens to protein carriers, show improved immunogenicity in children under two and hold greater promise for preventing *H. influenzae* disease in the very young. Although experience with use of diphtheria toxoid as a conjugate has been mixed, tetanus toxoid carriers may be more effective (Eskola and others 1990; Siber and others 1990; Ward and others 1990; Wanger and others 1991). Formulations for developing countries will need to include additional types (that is, non-b and nonserotypable *H. influenzae*) which are not a prominent cause of invasive disease in the industrialized world (Funkhouser, Steinhoff, and Ward 1991). Recent studies in Papua New Guinea (Weinberg and others 1990), Pakistan (Ghafoor and others 1990), and the Gambia have shown that approximately half of all invasive *H. influenzae* disease is due to nonserotypable or non-b strains.

The costs of the current conventional Hib vaccine is $2.19 per dose, while the conjugate vaccine is $14.00 per dose. Hay and Daum (1987) compared the costs and benefits of rifampin prophylaxis of exposed contacts to immunization with the currently available unconjugated vaccine. Vaccination was predicted to be the most cost-effective strategy with a calculated overall net savings of $64.8 million, in the setting of an anticipated social cost of $1.94 billion for *H. influenzae* disease in the 1984 birth cohort. Because of the paucity of data on Hib vaccine effectiveness in developing countries, no estimates of cost-effectiveness have been included in table 4-3.

OTHER IMMUNIZATIONS. Vaccination to induce immunity to organisms which cause ARI mortality is clearly an effective preventive intervention. There is good evidence to support the use of vaccines against measles and pertussis, both in the documented importance to public health of these problems and the effectiveness of immunization. Although the expected effect of diphtheria vaccine is difficult to predict because of the lack of information regarding diphtheria morbidity and mortality, marginal costs of including the vaccine with pertussis and tetanus (in DPT vaccine) are nearly negligible.

Effective vaccines against the viral causes of pneumonia and bronchiolitis would likely avert additional mortality. Attempts to develop effective vaccines against the two most important causes of mortality, RSV and parainfluenza viruses, however, have been frustrating. Still, the mechanism for the adverse hypersensitivity responses to RSV antigens has recently been identified, so that purified antigen and recombinant vaccines currently under development should offer greater hope for these important causes of respiratory mortality (Pringle 1987). Influenza vaccines have been effective in preventing infections, particularly among the elderly, but the "antigenic drift," or frequent changes in surface proteins which characterize these viruses make vaccine production and distribution more costly. Such immunization programs for adults have also been poorly received and achieve limited coverage.

ENVIRONMENTAL AND NUTRITIONAL RISK REDUCTION. Alteration of other documented and suspected risk factors for ARI mortality, such as poor nutritional status (including low birth weight, poor infant-feeding practice, undernutrition, and vitamin A deficiency) and exposure to smoke (including smoke from active and passive cigarette smoking and from organic-fuel cookfires), have been suggested as additional strategies for the prevention of ARI deaths. Although the association of some of these risk factors with disease is strong, few studies support the feasibility of programs using these interventions or their effectiveness in preventing ARI. The data show as far more feasible and effective the promotion of breastfeeding and reduction of malnutrition.

Good Practice and Actual Practice: Are There Gaps?

Correct case management is the central strategy of WHO's Programme for the Control of Acute Respiratory Infections. One of the four objectives, however, is "to reduce the incidence of acute lower respiratory infection" (WHO/ARI 1991). Although intervention to alter some of the nonspecific risk factors for ARI (table 4-2) is an intriguing possibility for prevention of pneumonia, immunization remains the only strategy known to be effective in the prevention of morbidity and mortality due to pneumonia.

Even this proven technology, however, has not been fully exploited to prevent ARI mortality. As of 1988, many of the 97 countries with an Expanded Programme on Immunization still had subnational coverage, often neglecting the neediest children in the most remote areas (Keja and others 1988). Vaccination efforts are most appropriately integrated with the primary health care system, avoiding duplication of necessary management, supervision, training, and logistical resources. Immunization campaigns, although they result in high short-term coverage, may compromise sustainability and divert resources from the development of the rest of the primary health care infrastructure.

Global coverage estimates for children immunized during the first year of life are 50 percent for measles and 55 percent for the DPT series of three doses (Keja and others 1988), although figures are considerably lower in Africa. Barriers to achieving improved coverage with the EPI vaccines include difficulties with supply and management systems and the practical problems of maintaining the cold chain. High drop-out rates for immunization series are partly the result of limitations of resources for social mobilization, the opportunity costs to the family in obtaining immunizations, failure of health workers to profit from clinic visits by giving immunizations (Keja and others 1988), and adverse effects of current vaccine preparations.

Increasing attention, especially in Africa, has been paid to the reuse of syringes and needles in immunizations. These unsafe immunization practices introduce the risk of transmission of blood-borne diseases such as hepatitis and AIDS.

Efforts to prevent ARI mortality through reduction of the prevalence of malnutrition and low birth weight are hampered by the obvious social, economic, and political barriers to development. Promotion of appropriate infant-feeding practice, including breastfeeding, represents an opportunity to reduce ARI morbidity and mortality that deserves greater emphasis.

Table 4-4. Diagnosis and Treatment of Pneumonia in Children Aged Two Months to Five Years

Disease	Signs	Treatment
Very severe disease	Unable to drink Convulsions Abnormally sleepy or hard to wake Stridor in calm child Severe undernutrition	Refer urgently to hospital Give first does of antibiotic Treat fever, if present Treat wheezing, if present If cerebral malaria possible, give antimalarial drug
Severe pneumonia	Chest indrawing	Refer urgently to hospital[a] Give first dose of antibiotic Treat fever, wheezing if present
Pneumonia	No chest indrawing Fast breathing[b]	Advise parent for home care Give antibiotic Treat fever, wheezing if present Reassess in two days; if child getting worse (unable to drink, chest indrawing, other danger signs), refer urgently to hospital; if child the same, change antibiotic or refer; if child improving (breathing slower, less fever, eating better), finish five days of antibiotic
No pneumonia: cough or cold	No chest indrawing No fast breathing	If coughing more than thirty days, refer for assessment Assess and treat ear problem or sore throat, if present Advise parent for home care Treat fever, wheezing, if present

a. If referral not feasible, treat with antibiotic and follow closely.
b. Fast breathing defined as fifty breaths per minute or more in infant age two to twelve months, forty breaths per minute or more in child age one to five years.
Source: WHO/ARI 1991b.

Table 4-5. Diagnosis and Treatment of Pneumonia in Infants Less than Two Months Old

Disease	Signs	Treatment
Very severe disease	Not feeding well Convulsions Abnormally sleepy or hard to wake Stridor in calm child Wheezing Fever or low body temperature	Refer urgently to hospital Keep infant warm Give first dose of antibiotic
Severe pneumonia	Severe chest indrawing Fast breathing[a]	Refer urgently to hospital[b] Keep infant warm Give first dose of antibiotic
No pneumonia: cough or cold	No severe chest indrawing No fast breathing	Advise parent to give following home care: Keep infant warm Breastfeed frequently Clear nose if it interferes with feeding Return quickly if breathing becomes fast or difficult, feeding becomes a problem, or infant becomes sicker

a. Fast breathing defined as sixty breaths per minute or more.
b. If referral not feasible, treat with antibiotic and follow closely.
Source: Authors' data.

Case Management

Although research must continue to improve preventive technologies for the primary causes of ARI mortality, ARI control programs for the near future will rely principally on improved case management.

Elements of the Case Management Strategy

The World Health Organization's ARI control program has taken the lead in promoting intervention to address the problem of ARI in children. The primary objective of the program is the reduction of ALRI mortality through effective case management. Secondary objectives include the reduction of (a) the severity and complications of acute upper respiratory tract infections, (b) the inappropriate use of antibiotics and other drugs for the treatment of ARI, and (c) the incidence of pneumonia. To improve the case management of pneumonia, WHO has developed guidelines for standard treatment at the most peripheral and referral health facilities and at the community level.

In countries with a high incidence of bacterial pneumonia (generally those with an infant mortality rate greater than 40 per 1,000), pneumonia may be relatively reliably diagnosed on the basis of simple clinical criteria alone. For any child under five with cough or difficult breathing, tachypnea (rapid breathing) appears to be the best single predictor of pneumonia and the need for antibiotic treatment (Shann, Hart, and Thomas 1982; Campbell, Byass, and Greenwood 1988; Cherian and others 1988; Campbell, Armstrong, and Byass 1989; Campbell and others 1989; Lucero and others 1990). In view of the variation of normal respiratory rates with age, WHO guidelines recommend a threshold rate of sixty or more per minute in young infants (under two months), fifty or more for older infants (two months through eleven months), and forty or more for children one through four years of age (WHO 1990).

Chest indrawing (retraction of the lower part of the chest wall on inspiration) detected in children two months to four years of age indicates the presence of severe pneumonia requiring hospitalization. The algorithms used for diagnosis and treatment of childhood pneumonia, including additional criteria for referral for hospitalization, are summarized in tables 4-4 and 4-5 (WHO/ARI 1991b). Any of four inexpensive antibiotics may be recommended for the home care of uncomplicated pneumonia, including co-trimoxazole (trimethoprim-sulfamethoxazole), amoxycillin, ampicillin, and procaine penicillin.

Although wheezing (including asthma) is managed within this algorithm, there are separate guidelines for care of sore throats and ear infections. All cases receive general supportive care, including fluids, continued feeding, treatment of fever, and clearing of nasal or ear discharge as needed. Although these findings require further confirmation, studies in Pakistan have suggested that such supportive measures may actually reduce the likelihood of progression of uncomplicated coughs and colds to life-threatening pneumonias (Khan, Addiss, and Rizwan-Ullah 1990).

There is no doubt about the importance of bacterial pneumonia as a cause of mortality or about the effectiveness of antimicrobials in reducing case-fatality ratios. But to address concerns about whether peripheral health care workers with limited training could identify and treat cases appropriately, several intervention studies were conducted to test the algorithm for case management in an operational setting in several developing countries. These and another study conducted in Jumla, Nepal, were recently reviewed (WHO/ARI 1988). Although each of the studies suffered from design flaws or confounding as a result of simultaneous introduction of other interventions, taken as a whole they present strong evidence of the effectiveness of case management by peripheral health care workers. It was found that ARI-specific mortality declined by an average of 41.6 percent (range 18–65 percent), whereas overall mortality was reduced in the same five study areas by an average of 22.2 percent (range 11.5 to 40 percent). These studies, for which further details are presented in table 4-6, confirmed the feasibility and efficacy of providing case management of pneumonia through peripheral health workers with limited training.

These results compare favorably with earlier, more theoretical calculations of the expected effectiveness of pneumonia case management interventions. For example, Tugwell and others (1985) assumed an efficacy of co-trimoxazole in treatment of community-acquired pneumonia of 80 percent, a diagnostic accuracy of 80 percent by the health workers, a correct treatment rate of 90 percent, 80 percent patient compliance with the medication regimen, and 80 percent access to appropriate treatment, calculating an expected program effectiveness of 37 percent.

Lessons learned from the case management intervention trials must be taken into account in program design and selection of research priorities. For example, the Jumla study documented a mean duration of fatal episodes of pneumonia of three and one-half days (Nils Daulaire, personal communication, 1990). Under these circumstances, active surveillance by health workers is unlikely to detect an adequate proportion of cases. Control programs for ARI must rely on families to detect signs and symptoms of pneumonia and bring suspected cases to a health worker for evaluation and treatment. Reductions in deaths due to diarrhea were observed in Jumla, where only pneumonia cases were treated (WHO/ARI 1988), raising the important question of the effect of antibiotic treatment on concurrent infections such as diarrhea or malaria.

Few operational programs for pneumonia case management have measured cost per case treated or death averted. The figures which are available have been obtained in research settings, where expenditure may not be representative. Costs per case treated in the Philippines have been estimated at $5.15 and $4.37 (Brenzel 1990). Costs per death averted have ranged from $200 in Indonesia to $350 in Nepal (Brenzel 1990). Using a model to estimate cost-effectiveness outlined in the appendix to this chapter, we have calculated an expected cost per death averted of $926, and a cost per discounted healthy year of life saved of $37.

Good Practice and Actual Practice: Are There Gaps?

By the end of 1990, fifty-four countries had prepared plans of operation for ARI control programs and forty-seven had functioning programs (WHO/ARI, 1991a). Eighteen additional countries had designated a national program manager and issued technical guidelines for case management. Therefore, a total of fifty-nine countries, most of which are in the Americas and Western Pacific, had taken some steps to establish a national ARI control program.

Yet it is clear that the intrinsic complexity of the management of ARI will present great challenges in the implementation of control programs. The significant operational problems encountered in immunization and diarrheal disease control programs, for example, are likely to be dwarfed by the obstacles

to successful implementation of an ARI control program. Appropriate case management requires that each of many difficult conditions be met, including the design and communication of culturally appropriate and effective health education for family recognition of suspected pneumonia, prompt presentation to an effectively trained and carefully supervised health worker, correct diagnosis and selection of treatment, development and maintenance of reliable logistical systems to ensure adequate supplies of antibiotics, family compliance with appropriate instructions for care, and access to competent referral care as required.

These prerequisites for effective case management of pneumonia are inextricably linked to the basic infrastructure for primary health care. Although ARI control may be introduced as another "vertical" program, it is less conveniently addressed outside the context of the health care delivery system as a whole. Strengthening of systems to reduce pneumonia mortality therefore requires a more comprehensive approach to improving access and quality of care.

It will be important, for example, to rationalize the use of antibiotics for other health problems in order to ensure that adequate supplies remain to treat cases of pneumonia. Even when basic antibiotics are unavailable in peripheral health centers, the presence of antibiotics in remote markets provides evidence of the effectiveness of informal systems of distribution. Such sales of antimicrobials in the informal sector likely leads to their inappropriate use in even more than the 50 to 95 percent of cases in which inappropriate use is observed in health centers (Chaulet and Khaled 1982; Hossain, Glass, and Khan 1982; Gutierrez and others 1986). Reduction of the inappropriate use of these supplies may actually avert pneumonia deaths at no increased cost, both through increasing effective use and reducing adverse effects and the evolution of antimicrobial resistance (Stansfield 1990). Although the feasibility of labeling antibiotics in special packages (as solely for use in the treatment of pneumonia in children) is being assessed (WHO 1990), the inevitable discovery of the alternative uses of these powerful pharmaceuticals will likely render such practices ineffective.

Another obstacle to be anticipated is the resistance of physicians to empowering other health care workers with training to diagnose and treat with antibiotics. Narain and Sharma (1987), for example, have presented evidence that over 90 percent of physicians do not agree that nonphysician health workers should be provided with antibiotics to treat children suffering from pneumonia. Vigilance will also be required to prevent commercial drug companies from exploiting new markets by extracting inflated prices for basic pharmaceutical supplies.

Many countries will require assistance in the development of laboratory capability to ensure the correct selection of antibiotics (at least in reference centers), particularly for referral patients who have failed treatment with first-line antibiotics, through basic bacterial cultures and tests for antibiotic sensitivity. These capabilities are also required to maintain the necessary surveillance for the emergence of significant antibiotic resistance patterns, as is evidenced by the alarming resis-

Table 4-6. *Case Management of* ARI *in Children: Summary of Intervention Studies*

Location (dates)	Study design	Baseline data		Case detection		Pneumonia treatment			Mortality reduction	
		IMR [a] (per 1,000)	Measles immunization coverage (percent)	Case-finding	Maternal education	Source	First-line antimicrobial	Referral care	ALRI-specific (percent)	Overall (percent)
Haryana, India (1982–84)	Concurrent control; low birth weight only	210–275	0	Active (weekly)	Yes	Community health worker	Penicillin (oral)	None	42	24
Abbottabad, Pakistan (1985–87)	Concurrent control, subsequent intervention in control area	90–100	5.4	Active (every 10–14 days)	Yes	Community health worker or clinic	Co-trimoxazole	Poor access	56	55
Bohol, Philippines (1984–87)	Concurrent control	49–63	58–60	Passive	No	Clinic	Co-trimoxazole	Yes	25	13
Bagamoyo, Tanzania (1985–87)	Concurrent control; subsequent intervention in control area	137	53	Passive	No	Community health worker or clinic	Co-trimoxazole	Yes	30	27
Kathmandu, Nepal (1984–87)	Before and after	162	11	Active (every 2 weeks)	Yes	Community health worker	Ampicillin	Poor utilization	62	40
Kediri, Indonesia (1986–87)	Before and after	154	1.5	Active (every 2 weeks)	Yes	Community health worker	Co-trimoxazole	Poor access	67	41

a. Infant mortality rate.
Source: WHO/ARI/88.2 and WHO/ARI/91.20.

tance to commonly used antimicrobials in several countries (El-Mouza and others 1988; Lataorre Otin, Juncosa Morros, and Sanfeliu Sala 1988; Mastro and others 1991).

Donor agencies must recognize these gaps when allocating resources for ARI control program development. Although the historical lack of donor support in this area has also been an important obstacle to ARI control, the donor community has recently shown increased interest in strengthening pneumonia case management. Reduction in pneumonia deaths by 25 percent was included among targets established for the 1990s by the World Health Organization and United Nations Children's Fund (UNICEF) Joint Committee on Health Policy. This commitment is only beginning to be reflected in increased levels of national, bilateral, and multilateral funding to ARI control programs.

Priorities for ARI Control

The many national health plans which emphasize the priority of interventions to reduce infant and child mortality cannot long ignore pneumonia which is often a primary cause of this mortality. Global commitment to addressing this problem was reflected in the adoption, at the World Summit for Children in September 1990, of a resolution to reduce deaths due to ARI by one-third during the final decade of this century (UNICEF 1991).

Priorities for Resource Allocation

In view of the effectiveness of the vaccines and of antibiotic therapy for pneumonia, it is probable that more than half of ARI deaths could be averted through use of only the currently available technologies of immunization and improved case management. Breastfeeding promotion and reduction of the prevalence of malnutrition are also likely to be cost-effective in reducing mortality due to ARI. Interventions for the promotion of breastfeeding, reduction of malnutrition, and immunization with EPI vaccines will have a broader effect on child survival through their effectiveness in prevention of mortality due to diseases other than ARI. These three interventions, along with appropriate case management, should be given high priority for implementation, particularly in countries with high infant mortality. Such a combined curative-preventive approach is likely to be the most effective as a strategy to reduce mortality (Mosley and Becker 1988).

National ARI control programs should be developed or accelerated according to the guidelines recently refined by WHO's Programme for the Control of Acute Respiratory Infections. Intervention studies have provided adequate evidence among children under five that improved case management of pneumonia will reduce mortality due to ARI and, possibly, overall mortality in that population. As WHO has pointed out (WHO/ARI 1988), "there is no technical justification in delaying any further the expansion of ARI control programmes as an essential component of child survival efforts, and with the same priority attached to the Expanded Programmes on Immunization (EPI) and the diarrheal disease control (CDD) programmes." Al-

though most countries have active EPI programs, these programs must also be strengthened to ensure improved coverage (Poore 1988).

Referral care for pneumonia in persons who have responded poorly to antibiotic treatment requires adequate laboratory support to obtain bacteriologic cultures, identify organisms, and determine antibiotic sensitivities. Any national ARI control program must, therefore, allocate adequate resources to monitor antibiotic resistance competently in at least one national reference center. Ability to conduct vaccine trials will also depend on laboratory capability in the identification of specific serotypes for the main pathogens.

Research Priorities

During program design and implementation, high priority should also be assigned to establishing a strong evaluation or applied research component to aid in assessing the effectiveness of operational programs, refining program priorities, and addressing the many questions which remain regarding optimal strategies for prevention and case management. The World Health Organization recently reviewed research priorities for ARI control (WHO/ARI 1989a, 1990), preparing a list which we have adapted and present below.

- Assess the effectiveness of interventions and programs to modify the risk of pneumonia, especially through reduction of exposure to biomass fuel emissions.
- Document the epidemiology of invasive strains of *Hemophilus influenzae* and *Streptococcus pneumoniae* to guide the development of effective vaccines.
- Define the relative prevalence and etiologies of pneumonia, sepsis, and meningitis in less immunocompetent groups such as young infants (less than three months of age) and undernourished children.
- Identify the signs and symptoms which indicate the need for hospital care.
- Evaluate the performance of the treatment protocols, including for wheezing, at first-level referral facilities.
- Explore the most effective ways to define and teach the reliable distinction between clinical presentations of pneumonia and malaria and to determine the effectiveness of co-trimoxazole in treatment of malaria.
- Define the clinical features and optimal treatment of serious bacterial infections (pneumonia, sepsis, and meningitis) in young infants (less than three months of age).
- Determine the special needs of undernourished children, including defining the clinical features and causes of pneumonia and the optimal treatment for these children.
- Examine cultural and other factors which determine the ability of families to recognize signs of pneumonia, seek appropriate care, and comply with treatment regimens.
- Identify optimally effective strategies for the design of appropriate health education programs, including strategies for the modification of risk factors for pneumonia.

- Develop inexpensive, simple, and reliable diagnostic technologies to aid in counting respiratory rate and determining the etiology of pneumonia, such as by identifying viral or bacterial antigens in urine or blood.
- Perform field trials of the available polysaccharide pneumococcal vaccine and conjugate vaccines for *H. influenzae* type b and for nonserotypable *H. influenzae*, RSV, and parainfluenza viruses, when available.

Additional research needs that must be addressed include the development and validation of survey techniques for detection of ARI episodes and pneumonia deaths for use in program evaluation. Studies are also needed to determine the effect of antibiotic use on the incidence of and mortality from other diseases (especially malaria and diarrhea) and the sociocultural factors which modulate the effectiveness of programs. Vaccine research issues, in addition to those detailed in the list above, should include additional efficacy trials of the newer measles vaccines and two-dose schedules of administration.

Another issue for operational research will be the effect of current program emphasis on children under five. Promoting the recognition of the need and increasing the demand for health services will be essential to the success of ARI control programs. Although the opportunity to have an effect is greatest among the program's target group, it will be important to assess the benefits and costs to national programs which attempt to reserve the attention of health workers and the supplies of antibiotics for children at the perceived expense of the communities' adult decisionmakers and opinion leaders.

Opportunities to explore mechanisms to achieve financial sustainability may be limited for the immunization interventions designed to prevent ARI. For the curative care provided in the case management of ARI, however, it will be important to explore mechanisms for cost recovery, such as health insurance schemes, taxation, and user fees, to increase the financial sustainability of national programs.

Appendix 4A. Sources of Data and Method Used to Obtain Cost-Effectiveness Estimates Summarized in Table 4-3

Since no prospective data are available for the effectiveness of preventive interventions in the reduction of ARI mortality among children under five, the estimates used in table 4-3 are obtained primarily from retrospective observations of relative risk. These figures, therefore, represent indirect estimates of the potential effectiveness of the intervention rather than a measure of effectiveness achieved in an operational setting. Cost estimates for these preventive interventions are also obtained indirectly, through review of data for similar programs. Cost estimates for case management interventions are similarly derived from data available from other programs with similar interventions.

Estimates assume a standard population of 1 million persons, with 15 percent of the population being children under five (approximately 3 percent infants) and 8 percent mothers of

children under five. Estimates of cost and effectiveness for immunization interventions are made using a coverage range of 45 to 90 percent, as used by Feachem and Koblinsky (1983). "Most likely" values for immunization interventions are calculated assuming an immunization coverage of 80 percent, the target specified for UNICEF's goal of universal childhood immunization. Calculations of deaths averted are based on preintervention ARI-specific mortality rates of 5 to 20 per 1,000 (with a most likely value of 10 per 1,000), which yields an expected 750 to 3,000 (most likely 1,500) deaths among the 150,000 children under five in the standard population of 1 million.

The effect of implementing multiple interventions to prevent ARI mortality is unlikely to be simply additive. Many children who die with ARI suffer from several risk factors, such as the malnourished child who dies of pneumococcal pneumonia during or within one month of an episode of measles. One possibility is that such competing risks of mortality may operate on the same children, so that prevention of one potentially mortal event may only leave children vulnerable to other causes of so-called "replacement mortality" (WHO/EPI 1987).

Another possibility is that prevention of ARI is actually synergistic with other preventive interventions through reducing the cumulative contributions to the frailty (Mosley 1985) of the child, such as is observed in the growth faltering that occurs with recurrent infection. An example of the potential for synergism among interventions has been suggested by recent observations of a reduction of mortality from diarrheal disease in a program which treats only childhood pneumonias (WHO 1988).

The calculations presented below consider only the short-term effects of these interventions upon mortality. It is not known whether the long-term effect of these preventive and curative interventions would be augmented by reduction in the frailty of these children, or offset by replacement mortality. Because of these theoretical problems and the many operational problems associated with predicting the effects of multiple health interventions, the figures presented in table 4-3 are of use primarily as estimates of the relative cost-effectiveness of interventions when implemented alone to reduce ARI mortality.

Expanded Programme on Immunization

Most of the ARI mortality prevented by the EPI vaccines is due to measles and pertussis. Feachem and Koblinsky (1983) estimate that measles immunization between the ages of nine months and twelve months, with an ideal effectiveness of 90 percent and a coverage of between 45 and 90 percent, can avert 44 to 64 percent of measles cases. In anticipation of the improved effectiveness of the higher-potency vaccines and immunization before nine months of age, the upper limit of the proportion of cases averted was adjusted to 80 percent. Since pertussis vaccine has a similar ideal effectiveness, it is assumed that a similar proportion of cases would be averted at the same coverage rates of 45 to 90 percent. Therefore, for pertussis and measles, an effectiveness range of 44 to 80 percent has been used for the model, with an intermediate most likely value of 65 percent.

It has been estimated that up to 2,596 of ARI mortality may be preventable if current EPI vaccines are used. Mortality among children under five due to measles-associated ARI accounted for approximately 20 percent of all ARI mortality (1.8 per 1,000 out of 9.1 per 1,000) in seventeen study areas during case management trials for WHO (WHO/ARI 1988). It is therefore assumed that 20 to 25 percent of ARI mortality would be addressed through use of current EPI vaccines. An expected ARI-specific mortality reduction of 8.8 to 20 percent (most likely 14.6 percent) may be calculated from these figures. These estimates are comparable to the ARI mortality reduction figures of 5 to 20 percent calculated by Singhi and Singhi (1987), although it was observed that measles vaccine provided an effective protection of 22 percent against respiratory deaths in Bangladesh. Based on the expected number of deaths of 750 to 3,000, the number of deaths averted may be calculated to range from 66 to 600, with a most likely value of 219.

The cost per child served for EPI immunization interventions to prevent ARI mortality is calculated as that portion of the cost of delivering all EPI vaccines, which is proportional to the benefit achieved in averting ARI deaths. Tetanus is the only non-ARI EPI disease which is a significant cause of infant and child mortality. Since tetanus accounts for up to 40 percent of the overall mortality prevented through EPI vaccines, 60 percent ($9.08) of the $15.13 average cost per fully immunized child (Brenzel 1989) was ascribed to ARI prevention. The cost per ARI death averted (achieving coverage levels of 45 to 90 percent among the 30,000 infants in the target age group) may, therefore, be calculated at $409 to $1,857, with a most likely value of $995.

Pneumococcal Immunization

The effectiveness of pneumococcal vaccine, particularly among the youngest children, has not been clearly demonstrated in the developing world. The reported effective range in adults of 0 to 80 percent and the effectiveness of 69 percent noted among children in the United States suggest a range of 0 to 70 percent. Still, because the vaccine is less immunogenic among children under two (who constitute approximately 40 percent of children under five), an estimated 20 percent of invasive, pneumococcal infections in developing countries are caused by serotypes not included in the vaccine, and assuming a 45 to 90 percent coverage (as for the EPI vaccines), the expected disease-specific mortality reduction may be in the range of 0 to 30 percent. An intermediate most likely value of 15 percent has been selected.

Since pneumococcal disease accounts for less than one-third to one-half of pneumonia cases (WHO/RSD 1986), the maximal reduction in pneumonia mortality with the presently available vaccine is likely about 0 to 15 percent, with a most likely value of 7 percent. Although this range does not include the greater reductions in ARI-specific mortality observed among children six months through fifty-nine months of age in Papua New Guinea (Riley and others 1986), the epidemiology of pneumo-

coccal disease in that country is probably not typical of that in most developing countries. On the basis of the 750 to 3,000 expected deaths among children under five, the number of deaths averted may be calculated to be from 0 to 450, with a most likely value of 105.

The estimated cost per child vaccinated is calculated by reducing the current price of the vaccine ($9.69 per dose) by one-half (assuming that the cost will be reduced for the international market in exchange for waiver of liability and once research and development costs are recovered) and adding the cost per dose delivered for the EPI vaccines ($2.44 average), since the costs of EPI vaccines ($0.04–$0.15 per dose) are small in relation to the cost of the pneumococcal vaccine. The resulting estimated cost per dose delivered of $7.28 suggests that (at coverage levels of 45 to 90 percent) the cost per death averted would be greater than $437, with a most likely value of $1,664.

Breastfeeding Promotion

Reductions in incidence of and case-fatality ratios for pneumonia that have been noted with breastfeeding (Chandra 1979; LePage, Munyakazi, and Hennart 1981; Victora and others 1987) suggest that a 50 to 80 percent ARI-specific mortality reduction might be realized among breastfed infants. The protective effect is observed, however, only below twelve months of age (approximately 20 percent of children under five), and actual prevalence of breastfeeding among infants is generally over 80 percent in high-mortality countries, such that only about 4 percent of children under five would benefit from a program to promote breastfeeding. Even assuming 100 percent effectiveness in changing breastfeeding practice, the reduction of ARI-specific mortality among children under five resulting from such promotion would be only 2 to 3.2 percent (with, on the basis of Victora's observation of over 70 percent reduction in relative risk, a most likely value of 2.8 percent). The end result would be an estimated fifteen to ninety-six (most likely forty-two) deaths averted through promotion of breastfeeding.

The average cost of a program to promote breastfeeding has been estimated at $5 (Feachem and Koblinsky 1984; Feachem 1986; Phillips, Feachem, and Mills 1987) per mother. Even if targeting of services is only adequate to identify the subset of 50 percent of the mothers who are "at risk" of not breastfeeding, the population served might be reduced to half of the mothers with infants (8,000 in the standard population of 1 million). The estimated cost per ARI death averted for an educational program to promote breastfeeding may be calculated to be $417 to $2,667, with a most likely value of $952.

Reduction of Malnutrition

Expected mortality reduction with improved nutritional status was estimated on the basis of mortality two to twenty times higher observed in malnourished children (Kielmann and McCord 1978; Tupasi and others 1988). Successful improvement of nutritional status might be expected to result in a 50 to 95 percent reduction in the risk of ARI-mortality among malnourished children. A most likely value of 80 percent reflects the modest estimate of a fivefold higher relative risk of pneumonia deaths among these malnourished children. Since 70 to 90 percent of all pneumonia deaths occur among the malnourished, expected ARI-specific mortality reductions of 35 to 85 percent (most likely 64 percent) might be expected with successful improvement of nutritional status. Support for these estimates is provided by the results of a nutritional intervention program in Tanzania (UNICEF 1988b), where a 23 percent reduction (from 48 to 37 percent) in the prevalence of mild to moderate malnutrition (less than 80 percent weight-for-age) and a 60 percent reduction (from 5 to 2 percent) in the prevalence of severe malnutrition (less than 60 percent weight-for-age) were associated with a 64 percent reduction in ARI-specific mortality. The expected number of ARI deaths averted at this level of effectiveness would be 263 to 2,550, with a most likely value of 960, although these figures would be highly dependent on the initial prevalence of undernutrition.

The lower estimate for the cost of such a program to improve nutritional status is based on expenditure of $15.00 per year per malnourished child under five (Ashworth and Feachem 1986), although effective targeting of the malnourished children would be difficult to achieve. The Joint Nutrition Support Program in Tanzania (UNICEF 1988b) estimated its costs at $10.05 per child per year (from both national and donor sources), with the addition of $9.00 per child for start-up costs. Annual costs may be estimated at $11.85 per child if the initial program start-up costs can be spread over five years. On the basis of this model, therefore, the cost per million population would likely be between $810,000, for the targeted program for the expected 54,000 children (36 percent, on the basis of 1990 UNICEF data) (UNICEF 1991) who are malnourished, and

$1,777,500, to serve all 150,000 children expected in the sample population. The use of the most likely value of $1,500,000 reflects the better credibility of the figures from Tanzania. Final evaluation of the Joint Nutrition Support Program may yield costs per child as low as $2.50 per year (UNICEF, personal communication, June 1991). On the basis of the less favorable preliminary figures, however, the cost per death averted is calculated to be $697 to $3,080, with a most likely value of $1,563.

Case Management

There is little information available to date regarding the cost of operational programs for ARI case management for which effectiveness has also been assessed. Cost per child treated and death averted may, however, be estimated from drug costs and costs for implementing other programs with similar interventions. The following model was constructed to provide an estimate of the cost of case management for cost-effectiveness calculations.

The cost per million population of appropriate case management for ARI is equal to the sum of the costs of the following:

- Health education or sensitization regarding program interventions (E).
- Outpatient care for coughs and colds ($U \cdot C_u \cdot (V + M + Z \cdot A)$), where U = the incidence of coughs and colds (per 1,000), C_u = the coverage or proportion of coughs and colds in the community which come to the attention of the health care system, V = the average cost of an ambulatory care visit or consultation, M = the cost of nonantimicrobial medications, Z = the proportion of URI cases inappropriately treated with antimicrobials, and A = the average cost of a course of antimicrobials).

Table 4A-1. Range of Values for Variables in Model of Cost-Effectiveness of ARI Case Management

Symbol	Variable	Least favorable	Most likely	Most favorable
E	Sensitization cost	$800,000	$400,000	$80,000
V	Cost of one outpatient consultation	$2.00	$1.50	$1.00
M	Cost per episode of non-antimicrobial pharmaceuticals	$3.20	$0.08	0
A	Cost per episode of antimicrobials	$7.00	$0.80	$0.16
H	Cost of inpatient or referral care	$135	$45	$6
N	Average number of visits per episode	2	1.5	1
U	Cases of coughs and colds	1,500,000	1,050,000	600,000
P	Cases of uncomplicated pneumonia	5,000	7,500	10,000
S	Cases of severe or complicated pneumonia	1,000	1,500	2,000
C_u	Proportion of URI cases seen and treated by health worker	0.10	0.05	0.02
Z	Proportion of URI cases seen and treated with antibiotics	0.50	0.10	0
C_p	Proportion of uncomplicated pneumonia cases appropriately diagnosed and treated	0.10	0.40	0.70
C_s	Proportion of severe pneumonia cases appropriately diagnosed and treated	0.40	0.65	0.90
F_p	Case-fatality ratio for untreated uncomplicated pneumonia	0.10	0.13	0.20
F_s	Case-fatality ratio for untreated severe or complicated pneumonia	0.25	0.35	0.50
R_s	Percent reduction in mortality with appropriate antibiotic treatment	0.60	0.80	0.90

Source: See text of appendix.

Table 4A-2. Derived Variables and Their Most Likely Values

Symbol	Variable	Derivation[a]	Most likely value (U.S. dollars)
C	Cost per capita of ARI care	$E + U \cdot C_u \cdot (V + M + Z \cdot A) + P \cdot C_p$ $(M + A + N \cdot V) + S \cdot C_s (V + H)$	0.54
T_p	Number of uncomplicated pneumonia cases treated	$P \cdot C_p$	3,000
T_s	Number of complicated or severe pneumonia cases treated	$S \cdot C_s$	975
D	Number of ALRI deaths averted	$(T_p \cdot F_p + T_s \cdot F_s) \cdot R$	585
CE	Cost-effectiveness, or cost per ALRI death averted	C, D	926
CE_{DALY}	Cost per disability-adjusted life-year saved	CE/25	37

a. For symbols not defined in this table, see table 4A-1.

- Outpatient care for pneumonia ($P \cdot C_p \cdot (M + A + N \cdot V)$), where P = the incidence of pneumonia (per million), C_p = the coverage or proportion of pneumonia cases in the community which are diagnosed and treated appropriately (that is, given antimicrobials with or without other medications for supportive care), and N = the number of consultations per episode).

- Inpatient care for severe pneumonia ($S \cdot C_s \cdot (H + V)$), where S = the incidence of severe pneumonia (per million), C_s = the coverage or proportion of severe pneumonia in the community which is diagnosed and treated appropriately (that is, given antimicrobials and referred for more specialized care), and H = the cost of referral, generally including impatient hospital care).

Therefore, the total cost of case management per million population is:

$$E + U \cdot C_u \cdot (V + M + Z \cdot A) + P \cdot C_p \cdot (M + A + N \cdot V) + S \cdot C_s \cdot (H + V)$$

Clearly, each of the variables in the model has a range of values. Calculations of cost and effectiveness were made using a range of values including "most favorable," for the effect on cost-effectiveness, "least favorable," and "most likely." The specific values used for each variable are listed in table 4A-1 and the "most likely" values for the derived variables in table 4A-2.

Sensitization costs (E) are derived from estimates by Phillips, Feachem, and Mills (1987), including a low-cost option, which used person-to-person communications at a cost of $1 per mother (in groups of ten), and a high-cost program, which used mass media at a cost of $10 per mother (assuming that there are 80,000 mothers of children under five). The intermediate cost program estimate of a cost of $5 per mother equals those estimates used for breastfeeding promotion and weaning education programs (Feachem 1986; Phillips, Feachem, and Mills 1987).

The cost of one outpatient consultation (V) has been derived from figures for diarrheal disease and immunization consultations (Phillips, Feachem, and Mills 1987), under the assumption that the time spent by the health worker is comparable. A high-cost figure of $2.00 reflects average costs per visit in many Latin American countries, the intermediate cost of $1.50 and low cost of $1.00 are more typical of costs per outpatient consultation in Asia and Africa. Costs for non-antimicrobial pharmaceuticals (M), which are optional in the management of ARI, are estimated at zero for the low-cost figure, $0.08 for intermediate costs typical of five days supply of a locally made cough syrup, and $3.20 to reflect the often larger expenditure on nonantimicrobial pharmaceuticals in many developing countries (Quick and others 1988).

The values selected for the cost per episode of antimicrobials (A) were based on UNICEF prices in 1988 for a five-day course for a child weighing ten kilograms. These figures were doubled to include costs for transport, packaging, and dispensing these medications. Basic prices included a low-cost figure of $0.08 for five days of co-trimoxazole for a ten-kilogram child, $0.40 for the intermediate figure (Bates and others 1987; Quick and others 1988), and $3.50 for intramuscular penicillin and chloramphenicol for the high-cost program. Costs for referral care with hospitalization (H) used in the model include a high-cost figure of $135 (three days at $45 per day) from Brazil, an intermediate figure of $45 (three days at $15 per day) from Rwanda (Shepard 1989), and a low-cost figure of $6 (three days at $2 per day). The ideal number of visits per episode (N) is 2, although a lower average value of 1 is used, because some programs require no follow-up visit (WHO 1988). The intermediate figure of 1.5 reflects probable level of compliance with the recommended follow-up visit.

The values used for high, intermediate, and low incidence of coughs and colds among children under five (U) are ten, seven, and four per child per year (Datta Banik, Krishna, and Mane 1969; Kamath and others 1969; Friej and Wall 1977; Foreit and Lesevic 1987), yielding the numbers of episodes specified in table 4A-1 among the 150,000 children under five in the standard population. For pneumonia incidence (P), the figures selected were 100, 50, and 25 per 1,000 (Riley and Douglas 1981; Pio, Leowski, and Luelmo 1982; WHO/ARI 1989b), suggesting a range of 5,000 to 10,000 cases of uncomplicated pneumonia. For severe pneumonia (S), the figures are 25, 10, and 5 per 1,000 (Chen and others 1980; Riley and others 1983; WHO 1984), implying a range of 1,000 to 2,000 cases of severe pneumonia, with a most likely value of 1,500.

Although ideally fewer than 2 percent of coughs and colds will be brought to the attention of and diagnosed by the health worker (C_u), a likelier figure is 5 percent, and more than 10 percent has been observed in some programs (Foreit and Lesevic 1987). The cost of inappropriate treatment of coughs and colds with antibiotics is included in the model, since this may be a source of excess costs and of potential savings in improving case management practices (Stansfield 1990). The percentage of coughs and colds seen by a health worker and treated inappropriately with antibiotics (z) will ideally be zero, although in many programs up to half of such cases receive antimicrobials. A most likely value of 10 percent should be achievable with careful training and supervision of health workers. A study in Lesotho (Redd, Moteetee, and Waldman 1990) found that 6 to 15 percent of practitioners (before being retrained under WHO guidelines) reported that they would treat a cough or cold with antimicrobials, so it is likely that observed rates of inappropriate use of antimicrobials would exceed these reported rates.

For pneumonia coverage (c_p), the figures selected for the model are 70 percent, 40 percent, and 10 percent. The World Health Organization estimates that 12 percent of all childhood pneumonias were treated with antibiotics in 1990, and it projects increases to 40 percent in 1995 and 60 percent by 2000 (WHO/ARI 1991a). Although there are no good data from operational setting, it has been estimated that from 40 to 90 percent (with a most likely value of 65) of severe pneumonias may be seen and diagnosed by a health care worker (c_s). Incidence and coverage figures selected for URI and pneumonias suggest that 4 percent (least favorable) to 50 percent ("most favorable")— with a most likely value of 17 percent—of all cases of ARI presenting to health facilities would be diagnosed as pneumonia. These figures reflect such measurements made in operational settings (WHO/ARI 1990; Foreit and Lesevic 1987; Quick and others 1988). The incidence (P and S) and case-fatality

ratios (F_p and F_s) specified in table 4-6 yield ARI-specific mortality values of 5 per 1,000, 10 per 1,000, and 20 per 1,000, reflecting probable levels of ARI mortality (UNICEF 1991; WHO/ARI 1991b) among children under five in middle-mortality, high-mortality, and very high mortality countries. Numbers of deaths averted were, therefore, calculated on the basis of expected numbers of deaths of 750 (5 per 1,000), 1,500 (10 per 1,000), and 3,000 (50 per 1,000) for moderate-, high-, and very high mortality countries, respectively. The range of assumptions for effectiveness of treatment (R) includes 90 percent for a highly efficacious program (Berman and McIntosh 1985), 80 percent for the intermediate level of effectiveness (Institute of Medicine 1986), and 60 percent for the lower level of effectivenesss, such as may be seen in settings where compliance is poor.

The additional variables defined in table 4A-2 were derived from the values for each variable specified in table 4A-1. Calculation of the cost per capita of ARI care (C) using these figures yields a most likely per capita value of $0.54, or $541,877 for the sample population of 1 million. The ranges for total cost (of $220,000 to $940,000) and for the cost-effectiveness figures used in table 4-3 reflect values obtained from the sensitivity analysis, which is summarized in table 4A-3, obtained by varying one parameter at a time. The sensitivity analysis data indicate that program costs and cost-effectiveness are most sensitive to the costs for health education, or "sensitization." The program effectiveness (as measured by deaths averted) is most sensitive to the proportion of uncomplicated pneumonia cases appropriately diagnosed and treated.

A most likely value for cost-effectiveness for ARI case management of $926 (per death averted) was calculated. Use of the extreme figures for incidence and case-fatality ratios (rather

Table 4A-3. Least and Most Favorable Costs, Effectiveness, and Cost-Effectiveness for Each Variable in Case Management Model for ARI

Variable[a]	Cost per capita (U.S. dollars)		Deaths averted		Cost-effectiveness (cost per death averted, U.S. dollars)	
	Least favorable	Most favorable	Least favorable	Most favorable	Least favorable	Most favorable
E	0.94	0.22	585	585	1,610	379
V	0.57	0.51	585	585	976	877
M	0.72	0.54	585	585	1,222	919
A	0.59	0.54	585	585	1,014	917
H	0.63	0.50	585	585	1,076	861
N	0.54	0.54	585	585	930	922
U	0.58	0.50	585	585	990	862
P	0.54	0.55	481	689	1,120	791
S	0.53	0.56	494	676	1,066	824
C_u	0.63	0.49	585	585	1,075	837
Z	0.56	0.54	585	585	955	919
C_p	0.53	0.55	351	819	1,524	670
C_s	0.52	0.56	480	690	1,093	811
F_p	0.54	0.54	513	753	1,056	720
F_s	0.54	0.54	585	702	926	772
R	0.54	0.54	439	658	1,235	823

Note: Figures enclosed in boxes represent the minimum and maximum values for cost, effectiveness, and cost-effectiveness.
a. For definition of symbols, see table 4A-1.
Source: Authors' data.

Table 4A-4. Cost-Effectiveness of ARI Case Management for Low- and High-Mortality Countries

Mortality	Low-mortality country	High-mortality country
Cost per capita of ARI care	$0.52	$0.56
Cost per target population	$3.49	$3.61
Deaths averted	338	1,160
Cost per death averted	$1,152	$483
Cost per disability-adjusted life-year saved	$46	$19

Source: See text of appendix.

than varying one parameter at a time, as in the sensitivity analysis), such as may be observed in high- and low-mortality countries, yields cost and effectiveness figures specified in table 4A-4. These figures underline the fact that interventions to improve ARI case management are of highest priority in the countries with high overall and ARI-specific infant and child mortality rates. These estimates are higher than the estimates of $350 per death averted obtained in a field study in Nepal and $131 per death averted obtained in the Philippines (John Snow International, unpublished data).

Calculations of cost per discounted healthy year of life saved are made using a life expectancy of fifty years, an average age at death of two years, and a discount rate of 3 percent per annum. Ranges for the intermediate variables and a summary of the cost-effectiveness calculation are presented in table 4-3, in a format for comparison with the analogous figures for the other ARI interventions.

Notes

The authors would like to express their gratitude for the invaluable contributions of the many colleagues and friends who reviewed and commented on drafts of this chapter, with special recognition of assistance provided by C. J. Clements, Nils M. P. Daulaire, Floyd W. Denny, Don de Savigny, Ralph R. Frerichs, Y. Ghendon, Sandy Gove, Davidson Gwatkin, Dean Jamison, Joel A. Lamounier, Nancy Pielemeier, Antonio Pio, Mark C. Steinhoff, Tessa L. Tan-Torres, and James Tulloch.

References

Aaby, Peter. 1988. "Malnutrition and Overcrowding/Intensive Exposure in Severe Measles Infection: Review of Community Studies." *Reviews of Infectious Diseases* 10:478–91.

Armstrong, J. R. M., and H. Campbell. 1991. "Indoor Air Pollution Exposure and Lower Respiratory Infections in Young Gambian Children." *International Journal of Epidemiology* 20(2):424–29.

Ashworth, Ann and Richard G. Feachem. 1986. *Interventions for the Control of Diarrhoeal Diseases among Young Children: Growth Monitoring Programmes.* Geneva: World Health Organization.

Balint, O., and K. Anand. 1979. "Infectious and Parasitic Diseases in Zambian Children." *Tropical Doctor* 9:99–103.

Barclay, A. J. G., A. Foster, and A. Sommer. 1987. "Vitamin A Supplementation and Mortality Related to Measles: A Randomised Clinical Trial." *British Medical Journal* 294:294–96.

Bates, J. A., Bimo, P. Tengko, P. Foreman, B. Santoso, D. Adi, D. Ross-Degnan, and J. D. Quick. 1987. "Child Survival Pharmaceuticals in Indonesia: Opportunities for Therapeutic and Economic Efficiencies in Pharmaceutical Supply and Use." Management Sciences for Health, Yayasan Indonesia Sejahtera, Ministry of Health. Boston, Mass.

Berman, Stephen. 1991. "Epidemiology of Acute Respiratory Infections in Children of Developing Countries." *Reviews of Infectious Diseases* 13(Supplement 6):S454–62.

Berman, Stephen, A. Duenas, A. Bedoya, and others. 1983. "Acute Lower Respiratory Tract Illnesses in Cali, Colombia: A Two-Year Ambulatory Study." *Pediatrics* 71:210–18.

Berman, Stephen, and Kenneth McIntosh. 1985. "Selective Primary Health Care: Strategies for Control of Disease in the Developing World. XXI. Acute Respiratory Infections." *Reviews of Infectious Diseases* 71(5):674–91.

Black, F. L. 1982. "The Role of Herd Immunity in Control of Measles." *Yale Journal of Biology and Medicine* 55:351–60.

Black, S. B., H. R. Shinefield, R. A. Hiatt, B. H. Fireman, and the Kaiser Permanente Pediatric Vaccine Study Group. 1988. "Efficacy of *Haemophilus influenzae* Type B Capsular Polysaccharide Vaccine." *Pediatric Infectious Disease* 7:149–56.

Bloem, M. W., M. Wedel, R. J. Egger and others. 1990. "Mild Vitamin A Deficiency and Risk of Respiratory Tract Diseases and Diarrhea in Preschool and School Children in Northeastern Thailand." *American Journal of Epidemiology* 131:332–39.

Borrero, I., L. Farjardo P., A. Bedoya M., A. Zea, F. Carmona, and M. F. de Borrero. 1990. "Acute Respiratory Tract Infections among a Birth Cohort of Children from Cali, Colombia, Who Were Studied through 17 Months of Age." *Reviews of Infectious Diseases* 12(Supplement 8):S950–56.

Brahmans, D. 1986. "Does Pertussis Vaccine Cause Brain Damage?" *Lancet* 2:286.

Brenzel, Logan. 1989. "The Costs of EPI: A Review of Cost and Cost-Effectiveness Studies (1979–1987)." Resources for Child Health (REACH) Project, Rosslyn, Va.: John Snow, Inc., April.

———. 1990. "Cost and Cost-Effectiveness Issues for ARI Case Management." In *ALRI and Child Survival in Developing Countries: Understanding the Current Status and Directions for the 1990s.* Proceedings of a workshop given by the Johns Hopkins University School of Hygiene and Public Health. Washington, D.C.: Institute for International Programs, and the U.S. Agency for International Development, August 2–3.

Broome, C. V. 1981. "Epidemiology of Pertussis, Atlanta, 1977." *Journal of Pediatrics* 98:362–67.

Bulia, A., and K. L. Hitze. 1978. "Acute Respiratory Infections: A Review." *Bulletin of the World Health Organization* 56:481–98.

Burchfiel, C. M., M. W. Higgins, J. B. Keller, W. F. Howatt, W. J. Butler, and I. T. T. Higgins. 1986. "Passive Smoking in Childhood." *American Review of Respiratory Diseases* 133:966–73.

Bwibo, N. O. 1971. "Whooping Cough in Uganda." *Scandinavian Journal of Infectious Diseases* 3:41–43.

Byass, P., H. Campbell, T. J. O'Dempsey, and B. M. Greenwood. 1991. "Coincidence of Malaria Parasitemia and Abnormal Chest X-ray Findings in Young Gambian Children." *Journal of Tropical Medicine and Hygiene* 94:22–23.

Camargos, P. A., M. D. Guimaraes, and E. de F. Drummond. 1989. "Mortalidade por pneumonia em crianças menores de conco anos de idade em localidade do estado de Minas Gerais (Brasil), 1979–1985." *Revue de Saude Publica* 23(5):398–94.

Campbell, H., J. R. M. Armstrong, and P. Byass. 1989. "Indoor Air Pollution in Developing Countries and Acute Respiratory Infection in Children." *Lancet* 1:1012.

Campbell, H., P. Byass, and B. Greenwood. 1988. "Simple Clinical Signs for Diagnosis of Acute Lower Respiratory Tract Infections." *Lancet* 1:742–43.

Campbell, H., P. Byass, I. M. Forgie, and N. Lloyd-Evans. 1989. "Clinical Signs of Pneumonia in Children." *Lancet* 1:899–900.

Campbell, H., P. Byass, A. C. Lamont, and others. 1989. "Assessment of Clinical Criteria for Identification of Acute Lower Respiratory Tract Infections in Children." *Lancet* 1:297–99.

Chandra, R. K. 1979. "Prospective Studies of the Effect of Breastfeeding on the Incidence of Infection and Allergy." *Acta Pediatrica Scandinavica* 68:691–94.

Chaulet, P., and N. Ait Khaled. 1982. "Enquête sur les infections respiratoires aiguës et la prescription d'antibiotiques dans les unités sanitaires de base en Algeria, au cours de l'année 1980." *Revue Français des Maladies Respiratoires* 10(1):45–52.

Chen, B. H., C. J. Hong, M. R. Pandey, and K. R. Smith. 1990. "Indoor Air Pollution in Developing Countries." *World Health Statistics Quarterly* 43:127–38.

Chen, Lincoln C., Mizanur Rahman, and A. M. Sarder. 1980. "Epidemiology and Causes of Death among Children in a Rural Area of Bangladesh." *International Journal of Epidemiology* 9:25–33.

Chen Yue, Wanxian Li, and Shunzhang Yu. 1986. "Influence of Passive Smoking on Admissions for Respiratory Illness in Early Childhood." *British Medical Journal* 293:303–6.

Cherian, Thomas, T. Jacob John, Eric Simoes, Mark C. Steinhoff, and Meray John. 1988. "Evaluation of Simple Clinical Signs for the Diagnosis of Acute Lower Respiratory Tract Infections." *Lancet* 2:125–28.

Cherian, Thomas., Eric A. F. Simoes, Mark C. Steinhoff, K. Chitra, Meray John, P. Raghupathy, and T. Jacob John. 1990. "Bronchiolitis in Tropical South India." *American Journal of Diseases of Children* 144.

Cherry, J. D. 1984. In *Current Problems in Pediatrics* 14:68.

Church, M. A. 1979. "Evidence of Whooping Cough Vaccine Efficacy from the 1978 Whooping Cough Epidemic in Hertfordshire." *Lancet* 2:188–90.

Cohen, Sheldon, David Tyrell, and Andrew Smith. 1991. "Psychological Stress and Susceptibility to the common cold." *The New England Journal of Medicine* 325(9):606–12.

Crofton, J., and A. Douglas. 1975. *Respiratory Diseases.* Oxford: Blackwell.

Dabis, François, A. Sow, Ronald Waldman, and others. 1988. "The Epidemiology of Measles in a Partially Vaccinated Population in an African City: Implications for Immunization Programs." *American Journal of Epidemiology* 127:171–78.

Datta, Neena 1987. "Acute Respiratory Infection in Low Birth Weight Infants." *Indian Journal of Pediatrics* 54:171–76.

Datta Banik, N. D., R. Krishna, and S. I. S. Mane. 1969. "A Longitudinal Study of Morbidity and Mortality Pattern of Children under Age of Five Years in an Urban Community." *Indian Journal of Medical Research* 57:948–57.

de Koning, H. W., K. R. Smith and J. R. Last. 1985. "Biomass Fuel Consumption and Health." *Bulletin of the World Health Organization* 63(1):11–26.

Denny, F. W., and W. A. Clyde. 1983. "Acute Respiratory Tract Infections: An Overview." *Pediatric Research* 17:1026–29.

Douglas, R. G., K. M. Lindgram, and R. B. Cough. 1968. "Exposure to Cold Environment and Rhinovirus Cold: Failure to Demonstrate an Effect." *New England Journal of Medicine* 279:742–47.

Ekwo, E. E., M. W. Weinberger, P. A. Lachenbruch, and W. H. Huntley. 1983. "Relationship of Parental Smoking and Gas Cooking to Respiratory Disease in Children." *Chest* 84:662–68.

El-Mouza, M. I., K. Twan-Danso, B. H. Al-Awamy, G. A. Niazi, and M. T. Altork. 1988. "Pneumococcal Infections in Eastern Saudi Arabia: Serotypes and Antibiotic Sensitivity Patterns." *Tropical and Geographic Medicine* 40:213–17.

Escobar, J. A., A. S. Dover, and A. Duenas. 1976. "Etiology of Respiratory Infections in Children in Cali, Colombia." *Pediatrics* 57:123–30.

Escola, J. H. Kiyhty, A. K. Takala, H. Peltola, P.-R. Ronnberg, E. Kela, E. Pekkanen, P. H. McVerry, and P. H. Makela. 1990. "A Randomized, Prospective Field Trial of a Conjugate Vaccine in the Protection of Infants and Young Children against Invasive *Haemophilus influenzae* Type B Disease." *New England Journal of Medicine* 323(20):1381–87.

Fine, P. E., and J. A. Clarkson. 1987. "Reflections on the Efficacy of Pertussis Vaccine." *Reviews of Infectious Diseases* 9(5):866–83.

Feachem, R. G. A. 1986. "Preventing Diarrhoea: What Are the Policy Options?" *Health Policy and Planning* 1(2):109–17.

Feachem, R. G. A., and M. A. Koblinsky. 1983. "Interventions for the Control of Diarrhoeal Diseases among Young Children: Measles Immunization." *Bulletin of the World Health Organization* 61(4):641–52.

———. 1984. "Interventions for the Control of Diarrhoeal Diseases among Young Children: Promotion of Breastfeeding." *Bulletin of the World Health Organization* 62(2):271–91.

Foreit, Karen G., D. Haustein, M. Winterhalter, and E. La Mata. 1991. "Costs and Benefits of Implementing Child Survival Services at a Private Mining Company in Peru." *American Journal of Public Health* 81(8):1055–57.

Foreit, Karen G., and B. Lesevic. 1987. "Business Analysis: Implementing Child Survival Services at a Private Mining Company in Peru." Technical Information on Population and the Private Sector (TIPPS) Project, John Short and Associates and the U.S. Agency for International Development. Sponsored by USAID, Washington, D.C.

Foulke, F. G., K. G. Reeh, A. V. Graham, and others. 1988. "Family Function, Respiratory Illness and Otitis Media in Urban Black Infants." *Family Medicine* 20:128–32.

Freij, L., and S. Wall. 1977. "Exploring Child Health and Its Ecology: The Kirkos Study in Addis Ababa: An Evaluation of Procedures in the Measurement of Acute Morbidity and a Search for Causal Structure." *Acta Pediatrica Scandinavica* 5:267.

Funkhouser, A., M. C. Steinhoff, and J. Ward. 1991. "*Haemophilus influenzae* Disease and Immunization in Developing Countries." *Reviews of Infectious Diseases* 13(Supplement 6):S542–54.

Garenne, Michel, Odile Leroy, Jean-Pierre Beau, and Ibrahima Sene. 1991. Child Mortality after High-Titre Measles Vaccines: Prospective Study in Senegal. *Lancet* 338(2):903–6.

Ghafoor, A., N. K. Nomani, Z. Ishaq, S. Z. Zaidi, F. Abnwar, M. I. Burney, A. W. Oureshi, and S. A. Ahmad. 1990. "Diagnoses of Acute Lower Respiratory Tract Infections in Children in Rawalpindi and Islamabad, Pakistan." *Reviews of Infectious Diseases* 12(Supplement 8):S907–14.

Ghana Health Assessment Project Team. 1981. "A Quantitative Method of Assessing the Health Impact of Different Diseases in Less Developed Countries." *International Journal of Epidemiology* 10:73–80.

Gilsdorf, J. R. 1988. "*Haemophilus influenzae* Type B Vaccine Efficacy in the United States." *Pediatric Infectious Disease* 7:147–48.

Graham, N. M. H., A. J. Woodward, P. Ryan, and R. M. Douglas. 1990. "Acute Respiratory Illness in Adelaide Children. 11: The Relationship of Maternal Stress, Social Supports and Family Functioning." *International Journal of Epidemiology* 19(4):937–44.

Granoff, D. M., P. G. Shackelford, B. K. Suarex, and others. 1986. "*Haemophilus influenzae* Type b Disease in Children Vaccinated with Type B Polysaccharide Vaccine." *New England Journal of Medicine* 315:1583–90.

Greenwood, B. M., A. M. Greenwood, A. K. Bradley, S. Tulloch, R. Hayes, and F. S. J. Oldfield. 1988. "Deaths in Infancy and Early Childhood in a Well-Vaccinated, Rural, West African Population," *Annals of Tropical Paediatrics* 7:91–99.

Gutiérrez, G., M. C. Martínez, H. Guiscafre, G. Gómez, A. Peniche, and O. Muñoz. 1986. "Encuesta sobre el uso de antimicrobianos en las infecciones repiratorias agudas en la población rural mexicana." *Boletín Medico-Hospital Infantil de México* 43(12):761–68.

Harlap, S., and A. M. Davies. 1974. "Infant Admissions to Hospital and Maternal Smoking." *Lancet* 1(875):529–32.

Harrison, L. H., A. W. Hightower, S. Gaventa, and others. 1987. "Case-Control Efficacy Study of the Polysaccharide *Haemophilus influenzae* Type B (Hib) Vaccine." Abstract 317, presented at the 27th Interscience Conference on Antimicrobial Agents and Chemotherapy, New York, October 5.

Hay, J. W., and R. S. Daum. 1987. "Cost-Benefit Analysis of Two Strategies for Prevention of *Haemophilus influenzae* Type B Infection." *Pediatrics* 80(3):319–29.

Hayes, Richard, Thierry Mertens, Geraldine Lockett, and Laura Rodrigues. 1989. "Causes of Adult Deaths in Developing Countries: A Review of Data and Methods." PPR (Policy, Planning and Research) Working Paper. World Bank, Population Health and Nutrition, Population and Human Resources Department. July.

Heymann, David L., G. K. Mayben, K. R. Murphy, B. Guyer, and S. O. Foster. 1983. "Measles Control in Yaounde: Justification of a One Dose, Nine-Month Minimum Age Vaccination Policy in Tropical Africa." *Lancet* 127:788–94.

Honicky, R. E., J. S. Osborne, and C. A. Akpom. 1985. "Symptoms of Respiratory Illness in Young Children and the Use of Wood-Burning Stoves for Indoor Heating." *Pediatrics* 75(3):587–93.

Hossain, M. M., R. I. Glass, and M. R. Khan. 1982. "Antibiotic Use in a Rural Community in Bangladesh." *International Journal of Epidemiology* 11(4):402–5.

Hull, Harry F., J. W. Pap, and F. Oldfield. 1983. "Measles Mortality and Vaccine Efficacy in Rural West Africa." *Lancet* 1:972–75.

Hussey, G. D., and M. Klein. 1990. "A Randomized, Controlled Trial of Vitamin A in Children with Severe Measles." *New England Journal of Medicine* 323(3):160–64.

Ikejani, O. 1966. "Immunity against Diphtheria in Nigerian Children." *West African Medical Journal*:272–77.

Institute of Medicine. 1986. "The Burden of Disease Resulting from Acute Respiratory Illnesses." In *New Vaccine Development: Establishing Priorities* Volumes 1 and 2. Washington, D.C.: National Academy Press.

Jackson, G. G., R. L. Muldoon, G. C. Johnson, and others. 1963. "Contribution of Volunteers to Studies of the Common Cold." *American Review of Respiratory Diseases* 88(Supplement):120–27.

James, J. W. 1971. "Longitudinal Study of the Morbidity of Diarrheal and Respiratory Infections in Malnourished Children." *American Journal of Clinical Nutrition* 25:690–94.

Jason, Janine M., Philip Nieburg, J. S. Marks, and others. 1984. "Mortality and Infectious Disease Associated with Infant Feeding Practices in Developing Countries." *Pediatrics* 74(Supplement):702–27.

Kamat, S. R., K. D. Godkhindi, B. W. Shah, and others. 1980. "Correlation of Health Morbidity to Air Pollution Levels in Bombay City: Results of a Prospective 3 Year Survey at One Year." *Journal of Postgraduate Medicine* 26:45–62.

Kamath, K. R., R. A. Feldman, P. S. S. Sundar Rao, and others. 1969. "Infection and Disease in a Group of South Indian Families." *American Journal of Epidemiology* 89:375–83.

Keja, K., C. Chan, G. Hayden, and R. H. Henderson. 1988. "Expanded Programme on Immunization." *World Health Statistics Quarterly* 41:59–63.

Khan, J. A., D. G. Addiss, and Rizwan-Ullah. 1990. "Pneumonia and Community Health Workers." *Lancet* 336(8720):939.

Kiecolt-Glaser, J. K., and R. Glaser. 1986. "Psychological Influences on Immunity." *Psychosomatics* 27:621–24.

Kielmann, Ainfried Arndd, and Colin McCord. 1978. "Weight-for-Age as an Index of Risk of Death in Children." *Lancet* 1:1247–350.

Koplan, J. P., S. C. Schoenbaum, M. C. Weinstein, and D. W. Fraser. 1979. "Pertussis Vaccine—An Analysis of Benefits, Risks and Costs." *The New England Journal of Medicine* 301(17):906–11.

Kossove, D. 1982. "Smoke-Filled Rooms and Lower Respiratory Disease in Infants." *Sa Mediese Tydskri* 24 April:622–23.

Lataorre Otin, C., T. Juncosa Morros, and I. Sanfeliu Sala. 1988. "Antibiotic Susceptibility of *Streptococcus pneumoniae* Isolates from Pediatric Patients." *Journal of Antimicrobial Chemotherapy* 22:659–65.

Leeder, S. R., R. Corkhill, L. M. Irwig, W. W. Holland, and J. R. T. Colley. 1976. "Influence of Family Factors on the Incidence of Respiratory Infections in the First Year of Life." *British Journal of Preventive and Social Medicine* 30(4):203–12.

Leowski, Jerzy 1986. "Mortality from Acute Respiratory Infections in Children under Five Years of Age: Global Estimates." *World Health Statistics Quarterly* 39:138–44.

Lepage, P., C. Munyakazi, and P. Hennart. 1981. "Breastfeeding and Hospital Mortality in Children in Rwanda." *Lancet*: 409–11.

Linnemann, C. C., M. S. Yine, G. A. Roselle, and others. 1982. "Measles Immunity after Revaccination: Results in Children Vaccinated before 10 Months of Age." *Pediatrics* 69:332–35.

Lipsky, Benjamin A., E. J. Boyko, Thomas S. Inui, and others. 1986. "Risk Factors for Acquiring Pneumococcal Infections." *Archives of Internal Medicine* 146:2179–85.

Lucero, M. G., T. E. Tupasi, M. L. O. Gómez, G. L. Beltrán, A. U. Crisóstomo, V. V. Romano, and L. M. Rivera. 1990. "Respiratory Rate Greater than 50 per Minute as a Clinical Indicator of Pneumonia in Filipino Children with a Cough." *Reviews of Infectious Diseases* 12(Supplement 8):S1081–83.

McConnochie, K. M., C. B. Hall, and W. H. Barker. 1988. "Lower Respiratory Tract Illness in the First Two Years of Life: Epidemiologic Patterns and Costs in a Suburban Pediatric Practice." *American Journal of Public Health* 78(1):34–39.

McLean, A. R., and R. M. Anderson. 1988. "Measles in Developing Countries. Part II. The Predicted Impact of Mass Vaccination." *Epidemiology and Infection* 100:419–44.

Markowitz, Milton. 1981. "Observations on the Epidemiology and Preventibility of Rheumatic Fever in Developing Countries." *Clinical Therapeutics* 4(4):240–51.

Martin, T. R., and M. D. Bracken. 1986. "Association of Low Birth Weight with Passive Smoking in Pregnancy." *American Journal of Epidemiology* 124:633–42.

Mastro, Timothy D., Abdul Ghafoor, Nasreen Khalir Nomani, Zahir Ishaq, Favzal Anwar, Dan M. Granoff, John S. Spika, Clyde Thornsberry, and Richard R. Facklam. 1991. "Antimicrobial Resistance of Pneumococci in Children with Acute Lower Respiratory Tract Infection in Pakistan." *Lancet* 337:156–59.

Mata, Leonardo J. 1978. *The Children of Santa Maria Cauque: A Prospective Field Study of Health and Growth.* Cambridge, Mass.: MIT Press.

Miller, E., L. A. E. Ashworth, A. Robinson, P. A. Wright, and L. I. Irons. 1991. "Phase II Trial of Whole-Cell Pertussis Vaccine vs. an Acellular Vaccine Containing Agglutinogens." *Lancet* 337:70–73.

Mohs, Edgar. 1985. "Acute Respiratory Infections in Children: Possible Control Measures." PAHO *Bulletin* 19:82–87.

Monto, A. S., and B. M. Ullman. 1974. "Acute Respiratory Illness in an American Community: The Tecumseh Study." *Journal of the American Medical Association* 227:164–69.

Mosley, W. Henry. 1985. "Child Survival Research and Policy." *World Health Forum* 6:352–60.

Mosley, W. Henry, and S. Becker. 1988. "Demographic Models for Child Survival: Implications for Program Strategy." Paper presented at the seminar Child Survival Programs: Issues for the 1990s, Johns Hopkins University School of Hygiene and Public Health. Washington, D.C.: Institute for International Programs, November 21.

Muller, A. S., J. Leeuwenburg, and D. S. Pratt. 1986. "Pertussis: Epidemiology and Control." *Bulletin of the World Health Organization* 64(2):321–31.

Muyembe, J. J., F. Gatti, J. Spaepen, and J. Vandepitte. 1972. "L'épidémiologie de la diphtérie en la République du Zaire: le rôle de l'infection cutanée." *Annales de la Société Belge de Médecine Tropicale* 52:141–52.

Narain, J. P., and T. D. Sharma. 1987. "Acute Respiratory Infections in Kangra District: Magnitude and Current Treatment Practices." *Indian Journal of Pediatrics* 54(3):441–44.

Ngalikpima, V. F. 1983. "Review of Respiratory Infections in a Developing Country." *European Journal of Respiratory Diseases* 64:481–86.

Osterholm, M. T., J. H. Rambeck, K. E. White, and others. 1987. "Lack of Protective Efficacy and Increased Risk of Disease within 7 Days after Vaccination Associated with *Haemophilus influenzae* Type B (Hib) Polysaccharide (PS) Vaccine Use in Minnesota." Abstract 318, presented at the 27th Interscience Conference on Antimicrobial Agents and Chemotherapy, New York, October 5.

PAHO (Pan-American Health Organization). 1980. "Acute Respiratory Infections in the Americas." PAHO *Epidemiological Bulletin* 1(5):1–4.

Pandey, M. R., and ARI Study Team. 1988. "Acute Respiratory Infections in Rural Hill Region of Nepal: A Prospective Pilot Intervention Study." Mrigendra Medical Trust, Kathmandu.

Pandey, M. R., J. S. M. Boleij, K. R. Smith, and E. M. Wafula. 1989. "Indoor Air Pollution in Developing Countries and Acute Respiratory Infection in Children." *Lancet* 1:427–29.

Pandey, M. R., R. P. Neupane, A. Gautam, and I. B. Shrestha. 1989. "Domestic Smoke Pollution and Acute Respiratory Infections in a Rural Community of the Hill Region of Nepal." *Environment International*.

Pedreira, F. A., V. L. Guandolo, E. F. Feroli, G. W. Mella, and I. P. Weiss. 1985. "Involuntary Smoking and Incidence of Respiratory Illness during the First Year of Life." *Pediatrics* 75:594–97.

Penna, M. L. F., and M. P. Duchiade. 1991. "Air Pollution and Infant Mortality from Pneumonia in Rio de Janeiro Metropolitan Area." PAHO *Bulletin* 25(1):47–54.

Phillips, M. A., R. G. A. Feachem, and A. Mills. 1987. "Options for Diarrhoea Control: The Cost-Effectiveness of Selected Interventions for the Prevention of Diarrhoea." Publication 13, EPC (Evaluation and Planning Centre for Health Care), London School of Hygiene and Tropical Medicine and the Diarrhoeal Diseases Control Division, WHO (World Health Organization).

Pio, A., J. Leowski, and F. Luelmo. 1982. "Bases for WHO Programme on Acute Respiratory Infections in Children." 25th World Conference on Tuberculosis, Buenos Aires, December 15–18.

Pio, A., J. Leowski, and H. G. ten Dam. 1985. "The Magnitude of the Problem of Acute Respiratory Infection." In R. M. Douglas and E. Kerby-Eaton, eds., *Acute Respiratory Infections in Childhood. Proceedings of an International Workshop*. Adelaide: University of Adelaide.

Poore, P. 1988. "Vaccination Strategies in Developing Countries." *Vaccine* 6:393–98.

Pringle, C. R. 1987. "Progress towards Control of the Acute Respiratory Viral Diseases of Childhood." *Bulletin of the World Health Organization* 65(2):133–37.

Quick, Jonathan D., P. Foreman, D. Ross-Degnan, and others. 1988. "Where Does the Tetracycline Go?: Health Center Prescribing and Child Survival in East Java and West Kalimantan, Indonesia." Report of Consultation. Drug Management Program, Management Sciences for Health, Boston.

Rahmathullah, L., B. A. Underwood, R. D. Thulasiraj, and R. C. Milton. 1991. "Diarrhea, Respiratory Infections and Growth Are Not Affected by a Weekly Low-Dose Vitamin A Supplement: A Masked, Controlled Field Trial in Children in Southern India." *American Journal of Clinical Nutrition* 54:568–77.

Rahmathullah, L., B. A. Underwood, R. D. Thulasiraj, R. C. Milton, K. Ramaswamy, R. Rahmathullah, and G. Babu. 1990. "Reduced Mortality among Children in Southern India Receiving a Small Weekly Dose of vitamin A." *New England Journal of Medicine* 323(14):929–35.

Redd, Stephen, Mpolai Moteetee, and Ronald Waldman. 1990. "Diagnosis and Management of Acute Respiratory Infections in Lesotho." *Health Policy and Planning* 5(3):255–60.

Riley, Ian D., and R. M. Douglas. 1981. "An Epidemiologic Approach to Pneumococcal Disease." *Reviews of Infectious Diseases* 3:233–45.

Riley, Ian, Emmanuel Carrad, Helen Gratten, and others. 1983. "The Status of Research on Acute Respiratory Infections in Children in Papua New Guinea." *Pediatric Research* 17:1041–43.

Riley, Ian D., Deborah Lehmann, M. P. Alpers, and others. 1986. "Pneumococcal Vaccine Prevents Death from Acute Lower Respiratory Tract Infections in Papua New Guinea Children." *Lancet* 2:877–81.

Rowland, M. G. M., S. G. H. G. Rowland, and T. J. Cole. 1988. "Impact of Infection on the Growth of Children from 0 to 2 Years in an Urban West African Community." *American Journal of Clinical Nutrition* 47:134–38.

Ruben, D. H., J. M. Leventhal, P. A. Krasilnikoff, B. Weile, and A. Berget. 1986. "Effect of Passive Smoking on Birth Weight." *Lancet* 2:415–17.

Salih, M. A., F. El Hakim, G. I. Suliman, S. A. Hassan, and A. El Khatim. 1985. "An Epidemiological Study of the 1978 Outbreak of Diphtheria in Khartoum Province." *Journal of Tropical Pediatrics* 31:812.

Samet, J. M., M. C. Marbury, and J. D. Spengler. 1987. "Health Effects and Sources of Indoor Air Pollution." *American Review of Respiratory Diseases* 136:1486–1508.

Selwyn, B. J., on behalf of the Coordinated Data Group of BOSTID Researchers. 1990. "The Epidemiology of Acute Respiratory Tract Infection in Young Children: Comparison of Findings from Several Developing Countries." *Reviews of Infectious Diseases* 12(Supplement 8):S870–88.

Shann, F., M. Gratten, S. Germer, and others. 1984. "Aetiology of Pneumonia in Children in Goroka Hospital, Papua New Guinea." *Lancet* 2:537–41.

Shann, F., K. Hart, and D. Thomas. 1982. "Acute Lower Respiratory Infections in Children: Possible Criteria for Selection of Patients for Antibiotic Therapy and Hospital Admission." *Bulletin of the World Health Organization* 62:749–53.

Shepard, D. S., R. Robertson, C. Cameron, P. Satarus, M. Pollock, J. Manceau, P. Meissner, and J. Perroni. 1989. "Cost Effectiveness of Routine and Campaign Vaccination Strategies in Ecuador." *Bulletin of the World Health Organization* 67:649–62.

Siber, G. R., M. Santosham, G. R. Reid, C. Thompson, J. Almeido-Hill, A. Morell, G. DeLange, J. K. Ketcham and E. H. Callahan. 1990. "Impaired Antibody Response to *Haemophilus influenzae* Type B Polysaccharide and Low IgG2 and IgG4 Concentrations in Apache Children. *New England Journal of Medicine* 323(20):1387–92.

Simberkoff, M. S., A-P. Cross, M. Al-Ibrahim, and others. 1986. "Efficacy of Pneumococcal Vaccination in High Risk Patients." *New England Journal of Medicine* 315:1318–27.

Singhi, S., and P. Singhi. 1987. "Prevention of Acute Respiratory Infections." *Indian Journal of Pediatrics* 54:161–70.

Sofoluwe, G. O. 1968. "Smoke Pollution in Dwellings of Infants with Bronchopneumonia." *Archives of Environmental Health* 16:670–72.

Sommer, Alfred. 1983. "Mortality Associated with Mild Untreated Xerophthalmia." *Transactions of the American Ophthalmological Society* 81:825–53.

Sommer, Alfred, J. Katz, and I. Tarwotjo. 1984. "Increased Risk of Respiratory Disease in Children with Preexisting Mild Vitamin A Deficiency." *American Journal of Clinical Nutrition* 40:1090–95.

Spika, John S., M. H. Munshi, B. Wojtyniak, D. A. Sack, A. Hossain, M. Rahman, and S. K. Saha. 1989. "Acute Lower Respiratory Infections: A Major Cause of Death in Children in Bangladesh." *Annals of Tropical Paediatrics* 9:33–39.

Stansfield, S. K. 1987. "Acute Respiratory Infections in the Developing World: Strategies for Prevention, Treatment and Control." *Pediatric Infectious Diseases* 61:624–29.

———. 1990. "Potential Savings through Reduction of Inappropriate Use of Pharmaceuticals in the Treatment of Acute Respiratory Infections." In *ALRI and Child Survival in Developing Countries: Understanding the Current Status and Directions for the 1990s*. Proceedings of a workshop given by the Johns Hopkins University School of Hygiene and Public Health, Institute for International Programs, and the U. S. Agency for International Development. Washington, D.C., August 2–3.

Stein, C. M., W. T. A. Todd, D. Parirenyatwa, J. Chakonda, and A. G. M. Dizwani. 1984. "A Survey of Antibiotic Use in Harare Primary Care Clinics." *Journal of Antimicrobial Chemotherapy* 14:149–56.

Stetler, H. C., W. A. Orenstein, R. H. Bernier, and others. 1986. "Impact of Revaccination of Children Who Initially Received Measles Vaccine before 10 Months of Age." *Pediatrics* 77:471–76.

Taylor, W. R., Ruti-Kalisa, Mambu ma-Disu, and J. M. Weinman. 1988. "Measles Control Efforts in Urban Africa Complicated by High Incidence of Measles in the First Year of Life." *American Journal of Epidemiology* 127(4):788–94.

Tracey, V. V., N. C. De, and J. R. Harper. 1971. "Obesity and Respiratory Infections in Infants and Young Children." *British Medical Journal* 11:16–18.

Tugwell, Peter, Kathryn J. Bennett, D. L. Sackett and R. B. Haynes. 1985. "The Measurement Iterative Loop: A Framework for the Critical Appraisal of Need, Benefits and Costs of Health Interventions." *Journal of Chronic Diseases* 38:339–51.

Tupasi, Thelma E., 1985. "Nutrition and Acute Respiratory Infections." In R. M. Douglas and E. Kerby-Eaton, eds., *Acute Respiratory Infections in Childhood. Proceedings of an International Workshop*. Adelaide: University of Adelaide.

Tupasi, Thelma E., M. G. Lucero, D. M. Magdangal, N. V. Mangubat, M. E. S. Sunico, C. U. Torres, Lillian E. de Leon, J. F. Paladin, L. Baes, and M. C. Javato. 1990. "Etiology of Acute Lower Respiratory Tract Infections in Children from Alabang, Metro Manila." *Reviews of Infectious Diseases* 12(Supplement 8):S929–39.

Tupasi, Thelma E., Melicia A. Velmonte, Maria Elinor G. Sanvictores, Leticia Abraham, Lillian E. de Leon, Susan A. Tan, Cynthia A. Miguel, and Mediadora C. Saniel. 1988. "Determinants of Morbidity and Mortality due to Acute Respiratory Infections: Implications for Intervention." *Journal of Infectious Diseases* 157(4):615–23.

UNEP/WHO (United Nations Environment Program/World Health Organization). 1988. "Global Environment Monitoring System: Assessment of Urban Air Quality." Geneva.

UNICEF (United Nations Children's Fund) 1988. Essential Drugs Price List. Copenhagen.

———. 1988b. *Joint WHO/UNICEF Nutrition Support Programme in Iringa, Tanzania: 1983–1988 Evaluation Report*. Dar es Salaam: Government of the Republic of Tanzania, World Health Organization.

———. 1991. *The State of the World's Children*. Oxford: Oxford University Press for UNICEF.

USDHHS (U. S. Department of Health and Human Services). 1989. "Reducing the Consequences of Smoking: 25 Years of Progress." Publication CDC89–8411. Atlanta: Public Health Service, Centers for Disease Control.

Vathanophas, K., R. Sangchai, S. Raktham, A. Pariyanonda, J. Thangsuvan, P. Bunyaratabhandu, S. Athipanyakom, S. Suwanjutha, P. Jayanetra, C. Wasi, M. Vorachit, and P. Puthavathana. 1990. "A Community-Based Study of Acute Respiratory Tract Infection in Thai Children." *Reviews of Infectious Diseases* 12(Supplement 8):S957–65.

Verma, I. C., and P. S. N. Menon. 1981. "Epidemiology of Acute Respiratory Disease in North India." Indian Journal of Pediatrics 48:37–40.

Victora, Cesar G., P. G. Smith, J. P. Vaughn, L. C. Nobre, C. Lombardi, A. M. B. Teixeira, S. M. C. Fuchs, L. B. Moreiral, L. P. Gigante, and F. C. Barros. 1987. "Evidence for Protection by Breastfeeding against Infant Deaths from Infectious Disease in Brazil." *Lancet* 2:319–21.

Vijayaraghavan, K. G. Radhaiah, B. S. Prakasam, K. V. R. Sarma, and V. Reddy. 1990. "Effect of Massive Dose Vitamin A on Morbidity and Mortality in Indian Children." *Lancet* 336:1342–45.

Voorhoeve, A. M., A. S. Muller, T. W. I. Shulpen, W. Manetje, and M. Vangens. 1977. "The Epidemiology of Pertussis." *Tropical and Geographic Medicine* 30:121–24.

Wanger, J. D., Richard Pierce, Katharine A. Deaver, Brian D. Phkaytis, Richard R. Facklam, Claire V. Broome, and the *Haemophilus influenzae* Vaccine Efficacy Study Group. *Lancet* 338(8764):395–98.

Ward, J., G. Brenneman, G. W. Letson, W. L. Heyward, and the Alaska *H. influenzae* Vaccine Study Group. 1990. "Limited Efficacy of a *Haemophilus influenzae* Type B Conjugate Vaccine in Alaska Native Infants." *New England Journal of Medicine* 323(20):1393–1401.

Ware, J. H., D. W. Dockery, A. Spiro III, F. E. Spaizer, and B. G. Ferris, Jr. 1984. "Passive Smoking, Gas Cooking, and Respiratory Health of Children Living in Six Cities." *American Review of Respiratory Diseases* 129:366–74.

Weinberg, G. A., D. Lehmann, T. E. Tupasi. and D. M. Granoff. 1990. "Diversity of Outer Membrane Protein Profiles of Nontypeable *Haemophilus influenzae* Isolated from Children from Papua New Guinea and the Philippines." *Reviews of Infectious Diseases* 12(Supplement 8):S1017–20.

Weiss, S. T., I. B. Tager, M. Schenker, and F. E. Spaizer. 1983. "The Health Effects of Involuntary Smoking." *American Review of Respiratory Diseases* 128:933–42.

Wilkins, J., and P. F. Wehrle. 1979. "Additional Evidence against Measles Vaccine Administration to Infants Less than 12 Months of Age: Altered Immune Response Following Active/Passive Immunization." *Journal of Pediatrics* 94:865–69.

Williams, P. J., and F. H. Hull. 1983. "Status of Measles in the Gambia, 1981." *Reviews of Infectious Diseases* 5:391–95.

WHO (World Health Organization). 1984. "A Programme for Controlling Acute Respiratory Infections in Children: Memorandum from a WHO Meeting." *Bulletin of the World Health Organization* 62:47–58.

———. 1988. "Rheumatic Fever and Rheumatic Heart Disease." Technical Report Series, 764. Geneva.

———. 1990. "Respiratory Infections in Children: Management at Small Hospitals." Draft. Geneva.

WHO/ARI (World Health Organization/Programme for Control of Acute Respiratory Infections). 1988. "Case Management of Acute Respiratory Infection in Children: Intervention Studies." Publication 88–2. Geneva.

———. 1989b. "Programme for Control of Acute Respiratory Infections: Programme Report, 1988." Publication 89–3. Geneva.

———. 1990. "Programme for the Control of Acute Respiratory Infections: Case Management Research Priorities." Publication 90–1. Geneva.

———. 1991a. "Programme for Control of Acute Respiratory Infections: Interim Programme Report." Publication 91–19. Geneva.

———. 1991b. "Technical Bases for the WHO Recommendations on the Management of Pneumonia in Children at First-Level Health Facilities." Publication 91–20. Geneva.

WHO/EPI (World Health Organization/Expanded Programme on Immunization). 1982. "The Optimal Age for Measles Vaccination." *Weekly Epidemiologic Record* 57:21–31.

———. 1987. "Key Issues in Measles Immunization Research: A Review of the Literature." Report of the Global Advisory Group Meeting, November.

———. 1990. "Measles Control in the 1990s: Immunization before 9 Months of Age." Publication 90–3. Geneva.

WHO/EPP (World Health Organization). 1984. "Biomass Fuel Consumption and Health." Geneva.

WHO/RSD (World Health Organization). 1986. "Respiratory Infections in Children: Management at Small Hospitals, Background Notes and a Manual for Doctors." Publication 86–26. Geneva.

Yurdakok, K., T. Yavuz, and C. E. Taylor. 1990. "Swaddling and Acute Respiratory Infections." *American Journal of Public Health* 80(7):873–75.

Zimicki, Susan. 1988. "L'enregistrement des causes de décès par des non-médecins: deux expériences au Bangladesh." In J. S. Vallin and A. Palloni, eds., *Mesure et analyse de la mortalité: nouvelles approches*. Paris: Presses Universitaires de France.

5

Diarrheal Diseases

José Martines, Margaret Phillips, and Richard G. A. Feachem

Diarrhea is a complex of symptoms and signs, usually defined as an increased number of stools of liquid or semiliquid consistency passed during a twenty-four-hour period. Although a considerable variety of definitions can be found in the literature (Snyder and Merson 1982), recent studies have tended to consider more than three stools passed in twenty-four hours of observation as an indication of diarrhea after the age of three months (WHO 1988c). The word "diarrhea" is also used in programmatic and public health contexts, although not typically in clinical contexts, to embrace dysentery. Dysentery is usually characterized by the presence of blood in the stools, with or without excessive looseness or frequency.

Considerable differences of opinion still exist as to the minimum number of healthy days that marks the end of a diarrheal episode, ranging from forty-eight hours (WHO 1988c) to two weeks (Scrimshaw and others 1961). Episodes tend to be self-limiting, generally lasting for less than seven days. Studies in several developing countries have shown that 3 to 20 percent of acute diarrheal episodes in children under five may become persistent, lasting for at least fourteen days (WHO 1988b).

A variety of enteric pathogens—including bacteria such as enterotoxigenic *Escherichia coli*, enteropathogenic *E. coli*, *Salmonella*, *Shigella*, *Vibrio cholerae*, and *Campylobacter jejuni*; viruses such as rotavirus; and protozoa such as *Giardia lamblia*, *Entamoeba hystolytica*, and *Cryptosporidium*—can cause diarrhea (Farthing and Keusch 1989). The specific pathogens of greatest importance to public health vary according to age of the patient and the geographical setting. For example, rotavirus is a significant cause of severe diarrhea in children under two years of age in developing countries, and *Salmonella* and *Campylobacter* are primary causes among adults in industrialized countries who consume poultry raised in factory-farming conditions.

Other causes of diarrhea, considered to be relatively unimportant in developing countries, include food intolerance, especially lactase deficiency and allergies to animal protein, granulomatous diseases of the gut, and tumors elaborating gastrointestinal hormones (Rohde 1986). Diarrhea may also be associated with infections outside the intestinal tract, such as malaria, measles, and respiratory infections and is a prominent feature in acquired immunodeficiency syndrome (AIDS).

The pathogenesis of infectious diarrhea has been extensively studied, and the primary pathogenic mechanisms are summarized in figure 5-1. Some of these pathogenic processes, especially those relating to the production and action of the enterotoxins of *E. coli* and *V. cholerae*, are understood in great detail. This understanding has opened the way to the production of sophisticated vaccines, including the live, genetically engineered, vaccine strains.

The risk of diarrheal morbidity and mortality is greater among families of lower socioeconomic status and in conditions of poor personal and domestic hygiene. Low family income (Manderson 1981; Stanton and Clemens 1987b), lack of luxury items (Huttly and others 1987), living in a one-room house (Stanton and Clemens 1987b), living in a house with an earthen floor (Bertrand and Walmus 1983), lower maternal education (Bertrand and Walmus 1983), lower occupational status of the head of the family (Islam, Bhuiya, and Yunus 1984), and unclean living conditions (Bertrand and Walmus 1983; Huttly and others 1987; Taylor and others 1986) have all been associated with increased risk of diarrheal morbidity and mortality.

The risk of diarrheal morbidity and mortality is higher among infants who are not breastfed (Feachem and Koblinsky 1984). More recent studies in developing countries have confirmed the very substantial role of breastfeeding in protecting infants against diarrheal incidence, severity, and mortality (Briend, Wojtyniak, and Rowland 1988; Clemens and others 1986; Huttly and others 1987; Mahmood, Feachem, and Huttly 1989; Martines 1988; Victora and others 1987). Several studies indicate a risk of increased diarrheal duration and severity among the malnourished (Bairagi and others 1987; Black, Brown, and Becker 1984a; Black and others 1984; Chen, Huq, and Huffman 1981; Palmer and others 1976). Recent studies in Sudan and Mexico have suggested that malnutrition also increases the risk of frequent diarrheal episodes (Samani, Willet, and Ware 1988; Sepúlveda, Willet, and Muñoz 1988). Although information is scarce on the role of low birth weight as a determinant of diarrheal morbidity (Ash-

Figure 5-1. Primary Pathogenic Mechanisms for Infectious Diarrheal Diseases

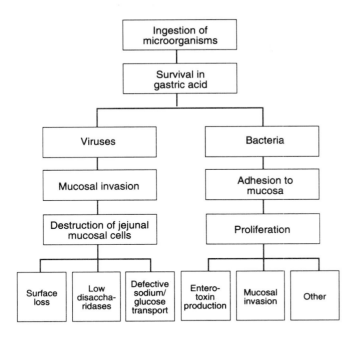

Source: Candy and Phillips 1986.

worth and Feachem 1985b), the association between intrauterine growth retardation and impaired immunocompetence, and the strong association between low birth weight and diarrheal mortality in infancy in developing countries (Barros and others 1987), suggest that low birth weight is a risk factor for diarrheal severity and mortality.

Diarrhea can lead to dehydration and early death, particularly in young children (Gordon and others 1968; Snyder and Merson 1982), and to impaired growth and nutritional status among the survivors. The effect of diarrhea on infant and child growth and nutritional status is the outcome of a complex interplay of host, pathogen, and sociocultural factors, which may cause decreased food intake (Briscoe 1979; Brown and others 1985; Hoyle, Yunus, and Chen 1980; Khan and Ahmad 1986; Martorell and others 1980; Mata and others 1977; Nabarro and others 1988), malabsorption (Chen 1983; Molla, Molla, and Khatun 1986; Rosenberg, Solomons, and Schneider 1977; Scrimshaw 1977), loss of endogenous nutrients (Chen 1983; Sarker and others 1986), and increased metabolic rate (Beisel 1977; Chen 1983; Keusch and Katz 1979; Keusch and Scrimshaw 1986).

Longitudinal studies have detected a significant effect of diarrheal episodes on the growth of infants and children (Bairagi and others 1987; Black, Brown, and Becker 1984b; Cole and Parkin 1977; Condon-Paoloni and others 1977; Guerrant and others 1983; Martorell and others 1975; Martorell and others 1977; Nabarro and others 1988; Rowland, Rowland, and Cole 1988; Zumrawi, Dimond, and Waterlow 1987). The wide range of effects recorded have been variously

attributed to the severity or duration of diarrheal episodes, the nutritional effectiveness of case management, and the extent of catch-up growth (Black, Brown, and Becker 1983; Brown and others 1985; Keusch and Scrimshaw 1986; Khan and Ahmad 1986; Miall, Desai, and Standard 1970; United Nations University 1979; Whitehead 1977).

Despite diarrheal incidence and severity being lower among adults, diarrhea may still represent a significant portion of total adult morbidity in developing countries. In Nigeria, diarrhea was associated with 20 percent of all illnesses in adults (Huttly and others 1987) and accounted for a median of 23 percent (range 5–41 percent) of disability days per year among adults age fifteen through forty-four in Pakistan, Indonesia, Nepal, and Ghana (Grosse 1980). In rural Bangladesh, diarrhea accounted for 14 percent of the total mortality among the population over forty-five years old surveyed between 1980 and 1983 (BRAC, 1987).

The Public Health Significance of Diarrhea

The current levels and trends of diarrhea morbidity and mortality in the developing world, and the probable patterns of morbidity and mortality in the next century are examined in this section.

Current Levels and Trends in the Developing World

Information on the current levels and trends in the incidence and mortality due to diarrhea is reviewed in the following paragraphs.

MORBIDITY. Measurements of diarrheal incidence depend on such factors as what definition of diarrhea is used, the frequency of surveillance, and the location of the study population (Snyder and Merson 1982). Since 1981, the Diarrhoeal Diseases Control Programme of the World Health Organization (WHO/CDD) has promoted a series of surveys to measure diarrheal morbidity and mortality rates using a consistent methodology (WHO 1987b, 1988c). Results from 276 surveys conducted in sixty countries between 1981 and 1986 are summarized in table 5-1. They indicate that, on average, children under five years of age in developing countries suffer 3.5 episodes of diarrhea per year. Excluding the Americas, where relatively few surveys have been undertaken, the highest rates were found in Sub-Saharan Africa and the lowest in Asia, especially in China and other countries in the Western Pacific region.

In order to estimate diarrheal morbidity rates among older age groups, for which information is scarcer, the estimates of relative incidence of diarrheal episodes in the older age groups adopted by the Committee on Issues and Priorities for New Vaccine Development of the Institute of Medicine of the United States (U.S. Institute of Medicine 1986) were applied to the WHO/CDD morbidity rates. Diarrheal incidence was estimated to be four to six times lower for those between five and fourteen years old, and thirteen to sixteen times lower for those

Table 5-1. Morbidity in 276 Surveys in Children Aged Four Years and Younger Using the WHO/CDD Methodology, 1981–86

Region	Surveys	Countries	Annual incidence (episodes/child/year)[a] Median	Range
Latin America and the Carribean	12	8	4.9	0.8–10.4
Sub-Saharan Africa	67	22	4.4	1.6–9.9
Middle East and North Africa	47	10	2.7	2.1–10.8
Asia and the Pacific	150	20	2.6	1.1–5.7
India	—	1	2.7	—
China	—	1	1.2	—
Other	—	1	2.6	—
All regions	276	60	3.5	0.8–10.8

— Not available.

Note: Surveys were conducted mainly in geographically limited areas. If more than one survey was conducted in any country, the median for the country was used to calculate the regional and global medians.

a. Survey estimate was adjusted for seasonality when appropriate data were available.

Source: Unpublished World Health Organization data.

beyond the age of fourteen years, than that observed among children under five (table 5-2).

Independent longitudinal studies largely confirm these estimates of diarrhea incidence in Latin America presented in table 5-2. In a poor periurban population in the north of Brazil, Giugliano and others (1986) recorded 4.8 episodes per year for children from birth to thirty-five months and 0.2 episodes per year for adults. Guerrant and others (1983), studying a poor urban group in northeast Brazil, found similar rates for young children but substantially higher ones for adults, for whom they estimated more than one episode per adult per year.

Diarrheal rates presented for Sub-Saharan Africa (table 5-2) are substantially lower than those estimated from cross-sectional surveys by Huttly and others (1987) in Nigeria (14 episodes per year among children six months through eleven

Table 5-2. Estimated Annual Diarrheal Morbidity Rates Region and Age, 1985

Region	Age (years) 0–4	5–14	15–59	> 59
Latin America and the Carribean	4.9	1.2	0.3	0.3
Sub-Saharan Africa	4.4	0.9	0.3	0.3
Middle East and North Africa	2.7	0.5	0.2	0.2
Asia and the Pacific	2.6	0.4	0.2	0.2
All regions (median)	3.5	0.7	0.2	0.2

Note: Rates were calculated as episodes per person per year. Rates for children aged four years and younger were derived from CDD mobidity survey (table 5-1). Other rates were estimated according to relative incidence rates by age adopted by the Institute of Medicine 1986.

Source: Unpublished World Health Organization data. Rates were calculated by the authors.

months and 2.5 episodes per year among adults). Diarrheal rates described by Georges and others (1987) in the Central African Republic (7 episodes per child per year among children under five), although higher than the average of those presented for the region, were still within the range of the WHO/CDD survey findings from which the presented values were derived. A lower incidence (1.9 episodes per child per year)—but also within the range measured in the WHO/CDD surveys—was described among children under four years of age in rural Ghana (Biritwun and others 1986). Kirkwood (1991) provides a comprehensive review of knowledge of diarrhea epidemiology in Sub-Saharan Africa. Incidence rates presented for North Africa and the Middle East are similar to those described by el-Alamy and others (1986) among adults and children in rural Egypt.

Recently the epidemiology of persistent diarrhea (diarrhea lasting at least fourteen days) has been the focus of particular investigation. In rural northern India, Bhan and others (1989) report a low incidence of persistent diarrhea of 0.06 episodes per child per year in children under six years of age, with a peak incidence of 0.3 episodes per child per year in infants. Persistent episodes made up 10 percent of all episodes in children under six years and 22 percent of all episodes in infants under one year. In rural Bangladesh, Huttly and others (1989) report an incidence of persistent diarrhea of 0.6 episodes per child per year in children under five years of age (16 percent of all episodes). In the first half of infancy, persistent episodes comprised one-quarter of all episodes.

No evidence could be found in the literature of a fall in incidence rates of diarrhea during the past fifteen years. Snyder and Merson (1982), using active surveillance studies conducted between 1954 and 1979, estimated that diarrheal incidence in developing countries averaged 2.2 episodes per child per year. Comparing this value with the 3.5 episodes per child per year derived from cross-sectional survey data collected between 1981 and 1986, we must conclude that it is unlikely that any significant reduction in diarrheal incidence has occurred in the period between 1970 and 1985, particularly as cross-sectional surveys are likely to underestimate morbidity rates.

MORTALITY. Available data on diarrheal mortality tend to be less reliable than those on morbidity. The only global data source available was generated during the WHO/CDD morbidity and mortality surveys (table 5-3). Some of the information on mortality was considered implausible by WHO, a situation that was attributed to lack of training or supervision of the surveyors (WHO 1988c). In addition, the survey method used, the interviewing of heads of households, who were asked to recall the deaths of family members in the past year, is regarded skeptically by some demographers and may greatly underestimate mortality rates (Timaeus and Graham 1989). The information in table 5-4, although the best presently available, should be regarded with caution. Estimates of diarrhea case-fatality rates by age that were made by the U.S. Institute of Medicine (1986) were used to calculate mortality rates of those beyond the age

Table 5-3. Mortality in 276 Surveys in Children Aged Four Years and Younger, Using WHO/CDD *Methodology, 1981–86*

Region	Surveys	Countries	Diarrhea Mortality Rate (deaths/1,000 children/year) Median	Diarrhea Mortality Rate (deaths/1,000 children/year) Range	Diarrhea deaths as percentage of total deaths (median)
Latin America and the Carribean	12	8	4.2	1.2–9.2	35
Sub-Saharan Africa	67	22	10.6	3.1–54.9	38
Middle East and North Africa	47	10	5.8	1.0–25.3	39
Asia and the Pacific	150	20	3.2	0.0–17.2	29
India	—	1	3.2	—	—
China	—	1	0.0	—	—
Other	—	18	3.3	—	—
All regions	276	60	6.5	0.0–54.9	36

— Not available.

Note: Surveys were conducted mainly in geographically limited areas. If more than one survey was conducted in any country, the median for the country was used to calculate the regional and global medians.

Source: Unpublished World Health Organization data.

of four years shown in the table. Case-fatality rates were estimated to fall from 2 per 1,000 among children under five, to 0.4 per 1,000 among those between five and fourteen years and 0.3 per 1,000 among persons between fifteen and fifty-nine years. A slight increase, to 0.5 per 1,000, was estimated for members of the population age sixty years and older.

Estimates of adult mortality due to diarrhea for developing countries with adequate vital registration systems are reported by Feachem and others (1992). Estimates of the risk of death from diarrhea between ages fifteen and fifty-nine vary from 0.01 percent (for example, in Argentina) to 3 percent in Guatemala. The proportion of deaths due to diarrhea was reported to be roughly 4 percent in India in persons aged fifteen through fifty-four years and 2 percent in Kenya in persons aged fifteen through sixty-four years (Feachem and others 1992).

Diarrheal mortality appears to have fallen substantially in many areas during the past fifteen years. Indications of this trend are reported from Egypt (el-Rafie and others 1990; Egypt, National Control of Diarrheal Diseases Project 1988), Thailand (Phonboon and others 1986), Brazil (Benicio and others 1987; Monteiro and Benicio 1989), Cuba (Riveron-Corteguera and Muñoz 1982) and Costa Rica (Mata 1981).

The data from Egypt and Costa Rica indicate that this reduction in diarrheal mortality rates has been accompanied by reductions in general childhood mortality rates during the same period, in a way that suggests that diarrhea has not been replaced by other causes of death.

Diarrheal mortality in children under five was calculated by Snyder and Merson (1982) to be 13.6 deaths per 1,000 from data collected between 1956 and 1979, whereas a median value of 6.5 deaths per 1,000 was estimated by the WHO/CDD morbidity-mortality surveys (table 5-3). These latter data may, as explained above, be substantial underestimates. The case-fatality rates in children under five years old used by the U.S. Institute of Medicine (1986) increases the mortality rate to 7.1 per 1,000, still 48 percent lower than that calculated by Snyder and Merson (1982) for the period 1956–79. This fall in diarrheal mortality can be attributed reasonably to a fall in the case-fatality rate during the time. Current case-fatality rates vary widely: for children under five years they were found to be 0.8 per 1,000 in Bangui, Central African Republic (Georges and others 1987), 3 per 1,000 in rural Egypt (el-Alamy and others 1986), 3.6 per 1,000 in rural northern India (Kumar, Kumar, and Dutta 1987), and 5.4 per 1,000 in rural Indonesia (Nazir, Pardede, and Ismail 1985). Nevertheless, these values

Table 5-4. Estimated Annual Diarrhea Mortality Rates, by Region and Age, 1986

Region	Age (years) 0–4[a]	5–14	15–59	> 59
Latin America and the Carribean	4.2	0.5	0.1	0.1
Sub-Saharan Africa	10.6	0.4	0.1	0.1
Middle East and North Africa	5.8	0.2	0.1	0.1
Asia and the Pacific	3.2	0.2	0.1	0.1
All regions (median)	6.5	0.3	0.1	0.1

Note: Rates were calculated as deaths per 1,000 persons per year. Rates for children aged four and younger were derived from CDD mortality surveys (table 5-3). Other rates were estimated according to case-fatality rates by age adopted by the Institute of Medicine 1986.

a. Mortality rates (per 1,000 children) estimated according to the Institute of Medicine's (1986) case-fatality ratios are as follows: Latin America, 9.8; Sub-Saharan Africa, 8.8; North Africa, 5.4; Asia, 5.2.

Source: Unpublished World Health Organization data. Ratios were calculated by the authors.

are all lower than the 6 per 1,000 estimated by Snyder and Merson (1982) from data collected before 1980.

In summary, therefore, there is evidence of a fall in diarrheal mortality rates in children in recent years, but little evidence of a parallel fall in incidence rates. This implies, on the one hand, falling case-fatality rates and, on the other, stagnating levels of the key risk factors for diarrhea morbidity. Central questions for policy that emerge are, first, to what extent the declining case-fatality rates have been created by the interventions of national CDD programs and, second, whether there are reasonable prospects for reducing morbidity over the next decade. We return to these questions later in this chapter.

Likely Morbidity and Mortality Patterns—Next Century

Although risk factors for diarrhea morbidity and mortality have been identified, and in some cases quantified, and the effects of certain interventions to control diarrheal diseases measured, only very general predictions of the likely future pattern of diarrheal morbidity and mortality are possible. In the first place, explorations of many of the relationships between risk factors and diarrhea outcome have been conducted at a relatively simplistic level—ignoring, for example, interactions between various causes—and in relatively few locations. Second, it is not clear how or how much various factors influencing diarrhea morbidity or mortality will change in the future. Evidence of past trends suggests, although only weakly, that morbidity levels have remained stagnant over the last fifteen years (see previous section), despite changes at the global level in several of the risk factors, such as substantial increases in measles immunization coverage and more modest increases in the proportion of households having improved water supply and sanitation. These global trends, however, disguise what are probably considerable variations within regions and countries, and not all these risk factors have moved in a direction associated with reductions in diarrhea rates. For example, breastfeeding rates in rural areas in developing countries have tended to decline and are unlikely to have increased significantly during the period in urban areas (Popkin and Bisgrove 1988), and nutritional status has remained stagnant in many countries, especially in Sub-Saharan Africa (Ashworth and Dowler 1991).

Nevertheless, diarrheal mortality rates in children have fallen in the last fifteen years. In the same period, overall infant and child mortality rates have also fallen throughout the developing world for reasons that are not entirely understood (Feachem, Timaeus, and Graham 1989). It is not clear how much of the diarrhea mortality decline has been brought about by increased use of oral rehydration therapy (ORT); how much by general improvement, access to, and quality of health care services at the periphery; and how much by nonspecific factors such as improving parental education (leading to more prompt attention to worsening symptoms of a sick child).

Present coverage rates and estimated use rates suggest that there is potential for mortality to decline through more effective delivery of CDD programs. Although global access to oral rehydration salts (ORS) has increased from less than 10 percent in 1982 to 51 percent in 1985 (WHO 1988c) and to 63 percent in 1989 (WHO 1991), nearly 40 percent of the population remain uncovered. The level of mortality decrease that can be expected from expanding ORT programs will depend on the risk of diarrheal death from dehydration among those as yet without access to ORS and on the potential for improvement in the quality of case management required to make a difference. Boosting coverage from current levels and, even more so, improving the correctness of ORT use, may be difficult. The CDD program has recently instituted a new applied research initiative to deal with these issues and has intensified efforts to train health care providers (doctors, nurses, paramedical staff, pharmacists, traditional healers) in diarrhea case management (WHO 1989). This will require, nevertheless, that governments or agencies be prepared to devote the necessary financial and manpower resources for it.

Improvement in the rates of use of ORT is unlikely to reduce mortality due to persistent or dysenteric diarrhea. Better overall case management is necessary and may require new methods, with special attention to feeding during the episode and recovery. The same points apply to complicated diarrheas, such as diarrheas accompanied by measles, acute respiratory infections, or malaria. These complicated diarrheas represent a considerable proportion of all inpatient diarrhea cases in some hospitals; the more so since the establishment of ORT-based outpatient facilities for the treatment of uncomplicated acute watery diarrheas.

Summary of the Public Health Significance of Diarrhea

Despite developments in the last decades in the understanding of the etiology and pathogenesis of diarrheal diseases and the discovery of an effective oral rehydration solution to treat the majority of the patients with watery diarrhea, morbidity rates among young children are still high, and diarrhea remains a significant cause of adult illness. In 1985, nearly 3 billion diarrheal episodes are estimated to have occurred in the developing world, leading to the death of 5 million persons, 80 percent of them under five years of age (see Lopez, chapter 2, this collection). Although evidence exists of a reduction in diarrheal mortality during the past fifteen years, no indication has been found of reductions in diarrheal incidence during the same period. This lack of decline points to the need for the development, implementation, and evaluation of effective measures to lower diarrheal morbidity.

Lowering Disease Incidence

The promotion of ORT for the case management of acute diarrheal diseases may have contributed to the reduction of diarrheal mortality rates observed in developing countries in the last fifteen years. Still, ORT cannot be expected to have a significant effect on the incidence of diarrhea. If morbidity rates are to be reduced, primary preventive strategies must be identified and implemented.

Elements of a Preventive Strategy

A systematic study of interventions, excluding case management, that might play a role in diarrhea control was initiated in 1982 by the Diarrhoeal Diseases Control Programme of WHO (Feachem, Hogan, and Merson 1983). Eighteen interventions were evaluated, with particular emphasis on their effectiveness and feasibility (table 5-5). Of these, four interventions—improving lactation, supplementary feeding programs, chemoprophylaxis, fly control—were found to be either ineffective or too costly for incorporation in programs of diarrheal diseases control in developing countries. Seven other interventions—prevention of low birth weight, use of growth charts, increase in child spacing, vitamin A supplementation, improvement of food hygiene, control of zoonotic reservoirs, epidemic control—were considered of uncertain effectiveness, feasibility, or cost and required further research before their potential role could be properly assessed. Two of these potential interventions—increase in child spacing and control of zoonotic reservoirs—are still under review.

Seven interventions were identified for which evidence of adequate effectiveness and feasibility were reasonably strong:

- Promotion of breastfeeding
- Improvement in weaning practices

- Rotavirus immunization (when an effective vaccine becomes available)
- Cholera immunization (in selected countries, when a more effective new vaccine becomes available)
- Measles immunization
- Improvement of water supply and sanitation facilities
- Promotion of personal and domestic hygiene

These interventions, except for improved water and sanitation, were the object of more detailed analysis of cost-effectiveness (Phillips, Feachem, and Mills 1987). Information regarding the potential effectiveness and cost-effectiveness of these interventions is summarized in table 5-6.

PROMOTION OF BREASTFEEDING. The hypothesis that breastfed infants may have a reduced risk of diarrheal morbidity and mortality is supported by evidence indicating the immunological and antimicrobial properties of breast milk, its contribution to good nutritional status during the first few months of life, and the risk associated with contaminated feeds. The literature on the risks of diarrheal morbidity and mortality among children, according to mode of feeding, was reviewed by Feachem and Koblinsky (1984). More recent studies, in which confounding was carefully controlled, have shown even higher relative risks of severe diarrhea and diarrhea mortality associ-

Table 5-5. Potential Nonclinical Interventions for Control of Diarrhea among Young Children

Strategy	Intervention	Reference[a]
Maternal Health	Preventing low birth weight	Ashworth and Feachem 1985[b]
	Improving Lactation	Ashworth and Feachem 1985[a]
Child health	Promoting breastfeeding	Feachem and Koblinsky 1984
	Improving weaning practices	Ashworth and Feachem 1985[c]
	Supplementary feeding programs	Feachem 1983
	Using growth charts	Ashworth and Feachem 1986
	Increasing child spacing	n.a.
	Vitamin A supplementation	Feachem 1987
Immunization and chemoprophylaxis	Rotavirus immunization	de Zoysa and Feachem 1985
	Cholera immunization	de Zoysa and Feachem 1985
	Measles immunization	Feachem and Koblinsky 1983
	Chemoprophylaxis	de Zoysa and Feachem 1985
Interrupting transmission	Improving water supply and sanitation facilities	Esrey, Feachem, and Hughes, 1985
	Promoting personal and domestic hygiene	Feachem 1984
	Improving food hygiene	Esrey and Feachem 1989
	Controlling zoonotic reservoirs	n.a.
	Controlling flies	Esrey 1991
Epidemic control	Epidemic surveillance, investigation, and control	n.a.

n.a. Not applicable.
Note: The general rational for the review series is described in Feachem, Hogan, and Merson, 1983. Policy conclusions are discussed in Feachem, 1986. Cost-effectiveness analysis of selected interventions is presented in Phillips, Feachem, and Mills, 1987.
a. Some of these publications are also available in French and Spanish.
Source: See table (last column) and note above.

ated with nonbreastfeeding. For example, in Basrah, Iraq, for the nonbreastfed infant the risk of hospitalized diarrhea was thirty-seven times greater than for the exclusively breastfed infant in the first three months of life and twenty-four times greater in the second three months (Mahmood, Feachem, and Huttly 1989). In Brazil in 1985, the risk of diarrheal mortality was found to be fourteen times greater for nonbreastfed infants than for exclusively breastfed infants in the first year of life. The risk of infant mortality was highest among the nonbreastfed during the first two months of life, being twenty-three times greater than among the exclusively breastfed (Victora and others 1987). No evidence could be found by Feachem and Koblinsky (1984) that indicated that protection against diarrhea extended after the termination of breastfeeding (a conclusion supported by Mahmood, Feachem, and Huttly 1989) or after the first year of life. Recent studies have suggested, however, significant protection from breastfeeding against the severity of diarrhea even during the third year of life (Briend, Wojtyniak, and Rowland 1988; Clemens and others 1986).

Breastfeeding promotion projects have been shown to be effective in increasing the number of women initiating breastfeeding and the total duration of exclusive or partial breastfeeding (Hardy and others 1982; Huffman and Combest 1988; Winikoff and Baer 1980). Methods of breastfeeding promotion have included the training and education of health professionals; the changing of hospital practices to facilitate early suckling following birth, rooming-in, limited supplementary and glucose-water feeds, and restrictions on the distribution of formula samples; and the provision of assistance to breastfeeding support groups. Large-scale projects in Brazil, Honduras, Indonesia, Panama, and Thailand were reviewed by Huffman and Combest (1988). Although few adequately designed evaluations have been carried out, the results point consistently to the success of these promotional programs in decreasing rates of nonbreastfeeding.

Theoretical calculations based on the above data (Feachem and Koblinsky 1984) indicate that promotion of breastfeeding can reduce diarrhea morbidity by 8 to 20 percent in the first six months of life and by 1 to 4 percent for children under five

Table 5-6. *Effectiveness and Cost-Effectiveness of Interventions for Diarrhea Control among Young Children*

Strategy	Intervention	Effectiveness[a] (percent)	Cost-effectiveness[b] range (median) (1982 U.S. dollars)	
Child health	Promoting breastfeeding	Reduction in nonbreastfeeding 0–2 months: 40 3–5 months: 30 6–11 months: 10	—	
		Reduction in diarrhea morbidity 0–6 months: 8–20 0–59 months: 1–4	10–75	45
		Reduction in diarrhea mortality 0–6 months: 24–27 0–59 months: 8–9	400–10,750	1000
	Improving weaning practices	Reduction in percentage of children < 75 percent weight-for-age 6–59 months: 50 Reduction in diarrhea mortality 6–59 months: 2–12	50–2000	1070
Immunization	Rotavirus immunization[c]	Reduction in diarrhea incidence: 4	3–30	5
		Reduction in diarrhea mortality: 13	140–1400	220
	Cholera immunization[f]	Reduction in diarrhea incidence: 0.2[e]	90–1450	174
		Reduction in diarrhea mortality: 2.8[e]	1,075–16,710	2,000
	Measles immunization	Reduction in diarrhea incidence: 3	3–60	7
		Reduction in diarrhea mortality: 22	66–1,156	143
Interrrupting transmission	Improving water supply and sanitation	Reduction in diarrhea incidence: 27 Reduction in diarrhea mortality: 30	No meaningful estimates; multiple benefits	
	Promoting personal and domestic hygiene	Reduction in diarrhea incidence: 14–48	5–500	10

— Not available.

a. For children from birth to age fifty-nine months, unless otherwise specified.

b. Only considers diarrhea deaths or episodes averted in children under age five years.

c. Assumes 100 percent coverage with 80 percent vaccine efficiency.

d. Assumes 100 percent coverage with 70 percent vaccine efficiency.

e. In Bangladesh.

f. Assumes 100 percent coverage with 85 percent vaccine efficiency.

Source: See table 5-5.

years. Mortality rates can be reduced by 24 to 27 percent in the first six months, and by 8 to 9 percent for children under five years. Results from more recent studies indicate that these calculations are conservative, especially with reference to the prevention of diarrheal mortality, and that breastfeeding provides greater and more extended protection against diarrheal deaths and severe diarrheal episodes, even up to the third year of life (Briend, Wojtyniak, and Rowland 1988; Clemens and others 1986; Mahmood, Feachem, and Huttly 1989; Martines 1988; Victora and others 1987).

Phillips, Feachem, and Mills (1987) constructed a range of plausible costs for a variety of different breastfeeding promotion strategies (changes in hospital routine, face-to-face education, mass media campaigns, discouragement of breastfeeding alternatives, provision of facilities for working women), using information on the characteristics of these interventions, their likely resource requirements (principally in terms of staff time), and salary estimates. Even with salaries set at a constant average level and the use of a standard input package (except for mass media campaigns), the cost per child affected varied considerably within each strategy, depending on such factors as scale (hospital size in the case of hospital-based interventions; population size in the case of mass media campaigns) and on assumptions concerning the coverage of the intervention and the degree of secondary effect. Phillips, Feachem, and Mills concluded that, with a judicious selection of interventions (excluding the relatively costly strategies involving the provision of facilities for working women), it should be possible in most countries to provide a breastfeeding promotion package for about $5 per infant exposed.[1] Using this estimate and adopting conservative estimates of effectiveness based on Feachem and Koblinsky (1984), we estimated the cost-effectiveness of breastfeeding promotion to range between $10 and $75 (median $45) per diarrheal episode averted and between $400 and $10,750 (median $1,000) per diarrheal death averted in children under five years of age.

IMPROVED WEANING PRACTICES. The hypothesis that underweight children may be predisposed to diarrhea is supported by evidence suggesting that protein-energy malnutrition causes impaired cellular (Chandra 1986) and secretory immune responses (Sirisinha and others 1975). This hypothesis is further corroborated by evidence from patients with congenital or acquired immunodeficiency syndromes, who have increased diarrheal risk (Arbo and Santos 1987). Nonspecific protective mechanisms, such as gastric acid production and intestinal mucosal renewal, may also be affected by malnutrition (Brunser and others 1968; Guiraldes and Hamilton 1981). Increased risk of diarrhea has been described in hypochlorhydric individuals (Gianella, Broitman, and Zamcheck 1973), and recovery from diarrhea may be delayed by an impaired mucosal renewal (Butzner and others 1985).

Epidemiological studies conducted in Bangladesh indicate that protein-energy malnutrition is a significant determinant of diarrhea severity and duration in infancy and childhood, but not of its incidence (Bairagi and others 1987; Black, Brown,

and Becker 1984a; Chen, Huq, and Huffman 1981; Palmer and others 1976). Studies in Nigeria (Tomkins 1981), Mexico (Sepúlveda, Willet, and Muñoz 1988), and the Republic of the Sudan (Samani, Willet, and Ware 1988) suggest that malnourished children may also experience increased incidence of diarrhea. The effect of nutritional status on the severity (degree of dehydration and purging rate) of diarrhea has also been investigated in clinical studies (Black and others 1981; Black and others 1984). Diarrheal mortality has also been shown to be higher in malnourished children.

In Bangladesh, children who had diarrheal episodes and whose weight-for-age was below 65 percent of the expected were 3.7 times more likely to die during the subsequent twenty-four months than their better-nourished counterparts (Chen, Chowdhury, and Huffman 1980). In northern India, case-fatality rates in children with diarrhea were significantly greater among those who were severely malnourished (7.7 percent) than among moderately malnourished (2.2 percent) or well-nourished children (0.3 percent) (Bhan and others 1986).

Poor weaning practices can be the result of lack of access to appropriate foods. Such practices, however, also appear to derive from food taboos or ignorance and to be potentially susceptible, therefore, to education. Few weaning education programs have been evaluated in terms of improvement produced in nutritional status (Ashworth and Feachem 1985c). The information available suggests that a weaning education program can halve the proportion of children who are less than 75 percent weight-for-age, children who are likely to have a diarrheal mortality rate twice as high as other children (Ashworth and Feachem 1985c). If the effect of weaning education is manifest only during the weaning period, eighteen months to twenty-three months of age marking its upper limit, reductions in diarrhea mortality in children under five years old of 2 to 8 percent may be expected when the prevalence rates of moderate and severe malnutrition in the community, before the intervention, range from 10 to 50 percent of children. If the effect of weaning education can be extended to 59 months, and indeed a high proportion of undernutrition up to this age may be the result of failure to catch up after the weaning period, reductions of diarrheal mortality of 2 to 12 percent may be expected. According to most of the evidence available, the risk of diarrheal incidence is not likely to be reduced with improvements in the child's nutritional status, although more recent studies challenge these conclusions (Samani, Willet, and Ware 1988; Sepúlveda, Willet, and Muñoz 1988). Improvements in food hygiene resulting from weaning education are likely to increase the effect of the intervention, reducing diarrheal incidence and, possibly, the severity of episodes (Esrey and Feachem 1989).

From the few available data on the cost of implementing weaning education programs, Phillips, Feachem, and Mills (1987) found that weaning education activities have been mounted for between $0.50 and $10.00 per child benefiting, though these estimates are very sensitive to assumptions concerning the number of children benefiting and the comprehensiveness of the costings. The cost to the family, in the form of purchase and preparation of food, which may be substantial, is not included in these estimates. Using effectiveness data from Ashworth and Feachem (1985c), the cost-effectiveness of weaning education was estimated to range between $50 and $2,000 per diarrhea death averted, with a median estimate of $1,070.

ROTAVIRUS IMMUNIZATION. Rotavirus is the most frequent etiological agent isolated in children under two years who attend treatment centers for diarrheal diseases in developing countries (Black and others 1980; Levine and others 1986; Mata and others 1983; Stoll and others 1982). Rotavirus vaccines can thus be expected to have a role in reducing diarrheal incidence and mortality among young children in the developing world (de Zoysa and Feachem 1985b).

No vaccine is currently available for full-scale application. Attempts are under way to develop live, attenuated, oral vaccines against disease caused by human rotavirus (Flores and Kapikian 1989) and reassortant rotaviruses that incorporate in an animal rotavirus a gene segment encoding for the VP7 surface antigen of human rotavirus serotypes 1, 2, and 4. More recently, the naturally attenuated human "nursery strain" rotavirus has also been considered for use as an oral vaccine.

Field trials conducted to date have shown that vaccination with live rotavirus vaccines, in industrial countries, can reduce the incidence of clinically significant rotavirus diarrhea by nearly 80 percent. Vaccine efficacy in developing countries, for reasons that are not fully understood, has been much lower. The level of protection against all rotavirus diarrhea has in most studies been lower than that against severe rotavirus diarrhea (de Zoysa and Vesikari 1990).

Exploring the potential of rotavirus vaccines, de Zoysa and Feachem (1985b) suggested that a rotavirus vaccine of 80 percent efficacy given to children whose average age at full vaccination was six months could achieve reductions of 4 percent in diarrheal incidence and 13 percent in diarrheal deaths among children under five.

On the basis of actual cost data available for several national vaccination programs conducted in nine developing countries, and taking into account various features of the vaccines used in those programs (whether orally administered or injected, with another vaccine at the same visit or in the same injection, and the number of doses), Phillips, Feachem, and Mills (1987) calculated an average cost per "injected dose equivalent." They then applied this cost unit to the rotavirus vaccine (as well as to the measles and cholera vaccines discussed in the following sections). Taking account of the relevant characteristics of that vaccine and assuming the presence of an ongoing vaccination program, they derived estimated costs per child fully vaccinated of between $1.20 and $12.00, with a median of $1.90. Employing effectiveness results presented by de Zoysa and Feachem (1985b), they calculated the cost per diarrhea episode averted in children under five to lie in the range $3 to $30 (median $5) and the cost per diarrheal death averted to be between $140 and $1,400 (median $220).

CHOLERA IMMUNIZATION. Intestinal infections with *Vibrio cholerae* 01 are associated with especially severe diarrheal disease that occurs in both epidemic and endemic form (Feachem 1981; Miller, Feachem, and Draser 1984). In recent years, strains resistant to multiple antibiotics have been described in Bangladesh and East Africa.

The cholera vaccines that are available at present need to be given parenterally and are of low efficacy (WHO 1986c). Current research on cholera vaccines is directed toward the development of an effective oral vaccine that uses either nonliving bacteria and purified bacterial antigens or living avirulent mutants or genetically engineered strains. The hope is that these will stimulate the substantial immunity that is known to follow clinical cholera (WHO 1986c). Field trials of new nonliving oral vaccines in Bangladesh indicated overall protection for three years of 50 percent—but only 23 to 26 percent protection for children under six years (WHO 1989). The field is controversial and fast moving, and it remains unclear which type of vaccine for widespread application will emerge from the field trials (Levine 1989).

The administration schedule for the new cholera vaccines is still tentative. Two or three oral doses in the second year of life is one possible schedule. The vaccine is likely to be administered at a new contact and at an age when healthy children are not normally brought to health services, which may increase costs and decrease coverage. De Zoysa and Feachem (1985b) investigated the potential of cholera vaccination in Bangladesh, which has relatively high rates of endemic cholera. For a cholera vaccine of 70 percent efficacy and an average age at full vaccination of two years, 0.21 percent of diarrhea episodes and 2.8 percent of diarrheal deaths in vaccinated children under five years could be averted. In countries that had a lower proportion of diarrhea episodes and deaths caused by cholera, the effects would be less.

Phillips, Feachem, and Mills (1987) calculated costs using the methodology described for rotavirus and assuming a vaccination schedule of three doses given in the second year of life, a constant dropout rate between each contact of 10 percent, and a vaccine cost per dose similar to that of measles ($0.20). The results suggested that the cost per child fully vaccinated with a new oral cholera vaccine would range from $1.70 to $27.00, with a median value of $3.20. The cost per diarrhea episode and diarrhea death averted through cholera vaccinations, assuming 70 percent efficacy of the vaccine and cost of $4.00 per child fully vaccinated, was calculated to be $174.00 per diarrhea episode and $2,000.00 per diarrhea death averted in children under five years of age in Bangladesh. This estimate, however, relates only to routinely administered vaccination and not to vaccination in the presence of epidemics, when the cost-effectiveness would probably improve. The cost of vaccination is the highest of the vaccines evaluated, possibly twice as expensive as rotavirus or measles. The relatively poor performance of cholera vaccination in terms of cost-effectiveness is largely attributable to the rarity of the disease. Cholera constitutes a small proportion of the total diarrheal cases, even in Bangladesh, and even with equal costs per child vaccinated its cost-effectiveness would be about five times lower than that of measles or rotavirus vaccines.

MEASLES IMMUNIZATION. A marked association between measles and diarrhea has been described in developing countries (Koster and others 1981; Morley, Woodland, and Martin 1963; Scrimshaw and others 1966), and measles immunization has been considered a potential intervention for diarrhea control (Feachem and Koblinsky 1983). It is the only one of the three vaccines discussed here that is already commercially available and widely used. A single injected dose at the age of nine months is recommended in most developing countries. This is an age at which children are likely to be brought to the health services for various reasons, though no other vaccines are scheduled for this age.

Feachem and Koblinsky (1983), on the basis of the proportion of diarrheal episodes and diarrheal deaths that are measles-associated and the proportion of measles cases averted in the first five years of life by measles immunization, suggest that a measles vaccine that is 85 percent efficacious, given at the age of nine months through eleven months, with coverage of between 45 and 90 percent, can prevent 44 to 64 percent of measles cases, 0.6 to 3.8 percent of diarrheal episodes, and 6 to 26 percent of diarrheal deaths among children under five years of age. This estimate may be too conservative, however, as indicated by recently reported reductions of over 80 percent in total mortality among children nine months through thirty-nine months in Haiti (Holt and others 1990) and of 59 percent in diarrheal mortality among vaccinated children age ten months to sixty months in Bangladesh (Clemens and others 1988).

Phillips, Feachem, and Mills (1987) estimated the cost per child vaccinated against measles to range from $0.60 (Indonesia, mixed strategy: static/mobile delivery) to $12.00 (Ghana, outreach delivery strategy), with a median of $1.40. The cost per diarrheal episode averted in children under five through measles vaccination was calculated as $7.00, and the cost per diarrheal death averted as $143.00. Discounting diarrhea episodes and deaths averted in years following vaccination makes relatively little difference to the results, because the primary effect of the vaccine on diarrhea in children under five occurs within two years of vaccination. These values are roughly similar to that of rotavirus vaccine, which is more cost-effective in terms of diarrheal morbidity but less cost-effective in terms of diarrheal mortality.

IMPROVED WATER SUPPLY AND SANITATION FACILITIES. All major infectious agents that cause diarrhea are transmitted by the fecal-oral route. These enteric pathogens can be transmitted via contaminated water, and water-borne transmission has been documented for most of them. Improvement in water quality is, therefore, a potentially important intervention. Improvement in water quantity and availability is also important as an aid to hygienic practices which may interrupt the fecal-oral transmission. As all principal infectious agents of diarrhea are shed by infected persons via the feces, hygienic

disposal of excreta has the potential to play a role in controlling their transmission. Environmental improvements of these kinds probably contributed to the reduction in diarrheal morbidity and to the control of epidemic cholera and typhoid in Europe and North America between 1860 and 1920.

A review of sixty-seven studies from twenty-eight countries on the effect of water supply and sanitation on diarrhea, related infections, nutritional status, and mortality was conducted by Esrey, Feachem, and Hughes (1985). A median reduction of 27 percent in diarrhea morbidity and 30 percent in diarrheal mortality with the provision of improved water supply and excreta disposal was found in a subset of studies selected for their better design. Improvements in water quality appeared to have a lower effect than improvements in water availability or excreta disposal. No adequate data could be located, however, on the effect of improvements in water quality and availability together with excreta disposal. It is possible that well-designed projects combining water supply, excreta disposal, and hygiene education may achieve reductions of 35 to 50 percent in diarrheal morbidity (Esrey, Feachem, and Hughes 1985). It is expected that, except in areas where other interventions have substantially reduced diarrheal mortality, the effect will be larger on mortality rates than on morbidity.

A recent case-control study in the south of Brazil found that those infants whose homes had piped water had a diarrhea mortality rate 80 percent lower than those from homes with no easy access to piped water. No difference in mortality rates was detected, however, between infants receiving treated or untreated water, suggesting that beneficial effects of piped water may be related to the easy availability rather than its quality (Victora and others 1988). In addition to this Brazilian study, roughly a dozen studies of the effect of water and sanitation on diarrhea have been conducted since the review by Esrey, Feachem, and Hughes (1985). They were conducted in Bangladesh, the Gambia, Lesotho, Malawi, Nicaragua, Nigeria, the Philippines, and Sri Lanka. Half of them employed a case-control methodology. The studies have been reviewed recently by Cairncross (1990) and Huttly (1990).

Analysis of cost data from eighty-seven developing countries suggests median annual costs of $14 per capita for rural water supply and latrine projects and $46 per capita for a combination of in-house water supply and sewerage in an urban area (Esrey, Feachem, and Hughes 1985). The multiple benefits deriving from water-supply and sanitation interventions, including the reduction of diarrheal morbidity and mortality in other age groups, the reduction of the incidence of other infections, and other benefits not directly related to health (Briscoe 1984), make interpretation of simple cost per diarrhea death or episode averted problematic (Okun 1988). Further studies on ways to overcome these analytical difficulties are needed.

IMPROVED DOMESTIC AND PERSONAL HYGIENE. Poor personal hygiene of food handlers, inadequate cooking, and storage of food at incorrect temperatures for long periods are the most common contributing factors to food-borne diarrheal outbreaks in industrial countries (Frank and Barnhart 1986). Similar factors probably apply to food contamination in developing countries, where personal hygiene is likely to be markedly impaired by restricted water availability, overcrowding, and poor sanitation. Shortages of fuel, heavy workloads, and lack of access to refrigerators are probably additional contributory factors in developing countries (Esrey and Feachem 1989).

Unclean living conditions have been found to be associated with an increased risk of diarrheal incidence in children and adults (Bertrand and Walmus 1983; Huttly and others 1987; Taylor and others 1986). Infant-feeding bottles and bottle nipples are often highly contaminated (Elegbe and others 1982; Hibbert and Golden 1981; Phillips and others 1969; Surjono and others 1980), especially in lower-income households (Mathur and Reddy 1983). Feeding bowls and other feeding utensils have been found contaminated with *Escherichia coli* (Rowland, Barrell, and Whitehead 1978). Storage of food at high ambient temperatures increases the risk of contamination with fecal organisms (Barrell and Rowland 1979, 1980; Black and others 1982; Capparelli and Mata 1975). In these conditions, bacterial counts increase substantially with length of storage (Black and others 1982; Rowland, Barrell, and Whitehead 1978).

Few studies have been found that quantify the effectiveness of hygiene education interventions on diarrheal morbidity. Those that have been located (Bartlett and others 1985; Black and others 1981; Khan 1982; Stanton and Clemens 1987a; Torun 1982) focus mainly on the promotion of handwashing. Reductions of diarrheal incidence ranged from 14 to 48 percent, suggesting that hygiene education, and handwashing promotion in particular, has a marked effect on diarrheal rates.

Information on the cost of hygiene education is scarce. Costs are lower than for the provision of water supply and excreta disposal facilities, but the success of the promotion of handwashing may depend on the presence of these improved facilities (Feachem 1984). Analysis of three educational interventions for which data are available reveals a range of cost-effectiveness of under $20 per childhood case averted for village-based group education and supervision of day-care centers, to $300 to $500 per case averted for individual education of families presenting one or more cases of shigellosis (Phillips, Feachem, and Mills 1987).

Development of a Preventive Strategy in the Next Decade

During the next decade, the mainstay of diarrhea prevention will probably continue to be the interventions discussed above and listed in table 5-6. The change that can be expected is in the effectiveness (and the cost-effectiveness) of these interventions. The goal pursued in the use of the interventions, except for the immunizations, is substantial behavior change through education. Public health education is a relatively new field, and most countries currently lack the ability to deliver health education messages effectively to appropriate target groups. As experience grows and technology improves, these

antidiarrhea programs can be expected to yield greater benefits. The emphasis on education in the current AIDS-control strategy can only accelerate this process. The only new interventions that are expected are new vaccines. The next decade may see the incorporation into immunization programs of new vaccines against *Escherichia coli* and *Shigella*, besides the vaccines against *Vibrio cholerae* and rotavirus that were reviewed earlier in the chapter.

ESCHERICHIA COLI VACCINES. The incidence of diarrhea associated with enterotoxigenic *E. coli* in developing countries appears to be highest in children under two years, in which one or even two episodes per year have been noted. The incidence remains high in older children. Because partial immunity appears to develop after childhood, the target population for vaccination would be children during the first six months of life. It is difficult to estimate the number of strains the vaccine would need to cover, and a small proportion of disease would still occur at an early age, before vaccination could confer full protection.

Taking these two factors into account, the U.S. Institute of Medicine (1986) estimated that 50 to 60 percent of enterotoxigenic *E. coli* episodes would be vaccine preventable. Recent advances in the development of vaccines against diarrhea due to enterotoxigenic *E. coli* were reviewed by Levine (1989, 1990). The first experimental vaccines were expected to be ready for testing in human volunteers in 1990 (WHO 1989). Studies in Swedish volunteers have shown that the prototype *E. coli* vaccine is safe and immunogenic. At least 80 percent of the volunteers developed intestinal antibody response to the antigens after receiving two or three doses of vaccine. (WHO 1992)

SHIGELLA VACCINES. The development of effective *Shigella* vaccines deserves special priority. Of all the diarrhea-causing agents, it is the most life-threatening. *S. dysenteriae* is responsible for an especially serious form of dysentery which can prove difficult to manage, even in sophisticated clinical settings. Major outbreaks of drug-resistant *S. dysenteriae* have occurred in the past thirty years in Central America, Central Africa, and Bengal (East and West) and have resulted in hundreds of thousands of deaths in all age groups. Nalidixic acid was the antibiotic of choice in these circumstances, but resistance to this product is now reported.

The incidence of shigellosis in developing countries is highest for children age two to four years, but it is already a problem from six months of age. All age groups are susceptible and could benefit from immunization. A vaccine incorporating protective antigens from the most common infecting strains in a given geographic area should prevent 80 to 90 percent of the *Shigella* infections, depending on the prevalence of these strains and assuming total coverage of the target population with a vaccine that is 100 percent effective and is delivered at the earliest feasible age (U.S. Institute of Medicine 1986). *Shigella* vaccines are reviewed by Levine (1989). A candidate vaccine, developed from a live attenuated *S. flexneri* strain, is being tested for safety and immunogeneity in the United States. Other efforts are under way in France and Sweden (WHO 1989).

Ideal Prevention and Current Prevention: Closing the Gaps

The following section describes the technical and institutional aspects involved in closing the gap between current preventive practices and ideal prevention.

TECHNICAL ASPECTS. Although a set of behaviors associated with lower diarrheal incidence and reduction of severity has already been identified, there is still a long way to go before these desirable behaviors are widespread and commonplace and before the necessary improvements in water, sanitation, and kitchen equipment are available to most families. Exclusive breastfeeding during the first four to six months of life, followed by partial breastfeeding during the remainder of the first year of life, can be expected to reduce infant diarrheal morbidity and mortality significantly. Trends in developing countries have, however, been toward lower prevalence and duration of breastfeeding in urban areas (Popkin, Bilsborrow, and Akin 1982; Popkin and Bisgrove 1988), and early food supplementation for breastfed infants is the rule, rather than the exception. Early weaning and inadequate supplementation, the use of foods of low energy and nutrient concentration, the selection of single foods of low nutritional value, the use of contaminated foods, feeding at infrequent intervals, and giving infants a disproportionately small share of the family food are still common practices in developing countries (Ashworth and Feachem 1985c).

Measles vaccination should reduce diarrheal mortality in children under five. Coverage, however, remains low in some regions, averaging 46 percent in Africa and 51 percent in Southeast Asia (WHO 1990a), and the effectiveness of vaccines may be reduced by an inadequate "cold chain." Improvements in water supply and sanitation can lead to reductions in diarrheal morbidity and mortality in children under five of about 30 percent. Access to better facilities does not imply improved use, however, and water and sanitation interventions have failed to reduce diarrheal rates in some settings (Nigeria, Imo State Evaluation Team 1989; Ryder, Reeves, and Sack 1985). Personal and domestic hygiene behaviors that may reduce diarrheal incidence have been identified. Handwashing before preparing and offering food and careful disposal of child feces, two potentially effective practices, may depend on changes in attitudes and in the availability of water and soap. In Bangladesh, for example, it was observed that mothers washed their own hands before offering food to young children in 53 percent of feedings but in almost all cases without using soap. Other caretakers were observed washing their hands when offering the food in only 11 percent of the feeds (Guldan 1988).

INSTITUTIONAL ASPECTS. The WHO/CDD program has played a major role since 1980 in promoting research on diarrhea epidemiology, vaccine development, and the cost-effectiveness of specific interventions. Much of the work reported in this chapter on diarrhea prevention has been initiated or influenced by WHO/CDD. It is important that this effort continue with an increased focus on research that will assist in the design and delivery of cost-effective interventions.

The WHO/CDD program is taking substantial steps to influence the ability and commitment of governments to implement these known effective interventions. Measles immunization and improvements in water supplies and sanitation are under way in any case and are not the responsibility of national CDD programs. The other interventions discussed here (table 5-6) exist in a very limited fashion in most countries. A great challenge for the WHO/CDD program during the next decade lies in rectifying this situation. Promotion of exclusive breastfeeding in the first four to six months of life is the first preventive intervention chosen by WHO/CDD for implementation efforts, which started in 1990.

Defining the Optimal Preventive Strategy

What preventive measures should reasonably be taken for any particular population will depend on a range of factors—the relative and absolute importance of diarrhea morbidity and mortality; the relative importance of different etiologies and of the risk factors that predispose children and adults to diarrhea; the nature and extent of the existing infrastructure; government priorities for development and ongoing interventions; relative and absolute price levels; and, very important, the level of relevant budgetary constraints.

Several of the preventive strategies, in addition to being relatively cost-effective in preventing diarrhea (still one of the most important causes of death in many developing countries), have important additional potential health benefits beyond diarrhea control. It would seem reasonable, therefore, that at least one-twentieth of a country's health budget be spent on efforts to prevent diarrhea—say $1 per head for high-mortality countries (whose health budgets are generally small) and $3 per head for lower-mortality (and generally higher-income) countries. A rough order of priorities for preventive interventions, based substantially on the cost-effectiveness of currently available technology, is set out below:

• Measles vaccination for at least 80 percent of the nine-to-twelve-month-old population. At a cost of about $2.00 per additional child vaccinated (assuming a vaccination program is already in place), and possibly double that to cover the least accessible final 20 percent, this amounts to some $0.10 per head, or up to 10 percent of the proposed budget allocation for diarrhea prevention in high-mortality countries. Such a vaccination program would be expected to avert 23 percent to 29 percent of diarrheal deaths in those under five years of age. It would also avert substantial measles mortality and, in areas where measles is severe and associated with high risks of xerophthalmia, an additional benefit would be the prevention of a substantial proportion of blindness.

- For areas where breastfeeding rates are low or early supplementation is a common practice, investment in breastfeeding promotion aimed at achieving exclusive breastfeeding up to four or six months should also be a priority. Some interventions, such as changing hospital routines, can be implemented relatively cheaply (under $1.00 per delivery—or less than $0.05 per head even if all children were delivered in a hospital and routines changed in all hospitals). For about $0.20 per head per year it should be possible to implement a package of hospital-based, legislative, and mass media measures designed to improve breastfeeding rates.

- With the remaining funds available, promotion of improved weaning and hygiene practices for mothers (both feasible for about $0.30 per head each), should be next on the agenda (the former particularly for high-mortality countries), although adoption of hygiene practices may be constrained by water availability.

- Improvements in water and sanitation facilities are relatively expensive, estimated at between $14 to $46 per head annually. Even if the whole of the $1 to $3 per head notionally set aside for diarrhea prevention were allocated to water supply, only one-fifth to one-forty-fifth of individuals would be covered by the interventions. Some countries could partially overcome this difficulty by requiring that individual consumers be responsible for some or all of the costs of these services, which they may, indeed, provide for themselves. Self-provision of Ventilated Improved Pit latrines in Lesotho is a case in point and has achieved notable health benefits (Daniels and others 1990).

Case Management

The elements of the current case management strategy, its likely development over the next decade, the gap between good and actual case management, and the definition of an optimal case management strategy are examined in this section.

Elements of a Case Management Strategy

Case management involves several dimensions: the way diagnoses are made, the nature of medication and advice offered, and the level and location of services. We concentrate principally on the effectiveness and costs of medication options, referring more briefly to the way these are influenced by various options for making diagnoses and for providing services.

A serious complication of some diarrhea episodes is dehydration, which can lead to death, particularly in small children. Correct case management involves, at a minimum, the prevention and correction of dehydration. Considerable effort has been devoted in the last twenty years to the development and promotion of rehydration solutions which can be taken orally. These advances, and the effectiveness and cost of the alternative methods of prevention and correction of dehydration, are outlined below. We follow this with a discussion of antibiotics and antidiarrheals and their limited role in curative and palliative treatment of diarrhea.

SECONDARY PREVENTION: REHYDRATION. Until the late 1960s the primary medical method of rehydration was intravenous (IV) therapy. The development of oral rehydration solutions, combining electrolytes and glucose, sucrose, or rice powder, has been an important breakthrough (Darrow and others 1949; Nalin and others 1968; Pierce and others 1968; *Lancet* 1981). The composition for ORS recommended currently by WHO is 3.5 grams of sodium chloride, 2.9 grams of trisodium citrate dihydrate, 1.5 grams of potassium chloride, and 20 grams of glucose (WHO 1987c). Clinical studies have shown that ORS can successfully rehydrate 90 to 95 percent of cases of acute watery diarrhea, substantially reducing the requirements for IV rehydration (Hirschhorn 1980; Levine and others 1986). Not only are ORS as effective as intravenous rehydration in the vast majority of cases, they are also less hazardous, especially in settings in which the risk of infection in the hospital is high.

In efforts to identify ways of promoting early and increased use of rehydration therapy, researchers have explored the efficacy of fluids which can be prepared with ingredients available in the home. Solutions of sugar and salt (SSS) have been shown to correct fluid volume deficits in noncholera diarrhea in adults and children (Clements and others 1981; Islam and others 1980). They correct acidosis slowly, however, and are not adequate for the correction of hypokalemia or the replacement of electrolyte losses in cholera (Islam and Bardhan 1985). Home-based fluids (such as gruels, soups, and diluted yoghurt drinks) which contain some salt and a source of glucose, can be effective in preventing dehydration as long as the sodium concentration lies in the range of 30 to 80 millimolars, and the osmolarity is less than 300 milliosmoles per kilogram of water (WHO 1987a). The glucose range is not relevant if a complex carbohydrate is used.

Studies of the effectiveness of ORT promotion under field conditions are not uniformly positive in their findings (for example, Tekce 1982). This is small wonder, given the reliance on adequate supplies of ORS and the multiple steps required by caretakers in the preparation and use of ORT, where practice can readily stray from the ideal. In a later section we provide some evidence of the extent to which practice diverges from the ideal. Nevertheless, the overall findings on effectiveness tend to be positive. Studies in Egypt (Kielman and others 1985) and India (Kielman and McCord 1977) described marked decreases in diarrhea-associated mortality rates with the use of SSS by village health workers for the treatment of diarrhea. It is not clear, however, if the results were due to the use of SSS at home, an increase in the use of ORS in the treatment of more severe cases, or the repeated home visits by health workers. Recent evaluations of the effect of oral rehydration therapy in Egypt associate a sharp reduction in diarrheal mortality rates among children under five with improved diarrheal case management by mothers and doctors (Egypt, National Control of Diarrheal Diseases Project 1988; el-Rafie and others 1990). The constancy of death rates from other causes, the nature of the change in the seasonal pattern of total mortality, and the lack of change in diarrhea incidence or nutritional status are all compatible with the hypothesis that improved case management is the explanation for the reduction in diarrhea mortality. Nevertheless, uncertainty as to the accuracy of mortality statistics may indicate a need for caution in the evaluation of these results.

Data on the effect of ORT in a hospital setting summarized by WHO/CDD from twenty-eight reports from twenty-one countries indicate median reductions of 61 percent in diarrhea admission rates, 71 percent in overall diarrhea case-fatality rates, and 41 percent in inpatient diarrhea case-fatality rates. Reductions of nearly 70 percent in the proportion of hospitalized cases treated with IV fluids after the introduction of ORT were reported from Malawi and Tanzania. In Stanley Hospital, Madras, India, the average number of days of hospital stay decreased from 6 to 1.5 in association with the gradual increase of ORT use in a period of seven years (WHO 1988a). In a hospital in Haiti, for example, diarrhea mortality fell from 35 percent to 14 percent and then to less than 1 percent with the creation of an ORT unit (Allman and Rohde 1985).

The effectiveness of ORT, high in preventing death from dehydration caused by acute watery diarrheal episodes and, possibly, in aiding recovery of appetite and thus increasing food intake, is probably low in the prevention of death from persistent and dysenteric episodes.

The cost of ORS is low; UNIPAC (the central warehouse of UNICEF in Copenhagen) provides 1-liter sachets for $0.07. A course of treatment using 2 to 3 liters would cost $0.14 to $0.21 per episode. The cost of the ingredients for home-based solutions is likely to be lower than the cost of packaged ORS, and certainly the cost is lower for the health services if ORS are otherwise supplied free or at a subsidized rate. Still, other costs to the health services may be greater when home-based solutions rather than ORS are used. The effectiveness and safety of SSS depend, for example, on the ability of mothers to learn and retain the skills required in its preparation. This calls for educational interventions which may need to be more substantial than those required for ORS. Education of mothers on the use of SSS has been shown to be short-lived in its effect on behavior (AED 1985; Chowdhury, Vaughan, and Abed 1988; WHO 1986b), which suggests the need for more effective or repeated education. How this compares with the kind of effort required to educate mothers about ORS is, however, not documented.

Oral rehydration salts and home-based fluids differ in their cost implications for families, and the net result is difficult to judge. On the one hand, ingredients for home-based fluids are likely to be fully paid for by the family, whereas ORS may well be wholly or partly subsidized. Household costs for preparing food-based fluids may be particularly high if regular preparation of small quantities (with the associated time and fuel demands) is required in order to avoid spoilage. On the other hand, if ingredients are at hand, home-based fluids may be more convenient to mothers, reducing costs in time and transportation associated with visits to health facilities. Treatment-

associated household costs in using ORS could, however, be reduced by regular stocking of household or neighborhood supplies. Both ORS and home-based fluids probably place considerable time demands on mothers. Evidence is scarce, but a rough calculation suggests that a mother with young children could spend 10 percent of the year treating diarrhea in her children with ORT (Leslie 1989).

Oral rehydration therapy is considerably less costly than intravenous rehydration, not only in terms of the ingredients and equipment but, more important, because of the reduced demand for hospital beds and all the associated inpatient costs. Oral rehydration therapy can generally be provided at the lowest level of health facility or in the home, as can the clinical diagnosis required both to distinguish watery from other diarrheas and to identify the degree of severity of dehydration. At Safdargang Hospital in New Delhi, India, diarrhea treatment costs were reduced by 69 percent and at San Lazaro Hospital, Manila, the Philippines, by 62 percent, when ORT was introduced (WHO 1988c). In a children's hospital in Mexico City, the opening of an oral rehydration unit reduced the number of inpatients with diarrhea by 25 percent, giving rise to considerable potential savings, (Phillips, Kumaté-Rodrígues, and Mota-Hernández 1989). Another study in Mexico City also identified savings as a result of the introduction in two clinics of therapeutic norms stressing the importance of ORT (Castro and others 1988). In the first two years following staff training and the establishment of an ORT unit at the Kamuzu Central Hospital, Lilongwe, Malawi, there was a 50 percent decrease in the number of children admitted to the pediatric ward with diarrhea, a 56 percent decrease in the use of intravenous fluids to rehydrate such children, and a 32 percent reduction in recurrent hospital costs attributable to pediatric diarrhea (Heymann and others 1990). The results, however, are not uniformly positive. In a study in Indonesia, neither hospitalization rate nor intravenous fluid expenditure were related to the rate of ORS use in the community (Lerman, Shepard, and Cash 1985). The time demands of ORT probably remain higher than for IV rehydration, which may partly explain why in many cases children hospitalized with diarrhea who could be treated with ORT receive IV therapy instead.

Relatively few studies have attempted to measure both the costs and the effectiveness of field-based ORT programs, and with few exceptions measures of health effects (for example, deaths averted) have not been used. "Diarrhea cases treated" is the most common direct measure of effectiveness. The nature of the cost analysis in these studies has not been consistent. Shepard, Brenzel, and Nemeth (1986) identified studies with adequate cost data in only four countries and reanalyzed the cost data to generate reasonably compatible estimates of full economic costs. The results from these studies and three additional ones are shown in table 5-7 and reveal costs per child treated in the range of approximately $1 to $10. Much of the variation in cost between countries can be explained by differences in gross national product per capita. The rest is probably the result of (a) differences in the level of services provided (Horton and Claquin [1983] found an ap-

Table 5-7. Cost of Treatment with ORT

Location	Average cost per child treated (1982 U.S. dollars)	Reference
The Gambia	0.70	Shepard, Brenzel, and Nemeth, 1986
Indonesia	0.77	Shepard, Brenzel, and Nemeth, 1986
Malawi	1.86	Qualls and Robertson, 1989[a]
Honduras	2.94	Shepard, Brenzel, and Nemeth, 1986
Bangladesh	3.30	Horton and Claquin, 1983
Egypt	5.56[b]	Shepard, Brenzel, and Nemeth, 1986
Swaziland	6.28	Qualls and Robertson, 1989[a]
Turkey	9.66	Brenzel, 1987

a. Study reports data collected in 1984.
b. Cost per child in the population.
Source: See last column of table.

proximately tenfold difference in cost between treatment in basic facilities and that in relatively sophisticated facilities in Bangladesh); (b) the scale of the operation's fixed costs, which tends to be relatively high (for example, 96 percent of the Turkish ORT program costs were fixed [Brenzel 1987]), giving rise to substantial changes in average costs as the program expands; (c) the efficiency with which the program is conducted; and (d) the costing methodology employed, particularly with respect to the measurement of personnel costs, which are often the largest component and the least straightforward to measure.

The effectiveness of the programs in averting deaths is likely to vary, depending on the nature and severity of all the diarrhea cases, the degree of selectivity in treatment, how well the intervention is delivered, and the extent of use and effectiveness of alternative treatments. Case-fatality rates prior to the widespread use of ORT were estimated to be of the order of 6 per 1,000 (Snyder and Merson 1982). If ORT were 100 percent effective and targeted at the diarrhea group with a case-fatality ratio of 10 per 1,000, then deaths averted would be 1 percent of treated cases. If case-fatality ratios were higher or ORT programs were successfully targeted at those with even more

Table 5-8. Cost per Death Averted for Different Treatment Costs and ORT Effectiveness

Costs per episode treated (U.S. dollars)	Cases treated that prevented one death			
	0.05	0.10	0.50	1.00
0.50	1,000	500	100	50
1.00	2,000	1,000	200	100
5.00	10,000	5,000	1,000	500
10.00	20,000	10,000	2,000	1,000

Source: Authors' calculations from assumptions based on figures of table 5-7.

severe diarrhea, then effectiveness would increase. If the pre-ORT case-fatality rates were lower, 1 per 1,000, for example, and ORT were only 50 percent effective, deaths would be averted in 0.05 percent of the treated cases. Table 5-8 shows how costs per death averted vary for different costs per episode treated and deaths averted per case treated. The range of most likely estimates appears to be between $1,000 and $10,000. Most of the estimates of Shepard, Brenzel, and Nemeth (1986) lie below $10,000, and some below $1,000.

CURE AND PALLIATIVE TREATMENT—DRUGS. A large variety of drugs is currently promoted commercially for the management of diarrhea. They include antimotility drugs, antisecretory drugs, adsorbents, and antibiotics. The majority of these drugs have no proven benefit and can be positively dangerous, particularly for small children. Most have a minimal effect on the clinically important aspects of diarrhea, some have negative side effects, and all are suspected of diverting attention away from life-saving rehydration therapies. Table 5-9 outlines the evidence on the efficacy of selected drugs commonly promoted as antidiarrheals.

Case management for adult sufferers of diarrhea poses different challenges from those of childhood diarrhea. Not only are there differences in the relative incidence of different etiologies of diarrhea and in the average severity and length of episodes (U.S. Institute of Medicine 1986) but also in the significance of different characteristics of diarrhea. For example, the inconvenience of poor control over defecation is likely to be an important motivation for adults seeking treatment for diarrhea. Furthermore, the negative side effects of antidiarrheals are generally less severe for adults. Palliative treatment, strongly discouraged for young children, given the currently available selection of drugs, has a role to play in adult treatment.

Patients with AIDS commonly suffer from severe and chronic watery diarrhea, associated variously with protozoan organisms such as *Isospora belli* and *Cryptosporidium* (Young 1987), with mycobacterial organisms such as *Mycobacterium avium intracellulare* (Carswell 1988), and occasionally with well-recognized agents such as *Giardia, Salmonella, Shigella,* and *Campylobacter.* Some reports have suggested improvements of diarrhea in patients who have been treated with either spiramycin or α-eflornithine, though the evidence is not consistent (Kaplan, Wofsy, and Volberding 1987). At the present time maintenance of hydration and, in adult patients, symptomatic control with opiate derivative antidiarrheals are the only helpful interventions (Kaplan, Wofsy, and Volberding 1987), though a role for prostaglandin inhibitors has been suggested (Young 1987).

For all ages there is a legitimate, though limited, role for antibiotics in the treatment of diarrhea: antibiotics can significantly diminish the severity and duration of diarrhea due to cholera and *Shigella* and shorten the period of pathogen excretion in the case of dysenteric episodes. Antibiotics have no proven value for the routine treatment of acute watery diarrhea, however, and their use, besides being inappropriate, may

Table 5-9. Efficacy and Side Effects of Selected Drugs Promoted for Treatment of Diarrhea

Drug	Efficacy	Side effects
Antimotility		
Loperamide (Imodium)	Trials have failed to demonstrate clinically significant effects on daily stool volume or rehydration requirements	Can prolong infectious diarrhea, cause toxic megacolon, central nervous system toxicity
Diphenoxylate (Lomotil)	No clinically important reduction in number or volume of stools, length of episode, or intravenous liquids required	Can worsen clinical course (prolong fever and Shigella excretion); central nervous system toxicity at recommended doses
Antisecretory		
Bismuth subsalicylate (Pepto–Bismol)	No effect on quantity of liquid or total stool weight; diminished number of liquid stools and subjective complaints in young adults with travelers' diarrhea	Required doses too large to be practical or safe
Aciduric bacteria	No therapeutic or prophylactic benefits demonstrated	—
Adsorbents		
Kaolin	Can increase consistency of stool; no effect on weight, liquid content, or frequency of stools	May interfere with efficacy of antibiotics
Charcoal	Ineffective	Interferes with effects of tetracycline
Attapulgite and Smectite	Can increase consistency of stools; no conclusive evidence of effect on fluid or electrolyte losses	May bind and inactivate other drugs
Cholestyramine	Conflicting evidence; not recommended	Interferes with fat and vitamin absorption

— Not available.
Source: WHO 1986 and 1990.

even be dangerous (WHO 1986a). In Basrah, for example, Mahmood and Feachem (1987) found that antibiotic therapy was significantly associated with prolonged hospitalization of infants with diarrhea caused by enteropathogenic *Escherichia coli*. In table 5-10 it is noted which antibiotics are recommended for the treatment of diarrhea associated with specific pathogens.

On grounds of efficacy alone many of the drugs marketed as antidiarrheals can be dismissed. Furthermore, they can be quite costly: a bottle of tetracycline syrup, for example, costs more than six times that of a liter-size package of ORS in Indonesia. This, together with the high rate of use of antibiotics and antidiarrheals (discussed later), accounts for the substantial levels of expenditure on these drugs. Sixty percent of drug costs for treating simple diarrhea were spent on antimicrobials in one area of Indonesia (Quick and others 1988). In another study in Indonesia (Lerman, Shepard, and Cash 1985), more than five times as much was spent on antimicrobials and antidiarrheals as on ORS ($1.01 compared with $0.18 per child).

For the relatively few cases of diarrhea in which antibiotics can appropriately be prescribed, recommendations concerning the preferred choice from the range of available drugs have largely been based on relative efficacy (taking into account the problem of resistance) and severity of side effects. Costs have

Table 5-10. Antibiotic Treatment for Specific Diarrheal Diseases

Disease	Recommended treatment	Alternatives
Cholera (proven or suspected)	Tetracycline or doxycycline	Furazolidone or sulamethoxazole-trimethoprim
Dysentery (no coproculture necessary)	Sulfamethoxazole-trimethoprim	Nalidixic acid or ampicillin
Amebiasis (trophozoite in stool)	Metronidazole	In severe cases, dehydroemetine hydrochloride
Giardia lamblia (trophozoite or giardial antigen in stool)	Metronidazole	Quinacrine
Campylobacter	Erythromycin[a]	None
Severe *Yersinia*	Chloramphenicol	None
Escherichia coli rotavirus	No antibiotics[b]	None

a. Antibiotic treatment is recommended only if rapid diagnosis is possible and treatment can begin on the first day.
b. Antibiotics can lead to harmful overgrowth of organisms such as *Clostridium difficile*, with attendant necrotizing colitis.
Source: WHO 1986c and 1990b.

not been an important consideration. That the cost of alternative regimens can be significant is illustrated by *Giardia*, for which no treatment is usually required: the cheapest recommended treatment (quinacrine) costs less than one-eighth of the most expensive recommended treatment (furazolidone) (Stevens 1986).

Laboratory tests are often used to discriminate between different etiologies of diarrhea. These tests are of very limited value for guiding therapy, however, and their costs can be high. It is claimed, for example, that routine stool culture has been one of the most costly and ineffective microbiological tests, with the costs per positive result exceeding $1,000 in the United States (Guerrant and others 1985).

REHABILITATION—CONTINUED FEEDING. Among infectious diseases, diarrhea is probably the most common contributor to malnutrition in developing countries. Malnourished children are particularly prone to more persistent and severe diarrheal episodes, and possibly they are at higher risk of frequent episodes, leading to further nutritional deterioration and allowing less time for recovery and catch-up growth. The need to prevent and offset the deterioration of the nutritional status, and the evidence that recovery is accelerated with continued feeding during diarrhea, make nutritional care of acute and persistent diarrhea episodes a key element of case management (United States, National Research Council 1985; WHO 1988b). Despite efforts at continued feeding during diarrhea episodes, the reduced food intake (due to anorexia or food withholding), malabsorption, and increased catabolism are likely to result in net nutritional losses. This leads to weight loss and growth retardation. Increased consumption is required, therefore, during convalescence to compensate for weight loss and to allow catch-up growth.

Continued feeding during the active and early convalescence phases of diarrhea has been recommended by the Subcommittee on Nutrition and Diarrheal Diseases Control of the United States National Research Council (1985). Two important objectives are addressed through continued feeding: to minimize the nutritional effect of the illness and to promote normal intestinal mucosal renewal and absorptive and digestive functions. These objectives are the same whether the treatment is being carried out in a hospital or at home. Choice of foods, modes of preparation, and frequency of feeding depend on the child's age, feeding history, and physiological status. Feeding recommendations should take into account the cultural norms and practices, food availability, economic constraints, and the difficulty of preparation of the foods in the home. Breastfeeding should be continued and, for children less than six months, breast milk alone given at adequate frequency is likely to offset the effect of diarrhea on nutritional status. For infants older than six months, breastfeeding should be continued but supplemented with other foods.

The selection of weaning foods to be recommended by health authorities should take into account the fat-to-energy ratio, the quality of the mixture of dietary proteins, and the carbohydrate content. Fat should supply 40 to 50 percent of the dietary energy during the first six months of life and 34 to 40 percent for the remainder of early childhood, lower ratios being associated with increased bulk and higher risk of inadequate energy intake. A combination of unsaturated fats and mixed long-chain saturated fats is likely to lead to better absorption than saturated fats alone. Malabsorption of fats does not appear to exacerbate diarrhea, but it does prolong nutritional rehabilitation and, if protein intake is marginal, adversely affects nitrogen retention (United States, National Research Council 1985). Animal protein is generally more digestible and of higher biological quality than plant protein. Plant proteins can be mixed, however, to improve their biological quality. Carbohydrates, mostly starches, sucrose, and lactose, usually account for 35 to 55 percent of energy intake in early infancy. Although feeding of lactose to infants with diarrhea may be considered unwise, given the recognized reduction in intestinal lactase during illness, this type of acquired lactase deficiency is seldom total. Concentrations of lactose equivalent to those found in half-strength cow's milk are generally well tolerated in diarrhea, especially in mixed foods, such as milk-cereal combinations (United States, National Research Council 1985). Sucrose and processed vegetable starches are usually easily digested and absorbed in children with diarrhea. Misconceptions concerning the significance of transient intolerance to carbohydrates too often lead to unnecessary food withholding. The risk of intolerance can be minimized by multiple feeding of small amounts of mixtures of carbohydrates. If single trials with foods that contain lactose do not aggravate clinical symptoms, continued tolerance during convalescence may be assumed (United States, National Research Council 1985).

Food preparation should take into account its energy density, consistency, digestibility, and acceptability. Energy density can be enhanced by increasing the fat content. Watery paps and soups should not comprise the entire diet, given their low energy concentrations. Meals should be small and frequent (at least once every three to four hours), especially in early treatment. During convalescence, increased intake of food (at least 25 percent higher than levels before the illness) should be ensured for more than two weeks, because early resumption of usual feeding patterns will probably be inadequate for full recovery in a reasonable period.

Case Management Strategy for the Next Decade

Case management of diarrheal diseases is likely to become more effective and to reach a greater proportion of the population in the next decade. More attention will probably be paid to the maintenance of the nutritional status of diarrheal patients, the use of improved oral rehydration solutions that will actually decrease stool losses, and the control of persistent and dysenteric episodes, possibly through the use of newly developed drugs together with adequate nutritional support.

SECONDARY PREVENTION—IMPROVED ORS. Intense research efforts have been dedicated to the development of oral rehydration solutions that might correct dehydration and decrease stool output. The basic principle is to increase intestinal sodium absorption by providing larger amounts of different types of organic carriers than those present in the glucose-based ORS. The most promising of the improved ORS formulations studied to date is rice-based ORS. Results of clinical trials performed with rice-based ORS indicate that the rate of stool loss is significantly reduced (33 to 42 percent during the first twenty-four hours of treatment) in patients with rapidly purging diarrhea who are given rice-based ORS solution, as compared with patients given glucose-ORS solution. Treatment with rice-based ORS in such patients also reduces the duration of diarrhea. These reductions in the rate of stool loss and in the duration of diarrhea combine to cause an even greater reduction in total stool output during the entire illness. Feeding rice to patients given glucose-based ORS solution does not appear to cause the same reduction in stool output as treatment with rice-based ORS solution (WHO 1990c). The results summarized above indicate that rice-based ORS can be recommended in the treatment of patients with rapidly purging diarrhea. Its role in the treatment of less severe diarrhea, however, is still unclear and is the subject of ongoing research.

CURE AND PALLIATIVE TREATMENT—NEW DRUGS. As the understanding of secretory physiology increases, new methods of controlling watery diarrhea may be developed, and both improved antibiotics in the treatment of dysenteric episodes and drugs able to reverse the derangements caused by bacterial toxins may be produced (Guerrant 1986). Advances are also to be expected in drugs that are useful in persistent diarrheas. The interested reader should refer to Kandel and Donowitz (1989) and Murray and DuPont (1989).

REHABILITATION—CONTINUED FEEDING. Increasing attention has been paid to continued feeding during diarrheal episodes as a way of reducing the negative effects of the disease on child growth and the nutritional status of adults and children. More and more evidence indicates that continued feeding has no negative effects on the severity or duration of the disease and that it significantly improves nutritional outcomes (Brown and others 1988). Lactose intolerance has been found to be a minor problem among infants older than six months (WHO 1988b). Studies are being conducted to evaluate the effectiveness and safety of lactose-containing diets for feeding young infants suffering with diarrhea.

Good and Actual Case Management: Closing the Gap

The following section describes the technical and institutional aspects involved in closing the gap between good case management and actual case management practices.

TECHNICAL ASPECTS. It is unfortunately true that the usual management of diarrhea patients is markedly at odds with recommended methods. Secondary prevention in the form of the prevention and treatment of dehydration, although acknowledged to be the crucially important element in the case management of diarrhea, is not common practice everywhere. However, antibiotic and palliative treatment is frequent, despite substantial evidence of its inefficacy and risk, particularly for children. Rehabilitation through the adoption of appropriate feeding practices following a diarrhea episode is less likely to take place among the groups at higher risk of diarrheal incidence or severity and has been promoted less strenuously than the prevention and treatment of dehydration.

Table 5-11 shows the nature of treatment provided to children under five years of age with diarrhea according to a set of WHO/CDD surveys in sixty countries. Although the median of use of some form of oral rehydration therapy was more than 50 percent of cases, ranges were very wide. "Other medicine," often indicating antibiotics or antimotility drugs, was reported to have been used in nearly 50 percent of cases. This general picture is fleshed out by more detailed studies in specific settings. In a household survey in four subdistricts in Indonesia, Lerman, Shepard, and Cash (1985) found that almost three-quarters of all episodes of diarrhea were treated with another agent, either alone or in combination with ORS (which were received by about 50 percent of the patients): 34 percent were treated with tetracycline, 27 percent with iodochlorhydroxyquin, and 23 percent with sulphaguanidine. Another study in Indonesia (Quick and others 1988) supported these general findings: antibiotics were prescribed in over 90 percent of cases, more than twice as frequently as ORS (with children under five receiving an average of five drugs per episode), and vitamins and minerals were prescribed more often than ORS. Furthermore, the antibiotics were often prescribed in inadequate quantities. There was no evidence that prescribers distinguished diarrheas benefiting from antibiotics from those worsened or unaffected by antibiotics. A study in Nepal found that despite extensive ORT education of families, only 8 percent of diarrhea patients received ORS or home fluids (Wornham 1987).

A small hospital-based study in Mexico City found that although hospital treatment was reasonably satisfactory, prehospital treatment involved very high antibiotic and antidiarrheal use (Phillips, Kumaté-Rodrígues, and Mota-Hernández 1989). A study of hospitalized infants with diarrhea in Iraq found that intravenous rehydration was given in 94 percent of cases and antibiotics in 50 percent (Mahmood and Feachem 1987). The authors judged that most of this IV and drug use was unnecessary.

Evidence from the pharmaceutical industries supports the suggestion of substantial use of largely ineffective or dangerous drugs: the antidiarrheal with the largest turnover in 1984 was Imodium, which had over 10 percent of the market for antidiarrheals. Lomotil, Kaopectate, and Entero-Vioform made up another 10 percent (Health Action International 1986). A survey of dispensing patterns of seventy-five pharmacists in Bangladesh, Sri Lanka, and Yemen found that only 25 percent of pharmacies recommended ORS or referral to a health worker, but 65 percent dispensed drugs with or without ORS (Thomson and Sterkey 1986).

Treatment with ORT that is recorded cannot automatically be taken to mean ideal treatment. Rehydration solutions are normally prepared in the home—their effectiveness and safety

Table 5-11. Treatment Rates of Diarrhea Episodes in Children under Age Five in 276 Studies in 60 Countries
(percent)

Treatment	Treatment rates	
	Median	Range
ORS	26.4	0.0–53.0
Sugar-salt solutions	7.0	0.7–43.4
Home fluids	25.3	6.0–82.1
IV fluids	1.5	0.0–7.1
"Traditional" medicines	21.3	2.1–69.1
Other medicines	48.3	7.4–71.0
No treatment	15.3	5.0–64.1

Source: Unpublished World Health Organization data.

are highly dependent on how well informed and motivated mothers are, on their time availability, and on their access to the correct ingredients and utensils. Not all marketed oral rehydration fluids have the WHO-recommended composition and not all ORT is properly prepared or administered. Several studies have highlighted the difficulty of ensuring the correct preparation of SSS: 25 percent of samples prepared in Nepal (using the pinch-and-scoop method of measuring ingredients), 24 to 48 percent in Bangladesh, and 40 percent in Nigeria were found to be hypertonic, with sodium levels greater than 90, 100, and 80 millimolars, respectively (Poudayl and Thapa 1980; Chowdhury, Vaughan, and Abed 1988; and Nwoye, Uwagboe, and Madubuko 1988). There are also problems with incorrect use of solutions once they have been prepared, most commonly their underuse: in a study in Pakistan, 19 percent of mothers who used ORS stated that the dose should be one to two teaspoons given two to three times a day (Mull and Mull 1988). Similar findings were reported from Mozambique (Mozambique Ministry of Health and Eduardo Mondlane University Faculty of Medicine 1988).

These less-than-ideal practices (inadequate and incorrect use of ORT and use of other inappropriate treatments) contribute to the continuing high levels of death from diarrhea in children and give rise to unnecessarily high levels of side effects: 15 percent of diarrhea patients hospitalized in one children's hospital in Mexico City suffered from side effects associated with medication received prior to hospitalization (Phillips, Kumaté-Rodrígues, and Mota-Hernández 1989). They also contribute to a financial outlay that is higher than necessary: the annual global sale's value of "diarrhea drugs" is estimated at some $438 million (Health Action International 1986).

INSTITUTIONAL ASPECTS. Although, by and large, conclusions as to what constitutes appropriate case management are fairly straightforward, what governments and international organizations should be doing to ensure their adoption is less obvious. The fact that poor management of diarrhea cases continues in some areas points to the potential for improvement through the action of health and other ministries or international organizations. Governments have already made considerable progress. National diarrheal disease control pro-

grams, with the priority of implementing oral rehydration therapy as part of primary health services, are operational at various states of advancement in 100 countries, which include over 98 percent of the total population in the developing countries (WHO 1991).

Production and availability of ORS have increased rapidly during the past few years. The world supply of ORS reached the equivalent of about 350 million liters in 1989, over 70 percent of this quantity being locally produced in sixty-four developing countries (WHO 1991). The global rate of access to ORS has been estimated by WHO to have reached 63 percent in 1989. Training in diarrhea case management has also been supported. Data from developing countries indicate that 14 percent of community health workers have been trained in case management (WHO 1991). Most countries have legislation relating to the import, manufacture, and prescription of pharmaceuticals.

Although there is evidence that governments have made efforts to promote appropriate case management, there is clearly room for improvement. The World Health Organization (WHO 1991) has reported that the rate of use of ORS is still low in some countries (less than 20 percent in Sub-Saharan Africa), and there is evidence of inefficiency in the purchase, production, storage, and distribution of ORS. Soeters and Bannenberg (1988), for example, estimate that purchase through UNIPAC rather than currently used commercial sources would have allowed Gabon substantial savings in its drug bill. Even countries with pharmaceutical legislation rarely have the capacity to enforce it (WHO 1987d).

Unfortunately, it is not always clear what strategies are the most appropriate for governments to adopt. Although some studies have measured the costs and effectiveness of selected interventions, there is no comparable body of data that allows one, for example, to explore readily the relative merits of different methods of training staff, or of different pricing and legislative policies to control the production, importation, and marketing of, and the demand for, ineffective or dangerous drugs.

To date, international efforts have focused principally on attempts to promote ORT widely: ORT use rates have increased from below 1 percent in 1980 to 35 percent in 1989. This emphasis on a crucial life-saving intervention was an appropriate first priority and may have contributed to the decline in mortality. More attention needs to be paid to complementary efforts to discourage the use of costly, largely ineffective, and sometimes dangerous drugs. In addition, much greater efforts are needed to promote effective use of ORS, and effective ORT in general, with increased attention to feeding during diarrhea episodes and in the recovery period and the development of effective strategies of case management of dysenteric and persistent diarrheas. This constitutes the second most important priority for the WHO/CDD program (see also the subsection entitled "Institutional Aspects," under "Lowering Disease Incidence," above).

Defining an Optimal Strategy of Case Management

An optimal strategy of the case management of diarrhea in children should include correct fluid therapy, correct feeding therapy, appropriate use of antibiotics, no use of antidiarrheals, and effective education of the mother or caretaker. Correct fluid therapy should start at home. The mother or caretaker is the person available to initiate treatment when diarrhea begins. Home fluids, preferably containing sodium and a source of glucose and an osmolarity below 300 milliosmoles per liter, are recommended for the prevention of dehydration. If vomiting is present, more fluid should be offered, given in spoonfuls every three to five minutes. Dehydrated patients should be referred to a health facility and treated with ORS or, if severely dehydrated, with intravenous fluids. Feeding should be continued—breast milk for infants and nutrient-dense weaning foods for children who are already weaned. Food intake should be increased during the recovery period for nutritional rehabilitation. Antibiotics have a limited role in the treatment of diarrhea, being recommended only for the treatment of cholera and *Shigella* (visible blood in the stools is an adequate sign to indicate antimicrobial therapy against shigellosis, being more than 40 percent specific). Antidiarrheals should not be used in children. Effective case management also includes the education of the caretaker (a) to carry out fluid therapy; (b) to continue feeding during diarrhea and to increase feedings in the recovery period; (c) to avoid the use of antidiarrheal drugs; (d) to use antimicrobials correctly, if recommended; (e) to identify signs of severity of the disease, for rapid referral to health services; and (f) to prevent further diarrheal episodes, through breastfeeding, measles immunization, improved personal and domestic hygiene, and improved weaning practices.

Strategies which governments could consider in attempts to encourage optimal treatment practices include education (for example, training pharmacists, changing medical curricula, initiating workshops for private medical practitioners), legislation to control the use of antidiarrheal drugs, and pricing policies that make prescribing of ORT financially attractive.

Priorities and Policies

Until now the emphasis of both international efforts and national programs in the field of diarrhea control has been almost exclusively on ORT. It has been widely claimed that, because dehydration is a primary cause of death in children with acute watery diarrhea, ORT programs can greatly reduce diarrhea mortality rates, and, because diarrhea accounts for 20 to 40 percent of all child deaths, ORT programs will also have a significant effect on overall child mortality rates.

With a decade of accumulated experience to draw upon, it is time to question these assumptions. At the heart of the issue is the estimate of the effect on child mortality from diarrhea or all causes that can be expected realistically from a good ORT program. Empirical evidence is very scarce and not easy to collect. Figure 5-2 presents a schematic view of the steps involved. Childhood diarrheas are first divided into those that are life-threatening and those that are not. The life-threatening diarrheas are made up of acute watery cases, persistent cases, dysenteric cases, and complicated cases (those with accompanying problems such as measles, malaria, or

respiratory infection). The distribution of life-threatening cases among these four types is not documented. Oral rehydration therapy has its effect almost exclusively on the acute watery episodes. Figure 5-2 then distinguishes between those acute watery episodes that were effectively treated (for example, episodes in which the patient did not die) prior to ORT programs and those that were not. This is relevant to the effect on diarrhea and mortality from all causes that ORT programs will have. To have a greater effect on mortality, ORT must avert mortality not previously averted by other methods. Figure 5-2 then contrasts those effectively treated with those not effectively treated with ORT. As discussed previously, ineffective treatment may be rather common at present in many countries and may be amenable to substantial reduction. Finally, some of those effectively treated will die soon anyway from other causes (replacement or substitution mortality) and so will not contribute to reduction in mortality from all causes. The reader may substitute different speculative numbers in figure 5-2 to arrive at an estimate of the proportion of life-threatening diarrhea episodes averted or potentially averted by ORT. Even with the most optimistic assumptions, it is hard to produce a figure of more than 40 percent. The policy conclusions are clear: namely, much more emphasis should be

Figure 5-2. Role of ORT in Averting Mortality from Diarrhea

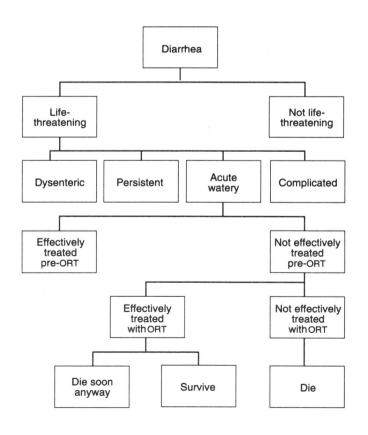

Source: Authors' design.

placed on primary prevention and on more comprehensive case management that would encompass all life-threatening episodes, including those that are persistent, dysenteric, and complicated.

In operational terms there are two important challenges for the 1990s. The first challenge is to put in place in all developing countries an effective system of case management for all diarrheas. This will involve going well beyond the focus on ORT to embrace nutritional management and correct use of drugs. Education of parents and training of health personnel will be key elements in any national program. For some dysenteric, persistent, and complicated diarrheas the results of research will be required before effective recommendations on case management can be made. The second challenge, and perhaps of as great priority, is the vigorous implementation of the available cost-effective preventive interventions. In particular these include measles vaccination, promotion of breastfeeding, improved hygiene and weaning practices, improved water and sanitation facilities, and the delivery of new vaccines as they become available.

For research, the priority is to support the operational priorities described above. Effective use of ORT, in both home and hospital settings, remains a poorly documented problem. The broader approach to case management requires a vigorous research agenda, ranging from the development of new drugs and studies on clinical efficacy to applied work on delivery and cost-effectiveness. For the preventive interventions we still need to know much more about design, delivery, sustainability, effectiveness, and costs. Research resources to date have focused largely on the development of technologies for diarrhea prevention and treatment. Additional attention needs to be given in the future to the means of application of these technologies. These research challenges can be met only from a strongly multidisciplinary perspective.

Notes

The authors are grateful for the comments and suggestions provided on earlier versions of this chapter by Robert Black, Isabelle de Zoysa, Richard Guerrant, Judith McGuire, Michael Merson, James Tulloch, and Ann Van Dusen.

1. All dollar amounts are 1982 U.S. dollars.

References

AED (Academy for Educational Development). 1985. "Lessons from Five Countries: Honduras, The Gambia, Swaziland, Ecuador, Peru." Report on the Communication for Child Survival Project. Washington, D.C.

Allman, J., and Jon E. Rohde. 1985. "Implementing Primary Health Care in Developing Countries." In J. Vallin and A. D. Lopez, eds., *Health Policy, Social Policy and Mortality Prospects*. Liège: Ordina Editions.

Arbo, Antonio, and J. I. Santos. 1987. "Diarrhoeal Diseases in the Immunocompromised Host." *Paediatric Infectious Disease Journal* 6:894–906.

Ashworth, Ann, and Elizabeth Dowler. 1991. "Malnutrition." In R. G. A. Feachem and D. T. Jamison, eds., *Disease and Mortality in Sub-Saharan Africa*. New York: Oxford University Press.

Ashworth, Ann, and R. G. A. Feachem. 1985a. "*Interventions for the Control of Diarrhoeal Diseases in Young Children: Improving Lactation*. Document CDD/85.2. Geneva: World Health Organization.

———. 1985b. "Interventions for the Control of Diarrhoeal Diseases in Young Children: Prevention of Low Birth Weight." *Bulletin of the World Health Organization* 63:165–84.

———. 1985c. "Interventions for the Control of Diarrhoeal Diseases in Young Children: Weaning Education." *Bulletin of the World Health Organization* 63:1115–27.

———. 1986. *Interventions for the Control of Diarrhoeal Diseases in Young Children: Growth Monitoring Programmes*. Document CDD/86.1. Geneva: World Health Organization.

Bairagi, Radheshyam, M. K. Chowdhury, Young J. Kim, George T. Curlin, and Ronald Gray. 1987. "The Association between Malnutrition and Diarrhoea in Rural Bangladesh." *International Journal of Epidemiology* 16:477–81.

Bangladesh Rural Advancement Committee. *See* BRAC.

Barrell, R. E., and M. G. M. Rowland. 1979. "Infant Foods as Potential Source of Diarrhoeal Illness in Rural West Africa." *Transactions of the Royal Society of Tropical Medicine and Hygiene* 73:85–90.

———. 1980. "Commercial Milk Products and Indigenous Weaning Foods in Rural West African Environment: A Bacteriological Perspective." *Journal of Hygiene* 84:191–202.

Barros, F. C., C. G. Victora, J. P. Vaughan, H. J. Estanislaw. 1987. "Infant Mortality in Southern Brazil: A Population Based Study of Causes of Death." *Archives of Disease in Childhood* 62:487–90.

Bartlett, A. V., Melinda Moore, G. W. Gary, Karen M. Starko, John J. Erben, and Betty A. Meredith. 1985. "Diarrhoeal Illness among Infants and Toddlers in Day Care Centres: I. Epidemiology and Pathogens." *Journal of Paediatrics* 107:495–502.

Beisel, W. R. 1977. "Magnitude of the Host Nutritional Responses to Infection." *American Journal of Clinical Nutrition* 30:1236–47.

Benicio, M. H. A, C. A. Monteiro, H. P. P. Zuñiga, Evany Margazao, and Beringhs Rio. 1987. "Estudo das condiçoes de saude das crianças do municipio de São Paulo, SP (Brasil), 1984–1985." *Revista de Saude Publica* 21:23–28.

Bertrand, W. E., and B. F. Walmus. 1983. "Maternal Knowledge, Attitudes and Practice as Predictors of Diarrhoeal Disease in Young Children." *International Journal of Epidemiology* 12:205–10.

Bhan, M. K., N. K. Arora, O. P. Ghai, K. Ramchandran, V. Khoshoo, and Nita Bhandari. 1986. "Major Factors in Diarrhoea Related Mortality among Rural Children." *Indian Journal of Medical Research* 83:9–12.

Bhan, M. K., Nita Bhandari, Sunil Sazawal, John Clemens, P. Raj, M. M. Levine, and J. B. Kaper. 1989. "Descriptive Epidemiology of Persistent Diarrhoea among Young Children in Rural Northern India." *Bulletin of the World Health Organization* 67:281–88.

Biritwum, R. B., S. Isomura, A. Assoku, and S. Torigoe. 1986. "Growth and Diarrhoeal Disease Surveillance in a Rural Ghanaian Pre-school Child Population." *Transactions of the Royal Society of Tropical Medicine and Hygiene* 80:208–13.

Black, R. E., K. H. Brown, and Stan Becker. 1983. "Influence of Acute Diarrhoea in the Growth Parameters of Children." In J. A. Bellanti, ed., *Acute Diarrhoea: Its Nutritional Consequences in Children*. Nutrition Workshop Series. New York: Raven Press.

———. 1984a. "Effects of Diarrhoea Associated with Specific Enteropathogens on the Growth of Children in Rural Bangladesh." *Paediatrics* 73:799–805.

———. 1984b. "Malnutrition Is a Determining Factor in Diarrhoeal Duration, but Not Incidence, among Young Children in a Longitudinal Study in Bangladesh." *American Journal of Clinical Nutrition* 37:87–94.

Black, R. E., K. H. Brown, Stan Becker, A. R. M. Abdul Alim, and M. H. Merson. 1982. "Contamination of Weaning Foods and Transmission of Enterotoxigenic *Escherichia coli* Diarrhoea in Children in Rural Bangladesh." *Transactions of the Royal Society of Tropical Medicine and Hygiene* 76:259–64.

Black, R. E., A. C. Dykes, K. E. Anderson, J. G. Wells, S. P. Sinclair, G. William Garry, M. H. Hatch, and E. J. Gangarosa. 1981. "Handwashing to Prevent Diarrhoea in Day-care Centres." *American Journal of Public Health* 113:445–51.

Black, R. E., M. H. Merson, Abu Eusof, Imdadul Huq, and Robert Pollard. 1984. "Nutritional Status, Body Size and Severity of Diarrhoea Associated with Rotavirus or Enterotoxigenic *Escherichia coli*." *Journal of Tropical Medicine and Hygiene* 87:83–89.

Black, R. E., M. H. Merson, A. S. Rahman, and others. 1980. "A Two Year Study of Bacterial, Viral and Parasitic Agents Associated with Diarrhoea in Rural Bangladesh." *Journal of Infectious Diseases* 142:660–64.

Black, R. E., M. H. Merson, P. R. Taylor, R. H. Yolken, M. Yunus, A. R. M. Abdul Alim, and D. A. Sack. 1981. "Glucose vs. Sucrose in Oral Rehydration Solutions for Infants and Young Children with Rotavirus-Associated Diarrhoea." *Paediatrics* 67:79-83.

BRAC (Bangladesh Rural Advancement Committee). 1987. "Mortality Effects of the B.R.A.C. O.R.T. Programme in Rural Bangladesh: An Assessment of the First Phase Experience." Dhaka.

Brenzel, L. 1987. "Cost Analysis of the National Immunisation and Control of Diarrhoeal Diseases Programmes in the Republic of Turkey." Report prepared by Resources for Child Health with USAID support.

Briend, André., Borgdan Wojtyniak, and M. G. M. Rowland. 1988. "Breastfeeding, Nutritional State and Child Survival in Rural Bangladesh." *British Medical Journal* 296:879–82.

Briscoe, John. 1979. "The Quantitative Effect of Infection on the Use of Food by Young Children in Poor Countries." *American Journal of Clinical Nutrition* 32:648–76.

———. 1984. "Water and Health: Selective Primary Health Care Revisited." *American Journal of Public Health* 74:1009–13.

Brown, Kenneth H., R. E. Black, A. D. Robertson, and Stan Becker. 1985. "Effects of Season and Illness on the Dietary Intake of Weanlings during Longitudinal Studies in Rural Bangladesh." *American Journal of Clinical Nutrition* 41:343–55.

Brown, Kenneth H., Arturo S. Gastañaduy, J. M. Saavedra, Jorge Lembcke, Diana Rivas, A. D. Robertson, Robert Yolken, and R. Bradley Sack. 1988. "Effect of Continued Oral Feeding on Clinical and Nutritional Outcomes of Acute Diarrhoea." *Journal of Paediatrics* 112:191–200.

Brunser, Oscar, Alejandro Reid, Fernando Monckeberg, Alejandro Manccioni, and Iván Contreras. 1968. "Jejunal Mucosa in Infant Malnutrition." *American Journal of Clinical Nutrition* 21:976–83.

Butzner, D., D. G. Butler, P. Miniats, and J. R. Hamilton. 1985. "Impact of Chronic Protein-Calory Malnutrition on Small Intestinal Repair after Acute Viral Enteritis: A Study in Gnotobiotic Piglets." *Paediatric Research* 19:476–81.

Cairncross, A. M. 1990. "Health Impact in Developing Countries: New Evidence and New Prospects." *Journal of the Institution of Water and Environmental Management* 4:571–77.

Candy, D., and A. D. Phillips. 1986. "Pathophysiology of Bacterial and Viral Diarrhoea." In P. D. Manuel, J. A. Walker-Smith, and Andrew Tomkins, eds., *Infections of the Gastrointestinal Tract*. London: Churchill Livingstone.

Capparelli, Edward, and Leonardo Mata. 1975. "Microflora of Maize Prepared as Tortillas." *Applied Microbiology* 29:802–6.

Carswell, J. W. 1988. "Clinical Manifestations of AIDS in Tropical Countries." *Tropical Doctor* 18:147–50.

Castro, Roberto, Mario Bronfman, Victoria Castro, Hector Guiscafre, and Gonzalo Gutierres. 1988. "Análisis del impacto económico de la estratega utilizada." *Archivos de Investigación Médica* (Mexico) 19:427–36.

Chandra, R. K. 1986. "Nutritional Regulation of Immunity and Infection: From Epidemiology to Phenomenology to Clinical Practice." *Journal of Paediatric Gastroenterology and Nutrition* 5:844–52.

Chen, L. C. 1983. "Planning for the Control of the Diarrhoea-Malnutrition Complex." In D. S. McLaren, ed., *Nutrition in the Community*. Chichester: John Wiley and Sons.

Chen, L. C., A. K. M. Chowdhury, and S. L. Huffman. 1980. "Anthropometric Assessment of Energy-Protein Malnutrition and Subsequent Risk of Mortality among Pre-school Aged Children." *American Journal of Clinical Nutrition* 33:1836–45.

Chen, Lincoln C., Emdadul Huq, and S. L. Huffman. 1981. "A Prospective Study of the Risk of Diarrhoeal Diseases According to the Nutritional Status of Children." *American Journal of Epidemiology* 114:284–92.

Chowdhury, A. M. R., J. P. Vaughan, and F. H. Abed. 1988. "Use and Safety of Home-made Oral Rehydration Solutions: An Epidemiological Evaluation from Bangladesh." *International Journal of Epidemiology* 17:655–65.

Clemens, John D., Bonita Stanton, J. Chakraborty, Shahriar Chowdhury, Malla R. Rao, Mohammed Ali, Susan Zimicki, and Bogdan Wojtyniak. 1988. "Measles Vaccination and Childhood Mortality in Rural Bangladesh." *American Journal of Epidemiology* 128:1330–39.

Clemens, John D., Bonita Stanton, Barbara Stoll, N. S. Shahid, Hasina Banu, and Alauddin Chowdhury. 1986. "Breastfeeding as a Determinant of Severity of Shigellosis." *American Journal of Epidemiology* 123:710–20.

Clements, M. L., M. M. Levine, F. Cleaves, and others. 1981. "Comparison of Simple Sugar/Salt versus Glucose/Electrolyte Oral Rehydration Solutions in Infant Diarrhoea." *Journal of Tropical Medicine and Hygiene* 84:189–94.

Cole, T. J., and J. M. Parkin. 1977. "Infection and Its Effect on the Growth of Young Children: A Comparison of The Gambia and Uganda." *Transactions of the Royal Society of Tropical Medicine and Hygiene* 71:196–98.

Condon-Paoloni, Deanne, Joaquin Cravioto, F. E. Johnston, E. R. de Licardie, and T. O. Scholl. 1977. "Morbidity and Growth of Infants and Young Children in a Rural Mexican Village." *American Journal of Public Health* 67:651–56.

Cutts, Felicity, Julie Cliff, R. Reiss, and Julia Stuckey. 1987. "Evaluating the Management of Diarrhoea in Health Centres in Mozambique." Internal study, government of Mozambique, Ministry of Health.

Daniels, D. L., S. N. Cousens, L. N. Makoae, and R. G. A. Feachem. 1990. "A Case Control Study of the Impact of Improved Sanitation on Diarrhoea Morbidity in Lesotho." *Bulletin of the World Health Organization* 68:455–63.

Darrow, D. C., E. L. Pratt, J. Flett, Jr., and others. 1949. "Disturbances of Water and Electrolytes in Infantile Diarrhoea." *Paediatrics* 3:129–56.

de Zoysa, Isabelle, and R. G. A. Feachem. 1985a. "Interventions for the Control of Diarrhoeal Diseases in Young Children: Chemoprophylaxis." *Bulletin of the World Health Organization* 63:295–315.

———. 1985b. "Interventions for the Control of Diarrhoeal Diseases in Young Children: Rotavirus and Cholera Immunisation." *Bulletin of the World Health Organization* 63(3):569–83.

de Zoysa, Isabelle, and T. Vesikari. 1990. "Cost Effectiveness of Rotavirus Immunization in the Control of Diarrhoeal Diseases in Developing Countries." In D. A. Sack and L. Freij, eds., *Prospects for Public Health Benefits in Developing Countries from New Vaccines against Enteric Infections*. Gothemburg, Sweden: SAREC (Swedish Agency for Research Cooperation).

Egypt, National Control of Diarrheal Diseases Project. 1988. "Impact of the National Control of Diarrhoeal Diseases Project on Infant and Child Mortality in Dakahlia, Egypt." *Lancet* 2:145–48.

el-Alamy, M. A., S. B. Thacker, R. R. Arafat, C. E. Wright, and A. M. Zaki. 1986. "The Incidence of Diarrhoeal Disease in a Defined Population in Rural Egypt." *American Journal of Tropical Medicine and Hygiene* 35:1006–12.

Elegbe, I. A., O. O. Ebenezer, I. Elegbe, and M. O. Akinola. 1982. "Pathogenic Bacteria Isolated from Infant Feeding Teats." *American Journal of Diseases of Children* 136:672–74.

Esrey, S. A., and R. G. A. Feachem. 1989. *Interventions for the Control of Diarrhoeal Diseases among Young Children: Promotion of Food Hygiene*. Document CDD/89.30. Geneva: World Health Organization.

el-Rafie, M., W. A. Hasouna, Norbert Hirschhorn, and others. 1990. "Effect of Diarrhoeal Disease Control on Infant and Childhood Mortality in Egypt." Report from the National Control of Diarrhoeal Diseases Project. *Lancet* 1:334–38.

Esrey, S. A., R. G. A. Feachem, and J. M. Hughes. 1985. "Interventions for the Control of Diarrhoeal Diseases among Young Children: Improving Water Supplies and Excreta Disposal Facilities." *Bulletin of the World Health Organization* 63:757–72.

Farthing, M. J. G., and G. T. Keusch, eds. 1989. *Enteric Infection: Mechanisms, Manifestations and Management.* London: Chapman and Hall Medical.

Feachem, R. G. A. 1981. "Environmental Aspects of Cholera Epidemiology: I. A Review of Selected Reports of Endemic and Epidemic Situations during 1961–1980." *Tropical Diseases Bulletin* 78:675–98.

———. 1983. "Interventions for the Control of Diarrhoeal Diseases among Young Children: Supplementary Feeding Programmes." *Bulletin of the World Health Organization* 61:967–79.

———. 1984. "Interventions for the Control of Diarrhoeal Diseases among Young Children: Promotion of Personal and Domestic Hygiene." *Bulletin of the World Health Organization* 62:467–76.

———. 1986. "Preventing Diarrhoea: What Are the Policy Options?" *Health Policy and Planning* 1:109–17.

———. 1987. "Vitamin A Deficiency and Diarrhoea: A Review of Interrelationships and Their Implications for the Control of Xerophthalmia and Diarrhoea." *Tropical Diseases Bulletin* 84:R1–R16.

Feachem, R. G. A., R. C. Hogan, and M. H. Merson. 1983. "Diarrhoeal Diseases Control: Reviews of Potential Interventions." *Bulletin of the World Health Organization* 61:637–40.

Feachem, R. G. A., Tord Kjellstrom, C. T. L. Murray, Mead Over, and M. A. Phillips. 1991. *The Health of Adults in the Developing World.* New York: Oxford University Press.

Feachem, R. G. A., and M. A. Koblinsky. 1983. "Interventions for the Control of Diarrhoeal Diseases among Young Children: Measles Immunisation." *Bulletin of the World Health Organization* 61:641–52.

———. 1984. "Interventions for the Control of Diarrhoeal Diseases among Young Children: Promotion of Breastfeeding." *Bulletin of the World Health Organization* 62:271–91.

Feachem, R. G. A., I, M. Timaeus, and W. J. Graham. 1989. "Identifying Health Problems and Health Research Priorities in Developing Countries." *Journal of Tropical Medicine and Hygiene* 92:133–91.

Flores, J., and A. Z. Kapikian. 1989. "Rotavirus Vaccines." In Farthing and Keusch 1989.

Frank, J. F., and H. M. Barnhart. 1986. "Food and Dairy Sanitation." In J. M. Last, ed., *Public Health and Preventive Medicine*, 12th ed. Norwalk, Conn.: Appleton-Century-Crofts.

Georges, M. C., C. Roure, R. V. Tauxe, D. M. Y. Meunier, M. Merlin, J. Testa, C. Baya, J. Limbassa, and A. J. Georges. 1987. "Diarrhoeal Morbidity and Mortality in Children in the Central African Republic." *American Journal of Tropical Medicine and Hygiene* 36:598–602.

Gianella, Ralph A., Selwyn A. Broitman, and Norman Zamcheck. 1973. "Influence of Gastric Acidity on Bacterial and Parasitic Enteric Infections: A Perspective." *Annals of Internal Medicine* 78:271–76.

Giugliano, L. G., M. G. P. Bernardi, J. C. Vasconcelos, C. A. Costa, and R. Giugliano. 1986. "Longitudinal Study of Diarrhoeal Incidence in a Peri-urban Community in Manaus (Amazon—Brazil)." *Annals of Tropical Medicine and Parasitology* 80:443–50.

Gordon, J. E., Werner Ascoli, L. J. Mata, M. A. Guzmán, and Nevin S. Scrimshaw. 1968. "Nutrition and Infection Field Study in Guatemalan Villages, 1959–1964: VI. Acute Diarrhoeal Disease and Nutritional Disorders in General Disease Incidence." *Archives of Environmental Health* 16:424–37.

Grosse, R. N. 1980. "Interrelation between Health and Population: Observations Derived from Field Experiences." *Social Sciences and Medicine* 14C:99–120.

Guerrant, R. L. 1986. "Unresolved Problems and Future Considerations in Diarrhoeal Research." *Paediatric Infectious Disease Journal* 5:S155–61.

Guerrant, R. L., L. V. Kirchoff, D. S. Shields, M. K. Nations, J. Leslie, M. A. de Souza, J. G. Araugo, L. L. Coreia, K. T. Sauer, K. E. McClelland, F. L. Trowbridge, and J. M. Hughes. 1983. "Prospective Study of Diarrhoeal Illnesses in Northeastern Brazil: Patterns of Disease, Nutritional Impact, Etiologies and Risk Factors." *Journal of Infectious Diseases* 148:986–97.

Guerrant, R. L., D. S. Shields, S. M. Thorson, J. B. Schorling, and D. H. Gröschel. 1985. "Evaluation and Diagnosis of Acute Infectious Diarrhoea." *American Journal of Medicine* 78(supplement 6B):91–8.

Guiraldes, E., and J. R. Hamilton. 1981. "Effect of Chronic Malnutrition on Intestinal Structure, Epithelial Renewal and Enzymes in Suckling Rats." *Paediatric Research* 15:930–34.

Guldan, G. S. 1988. "Maternal Education and Child Caretaking Practices in Rural Bangladesh: Part 2, Food and Personal Hygiene." Thesis, Tufts University, School of Nutrition.

Hardy, Ellen E., Anna M. Vichi, Regina C. Sarmento, Lucila Moreira, and Celia M. Bosqueiro. 1982. "Breastfeeding Promotion: Effect of an Educational Programme in Brazil." *Studies in Family Planning* 13:79–86.

Health Action International. 1986. "Antidiarrhoeals." In International Organization of Consumers Union, *Problem Drugs.* The Hague.

Heymann, D. L., M. Mbvundula, A. Macheso, D. A. McFarland, R. V. Hawkins. 1990. "Oral Rehydration Therapy in Malawi: Impact on the Severity of Disease and on Hospital Admissions, Treatment Practices, and Recurrent Costs." *Bulletin of the World Health Organization* 68:193–97.

Hibbert, J. M., and M. H. N. Golden. 1981. "What Is the Weanling's Dilemma? Dietary Faecal Bacterial Ingestion of Normal Children in Jamaica." *Journal of Tropical Paediatrics* 27:225–58.

Hirschhorn, Norbert. 1980. "The Treatment of Acute Diarrhoea in Children: An Historical and Physiological Perspective." *The American Journal of Clinical Nutrition* 33:637–63.

Holt, E. A., R. Boulos, N. A. Halsey, L. M. Boulos, C. Boulos. 1990. "Childhood Survival in Haiti: Protective Effect of Measles Vaccination." *Pediatrics* 85:188–94.

Horton, S., and P. Claquin. 1983. "Cost-Effectiveness and User Characteristics of Clinic-Based Services for the Treatment of Diarrhoea: A Case Study in Bangladesh." *Social Science and Medicine* 17:721–29.

Hoyle, Bruce, M. Yunus, and Lincoln C. Chen. 1980. "Breastfeeding and Food Intake among Children with Acute Diarrhoeal Disease." *American Journal of Clinical Nutrition* 33:2365–71.

Huffman, Sandra L., and Cheryl Combest. 1988. *Promotion of Breastfeeding: Yes, It Works.* Bethesda, Md.: Center to Prevent Childhood Malnutrition.

Huttly, S. R. A. 1990. "The Impact of Inadequate Sanitary Conditions on Health in Developing Countries." *World Health Statistics Quarterly* 43:118–26.

Huttly, S. R. A., Deborah Blum, B. R. Kirkwood, R. N. Emeh, R. G. A. Feachem. 1987. "The Epidemiology of Acute Diarrhoea in a Rural Community in Imo State, Nigeria." *Transactions of the Royal Society of Tropical Medicine and Hygiene* 81:865–70.

Huttly, S. R. A., B. A. Hoque, K. M. Aziz, K. Z. Hasan, M. Y. Patwari, M. Mujibur Rahaman, R. G. A. Feachem. 1989. "Persistent Diarrhoea in a Rural Area in Bangladesh: A Community-Based Longitudinal Study." *International Journal of Epidemiology* 18:964–69.

Islam, M. R., and P. K. Bardhan. 1985. "A Comparison of Oral Solutions from Common Salt and Crude Sugar (Molasses) with and without Bicarbonate in Severe Paediatric Diarrhoea." *Asian Medical Journal* 27:243–49.

Islam, M. R., W. B. Greenough III, M. Mujibur Rahaman, Akazad Chowdhury, and D. A. Sack. 1980. "Labon-gur (Common Salt and Brown Sugar) Oral Rehydration Solution in the Treatment of Diarrhoea in Adults." *Journal of Tropical Medicine and Hygiene* 83:41–45.

Islam, M. S., A. Bhuiya, and M. D. Yunus. 1984. "Socioeconomic Differentials of Diarrhoea Morbidity in Selected Villages of Bangladesh." *Journal of Diarrhoeal Disease Research* 2:232–37.

Kandel, G., and M. Donowitz. 1989. "Antidiarrheal Drugs for the Treatment of Infectious Enteritis." In M. J. G. Farthing and G. T. Keusch, eds., *Enteric Infection: Mechanisms, Manifestations and Management.* London: Chapman and Hall Medical.

Kaplan, L. D., C. H. Wofsy, and P. A. Volberding. 1987. "Treatment of Patients with Acquired Immunodeficiency Syndrome and Associated Manifestations." JAMA 257:1367–74.

Keusch, Gerald T., and Michael Katz. 1979. "Malnutrition and Infection." In R. B. Alfin-Slater, and D. Kritchevsky, eds., *Human Nutrition: A Comprehensive Treatise*. New York: Plenum Press.

Keusch, G. T. and Nevin S. Scrimshaw. 1986. "Selective Primary Health Care: Strategies for Control of Disease in the Developing World—XXIII. Control of Infection to Reduce the Prevalence of Infantile and Childhood Malnutrition." *Reviews of Infectious Diseases* 8:273–87.

Khan, Moslem Uddin. 1982. "Interruption of Shigellosis by Handwashing." *Transactions of the Royal Society of Tropical Medicine and Hygiene* 76:164–68.

Khan, Moslem Uddin, and Kamal Ahmad. 1986. "Withdrawal of Food during Diarrhoea: Major Mechanism of Malnutrition Following Diarrhoea in Bangladesh Children." *Journal of Tropical Paediatrics* 32:57–61.

Kielman, Arnfried A., and Colin McCord. 1977. "Home Treatment of Childhood Diarrhoea in Punjab Villages." *Journal of Tropical Paediatrics and Environmental Child Health* 23:197–201.

Kielman, Arnfried A., A. B. Mobarak, M. T. Hammamy, A. I. Gomas, S. Abou-el-Saad, R. K. Lotfi, I. Mazen, and A. Nagaty. 1985. "Control of Deaths from Diarrhoeal Disease in Rural Communities: I. Design of an Intervention Study and Effects on Child Mortality." *Tropical Medical Parasitology* 36:191–98.

Kirkwood, Betty R. 1991. "Diarrhea." In R. G. A. Feachem and D. T. Jamison, eds., *Disease and Mortality in Sub-Saharan Africa*. New York: Oxford University Press.

Koster, F. T., G. C. Curlin, K. M. A. Aziz, and A. Haque. 1981. "Synergistic Impact of Measles and Diarrhoea on Nutrition and Mortality in Bangladesh." *Bulletin of the World Health Organization* 59:901–8.

Kumar, V. J., R. Kumar, and N. Dutta. 1987. "Oral Rehydration Therapy in Reducing Diarrhoea-Related Mortality in Rural India." *Journal of Diarrhoeal Diseases Research* 5:159–64.

Lancet. 1981. "Oral Therapy for Acute Diarrhoea." 2:615–16.

Lerman, S. J., D. S. Shepard, and R. A. Cash. 1985. "Treatment of Diarrhoea in Indonesian Children: What It Costs and Who Pays for It." *Lancet* 2:651–54.

Leslie, J. 1989. "Women's Time: A Factor in the Use of Child Survival Technologies." *Health Policy and Planning* 4(1):1–16.

Levine, M. M. 1989. "Development of Vaccines against Bacteria." In M. J. G. Farthing and G. T. Keusch, eds., *Enteric Infection: Mechanisms, Manifestations and Management*. London: Chapman and Hall Medical.

————. 1990. "Modern Vaccines—Enteric Infections." *Lancet* 1:958–61.

Levine, M. M., Gevevoeve Losonsky, Deidre Herrington, J. B. Kaper, Carol Tacket, M. B. Rennels, and J. G. Morris. 1986. "Paediatric Diarrhoea: The Challenge of Prevention." *Paediatric Infectious Disease Journal* 5:S29–S43.

Mahmood, D. A., and R. G. A. Feachem. 1987. "Clinical and Epidemiological Characteristics of Rotavirus and EPEC-Associated Hospitalised Infantile Diarrhoea in Basrah, Iraq." *Journal of Tropical Paediatrics* 33:319–25.

Mahmood, D. A., R. G. A. Feachem, and S. R. A. Huttly. 1989. "Infant Feeding and Risk of Severe Diarrhoea in Basrah City, Iraq: A Case Control Study." *Bulletin of the World Health Organization* 67:701–6.

Manderson, Lenore. 1981. "Socioeconomic and Cultural Correlates of Gastroenteritis among Infants and Small Children in Malaysia." *Journal of Tropical Paediatrics* 27:166–76.

Martines, J. C. 1988. "The Interrelationships between Feeding Mode, Malnutrition and Diarrhoeal Morbidity in Early Infancy among the Urban Poor in Southern Brazil." Ph.D. thesis, University of London.

Martorell, Reynaldo, Jean-Pierre Habicht, Charles Yarbrough, Aaron Lechtig, Robert E. Klein, Karl A. Western. 1975. "Acute Morbidity and Physical Growth in Rural Guatemalan Children." *American Journal of Diseases in Childhood* 129:1296–1301.

Martorell, Reynaldo, Aaron Lechtig, Charles Yarbrough, S. Yarborough, Hernán Delgado, and R. E. Klein. 1977. "Efecto de las diarreas sobre el retardo en crecimiento físico de niños guatemaltecos." *Archivos Latinoamericanos de Nutrición* 27:311–24.

Martorell, R., Charles Yarbrough, S. Yarbrough, and R. E. Klein. 1980. "The Impact of Ordinary Illnesses on the Dietary Intakes of Malnourished Children." *American Journal of Clinical Nutrition* 33:345–50.

Mata, Leonardo. 1981. "Epidemiologic Perspective of Diarrhoeal Disease in Costa Rica and Current Efforts in Control, Prevention and Research." *Revista Latinoamericana de Microbiologia* 23:109–19.

Mata, Leonardo, Richard A. Kronmal, Juan J. Urrutia, and Bertha Garcia. 1977. "Effect of Infection on Food Intake and the Nutritional State; Perspectives as Viewed from the Village." *American Journal of Clinical Nutrition* 30:1215–27.

Mata, Leonardo, A. Simhon, J. J. Urrutia, Richard A. Kronmal. 1983. "Epidemiology of Rotavirus in a Cohort of 45 Guatemalan Mayan Indian Children Observed from Birth to the Age of Three Years." *Journal of Infectious Diseases* 148:452–61.

Mathur, Rita., and Vinodini Reddy. 1983. "Bacterial Contamination of Infant Foods." *Indian Journal of Medical Research* 77:342–46.

Miall, W. E., P. Desai, and K. L. Standard. 1970. "Malnutrition, Infection and Child Growth in Jamaica." *Journal of Biosocial Science* 2:31–44.

Miller, C. J., R. G. A. Feachem, and B. S. Draser. 1984. "Cholera Epidemiology in Developed and Developing Countries: New Thoughts on Transmission, Seasonality and Control." *Lancet* 1:261–63.

Molla, A. M., Ayesha Molla, and Naseha Khatun. 1986. "Absorption of Macronutrients in Children during Acute Diarrhoea and after Recovery." In T. G. Taylor and N. K. Jenkins, eds., *Proceedings of the XIII International Congress of Nutrition*. London: John Libbey.

Monteiro, C. A., and M. H. D. A. Benicio. 1989. "Determinants of Infant Mortality Trends in Developing Countries—Some Evidence from São Paulo City." *Transactions of the Royal Society of Tropical Medicine and Hygiene* 83:5–9.

Morley, David C., M. Woodland, and W. J. Martin. 1963. "Measles in Nigerian Children: A Study of the Disease in West Africa and its Manifestations in England and Other Countries during Different Epochs." *Journal of Hygiene* 61:115–35.

Mozambique Ministry of Health and Eduardo Mondlane University Faculty of Medicine. 1988. "Evaluating the Management of Diarrhoea in Health Centres in Mozambique." *Journal of Tropical Medicine and Hygiene* 91:61–6.

Mull, J. D., and D. S. Mull. 1988. "Mothers' Concepts of Childhood Diarrhoea in Rural Pakistan: What ORT Programme Planners Should Know." *Social Sciences and Medicine* 27:53–67.

Murray, B. E., and H. L. DuPont. 1989. "New Antimicrobial Agents and Drug Resistance." In M. J. G. Farthing and G. T. Keusch, eds., *Enteric Infection: Mechanisms, Manifestations and Management*. London: Chapman and Hall Medical.

Nabarro, David, Peter Howard, Claudia Cassels, Mahesh Pant, Alet Nijga, and Nigel Padfield. 1988. "The Importance of Infections and Environmental Factors as Possible Determinants of Growth Retardation in Children." In J. C. Waterlow, ed., *Linear Growth Retardation in Less Developed Countries*. New York: Raven Nutrition Workshop Series.

Nailin, D. R., R. A. Cash, R. Islam, and others. 1968. "Oral Maintenance Therapy for Cholera in Adults." *Lancet* 2:370–72.

Nazir, Mohammed., Nancy Pardede, and Rudi Ismail. 1985. "The Incidence of Diarrhoeal Diseases and Diarrhoeal Diseases–Related Mortality in Rural Swampy Low-land Area of South Sumatra." *Journal of Tropical Paediatrics* 31:268–72.

Nigeria, Imo State Evaluation Team. 1989. "Evaluating Water and Sanitation Projects: The Lessons from Imo State, Nigeria." *Health Policy and Planning* 4:40–49.

Nwove, L. O., P. E. Uwagboe, and G. U. Madubuko. 1988. "Evaluation of Home-made Salt-Sugar Oral Rehydration Solution in a Rural Nigerian Population." *Journal of Tropical Medicine and Hygiene* 91:23–27.

Okun, D. A. 1988. "The Value of Water Supply and Sanitation in Development: An Assessment." *American Journal of Public Health* 78(2):1463–67.

Palmer, D. L., F. T. Koster, A. K. M. J. Alam, and M. R. Islam. 1976. "Nutritional Status: A Determinant of Severity of Diarrhoea in Patients with Cholera." *Journal of Infectious Diseases* 134:8–14.

Phillips, I., S. K. Lwanga, W. Lore, and D. Wasswa. 1969. "Methods and Hygiene of Infant Feeding in an Urban Area of Uganda." *Journal of Tropical Paediatrics* 15:167–71.

Phillips, M. A., R. G. A. Feachem, and Anne Mills. 1987. *Options for Diarrhoeal Diseases Control: The Cost and Cost-Effectiveness of Selected Interventions for the Prevention of Diarrhoea.* London: Evaluation and Planning Centre for Health Care.

Phillips, M. A., J. Kumaté-Rodrígues, and F. Mota-Hernández. 1989. "The Cost of Diarrhoea Treatment in a Children's Hospital in Mexico City." *Bulletin of the World Health Organization* 67:273–80.

Phonboon, K., P. Kunasol, T. Chayaniyayodhin, and D. Srisomporn. 1986. "Surveillance of Diarrhoeal Diseases in Thailand." *Bulletin of the World Health Organization* 64:715–20.

Pierce, N. F., J. G. Banwell, R. C. Mitra, and others. 1968. "Oral Replacement of Water and Electrolyte Losses in Cholera." *Indian Journal of Medical Research* 57:848–55.

Popkin, B. M., R. E. Bilsborrow, and J. S. Akin. 1982. "Breastfeeding Patterns in Low-Income Countries." *Science* 218:1088–93.

Popkin, B. M., and E. Z. Bisgrove. 1988. "Urbanisation and Nutrition in Low-Income Countries." *Food and Nutrition Bulletin* 10:3–23.

Poudayl, L., and R. Thapa. 1980. "Home-made Oral Rehydration Solutions: Feasibilty Study in Nepal." *WHO Chronicle* 34:496–500.

Qualls, N., and R. Robertson. 1989. "Potential Uses of Cost Analyses in Child Survival Programmes: Evidence from Africa." *Health Policy and Planning* 4(1):50–61.

Quick, J. B., P. Foreman, D. Ross-Degnan, and others. 1988. "Where Does Tetracycline Go? Health Center Prescribing and Child Survival in East Java and West Kalimantan, Indonesia." Drug Management Program, Management Sciences for Health, Boston.

Riveron-Corteguera, Raúl, and José. A. Gutiérrez Muñoz. 1982. "Enfermedades diarreicas agudas en América Latina, 1970–1979: La situación en Cuba." *Boletín de la Oficina Sanitaria Panamericana* 92:508–19.

Rohde, Jon E. 1986. "Acute Diarrhoea." In J. A. Walsh and K. S. Warren, eds., *Strategies for Primary Health Care: Technologies Appropriate for the Control of Disease in the Developing World.* Chicago: University of Chicago Press.

Rosenberg, I. H., N. W. Solomons, and R. E. Schneider. 1977. "Malabsorption Associated with Diarrhoea and Intestinal Infections." *American Journal of Clinical Nutrition* 30:1248–53.

Rowland, M. G. M., R. A. E. Barrell, and R. G. Whitehead. 1978. "Bacterial Contamination in Traditional Gambian Weaning Foods." *Lancet* 1:136–38.

Rowland, M. G. M., S. G. J. G. Rowland, and T. J. Cole. 1988. "Impact of Infection on the Growth of Children from 0 to 2 Years in an Urban West African Community." *American Journal of Clinical Nutrition* 47:134–38.

Ryder, R. W., W. C. Reeves, and R. B. Sack. 1985. "Risk Factors for Fatal Childhood Diarrhoea: A Case-Control Study from Two Remote Panamanian Islands." *American Journal of Epidemiology* 121:605–10.

Samani, E. F. Z., W. C. Willet, and J. H. Ware. 1988. "Association of Malnutrition and Diarrhoea in Children Aged under Five Years: A Prospective Follow-up Study in a Rural Sudanese Community." *American Journal of Epidemiology* 128:93–105.

Sarker, S. A., M. A. Wahed, M. M. Rahaman, A. N. Alam, A. Islam, and F. Jahan. 1986. "Persistent Protein-Losing Enteropathy in Post-Measles Diarrhoea." *Archives of Diseases in Childhood* 61:739–43.

Scrimshaw, Nevin S. 1977. "Effect of Infection on Nutrient Requirements." *American Journal of Clinical Nutrition* 30:1536–44.

Scrimshaw, Nevin S., Hans A. Bruch, Werner Ascoli, and John E. Gordon. 1961. "Studies of Diarrhoeal Disease in Central America: IV. Demographic Distributions of Acute Diarrhoeal Disease in Two Rural Populations of the Guatemalan Highlands." *American Journal of Tropical Medicine and Hygiene* 11:401–9.

Scrimshaw, Nevin S., J. B. Salomon, Hans A. Bruch, and others. 1966. "Studies of Diarrhoeal Disease in Central America: VIII. Measles, Diarrhoea and Nutritional Deficiency in Rural Guatemala. *American Journal of Tropical Medicine and Hygiene* 15:625–31.

Sepúlveda, Jaime, Walter Willet, and Alvaro Muñoz. 1988. "Malnutrition and Diarrhoea: A Longitudinal Study among Urban Mexican Children." *American Journal of Epidemiology* 27:365–76.

Shepard, D. S., L. E. Brenzel, and K. T. Nemeth. 1986. "Cost-Effectiveness of Oral Rehydration Therapy for Diarrhoeal Diseases." PHN Technical note 86–26, World Bank, Population, Health and Nutrition Department, Washington, D.C.

Sirisinha, Stitaya, Robert Suskind, Robert Edelman, Chairat Asvapaka, and Robert E. Olson. 1975. "Secretory and Serum IgA in Children with Protein-Calory Malnutrition." *Paediatrics* 55:166–70.

Snyder, J. D., and M. H. Merson. 1982. "The Magnitude of the Global Problem of Acute Diarrhoeal Disease: A Review of Active Surveillance Data." *Bulletin of the World Health Organization* 60:605–13.

Soeters, R., and W. Bannenberg. 1988. "Computerized Calculation of Essential Drug Requirements." *Social Sciences and Medicine* 27:955–70.

Stanton, B. F., and J. D. Clemens. 1987a. "An Educational Intervention for Altering Water-Sanitation Behaviours to Reduce Childhood Diarrhoea in Urban Bangladesh: II. A Randomised Trial to Assess the Impact of the Intervention on Hygienic Behaviours and Rates of Diarrhoea." *American Journal of Epidemiology* 125:292–301.

———. 1987b. "Socioeconomic Variables and Rates of Diarrhoeal Disease in Urban Bangladesh." *Transactions of the Royal Society of Tropical Medicine and Hygiene* 81:278–82.

Stevens, D. P. 1986. "Giardiasis." In J. A. Walsh and K. S. Warren, eds., *Strategies for Primary Health Care: Technologies Appropriate for the Control of Disease in the Developing World.* Chicago: University of Chicago Press.

Stoll, Binita J., R. I. Glass, M. I. Huq, M. U. Khan, H. Banu, and J. Holt. 1982. "Surveillance of Patients Attending a Diarrhoeal Diseases Hospital in Bangladesh." *British Medical Journal* 285:1185–88.

Surjono, Dani, S. D. Ismadi, Swardji, and Jon E. Rohde. 1980. "Bacterial Contamination and Dilution of Milk in Infant Feeding Bottles." *Journal of Tropical Paediatrics* 1:58–61.

Taylor, S. M., J. Frank, N. F. White, and J. Meyers. 1986. "Modelling the Incidence of Childhood Diarrhoea." *Social Science and Medicine* 10:995–1002.

Tekce, B. 1982. "Oral Rehydration Therapy: An Assessment of Mortality Effects in Rural Egypt." *Studies in Family Planning* 13:315–27.

Timaeus, Ian, and Wendy Graham. 1989. "Measuring Adult Mortality in Developing Countries: A Review and Assessment of Methods." Planning, Policy and Research Working Paper 155. World Bank, Population, Health and Nutrition Department, Washington, D.C.

Tomkins, Andrew. 1981. "Nutritional Status and Severity of Diarrhoea among Pre-school Children in Rural Nigeria." *Lancet* 1:860–62.

Thomson, G., and G. Sterkey. 1986. "Self-Prescribing by Way of Pharmacies in Three Asian Developing Countries." *Lancet* 2:620–21.

Torún, Benjamin. 1982. "Environmental and Educational Interventions against Diarrhoea in Guatemala." In L. C. Chen and N. S. Scrimshaw, eds., *Diarrhoea and Malnutrition: Interactions, Mechanisms and Interventions.* New York: Plenum Press.

United Nations University. 1979. "Nutrient Requirements for Catch-up Growth and Tissue Repletion." In *Protein-Energy Requirements under Conditions Prevailing in Developing Countries: Current Knowledge and Research Needs.* WHTR-l/UNUP-18:34–38.

United States, National Research Council. 1985. *Nutritional Management of Acute Diarrhoea in Infants and Children.* Washington, D.C.: National Academy Press.

U.S. Institute of Medicine. 1986. *New Vaccine Development: Establishing Priorities.* Vol. 2, *Diseases of Importance in Developing Countries.* Washington, D.C.: National Academic Press.

Victora, C. G., P. G. Smith, J. P. Vaughan, L. C. Nobre, Cintia Lombardi, A. M. B. Teixera, S. M. C. Fuchs, L. B. Moreira, L. P. Giganta, and F. C. Barros. 1987. "Evidence for Protection by Breastfeeding against Infant Deaths from Infectious Diseases in Brazil." *Lancet* 2:319–22.

————. 1988. "Water Supply, Sanitation and Housing in Relation to the Risk of Infant Mortality from Diarrhoea." *International Journal of Epidemiology* 17:651–54.

Whitehead, R. G. 1977. "Protein and Energy Requirements of Young Children Living in the Developing Countries to Allow for Catch-up Growth after Infections." *American Journal of Clinical Nutrition* 30:1545–47.

Winikoff, Beverly, and E. C. Baer. 1980. "The Obstetrician's Opportunity: Translating 'Breast Is Best' from Theory to Practice." *American Journal of Obstetrics and Gynaecology* 138:105–17.

WHO (World Health Organization). 1986a. *Drugs in the Management of Acute Diarrhoea in Infants and Young Children.* Document CDD/CMT/86.1. Geneva.

————. 1986b. *Oral Rehydration Therapy for Treatment of Diarrhoea in the Home.* Document CDD/SER/86.9. Geneva.

————. 1986c. *Research on Vaccine Development.* Document CDD/IMV/86.1. Geneva.

————. 1987a. *A Decision Process for Establishing Policy on Home Therapy for Diarrhoea.* Document CDD/SER/87.10. Geneva.

————. 1987b. "Diarrhoeal Diseases Morbidity, Mortality and Treatment Surveys." *CDD Update* 1:1–3.

————. 1987c. "Oral Rehydration Salts (ORS)." *CDD Update* 2:1–3.

————. 1987d. *Use of Drugs in the Treatment of Diarrhoea.* Document CDD/TAG/87.5. Geneva.

————. 1988a. "Impact of Oral Rehydration Therapy on Hospital Admission and Case-Fatality Rates for Diarrhoeal Disease: Results from 11 Countries." WHO *Weekly Epidemiological Record* 8:49–52.

————. 1988b. *Persistent Diarrhoea in Children in Developing Countries.* Report of a WHO meeting. Document CDD/88.27. Geneva.

————. 1988c. *Sixth Programme Report 1986–1987.* Document CDD/88.28. Geneva.

————. 1989. *Interim Programme Report 1988.* Document CDD/89.31. Geneva.

————. 1990a. "Global Situation—Immunization Coverage." *EPI Update* 16:1.

————. 1990b. *The Rational Use of Drugs in the Management of Acute Diarrhoea in Children.* Geneva.

————. 1990c. *Seventh Programme Report.* Document CDD/90.34.

————. 1991. *Interim Programme Report 1990.* Document CDD/91.36. Geneva.

————. 1992. *Eighth Programme Report 1990–1991.* Document CDD/92.38 Geneva.

Wornham, W. 1987. "Development and Field Testing of a Method for Assessing the Effectiveness of Diarrhoea Case Management by Mothers." World Health Organization, Geneva.

Young, L. S. 1987. "Treatable Aspects of Infections Due to Human Immunodeficiency Virus." *Lancet* 2:1503–6.

Zumrawi, F. Y., H. Dimond, and J. C. Waterlow. 1987. "Effects of Infection on Growth in Sudanese Children." *Human Nutrition: Clinical Nutrition* 41C:453–61.

6

Poliomyelitis

Dean T. Jamison, Alberto M. Torres, Lincoln C. Chen, and Joseph L. Melnick

Aware that poliomyelitis is the [Expanded Programme on Immunization] target disease most amenable to global eradication, and that regional eradication goals by or before the year 2000 have already been set in the regions of the Americas, Europe and the Western Pacific, [the Forty-first World Health Assembly] DECLARES *the commitment of* WHO *to the global eradication of poliomyelitis by the year 2000.*

Geneva, 13 May 1988

Poliomyelitis is a viral disease conveyed through fecal-oral and pharyngeal-oral transmission. In unhygienic environments with unvaccinated populations, transmission is widespread, and virtually everyone will be infected (and thereby suffer illness or become immune) prior to age five. Only about 1 percent of those infected experience symptoms, but for that 1 percent the consequences may be death or permanent paralysis. Improving hygiene retards transmission, thereby increasing the average age of disease onset; this leads to epidemics among older children and young adults. As polio paralysis increases in severity with the age of onset, the effect of improved hygiene, in the absence of effective immunization programs, may well be perverse. Highly effective vaccines against polio were developed in the 1950s, however, and the disease is now completely controlled in high-income countries. In low-income countries, polio's inclusion as a target disease in the World Health Organization's (WHO's) Expanded Programme on Immunization (EPI), as well as many strong national efforts, has resulted in progress in reducing disease incidence.

Despite this progress, during the 1980s paralytic polio affected more than 200,000 to 250,000 children per year in the period 1986–88 (Robertson and others 1990). Paralytic poliomyelitis leads to lifelong disability, and the sequelae of past disease has left between 10 million and 20 million youth and adults crippled today. In contrast to its significance as a cause of disability, the contribution of polio to mortality of children under five is relatively modest. Direct evidence from a survey of causes of childhood death in Senegal (Goldberg and McBodji 1988) suggests a contribution to deaths of children under five years old of perhaps 2 per 1,000 live births in an essentially preimmunization environment. This number would

constitute about 1 percent of all deaths of those under five years. If applied globally, these figures would suggest that, in the absence of immunization, polio would account for about 150,000 child deaths per year. Lopez (forthcoming) estimates that, in fact, there may currently be about 25,000 deaths per year from polio, although current WHO estimates are somewhat lower at 10,000 (WHO 1990). Polio-related disability in older children and adults is, very plausibly, a risk factor for premature mortality in those age groups, but quantitative assessment of this effect remains to be undertaken. Likewise, we are unaware of studies relating the extent of polio paralysis to earnings or productivity losses, although there is indirect evidence of the importance of these effects. A study from southern India (Max and Shepard 1988) found earning losses of two-thirds and more of annual income associated with moderate degrees of disability resulting from leprosy. This suggests that significant economic benefits (in addition to reduction in suffering) could be derived from prevention. It also suggests that rehabilitation programs could be justified on economic grounds alone if they could reduce a fraction of the earnings disadvantage from paralysis while having costs less than a small multiple of annual earnings.

For polio, the possibility of eradication shapes the discussion of prevention. The quote at the beginning of this chapter from a resolution of the 1988 World Health Assembly states the global goal of eradicating polio by the year 2000. Indeed, polio is one of two diseases—the other is Guinea worm disease—that the International Task Force for Disease Eradication has concluded could be eradicated in this decade. The next section of this chapter deals with several of the most important issues concerning polio eradication; these include questions of feasibility, of the extent to which eradication efforts could divert resources from interventions that would have greater effect on health, and of the extent to which existing immunization schedules could be redesigned to respond more effectively to region-specific conditions. The next main section discusses the generally neglected issue of rehabilitation; although the evidence is sparse, it appears likely that serious attention to and investment in rehabilitation could prove quite cost-effective.

Prevention and Eradication

Immunization is the only primary preventive measure for polio paralysis. Improvement in hygiene, in the absence of immunization programs, can, by raising the average age of disease incidence and hence severity, actually have a deleterious effect, as noted earlier. Sanitation, however, should accompany vaccination. Not only will a more sanitary environment protect children prior to their being immunized, but also, after immunization coverage is relatively high, a sanitary environment will stop or delay transmission and allow more time for an effective response to occasional outbreaks. It is the experience of industrial countries that a moderate vaccination level can interfere with transmission if sanitation is high (Horstmann 1982). Table 6-1 provides a qualitative summarization of how patterns of polio in a population respond to the hygienic environment and vaccination coverage levels.

Immunization

There are currently two highly effective vaccines—the injectable polio vaccine (IPV) and the oral polio vaccine (OPV)—and vaccines with improved characteristics are being developed (Melnick 1988b). Each has been successfully used in high-income countries virtually to eliminate polio, although OPV is much more widely used (Hinman and others 1988). Both vaccines have advantages and limitations for developing countries. When given at the same time, both OPV and IPV are effective, and they do not interfere with each other. In table 6-2 we summarize the characteristics of OPV and compare them with those of IPV. The oral vaccine itself is much cheaper than the injectable vaccine, and it may provide secondary immunization to those in contact with the person who has been vaccinated. The oral vaccine also produces local intestinal immunity, and so it inhibits the transmission of wild polioviruses in a community, although the duration of local immunity is unclear (Beale 1990; Nishio 1984). Additional factors that may favor OPV are that it may be more

easily accepted by the population than an injected vaccine (although this is only relevant if polio vaccine is being delivered independently of diphtheria-pertussis-tetanus [DPT] vaccine), and it also simplifies vaccination days or mop-up operations since revaccination is easy and verification of immunization status is not important. The rapid progress to effective control achieved in the Americas is a powerful argument for the effectiveness of OPV in an eradication program. The constraints imposed by use of OPV are the necessity for three or more immunization contacts with the target children, stricter "cold-chain" requirements due to greater heat sensitivity, and an uncertain effectiveness in some tropical settings in which other enteroviruses are present in the environment.

The injectable vaccine protects against poliomyelitis by inducing humoral immunity in vaccinated individuals (Salk 1984). Although it does not induce local immunity, it may reduce the likelihood of polio transmission by preventing pharyngeal excretion of the virus, and, possibly, by reducing virus excretion in stools. The number of IPV injections needed to maintain an enduring immunity has not been established, but two doses appear sufficient to establish initial immunity (Robertson 1988). In European countries such as Sweden and Holland, where IPV alone has been successful in eliminating polio, three injections are given in the primary series, followed by at least two or three booster injections in childhood.

In light of the difficulties of seroconversion using OPV in tropical countries and of interrupting transmission using IPV alone in the same environments, recommendations and testing have been made of a combined IPV-OPV schedule in some developing countries (Melnick 1988b; Tulchinsky 1989), particularly in Asia and Africa. Combined strategies have been successfully used in the West Bank and the Gaza Strip, and they show particular promise in those environments where—for reasons of cost and logistics—many children are still receiving fewer than the recommended numbers of immunizations. Combined strategies would likely rely on OPV for administra-

Table 6-1. Determinants of Patterns of Poliomyelitis

Vaccination coverage	Level of hygiene	
	Low	High
Low	Polio endemic Infection universal at early age Cases usually less severe than when polio is epidemic 1 percent of all births may result in death or permanent paralysis from polio	Polio endemic Most of population eventually infected Average age of infection may be in teens or young adulthood Cases usually relatively serious
High	Polio may become epidemic unless high OPV coverage is reached Infection levels and average age of onset depend on degree of vaccine coverage May be susceptible population if unvaccinated pockets	Polio controlled Circulation of wild virus interrupted Paralytic polio extremely rare; cases are imported or vaccine associated

Source: Authors.

Table 6-2. Characteristics of Attenuated and Inactivated Poliomyelitis Vaccines

Characteristics	Attenuated OPV	Inactivated IPV
Protects against disease	Yes	Yes
Neutralizing antibodies	Yes	Yes
Vaccine virus		
Excretion	Yes	No
Mutations	Yes	No
Vaccine-induced paralysis	Very rare	None
Mucosal and gut immunity to wild virus	Very high	Very low
Potential for circulation of wild virus in vaccinated population	No	Yes
Number of doses required for initial immunity	Three	Two
Vaccine boosters needed	Yes[a]	Yes[a]
Cost of vaccine dose ($)	0.01–0.05	0.50
Cost of delivery per child contacted for vaccination ($)	1–10	1–10

a. Precise schedules remain to be determined.
Source: Modified and updated from Melnick 1978.

tion at birth when feasible (the so-called OPV-zero) and for occasional mass vaccination days; IPV would be formulated with the DPT shot into a single injection.

Taking all these factors into account, EPI "continues to recommend OPV as the standard EPI antigen for the control of poliomyelitis because of its low cost, dissemination within a community and its record of efficacy" (WHO n.d., p. 11). Nonetheless, it might be more cost-effective to add IPV selectively into the immunization schedule in some geographical areas (Martin 1984). Research is continuing into the effectiveness of schedules combining OPV and IPV compared with those that rely entirely on IPV.

The Cost-Effectiveness of Immunization

The World Bank's Health Sector Priorities Review, of which this chapter is a part, is using two model populations of 1 million to illustrate the magnitude of problems and the cost and effectiveness of interventions. In this subsection we provide estimates of the cost-effectiveness of immunization in these two populations. (The high-mortality population is assumed to have a life expectancy of fifty-one years and an infant mortality rate (IMR) of 129 per 1,000; the low-mortality developing country has a life expectancy of sixty-four years and an IMR of 51 per 1,000.)

Because the timing of administration of polio vaccine corresponds closely to that for DPT, and because the probable administration of IPV should actually be combined with DPT into a four-antigen formulation, the economics of polio vaccination cannot be separated from that of DPT. Underlying this conclusion is the assumption that when polio vaccination costs and effects are considered marginal to those of DPT, the cost-effectiveness of including polio will be very high; calculations strongly support this assumption.[1] Table 6-3 shows illustrative (but plausible) mortality in cohorts of 10,000 births in high- and low-mortality environments, with and without effective vaccination programs. The data in the table suggest that full immunization of the cohort in a high-mortality envi-

ronment might avert between 170 and 180 deaths in the cohort of 10,000; that is, it might reduce the IMR by 17 or 18 from the the initial level of 129; in the low-mortality environment, the reduction might be about 7 or 8 from 51. These are, of course, highly significant mortality reductions; in addition, assuming an 85 percent effectiveness for polio vaccination, perhaps 50 cases of paralytic polio would be averted (in each environment). After several years of this level of coverage, eradication of local polio could be expected; new cases of disease would drop to zero.

Under conservative assumptions about vaccination program costs (that is, assuming that three contacts per child are required at a cost of $4 each for a total of $12 to immunize against DPT and polio), the cost per child death averted in an immunization effort that covers DPT plus polio is about $670 in a high-mortality environment and about $1,600 in a low-mortality environment. If we assume a 3 percent discount rate, a loss of 0.2 healthy life-years per affected person per year resulting from mild-to-moderate paralysis, and a loss of 0.6 healthy life-years per person per year resulting from severe paralysis, it becomes possible to combine the effects of polio disability averted with the mortality reduction effects of vaccination. The cost per healthy life-year gained is, then, about $20 in the high-mortality environment and about $42 in the low-mortality environment; these costs would go up by about 10 percent and 25 percent, respectively, if polio disability were not considered. Other causes of mortality would, of course, reduce the gains from vaccination; the effect is probably small—perhaps a 10 percent increase in cost per year of healthy life gained in a high-mortality environment and 5 percent in a low-mortality one.

We stress that the numbers in these examples are illustrative and would, most obviously, vary from country to country for many reasons. In particular, as program coverage expands, one expects rising marginal costs, and different countries will be at different levels of current coverage and will be facing different environments. These numbers do give a sense of typical marginal cost-effectiveness in two environments, though, and the

Table 6-3. **Effects of** DPT **and Polio Vaccination on Deaths in High- and Low-Mortality Environments**
(per 10,000 births)

Disease	Deaths in high-mortality environment[a]		Deaths in low-mortality environment[a]	
	Without vaccination[b]	With vaccination[c]	Without vaccination[b]	With vaccination[c]
Polio	15	0–1	15	0–1
Diphtheria	12	1	5	0
Pertussis	110	11	55	11
Tetanus[d]	60	3	15	1
Total	197	26–27	90	12–13

a. The high- and low-mortality environments are characterized by infant mortality rates of 129 per 1,000 and 51 per 1,000, respectively.

b. Estimates come from various sources, including EPI program documents, and are approximate.

c. Estimates assume complete coverage with recommended doses of potent vaccine. The assumed efficacies of the vaccines are: polio, 85 percent; diphtheria, 95 percent; pertussis, 80 percent; tetanus, 95 percent.

d. Excludes neonatal tetanus.

Source: Authors.

cost-effectiveness conclusions serve to give a rough sense of the attractiveness of vaccination against these conditions. Findings from other chapters of this collection allow these estimates of the cost-effectiveness of DPT-plus-polio immunization programs to be placed in perspective. Although noticeably less cost-effective than immunization to prevent neonatal tetanus or measles, say, immunization for DPT and polio is solidly among the most cost-effective interventions for children (Jamison, chapter 1, this collection).

Global Eradication

In May 1988 the Forty-first World Health Assembly declared the goal of global eradication of poliomyelitis by the year 2000 (World Health Assembly 1988). An international consensus for the global eradication of poliomyelitis had been building for some time, spurred on by the successful eradication of smallpox in 1977. Similarities in the epidemiologic characteristics of the diseases (spread by human contact) and the availability of effective vaccines suggested that poliomyelitis, like smallpox, was eradicable (Hinman and others 1987). In the 1980s the intensification of immunizations as part of primary health care and the Expanded Programme on Immunizations stimulated marked improvements in polio vaccine coverage, and recent estimates (WHO 1990) suggest that coverage with the third dose of OPV ranges from 47 percent in Africa to 91 percent in the western Pacific region. By 1985 the Pan-American Health Organization (PAHO) and the regional offices of the World Health Organization for Europe and for the western Pacific had declared regional polio elimination targets for the years 1990 and 2000, respectively, and enormous progress has been made toward this goal. In the Americas, there were only 130 cases of paralysis in 1989 that were confirmed as polio-related (MMWR 1990); preliminary estimates for 1990 suggest that this number had dropped to 10. Sufficient progress had been made by March of 1988 that the Child Survival Task Force meeting at Talloires in France declared the target of global eradication of polio by the year 2000, preparatory to the World Health Assembly resolution.

What are the implications of an eradication strategy, in comparison with current control strategies? What lessons can be drawn from biologic and epidemiologic similarities (and differences) between polio and smallpox? Is global eradication of polio technically feasible? If so, what are the operational and program design issues associated with the adoption of such a strategy? These questions are addressed in turn.

SPECIFYING ERADICATION STRATEGIES. Stages of control of infectious agents range from effective control to regional elimination to global eradication. In effective control polio immunization EPI is aimed at reducing disease incidence. Regional elimination, the goal in Europe and the Americas, aims at complete cessation of continuous indigenous transmission of wild virus within a specific region. After regional elimination, certain control measures may be dropped and others relaxed; but immunization, plus detection and control of imported cases, must be continued. Global eradication of a disease like polio is the complete and permanent cessation of the natural transmission of the wild virus. After certification of eradication of the disease, vaccinations cannot be stopped permanently until further studies prove the wild virus and virulent strains of the OPV virus are no longer present in the world. It should be emphasized that the World Health Assembly's goal for the year 2000 does not go as far as proven elimination of wild virus; rather, with continued immunization and containment programs, EPI hopes, in the next decade, to reduce to zero the actual incidence of disease. The cost savings associated with being able to cease control efforts, which were an important consequence of smallpox eradication, cannot, however, be expected for polio until, perhaps, substantially after the year 2000.

It is important to recognize that although these programs represent a spectrum of goals, the strategies are fundamentally different in ultimate objective, time frame, and operational translation. Effective control has the modest goal of reduction of the disease burden, and, in the case of polio, the strategy is broad immunization coverage. Regional elimination requires extremely high immunization coverage to levels in which natural transmission is interrupted completely. The strategy is the maintenance of high vaccine coverage with concurrent surveillance, detection, and control of imported cases. The goal of eradication is to interrupt natural transmission worldwide completely and permanently. The time dimension is critical because there is both the need to attain interruption of transmission as well as the need to achieve complete eradication before political and popular support wane from fatigue or decreasing awareness of the threat of the disease. Even after complete eradication of polio as a disease has been certified, vaccination will have to be continued and the situation evaluated for years before all control measures can be dropped.

IS ERADICATION FEASIBLE? Success with eradication of smallpox raises the question of whether polio has similar characteristics that also make it amenable for potential eradication (Fenner and others 1988). The main similarities between smallpox and polio viruses are the limitation of the virus to human hosts, and that there are no long-term carriers. Several features of poliomyelitis epidemiology suggest that eventual eradication of polio is technically feasible. Effective and cheap vaccines are readily available, and recent experience suggests that complete interruption of natural transmission is feasible (Sabin 1984). In the United States, where nearly 97 percent of school-age children are immunized, naturally acquired indigenous polio has not been reported since 1979. Similar effects of mass vaccine coverage have been observed in Western Europe. Considerable success has also been achieved in certain developing countries, for example, in Chile (no cases since 1975), Cuba (one case since 1973), Costa Rica (no cases), and Brazil (a tenfold reduction of cases since 1980 as a result of mass campaigns during national vaccination days) (PAHO 1985). Indeed, as of April 1989, for the Americas as a whole, "the data appear to indicate that circulation of the wild virus is limited to a few areas of the Andean region (Columbia, Peru, and Venezuela), the Northeastern region of Brazil, and a few areas of Mexico" (PAHO 1989, p. 1). De Quadros and others (1991) provide an overview of recent progress in the Americas and describe the strategies responsible for success.

The biologic differences are numerous, however. These include the existence of three serotypes of poliovirus (rather than one), although the three types have proven to be stable for the past fifty years, so no change in vaccine composition

has been necessary. In addition, polio differs markedly in its high ratios of asymptomatic infection.

Not only are there biologic differences between these viruses, but these differences have important implications for the programmatic control of the viral diseases (table 6-4). First, controlling the transmission of poliovirus is far more difficult than controlling the spread of smallpox. The ease of poliovirus transmission and the fact that the overwhelming proportion of infections are asymptomatic render containment much more difficult. Since the fecal-oral route is the primary mode of spread of poliovirus, improved sanitation should help to interrupt transmission.

Second, vaccination around a case of paralytic poliomyelitis would require mop-up operations in whole areas and may not be as effective as vaccination around index smallpox cases. Effectiveness depends, however, on the geographical mobility of the virus, which recent experience suggests is limited. Paralysis is a rare consequence of polio infection, and by the time paralytic cases are recognized, poliovirus may have been widely transmitted. Ultimately, polio eradication may be far more dependent upon mass vaccination than on focused immunization efforts around index cases. Worthy of note is that the mass immunization strategy undertaken in the attempt to eradicate smallpox was extraordinarily difficult and failed in many developing countries.

Third, persons not vaccinated against polio are not as easy to identify as those without smallpox vaccinations. This constraint becomes particularly important for a vaccine which requires multiple doses for effective protection, since partially immunized subjects require identification and revaccination. Consequently, mass vaccination for polio at certain times of the year has been recommended, with OPV being given to all young children. This strategy has been used by PAHO in the Americas and constitutes a definite advantage of OPV over IPV for polio-only vaccination days.

Finally, although the smallpox and the oral and injectable polio vaccines are biologically effective, the polio vaccines are less stable than the smallpox vaccine, especially in tropical climates; they require multiple doses to achieve protective antibody levels; and the cost-effectiveness of a containment strategy of immunizing around index paralysis cases remains uncertain, although recent experiences in the Americas are very encouraging.

Table 6-4. Criteria and Methods of Assessment for Smallpox and Poliomyelitis

Assessment criterion	Assessment method	
	Smallpox	*Poliomyelitis*
Virus in environment	No environmental tests required; only human-to-human spread	Test sewage or fecal samples for virus carriage
Immunity in population	Scar good indicator	Serosurveys
Subclinical infections	None; unusual	Viral isolation or serologic tests
Clinical disease	Characteristic rash; sometimes confused with chickenpox	Persistent flaccid paralysis; other viruses can cause paralysis, but rarely this type
Prevalence of clinical disease in area	Presence of clinical cases	Lameness survey

Source: Modified from Evans 1984.

For all these reasons, then, eradication of poliomyelitis will prove more difficult than was eradication of smallpox. Nevertheless, the efforts to eradicate polio benefit from (and contribute to) a massive global immunization program that was totally lacking when smallpox eradication commenced. And in all, vaccination trends plus current and past experiences in polio control suggest that if success is not attained by the year 2000, it should come soon thereafter.

IMPLEMENTATION AND PROGRAM DESIGN. The 1988 World Health Assembly resolution that declared the commitment of WHO and its member states to global eradication of polio recommended a three-pronged attack: (a) achievement and maintenance of high immunization levels, (b) effective surveillance to detect all new cases, and (c) rapid and vigorous response to the occurrence of cases. Countries which have over 70 percent vaccine coverage are encouraged to focus on the elimination of natural transmission, whereas countries with lower vaccine coverage are encouraged to accelerate immunization delivery. Wherever natural transmission has ceased, it should be so confirmed. The director-general of WHO was requested to strengthen planning, training, and supervision within national programs; to enhance monitoring and evaluation; and to improve disease surveillance, clinical laboratory, and vaccine production and quality services. Close cooperation with UNICEF (United Nations Children's Fund) and the Rotary International (*Polio-Plus*) was recommended, and a major resource mobilization effort to seek "extrabudgetary contributions" was mandated.

In pursuing this strategy, certain impediments to eradication were identified. These are political and social will; management constraints; vaccine effectiveness, stability, and cost; and adequacy of surveillance.

The lessons learned from smallpox eradication suggest certain areas that deserve attention. First, the polio eradication effort will be an integral part of EPI and not an entirely separate effort. The smallpox program, in contrast, was greatly facilitated by its organization as a special program with specific targets and a limited time frame. To fulfill its goals, it had a full-time technical staff, at one stage numbering more than 100, and earmarked resources and internally established working procedures. The WHO resolution specifically emphasizes the importance of strengthening EPI and primary health care through polio eradication activities, and the key role of increasing vaccination coverage (including all EPI antigens) is stressed in recent program descriptions. Given the polio eradication effort as currently articulated, there should be no competition between polio eradication and other EPI or primary health care objectives.

Second, plans for polio eradication implicitly call for an articulated strategy that emphasizes both general health service objectives (higher general vaccine coverage) as well as special vertical efforts (surveillance, special immunization efforts around index cases, and national polio vaccination days). Experience from industrial countries has demonstrated that high levels of general coverage are feasible, assuming strong health infrastructure, and can lead to the interruption of natural transmission. In many developing countries, however, the maintenance of high levels of general vaccine coverage may be operationally difficult or unsustainable at present. Understandably, vertical efforts such as national vaccine days have encountered some success. The implication of larger-scale, vertical efforts such as these on the existing health care system will vary considerably between countries. The experience of PAHO in the Americas is very illustrative. Polio vaccination has been used as the leading edge for EPI, and the use of all vaccines has been encouraged on immunization days.

Third, the smallpox program had built-in applied research with sufficient programmatic flexibility to adapt management of program structures to specific country situations. Indeed, the smallpox experience demonstrated that research and learning led to many programmatic modifications. Such research and adaptive managerial responses are being developed and successfully used in the Americas, where the global effort has recently articulated a research program.

Case Management

The true dimensions of the tragedy of poliomyelitis worldwide can be understood, not from the incidence figures given earlier in this chapter, but only by the realization that poliomyelitis will lead each one of the paralyzed individuals to a lifetime of disability. A child that suffers polio in 1990 and who lives sixty years will still be a member of the disabled population in the year 2050. Even if polio were eradicated by the year 2000, there would still remain well into the next century 10 million to 20 million persons paralyzed from poliomyelitis. The aims of rehabilitation are to facilitate integration of these people into the family and community of polio victims, transforming their personal and social expectations and contribution. In most developing countries, few individuals suffering disability from poliomyelitis receive treatment. This situation is not unique to polio. Probably no more than 1 or 2 percent of all disabilities in developing countries are actually treated (Shirley 1983).

There is a complex set of political, structural, and cultural reasons for this situation (Heim 1979; Vossberg 1985). First, rehabilitation and treatment of disabled individuals have been a low priority for governments because of a lack of recognition of the extent of the problem and an underestimation of the burden it poses. Incidence figures of poliomyelitis, when compared with those of acute diseases, underrepresent the true burden of the disease, which amounts to a life of disability, suffering, and lost productivity. Besides an underestimation of the true burden of the disease, another reason why governments have given low priority to rehabilitation programs is that disabled individuals are a marginal population and have little ability to influence policy. Second, there is a problem of access. Existing rehabilitation services tend to be located in urban areas and to be costly. Finally, there are cultural reasons: disabled individuals may be rejected by their communities, denied, or hidden. And in general there may be a fatalistic attitude that nothing can be done to improve the living conditions of persons with paralytic disabilities.

Despite this current inattention to rehabilitation, there is a wide range of interventions that can reduce the level of disability and improve the quality of life of persons suffering from paralytic polio (Ajao 1981; Huckstep 1970; Werner 1987; WHO 1982). Many of the needed interventions, with the exception of surgery, can be easily learned and practiced by family members of disabled individuals or by other disabled individuals themselves who are trained as rehabilitation, primary care, or other types of health workers. This is true for other motor disabilities as well, which suggests the value of an integrated approach to rehabilitation.

Rehabilitation of polio paralysis in the first few days after the onset of paralysis is oriented to reducing the pain associated with muscle spasm. Hot wet packs, warm baths, dry heat, changing the position of paralyzed limbs and moving the patient in the bed are all effective in reducing frequency and intensity of pain. In the weeks following the attack, and once pain has disappeared, physiotherapy can be initiated on a daily basis. The aims of physiotherapy are (a) to strengthen muscles, and (b) to limit deformities and contractures by putting limbs through a full range of passive movements. Physiotherapy needs to be continued for several months in order to be most effective (Coovadia 1984).

Once paralysis is established, usually one to two years after disease onset, rehabilitation, through physiotherapy, is oriented to overcome deformities resulting from rigidities and contractures. Severe or old deformities will often need surgery to be corrected, which suggests the secondary preventive value of early intervention. Once limbs are returned to their most functional positions, appliances are needed to correct residual lesions, like leg length inequalities, or to facilitate motion (Coovadia and Loening 1984).

Prostheses and aids can be cheaply and appropriately produced in developing countries, frequently with material available in the same communities where they are to be used (Barneji 1984; Eyre-Brook 1986; Sankaran 1984). Importation of orthopedic devices is costly and often inappropriate because of cultural differences and difficulties of maintenance (Abayoni 1981).

Rehabilitation programs in developing countries face many challenges. The most important ones are lack of trained professionals and a large, dispersed rural population with limited access to rural rehabilitation services. A number of programs in developing countries are successfully providing rehabilitation services to underserved populations. One of them is the Projimo project in Mexico (Werner 1987). This project is run by disabled individuals of the locality, whose education averages three years. In the experience of this project only 10 percent of the disabled individuals in the area needed specialized services that had to be provided outside at a referral center. The operating cost of this program is about $9 per patient per year.

This experience of those in this and other projects (Barneji 1984; Eyre-Brook 1986; Sankaran, 1984), points out that tertiary and secondary facilities can be effectively linked to community-based projects. Such linkage can widen the coverage that specialized programs offer and increase their effectiveness. The typical cost of operating a community-based project remains to be worked out. Although the cost of attending an individual patient will likely be low, the cost of effective supervision and training may well be important. Table 6-5 summarizes the nature of case management interventions that might be delivered at various levels of referral, including the household level.

Current experiences in developing countries provide some insight and guidance (often untapped) on ways to approach these problems. The main lesson is that viable options exist for the disabled, even in very poor countries. In this context, it is encouraging that WHO feels that "[p]olio eradication will provide a setting in which significant improvements in rehabilitation services can be undertaken" (WHO/EPI 1989). It is important that these sentiments be backed by resources.

Conclusions

Poliomyelitis has, historically, imposed a significant (but most often underrecognized) burden on the world's population. Prior to the development and introduction of vaccines, more than five out of every thousand children born would have been seriously affected by the disease, most typically with permanent lameness. Programs built around the highly effective and relatively low-cost vaccines now available have greatly reduced the global burden of poliomyelitis. Available technologies hold the promise of being able to eradicate poliomyelitis, and

Table 6-5. Management of Cases of Paralytic Poliomyelitis

Objective	Household	Primary facility	District hospital	Tertiary hospital
		Level of intervention		
Rehabilitation	Passive movements	Passive movements; functional postures	Physiotherapy; corrective surgery	Corrective surgery
Secondary prevention	Posture playing; passive movements	Appliances; passive movements; social integration	Physiotherapy; corrective surgery	Corrective surgery
Palliation	Pain reduction with hot wet packs and warm baths	Painkillers and pain reduction with hot wet packs and warm baths	Painkillers and pain reduction with hot wet packs and warm baths	Painkillers and pain reduction with hot wet packs and warm baths

Note: Cure is not an objective at any level of intervention.
Source: Authors.

the World Health Organization is providing global leadership to achieve this goal by the year 2000. Yet moving toward eradication raises difficult economic and managerial issues, particularly for the poorest countries; and the question of how to provide minimally adequate rehabilitation for the hundreds of thousands of new cases every year, and the 10 million to 20 million existing cases, remains to be addressed.

Our main conclusions deal with these issues:

- The commitment to polio eradication by the year 2000, within the context of EPI, deserves strong national and international financial and technical support. With such support, sustained throughout the 1990s, it is reasonable to hope that polio will be eradicated by the year 2000 or soon thereafter. It will probably prove unwise to advance eradication through substantial expenditure on polio-only activities; although such a less-focused, broader approach may delay eradication somewhat, it will maximize the cross-benefits of political concern for polio by increasing the efforts put forth generally to strengthen EPI and primary health care.

- There are now available, in OPV and IPV, two highly effective vaccines; the choice of OPV or IPV or a schedule that relies on both should consider the epidemiological, economic, and logistic realities of each country. At present, schedules based on OPV are recommended by WHO as globally most desirable; a careful assessment, by country or by region, of the effectiveness of alternative vaccination schedules, given their costs, might suggest the desirability of different schedules for different environments.

- Effective interventions exist both to reduce disability from paralytic polio and to (partially) rehabilitate the already disabled. Little, concretely, is known about the costs, short-term effectiveness, or long-term benefits of programs based on these interventions. Yet the available evidence strongly suggests that much more should be done and could be done at modest cost; there is no justification for continued neglect of rehabilitation.

Appendix 6A. Epidemiology of Polio

In this appendix we first discuss the general characteristics of polio and then turn to several specific aspects of descriptive gender differences in epidemiology, results form lameness surveys, and incidence trends.

General Characteristics

Poliovirus belongs in the family Picornaviridae, genus *Enterovirus*. They are small icosahedron-shaped viruses with a protein coat and an RNA core and do not contain lipids. There are three main antigenic types, with many intratypic differences, and they are identified by type, place, strain number, and year of isolation. Poliovirus 1 predominates in unvaccinated communities, and types 2 and 3 are responsible for most outbreaks in vaccinated populations (Assaad and Ljungars-Esteves 1984).

The poliovirus enters the body through oral ingestion and initially multiplies in the lymphoid tissue. The incubation period is usually seven to fourteen days, but it may range from three to thirty-five. Through dissemination in the blood stream, the virus may invade anterior horn cells (motor neurons) of the spinal cord, and in the process of intracellular replication, poliovirus may cause temporary or permanent loss of neurologic function due to inflammation. Following the attack, most individuals will recover completely. In rare cases, permanent damage or complete destruction of the nerve cell leads to irreversible paralysis. The infection stimulates permanent local and serum immunity to the viral type causing the infection (Paul, Riordan, and Melnick 1951). Local immunity prevents reinfection in the gastrointestinal tract (Melnick 1982).

Only about 1 percent of the total infections will produce clinical symptoms. The most common form of poliovirus infection is asymptomatic. Severe illness may follow nonspecific symptoms of infection—fever, malaise, sore throat, and symptoms of aseptic meningitis—but most often, severe disease is preceded by no manifestations of disease. Characteristic signs of severe disease are a flaccid paralysis—due to lower motor neuron damage—typically asymmetric for limbs and with no loss of sensation. In table 6A-1 we show a hypothetical pattern of outcomes for 10,000 cases of infection with poliovirus.

Besides the immediate paralysis, affected persons suffer in subsequent years or decades an aggravation of paralysis and intense symptoms of asthenia, fatigue, or pain. These late effects of poliomyelitis typically manifest themselves several decades after the onset of primal paralysis, sometimes leading to a severe incapacitation of individuals who were previously only moderately affected. Two factors may play a predisposing role to late effects of poliomyelitis: older ages at polio onset and an initially severe presentation of the disease (Halstead 1985).

Polioviruses can maintain their infectivity in water, unpasteurized milk, and other food products (Robbins and Nightingale 1986). Polioviruses replicate, however, only in human beings, and man is the only known reservoir. The viruses multiply in the alimentary track—throat and lower intestine—and are eliminated with feces. The virus can then be found in the stools of infected persons for a period of one or two months. Contaminated water may be an important route

Table 6A-1. Typical Outcomes among 10,000 Cases of Poliomyelitis

Outcome	Number
Asymptomatic	9,900
Symptomatic	100
Death	15
Complete recovery	25
Mild paralysis	30
Moderate paralysis	15
Severe Paralysis	15

Source: Authors' estimation from epidemiologic findings; Basu and Soc Khey 1984.

of transmission in most developing countries (Evans 1984), and although polioviruses are resistant to the action of lipid solvents, they can be rendered inactive by chlorination of water. Standard sewage treatment does not usually eliminate poliovirus from the effluent (Melnick 1982). Besides stools, droplets from coughing or sneezing can also be a source of transmission in the early stages of the infection. Increased risk of paralysis has been reported following intramuscular inoculations (Guyer 1980; Wyatt 1985).

Hygiene, sanitation, and poverty are primary determinants of the environmental prevalence of the viruses and consequently of the average age at first infection (Horstmann 1982). In unvaccinated populations of developing countries almost all children are exposed to polioviruses before five years of age. Given the low mortality rate from infection (indicated in table 6A-1), the contribution of polio to mortality of children under the age of five years would be very modest—only 1.5 per 1,000, out of the approximately 90 per 1,000 in Asia, or the 170 per 1,000 in Sub-Saharan Africa. That figure was found to be about 2 per 1,000 in a preimmunization environment in West Africa (Goldberg and McBodji 1988).

The pattern of polio transmission in now-industrial countries before the advent of mass vaccination provides excellent evidence of changes in epidemiologic patterns related to environmental conditions, mainly hygiene and sanitation. In the epidemic of 1916 in the United States, 80 percent of the cases were in children below five years of age. A few decades later, before vaccination was started, the average age had moved higher, to five to nine years, with one-third of the cases above fifteen years. In both the 1916 and 1950 epidemics, children from higher socioeconomic classes, who, presumably, were less exposed at young ages, experienced a higher mean age of disease and, consequently, more severe cases. Historically, in industrial countries, before mass vaccination, children of higher economic groups were infected at older ages than those

of lower socioeconomic ones. Those stricken at older ages are more likely to develop more severe forms of disease.

Traditionally, in tropical countries poliomyelitis has been an infection of infants. In those countries, the virus has been widely distributed in the environment, and passive immunity conferred by the mothers to the newborns may have provided some early protection in infants that reduced the presentation of severe forms of disease. Among the nonimmunized, infection would have invariably occurred early in life (Melnick 1988a and 1988b). As sanitation and general development improves, a shift from endemic to epidemic patterns of polio transmission is observed. The overall incidence of severe paralytic disease appears to increase along with older mean age of infection and the transition from endemic to epidemic disease transmission (Fang-Chou and others 1982; Goldblum and others 1984).

The experience of industrial countries is that the incidence of disease drops soon after mass immunization is introduced (Kim-Farley, Rutherford, Lichfield, and others 1984). Except for some imported strains, wild polioviruses for the most part either have been eradicated or are in the process of being eradicated from most industrial countries. The experience of some countries, such as the Netherlands, the United States, Spain, China, and Taiwan, demonstrates that, even with high vaccination coverage, there are opportunities for occasional epidemics in unvaccinated segments of the population; for discussion of a relevant outbreak in Taiwan, see Kim-Farley (1984b). Those experiences underscore the need for good surveillance and rapid interventions as essential features of control and eradication strategies.

Gender Differences

Table 6A-2 is a summary of reported gender differences in the prevalence of paralytic poliomyelitis. The figures suggest that

Table 6A-2. Studies Indicating Prevalence of Paralytic Poliomyelitis by Gender

Country (year)	Number of cases	Male-female prevalence	Description of study	Source
Senegal (1986–87)	89	1.7:1	Postoutbreak study to assess effectiveness of new IPV; 85 cases were in children under age five; 63 percent were male	MMWR 1988
Senegal (1986)	60	1.2:1	Preliminary phase of above study	MMWR 1987
The Gambia (1986)	305	1.3:1	Investigation of outbreak to assess effectiveness of OPV	Global Advisory Group 1987
Yemen, Rep. of (1980–81)	40	2.5:1	School and community survey of lameness in children aged five to thirteen	Hajar 1983
Jordan (1978–80)	90	2.7:1	Hospital admissions following poliomyelitis outbreak	Khuri-Bulos and others 1984
Germany (1964–82)	27	1.7:1	Reports of paralytic poliomyelitis in recipients of OPV (21) or in contacts (6)	Maass and Quast 1987
United States (1969–81)	203	1.2:1[a]	Cases reported to Centers for Disease Control (CDC)	Moore and others 1983
India (1984)[b]	82	1.5:1	Community lameness survey in Bombay slums in children younger than six years	Tidke, Joshi, and Patel 1986
India (1978)	416	1.5:1	Hospital admissions of children following outbreak	Saeed and others 1980
India (1976–80)	2,953	1.7:1	Assessment of paralytic poliomyelitis victims, including vaccination history and prognosis	Strivastava and others 1983

a. 2.7:1 in vaccinees.
b. Date uncertain.
Source: See table (last column).

Table 6A-3. Prevalence of Poliomyelitis in Population-Based Lameness Surveys

Country	Year	Ages (years)	Children surveyed	Population[a]	Prevalence
Asia					
Indonesia	1977	0–20	57,000	Mixed	0.9
	1978	0–14	10,000	Rural	3
Bangladesh	1979	5–14	25,000	Rural	1
	1983	5–9	35,000	Mixed	2–3
Philippines	1980	0–14	12,000	Mixed	3
India	1981	5–9	358,000	Rural	6 (2–9)[b]
	1981	5–9	357,000	Urban	7 (2–9)[b]
	1985	5–15	6,000	Urban	17
	1986	0–4	27,000	Rural	5
	1987	0–5	10,000	Rural	3
Nepal	1982	5–9	6,000	Rural	2
	1982	5–9	5,000	Mixed	1
	1983	5–9	2,000	Mixed	3
Sri Lanka	1982	5–9	7,000	Rural	0.9
Viet Nam	1983	5–15	5,000	Mixed	1
	1985	5–15	43,000	Mixed	0.6
	1985	0–15	68,000	Mixed	0.5
	1987	0–14	340,000	Rural	0.4
Lao PDR	1985	5–14	27,000	Rural	3
Sub-Saharan Africa					
Ghana	1974	6–15	7,000	Rural	8
Cameroon	1978	5–11	4,000	Mixed	5
	1978	5–11	8,000	Rural	8.5
	1978	5–11	5,000	Urban	8
Côte d'Ivoire	1979	5–14	6,000	Rural	8
	1980	8–12	6,000	Mixed	12
	1980	6–15	5,000	Urban	7
Kenya	1979	5–14	7,000	Rural	0.7
Malawi	1979	0–15	35,000	Mixed	6.5
Swaziland	1979	0–10	6,000	Rural	3
Niger	1981	5–19	14,000	Rural	7
	1981	10–14	10,000	Rural	6
Sudan	1982	5–9	18,000	Mixed	5
Somalia	1982	5–13	51,000	Mixed	10 (6–20)[b]
Ethiopia	1983	5–9	18,000	Mixed	7
Tanzania	1984	0–4	4,000	Rural	0
	1984	5–9	4,000	Rural	2
	1984	10–14	3,000	Rural	5
Middle East and North Africa					
Egypt	1976	0–10	525,000	Urban	2
Morocco	1980	0–4	7,000	Urban	2
	1980	5–9	8,000	Urban	3
	1980	10–14	8,000	Urban	5
Yemen, Rep. of	1981	5–13	6,000	Rural	3
	1981	5–13	6,000	Urban	4
Jordan	1983	0–10	28,000	Mixed	1 (0.4–2)[b]
Pakistan	1984	0–5	10,000	Mixed	8
Iran, Islamic Rep. of	1986	0–15	15,000	Rural	4
	1986	0–15	15,000	Urban	3.8 (2–6)

a. Mixed population is both rural and urban.
b. Prevalence ranges.
Source: Adcock 1982; Bernier 1983; Bernier 1984; Basu 1986; WHO/EPI 1988; Heymann and others 1983; Nicholas and others 1977; Snyder and others 1981; Thuriaux 1982; Ulfah and others 1981.

Table 6A-4. Regional Variation in Vaccination Coverages, Cases of Poliomyelitis, and Mortality, 1985

Parameter	Global	Industrialized market economies	Industrialized transition economies	Latin America	Middle East and North Africa	Africa	Asia
Vaccination coverage[a] (percent)	50	90	85	85	20	50	60
Incidence (per thousand school-age children)	10	0	0	0.25	43	23	11
New cases (thousands)	500	0.1	0.3	0.8	183	81	283
Deaths (thousands)							
Age 0–1 year	24	0	0	0	9	4	11
Age 1–4 years	53	—	—	—	17	7	29
Age 5–14 years	4	—	—	—	1	1	2
Age 15–44 years	—	—	—	—	—	—	—
Age 45–64 years	—	—	—	—	—	—	—
Age 65 years and older	—	—	—	—	—	—	—
Total	81	—	—	—	27	12	42
Percentage of all deaths	0.16	—	—	—	0.37	0.25	0.1
Death rate (per ten thousand)	1.7	—	—	—	5.9	3.1	1

a. For children age five years and younger.
— Not available.
Source: Basu and Soc Khey 1984; Bernier 1984; Fang-Chou and others, 1982; Foster 1984; Hajar and others 1983; Heymann and others 1983; John 1984; LaForce and others 1980; MMWR 1987; PAHO 1985; Ramia and others 1987; Ulfah and others 1981; WHO/EPI 1987.

paralytic poliomyelitis tends to occur more frequently in males than in females. The reported effect varies from a ratio of 1.5 to 1 of males to females, to a ratio of 2.5 to 1, the latter being found in the Republic of Yemen and Jordan. There is no clear explanation for these reported differences, although there are several possibilities. First, since not all prevalence studies report ratios of paralysis between males and females, isolated findings could be attributed to chance alone. Although that is theoretically possible, it is unlikely. It must also be noticed that there are no similar reports showing higher rates of disease in females than in males. Second, the figures could be attributed to biased population reporting of polio paralysis. That could explain some of the extreme ratios reported, but Germany and the United States, both of which have good reporting and recording systems, still show a higher prevalence of polio paralysis in males than in females. Third, some unknown factors may lead to (a) higher fatality rates in girls or (b) to a greater severity of the disease in boys. The male-to-female ratio in prevalence of polio paralysis suggested by the literature— excluding extreme values—would be about 1.4, between 1.2 and 1.7 to 1.

Prevalence of Lameness by Region

Paralytic poliomyelitis leads to significant life-long disability and handicap in affected persons. Surveys have been done all over the world to estimate the prevalence of lameness due to poliomyelitis in developing countries. Important differences have been found not just from one country to another, but within the same country between rural and urban areas. The prevalence of paralytic poliomyelitis in developing countries is, on average, higher than the 3 cases per 1,000 population reported for the United States in 1936. On average, the re-ported prevalence of disability is about 5 cases per 1,000 school-age children in developing countries, ranging from 0.5 to 19 (Bernier 1984). Most lameness surveys, however, have been based on school-age children, which holds the potential of underestimation of the true burden of the disease. For this report, we have considered population-based surveys and surveys that included the school catchment area. Table 6A-3 shows the prevalence of poliomyelitis detected by lameness surveys in Sub-Saharan Africa, Asia, and the Middle East and North Africa region. If several surveys were carried out simultaneously, prevalence figures reflect average reported figures; if the reported prevalences differ by more than 20 percent, however, the range of reported prevalences is given.

Declining Trends in Polio Incidence

The actual incidence or prevalence of poliomyelitis in the world is not known, but indirect estimates of incidence derived from lameness surveys have suggested a much heavier disease burden than reported cases would suggest. The World Health Organization estimated that almost 250,000 new cases of poliomyelitis paralysis occurred each year from 1984 to 1988. It is unlikely that actual figures will currently be higher than that. On the contrary, there are strong indications that the number of new cases of polio paralysis has declined significantly in the last decade. Table 6A-4 shows our estimation of new cases that would have occurred about 1985 if disease incidence had been the same as estimated from lameness surveys. More than half a million cases of permanent polio paralyses would have occurred if disease incidence had remained unchanged and similar to that of one or two decades earlier. That figure doubles the estimated number of cases for that year and is comparable to the one estimated by WHO for the late 1970s or early 1980s.

Notes

The authors are grateful for having received numerous helpful comments on earlier drafts of this chapter. Donald A. Henderson provided extensive critical reactions, and valuable comments were also received from Howard Barnum, Logan Brenzel, Ann Goerdt, Mark Grabowski, John Haaga, Ralph Henderson, Peter Patriarca, Ciro de Quadros, Susan Robertson, Nicholas Ward, and David Werner. Preparation of the chapter was supported by the World Bank as part of its Health Sector Priorities Review; the views expressed in the chapter are, however, those of the authors and do not, of course, necessarily reflect those of the World Bank or of any of the individuals who have commented on drafts. A shortened version of this chapter has been published elsewhere (Jamison, Torres, Chen, and Melnick 1991).

1. The calculations are reported in the unpublished versions of this chapter.

References

Abayoni, O. 1981. "Indigenous Substitutes for Modern Prostheses and Orthoses." *Prosthetics Orthotics International* 5:144–46.

Adcock, C. 1982. "Poliomyelitis in Sierra Leone." *British Medical Journal* 285:1031–32.

Ajao, S. A., and A. A. Oyeniade. 1981. "The Team Fights the Scourge of Poliomyelitis." *Prosthetics Orthotics International* 5:68–74.

Assaad, F., and K. Ljungars-Esteves. 1984. "World Overview of Poliomyelitis: Regional Patterns and Trends." *Review of Infectious Diseases* 6(Supplement 2):302–7.

Barneji, B., and J. B. Barneji. 1984. "A Preliminary Report on the Use of Cane and Bamboo as Basic Construction Materials for Orthotic and Prosthetic Appliances." *Prosthetics Orthotics International* 8:91–96.

Basu, R. N. and J. Soc Khey. 1984. "Prevalence of Poliomyelitis in India." *Indian Journal of Pediatrics*, 51:515–19.

Basu, S. N. 1986. "A Review of Paralytic Poliomyelitis Cases Occurring after Polio Vaccination." *Journal of the Indian Medical Association* 84(7):203–6.

Beale, A. J. 1990. "Polio Vaccines: Time for Change in Immunization Policy?" *Lancet* 335:839–42.

Bernier, R. H. 1983. "Prevalence Survey Techniques for Paralytic Polio: An Update." In WHO/EPI/GAG. *Expanded Programme on Immunization*. Document 83/WP10. Geneva.

———. 1984. "Some Observations on Poliomyelitis Lameness Surveys." *Review of Infectious Diseases* 6(Supplement 2):371–75.

Coovadia, H. M., and W. E. K. Loening, eds. 1984. *Pediatrics and Child Health*. Oxford: Oxford University Press.

Evans, A. S. 1984. "Criteria for Control of Infectious Diseases with Poliomyelitis as an Example." *Progress in Medical Virology* 29:141–65.

Eyre-Brook, A. 1986. "An Appropriate Approach to Orthopedics in Developing Countries." *International Orthopedics* 10:5–10.

Fang-Chou, K., D. De-Xiang, S. Ou-Sheng, N. Ji-Tian, and Y. Hong-Hui. 1982. "Poliomyelitis in China." *Journal of Infectious Diseases* 146(4):552–57.

Fenner, F., D. A. Henderson, I. Arita, Z. Jezek, and I. D. Ladnyi. 1988. *Smallpox and Its Eradication*. Geneva: World Health Organization.

Foster, S. O. 1984. "Control of Poliomyelitis in Africa." *Review of Infectious Diseases* 6(Supplement 2):433–37.

Global Advisory Group Meeting. 1987. *Epidemic Poliomyelitis in the Gambia, 1986: Report of Epidemiologic Findings*. Banjul: Gambian Ministry of Health, Labor, and Social Affairs.

Goldberg, H. I., and F. G. McBodji. 1988. "Infant and Early Childhood Mortality in the Sine-Saloum Region of Senegal." *Journal of Biosocial Sciences* 20:471–84.

Goldblum, N., T. Swartz, C. B. Gerichber, R. Handsher, E. E. Lascu, and J. L. Melnick. 1984. "The Natural History of Poliomyelitis in Israel, 1949–1982." *Progress in Medical Virology* 29:115–23.

Guyer, B., A. A. E. Bisong, J. Gould, M. Brigaud, and M. Aymard. 1980. "Infections and Paralytic Poliomyelitis in Tropical Africa." *Bulletin of the World Health Organization* . 58(2):285–91.

Hajar, M. M., A. S. Zeid, M. A. Saif, M. A. Parrez, R. C. Steinglass, and S. Crain. 1983. "Prevalence, Incidence, and Epidemiological Features of Poliomyelitis in the Yemen Arab Republic." *Bulletin of the World Health Organization* 61(2):353–59.

Halstead, L. S., D. O. Wiechers, and C. D. Rossi. 1985. "Late Effects of Poliomyelitis: A National Survey." In L. S. Halstead and D. O. Wiechers, eds., *Late Effects of Poliomyelitis*. Miami, Fla.: Symposia Foundation.

Heim, S. 1979. "The Establishment of Prosthetic Services in African Countries." *Prosthetics Orthotics International* 3:152–54.

Heymann, D. L., V. D. Floyd, M. Lichnevski, G. K. Maben, and F. Mvonbo. 1983. "Estimation of Incidence of Poliomyelitis by Three Survey Methods in Different Regions of the United Republic of Cameroon." *Bulletin of the World Health Organization* 61(3):501–7.

Hinman, A. R., W. H. Foege, C. A. de Quadros, P. A. Patriarca, W. A. Orenstein, and E. W. Brink. 1987. "The Case for Global Eradication of Poliomyelitis." *Bulletin of the World Health Organization* 65(6):835–40.

Hinman, A. R., J. P. Koplan, W. A. Orenstein, E. W. Brink, and B. M. Nkowane. 1988. "Live or Inactivated Poliomyelitis Vaccine: An Analysis of Benefits and Risks." *American Journal of Public Health* 78:291–95.

Horstmann, D. M. 1982. "Control of Poliomyelitis: A Continuing Paradox." *Journal of Infectious Diseases* 146(4):540–51.

Huckstep, R. L. 1970. "Poliomyelitis in Uganda." *Physiotherapy* 54:347–53.

Jamison, D. T., A. M. Torres, L. C. Chen, and J. L. Melnick. 1991. "Poliomyelitis: What Are the Prospects for Eradication and Rehabilitation?" *Health Policy and Planning* 6(2):107–18.

John, T. J. 1984. "Poliomyelitis in India: Prospects and Problems of Control." *Review of Infectious Diseases* 6(Supplement 2):438–41.

Khuri-Bulos, N., J. L. Melnick, M. H. Hatch, and S. T. Dawod. 1984. "The Paralytic Poliomyelitis Epidemic of 1978 in Jordan: Epidemiological Implications." *Bulletin of the World Health Organization* 62(1):83–88.

Kim-Farley, R. T., G. Rutherford, P. Lictfield, S. Hsu, L. B. Schonberger, K. Lui, and C. Lin. 1984. "Outbreak of Paralytic Poliomyelitis, Taiwan." *Lancet* 2:1322–24.

Kim-Farley, R. T., L. B. Schonberger, K. J. Bart, W. A. Orenstein, B. M. NRowane, A. R. Hinman, O. M. Kew, M. H. Hatch, and J. E. Kaplan. 1984. "Poliomyelitis in the U.S.A.: Virtual Elimination of Disease Caused by a Mild Virus." *Lancet* 2:1315–17.

LaForce, F. M., M. S. Lichnevski, J. Keja, and R. H. Henderson. 1980. "Clinical Survey Techniques to Estimate Prevalence and Annual Incidence of Poliomyelitis in Developing Countries." *Bulletin of the World Health Organization* 58:609–20.

Maass, G., and U. Quast. 1987. "Acute Spinal Paralysis after the Administration of Oral Poliomyelitis Vaccine in the Federal Republic of Germany (1963–1984)." *Journal of Biological Standardization* 15:185–91.

Martin, J. F. 1984. "Consequences of the Introduction of the New Inactivated Poliovirus Vaccine into the Expanded Programme on Immunization." *Review of Infectious Diseases* 6(Supplement 2):480–82.

Max, E., and D. S. Shepard. 1988. "Productivity Loss Due to Deformity from Leprosy in India." Research paper of the Takemi Program in International Health, Harvard School of Public Health.

Melnick, J. L. 1978. "Advantages and Disadvantage of Killed and Live Poliomyelitis Vaccines." *Bulletin of the World Health Organization* 56:21–38.

———. 1982. "Enteroviruses." In A. S. Evans, ed., *Viral Infections of Humans: Epidemiology and Control*. New York: Plenum Medical Book Company.

———. 1984. "Poliomyelitis." In K. S. Warren and A. A. F. Mahmoud, eds., *Tropical and Geographical Medicine*. New York: McGraw-Hill.

———. 1988a. "Poliomyelitis: A Vanishing but Not Vanished Disease." Paper presented at the First Asia-Pacific Congress of Medical Virology, Singapore, November.

———. 1988b. "Vaccination against Poliomyelitis: Present Possibilities and Future Prospects." *American Journal of Public Health* 78:304–5.

MMWR (*Morbidity and Mortality Weekly Report*). 1987. "Preliminary Report: Paralytic Poliomyelitis—Senegal 1986." 36(24):387–90.

———. 1988. "Paralytic Poliomyelitis: Senegal 1986–1987—Update on the N-IPV Efficacy Study." 37(16):257–79.

———. 1990. "Update: Progress toward Eliminating Poliomyelitis from the Americas." 39(33):557–61.

Moore, M., P. Katond, J. E. Kaplan, and M. H. Hatch. 1982. "Poliomyelitis in the United States: 1969–1981." *Journal of Infectious Diseases* 146(4):558–63.

Nicholas, D. D., J. H. Kratzer, S. Ofosu-Amaah, and D. W. Belcher. 1977. "Is Poliomyelitis a Serious Problem in Developing Countries? The Danfa Experience." *British Medical Journal* 1:1009–12.

Nishio, O., Y. Ishihara, K. Sakae, and others. 1984. "The Trend of Immunity with Live Polio Virus Vaccine and the Effect of Revaccination: Follow-up of Vaccinees for Ten Years." *Journal of Biological Standardization* 12:1–10.

PAHO (Pan-American Health Organization). 1985. "Poliomyelitis in the Americas 1969–1984." PAHO *Bulletin* 19(4):389–90.

———. 1989. *EPI Newsletter* 11(2).

Paul, J. R., J. T. Riordan, and J. L. Melnick. 1951. "Antibodies to Three Different Antigenic Types of Poliomyelitis Virus in Sera from North Alaskan Eskimos." *American Journal of Hygiene* 54:275–85.

Quadros, C. A. de, A. M. Andrus, J.-M. Olive, C. M. da Silveira, R. M. Eikhof, P. Carrasco, J. W. Fitzsimmons, and F. P. Pinheiro. 1991. "The Eradication of Poliomyelitis: Progress in the Americas." *Pediatric Infectious Disease Journal* 10(3):222–29.

Ramia, S., T. M. F. Bakir, A. R. Al-Frayk, and H. Bahakim. 1987. "Paralytic Poliomyelitis and Non-Polio Enteroviruses in Saudi Arabia." *Journal of Tropical Pediatrics* 33:166–67.

Robbins, F. C., and E. O. Nightingale. 1986. "Poliomyelitis." In J. A. Walsh and K. S. Warren, eds., *Strategies for PHC*. Chicago: University of Chicago Press.

Robertson, S. E., H. P. Traverso, J. A. Drucker, B. Fabre-Teste, M. N'Diaye, F. Dioug, E. Z. Rovira, A. Sow, and M. T. AbySy. 1988. "Clinical Efficacy of a New, Enhanced-Potency, Inactivated Polio Virus Vaccine." *Lancet* 1:897–99.

Robertson, S. E., C. Chan, R. Kim-Farley, and N. Ward. 1990. "Worldwide Status of Poliomyelitis in 1986, 1987, and 1988, and Plans for Its Global Eradication by the Year 2000." *World Health Statistics Quarterly* 43:80–90.

Rosenthal, Gerald. 1989. "The Economic Burden of Sustainable EPI." Presentation at the International Center for Children, Paris, June 28.

Sabin, A. B. 1984. "Strategies for Elimination of Poliomyelitis in Different Parts of the World with Use of Oral Poliovirus Vaccine." *Review of Infectious Diseases* 6(Supplement 2):391–96.

Saeed, A., R. Kumar, A. K. Srivastava, H. Rahman, and V. K. Agarwal. 1980. "An Outbreak of Poliomyelitis in Allahabad." *Indian Pediatrics* 17:757–61.

Salk, D., A. L. van Wezel, and J. Salk. 1984. "Introduction of Long-term Immunity to Paralytic Poliomyelitis by Use of Non-Infectious Vaccine." *Lancet* 2:1317–21.

Sankaran, B. 1984. "Prosthetics and Orthotics in Developing Countries." *International Rehabilitative Medicine* 6:85–101.

Shirley, O., ed. 1983. *A Cry for Health: Poverty and Disability in the Third World.* London: Third World Group for Disabled People.

Snyder, J. D., R. E. Black, A. H. Baqui, and A. M. Sarder. 1981. "Prevalence of Residual Paralysis from Paralytic Poliomyelitis in a Rural Population of Bangladesh." *American Journal of Tropical Medicine and Hygiene* 30:426–30.

Srivastava, A. K., R. Kumar, H. Rahman, R. Sharan, and V. K. Agarwal. 1983. "A Clinical Profile of Paralytic Poliomyelitis with Special Emphasis on Physical Therapy and Rehabilitation." *Indian Pediatrics* 20:415–19.

Thuriaux, M. C. 1982. "A Prevalence Survey of Lower Limb Motor Disorders in School Age Children in Niger and an Estimation of Poliomyelitis Incidence." *Tropical and Geographical Medicine* 34:163–68.

Tidke, R. W., U. Joshi, and R. B. Patel. 1986. "Paralytic Poliomyelitis in Slums of Bombay." *Indian Journal of Pediatrics* 53:109–13.

Tulchinsky, T., Y. Abed, S. Shaheen, N. Toubassi, Y. Sever, M. Schoenbaum, and R. Handsher. 1989. "A Ten-Year Experience in Control of Poliomyelitis through a Combination of Live and Killed Vaccines in Two Developing Areas." *American Journal of Public Health* 79:1648–52.

Ulfah, N. M., S. Parastho, T. Sadjimin, and J. E. Rohde. 1981. "Polio and Lameness in Yogyakarta, Indonesia." *International Journal of Epidemiology* 10(2):171–75.

Vossberg, A. 1985. "The Development of Orthopaedic Appliances and Low-Cost Aids in Least-Developed Countries." *Prosthetics Orthotics International* 9:83–86.

Werner, D. 1987. *Disabled Village Children.* Palo Alto, Calif.: Hesperian Foundation.

WHO (World Health Organization). 1982. *Community-Based Rehabilitation.* Report of a WHO Interregional Consultation, Columbo, Sri Lanka. Document RHB/IR/82.1. Geneva.

———. 1990. "World Immunization Update." WHO Features September 147.

WHO/EPI (World Health Organization/Expanded Programme on Immunization). N.d. *Immunization Policy.* Document GEN/86/7, Review 1. Geneva.

———. 1987. "Poliomyelitis: The Child Crippler." EPI Update 6.

———. 1988. "Polio Lameness Surveys by Regions." EPI Information System July (Section 3): Table 3.4.

———. 1989. *Poliomyelitis: Global Eradication by the Year 2000.* Geneva.

World Health Assembly. 1988. *Global Eradication of Poliomyelitis by the Year 2000.* World Health Assembly Resolution, May 13. Document WHA 41.28.

Wyatt, H. V. 1985. "Provocation of Poliomyelitis by Multiple Infections." *Transactions of the Royal Society of Tropical Medicine and Hygiene* 79:355–58.

7

Helminth Infection

Kenneth S. Warren, D. A. P. Bundy, Roy M. Anderson, A. R. Davis,
Donald A. Henderson, Dean T. Jamison, Nicholas Prescott, and Alfred Senft

In "This Wormy World," published in 1947, N. R. Stoll estimated that there were more than 2,200 million human helminthic infections (cestodes, 72 million; trematodes, 148 million; nematodes, 2,000 million) in a world which contained 2,166 million people. Since then the world's population has more than doubled, but the proportion infected with different worm species remains almost unchanged. Approximately twenty major helminth species infect humans; table 7-1 provides both the scientific and common names of the organisms as well as the mode of infection and the principal disease manifestations. An examination of the prevalence, mortality, and morbidity of the primary infectious diseases of Africa, Asia, and Latin America ranked schistosomiasis fifth, hookworm tenth, onchocerciasis twelfth, ascariasis fifteenth, trichuriasis twenty-first, and filariasis twenty-second (Walsh and Warren 1984).

Such has been the concern about these infections that the first significant global campaign to attempt to eradicate any infectious disease was focused on hookworm (Fosdick 1952). It was considered to be an "anemia-producing disease which sapped vitality and handicapped, crippled, and even killed millions of men, women, and children in the hot, moist regions of the world." When the campaign began in 1913 it soon became apparent that it would not be possible to eradicate infection or even to control transmission. As the campaign progressed, however, it was realized that although infection was uncontrollable, disease could be prevented simply and rapidly by the reduction of worm burdens, even with the poor anthelmintic drugs then available. Unfortunately, not only was this unique strategy forgotten, but hookworm infection remains uncontrolled, there being today approximately 900 million infections.

Seventy-five years later, in 1988, an international symposium on hookworm reexamined these issues and concluded with the question, What can we do now? (Warren 1989). It then became apparent that the ineffective, toxic drugs of the past have been superseded by effective nontoxic, oral, single-dose, broad-spectrum benzimidazole anthelmintics that can treat not only hookworm infection but the other main geohelminthiases, ascariasis and trichuriasis, as well. Furthermore, the multispecies approach could be extended by including other broad-spectrum anthelmintics, such as praziquantel (PZQ), which is effective against virtually all the trematode and cestode infections, and ivermectin (IVR) for the filariases and strongyloidiasis (Warren 1989). Thus, it has now become possible to treat virtually all the major helminthic infections with single-dose, orally administered, relatively nontoxic drugs.

Advances in our understanding of the transmission characteristics of these parasites have also made a significant contribution to the development of more rational control strategies. Helminths are unique among infectious agents, including protozoa, bacteria, viruses, and fungi, in that, with very few exceptions, they do not multiply in their human definitive hosts. As each worm is the result of a separate infection event, reducing the number of infections reduces the worm burden and hence the morbidity. Furthermore, helminths have a clustered, overdispersed distribution in human populations such that only a small proportion of infected individuals harbor heavy worm burdens; it is within this intensely infected group that most of the morbidity and mortality occur. These findings suggest that a strategy is feasible in which helminth-induced disease can be prevented merely by keeping worm burdens at a low level. Because in most cases the rate of acquisition of infection is low, it may take many months or years for the burdens to reach disease-producing levels. This implies that treatment can be administered to reduce disease at much less frequent intervals than to reduce infection. Thus, a form of mass prophylaxis can be instituted in which infection (transmission) is not specifically targeted but disease is largely eliminated.

Another aspect of this strategy is that prophylaxis can be directed toward those groups of individuals with the highest degree of exposure and the heaviest worm burdens. With many of the helminthic infections the most vulnerable group is school-age children. Treatment of this age group offers the possibility not only that concurrent disease manifestations may be prevented but also that future consequences of chronic childhood infection (such as hepatosplenic disease in schistosomiasis, elephantiasis in filariasis, and blindness in oncho-

Table 7-1. Major Helminth Infections in Humans

Organism	Common name	Means of infection	Major disease manifestation[a]
Nematodes (roundworms)			
Ancylostoma duodenale, Necator americanus	Hookworm	Skin	Anemia
Ascaris lumbricoides	Giant roundworm	Oral	Intestinal obstruction
Dracunculus medinensis	Guinea worm	Oral	Cutaneous lesions
Enterobius vermicularis	Pinworm	Oral	Anal pruritus
Onchocerca volvulus	River blindness	Insect	Blindness
Strongyloides stercoralis	Strongyloidiasis	Skin	Autoinfection
Trichinella spiralis	Trichinosis	Oral	Myositis
Trichuris trichiura	Whipworm	Oral	Rectal prolapse
Wuchereria bancrofti, Brugia malayi	Filariasis	Insect	Elephantiasis
Trematodes			
Clonorchis sinensis, Opisthorchis viverrini, O. felineus	Liver fluke	Oral	Biliary obstruction
Fasciola hepatica	Liver fluke	Oral	Hepatomegaly
Fasciolopsis buski	Intestinal fluke	Oral	Diarrhea
Paragonimus westermani	Lung fluke	Oral	Cough
Schistosoma hematobium	Blood fluke	Skin	Hydronephrosis
Schistosoma japonicum, S. mansoni	Blood fluke	Skin	Hepatosplenomegaly
Cestodes			
Diphyllobothrium latum	Fish tapeworm	Oral	Anemia
Echinicoccus granulosus	Hydatid	Oral	Cyst
Tenia saginata	Beef tapeworm	Oral	None
Tenia solium	Pork tapeworm	Oral	Cysticercosis

a. These manifestations are relatively infrequent and tend to be related to the intensity of infection. Exceptions are dracunculiasis, strongyloidiasis, and echinococcosis.
Source: Authors.

cerciasis) will be ameliorated. In addition, the reduction in worm burdens in a heavily infected group will often reduce the rate of infection to others and hence reduce overall parasite transmission in the community. Of those few helminths that are particularly resistant to pharmacological agents, *Trichinella spiralis*, *Fasciola hepatica*, and *Dracunculus medinensis*, the latter is particularly worthy of mention as a prime candidate for global eradication, in which effort a variety of public health measures would be used (Hopkins and Ruiz-Tiben 1990).

Recent advances in our understanding of the public health consequences of helminthic infections suggest that attempts to control morbidity are now urgently required. Contrary to the earlier perception, it is not the acute effects of infection which are the primary public health concern but the chronic and insidious effects of continuous infection throughout childhood. This has implications not only for the growth and intellectual development of the affected child, but also for the subsequent well-being of the adult.

It is timely, then, for these reasons, to reassess both the priority that disease control should claim and the nature of the control strategies to be employed. Our purpose in this chapter is to begin that reassessment. First we describe helminthic infections and then turn to an assessment of their global public health significance. We go on to present potential strategies for control (vaccination, vector control, improved hygiene, and chemotherapy and chemoprophylaxis), after which we

discuss the potential for an integrated strategy for chemoprophylactic control of helminthic infections; and finally, we present our conclusions.

Public Health Significance of Helminth Infections

This section describes the geographical distribution of helminthic infections and then examines the public health consequences of these infection patterns.

Geographical Distribution

Current estimates suggest that more than a third of the world's population is infected with one or several species of parasitic worm and that these are among the most prevalent infections of humans (table 7-2). Although it is clear that the number of infections is very large, the precision of such estimates is rather crude because information is lacking for many areas. An error of a few percentage points in estimating the prevalence of infection in China, for example, with approximately one-quarter of the world's population, may result in an over- or underestimate of tens of millions of cases (Young and Prost 1985).

This margin of error is even greater when morbidity is considered. Very few studies include estimates of the intensity of infection, yet it is primarily the size of the worm burden which determines the morbid consequences of infection. Data on morbidity are notoriously more difficult to obtain than on

Table 7-2. Estimates of Number of Helminth Infections
(millions)

	Market economies	Nonmarket economies	South and Central America	Middle East and North Africa	Sub-Saharan Africa	Indian subcontinent	China	Asia (excluding Indian subcontinent and China)	Total
Nematodes									
Ascaris	4	30	150	55	45	160	510	175	1,129
Brugia	0	0	0	0	0	10	55	35	100
Hookworm	0.7	6	95	50	60	160	325	180	876.7
Onchocerca	0	0	0.1	2	16	0	0	0	18.1
Trichinella	4	2	4	1	..	..	..	..	11
Trichuris	2	45	110	20	30	70	320	170	770
Wuchereria	0	0	4	15	30	40	45	50	184
Trematodes									
Clonorchis	0	0	0	0	0	0	0	0	32
Fasciolopsis	0	0	0	0	0	0	0	0	17
Paragonimus	0	0	..	0	0	0	0	..	6
Schistosoma hematobium	0	0	0	30	70	0	0	0	100
Schistosoma intercalatum	0	0	0	0	12	0	0	0	12
Schistosoma japonicum	0	0	0	0	0	0	10	85	95
Schistosoma mansoni	0	0	14	20	35	0	0	0	69
Schistosoma mekongi	0	0	0	0	0	0	0	0.6	
Cestodes									
Diphyllobothrium	0.1	5	..	0	0	0	0	4	9.1
Tenia saginata	1	30	2	0	30	0	0	10	73
Tenia solium	..	1	1	0	1	0	0	3	5

0 represents very low prevalence of helminths and no reports of high prevalence.
.. Focal records, low prevalence.
Note: Estimates of morbidity ae generally unavailable for helminthiases. Estimates from Walsh (1984) suggest the following number of clinical cases of schistosomiasis: S. mansoni, 3.3 million; S. hematobium, 4.9 million; S. japonicum, 4.7 million; S. intercalatum, 0.6 million; S. mekongi, 30,000. There are an estimated 336,400 cases of blindness from onchocheriasis (WHO 1987).
Source: The data for geohelminths, lymphatic filariasis, and schistosomiasis are derived from a survey of the original literature. Data on onchocerciasis are from WHO 1987. All other estimates are based on secondary sources (Stoll 1947; Le Riche 1967; Peters 1978; WHO 1981, 1984, 1987; Warren and Mahmoud 1984).

mortality. Carefully conducted studies, however, have shown a relationship between infection intensity and clinical effects.

The geohelminths are the most ubiquitous of the major human helminthiases. *Ascaris lumbricoides* and the slightly less prevalent *Trichuris trichiura* occur worldwide in almost any community which is socioeconomically depressed. The distribution is limited by extremes of temperature and humidity but extends well beyond the tropics into northern and southern temperate zones (Crompton 1989). Current estimates by the World Health Organization (WHO) are 1,000 million *Ascaris* and 750 million *Trichuris* infections. Although these estimates of infection in table 7-2 are probably low, diseases or morbidity are also believed to be significantly underestimated (Pawlowski and Davis 1989; Bundy and Cooper 1989), largely because the chronic effects on growth and development in children are grossly underreported. In one study of trichuriasis, for example, only 2 percent of actual cases were represented in health statistics (Cooper, Bundy, and Henry 1986). Such underreporting may have led to the commonly quoted misconception that trichuriasis is of public health significance only in restricted regions, a perception that has been refuted by the accumulation of evidence of morbidity from a broad range of tropical locations. The estimate that 10 percent of all infec-

tions are sufficiently intense to affect growth and development, although not necessarily to cause overt clinical signs, suggests that more than 100 million people may suffer some morbidity from geohelminthic infections alone.

The two important hookworm species *Ancylostoma duodenale* and *Necator americanus* together have a circumequatorial distribution. Still, this is more restricted than that of the other geohelminths, and the hookworms are less commonly found outside the true tropics. The World Health Organization estimates that there are currently 900 million infections. The main morbidity is associated with anemia, involving both adults and children (Migasena and Gilles 1987; Schad and Warren 1989).

The pinworm, *Enterobius vermicularis*, still occurs commonly in temperate regions, where it is the most prevalent helminthiasis. It is now recognized that this worm is also common in tropical regions, although its true prevalence is unknown, largely because diagnosis of infection requires a technique, anal swabbing, which is not often employed in mass surveys. Infection is rarely associated with significant morbidity.

The filarial nematodes are almost exclusively tropical, and only *Wuchereria bancrofti* has a global distribution. *Brugia malayi* is confined to Asia, where the infection occurs in the

Malaysian peninsula, some areas of the Philippines, and Indonesia, as well as in foci in India and China (CIBA Foundation 1987). The World Health Organization estimates that there are currently 90 million infections, almost half of which (40 million) occur in India. The estimates in table 7-2 are significantly higher, even if the data for China (see caveat above) are excluded. Morbidity refers mainly to adult disablement due to elephantiasis. The number of cases afflicted by the less obvious, but functionally disabling, effects of episodic filarial fever is unknown.

Onchocerca volvulus is focal in West and Central Africa, in northern South America, and in Central America. It is the subject of major control efforts in West Africa. Although the condition is rarely fatal, it is severely disabling, because the main morbid consequence is blindness.

The guinea worm, *Dracunculus medinensis*, occurs in limited foci in arid habitats in India, Pakistan, and (currently) seventeen countries of Sub-Saharan Africa. This infection may be declining as a result of control efforts. It is estimated by WHO that there are currently 10 million cases globally, all of which are potentially disabling and have an attendant risk of severe morbidity due to secondary infection.

Strongyloides stercoralis occurs circumglobally in tropical and subtropical areas but is also of importance in the temperate regions because of the persistence of chronic relapsing infection in cases acquired elsewhere and because of endemic infection in specific foci (particularly, institutions). The true prevalence is unknown because of the difficulty in diagnosing subclinical infection. The actual morbidity is also unknown but is likely to be considerable, because most of the reported infections represent clinical cases (Grove 1989).

Trichinella spiralis is primarily an infection of temperate regions and is one of the few human nematodiases which is declining in prevalence, primarily because of improved food hygiene. Infection may be associated with severe morbidity.

Of the schistosomes, only *Schistosoma mansoni* has spread into the Americas, where the infection is endemic in large tracts of Brazil and in limited foci in Venezuela and the Caribbean islands. *S. mansoni* also remains endemic in much of West and East Africa, overlapping throughout most of this area with *S. hematobium*, which has a range extending further to the northeast and southwest. The distribution of both parasites encompasses the limited foci of *S. intercalatum* in Central and West Africa. *S. japonicum* predominantly occurs in China, the Philippines, and Indonesia. There may also be small foci in Malaysia, Thailand, Laos, and Cambodia, where there is overlap with the distribution of *S. mekongi*. The distribution has recently been described in detail (WHO 1987a), and it is estimated that there are currently 200 million cases. The clinical consequences of the various forms of schistosomiasis are well established and may be associated with significant morbidity (WHO 1985; Mott 1988), although precisely defining the extent of the morbidity has proven problematical (Morrow 1984). The estimates in table 7-2 are based on those of Walsh and Warren (1984), which some consider an overestimate.

Other digenean parasites of human health importance are *Clonorchis sinensis*, *Fasciolopsis buski*, and *Paragonimus westermani*. These are confined largely to Asia, where they may be associated with significant disease (Rim 1986).

Tenia saginata infection is endemic in pastoral communities in Africa, in urban communities in the area that was formerly Eastern Europe, and in both in Latin America. Epizootics occur in North America. The clinical effects are mild. In contrast, *T. solium* infection is much less common, is more closely associated with socioeconomically depressed communities, and may result in severe neurological symptoms. The prevalence of this disease may be underestimated, because the foci in Latin America are now recognized to be larger than had been assumed.

The fish tapeworm, *Diphyllobothrium latum*, is characteristic of northern temperate regions. Control measures have achieved significant declines in prevalence.

Echinococcus granulosus infection occurs wherever there are suitable domestic animal hosts, and it therefore has a global distribution which includes both tropical and temperate regions. Global prevalence data are unavailable, but human infection is associated with severe, sometimes fatal, clinical effects.

Consequences of Helminthic Infections

Helminthic infections may produce a range of diverse consequences: from impairment of the growth and development of children, to reducing the functioning of schoolchildren in educational institutions, and even their ability to attend school; from very low levels of impairment of the day-to-day function of adults to significant inhibition of productivity; from mild to severe acute morbidity (for example, anemia) to death (from, for example, intestinal obstruction); and from severe chronic disability (for example, blindness and elephantiasis) to death (from, for example, bleeding esophageal varices). As to mortality per se, only schistosomiasis generates a substantial burden (Walsh 1990); even that burden, however, is but a fraction of deaths in the developing world due to diarrheal disease, acute respiratory infections, and measles. The principal public health significance of the helminthiases resides, then, not in their effect on mortality but, rather, in their consequences of impaired growth and development in children, chronic disability, and long-term impairment of function. These consequences, combined with the extremely high prevalence of many helminthic infections, suggest aggregate outcomes for these conditions that are very substantial from the standpoint of both economic productivity and general welfare.

Our purpose in this section is to point out the available literature on the effect of helminthiases on disability, malnutrition, and functional impairment. For a few of the topics to be reviewed there is substantial literature, sometimes with useful and up-to-date reviews—for example, the reviews by Stephenson (1987) and Holland (1987a, 1987b) of the effect of helminths on nutrition and the review by Andreano and

Helminiak (1988) of, among other things, the effect of schistosomiasis on labor productivity. By and large, however, the literature is more notable for its gaps than its well-defined conclusions. For that reason this summary will draw more than we would like on anecdotal and clinical accounts, on plausible inferences, and on reports of associations that are potentially confounded by a range of extraneous variables. This "soft" literature is importantly suggestive; it in no way replaces but rather underlines the need for harder research in the future. Before turning to that literature, however, we provide brief descriptions of the nature of the infections and the associated morbidity and mortality.

ACUTE MORBIDITY AND MORTALITY. The major helminthic parasites of humans enter the body in a variety of ways: orally, by direct penetration of the skin, and by injection by biting insects (table 7-3). The invading organisms may undergo a variety of metamorphoses while in the body and may migrate through multiple organ systems to reach their preferred sites (table 7-3). The metamorphoses and migration routes provide insight into the ways by which these parasites cause disease and into the localization of signs and symptoms. It must also be borne in mind that in many parts of the developing world, people, particularly children, harbor multiple parasitic worms simultaneously. Thus, on the east coast of Kenya, children will frequently carry Ascaris, Trichuris, hookworm (the geohelminths), schistosomes, filariae, and the beef

Table 7-3. Migration Pathways of Helminths in Humans

Organism	Pathway
Nematodes	
Ancylostoma (Necator)	Skin–lungs–small intestines
Ascaris	Mouth–intestines–lungs–small intestine
Dracunculus	Mouth–intestines–subcutaneous tissues
Onchocerca	Insect bite–connective tissues–skin and eyes
Strongyloides	Skin–lungs–small intestine
Trichinella	Mouth–small intestine musculature
Trichuris	Mouth–large intestine
Wuchereria (Brugia)	Insect bite–lymph nodes–blood
Trematodes	
Clonorchis (Opisthorchis)	Mouth–intestines–bile ducts
Fasciola	Mouth–intestines–liver–bile ducts
Fasciolopsis	Mouth–small intestine
Paragonimus	Mouth–small intestine–lung and brain
Schistosoma hematobium	Skin–lungs–vesical venules (bladder/ureters)
Schistosoma japonicum, S. mansoni	Skin–lungs–mesenteric venules (liver)
Cestodes	
Diphyllobothrium	Mouth–small intestine
Echinococcus	Mouth–small intestine–liver and lungs
Tenia saginata	Mouth–small intestine
Tenia solium	Mouth–small intestine

Source: Authors.

tapeworm. In western Africa, onchocerciasis and dracunculiasis may be added. In the northeast of Thailand, children will carry all the geohelminths, Opisthorchis, and perhaps Fasciolopsis. Colombians will harbor, in addition to the geohelminths, Onchocerca, the pork tapeworm with its attendant danger of cysticercosis and, possibly, Fasciola. Inuit children will often carry Trichinella, Diphyllobothrium, and Echinococcus. All the above individuals may also have enterobiasis and strongyloidiasis.

As previously observed, most helminths do not multiply in the human definitive host, and intensity of infection may vary from minimal numbers of worms to hundreds and, at times, thousands. Disease manifestations are closely related to intensity of infection; those with low worm burdens essentially have no signs or symptoms of infection.

When worm larvae penetrate through the skin or migrate within it they may cause a pruritic rash which can be quite severe (hookworm, Strongyloides, schistosomes). On oral ingestion and larval penetration into the bowel wall there may be transient intestinal symptoms (Ascaris, Trichinella, Fasciola, Paragonimus). During migration through the tissues eosinophilia will often occur (hookworm, Ascaris, Trichinella, filariae, Strongyloides, Fasciola, schistosomes). Migration through the lungs can lead to a transient pneumonitis (hookworm, Strongyloides, Ascaris).

The final site of the adult worms, however, plays the most important role in the development of most of the disease syndromes. These will now be described for each of the helminths found in table 7-1.

Nematodes

- A. duodenale, N. americanus. These organisms are attached to the mucosa of the small intestines and ingest 0.03–0.26 milliliters of blood per worm per day. The main manifestations of disease are iron-deficiency anemia and hypoalbuminemia. In heavy infections symptoms include fatigability, headache, numbness and tingling, dyspnea, palpitations, anorexia, dyspepsia, pedal edema, and sexual dysfunction. Signs include pallor and tachycardia.

- Ascaris. These large roundworms are free in the small intestines, and heavy worm burdens are associated with malnutrition, growth deficits, and impaired physical fitness. Masses of intertwined worms may cause intestinal obstruction, and single worms may obstruct the bile duct.

- Dracunculus. The long (30-centimeter), thin worms form burrows in the subcutaneous tissues, largely of the legs. When they reach maturity a blister occurs which bursts to release vast numbers of larvae. This is accompanied by itching and intense pain. Secondary bacterial infection of the worm tract is common.

- Enterobius. The main symptom of the presence of the worms in the perianal area is pruritis.

- Onchocerca. The adult worms are found in nodules in skin, muscles, and joint tissues. Larvae released from the female adults migrate in the skin, where they may cause severe pruritic dermatitis. Larval migration within the ocular tissues may result in keratitis and chorioretinitis, leading to blindness and often, therefore, to premature death.

• *Strongyloides.* Although these organisms reside in the small bowel, they may revert to infectious forms, penetrating the skin to initiate an autoinfectious cycle. Intestinal symptoms include epigastric pain and diarrhea. Skin manifestations include urticaria and a pruritic, papular, erythematous rash. The disseminated form of infection, often seen in immunocompromised hosts, may result in fatalities.

• *Trichinella.* During acute infection diarrhea may be present. Manifestations from the invasion of muscle include fever, periorbital edema, and myalgia.

• *Trichuris.* There are two manifestations; in heavy infections there is anemia, prolapse of the rectum, and chronic colitis; in more moderate infections the colitis is associated with growth stunting.

• *Wuchereria, Brugia.* Acute inflammatory reactions, including lymphangitis or lymphadenitis, funiculitis, epidi-

dymitis, and orchitis, may occur, accompanied by headache, backache, and nausea. In chronic infections there may be hydrocoeles and elephantiasis.

Trematodes

• *Clonorchis, Opisthorchis.* Manifestations due to bile duct obstruction include fever, abdominal pain, and jaundice.

• *Fasciola.* Acute manifestations include fever, abdominal pain, hepatomegaly, asthenia, and urticaria. Manifestations of bile duct obstruction are very rare.

• *Fasciolopsis.* In heavy infections abdominal pain, diarrhea, and facial edema may be present.

• *Paragonimus.* Cough and hemoptysis may be found, as well as chest pain and profuse expectoration. Cerebral involvement may be accompanied by epilepsy, and signs of space-occupying lesions.

• *Schistosoma.* In *S. hematobium* infections there may be hematuria, dysuria, and renal failure plus an increased risk of cancer of the bladder. In *S. japonicum* and *S. mansoni*

Table 7-4. *Disability and Nutritional Consequences of Helminth Infections*

Infection	Disability	Malnutrition	
		PEM *and growth retardation*	Anemia
Nematodes			
Hookworm	n.a.	Little effect on macronutrient absorption except, possibly, some protein loss[a]	Major consequence of hookworm infection
Ascaris	n.a.	Growth faltering, reversible by intervention. Mechanisms may include protein loss and lactose malabsorption[a]	n.a.
Dracunculus	Mobility constraints for up to thirty weeks	n.a.	n.a.
Onchocerca	Blindness; severe sustained itching	n.a.	n.a.
Strongyloides	n.a.	Suggestive studies point to growth retardation and, possibly, protein deficiency	n.a.
Trichuris	Persistent colitis in some cases	Can cause substantial (but reversible) growth retardation[a]	Probably important in heavy infections
Lymphatic filaria	Severe mobility constraints and discomfort from elephantiasis	n.a.	n.a.
Trematodes			
Schistosomes	Decreased work capacity in heavy infections	Growth faltering due to S. hematobium and S. japonicum; mechanisms may include protein loss and altered endocrine function	Some evidence that S. hematobium causes anemia; anecdotal accounts also implicate S. mansoni and S. japonicum
Cestodes			
Tenia solium	Long-term mental impairment, sometimes involving epilepsy, from neural cysticercosis	n.a.	n.a.

n.a. Not applicable.

a. Studies with broad-spectrum chemoprophylaxis for hookworm, *Ascaris,* and *Trichuris* infections have revealed marked increments in growth.

Source: Cooper and Bundy 1986, 1987, and 1988; Cooper and others 1989; Crompton 1986; El Karim and others 1980; Holland 1987a; Holland 1987b; McGarvey and others 1990; Smith and others 1989; Stephenson 1987; Stephenson and others 1989; Tanner and others 1987.

infections there may be hepatomegaly, splenomegaly, bleeding esophageal varices, and cor pulmonale.

Cestodes

• *Diphyllobothrium.* Diarrhea occasionally occurs. In cases where the worm is situated high in the small bowel, vitamin B$_{12}$ deficiency with a macrocytic anemia may be found.

• *Tenia saginata.* Passage of motile proglottids through the anus may be felt.

• *Tenia solium.* There are few symptoms from the adult form in the intestines. Larval cysticercosis can result in epilepsy, raised intracranial pressure, and psychotic change.

• *Echinococcus granulosus.* Large, space-occupying lesions may develop primarily in the liver, resulting in hepatomegaly, or in the lungs, leading to hemoptysis.

DISABILITY AND MALNUTRITION. Malnutrition may be an important accompaniment of the specific manifestations of parasitism by many of the helminths, particularly when there are multiple infections of relatively high intensity. The worms of the small bowel may impair digestion and absorption. Loss of nutrients may occur as a result of inflammation and toxic secretions, and the systemic consequences of infection such as fever may increase the catabolic rate. There may be a deficit of specific nutrients such as vitamins (B$_{12}$) and minerals (iron) as well as protein and calories. It must be remembered that children are also exposed to a wide variety of bacterial, viral,

and protozoan infections. Thus, the status of the individual is the outcome of all these infectious and nutritional forces. If virtually all the chronic helminthic infections could be eliminated as significant pathogenic factors, child health in the developing world would show clear improvement. Available findings of the literature on the chronic medical consequences of helminthiases—disability, developmental retardation, and malnutrition—are summarized in table 7-4.

The conditions resulting in serious disability—onchocerciasis, lymphatic filariasis, schistosomiasis, and cysticercosis—tend to be geographically focal. Nonetheless these conditions are of massive importance to the individuals affected and to communities of high endemicity. Given the control technologies to be discussed later in this chapter, the benefit-cost calculus in focal regions is likely to prompt the conclusion that control efforts are of very high priority.

The two main nutritional consequences of helminthiases are growth faltering and anemia, although other micronutrient deficiencies have been noted. Stephenson (1987, pp. 9–10) traces three channels that lead from infection to growth faltering—anorexia, nutrient losses through malabsorption, and decreased nutrient use because of impaired liver and spleen function. Whatever the mechanisms, a large and growing literature now provides some documentation of substantial growth impairment from the geohelminths and schistosomiasis. Figure 7-1 provides a dramatic illustration of both the magnitude of growth faltering which can result from moderate infection (in this case with *Trichuris*) and of its reversibility

Figure 7-1. *Growth Following Treatment for Trichuris Infection*

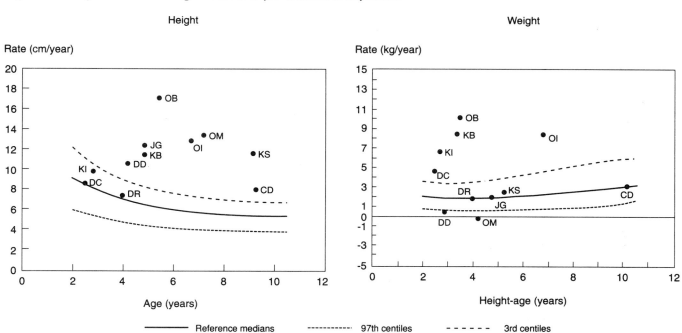

Note: Values for each child are shown (initials are for individual children). The reference medians and 97th and 3rd centiles are from the Tanner-Whitehouse data (sexes combined). The ages are shown at the mid-point of the interval over which average velocity was measured. Use of height-age rather than chronologic age standardizes for that component of weight increment attributable to increasing stature. A comparison between the chronologic age and the height-age of each child indicates the extent of initial stunting.
Source: Cooper and others 1989.

after anthelmintic treatment. The initialed points in the figure show the growth velocities for children four to eight months after worm expulsion, in relation to growth velocity norms (solid line) and the ninety-seventh percentile (upper dotted line). These effects are indeed dramatic, given that the children were returned to their previous (unhealthy) environment.

In chapter 18 of this collection, Pinstrup-Andersen and others discuss in detail the general causes and consequences of growth faltering and protein-energy malnutrition (PEM). Two further points are, however, worth noting here. First, the functional consequences of PEM are substantial in many domains (for example, mortality risk and mental development), making the nutritional consequences of helminthic infection an important concern. Second, although the attributable risk for growth faltering cannot, with available data, be divided among insufficiency of nutrient intake, viral and bacterial infection, and helminthic infection, it does increasingly appear that a significant proportion of attributable risk results from helminthiases.

The other main nutritional concern is anemia, the main functional significance of which is discussed at length in chapter 19 of this collection. Anemia, too, results from highly prevalent helminths. Levin (1988) has shown that control of anemia through dietary measures or supplementation can have very high ratios of benefits to cost; similar or better results would obtain from helminth control strategies in communities in which helminthic infections are important cofactors for anemia. It should be noted, however, that control of helminths is not a substitute for iron supplementation, because hemoglobin levels improve much more rapidly if iron is provided with an anthelmintic.

FUNCTIONAL CONSEQUENCES OF HELMINTH INFECTIONS. There are two main functional consequences of economic significance—reduced efficiency of education in imparting the general intellectual skills that are of far-reaching significance for economic development, and reduced productivity of labor (and, to a lesser extent, land) (World Bank 1980). Hayashi (1980); Rosenfield, Galladay, and Davidson (1984); and Andreano and Helminiak (1988) provide valuable discussion of the mechanisms of these effects. In table 7-5 we summarize available findings. With respect to both productivity and schooling the literature is weak—not only in the number and scope of states, but also in the (probably) systematic way in which the studies undertaken and the sampling procedures that were used were likely to underestimate effects (Andreano and Helminiak 1988; Prescott 1989; for education, see Pollitt and others 1989). No solid studies of determinants of school attendance were found, although an early literature in Japanese on the effect of helminthiases on school attendance does exist (Morishita 1980). Stephenson (1987, p. 87) provides a bibliography of relevant literature from Africa. It is also likely that adverse effects of infection on learning have been biased downward by failure to sample those not in school.

The magnitude of the documented functional consequences of the helminthiases is substantial. But the available literature probably underestimates effects and certainly fails to consider a broad range of significant conditions and environments.

Table 7-5. *Functional Consequences of Helminth Infections*

| | Productivity Loss | | Educational Impairment | |
Infection	Labor	Land	Reduced school attendance	Impaired learning
Nematodes				
Hookworm	Improved physical fitness after treatment	n.a.	Plausible effect	Definite effects, probably because of anemia
Ascaris	n.a.	n.a.	Plausible effect because of malnutrition	n.a.
Dracunculus	Substantial	n.a.	Elevated absenteeism and dropout rates reported among infected children	n.a.
Onchocerca	Important effects because of blindness	Important though often overstated effects	n.a.	n.a.
Trichuris	n.a.	n.a.	Plausible effect	Definite effects
Lymphatic filaria	Plausible effect	n.a.	n.a.	n.a.
Trematodes				
Schistosomes	Heavy infection clearly implicated	Retarded investment in land productivity because of concern for schistosomiasis and irrigation projects	n.a.	Probably important only in heavy infections

n.a. Not applicable.
Source: Andreano and Helminiak 1988; Edungbola and others 1988; El Karim and others 1980; Evans 1989; Ilegbodu and others 1986; Kvalsvig 1988; Pollitt 1989; Prescott 1989; Seim 1990; Stephenson and others 1990.

These functional consequences almost entirely are borne by the poor. What the available evidence does strongly suggest is that, as an investment in the improved productivity of the poor, control of helminthic infections has high priority.

Strategies for Control of Helminthic Infections

In this section we consider the range of practical techniques and strategies which are available for the control of helminthic infections, and we briefly examine their relative effectiveness and practicality (table 7-6). In a technical assessment of this type it is necessary to treat the procedures separately, although in practice a multidimensional strategy of control may be employed. Furthermore, it is inevitable that discussion of procedures will focus on practical interventions rather than their method of implementation; in practice the method of implementation, in particular its community acceptability, affordability, and sustainability, may prove more critical to

success in controlling infection than the intervention employed. The relative merits and costs of different strategies of implementation are discussed later.

Vector Control

The control of the snails that are the intermediate hosts of schistosomes and other trematodes traditionally has contributed to overall control measures. Three main strategies have been employed: chemical (molluscicides), environmental (removal of snail habitats), and biological (the use of natural predators or competitors). Although the latter two methods have a significant contributory role in control, molluscicides have been the most extensively used in practical control programs. Recent developments (the availability of safe drugs, rising environmental concerns, and the escalating costs of the only commercially available chemical molluscicide) have, however, tended to reduce the emphasis on this form of control

Table 7-6. *Primary Preventive Strategies for Helminth Infection*

Parasite	Immunization	Chemoprophylaxis	Hygiene	Vector control	Health education
Nematodes					
Ascaris Trichuris	Inadequately studied	Albendaxole; ivermectin	Sanitation	n.a.	Personal hygiene; latrine building; geophagia
Hookworm Strongyloides	No immediate prospects	Albendazole; ivermectin	Sanitation	n.a.	Personal hygiene; latrine building; soil contact
Enterobius	Inadequately studied	Albendazole; ivermectin	Perianal washing; clean bed linen	n.a.	Personal hygiene; family treatment; family transmission
Dracunuculus	Inadequately studied	none	Clean drinking water	Filter drinking water	Water source; water contact
Onchocerca	No immediate prospects	Ivermectin	n.a.	Larvicide	Vector avoidance; early treatment
Wuchereria/Brugia	No immediate prospects	Ivermectin	Mosquito nets; repellents	Larvicide; kill adults; bed nets; environmental changes	Early treatment; environment modification
Trematodes					
Clonorchis, Fasciola Fasciolopsis, Opisthorchis Pargonimus	Inadequately studied	Praziquantel	Sanitation	Molluscicide; environmental changes	Food preparation; latrine building
Schistosomes	No immediate prospects	Praziquantel	Sanitation	Molluscicide; environmental changes	Latrine building; water contact; water source
Cestodes					
Tenia	Inadequately studied	Praziquantel	Sanitation; meat inspection	n.a.	Food preparation; latrine building; livestock management; personal hygiene
Echinococcus	Inadequately studied	Albendazole	Meat inspection	n.a.	Food preparation; dog and livestock management
Diphylobothrium	Inadequately studied	Praziquantel	n.a.	n.a.	Food preparation

n.a. Not applicable.
Source: Authors.

(Cook 1987). Still, there may be an increasing role for naturally occurring molluscicides, because they can be produced locally, are affordable, and typically are biodegradable (Lemma 1987).

Control of the other significant trematode infections of humans is now largely focused on treatment (Rim 1986), combined with improvements in sanitation. The countries in Asia have found that the control of intermediate host snails in natural habitats or in aquacultural enclosures is not practically feasible or culturally acceptable. Cultural resistance has also inhibited the dietary modification required to prevent transmission by way of the second intermediate hosts.

Control of the lymphatic filarial infections has also traditionally depended upon vector control, in this case through the use of insecticides and larvicides and, perhaps most sustainably, through the environmental reduction of breeding sites. The main drug in current use (diethylcarbamazine) has proved to be of limited effectiveness as a control tool (Sasa 1977), although it has some effect on low-level transmission of *Brugia malayi* (Partono, Purnomo and Soewarta 1979; Partono 1985). The introduction of ivermectin may dramatically change the choice of control approach.

The control of onchocerciasis has also been dominated by strategies based on vectors, although it now appears that control of morbidity may be possible through use of the newly assessed drug ivermectin. The Onchocerciasis Control Programme in the Volta River basin is the largest example of a vector-control program for a helminthic infection. This program was initiated in 1975 in an area of 654,000 square kilometers and because of reinvasion of vectors from surrounding regions was expanded in 1978 to include another 110,000 square kilometers. Control is based on aerial spraying of the larvicide temefos on a seven-day cycle, which is possible only because of the large size of the vector-breeding habitats. The program is scheduled to run for at least twenty years, because of the longevity of the adult parasite, and has already achieved some success in disease and infection reduction. There are great concerns, however, about the development of resistance to the larvicide. It is also unclear whether the expense involved would permit the application of this method in other endemic areas.

Assessments of the cost-effectiveness of the Onchocerciasis Control Programme have been undertaken—initially by Prost and Prescott (1984) and, subsequently, by Evans and Murray (1987), who modified the parameter estimates of Prost and Prescott. We would conclude from these studies that the vector-control strategy of dealing with onchocerciasis might cost in the range of $100 to $500 per year of healthy life gained, considering only gains from reduction in blindness and discounting future benefits at about 3 percent.

Dracunculiasis has also proved susceptible to local eradication by control of the vector. The simple and economic procedure of filtering drinking water through cloth to remove the crustacean intermediate host has proved to be a culturally acceptable and effective method of control in many endemic areas, and it is the method of choice for controlling this helminthiasis until enclosed water supplies are available. Provision of such water supplies, combined with health education, has been shown capable of eradicating the disease within three years (Edungbola and others 1988, Paul, Isley, and Ginsberg 1986). Assuming that the cost of providing safe water is about $8 per capita per annum, that infection prevalence is reduced from 30 percent to negligible, that individuals are 50 percent disabled while infected, and that communities would be prepared to pay half of the cost of water supplies if there were no Guinea worm, it is estimated that provision of water costs about $25 per healthy life-year gained. Obviously variation in costs and prevalence will very much affect this estimate, but, very clearly, intervention is likely to be highly cost-effective in a broad range of conditions.

Because of the relatively limited geographical scope of dracunculiasis and the high effectiveness combined with low cost of control measures, it (along with poliomyelitis) has been judged eradicable by the International Task Force for Disease Eradication. African ministers of health have set 1995 as the target date for eradication from that continent. Hopkins and Ruiz-Tiben (1990) review these goals and the activities now under way for attaining them.

Improving Hygienic Facilities and Behavior

It is self-evident that the sanitary disposal of feces will break the life cycle of many helminths and prevent transmission. It is also true that the safe disposal of human waste will provide a significant measure of protection from a wide range of other human pathogens. Feachem and others (1983a) reviewed eight major studies of community-wide sanitation improvement and in seven cases there was evidence of a reduction in enteric helminth transmission. This does not mean, however, that merely providing a dwelling with a latrine will result in improvements in the health status of the household. In communities where only some of the dwellings have sanitation facilities there is rarely any correlation between the enteric helminthic infection status of a particular household and the presence of a latrine (Otto and others 1931). In some cases households with latrines actually have higher rates of infection than those that do not (Feachem and others 1983b), particularly if the latrine is poorly maintained. Sanitation programs have to be community-wide if they are to achieve full benefit.

Community-wide sanitational improvement is not without its problems, however. A study in Indonesia showed that the provision of latrines made no difference to local levels of soil contamination with geohelminth eggs, because children persisted in promiscuous defecation (Ismid and Rukmono 1980). Reduction in environmental contamination demands not merely the provision of latrines but also their use (Feachem and others 1983b). In Iran, it is claimed that the provision of latrines actually increased the incidence of enteric helminthic infection, since it made human excreta more readily available as a fertilizer for domestic vegetable gardens (Arfaa 1986). Clearly the implementation of sanitation programs demands parallel programs of health education and particularly careful attention to sociocultural acceptability (Kilama 1989).

In addition to these sociological problems there may be significant practical difficulties. Rural-urban migration has resulted in the development of unsanitary slums and shanty towns around and within the cities of the developing world (Harpham and others 1987). In Malaysia, where 36 percent of the total population live in such impermanent settlements, it has been shown that slum-dwelling children have very high rates of enteric helminthic infection (Bundy and others 1988a) and that these rates are much higher than those recorded for children living in the rural areas from which the children came (Kan and others 1989). Provision of even low-cost sanitation for such slum areas is compromised by practical limitations on space, the absence of community organization, and sociolegal constraints on land tenure (Harpham and others 1987).

The beneficial effects of improvements in sanitation may take a considerable period to become apparent. Pawlowski (1984) cites the example of Lombardy in Italy, where the prevalence of trichuriasis in schoolchildren took twenty-five years to decline from 65 percent to 5 percent. A reduction in parasitic infection as a result of sanitational improvement alone is likely to take decades before a significant change is apparent.

Sanitation offers the advantage over other control measures of providing a long-term solution. It has the disadvantage of requiring a large initial capital investment—although the actual cost varies a great deal, depending on the system selected (Cairncross and Feachem 1983)—and a recurrent cost for maintenance.

Improvement in sanitation is a desirable goal and should be a component of enteric helminth control. Because of cost and sociocultural constraints, however, such improvement is likely to be slow and capital-intensive to implement, and it is likely to take decades before significant reductions in infection levels are achieved. Upgrading of sanitation may be best perceived, therefore, as a means of consolidating the more immediate benefits of chemotherapy and as a program best developed as one part of an integrated strategy.

Vaccination

No vaccines against the helminthic infections of humans are currently available. Vaccine development is, however, the goal of a considerable body of current research, particularly research into schistosomiasis, and it is therefore worthwhile, considering the potential benefits which might derive from the availability of an effective vaccine. It is relevant to note that a vaccine has been developed to protect dogs from hookworm (Miller 1978) and that modern molecular and immunological strategies may accelerate the availability of vaccines against human helminths.

The effect of vaccination is to increase the size of the immune and uninfected class in an endemic population. The aim of vaccination, in population terms, is to reduce the basic reproductive rate, R_o, of the parasite population below unity in value (Anderson 1982; Anderson and May 1982). To achieve this, the proportion p of the population which must be effectively immunized (assuming that im-munized individuals do not contribute to transmission) at any one time is given by:

$$(1) \qquad p = 1 - (1/R_o)$$

The available evidence suggests, however, that the acquired protection is unlikely to be life-long, in which case the approximate criterion is:

$$(2) \qquad p = [1 - (1/R_o)] \, v^{-1},$$

where v is the period of vaccine-induced protection in years. This modification has important consequences. For example, if the vaccine provides life-long protection against a helminth such as hookworm or *Ascaris* (R_o approximately 3), the community could be protected by a single program of 67 percent vaccination in infancy. If protection lasts for only two years, then approximately 40 percent of the population would have to be vaccinated every year to achieve adequate community protection (Anderson and May 1985). Unfortunately it seems likely that such repetitive programs would be required, because the available evidence indicates that natural infection affords humans little protection against reinfection (Wakelin 1978; Bundy and others 1987).

These analyses suggest that a program to control human helminthiasis by vaccination would be logistically similar to a chemotherapeutic program in that both would require repeated intervention. The relative merits of the two strategies would therefore depend on the cost both of vaccines as compared with drugs and of delivery of vaccination as compared with delivery of treatment.

It is also relevant to note that vaccines which provide partial protection (that is, reduce the intensity of infection) may provide a significant measure of morbidity control when used against helminthic infections.

Chemotherapy

Advances in anthelmintic chemotherapy during the past twenty-five years have constituted the most important factor in the reformulation of strategies of disease control, in which emphasis is placed more on reduction and minimization of human morbidity and less on the concept of total eradication of infection (Davis 1986).

Some forty anthelmintics are available for use in human and veterinary medicine. Almost all of them originated from the classical screening mechanisms employed by industry. It is to be hoped that advances in biochemical, molecular, genetic, and parasitological technology will lead to a more rapid progression in "designer drugs" than has been the case to date.

For the treatment of helminthic infections in human beings, an impressive list of compounds exists. A recent review of selected drugs in frequent use against nematode infections at the community level included the benzimidazole carbamates, albendazole and mebendazole (with cyclobendazole or flubendazole as alternatives), levamisole, pyrantel, and the traditional piperazine salts (Davis 1985). Recent evidence suggests that ivermectin, the well-known macrocyclic lactone microfilaricide used in large-scale chemotherapy of onchocerciasis, is promising in use against the human intestinal nematodes (Naquira and others 1989). In worldwide use, these drugs are effective, in varying degrees, against *Ascaris lumbricoides*, the hookworms *Ancylostoma duodenale* and *Necator americanus*, *Trichuris trichiura*, *Strongyloides stercoralis*, and *Enterobius vermicularis*. Infection with multiple parasites is the general rule and thus anthelmintics possessing a broad spectrum of activity will invariably command a favored place in the strategy and tactics of chemotherapeutic control.

In infections other than those caused by the geohelminths, all of which are nematodes, praziquantel is the drug of choice in all forms of schistosomiasis, other snail-borne human trematode infections, and the common cestode infections, *Tenia solium*, *T. saginata*, *Diphyllobothrium latum*, and *Hymenolepis nana*. Ivermectin has some efficacy against the filarial nematodes, as well as several of the geohelminths, especially *Strongyloides*.

In any consideration of intervention programs against helminths it is essential to distinguish clearly between the meanings of the words "control" and "eradication." A control program is the implementation of specific measures to limit the incidence of an infection (Gemmell, Lawson, and Roberts 1986). It is taken for granted that any successes will produce, in parallel, a reduction in human morbidity and mortality from the conditions in question. In contrast, eradication implies the reduction of the incidence of a specific infection to the point of continued absence of transmission within a specific area through a time-limited campaign (Yekutiel 1980).

It is clear that for the immediate future and perhaps even for decades, emphasis in the control of intestinal helminthic infections in humans will be placed on the reduction of human morbidity and mortality implemented through population-based chemotherapy. Population-based chemotherapy is implemented in one of two main ways: through mass chemotherapy or through screening (often called selective) chemotherapy.

Mass chemotherapy is the treatment of a total population whether infected or not. Because it is rarely practicable to examine everyone in a population except in small or moderate-size villages or in school surveys, mass chemotherapy as a control tactic is usually applied after sampling procedures have revealed the levels of infection. Where prevalence or intensity of infection is high, or where there is clear evidence of associated morbidity or mortality, mass chemotherapy is a perfectly feasible tactic for morbidity control because the modern anthelmintic drugs are highly effective, their toxicity to humans is many orders of magnitude less than the compounds used even as recently as the 1950s and 1960s, and population acceptance is good. Furthermore, it may be wasteful of scarce and finite human, financial, and technical resources to continue sample examination programs when the epidemiological data indicate high prevalence and intensity of infection. This strategy is attractive to public health officials as the organization and implementation is easily managed by good planning.

Identifying which prevalence levels are sufficiently high to justify mass intervention is based on little more than intuition at present. Further broad-based research is urgently required to provide usable guidelines. One large question concerns the point at which the risks (apparently very small) associated with treating uninfected individuals exceed the benefits of treating those who are actually infected. Analogous considerations have been made in developing policy for vaccination strategies, where it is now generally held that the risks associated with vaccination are sufficiently low to justify vaccinating uninfected individuals even when the probability of infection is minimal. Similar analyses of anthelmintic risks and benefits may indicate that mass chemotherapy is appropriate and acceptable down to prevalence levels so low that intervention is unjustifiable on economic and health grounds.

The alternative strategy is screening chemotherapy: the treatment only of infected members of a population, where infection is demonstrated by standard diagnostic procedures (for example, Kato examination for geohelminths and enteric schistosomes; nucleopore filtration or hematuria for *S. hematobium*).

In certain situations, a combination of methods may constitute the most effective strategy: after mass chemotherapy has lowered prevalence and intensity rates, then screening chemotherapy could be used to treat those individuals exhibiting residual infection on follow-up examination. Such a strategy will, however, result in considerable additional cost (discussed later).

Chemoprophylaxis as a Primary Strategy

The terms "chemotherapy" and "chemoprophylaxis" refer to the resolution or prevention of disease and have no specific implications for infection. Drugs used in the prophylaxis of chronic, noninfectious disease (for example, antihypertensives) reduce the symptoms but do not solve the underlying problem. Chemoprophylaxis with chloroquine against chronic *Plasmodium vivax* infection also has the primary aim of avoiding disease, and only when so-called causal prophylactics such as primaquine are used is the infection removed. In an analogous manner, anthelmintic methods of reducing parasitic infection may be seen as aiming to avoid helminthic disease even though infection may persist.

Strategies of controlling parasitic infections within communities of people, as opposed to individual patients, have changed surprisingly little in the last sixty years. The control stratagems developed during the 1920s—principally as a result of the Rockefeller Foundation Hookworm Campaign (Cort 1922; Smillie 1924; Chandler 1925)—remain a dominant influence on the practical design of control programs.

In one sense this is a tribute to the earlier work. In another sense, however, it perhaps indicates a reluctance to apply new concepts, developed over the past few decades, to the practical problems of community-wide control. Considerable advances have been achieved in the development of safe and more effective anthelmintics and in the development of a global infrastructure for health delivery, but these advances have had relatively little effect on the prevalence of helminthic infection. In the almost four decades since Dr. Norman Stoll (1947) estimated that there were more helminth infections than people, the situation remains almost unchanged (Walsh and Warren 1979).

This situation undoubtedly reflects a complex of logistic constraints, ranging from lack of resources to lack of political will. It also indicates, however, a lack of appreciation of how to apply our rapidly improving understanding of the treatment of individuals to the development of programs for the treatment of communities (Walsh and Warren 1979).

A community strategy clearly depends on a thorough and detailed understanding of the population dynamics of the parasites of humans and an understanding of how an intervention in one component of the complex life cycle of a parasite might influence the overall pattern of transmission (Anderson 1988). Such understanding depends on precise assessment of the biological determinants of observed infection patterns (Warren 1973) and the development of a rigorous theoretical framework to describe the complexity of the multidimensional processes involved (Anderson and May 1985). The last decade has seen considerable development in both these areas, largely because population-based field study and the mathematical description of population dynamics have developed as a synergistic partnership. This linkage is perhaps best exemplified by age-group targeting, a strategy which was developed as a theoretical concept from mathematical analyses (Anderson and May 1982, 1985; Anderson and Medley 1985) developed from precise field studies (Croll and others 1982; Bundy and others 1985; Elkins, Haswell-Elkins, and Anderson 1986) and translated into successful, large-scale community control programs (Bundy and others 1989; Cabrera and others 1989).

The application of population dynamics to parasite epidemiology has shifted the focus of chemotherapy from the individual to the community. The principal area of progress has been in estimating the control effort (in treatment frequency, effectiveness, and coverage) required to achieve a given reduction in transmission (Anderson 1989; Anderson, May, and Gupta 1989). This permits the identification of chemotherapeutic regimens which are optimal, in dose minimization, both temporally and quantitatively, for controlling a specified level of parasite endemicity. Such an approach cannot alone define the overall strategy—there remains a major requirement to set these options within a context of broader logistic issues, particularly economic—but it can provide the decisionmaker with a range of quantitative estimates upon which strategic choices can be based.

Pharmacology

Although consideration of the pharmacology of a drug is essential whenever treatment or prophylaxis is considered, it is especially important when two or even three drugs may be used simultaneously. In attempting to control a broad range of parasitic infections concurrently it may be necessary to administer two or three medications to the same individual. In this section we examine these issues and briefly summarize what is known about the structure and modes of action of three of the most important anthelmintics.

BENZIMIDAZOLES. The first benzimidazole introduced commercially was thiabendazole. It proved to be an effective larvicide, and thus was useful in *Trichuris*, *Trichinella*, and *Strongyloides* infections (Prichard 1970). For the latter infection, thiabendazole proved to be 75 percent effective. The benzimidazoles continue to enjoy worldwide application in veterinary parasitology.

Mebendazole (Vermox) has had wide acceptance in clinical chemotherapy, and of late, albendazole (ABZ, Zentel) appears to be emerging as a compound of choice for treating nematodes in humans. It is of interest to note that the alkyl sulfide side chain of albendazole ($-S-CH_2-CH_2-CH_3$) favors the chemical reactivity of this sulfide *in vitro*. Thus, rapid sulfoxidation can occur *in vivo*. It is thought that this metabolite is the active moiety of this anthelmintic. However, the introduction of a bulky aromatic sulfide, as in mebendazole, fenbendazole, or oxfendazole, decreases the rate by which the sulfur is oxidized, and the metabolites of these later drugs appear more slowly.

It is widely accepted that the mode of action of the benzimidazoles is selective interference with polymerization of worm tubulin (Borges and others 1975). The observed inhibition of glucose uptake or of enzyme excretion is believed to be a secondary consequence. This view is strengthened by the finding that classical tubulin disrupters (colchicine and podophyllotoxin) can also inhibit fumarate reductase, as well as uptake of glucose in benzimidazole-susceptible *Haemonchus contortus* worms.

Interference with orderly cell development is nicely illustrated in parasites through the inhibition of *in vitro* egg hatches. It is interesting to note that drug concentrations which inhibit tubulin polymerization by 50 percent are about the same as those which inhibit 50 percent egg hatches in susceptible nematodes. This relationship has proved to be fairly constant for all the benzimidazoles described above.

PRAZIQUANTEL. Praziquantel is a polycyclic, mostly saturated, flat, planar compound, generically classed as a piperazinone-isoquinoline. The compound is chemically unique, quite unlike any other anthelmintic.

The most important effects of PZQ on trematodes or cestodes are the following, as described mainly in studies of *S. mansoni* or *S. japonicum*. Within less than thirty seconds after exposure to 10^{-7} molar PZQ, worms begin to contract, apparently as a result of a sudden tegumental leakiness, allowing the ingress of calcium ions. The muscles of the worms go into tetanus, they lose control of sucker action, and from their position in the mesenteric veins are swept into the liver. At low concentrations ($<10^{-7}$ M) the resultant inflooding of calcium also activates carbohydrate use through the second messenger-serotonin system.

Within minutes after exposure to PZQ, the surface of the worm, previously held in equilibrium, begins to undergo dramatic disintegration. This process has been called vacuolation, or "blebbing." The contraction of the worm is probably reversible and by itself might not be fatal to schistosomes. The tegumental damage, however, exposes heretofore inaccessible antigenic sites. These sites attract phagocytes and granulocytes, which release proteolytic enzymes and invade the worms. The worms are entrapped and encapsulated by fibroblasts and then totally destroyed. Whereas other antischistosomal drugs, such as hycanthone or oxamniquine, induce tegumental shredding and disruption, PZQ induces widespread surface changes within minutes and under conditions in which the host is not affected.

IVERMECTIN. Ivermectin (IVM) is a semisynthetic macrocyclic lactone which was first described about ten years ago (Albers-Schoenberg and others 1981). The basic substance is a fungal fermentation product derived from the coil-like actinomycete *Streptomyces avermitilis*, which was first isolated from a soil sample from a Japanese golf course. Ivermectin is derived from a chemical group of congeners, the avermectins (AVRs).

As potential bacteriocidal or antifungal agents, the avermectin compounds found no real chemotherapeutic application, but, in the early eighties (Mrozik and others 1982a), powerful anthelmintic properties were demonstrated. Many chemical alterations of the basic structure have been examined (Fisher and Mrozik 1989) in the course of pharmacological investigation of the AVR compounds, and IVM has been found to be the most active moiety against mammalian parasites.

Although IVM was initially believed to block the neurotransmitter gamma-aminobutyric acid (GABA) (Campbell and others 1983), a recent review (Turner and Schaeffer 1989) has postulated that in target organisms IVM may bind to specific high-affinity (of the order of 10^{-10} to 10^{-12}) sites. As the result of IVM binding, an increased permeability to chloride ions follows, and affected nerves are depolarized. The authors add that GABA-mediated chlorine channels may also react with IVM but at generally higher concentrations of the drug (about 10^{-7} M).

IVM can induce a variety of pharmacological responses which are influenced by many factors, such as variation in the GABA system (Soderlund, Adams, and Bloomquist 1987), drug penetration into membranes, and solubility in the test system. For instance, in *Ascaris suum*, IVM injection causes rapid paralysis, which is neither flaccid nor rigid (Kass and others 1980; Kass, Stretton, and Wang 1984). In the free-living nematode *Caenorhabditis elegans*, IVM induces rigid paralysis. Thus, specific worms react quite distinctly to this drug. In consequence, laboratory studies which employ traditional nerve-muscle preparations may not reliably describe what happens in those parasites which affect humans.

From field and laboratory studies it is known that IVM profoundly affects microfilariae, including those that are still developing in the female. The result is that normal larvation is halted, as dead or defective microfilariae accumulate in the uterus. The effect of the drug is quite stage-specific, involving early ("stretched") microfilariae in the distal uterus, and not the more mature coiled types (Albiez and others 1988; Lok, Harpaz, and Knight 1988). Peripheral migrating microfilariae, when observed in the anterior chamber of the human eye, showed "abnormal and reduced winding and coiling" (Sobaslay and others 1987). In patients that have been treated with the drug, progressively fewer microfilariae are recovered in skin snips. In one study, three days after therapy microfilariae were reduced to 14 percent of control numbers. Microfilariae that emerged from skin snips of treated patients, however, did not appear to be immobilized by IVM (Mossinger and others 1988).

The microfilaricidal effect of a single treatment is very persistent. A reduction of dermal microfilaria density both reduces skin pruritis and temporarily blocks transmission to the vector fly (Cupp and others 1989). Likewise, corneal and limbic invasion by microfilariae is decreased or halted. Dadzie and others (1987), Newland and others (1988), and Taylor and others (1989) all reported that annual treatment was very helpful for patients with light to severe onchocercal eye disease.

The disadvantage of IVM is that single-dose therapy regimens do not destroy adult filarial worms. Female *Onchocerca volvulus* (Greene, Brown, and Taylor 1989), *Loa*, and the oligo-pathologic agent *Mansonella perstans* (Richard-Lenoble and others 1988) as well as *Wuchereria bancrofti* (Kumaraswami and others 1988) all resume larvation within months after exposure to IVM. In the species mentioned above, the drug causes significant and long-term reduction in circulating microfilariae. Therefore, most recent reviews conclude that IVM is superior to, and safer to use than, diethylcarbamazine, a drug which has been used for half a century in the treatment of filariasis (Albiez and others 1988; Kumaraswami and others 1988; Ottesen and others 1990). Whether the combination of IVM with a benzimidazole (such as albendazole) will increase the filaricidal potential remains as yet undetermined.

Activity of IVM against intestinal nematodes is striking. According to recent field reports (Nalin and others 1987; Naquira and others 1989) a single or double dose of IVM will remove 100 percent of *Ascaris lumbricoides*, and 70 to 85 percent of *Strongyloides stercoralis*, *Enterobius vermicularis*, and *Trichuris trichiura*. Patients with hookworms achieved some benefit, since egg production was decreased by approximately 60 percent. A dosage of 200 micrograms per kilogram of IVM, however, resulted in only about 20 percent long-term cure at three months.

DRUG METABOLISM AND TOXICITY. Albendazole is poorly absorbed (less than 5 percent) by the gastrointestinal tract, which is appropriate because most nematodes that ABZ removes are enteric. Of the fraction of ABZ that is absorbed, essentially 100 percent is metabolized in the liver, yielding an albendazole sulfoxide. This metabolite may be the active moiety of the drug. The parent compound, ABZ, cannot be detected in the serum. The peak concentration is reached in about 2 hours, and the plasma half-life is about 8.5 hours. Hydroxylation and hydrolysis products of albendazole-sulfoxide have been found in the urine.

Praziquantel is extensively metabolized after oral administration, apparently in first-pass liver oxidation. Most (60 to 80 percent) of the hydroxylated PZQ products are excreted in the urine, as well as a small residue by way of the bile and feces. It has a very short half-life of 1 to 1.5 hours.

Ivermectin, when its pharmacokinetics were followed in humans, showed a rather complex excretion pattern. Its half-life, and that of the metabolites, is about 12 hours, and includes an enterohepatic recycling pathway. Only 1 percent of the metabolites are found in the urine; most of the excretion is by way of the bile. The degradation products may be fatty-acid ester conjugates, as well as the aglycon, that is, the basic structure stripped of the two oleandroses. Some IVM may be stored in body fat, and released slowly; this might explain why microfilaricide activity persists for months after medication.

In general these three drugs are not toxic to humans when administered as single-dosage agents. Those side effects which have been cataloged are restricted to what one might consider to be "mild" reactions. They tend to be symptoms of vertigo, nausea, or other gastrointestinal distress, evanescent skin pruritis, and orthostatic hypotension. Although such reactions are disturbing, they are not life-threatening.

Although the toxicity and side effects of the new broad-spectrum anthelmintics are rare enough and mild enough for their use in mass chemoprophylaxis, it is likely that these untoward reactions can be substantially reduced without compromising the goal of disease control. Recommended drug dosages are usually a compromise between the highest cure rates possible and the maximal acceptable level of side effects. Because cure, or as the pharmacologists put it, a 100 percent lethal dosage, is unnecessary in the context of helminth disease control, it is theoretically possible to reduce markedly the drug dosages and their attendant side effects while also decreasing intensity of infection below disease-producing levels.

Several dosage-ranging studies have been performed with antischistosomal drugs. Investigators in Saint Lucia (Cook, Jordan, and Armitage 1976) and Kenya (Warren and others 1978) examined the effects on prevalence, the intensity, and the side effects of a relatively toxic intramuscular drug, hycanthone, in patients with S. *mansoni* infections. In Saint Lucia it was observed that a reduction of the recommended dosage (3 milligrams per kilogram of body weight) to half that amount (1.5 milligrams per kilogram) reduced vomiting from 51 percent to 3 percent. In Kenya there was no vomiting at dosages of 1.5 milligrams per kilogram of body weight or lower. The total egg output was reduced by approximately 98 percent with both dosages in Saint Lucia and 96 percent with the lower dosage in Kenya. In the Saint Lucia study reductions in hepatomegaly and splenomegaly were similar at both dosages. Recently, Polderman, Gryseels, and DeCaluwe (1988), in studies of schistosomiasis mansoni in Zaire, found no difference in cure rate or egg

output with dosages of praziquantel of 40 and 30 milligrams per kilogram of body weight. King and others (1989), studying the treatment in Kenya of schistosomiasis hematobia with praziquantel at 40, 30 and 20 milligrams per kilogram showed a difference in cure rate ranging from 85 to 58 percent but no significant difference in reduction of egg counts (which ranged from 99.6 to 97.6 percent) and no difference in the marked decrease in morbidity as evinced by hematuria and proteinuria. Taylor, Murure, and Manomano (1988) in Zimbabwe showed similar results with praziquantel for both S. *mansoni* and S. *hematobium*. It should be noted that the original dosage recommended for albendazole was 200 milligrams per kilogram of body weight, or half the amount presently in use.

POTENTIAL USE OF THESE DRUGS IN MASS CHEMOTHERAPY. Because a substantial proportion of infections may involve more than one parasite species, there is often a need to treat the infection concomitantly with albendazole, ivermectin, and praziquantel. This raises the question of the effectiveness and safety of multiple treatment, particularly if it forms part of a community program. Note that these concerns are least severe for concomitant therapy that makes use of existing well-characterized anthelmintics. Combination of the anthelmintics into a single tablet, which might offer advantages in the logistics of delivery, would represent a new formulation and require extensive reassessment of toxicity.

A crucial aspect of the problem of anthelmintic therapy with multiple drugs is the issue of cross-interference or cross-reactivity. Because these agents have not been administered simultaneously to patients under controlled conditions, one can only speculate about the result. Fortunately, it seems that each of these three drugs acts at different biochemical points which do not overlap.

Therefore, an optimistic view is that these three broad-spectrum anthelmintics will be found to be mutually chemotolerant. Extensive clinical experience reveals limited toxicity and predominantly mild side effects for each of these compounds. When these drugs are taken together, will the side effects increase? Pilot trials are urgently needed before mass campaigns requiring two or three of the drugs are undertaken. In many areas, however, only one or two drugs will be necessary.

THE PROBLEM OF INDUCTION OF DRUG RESISTANCE. It has been suggested that in treatment of helminths one need not be concerned about the induction of drug resistance. In bacterial infections, the organisms have a short life span and a rapid rate of multiplication within the host. Thus, if bacteria are exposed to antibiotic drugs, they frequently undergo genetic selection which allows succeeding generations to circumvent the metabolic lesions caused by the antibiotics. When less-than-optimal concentrations of drugs are administered, succeeding generations with increasingly greater resistance are selected.

It has been asserted that this is less probable with most helminths, which have a much longer residence time in humans, and which, in any case, do not multiply within the host. But is the conclusion, that worms are unlikely to develop resistance, justified? Experience with both benzimidazoles and with ivermectin suggests that although the initial (P1) generation might be highly susceptible, succeeding generations (F1 through F20) can become less sensitive or altogether refractory to these drugs (Behm and Bryant 1985).

The phenomenon of resistance to the benzimidazoles has been most carefully studied in the veterinary field. Numerous strongyloid worms of domestic livestock have been found to be resistant to a spectrum of benzimidazoles (Lacey 1986). In fact, the development of resistance to thiabendazole was the basic reason for the introduction of other members of the benzimidazole series.

In assessing long-term effectiveness of IVM, Egerton, Suhayda, and Eary (1988) have reported decreasing sensitivity of *Haemonchus contortus* to the drug after only four generations of worms were exposed to drug concentrations designed to eliminate 95 percent of the parasites. By the seventh generation, a substantial increase of IVM was required to continue elimination of 95 percent of the worms. The induced resistance appeared to be stable through many generations.

Clearly, there are reasons to think that development of resistance to the drugs contemplated for mass chemotherapy will eventually occur. The onset of resistance is related to the dosage used for each treatment: adequate drug amounts with high killing indexes delay the onset of resistance.

In making a decision on the dosage recommended for a field campaign, answers to the following questions must be addressed:

- How important is it to treat patients under conditions in which side effects are either absent or extremely tolerable?
- How necessary is it to reduce the total amount of medication in order to control the cost of mass chemotherapy?
- How tolerable might it be to reduce the worm burden, while leaving a few viable (and egg-producing) worms behind? Could the surviving worms eventually produce a strain of offspring which are resistant to the chosen medication?

On an optimistic note, one may find that the combination of albendazole and ivermectin is particularly desirable in the sense that these two anthelmintics may potentiate each other. The combined use of levamisole and a benzimidazole against veterinary nematodes has an established history in veterinary practice. There is also evidence that mebendazole is useful in the treatment of onchocerciasis in cattle. Thus, combining ABZ and IVM might significantly reinforce a weak action of the latter on filaria, as well as on hookworms.

The Potential for a Multiple-Species Strategy

The traditional approach to developing a parasite control program has been to plan a specific strategy focused on a single parasite species. Although this has the advantage of simplicity, it ignores the reality that parasites have broadly overlapping geographical distributions and that multiple infection in the same individual is much more common than single infection. It also ignores the practical reality that a drug delivery system developed for one anthelmintic can readily deliver others (or even other agents such as vitamin A) for little additional cost. In this section we collate secondary data on the global distribution of geohelminthic, schistosomal, and filarial nematode infections in an attempt to identify which combinations occur most commonly in which geographical areas. The focus is on developing countries, and the analyses exclude North America, Europe, anglophone Australasia, and the former U.S.S.R.

The geographical distributions described in table 7-2 inevitably result in considerable areas of overlap. Because of the ubiquity of the geohelminthiases these can be perceived, to a large extent, as a broad background of geohelminthic infection on which are imposed areas of additional infection with the schistosomes, the filarial nematodes, and other helminths. This results in a complex distribution of multiple infections, involving three species of geohelminth, four species of schistosome, and three species of filarial nematode in more than fifteen different combinations.

Developing a chemotherapeutic intervention strategy for this complex of multiple infections, however, is considerably simplified by the availability of broad-spectrum anthelmintics. Single drugs are now available for treating all the most important geohelminthic infections (albendazole or mebendazole), all the schistosomes, all the significant digeneans, and all the main cestodes (praziquantel); and recent studies suggest that ivermectin is effective against the primary filarial nematode infections and *Strongyloides*.

The broad spectrum of activity of the available anthelmintics reduces to five the number of drug regimens required to treat the whole complex of multiple infections. In terms of global area, the largest requirements are for albendazole alone (in Central and South America, North Africa, and South Asia), or with praziquantel and ivermectin (in the north and east of South America, most of Sub-Saharan Africa, and in Southeast Asia). This is also the situation in terms of population density, as can be seen in table 7-7, although the relative importance of the parasites (and hence the drug regimens) varies regionally: in Central and South America, geohelminthiasis alone is the dominant infection except in Brazil; in Africa, geohelminthiasis is typically combined with both filariasis and schistosomiasis; and in Asia, no one combination is dominant. Table 7-7, however, does not take into consideration other predominantly Asian trematode infections such as *Opisthorchis*, *Clonorchis*, *Fasciolopsis*, and *Paragonimus*.

Further analyses of these data allow some estimates to be made of the proportion of the population requiring a particular anthelmintic. Table 7-8 indicates that the requirement for a drug against geohelminthiases is likely to be twice as great as for those against schistosomiasis or filariasis. This is a natural consequence of the ubiquity of geohelminthic infection; many

Table 7-7. Estimated Total Population in Areas Endemic for Various Combinations of Helminthiases
(millions)

Predominant helminthiasis	Central and South America	Africa	Asia	Total
Geohelminthiasis	210	128	801	1,139
Geohelminthiasis and filariasis	53	205	500	758
Geohelminthiasis, filariasis, and schistosomiasis	99	296	755	1,150
Geohelminthiasis and schistosomiasis	28	133	311	472
Schistosomiasis	0	44	0	44

Note: Total population does not necessarily reflect number of people infected or at known risk.
Source: Authors.

of those requiring treatment for gastrointestinal nematodes are likely to have concurrent infection with schistosomes or filarial nematodes, but not vice versa.

It should be stressed that these are crude estimates based on the total population of the endemic area and do not represent the population infected or the population at a known level of risk (calculation of these statistics was beyond the scope of the present study). The actual quantities of anthelmintics required will depend on data on the prevalence and intensity of the various infections in a particular area.

These studies suggest that control of multispecies helminthic infection will require specific combinations of anthelmintics. In the following section we consider how an understanding of the population dynamics of these infections can provide guidelines for developing control strategy.

Frequency of Treatment, Coverage, and Dosage

In the development of community-based programs for the control of helminthic infections, a sound understanding of epidemiological patterns forms a template for the use of scientific methods to calculate the intensity and frequency of anthelmintic treatment required to block transmission (community-wide) or to prevent morbidity (Anderson and May 1985). Ideally, a variety of types of information is required to assess epidemiological patterns and processes: age-stratified profiles of prevalence and intensity of infection; the distribu-

Table 7-8. Requirement for Anthelmintics Based on Proportion of Population Living in Areas Endemic for Various Combinations of Helminthiasis
(percentage)

Anthelmintic	Central and South America	Africa	Asia
Albendazole	58	44	50
Praziquantel	23	29	27
Ivermectin	19	27	23

Source: Authors.

tion of worm loads per person within an age class; and longitudinal (that is, through time) changes in intensity and prevalence following anthelmintic treatment (rates of reinfection). For the main helminths of humans, such information is available (although variable in quality) for many regions in developing countries. In this section we summarize the central features of the dynamics of helminth populations as they concern the control of helminthic infection.

Helminths are invariably aggregated in their distribution within human communities (or age or sex groups) such that most people harbor few worms and a few harbor many. It is typically the case, irrespective of helminth species, that more than 70 percent of the total population of worms are harbored by less than 30 percent of the human community. In addition, wormy people (who are more likely to show clinical symptoms and who are the primary contributors to morbidity statistics) are more frequently children than adults (Bundy and others 1988c).

Many recent studies of reinfection in individual patients following anthelmintic treatment show that those heavily infected prior to treatment tend, on average, to acquire heavy infection following a period of reinfection. Predisposition to heavy or light infection has been demonstrated for many geohelminth, schistosome, and filarial nematode species. The underlying mechanisms that generate predisposition are poorly understood at present, but some combination of behavioral, social, nutritional, and genetic factors is the likely cause.

In many rural and urban communities in developing countries, where social and economic conditions have changed little in many decades, changes in the prevalence and intensity of infection with age reflect changes through time. In other words, the rate of acquisition of infection (or exposure) as individuals age reflects the intensity of transmission in a defined area: the greater the transmission, the more rapidly infection prevalence and intensity rises with age. For helminthic infections, the intensity (usually measured indirectly by fecal egg counts) is a better reflection of this rate of transmission. Because of the highly aggregated distributions of worm numbers per person, large changes in mean worm burden may be accompanied by small changes in prevalence (Anderson 1982). As such, intensity is a much more sensitive indicator of both the rate of transmission and the effect of any given control program.

Typical age-intensity patterns for helminths in human communities are convex in form. Intensity usually rises from zero at birth to a peak in child, teenage, or adult age classes, depending on the intensity of transmission. In the case of some filarial infections, and perhaps hookworm, the intensity tends to plateau, without exhibiting a convex hump. Convex patterns with age may reflect age-dependent changes in exposure to infection or the slow build up of acquired resistance. In practice both are probably important, because behavioral studies of the acquisition of schistosomes and geohelminths point to the importance of behavior (Bundy and Blumenthal 1989), whereas the observation that increasing degrees of convexity in the age-intensity profile correlate positively with the intensity of transmission suggests a role for acquired immunity (Anderson 1987). Some typical profiles for various species of helminths are recorded in figure 7-2.

Following anthelmintic treatment, people in areas in which transmission is not interrupted reacquire worms at a rate dependent on the net force or intensity of transmission. The rate of reacquisition depends on the species of helminth (and its biological and life-cycle characteristics) as well as the intensity

of transmission within a given community. In table 7-9 we summarize typical return times to preinfection intensities of infection in areas of endemic infection with moderate to intense levels of transmission.

The implication of this trend for reinfection is that chemotherapy must be applied repeatedly to ensure low levels of infection and hence morbidity. If treatment is frequent enough, then transmission can in principle be blocked and the parasite

Figure 7-2. *Age Intensity Profiles for Common Helminthiases*

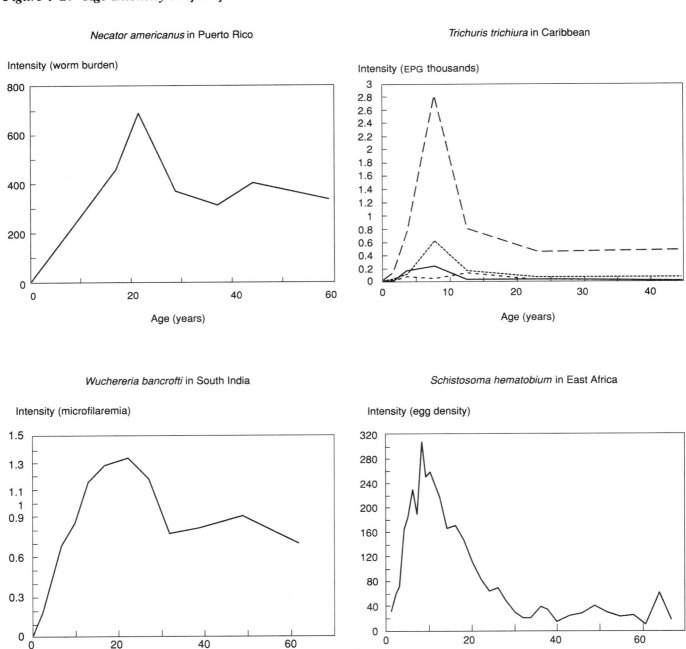

Source: (Left to right, top to bottom) Hill 1926; Bundy 1986; Rajagopalan and others 1989; Bradley and McCullough 1974.

Table 7-9. Time to Return to Pretreatment Levels of Infection after Anthelmintic Therapy, in Areas of Moderate to Intense Transmission, and the Life Expectancy in the Human Host

(years)

Parasite	Return time	Life expectancy
Trichuris trichiura	<1	<1
Enterobius vermicularis	1	<1
Ascaris lumbricoides	<1	1
Ancylostoma duodenale	2–3	2–3
Necator americanus	2–3	2–3
Schistosoma mansoni	3–5	3–5
Schistosoma hematobium	3–5	3–5
Schistosoma japonicum	3–5	3–5
Onchocerca volvulus	>5	>8
Wuchereria bancrofti	>5	>5

Source: Authors.

eradicated. In practice, however, spatial factors often result in reinvasion from neighboring areas where control effort is less effective.

Return times to pretreatment infection levels are inversely correlated with the life expectancy of the parasite in the human host (Anderson 1986; Anderson and May 1985; Bundy and others 1988b). If life expectancy is short, the return time is fast, and *vice versa.* Current estimates (often very crude and approximate) of the life expectancy of some important human helminths are given in table 7-9.

The intrinsic properties of a parasite to reproduce and transmit from host to host may be measured by reference to its basic reproductive rate, R_0. This quantity defines the average number of female worms (for a diecious species) produced by one female throughout her reproductive life span that themselves gain entry to a host and survive to reproductive maturity in a susceptible human population. Clearly if R_0 is less than one the parasite will not persist endemically in the human community. This constraint sets the target for control programs—the intensity of control (whether by chemotherapy or other methods) should aim to reduce reproductive success to less than unity in value (on average). If R_0 is greater than one the parasite will persist. The magnitude of R_0 for a given parasite

Table 7-10. Estimated Basic Reproductive Rate (R_0)

Parasite	R_0	Location	Source
Ascaris lumbricoides	4–5	Iran	Croll and others 1982
Necator americanus	2–3	India	Anderson 1980
Trichuris trichiura	4–6	St. Lucia	Bundy and Cooper 1989
Schistosoma mansoni	1–2	Egypt	Hairston 1965
Schistosoma hematobium	2–3	Egypt	Hairston 1965
Schistosoma japonicum	1–4	Philippines	Barbour 1982
Onchocerca volvulus	>9	Côte d'Ivoire	Dietz 1982

Source: See last column.

in a defined human community can be crudely measured by reference to the rapidity with which the average intensity of infection rises in infants and children as they age. The faster the rise, the higher the value of R_0 for that parasitic species, in a given situation. Some rough estimates of R_0 for various parasites in various settings are listed in table 7-10.

To block transmission of any given parasite effectively, the frequency of treatment required will depend not only on the ecological characteristics of the species (for example, life expectancy) but also on the intensity of transmission in that endemic locality (the magnitude of R_0). In order to generalize about the frequency of treatment it is necessary to assume a standard pattern for the transmission of a set of parasites (the species composition in a defined area or region). In what follows we assume that, prior to control, transmission was at moderate to intense levels.

Recent analytical work on the transmission dynamics of helminth parasites in human communities has led to the derivation of a "control criterion" of a fairly general character, which defines the frequency (in units of time) and the coverage (the proportion of the community treated during each intervention cycle) of treatment ideally required to reduce transmission, community-wide, to very low or negligible levels. This level of control should be significantly greater than that required to reduce morbidity. For an anthelmintic drug of effectiveness h, whose effectiveness defines the proportion of an individual's worm load killed by a single or a short course of treatment (for most drugs $h > 0.9$), the proportion of a human community, p, that must be treated per unit of time (for example, year or month) to block transmission is given approximately by the relationship

$$(3) \qquad p > \{1 - \exp{[(1 - R_0)/L]}\} / h$$

Here R_0 is the basic reproductive rate and L is parasite life expectancy in the human host (Anderson 1986). If effectiveness is less than 100 percent (that is, $h < 1$) and R_0 large, then it is possible that the value of p will be greater than one. In these cases the units of the life expectancy term, L, must be reduced (that is, years to months) such that the proportion to be treated is calculated on a more frequent cycle (shorter time interval).

In general, if we use the values of R_0 and L listed in table 7-11, for a drug that is 95 percent effective ($h = 0.95$) we can provide some rough guidelines on the coverage and frequency of treatment for the main helminths in areas of moderate to high transmission intensity. These guidelines are summarized in table 7-11.

In assessing the information presented in this table it must be noted that the parameter estimates (of R_0 and L) are rather crude at present. As a consequence of this, the estimates of frequency and coverage are very approximate and should only be viewed as rough guidelines.

The data in table 7-11 indicate that when considering single (or short course) treatment for multiple infections the interval between treatments will depend on the precise mix of parasite

Table 7-11. Estimated Ideal Coverage and Frequency of Drug Treatment to Reduce Parasite Transmission to Very Low Levels

Parasite	R_o[a]	L (years)[b]	Coverage (percent)	Frequency of treatment (years)
Trichuris trichiura	5	1	80–90	0.5–1
Ascaris lumbricoides	5	1	80–90	0.5–1
Necator americanus	2.5	2.5	70–80	2
Ancylostoma duodenale	2.5	2.5	70–80	2
Schistosoma mansoni	2	4	70–80	4
Schistosoma hematobium	2	4	70–80	4
Onchocerca volvulus	10	8	70–80	1
Wuchereria bancrofti	10	8	70–80	1

a. Basic reproductive rate.
b. Parasite life-expectancy.
Source: Authors.

species. In areas where filarial worms or geohelminths predominate, an ideal frequency is every year. For geohelminths, this interval might be slightly lengthened if treatment is targeted at schoolchildren, since this age group tends to be heavily infected. For hookworms the ideal interval is two years, whereas for schistosomes it is roughly four years.

These theoretical intervals are longer than those that are commonly applied in practice. There are two main reasons for this. First, current estimates of frequency are often based on time taken for prevalence, rather than intensity, to rebound to pretreatment levels. Because intensity is more closely correlated with transmission (and morbidity), it is the slow rebound in intensity which should more appropriately determine the frequency of treatment. Second, current estimates of the frequency of intervention are usually based on the rate of reinfection observed after the treatment of a few individuals living in an area of otherwise uncontrolled transmission. Reinfection rates under these conditions will be much higher than if the population were treated as part of a community-wide control program, thus giving a misleading impression of the frequency of treatment required. Examples of situations under which community-wide treatment results in slow rates of reinfection with schistosomiasis are described by Wilkins (1989).

In all cases, the coverage of treatment should be high: typically, 70 to 90 percent of the target community. In areas of high-intensity transmission, the intervals between treatments should be shorter and the population coverage greater, whereas in areas of low transmission, lower frequencies and coverage would be appropriate.

These preliminary analyses suggest two important conclusions of relevance to the development of a strategy of helminth control. First, they indicate that recent advances in anthelmintic development have made multispecies control of the main helminthiases a plausible option. Theoretically, the broad spectra of modern anthelmintics should permit the treatment of a complex range of infections using only five combinations of three anthelmintics. More precise estimation of the logistic implications of this strategy—in particular, finely stratified data on the global prevalence and intensity of infection—should be possible from existing data sources, but further studies are necessary to determine the effectiveness and pharmacodynamic properties of these drugs when used concomitantly.

Second, the analyses suggest that recent advances in the theory of population dynamics permit the estimation of "optimal" chemotherapeutic interventions (in frequency and coverage of treatment) for a given parasite species in a given locality. These estimates currently lack precision because of the absence of adequate data, but they may serve as broad guidelines for the development of control strategy. Further work is required to improve procedures for parameter estimation (particularly R_o), and to collect appropriate data for the range of parasite species in different epidemiological situations. These conclusions suggest that the study of parasite population dynamics and epidemiology has an important, and increasing, role to play in the development of policies of parasite control.

Cost and Effectiveness of Screening and Targeting

Many options are available for the delivery of chemotherapy to the community. Both economic and epidemiological factors determine which is the most cost-effective method in a given situation (Prescott 1987; Prescott and Bundy 1989: Prescott and Jancloes 1984). At the broadest level, there is an obvious choice between the treatment of children only (targeted chemotherapy) and the treatment of the whole population, including adults (population chemotherapy). For each of these options there is a choice between the treatment of all individuals, irrespective of infection status (mass chemotherapy), and the treatment of individuals shown to be infected after diagnostic testing (screening chemotherapy). In the latter case, treatment can be given to all infected persons (prevalence screening) or only to those individuals with "heavy" infections (intensity screening) (terminology adapted from WHO 1985). Each of these six different options (table 7-12) is associated with different costs and different levels of effectiveness, defined as reduction in prevalence, intensity, morbidity, or some other variable. Effectiveness should ideally also be defined per unit of time: because reinfection invariably occurs after treatment, the effective reduction in prevalence, intensity, and morbidity can be defined only for a particular observation or intervention period.

In this section we present an analysis of the cost-effectiveness of the alternatives outlined above in a standard population with defined epidemiological, economic, and behavioral parameters. The analyses are essentially static because, at this stage, they do not reflect parasite population responses to the various interventions. The more complex problem of dynamic economic analysis, taking account of differing reinfection patterns, is a subject for future research.

Table 7-12. Chemotherapeutic Strategies for Control of Helminthiasis

Targeted population	No screening		Screening for infection		Screening for intensity of infection	
	Population treated	*Control strategy*	*Population treated*	*Control strategy*	*Population treated*	*Control strategy*
None	All children and adults	Population mass (PM)	All infected children and adults	Population screening for prevalence (PSP)	All heavily infected children and adults	Population screening for intensity (PSI)
Children	All children	Targeted mass (TM)	All infected children	Targeted screening for prevalence (TSP)	All heavily infected children	Targeted screening intensity (TSI)

Source: Authors.

THE BASE CASE. Using representative data, we have simulated the costs and effectiveness of the chemotherapy options for a standardized population in the scenario for the base case shown in figure 7-3. The simulations model a chemotherapy program implemented for two years with six-month treatment cycles. Total costs per capita for the entire two-year program are estimated from unit cost data derived from an actual control program (Bundy and others 1989; Terry, Bundy, and Horton 1989). Because costs vary between countries, these data should be interpreted as comparative rather than absolute. Note that per capita costs refer to the cost of the entire program (two years) per person in the population ($N = 1$ million) whether or not infected. Effectiveness is measured by the proportion of total heavy infections (adults plus children) treated, assuming the epidemiological and behavioral parameter values summarized in table 7-13.

In considering effectiveness only, without regard to budget constraints, the main result in the base case is that the mass chemotherapy strategies are much more effective than any of the screening options. Population mass chemotherapy emerges as the best option, treating 94 percent of heavily infected cases, compared with 80 percent for targeted mass chemotherapy. By contrast the screening options are only about 60 percent effective. This result reflects the importance of compliance behavior: the effectiveness of mass interventions is modified only by compliance with treatment, whereas the effectiveness of screening-based interventions is also modified by compliance with the diagnostic screening test. Because screening compliance rates are typically much lower than treatment compliance, especially for adults, any screening approach must inevitably treat fewer infected individuals.

In the presence of a budget constraint, the screening options are not only less effective but also more costly than the mass chemotherapy alternatives. At lower budget levels, targeted mass chemotherapy is both more effective and less costly than targeted screening for prevalence. At higher budget levels, the more effective population mass chemotherapy becomes affordable and always dominates the more costly screening variants. This cost disadvantage of screening options occurs because the slightly lower treatment costs achieved by only treating infected cases are offset by the very high costs of the screening itself. This disadvantage is most acute with the screening for

intensity options, which are more costly than the equally effective screening for prevalence options. They have the highest screening costs because of lower technician productivity in assessing specimens for the intensity instead of the mere presence of infection, which implies higher technician and related cost requirements.

In examining the economic factors here and elsewhere in this collection, two standardized populations are considered: one has a low mortality rate and is at an intermediate level of development, and the other has high mortality and birth rates. These demographic differences influence only the overall costs of the various chemotherapy options, the populations with low mortality and low birth rate attracting lower costs because there are proportionately fewer children. The relative position of the different treatment options is unaffected, and the comments in this section apply equally to both types of population.

Increasing prevalence of infection does not change the main results illustrated by the base case. Figure 7-3 also shows the effect of increasing prevalence to 100 percent in both children and adults. The mass chemotherapy options continue to dominate both on effectiveness and on cost-effectiveness criteria. The only consequence of higher prevalence is to lower the effectiveness and raise the cost of all the screening options. In the targeted case this results from the smaller share of children in the total number of heavy infections. The graph in figure 7-3 showing 100 percent infection prevalence reflects the low screening compliance of adults who, in this scenario, have a larger share of the total heavy infections. Thus higher prevalence tends to make mass chemotherapy more attractive.

When screening compliance is raised from the low levels assumed in the base case to the hypothetical maximum of 100 percent both for adults and children, the screening options achieve the same effectiveness as the corresponding mass chemotherapy alternatives. The costs of screening also rise, however, because of the higher volume of postscreening treatment activity. As revealed in the graph showing 100 percent screening compliance in figure 7-3, the implications for optimal choice with a budget constraint are the same as in the base case. Thus even when effectiveness is maximized by the implausible assumption of 100 percent compliance with screening, the cost criteria make screening options unattractive.

Figure 7-3. Cost and Effectiveness of Different Approaches to Community Treatment

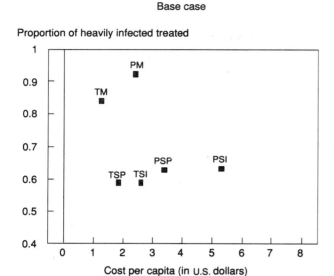

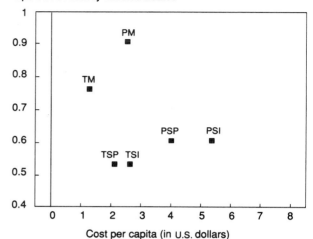

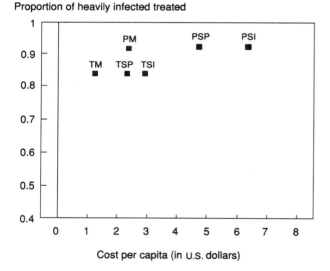

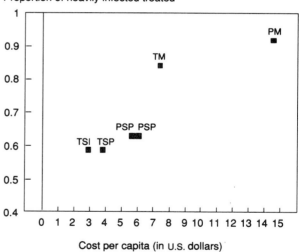

Note: Initials refer to the chemotherapy approaches detailed in table 7-12. Effectiveness is measured in terms of the percentage of heavy infections treated. Cost is given in U.S. dollars per person in a population of 1 million, whether or not infected, and are for the total program of two years (six-month cycles of treatment). Base case assumptions are listed in table 7-13.
Source: Authors.

Screening emerges as a preferred strategy only if drug costs are high in relation to screening costs and only in the presence of a budget constraint. The last graph in figure 7-3 illustrates this result in that drug costs are increased to US$4, which simulates the cost of praziquantel for the treatment of schistosomiasis. In this scenario, only the screening options are affordable at lower budget levels, initially on a targeted basis and then on a population basis. At these levels, screening for

intensity is less costly than screening for prevalence, although both options are equally effective. At higher budget levels, the more expensive but much more effective mass chemotherapy alternatives become affordable and preferred. An important factor here is that it is only at higher budgetary levels, and only with mass chemotherapy, that an acceptable level of effectiveness is achieved under the present assumptions. Note also that this model assumes a six-month cycle of treatment, whereas,

Table 7-13. Epidemiologic and Behavioral Parameters of the Base Case
(percent)

Parameter	Value[a]
Prevalence of infection	
Children	60
Adults	30
Children with heavy infections	15
Percentage of all heavy infections that occur in children	90
Reduction in prevalence due to each cycle of therapy	80
Compliance with treatment	
Children	95
Adults	75
Compliance with screening	
Children	70
Adults	50

a. Values are derived from empirical observation and broadly describe the patterns observed for *Ascaris, Trichuris,* and the schistosomes.
Source: Authors.

in practice, chemotherapy against schistosomiasis is delivered on cycles of twelve months or more, which would substantially reduce the costs of all the control programs.

In all the above scenarios we have assumed that intense infection is concentrated in children, as is the case for *Ascaris, Trichuris,* and schistosome infections. When it is assumed that intensity of infection rises to an asymptote in young adults, as appears to be the case for hookworm infection, the relative cost-effectiveness of targeted mass chemotherapy is reduced,

Figure 7-4. Cost Effectiveness of Various Approaches to Treatment when Intense Infection Occurs in Adults

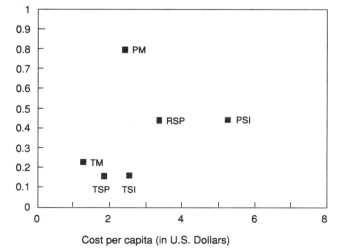

Proportion of heavy infections treated

Note: Abbreviated treatment strategies are described in table 7-12.
Source: Authors.

because it fails to treat the increased share of heavy infections in adults (figure 7-4). Even in this scenario, however, mass chemotherapy is more cost-effective than the screening equivalents. Note also that the age distribution described here is an extreme case and that in reality even hookworm infections may have a high proportion of intense infections in children, a situation that would favor targeted mass chemotherapy.

The main implications of these simulations are the following. First, if there is no budget constraint and the planning objective is simply to maximize the proportion of heavy infections treated, then population mass chemotherapy will always be the optimal intervention. Targeted mass chemotherapy will always be inferior because not all heavy infections occur in children. The higher the proportion of heavy infections in children, however, the greater will be the similarity in effectiveness between population mass and targeted mass chemotherapy. Screening options will generally be inferior because of attrition owing to imperfect screening compliance, but even if compliance were complete, these screening options would only be as good as, but never better than, mass chemotherapy.

Second, if there is a budget constraint the mass chemotherapy options will generally tend to be preferred, with targeted mass chemotherapy at lower budget levels and population mass chemotherapy at higher levels. For infections which tend to be most intense in children (such as *Ascaris, Trichuris,* and the schistosomes) the targeted option may provide similar levels of effectiveness to the population option. For infections such as hookworm, where intensity is high in adults, the effectiveness is reduced, although this may be outweighed by the beneficial reduction in morbidity in children.

Third, only in the particular case of drug costs that are high in relation to screening costs, and in the presence of a budget constraint, will screening options be more cost-effective. In these circumstances, higher drug costs will initially favor screening for prevalence, with screening for intensity taking over only when drug costs are high enough to offset the higher costs of screening.

Using the Educational System to Deliver Intervention

The massive prevalence of helminthic infection and the need to deliver treatment to a high proportion of infected individuals impose significant logistic constraints on the design of drug delivery systems. Parasite control programs share with vaccination programs the dubious distinction of being the most extensive health intervention programs ever attempted by humankind. Anthelmintics offer significant logistic advantages over vaccines, however: they are relatively thermostable and do not require a cold chain; they do not have specialized storage requirements; they have an extended shelf life; they do not require technical expertise for administration. Their disadvantage, when compared with most vaccines in current use, is the necessity for repeated delivery, although as discussed above, the putative antihelminth vaccines may require repeated administration and be more costly to deliver than anthelmintics.

The main logistic concern, therefore, is the development of methods to deliver anthelmintics to the community on a regular basis. One solution is to focus drug delivery on school-age children, using the existing educational infrastructure as a delivery mechanism. Treating schoolchildren for worms is not a new idea; it appears to be part of the traditional perception of worm infection in many communities that it is the children who should be treated. Recent research, however, has shown that school-based treatment offers a broad range of advantages, including the potential to achieve community-wide control. In this section we consider school-based treatment as a way of controlling geohelminthiasis and schistosomiasis. We take as given the finding of the preceding subsection that screening is likely to be economically unattractive and that the appropriate strategy will involve mass application to groups targeted by geography and age.

On therapeutic grounds, children are the natural targets for treatment because they tend to have the more intense infections and hence are at greater immediate risk of morbidity. It is now also recognized, however, that disease in childhood has potentially long-term consequences because the peaks of intensity, and thus morbidity, occur at an age which is crucial for physical and intellectual development. Recent studies have shown that the growth of children with intense worm infections may be seriously impaired; furthermore, they have shown that these effects are primarily due to worm infection, because they can be reversed by deworming (Stephenson 1987; Cooper and others 1990). It is particularly significant that deworming alone is sufficient to improve the nutritional status of the children and that great restoration of growth can be achieved without nutritional supplementation. This was graphically illustrated in a recent study showing a remarkable increase in height and weight in children treated for S. hematobium infection in Kenya (Stephenson and others 1989a). There is similar evidence that worm infection affects intellectual development (Nokes and others 1992), and the common physical consequences of infection, such as anemia and stunting, are significantly correlated with deficits in cognition and educational measures (Pollitt 1990). The potential effect of helminthiasis on intellectual development is a great cause for concern, because this may prevent children in many developing countries from benefiting from basic education—the only education they may ever receive. The United Nations Educational, Scientific, and Cultural Organization (UNESCO) has undertaken the important new initiative of assessing the effect of helminthiases on the intake of basic education.

Clearly the treatment of school-age children is beneficial in health and developmental terms. Repeated treatment of children also appears to offer benefits to the wider community by reducing the rate of transmission of infection to adults. A school-based chemotherapeutic program in the Caribbean not only achieved a substantial reduction in childhood infection with enteric nematodes, as might be expected, but also reduced infection in adults, less than 4 percent of whom were treated (Bundy and others 1989). It is probable that this effect was due to the significant reduction in contamination by infective

stages achieved by removing worms from the heavily infected children, an effect that had been predicted on theoretical grounds (Anderson and May 1982).

It is also now recognized that treatment of children has a long-term developmental effect on the whole community. Physical and intellectual retardation during childhood has consequences for the adult life of the affected individuals. Successful control of parasites in children would, therefore, be expected to provide tangible benefits into the next generation.

Targeting treatment at one specific age group obviously offers significant cost advantages over universal treatment. When the target is schoolchildren these advantages are further increased by the accessibility of the target group (King and others 1989; Wilkins 1989). Schools offer an existing infrastructure for low-cost delivery of anthelmintics and often have established mechanisms for clinical surveillance and community mobilization. They also offer the opportunity for long-term surveillance of randomly selected children with respect to reinfection rates and the effects of treatment of selected parasites on such indexes as height- and weight-for-age and hemoglobin level. Poor school attendance either generally or seasonally may vitiate the effectiveness of this approach.

Cost-Effectiveness of Mass Chemoprophylaxis

Earlier we assessed the economics of screening prior to treatment for various helminthiases and concluded that, for a robust range of assumptions concerning the costs of screening and treatment, mass treatment was a preferable population-based approach to use of diagnostic screening to ascertain which individuals required treatment. Mass treatment, however, could (and should) be targeted to specific geographical regions

Table 7-14. Costs of a Ten-Year School-Based Program Covering 1,000 Children with Chemoprophylaxis for Intestinal Helminthiasis and Schistosomiasis

Component	Cost (U.S. dollars)
Praziquantel (4,000 doses)	2,000
Albendazole (8,000 doses)	1,000
Delivery system	5,000–15,000
Total	8,000–18,000
Cost per child	8–18

Note: Program seeks to reach all children age five to fourteen through an annual school visit by a health team. In the ten years of the program, each child should receive praziquantel five times and albendazole ten times. It is assumed, however, that the program is 80 percent effective; on average each child will receive four doses of praziquantel and eight doses of albendazole.

The cost per child contact in WHO's Expanded Programme of Immunization averages about $2.50. That is an upper bound (probably a multiple) of what school-based systems are likely to cost.

The present value of costs would be slightly less than these estimates if costs over the ten-year period were discounted back to the initial year (at 3 percent), as should be done in principle. The effect is small, however, compared with the uncertainty in delivery system costs.

Source: UNICEF 1989.

Table 7-15. Estimated Gains in Healthy Life-Years from a School-Based Program of Chemoprophylaxis for Intestinal Helminthiasis and Schistosomiasis
(years)

Mechanism	Moderate estimate[a]	Low estimate[a]
Reduction in mild-to-moderate schistosomiasis[b]	225	90
Reduction in mild-to-moderate intestinal helminthiasis[b]	225	90
Reduction in heavy schistosomiasis[c]	300	150
Reduction in heavy intestinal helminthiasis[c]	300	150
Reduction in child mortality[d]	125	65
Post-intervention health benefits for target group[e]	150	0
During-intervention benefits for families of target group[f]	150	0
Total	1,475	545

Note: Gains in DALY over a ten-year period in a cohort of 1,000 school-age children, estimated from the program assumptions of table 7-14.

a. Intervention is assumed to result in a gain of 1.2 healthy life-years per year in moderate estimate and 0.1 life-year in low estimate for heavily infected children. Comparable figures for mild to moderate infection are 0.05 and 0.02 life-years.

b. Assumes that 45 percent of children are affected before intervention.

c. Assumes that 15 percent of children are affected before intervention.

d. Assumes 200,000 deaths in all age groups per year from schistosomiasis and all intestinal helminthiases for the low estimate and 400,000 for the moderate; 50 percent of these deaths occur in school-age children in the 40 percent most at risk (in which the cohort of 1,000 students occurs.) These assumptions posit the occurrence of an average of 2.3 deaths over ten years among 1,000 children in the low estimate and 4.6 deaths in the moderate estimate. Discounting at 3 percent from a life expectancy of sixty-five gives the estimates of life-years gained by averting these deaths.

e. In the moderate case, it is assumed that health benefits for each child from the ten-year intervention in the postintervention years would equal 15 percent of the benefits accruing during intervention.

f. In the moderate case, it is assumed that reducing infection in schoolchildren will partially interrupt transmission, thereby reducing morbidity in other members of the children's families. The effect is conservatively assumed to be 15 percent as important as the direct effect on schoolchildren.

Source: Authors.

and age groups. Given the substantially greater intensity of infection among school-age groups than others (figure 7-2), targeting this group becomes a natural priority; the attractiveness of this strategy is further increased by the (relative) logistic and cost attractiveness of intervention through the schools, as was discussed above. Our purpose in this section is to provide an extended hypothetical example of the cost-effectiveness of school-based intervention. Although hypothetical, the cost and effectiveness parameters used are intended to span a reasonable range of probable values; the range of cost-effectiveness estimates is likely, therefore, to provide a realistic sense of what can be achieved.

Given the inevitability of reinfection until high levels of hygiene are ultimately achieved, a strategy based on mass chemoprophylaxis requires periodic, repeated administration of anthelmintics. This is less desirable than prevention

achieved through sanitation and hygiene but far less costly. As an interim strategy, therefore, mass chemoprophylaxis is highly cost-effective and, at present, the case is strong for rapid and widespread adoption.

Because of the requirement for repeated drug administration, intervention is best considered as a long-term program. The example we take here assumes a ten-year intervention designed to control schistosomiasis and the intestinal helminthiases in the school-age population (age five to fourteen years). This combination would be appropriate for populations in Northern, Western, and Southern Africa, where a combination of albendazole and praziquantel is used. At low marginal cost, ivermectin could be added to the albendazole and praziquantel used in northern and eastern South America, Central Africa, and Southeast Asia; indeed, given that delivery costs are preponderant among all costs, the cost of serving any of the five groups depicted on the map would vary little from our cost estimates in table 7-14. In the table, we assume a school-based delivery system (probably provided by an annual visit to the school by a mobile team) that serves the entire school-age population. A more detailed discussion of school-based delivery systems for health intervention may be found in Jamison and Leslie (1990). The estimates in table 7-14 suggest that it would be likely to cost between $8.00 and $18.00 per child for a ten-year program (that is, between $0.80 and $1.80 per year) that provided, in that period, four administrations of praziquantel and eight of albendazole. This should control the schistosomes and hookworm very well and *Trichuris* and *Ascaris* moderately well (table 7-11).

Table 7-15 indicates both moderate and low estimates of the benefits of such an intervention for a population of 1,000 school-age children. There is, as shown in the table, a range of benefits; explicit assumptions are made about how these can be expressed in disability-adjusted life-years (DALYs) gained. These assumptions are, in our view, conservative; further, the results (at a broad level) are relatively insensitive to the assumptions. The implications of alternative assumptions, including assumptions about local epidemiology, can easily be assessed.

The cost estimates in table 7-14 and the effectiveness estimates in table 7-15 yield a range of cost-effectiveness estimates from $6 to $33 per DALY gained (table 7-16). Even the high end

Table 7-16. Cost-Effectiveness of a School-Based Program of Chemoprophylaxis for Intestinal Helminthiasis and Schistosomiasis
(U.S. dollars)

Cost per child for ten-year intervention[a]	Cost per disability-adjusted life-year gained	
	Moderate effect[b]	Low effect[b]
8	6	15
18	12	33

a. These costs are the low and high ends of the range reported in table 7-14.

b. The program effect cites the moderate and low estimates for table 7-15.

Source: Authors.

of this range of costs is relatively attractive—comparable to diphtheria-pertussis-tetanus (DPT)-plus-polio immunization (Jamison and others, chapter 6, this collection). At the low end of the range, the intervention becomes one of the most cost-effective means of promoting child health.

It is, in this context, worth recalling the estimates of cost-effectiveness of several preventive interventions that were previously presented. Although applicable in only limited foci, improved water supply to control dracunculiasis is also highly cost-effective—perhaps $25 per healthy life-year gained. Vector control for prevention of onchocerciasis is far less attractive at perhaps $300 per healthy life-year gained.

Priorities and Conclusion

The availability of a series of broad-spectrum anthelmintics which have minimal side effects and are administered orally in a single dosage has begun to be widely appreciated. Coupled with the unique biology, ecology, and epidemiology of the macroparasites (helminths) as compared with microparasites (viruses, bacteria, protozoa), these new anthelmintics allow a strategy of controlling disease, rather than infection, by maintaining worm burdens at low levels via chemoprophylaxis. How best the new drugs can be employed, with what effect, and at what cost are all questions which are beginning to be addressed. An important question is that, although the helminthiases are the most widespread infections in the developing world, is their control warranted in so many countries which today are operating under severe budget constraints and in an environment where prospects for significant assistance from donors for any health program are discouraging? The introduction of any new health intervention has to be weighed carefully, as to both the benefits and the costs, as well as to the prospects for obtaining needed resources.

Available data, as reviewed in this chapter, document the prevalence of helminthic infections, usually with several being present simultaneously. Substantial improvements in control through prevention is not an option in the short to medium term without unrealistically large investments in sanitation or vector control. (Dracunculiasis provides an important exception to this generalization; preventive measures appear both cost-effective and capable of eradicating the disease during the 1990s.) For the foreseeable future, therefore, chemotherapy is the dominant option in most countries. Traditional practice would call for evaluating the new chemotherapeutic agents by their ability to cure diagnosed infections in individuals. Diagnosis and treatment of infection in individuals, however, are not only costly procedures, but their application is beyond the capacity of most health services. Moreover, where infection is rife, amelioration of disease symptoms is apt to be of short duration because of rapid reinfection.

Given the fact that infections in many areas are so widespread, although not infrequently asymptomatic, alternative practices should be considered with two objectives in mind: to diminish the incidence of symptomatic infection and to provide for large-scale treatment without costly and time-consuming diagnostic procedures. The administration of lower dosages of certain of the drugs might reduce or eliminate symptoms without necessarily drastically reducing efficacy. Use of lower dosages might also be less costly.

The design, implementation, and evaluation of treatment regimens are complicated by the fact that most individuals in the tropics are infected with not one but several helminths. Symptomatic manifestations, not surprisingly, usually represent a cumulative burden of the effects of multiple infections. Studies which dissect out the proportionate contributions to illness of the different helminths are few indeed and often difficult to interpret. Even if done, it would be impossible to generalize results from one geographic area to another, given the array of variables which are present.

Given this quandary, and the immense global burden of multiple helminthic infection, it would be worthwhile to consider pilot programs in which two or even three chemotherapeutic agents are administered concomitantly at periodic intervals and on a large scale to selected population groups to evaluate the cost and effectiveness of such programs in diminishing symptomatic disease. Available data suggest that such programs should be cost-effective, but confirmation is required. Such a strategy would be consonant with a transformation which has begun to occur in the provision of a number of health services in developing countries. Community-wide programs for vaccination, oral rehydration therapy, vitamin A supplementation, and family planning have been growing in number and extent, proving to be far more effective than programs directed solely to individuals who present themselves at health centers or hospitals. Such community-based programs, directed to the control of helminthic diseases, have only begun to be explored but, where conducted, they have proved to be most successful. Community-wide programs for anthelmintic drug administration might be targeted at school-age children, for example, and be conducted simultaneously or at least in concert with other community-based programs for vitamin A administration or vaccination, at marginal additional cost.

Programs are needed to determine with certainty that two or three anthelmintic agents can be given concomitantly or within a circumscribed time period with safety and without loss of efficacy. Mechanisms for involving, motivating, and educating effectively the populations concerned are required, as they are with other community-based programs. High-risk populations requiring treatment would need to be identified. This could be done inexpensively by sample surveys rather than by a total screening of the population. Evaluation of selected regimens—for example, mass treatment of school-age children yearly—could be conducted in a similar manner.

The important departure, however, is to conceptualize the potential use and evaluation for these new chemotherapeutic agents in a new framework. Given their cost, particularly where therapeutic doses that are lower than usual could be employed, and given the burden of helminthic infection, large-scale mass treatment could represent an important and cost-effective health strategy in many parts of the world where improved sanitation and vector control are not presently feasible. Estimates of cost-effectiveness suggest that measures of this sort are likely to prove attractive within the present range of options for improving child health.

Notes

Preparation of this chapter was supported financially by the World Bank and by Global Health Partners, Inc. The views expressed do not, of course, necessarily reflect those of the sponsoring organizations. The authors wish to express their gratitude to the following individuals for valuable advice and comments on earlier drafts: J. Cook, C. Cruz, D. Evans, T. Evans, R. Feachem, D. Hopkins, J.-L. Lamboray, W. H. Mosley, M. Percopo, A. Seim, G. Torrigiani, and S. Van der Vynckt.

References

Albers-Schoenberg, G., B. H. Arison, J. C. Chabala, A. W. Douglas, P. Eskola, M. H. Fisher, A. Lusi, H. Mrozik, F. L. Smith, and R. L. Tolman. 1981. "Avermectins: Structure Determination." *Journal of the American Chemical Association* 102:4216–21.

Albiez, E. J., G. Walter, A. Kaiser, P. Ranque, H. S. Newland, A. T. White, B. M. Greene, H. R. Taylor, and D. W. Buttner. 1988. "Histological Examination of Onchocercomata after Therapy with Ivermectin." *Tropical Medicine Parasitology* 39:93–99.

Anderson, R. M. 1982. *Population Dynamics of Infectious Diseases: Theory and Applications.* London: Chapman and Hall.

———. 1986. "The Population Dynamics and Epidemiology of Intestinal Nematode Infections." *Transactions of the Royal Society of Tropical Medicine and Hygiene* 686–96.

———. 1987. "Determinants of Infection in Schistosomiasis." *Clinical Tropical Medicine and Communicable Diseases* 2:279–300.

———. 1988. "Determinants of Infection in Human Schistosomiasis." *Clinical Tropical Medicine and Communicable Diseases* 2:279–300.

———. 1989. "Transmission Dynamics of *Ascaris lumbricoides* and the Impact of Chemotherapy." In D. W. T. Crompton, M. C. Nesheim & Z. S. Pawlowski, eds., *Ascariasis and Its Prevention and Control.* London: Taylor and Francis.

Anderson, R.M. and R.M. May. 1982. "Population Dynamics of Human Helminth Infections: Control by Chemotherapy." *Nature* 297:557–63.

———. 1985. "Helminth Infections of Humans: Mathematical Models, Population Dynamics and Control." *Advances in Parasitology* 1–101.

Anderson, R. M., R. M. May, and S. Gupta. 1989. "Non-linear Phenomena in Host-Parasite Interactions." *Parasitology* 99:S59–S79.

Anderson, R. M. and G. F. Medley. 1985. "Community Control of Helminth Infections of Man by Mass and Selective Chemotherapy." *Parasitology* 90:629–60.

Andreano, R., and T. Helminiak. 1988. "Economics, Health and Tropical Disease: A Review." In H. N. Herrin, and P. Rosenfield, eds., *Economics, Health and Tropical Diseases.* Manila: University of the Philippines, School of Economics.

Arfaa, F. 1986. "Ascariasis and Trichuriasis." In J. A. Walsh and K. S. Warren, eds., *Strategies for Primary Health Care.* Chicago: University of Chicago Press.

Barbour, A. D. 1982. "Schistosomiasis." In R.M. Anderson, ed., *Population Dynamics of Infectious Diseases: Theory and Applications.* London: Chapman and Hall.

Behm, C. A., and C. Bryant. 1985. "The Modes of Action of Some Modern Anthelmintics." In Anderson and Waller, eds. *Resistance in Nematodes to Anthelmintic Drugs.* Glebe, Australia: CSIRO Publication.

Borgers, M., S. De Nollin, A. Verheyen, M. De Brabander, and D. Thienpont. 1975. "Influence of the Anthelmintic Mebendazole on Microtubules and Intracellular Organelle Movement in Nematode Intestinal Cells." *American Journal of Veterinary Research* 36:1153–66.

Bradley, D. J., and F. S. McCullough. 1974. "Egg Output Stability and the Epidemiology of *Schistosoma haematobium*." *Transactions of the Royal Society of Tropical Medicine and Hygiene* 80:706–18.

Bundy, D. A. P. 1986. "Epidemiological Aspects of *Trichuris* and Trichuriasis in Caribbean Communities." *Transactions of the Royal Society of Tropical Medicine and Hygiene* 80:706–18.

———. 1988. "Population Ecology of Intestinal Helminth Infections in Human Communities." *Philosophical Transactions of the Royal Society of London* 321:405–20.

Bundy, D. A. P., and U. Blumenthal. 1989. "The Impact of Human Behaviour on the Epidemiology of Schistosomiasis and Geohelminthiasis." In G. Bernard and J. Behnke, eds., *Behaviour and Parasitism.* London: Taylor and Francis.

Bundy, D. A. P., and E. S. Cooper. 1989. "Trichuris and Trichuriasis in Humans." *Advances in Parasitology,* 28:107–73.

Bundy, D. A. P., E. S. Cooper, D. E. Thompson, R. M. Anderson, and J. M. Didier. 1987. "Age-related Prevalence and Intensity of *Trichuris trichiura* Infection in a St. Lucian Community." *Transactions of the Royal Society of Tropical Medicine and Hygiene* 81:85–94.

Bundy, D. A. P., S. P. Kan, and R. Rose, and others. 1988a. "Age-related Prevalence, Intensity and Frequency of Distribution of Gastrointestinal Helminth Infections in Urban Slum Children from Kuala Lumpur, Malaysia." *Transactions of the Royal Society of Tropical Medicine and Hygiene* 82:289–94.

Bundy, D. A. P., E. S. Cooper, D. E. Thompson, J. M. Didier, and I. Simmons. 1988b. "Effect of Age and Initial Infection Status on the Rate of Reinfection with *T. trichiura* after Treatment." *Parasitology* 97:469–76.

Bundy, D. A. P., E. S. Cooper, D. E. Thompson, J. M. Didier, R. M. Anderson, and I. Simmons. 1988c. "Predisposition to *Trichuris trichiura* Infection in Humans." *Epidemiology and Infection* 98:65–71.

Bundy, D. A. P., D. E. Thompson, E. S. Cooper, M. H. N. Golden, and R. M. Anderson. 1985. "Population Dynamics and Chemotherapeutic Control of *Trichuris trichiura* Infection of Children in Jamaica and St. Lucia." *Transactions of the Royal Society of Tropical Medicine and Hygiene* 69:759–64.

Bundy, D. A. P., M. S. Wong, L. L. Lewis and J. Horton. 1989. "Control of Gastro-intestinal Helminths by Age-Group Targeted Chemotherapy Delivered through Schools." *Transactions of the Royal Society of Tropical Medicine and Hygiene* 8:115–20.

Cabrera, B. D., B. Caballero, L. Rampal, and W. de Leon. 1989. "The Philippines." In D. W. T. Crompton, M. C. Nesheim, and Z. S. Pawlowski, eds., *Ascariasis and Its Prevention and Control.* London: Taylor and Francis.

Cairncross, A. C., and R. G. Feachem. 1983. *Environmental Health Engineering in the Tropics.* Chichester, U.K.: John Wiley and Sons.

Campbell, W. C., M. H. Fisher, E. O. Stapley, G. Albers-Schoenberg, and T. A. Jacob. 1983. "Ivermectin: A Potent New Antiparasitic Agent." *Science* 221:823–28.

Chandler, A. C. 1925. "The Rate of Loss of Hookworms in the Absence of Reinfections." *Indian Journal of Medical Research* 13:625–34.

CIBA Foundation. 1987. *Filariasis,* ed. D. Everard and S. Cook. Chichester, U.K.: John Wiley and Sons.

Cook, J. A. 1987. "Strategies for Control of Human Schistosomiasis." *Clinical Tropical Medicine and Communicable Diseases* 2:449–63.

Cook, J. A., P. Jordan, and P. Armitage. 1976. "Hycanthone Dose-Response in Treatment of Schistosomiasis Mansoni in St. Lucia." *American Journal of Tropical Medicine and Hygiene* 25:602–7.

Cooper, E. S., and D. A. P. Bundy. 1986. "Trichuriasis." In A. S. McNeish and J. A. Walker-Smith, eds., *Diarrhoea and Malnutrition in Childhood*. London: Buttersworth.

——— 1987. "Trichuriasis: In Intestinal Helminthic Infections." *Baillière's Clinical Tropical Medicine and Communicable Diseases* 2:629–43.

———. 1988. "Trichuris Is Not Trivial." *Parasitology Today* 4:301–6.

Cooper, E. S., D. A. P. Bundy, and F. S. Henry. 1986. "Chronic Dysentery, Stunting, and Whipworm Infestation." *Lancet* (August 2):280–81.

Cooper, E. S., D. A. P. Bundy, T. T. Macdonald, and M. H. N. Golden. 1990. "Growth Suppression in the *Trichuris* Dysentery Syndrome." *European Journal of Clinical Nutrition* 44:138–47.

Cort, W. W. 1922. "A Graphic Analysis of Certain Factors in Hookworm Control." *American Journal of Tropical Medicine* 2:449–63.

Croll, N. A., R. M. Anderson, T. W. Gyorkos, and E. Ghadirian. 1982. "The Population Biology and Control of *Ascaris lumbricoides* in a Rural Community in Iran." *Transactions of the Royal Society of Tropical Medicine and Hygiene* 76:187–97.

Crompton, D. W. T. 1985. "Chronic Ascariasis and Malnutrition." *Parasitology Today* 1:47–52.

———. 1989. "The Prevalence of Ascariasis." In D. W. T. Crompton, M. C. Nesheim, and Z. S. Pawlowski, eds., *Ascariasis and Its Prevention and Control*. London: Taylor and Francis.

Cupp, E. W., A. O. Ochoa, R. C. Collins, F. R. Ramberg, and G. Zea. 1989. "The Effect of Multiple Ivermectin Treatments on Infection of *Simulium ochraceum* with *Onchocerca volvulus*." *American Journal of Tropical Medicine and Hygiene* 40:501–6.

Dadzie, K. Y., A. C. Bird, K. Awadzi, H. Schulz-Key, H. M. Gilles, and M. A. Aziz. 1987. "Ocular Findings in a Double-Blind Study of Ivermectin versus Diethylcarbamazine versus Placebo in the Treatment of Onchocerciasis." *British Journal of Ophthalmology* 71:78–85.

Davis, Andrew. 1986. "Available Anthelmintics and Future Needs." In H. Machleidt, ed., *Contributions of Chemistry to Health: Proceedings of the Fifth CHEMRAWN Conference*, vol. 2. Wernheim, Fed. Rep. Germany: VCH Verlagsgesellischaft mbH.

———. 1989. "Chemotherapy: Options for Delivery Systems." In Max J. Miller and E. J. Love, eds., *Parasitic Diseases: Treatment and Control*. Boca Raton, Fla.: CRC Press.

Degremont, A., G. K. Lwihula, C. Mayombana, E. Burnier, D. de Savigny, and M. Tanner. 1987. "Longitudinal Study on the Health Status of Children in a Rural Tanzanian Community: Parasitoses and Nutrition Following Control Measure against Intestinal Parasites." *Acta Tropica* 44:175–90.

Dietz, Klaus. 1982. "The Population Dynamics of Onchocerciasis." In R. M. Anderson, ed., *Population Dynamics of Infectious Diseases: Theory and Applications*. London: Chapman and Hall.

Edungbola, L. D., S. J. Watts, T. O. Alabi, and A. B. Bello. 1988. "The Impact of a UNICEF-Assisted Rural Water Project on the Prevalence of Guinea Worm Disease in Asa, Kwara State, Nigeria." *American Journal of Tropical Medicine and Hygiene* 39:79–85.

Egerton, J. R., D. Suhayda, and C.H. Eary. 1988. "Laboratory Selection of *Haemonchus contortus* for Resistance to Ivermectin." *Journal of Parasitology* 74:614–17.

el Karim, M. A., K. J. Collins, J. R. Brotherhood, C. Dore, J. S. Weiner, M. Y. Sukkar, A. H. Omer, and M. A. Amin. 1980. "Quantitative Egg Excretion and Work Capacity in a Gezira Population Infected with *Schistosoma mansoni*." *American Journal of Tropical Medicine and Hygiene* 29:54–61.

Elkins, D. B., M. Haswell-Elkins, and R. M. Anderson. 1986. "The Epidemiology and Control of Intestinal Helminths in the Pulicat Lake Region of Southern India: Study Design and Pre- and Post-treatment Observations on *Ascaris lumbricoides* Infection." *Transactions of the Royal Society of Tropical Medicine and Hygiene* 80:774–92.

Evans, T. G., and C. J. L. Murray. 1987. "A Critical Re-examination of Blindness Prevention under the Onchocerciasis Control Programme." *Social Science and Medicine* 25:241–49.

Feachem, R. G. A., D. J. Bradley, H. Garelick, and D. D. Mara. 1983a. *Sanitation and Disease*. Chichester, U.K.: John Wiley and Sons.

Feachem, R. G. A., M. W. Guy, S. Harrison, K. O. Wugo, T. Marshall, N. Mbere, R. Muller, and A. M. Wright. 1983b. "Excreta Disposal Facilities and Intestinal Parasitism in Urban Africa: Preliminary Studies in Botswana, Ghana and Zambia." *Transactions of the Royal Society of Tropical Medicine and Hygiene* 77:515–21.

Fisher, M. H., and H. Mrozik. 1989. "Chemistry." In W. C. Campbell, ed., *Ivermectin and Abamectin*. New York: Springer Verlag.

Fosdick, R. 1952. *The Story of the Rockefeller Foundation*. New York: Harper & Brothers.

Gemmell, M. A., J. R. Lawson, and M. G. Roberts. 1986. "Control of Echinococcosis/Hydatidosis: Present Status of World-Wide Progress." *Bulletin of the World Health Organization* 64:333–39.

Greene, B. M., K. R. Brown, and H. R. Taylor. 1989. "Use of Ivermectin in Humans." In W. C. Campbell, ed., *Ivermectin and Abamectin*. New York: Springer Verlag.

Grove, D. 1989. *Strongyloidiasis*. London: Taylor and Francis.

Hairston, N. G. 1965. "On the Mathematical Analysis of Schistosome Populations." *Bulletin of the World Health Organization* 33:45–62.

Harpham, T., T. Lusty, and P. Vaughan. 1987. *In the Shadow of the City: Community Health and the Urban Poor*. Oxford: Oxford University Press.

Hayashi, S. 1980. "Economic Loss from Parasites." *Collected Papers on the Control of Soil-Transmitted Helminthiases*. Tokyo: Asian Parasite Control Organization.

Hill, R. B. 1926. "The Estimation of the Number of Hookworms Harboured, by the Use of the Egg Dilution Method." *American Journal of Tropical Medicine* 6:19–41.

Holland, C. V. 1987a. "Hookworm Infection." In L. S. Stephenson, ed., *Impact of Helminth Infections on Human Nutrition*. London: Taylor and Francis.

———. 1987b. "Neglected Infections—Trichuriasis and Strongyloidiasis." In L.S. Stephenson, ed., *Impact of Helminth Infections on Human Nutrition*. London: Taylor and Francis.

Hopkins, D. R., and E. Ruiz-Tiben. 1990. *Dracunculiasis Eradication: Target 1995*. Atlanta: Carter Center. *American Journal of Tropical Medicine and Hygiene*. 43:296–300

Ilegbodu, V. A., O. O. Kale, R. A. Wise, B. L. Christensen, J. H. Steele, and L. A. Chambers. 1986. "Impact of Guinea Worm Disease on Children in Nigeria." *American Journal of Tropical Medicine and Hygiene* 35:962–94.

Ismid, I. S., and B. Rukmono. 1980. "The Effect of Latrine Provision and Health Education on Soil Pollution." In *Collected Papers on the Control of Soil-Transmitted Helminthiases*, vol. 1. Tokyo: Asian Parasite Control Organization.

Jamison, D. T., and J. Leslie. 1990. "Health and Nutrition Considerations in Educational Planning: The Cost and Effectiveness of School-based Intervention." *Food and Nutrition Bulletin* 12:204–14.

Kan, S. P., H. L. Guyatt, and D. A. P. Bundy. 1989. "Geohelminth Infection of Children from Rural Populations and Urban Slums in Malaysia." *Transactions of the Royal Society of Tropical Medicine and Hygiene* 83:817–21.

Kass, I. S., A. O. W. Stretton, and C. C. Wang. 1984. "The Effects of Avermectin and Drugs Related to Acetylcholine and 4-aminobutyric Acid on Neurotransmission in *Ascaris suum*." *Molecular and Biochemical Parasitology* 13:213–25.

Kass, I. S., C. C. Wang, J. P. Walrond, and A. O. W. Stretton. 1980. "Avermectin B_{1a}, a Paralyzing Anthelminthic that Affects Interneurons and Inhibitory Motor Neurons in *Ascaris*." *Proceedings of the National Academy of Science* 77:6211–15.

Kilama, W. L. 1989. "Sanitation in the Control of Ascariasis." In D. W. T. Crompton, M. C. Nesheim, and Z. S. Pawlowski, eds., *Ascariasis and Its Prevention and Control*. London: Taylor and Francis.

King, C. A., D. W. Wiper, K. V. Destigter, P. A. S. Peters, D. Koech, J. H. Ouma, T. K. A. Siongok, and A. A. F. Mahmoud. 1989. "Dose-finding Study for Praziquantel Therapy of *Schistosoma hematobium* in Coast Province, Kenya." *American Journal of Tropical Medicine and Hygiene* 40:507–13.

Kumaraswami, V., E. A. Ottesen, V. Vijayasekaran, S. Uma Devi, M. Swaminathan, M. A. Aziz, G. R. Sarma, R. Prabhakar, and S. P. Tripathy. 1988. "Ivermectin for the Treatment of *Wuchereria bancrofti* Filariasis: Efficacy and Adverse Reactions." *JAMA* 259:3150–53.

Kvalsvig, J. D. 1988. "The Effects of Parasitic Infection on Cognitive Performance." *Parasitology Today* 4:206–8.

Lacey, E. 1986. "The Biochemistry of Anthelmintic Resistance." In Anderson and Waller, eds., *Resistance in Nematodes to Anthelmintic Drugs*. Glebe, Australia: Commonwealth Scientific and Industrial Research Organization.

Lemma, A. 1987. "Overview of Endod Studies." In *Endod II: Report of the Second International Workshop on Endod*. New York: UNICEF CIPA.

Le Riche, W. H. 1967. "World Incidence and Prevalence of the Major Communicable Diseases." In G. Wolstenholme and M. O'Connor, eds., *Health of Mankind*. London: J. and A. Churchill.

Levin, N. 1988. "Controlling Iron-Binding Deficiency Anemia: A Cost-Benefit Analysis." *World Health* 27–29.

Lok, J. B., T. Harpaz, and D. H. Knight. 1988. "Abnormal Patterns of Embryogenesis in *Dirofilaria immitis* Treated with Ivermectin." *Journal of Helminthology* 62:175–80.

McGarvey, S. T., B. L. Daniel, M. Tso, G. Wu, S. Zhong, R. Olveda, P. M. Wiest, and G. R. Olds. 1990. "Child Growth and Schistosomiasis Japonica in the Philippines and China." Paper presented at the meeting of the American Society for Clinical Investigation, Washington, D.C. *Clinical Research* 38.

Migasena, S., and H. M. Gilles. 1987. "Hookworm Infections." *Clinical and Tropical Medicine and Communicable Diseases* 2:617–27.

Miller, T. A. 1978. "Industrial Development and Field Use of the Canine Hookworm Vaccine." *Advances in Parasitology* 16:333–42.

Morishita, K. 1980. "Japanese Literatures Concerning Influence of Parasites, Especially of Soil-Transmitted Helminths upon the Psychosomatic Condition in Maternity and Childhood." In *Collected Papers on the Control of Soil-Transmitted Helminthiases*. Tokyo: Asian Parasite Control Organization.

Morrow, R. H. 1984. "The Application of a Quantitative Approach to the Assessment of the Relative Importance of Vector and Soil-Transmitted Diseases in Ghana." *Social Sciences and Medicine* 19:1039–49.

Mossinger, J., H. Schulz-Key, and K. Dietz. 1988. "Emergence of *Onchocerca volvulus* Microfilaria from Skin Snips before and after Treatment of Patients with Ivermectin." *Tropical Medicine and Parasitology* 39:313–16.

Mott, K. E. 1988. "Schistosomiasis Control." In D. Rollinson and A. Simpson, eds., *The Biology of Schistosomes*. London: Academic Press.

Mrozik, H., P. Eskola, M. H. Fisher, J. R. Egerton, S. Cifelli, and D. A. Ostlind. 1982. "Avermectin Acyl Derivatives with Anthelminthic Activity." *J. Med. Chem.* 25:658–63.

Naquira, C., G. Jiminez, J. G. Guerra, R. Bernal, D. R. Nalin, D. Neu, and M. Aziz. 1989. "Ivermectin for Human Strongyloidiasis and Other Intestinal Helminths." *American Journal of Tropical Medicine and Hygiene* 40:304–9.

Newland, H. S., A. T. White, B. M. Greene, S. A. D'Anna, E. Keyvan-Larijani, M. A. Aziz, P. N. Williams, and H. R. Taylor. 1988. "Effect of Single-dose Ivermectin Therapy on Human *Onchocerciasis volvulus* Infection with Onchocercal Ocular Involvement." *British Journal of Ophthalmology* 72:561–69.

Nokes, C., S. M. Grantham-McGregor, A. W. Sawyer, E. S. Cooper, and D. A. P. Bundy. 1992. "Helminth Infection and Cognitive Function." *Proceedings of the Royal Society (London)* 247:77–81.

Ottesen, E. A., V. Vijayasekaran, V. Kumaraswami, S. V. Perumal Pillai, A. Sadanandam, S. Frederick, R. Prabhakar, and S. P. Tripathy. 1990. "A Controlled Trial of Ivermectin and Diethylcarbamazine in Lymphatic Filariasis." *New England Journal of Medicine* 322:1113–18.

Otto, G. F., W. W. Cort, and A. E. Keller. 1931. "Environmental Studies of Families in Tennessee Infested with Ascaris, Trichuris, and Hookworm." *American Journal of Hygiene* 14:156–93.

Partono, F. 1985. "Diagnosis and Treatment of Lymphatic Filariasis." *Parasitology Today* 1:52–57.

Partono, F., Purnomo, and A. Soewarta. 1979. "A Simple Method to Control *Brugia timori* by Diethylcarbamazine Administration." *Transactions of the Royal Society of Tropical Medicine and Hygiene* 73:536–42.

Paul, J. E., R. B. Isley, and G. M. Ginsberg. 1986. "Cost-Effective Approaches to the Control of Dracunculiasis." WASH Technical Report 38. USAID Office of Health, Washington, D.C.

Pawlowski, Z. S. 1984. "Ascariasis." *Annales de la Société Belge de Médecine Tropicale* 64:125–34.

Pawlowski, Z. S., and A. Davis. 1989. "Morbidity and Mortality in Ascariasis." In D. W. T. Crompton, M. C. Nesheim, and Z. S. Pawlowski, eds., *Ascariasis and Its Prevention and Control*. London: Taylor and Francis.

Peters, W. 1978. "The Relevance of Parasitology to Human Welfare Today." *Symposium of the British Society of Parasitology* 16:25–40.

Polderman, A. M., B. Gryseels, and P. DeCaluwe. 1988. "Cure Rates and Egg Reduction in Treatment of Intestinal Schistosomiasis with Oxamniquine and Praziquantel in Maniema, Zaire." *Transactions of the Royal Society of Tropical Medicine and Hygiene* 82:115–16.

Pollitt, E. 1990. *Malnutrition and Infection in the Classroom*. Paris: UNESCO.

Pollitt, E., P. Hathirat, and N. J. Kotchabharkdi. 1989. "Iron Deficiency and Educational Achievement in Thailand." *American Journal of Clinical Nutrition* 50:687–97.

Prescott, N. M. 1979. "Schistosomiasis and Development." *World Development* 7:1–14.

———. 1987. "The Economics of Schistosomiasis Chemotherapy." *Parasitology Today* 3:21–24.

———. 1989. "Economic Analysis of Schistosomiasis Control Projects." In M. W. Service, ed., *Demography and Vector-borne Diseases*. Boca Raton, Fla.: CRC Press.

Prescott, N. M., and M. F. Jancloes. 1984. "The Analysis and Assessment of Health Programs." *Social Science and Medicine* 19:1057–60.

Prichard, R. K. 1970. "Mode of Action of the Anthelmintic Thiabendazole in *Haemonchus contortus*." *Nature* 228:584–85.

Prost, A. and N. Prescott. 1984. "Cost Effectiveness of Blindness Prevention by the Onchocerciasis Control Programme in Upper Volta." *Bulletin of the World Health Organization* 62:795–802.

Rajagopalan, P. K., P. K. Das, S. Subramanian, P. Vanamail, and K. D. Ramaia. 1989. "Control of Bancroftian Filariasis in Pondicherry, South India. Precontrol Epidemiological Observations." *Epidemiology and Infection* 103:685–92.

Richard-Lenoble, D., M. Kombila, E. A. Rupp, E. S. Papayliuo, P. Gaxotte, C. Nguiri, and M. A. Aziz. 1988. "Ivermectin in Loiasis and Concomitant O. *volvulus* and M. *perstans* Infections." *American Journal of Tropical Medicine and Hygiene* 39:480–83.

Rim, H. J. 1986. "The Current Pathobiology and Chemotherapy of Clonorchiasis." *Korean Journal of Parasitology* 24:1–141.

Rosenfield, P. L., F. Galladay, and R. K. Davidson. 1984. "The Economics of Parasitic Diseases: Research Priorities." *Social Science and Medicine* 19:117–126.

Sasa, M. 1977. *Human Filariasis: A Global Survey of Epidemiology and Control.* Tokyo: University of Tokyo Press.

Schad, G. A., and K. S. Warren. 1989. *Hookworm Infection: Current Status and New Directions.* London: Taylor and Francis.

Seim, A. R. 1990. *Guinea Worm Disease Eradication Project.* Fagerstrand, Norway: Health and Development International.

Smillie, W. G. 1924. "Control of Hookworm Disease in South Alabama." *Southern Medical Journal* 17:494–99.

Smith, G. S., D. Blum, S. R. A. Huttly, N. Okeke, B. R. Kirkwood, and R. G. A. Feachem. 1989. "Disability from Dracunculiasis: Effect on Mobility." *Annals of Tropical Medicine and Parasitology* 83:151–58

Soboslay, P. T., H. S. Newland, A. T. White, K. D. Erttmann, E. J. Albiez, H. R. Taylor, P. N. Williams, and B. M. Greene. 1987. "Ivermectin Effect on Microfilaria of *Onchocerca volvulus* after a Single Oral Dose in Humans." *Trop. Med. Parasitol* 39:8–10.

Soderlund, D. M., P. M. Adams, and J. R. Bloomquist. 1987. "Difference in the Action of Avermectin B1a on the GABA Receptor Complex of Mouse and Rat." *Biochemical and Biophysical Research Communications* 146:692–98.

Stephenson, L. S. 1987. *Impact of Helminth Infections on Human Nutrition.* London: Taylor and Francis.

Stephenson, L. S., M. C. Latham, K. M. Kurz, and S. N. Kinotti. 1989a. "Single Dose Metrifonate or Praziquantel Treatment in Kenyan Children. Effects on Growth in Relation to *Schistosoma hematobium* and Hookworm Egg Counts." *American Journal of Tropical Medicine and Hygiene* 41: 445–53.

Stephenson, L. S., M. C. Latham, K. M. Kurz, S. N. Kinoti, and H. Brigham. 1989b. "Treatment with a Single Dose of Albendazole Improves Growth of Kenyan Schoolchildren with Hookworm, *Trichuris trichiura*, and *Ascaris lumbricoides* Infections." *American Journal of Tropical Medicine and Hygiene* 41:78–87.

Stephenson, L. S., S. N. Kinoti, K. M. Kurz, and H. Brigham. 1990. "Improvements in Physical Fitness of Kenyan Schoolboys Infected with Hookworm, *Trichuris trichuria* and *Ascaris lumbricoides* Following a Single Dose of Albendazole." *Transactions of the Royal Society for Tropical Medicine and Hygiene* 84:277–82.

Stoll, N. R. 1947. "This Wormy World." *Journal of Parasitology* 33:1–18.

Taylor, H. R., R. D. Semba, H. S. Newland, E. Keyvan-Larijani, A. White, Z. Dukuly, and B. M. Greene. 1989. "Ivermectin Treatment of Patients with Severe Ocular Onchocerciasis." *American Journal of Tropical Medicine and Hygiene* 40:494–500.

Taylor, P., H. M. Murure, K. Manomano. 1988. "Efficacy of Low Doses of Praziquantel for *Schistosoma mansoni* and *S. haematobium.*" *Journal of Tropical Medicine and Hygiene* 91:13–17.

Terry, C., D. A. P. Bundy, and J. Horton. 1989. "Relative Costs of Targeted, Selective, and Selected Chemotherapeutic Control of Geohelminths." PERG/SKF. Mimeo.

Turner, M. J., and J. M. Schaeffer. 1989. "Mode of Action of Ivermectin." In W. C. Campbell, ed., *Ivermectin and Avermectin.* New York: Springer Verlag.

UNICEF (United Nations Childrens Fund). 1989. *Essential Drugs Price List.* Copenhagen: Supply Division.

Wakelin, D. 1978. "Immunity to Intestinal Parasites." *Nature* 273:617–20.

Walsh, J. A. 1990. "Estimating the Burden of Illness in the Tropics." In K. S. Warren and A. A. F. Mahmoud, eds., *Tropical and Geographical Medicine.* New York: McGraw-Hill.

Walsh, J. A., and K. S. Warren. 1979. "Selective Primary Health Care: An Interim Strategy for Disease Control in Developing Countries." *New England Journal of Medicine* 301:967–74.

Warren, K. S. 1973. "Regulation of the Prevalence and Intensity of Schistosomiasis in Man: Immunology or Ecology?" *Journal of Infectious Diseases* 127:595–609.

———. 1989. "Selective Primary Health Care and Parasitic Diseases in McAdam, KPR." In K. P. R. McAdam, ed., *New Strategies in Parasitology.* London: Churchill Livingstone.

Warren, K.S., and A. A. F. Mahmoud. 1990. *Tropical and Geographical Medicine.* 2d ed. New York: McGraw Hill.

Warren, K. S., J. H. Ouma, T. Arap Siongok, and H. B. Houser. 1978. "Hycanthone Dose-Response in *Schistosoma mansoni* Infection in Kenya." *Lancet* 1:352–54.

WHO (World Health Organization). 1980. *Sixth Report on the World Health Situation.* Part 1, *Global Analysis.* Geneva.

———. 1985. "The Control of Schistosomiasis." Technical Report Series 728. Geneva.

———. 1987a. *Atlas of the Global Distribution of Schistosomes.* Geneva.

———. 1987b. "Prevention and Control of Intestinal Parasitic Infections." Technical Report Series 749. Geneva.

Wilkins, H. A. 1989. "Reinfection after Treatment of Schistosome Infections." *Parasitology Today* 3:83–88.

Yekutiel, P. 1980. "Eradication of Infectious Diseases." In M. A. Klinsberg, ed., *Contributions to Epidemiology and Biostatistics*, vol. 2. Basel: Karger.

Young, M. E., and A. Prost. 1985. "Child Health in China." World Bank Staff Working Paper. Washington, D.C.

8

Measles

Stanley O. Foster, Deborah A. McFarland, and A. Meredith John

Measles is a highly infectious disease transmitted person-to-person by way of the respiratory route; the severity of measles (morbidity, disability, and mortality) is affected by a wide range of epidemiologic, demographic, physiologic, socioeconomic, and behavioral determinants. Almost all children unprotected by immunization will be infected with measles; in the developing world, 1 to 5 percent will die of measles and its complications.

In 1954, Enders and Peebles isolated the measles virus, which paved the way for the development of an effective vaccine. Measles vaccine provides long-term protection to susceptible persons. Use of this vaccine has proved effective in reducing measles cases in both industrial and developing countries. With technical direction and leadership from the World Health Organization's (WHO's) Expanded Programme on Immunization (EPI), advocacy and financial support from the United Nations Children's Fund (UNICEF), and bilateral technical cooperation, national immunization programs have increased the global coverage of measles vaccine for children twelve months of age or younger from 20 percent in 1974 to 78 percent in 1990 (WHO 1991). Although global efforts effectively prevented an estimated 2.12 million measles deaths in 1990, an estimated 880,000 deaths were not prevented. In 1989 the WHO World Health Assembly established measles targets for achievement by the year 1995: a 95 percent reduction in measles mortality, a 90 percent reduction in measles incidence, and a measles vaccine coverage of 90 percent in the first year of life. In this chapter we review what is currently known about measles and its control and identify policies, strategies, and practices that will enable the achievement of the global objectives.

Epidemiology

Measles transmission occurs when an infectious individual comes into close contact with a susceptible individual. The probability that an individual will contract measles in a given time period depends upon his or her immune status (susceptibility to infection), the population size and density of the community, the frequency of the individual's contact with other population members, and the probability that such contacts are with an infectious person. Together, these factors determine not only the likelihood that an individual will be infected but also the age pattern of infection and whether measles is maintained endemically in the population or occurs only in sporadic outbreaks or epidemics.

Susceptibility to Infection

Measles transmission results from the exposure of a susceptible person to respiratory droplets or aerosolized droplet nuclei from a measles-infected person (Black 1982; Bloch and others 1985). The probability that an exposed, susceptible person in a household will be infected by the measles virus is 90 percent or higher.

Most infants are protected from measles at birth by passively acquired transplacental maternal antibodies. Breastfeeding practices affect neither the level nor the persistence of measles antibodies. Studies of 2,917 maternal blood samples from twenty different populations in thirteen countries demonstrated measles antibodies in 99.2 percent of samples (Black 1989), suggesting that a corresponding proportion of newborn infants have some degree of passively acquired antibody immunity. The mean duration of this protection varies considerably, however, ranging from three to six months in some populations to twelve months or more in others. Black identified three factors contributing to these interpopulation differences: (a) "the women of different countries have different amounts of measles antibody to pass to their children"—maternal titers as measured by hemagglutination inhibition in Gazankulu, South Africa, were eightfold higher than those from Taiwan; (b) "there are genetic or environmentally determined differences in the efficiency of the placenta in transporting IgG [immunoglobin G]"—that is, simultaneous collections of maternal and cord blood have shown maternal-infant differences in hemagglutination inhibition titer ranging from +0.86 $\log_2$ in New Haven, Connecticut, to -0.97 $\log_2$ in Kuala Lumpur, Malaysia; and (c) "there are differences in the rate at which children lose passively acquired antibody immunity"—for example, differences in the half-life of maternally acquired antibody (Black 1989, p. 19). These differences may be related to the rate of infection with other infectious agents, leading to increased catabolism of IgG, and higher rates of diarrhea, leading to increased loss of IgG into the interior lumen of the gut (Black 1989, p. 19). Geographic variations in the age at which infants lose passive immunity, as estimated by serologic studies, are consistent with observed patterns of immunologic response to vaccine or disease on exposure to infection.

Age of Infection in Four Populations

Individuals exposed to measles virus and not protected by either maternal or vaccine-acquired immunity usually develop infection. Age-specific rates of measles infection are determined by the number of infective measles cases in the population, the size and age composition of the pool of susceptibles, and the rate and age pattern of contact. Widely divergent age patterns of measles transmission are seen in the following four populations: (a) high-density urban populations in developing countries (for example, Kinshasa, Zaire); (b) rural populations in developing countries with low vaccine coverage (for example, Matlab, Bangladesh); (c) rural populations in developing countries with high vaccine coverage (for example, Lesotho); and (d) populations in industrial countries with high vaccine coverage such as the United States of America (figures 8-1–8-4).

HIGH-DENSITY URBAN—IN DEVELOPING COUNTRIES. In large cities in western and central Africa, an urban transmission pattern prevails; measles occurs primarily in the first two years of life. The early age of infection can be attributed to the high population density, the early exposure of infants to infectious individuals as mothers carry their babies on their backs on crowded public transport and in urban markets, and the early loss of maternally acquired antibody in relation to such loss in industrial countries. Measles is endemic in the population and

cases occur continuously. Data on 10,078 measles cases from the preimmunization era were collected from the Lagos Infectious Disease Hospital in Nigeria; they showed that 36 percent of hospitalized cases occurred in infants twelve months of age or younger (the median age of infection was fifteen months) and that 85 percent of admissions were of children less than thirty-six months old (Smith and Foster 1970). Moderate levels of vaccine coverage have not always changed this urban pattern of early infection. In Kinshasa, Zaire, where measles vaccine coverage during 1983 in children of twelve through fifty-nine months was 62 percent, a community survey showed high rates of measles transmission in infants and young children as indicated by the following age distribution of cases: six through eight months, 18 percent; nine through eleven months, 19 percent; one year, 40 percent; and two years, 10 percent (figure 8-1) (Taylor and others 1988). An estimated 77 percent of cases occurred prior to age three.

RURAL—IN DEVELOPING COUNTRIES WITH LOW VACCINE COVERAGE. In rural areas, where contact between young, susceptible children and infectious individuals is less frequent than in urban areas, measles is primarily a disease of childhood. Community surveillance data from Matlab, Bangladesh, collected prior to the introduction of measles vaccine, showed 23 percent of cases occurring in children under two years, 34 percent in children two and three years old, 22 percent in children four and five years old, and 22 percent in children six to ten years old (figure 8-2) (Koster and others 1981). Although the population density in Bangladesh is one of the highest in the world, the relative isolation of rural enclaves, the riverine geography, and the limited social mobility of the traditional Moslem culture result in a low probability that the measles virus will be introduced into a village and thus a low probability of exposure

Figure 8-1. Age Distribution of Measles, Kinshasa, Zaire, 1983

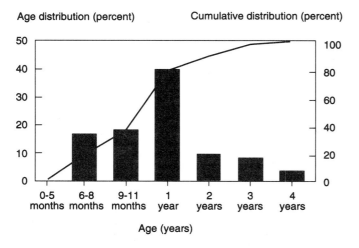

Source: Taylor and others 1988.

Figure 8-2. Age Distribution of Measles, Matlab, Bangladesh, 1975–76

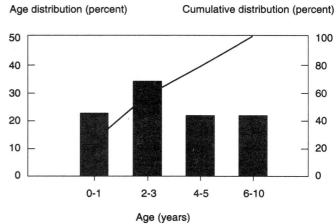

Source: Koster and others 1981.

Figure 8-3. Age Distribution of Measles, Lesotho, 1988

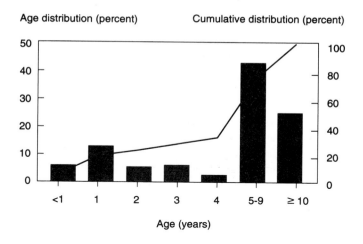

Source: Lesotho 1990.

Figure 8-4. Age Distribution of Measles, United States, 1989

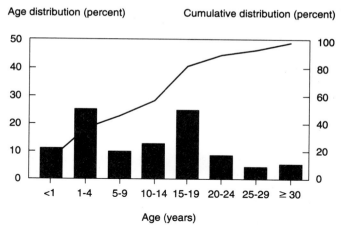

Source: MMWR 1990.

of susceptibles to measles infection. In such areas, measles occurs in sporadic epidemics and vanishes between outbreaks.

RURAL—IN DEVELOPING COUNTRIES WITH HIGH VACCINE COVERAGE. Many developing countries are achieving 80 percent measles immunization during the first year of life, the target established for 1990. In countries with low population density—for example, Lesotho—significant reductions in measles incidence and a corresponding change in the age pattern of disease have been documented. The age at onset of measles has increased; 60 percent of cases occur in children over five years of age (Lesotho 1990) (figure 8-3). This change is not being seen in the more densely populated developing countries with similar levels of vaccine coverage, such as Rwanda, Burundi, and Malawi.

INDUSTRIAL COUNTRIES WITH HIGH VACCINE COVERAGE. In the United States, where, in the prevaccine era, measles was primarily a disease of children, childhood immunization coupled with mandatory school immunization has reduced measles incidence by 98 percent (Markowitz and Orenstein 1990). The national goal of measles elimination has, however, been frustrated by outbreaks affecting urban preschoolers, who are primarily unvaccinated, and high school and college students, who, as a group, are highly vaccinated. The latter outbreaks represent transmission among the 2 to 5 percent who are not protected by a single dose of measles vaccine (United States, National Vaccine Advisory Committee 1991).

Measles Infection and Its Cost

While measles is recognized as an acute childhood infection, the long-term costs in terms of morbidity, disability, and mortality are less well understood.

Clinical Illness

Measles is a clinical illness easily recognized both by health workers and by experienced family members, and it frequently has a distinct name in the local language. The disease has been well described by Preblud and Katz: after an incubation period of ten to twelve days, "the prodromal stage is heralded by the onset of fever, malaise, conjunctivitis, coryza, and tracheobronchitis manifesting as cough, and it lasts for 2–4 days. . . . The temperature rises during the ensuing 4 days and may be as high as 40.6° C. . . . The rash is an erythematous maculopapular eruption that usually appears 14 days after exposure and spreads from the head to the extremities over 3–4 days. Over the next 3–4 days, the rash fades in the order of appearance. Desquamation can be detected in areas of greatest involvement" (Preblud and Katz 1988, p. 183).

Naturally occurring measles infection provides lifetime protection against reinfection. This was clearly demonstrated in the 1846 outbreak in the Faroe Islands, where infection was limited to those under age sixty-five, individuals born after the last measles epidemic in 1781 (Panum 1939).

In severe disease, a frequent occurrence in developing countries, the manifestations of clinical illness reflect the epithelial loci of infection as illustrated in Morley's classic diagram of severe measles: eyes (conjunctivitis), larynx (laryngitis), lungs (pneumonia), and gastrointestinal tract (diarrhea [Morley 1973, p. 214]; figure 8-5).

Complications

Most measles deaths are attributed to complications, which may be acute (within one month) or delayed (one month to one year). In industrial countries—for example, the United States—the most commonly cited complications are otitis

Figure 8-5. Clinical Manifestations of Severe Measles

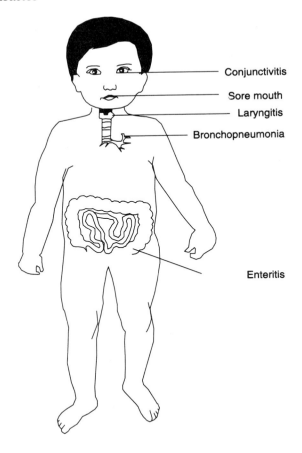

Conjunctivitis
Sore mouth
Laryngitis
Bronchopneumonia
Enteritis

Source: Morley 1979.

media (6 percent), diarrhea (6 percent), pneumonia (4 percent), measles encephalitis (0.2 percent), subacute sclerosing encephalitis (1 in 100,000 measles cases), and death (0.1–0.2 percent) (Preblud and Katz 1988; Atkinson and Markowitz 1991). Fifteen percent of the reported cases in the United States required hospitalization.

The distribution of complications in developing countries is somewhat different. Using active surveillance to identify measles cases in the community, investigators of 2,386 cases of measles in Sri Lanka documented complication frequencies as follows: diarrhea, 37 percent; respiratory infections, 30 percent; ear infections, 7 percent; and convulsions 2 percent (WHO/EPI Sri Lanka 1985). Fifty-seven percent of cases had medical care (Bloch, de Silva, and de Sylva 1983).

Morley's classic study from Imesi-Ile, Nigeria, was the first to document the long-term effect of measles on child health in developing countries. In that study, 25 percent of the children with measles lost 10 percent or more of body weight (Morley 1973). The time required to regain that weight ranged from 4.5 weeks for children with no diarrhea to 8.1 weeks for those with diarrhea. Further data on the relation between

diarrhea and measles come from Bangladesh, where a large outbreak of measles occurred in twelve villages among 5,775 children undergoing prospective surveillance for nutrition and diarrhea (Koster and others 1981). The frequency and duration of diarrheal episodes increased beginning one week before and lasting four weeks after the onset of rash. Fifty-one percent of the diarrheal episodes lasted longer than seven days compared with 25 percent of the diarrheal episodes of those who did not have measles. The case-fatality rate (CFR) for those with measles who had diarrhea episodes longer than seven days (11.9 percent) was significantly greater than the CFR for those with measles but without diarrhea (4.0 percent). Children with postmeasles diarrhea had a significant and prolonged (10 percent) deficit in weight-for-height. In a WHO-sponsored review assessing potential interventions to reduce diarrhea morbidity and mortality, it was projected that measles immunization could prevent 0.6 to 3.8 percent of all diarrheal episodes and 6 to 26 percent of all diarrheal deaths (Feachem and Koblinsky 1983).

Postmeasles pneumonia is the main cause of measles-associated mortality in the developing countries; 56 percent of measles-associated deaths in a community outbreak in Uttar Pradesh in India and 92.8 percent of measles-associated deaths in a hospital in Ilorin, Nigeria, were attributed to pneumonia (Fagbule and Orifunmishe 1988; Narain and others 1989). In the Sri Lanka community survey (CFR, 1.3 percent), 44 percent of measles-associated mortality was attributed to pneumonia, 25 percent to diarrhea, 19 percent to convulsions, and 9 percent to coma (Bloch, de Silva, and de Sylva 1983). Measles is responsible for a significant proportion of acute respiratory morbidity and mortality, 6 to 21 percent of the morbidity and 8 to 93 percent of the mortality (Markowitz and Nieburg 1991).

Studies have documented transient post-measles immunosuppression (Whittle and others 1973; Dossetor, Whittle, and Greenwood 1977; Kaschula, Druker, and Kipps 1983). Hussey and Simpson (1991) have identified immunosuppression as a probable cause of increased risk of nosocomial bacteremia in measles cases (3.37 per 100 hospital admissions), as compared with nonmeasles pediatric admissions (0.57 per 100 admissions). General immunosuppression following measles is an important factor in measles-associated mortality. Autopsy studies, which revealed serious nonbacterial bronchiolar and interstitial necrosis caused by adenovirus, measles virus, and herpes virus, indicate a failure of the immune mechanism in the postmeasles child (Kipps and Kaschula 1976).

The main causes of long-term disability following measles have been identified as blindness and malnutrition. In Africa, where the prevalence of blindness in preschool children is estimated at 1 in 1,000, measles has been identified as responsible for half of childhood blindness (Foster and Johnson 1988).

Mortality

In some developing countries, measles CFRs are 300 times those currently reported in industrial countries. Such rates were common in Europe in the 1800s. In the well-documented outbreak in Sunderland, England, in 1885, 25 of 311 measles patients died, a CFR of 8 percent (Drinkwater 1885). Community studies of measles outbreaks between 1961 and 1978 show CFRs from 1.5 to 15 percent (Walsh 1983; Cutts 1990; Cutts and others 1991). High mortality from measles was initially thought to occur only in Africa, but high CFRs from measles have also been reported in Asia and Latin America, for example, 7 percent in Tamil Nadu, 5.7 percent in Uttar Pradesh, and 4.5 percent in Guatemala (Gordon 1965; John and others 1980; Narain and others 1989).

Although measles outbreaks that result in high mortality are more likely to be investigated and reported, data from prospective surveillance among populations that have been studied in developing countries have also revealed high measles CFRs: 6.5 percent in Kenya; 6.1 percent in Zaire; 6.5 percent in Senegal; and 3.7 percent in Bangladesh (Voorhoeve and others 1977; Kasongo Project Team 1981; Koster and others 1981; Garenne and Aaby 1990). The World Health Organization estimates that 880,000 measles deaths occurred in 1990 (WHO 1991).

Mortality Risk Factors

High infant and child mortality in the developing world is usually attributed to the complex interaction of poverty, undernutrition, and infection. Mosley and Chen have proposed a child mortality proximate determinant model which emphasizes the importance of the complex interactions of maternal behavior, environmental contamination, nutritional deficiency, injury, and personal illness control action including preventive measures and seeking treatment at time of illness (Mosley and Chen 1984). Epidemiologic studies have documented a number of risk factors which explain, in part, the high rates of measles-associated mortality in the developing world.

AGE. Case-fatality rates exhibit substantial variations by age, the higher CFRs occurring in the younger age groups, usually six to eighteen months of age. The age pattern of mortality varies in different populations, reflecting both the epidemiology of the disease and the general health environment in which the child exists. In a recent outbreak in Rwanda, reported age-specific CFRs decreased with age: zero through eight months (3.0 percent); nine months through twenty-three months (1.4 percent); twenty-four months through fifty-nine months (1.0 percent); and sixty months and older (0.5 percent) (Weierbach 1989). In contrast, the Kasongo study from Zaire documented the highest rates in children of thirteen months to twenty-four months: one month to six months, 0 percent; seven months to twelve months, 6.2 percent; thirteen months to twenty-four months, 9.8 percent; twenty-five months to thirty-six months, 4.3 percent; and thirty-seven months to sixty months, 2.8 percent (Kasongo Project Team 1981). Data from Bangladesh show similar CFRs from measles in all age groups: one month to twenty-three months, 4.4 percent; twenty-four months to forty-seven months, 4.2 percent; and forty-eight months to seventy-one months, 4.2 percent (Koster and others 1981).

GENDER. In two studies from Asia, CFRs were higher for females than for males. In Bangladesh, the CFR among males (0.98 percent) was significantly less than for females (2.64 percent) (Bhuiya and others 1987). Similar results were reported from Varanasi in India: 1.3 percent for males and 3.3 percent for females (Chand and others 1989). Such differences have not been documented in African studies, suggesting that differences arise from sex-specific patterns of child care and response to illness rather than to biological differences between the sexes.

SOCIOECONOMIC STATUS. Using a multivariate logistic regression analysis of community data collected in the Matlab Bangladesh field area, Bhuiya and others (1987) identified low number of household articles owned (a proxy indicator of poverty) as a significant risk factor for measles mortality.

INTENSITY OF EXPOSURE: ACQUISITION OF MEASLES IN THE HOME. Aaby, in his studies in Guinea-Bissau, documented increased rates of measles mortality in secondary cases acquired in the home (Aaby 1988). Reexamination of the Machakos data from Kenya and ORSTOM data from Senegal has shown similar findings (Aaby and Leeuwenburg 1988; Garenne and Aaby 1990). In the Senegal data, odds ratios (OR) on mortality risk were related to the probable intensity of exposure: same hut (OR 3.8, 95 percent confidence interval CI, 1.7–8.4), same household (OR 2.3, 95 percent [CI], 1.0–5.7), and same compound (OR 1.9, 95 percent CI, 0.6–6.0).

NUTRITIONAL STATUS. Although high mortality from measles is seen in undernourished populations, individual nutritional status has not proved to be a reliable predictor of mortality in most studies (Aaby 1988; Koster and others 1981). During the last decade, vitamin A deficiency has been increasingly linked to higher child mortality and to high measles-associated mortality (Sommer 1990). In Tanzania, a clinical trial showed decreased measles mortality in hospitalized patients who received vitamin A (Barclay, Foster, and Sommer 1987). In Zaire, a multivariate logistic regression model of 283 measles patients admitted to two Kinshasa hospitals identified an increased mortality risk in children less than two years of age with a vitamin A level of less than 5 micrograms per deciliter (relative risk [RR] 2.9—CI 1.3–6.8 [Markowitz and others 1989]). In South Africa, a randomized double-blind trial using vitamin A in the treatment of 189 measles cases reduced measles mortality by half; the durations of pneumonia, diarrhea, croup, and hospitalization were shortened (Hussey and Klein 1990). Of historical note is Hussey's reference to a preantibiotic-era paper by Ellison (1932), in which intensive vitamin therapy reduced measles CFR from 8.7 percent to 3.7 percent and measles pneumonia CFR from 67.7 percent to 31.3 percent. Measles and its sequelae have also been identified as significant risk factors contributing to the development of protein-calorie malnutrition and kwashiorkor.

ABSENT OR DELAYED MEDICAL CARE. Most of the mortality associated with measles can be prevented through timely and appropriate medical care. In Senegal, early treatment of measles has resulted in the near elimination of measles mortality (Garenne and others 1992). Timely appropriate case management is rare in many developing countries because of lack of access to care, delayed seeking of care, lack of trained personnel, or lack of appropriate drugs. Contact with health facilities usually occurs late in the illness. In a hospital-based study from Burkina Faso, 55 percent of measles deaths occurred within twenty-four hours of admission (Sahuguede and others 1989). The symptoms upon admission to the hospital of 714 measles patients illustrate the seriousness of illness at the time of entry into the hospital: dehydration (91 percent), diarrhea (64 percent), conjunctivitis (56 percent), fever above 39.5° C (50 percent), respiratory infection (46 percent), and cardiovascular collapse (34.5 percent).

LOCAL TREATMENT. In many traditional cultures, measles is considered a normal event. In others, it has been attributed to the work of witches or sorcerers (Imperato and Traore 1969). Withholding food, especially protein, and fluids from measles cases has been reported (Morley 1973). In the Machakos data, measles was identified among "God's diseases" (Maina-Ahlberg 1979). Withholding of water and milk from children sick with measles was documented in 62 percent of 242 cases. Of cases reported, 50 percent received indigenous medicines and 98 percent also received Western medicine. Local treatments, restriction of fluids and food, delay in access to effective chemotherapy, and use of potential toxic substances have been identified as potential contributors to increased measles-associated mortality.

NONVACCINATION. The single most important determinant of measles morbidity and mortality is vaccination status. Almost all children unprotected by measles vaccine will eventually be infected with measles and 1 to 5 percent will die.

Economic Cost

The economic cost of a disease can be divided into direct and indirect costs. Direct costs are those borne by the health system in the prevention and treatment of the disease and by households or individuals in seeking preventive services or treatment. Indirect costs are usually measured in terms of lost productivity of workers as a result of their premature death or disability.

Few estimates of the costs for treatment of measles have been made in developing countries. Because care is generally delayed or absent, reliable data on costs of treatment for measles cases is not routinely available. In a study in Mexico, Cardenas-Ayala and others (1989) estimated the costs of medical care (hospitalization, physician's visits, medical treatment, and re-

habilitation) for measles patients; they also estimated the number of deaths that would have occurred in the absence of a measles immunization program. The analysis demonstrated large societal benefits of measles immunization with a benefit-to-cost ratio of 100 to 1. Indirect costs were estimated to be approximately 77 times the direct costs, but the authors acknowledge that the direct-cost measure represents a very low level of access to care and a severe underreporting of measles cases. A previous study (Verduzco, Calderon, and Velazquez-Franco 1974) of measles immunization in Mexico calculated a benefit-to-cost ratio of 27 to 1, although indirect costs (as measured by lost earnings) were not estimated.

Estimates of both direct and indirect costs attributable to measles were made in a study comparing Israel, the West Bank, and Gaza (Ginsberg and Tulchinsky 1990). Total costs for patients with simple cases of measles, patients requiring hospitalization, and patients with complications were estimated in each of the three regions. Estimates for a simple case of measles (treated in the outpatient setting) ranged from $13 in Gaza to $141 in Israel.[1] Costs of early mortality due to measles ranged from $11,628 in Gaza to $76,518 in Israel. The wide range in the latter estimates highlights one of the most difficult methodological issues in making estimates of premature mortality—that of placing a monetary value on life. Any of the available methods relates valuation of life to social productivity and is usually measured in discounted future expected earnings. Thus, the value of a life in Gaza, a region with low earnings and income, is valued below a life in Israel, an area with higher per capita income.

The economic cost of measles in industrial countries has been measured in more detail. Using 1983 data in the United States, White, Koplan, and Orenstein (1985) estimated a benefit-to-cost ratio for measles immunization of 11.9 to 1. Both direct and indirect costs were estimated with and without a vaccination program. Indirect costs were 3.2 times direct costs. The cost per measles case was estimated to be $209 (in 1983 dollars). Cost-benefit studies of measles immunization have consistently demonstrated large social benefits (Mast and others 1990) because of the high direct cost of treating complications of measles cases, the attendant indirect costs of work and productivity loss, and the relatively low cost of immunization programs.

The economic burden of measles can also be measured by days of healthy life lost as a result of premature mortality and disability. In Mali (Duflo and others 1986), measles ranked fifth among diseases in terms of days of healthy life lost, with 94.7 percent of the days lost because of premature death (as opposed to illness or disability). Losses resulting from measles accounted for 6.4 percent of the total days of healthy life lost in Mali. An earlier study in Ghana (Ghana Health Assessment Project Team 1981) ranked measles second, accounting for 7.3 percent of the total days of healthy life lost in the population.

Barnum (1989) notes the importance of applying a discount factor in order to account for the fact that the number of healthy life-years lost which are attributed to a disease each year do not actually occur in that year. The choice of discount factor is thus critically important when ranking diseases by productive life lost. Using the Ghana data, Barnum shows that the relative ranking of measles among diseases is second when the discount rate is zero but is fifteenth when the discount rate is 0.20. When the discount rate is zero, the diseases with the greatest cost in lost productivity are the diseases of childhood, such as measles, but as the discount rate rises, adult problems increase in importance and childhood diseases fall in significance.

Prevention of Measles

Measles can be prevented through immunization of the susceptible child with a potent live virus vaccine.

Vaccine

The history, uses, and effectiveness of measles vaccines are discussed below.

HISTORY. Measles virus was first isolated in the 1950s by Enders and Peebles (1954) from a child infected with measles and was attenuated through passage in tissue culture. Most of the vaccine strains used today (Schwarz, Moraten, Beckenham, Edmonston-Zagreb, EKC, and AIK-C) were developed from the original Edmonston isolation (Preblud and Katz 1988). The Leningrad-16 strain used in the former U.S.S.R. and eastern Europe, the strains used in China, and the CAM-70 strain were derived independently of the Edmonston isolation (Clements and others 1988). Heat stability of most strains has been increased through the addition of stabilizers. The minimum recommended dose of current standard measles vaccine applied at or after the age of nine months is 1,000 median tissue culture infective dose given subcutaneously in the arm.

AGE OF IMMUNIZATION. Because of differences in the duration of protection from passive maternal protection and differences in risk of exposure, selection of the age of immunization requires a balancing of two factors: "the earliest age at which high rates of seroconversion can be obtained, and the age group with the greatest risk of infection" (Orenstein and others 1986). On the basis of epidemiologic data on age-specific measles incidence and age-specific seroconversion data, WHO has recommended nine months as the optimal age for measles immunization in most developing countries (Kenyan Ministry of Health and WHO 1977; WHO/EPI Kenya 1979). In Haiti, seroconversion to a standard dose of Schwarz vaccine ranged from 45 percent in six-month-old children to 100 percent in children at twelve months of age (Halsey and others 1985). In some industrial countries, 100 percent seroconversion is not obtained until children are fifteen months of age. In the United States, policy recommendations regarding age for measles immunization have changed three times in response to field data on vaccine efficacy. Measles immunization was initially introduced in children at nine months of age. When challenge with wild virus identified vaccine failures in children

vaccinated at nine to eleven months and subsequently in those vaccinated at twelve to fourteen months, the minimum age of immunization was increased to twelve months in 1965 and then to fifteen months in 1976 (Orenstein and others 1986). In 1989, a two-dose measles vaccine schedule was recommended (ACIP 1989). The United States experience emphasizes the importance of epidemiology, disease surveillance, and outbreak investigation in setting and amending national vaccine policies.

In Lesotho, where the age for measles immunization is nine months and coverage has reached 80 percent, 60 percent of cases occur in school-age children. Serologic studies using enzyme-linked immunosorbent assay have documented 13.6 percent seronegativity in six- and seven-year-old children entering school (Lesotho 1990). When a policy of vaccinating all schoolchildren for the first time, regardless of vaccine history, proved difficult to maintain, a second dose of measles vaccine was added to the routine scheduled booster dose of the diphtheria-pertussis-tetanus (DPT) at fifteen months.

Immunization with potent vaccine administered at the recommended age does not ensure seroconversion or protection. Primary vaccine failures (the lack of a serologic and immunologic response to initial immunization) do occur. Secondary vaccine failures (the occurrence of disease in previously successfully immunized children) have been reported but are thought to be rare. In a vaccine study population in British Columbia, 93 percent of 188 children responded serologically to immunization. This percentage corresponds to a primary vaccine failure rate of 7 percent. In 1985–86 an outbreak of measles occurred in the same British Columbia study population; 9 of the 175 original seroconverters developed measles, corresponding to a secondary vaccine failure rate of 5 percent (Mathias and others 1989). Low rates (2 to 5 percent) of secondary vaccine failure have also been documented by other authors (Edmonson and others 1990; Markowitz, Preblud, Fine, and Orenstein 1990).

VACCINE EFFICACY. Orenstein and colleagues (1985) have outlined a range of methods for the field evaluation of vaccine efficacy (VE), including screening methods that can be used at health facilities, outbreak investigations, and case control studies. Several factors limit vaccine efficacy. They include the following:

- Interference with vaccine virus replication by prenatally acquired maternal antibody

- Exposure to wild virus infection prior to the recommended or actual time of immunization

- Impotent vaccine resulting from failure of the cold chain (the system designed to ensure vaccine potency from site of manufacture, through shipment, to central storage, to distribution, to peripheral storage, to dilution with cold diluent, to vaccine delivery)

- Incorrect administration of measles vaccine, for example, administration of less than the required 0.5 cubic centimeters or immunization at an inappropriate age

• Failure of immunologic response of a susceptible person to potent vaccine for unknown reasons

In industrial countries, vaccine efficacy in children vaccinated at twelve months to fifteen months of age is high. In Poland, measles vaccine efficacy has been estimated at 97 percent (WHO/EPI Poland 1986). In a measles outbreak investigated in Browning, Montana, vaccine efficacy was estimated at 96.9 percent (95 percent CI 89.5–98.2) (Davis and others 1987). Evidence to date indicates that live virus measles immunization also induces life-long immunity in most individuals (Markowitz, Preblud, Fine, and Orenstein 1990). In developing countries, where logistics and maintenance of the cold chain are difficult, seroconversion studies have occasionally documented low rates of seroconversion: 40 percent in Yaoundé, Cameroon, and 0 percent in Guinea-Bissau (McBean and others 1976; Aaby and others 1989). Most outbreak investigations in developing countries, however, document rates of vaccine efficacy in the range of 70 to 90 percent. Examples include community and hospital studies of urban measles in Point Noire, Congo, which reported vaccine efficacies of 78 percent and 87 percent, respectively; a Tanzanian case-control study in which card-documented records revealed a vaccine efficacy of 96 percent (95 percent confidence level 83–99 percent); and a recent study in rural Burundi that reported a vaccine efficacy of 72.4 percent (Dabis and others 1988; Chen 1990; Killewo and others 1991). Even under good cold-chain conditions, vaccine efficacy in developing countries is lower than in industrial countries because vaccine is applied at an age when 10 to 20 percent of children still have maternal antibody. Because of the risk of infection at an early age, vaccination cannot be delayed.

COST-EFFECTIVENESS: EPI. Total costs of the Expanded Programme on Immunization have been estimated in a number of countries (Brenzel 1990, 1991). Although the range is quite wide, the average cost of approximately $15.00 per fully immunized child (BCG vaccine, oral polio vaccine [OPV; four times], DPT [three times], and measles) appears to be indicative of true program costs. Comparisons of the cost per fully immunized child for alternative immunization strategies are approximately $11.00 for facility-based programs, $10.60 for mobile programs, and $15.60 for accelerated strategies.

Several crucial questions remain regarding the cost of immunization programs, including the relationship of costs to coverage, the effect of technology on costs, the current cost levels and the ability of countries to meet stated immunization targets (Rosenthal 1990), the distribution of costs between countries and donor groups, and the relative costs of alternative immunization strategies (for example, campaigns) and sustainable increases in coverage. Furthermore, all the EPI cost studies have been at one point in time; they have not been conducted in conjunction with coverage surveys over time. It is thus difficult to predict changes in cost per fully immunized child as coverage increases. The 1995 targets established by

WHO and endorsed at the 1990 World Summit for Children (90 percent reduction in measles morbidity and 95 percent reduction in measles mortality) were estimated for the Task Force on Child Survival at $15 per child for up to 80 percent coverage and then an additional $1 for each 1 percent increase in coverage up to $30 for 95 percent coverage (Forgy and others 1990). The authors of two studies conducted in Swaziland five years apart, 1984 and 1989, calculated a cost per fully immunized child of approximately $55 for coverage rates of 70 percent and 71 percent, respectively (Robertson 1985; McFarland and Kraushaar 1990). Although the costs are high in relation to other countries, they reflect the tradeoffs of achieving high coverage rates in a small population (approximately 700,000) with excellent access to health services and extensive surveillance and outbreak control activities. The Swaziland studies emphasize the importance of understanding the context in which health services are delivered and the fallacy of applying average cost figures for across all countries and all settings.

The cost of the measles component of the EPI total cost can be determined either as an incremental cost to the total or as the cost base of EPI to which other antigens are added. Using the first method, Phillips, Feachem, and Mills (1987) calculated the incremental cost of adding measles immunization to an existing EPI program as $1.35 (in 1982 dollars). Shepherd, Sanoh, and Coffi (1986) used the second method in Côte d'Ivoire, allocating 75 percent of EPI costs to the measles component. The cost per child vaccinated against measles was $12.30 (in 1980 dollars). The authors of an earlier study in Zambia, using slightly different methods, derived a cost of $8.00 to $14.00 (in 1982 dollars) per child vaccinated against measles in the rural areas and $2.00 to $5.00 in urban areas (Ponninghaus 1980). When estimating the cost of achieving the 1995 measles targets, Forgy and others (1990) attributed the entire cost of EPI ($15.00 per vaccinated child) to the measles component. Those who used UNICEF mortality figures estimated total worldwide costs for achieving the targets to be $5.707 billion; those who used World Bank mortality estimates arrived at a total worldwide cost of $8.517 billion.

Besides variation in methods used to assign costs to the measles component of EPI, several factors influence cost estimates, including the level of immunization activity (volume), the ratio of fixed costs to variable costs, prices of key inputs, the type of technology used, and the productivity of personnel providing services (Brenzel and Claquin 1991). Understanding cost behavior can assist program managers and donor agencies in controlling these factors and thus influencing the costs of measles immunizations.

Most cost studies of EPI and measles immunization focus on the direct cost to the system of providing the service rather than the cost to the family or household in seeking immunization services. Thus, cost figures routinely underestimate the full societal cost of an immunization program.

Given the range of cost and effectiveness estimates, it is not surprising that cost-effectiveness measures of measles immunization vary considerably. Several studies have attempted to measure cost-effectiveness of measles immunization by the number of measles cases prevented and measles deaths prevented. These estimates are compared in table 8-1.

Since measles contributes to morbidity and mortality from diarrhea, the same measures of cost-effectiveness can be calculated for diarrheal cases and deaths prevented as a result of measles immunization. Phillips, Feachem, and Mills (1987) estimate the cost per diarrheal case prevented at $7 (in 1982 dollars) and the cost per diarrheal death prevented at $143. Another measure of the cost-effectiveness of different diseases and interventions is the number of disability-adjusted life-years (DALYs) added for each intervention. Using data from Côte d'Ivoire and Zambia, Prescott, Prost, and Le Berre (1984) compared the cost-effectiveness of measles immunization with an onchocerciasis program in Upper Volta (now Burkina Faso) with regard to disability-adjusted life-years added. For measles immunization, the cost per DALY is $49 (in 1977 dollars) in Côte d'Ivoire and $56 in Zambia, compared with $150 for the onchocerciasis program.

Great care should be exercised in interpreting and extending the results of cost-effectiveness studies. As Brenzel and Claquin (1991) note, the most cost-effective intervention is not necessarily the most efficient; future costs of programs should cautiously be projected from cost-effectiveness studies because average costs do not remain the same over time; and overall cost savings do not necessarily accrue when the most cost-effective interventions are implemented, because resource allocation decisions are not made solely on the basis of cost-effectiveness results. Findings from cost-effectiveness studies are but one type of information for decisionmaking and must be weighed alongside political, ethical, organizational, managerial, and other factors.

Immunization programs have been the subject of many cost-effectiveness analyses, perhaps because of the large donor investment in such programs and because of the relatively straightforward measure of effectiveness employed. But immunization programs and other preventive interventions should not be subject to a standard which exceeds that of other services, in particular treatment and curative services. When cost-effectiveness analysis is employed, it should be applied to the whole range of services and interventions available in order to obtain a fairer assessment of how all resources are used and how such resources might be more effectively allocated.

Table 8-1. Costs per Measles Case and Death Prevented
(1980 U.S. dollars)

Country	Case prevented	Death prevented
The Gambia	1.96	41
Côte d'Ivoire	14.00	480
Cameroon	3.30	30–60

Source: Makinen 1980; Shepherd, Sanoh, and Coffi 1986; Robertson and others 1987.

EFFECT ON CHILD SURVIVAL. In 1981, *Lancet* published an article on measles in Zaire which questioned the effect of measles immunization on child survival: "In a zone with high measles case-fatality, the risk of dying between the ages of 7 and 35 months for a vaccinated population was compared with an unvaccinated control group. Life-table analysis for both groups showed that measles vaccination reduced the risk of dying at the age of maximum exposure to measles. The gain in survival probability, however, tended to diminish afterwards to approach that of the unvaccinated group" (Kasongo Project Team 1981, p. 33).

Although the interpretation of these data was questioned (Aaby and others 1981), the issue of replacement mortality has not, until recently, been adequately addressed. Several recent studies, however, have assessed the effect of measles immunization on child survival.

Because a definitive double-blind placebo control study would not be ethical, a variety of methods have been used in the following epidemiologic analyses to assess the effect of measles vaccine on child survival. In developing countries with high mortality in children under five, measles vaccine increases child survival.

• Bangladesh: Using a case-control methodology, Clemens and others matched 536 deaths of children ten to sixty months of age with two age and gender matched neighborhood controls. Measles immunization was associated with a 36 percent (95 percent CI 21–48 percent) proportionate reduction in overall mortality rate. For deaths plausibly associated with measles (measles, pneumonia, diarrhea, and malnutrition), vaccine effectiveness was estimated at 57 percent.

• Bangladesh: Using a cohort methodology and the same population described above, but with an additional year of follow-up, Koenig and others (1990) matched 8,135 vaccinated-unvaccinated pairs by month and year of birth. The mortality rate for the immunized children was 45 percent less than that of the controls ($P < .0001$, Gehan-Wilcoxon test $X^2 = 4.18$). Differences were significant for all children immunized under three years of age.

• Guinea-Bissau: Aaby and others (1989) found that, in a population in which serological data identified a subgroup of children not responding to measles vaccine, subsequent mortality among responders to vaccine (4.8 percent) was significantly less than among nonresponders (13.2 percent), a threefold difference in mortality.

• Haiti: Using a logistic regression model, Holt and colleagues (1990) followed up 1,381 children vaccinated to measure seroconversion rates; two and one half years later, infants who were seronegative at the time of vaccination had significantly lower mortality (1.27 percent) than that of nonvaccinated infants (6.62 percent). The adjusted odds ratio in a multivariate stepwise logistic regression associating measles vaccine with survival was 6.5 (95 percent CI 1.6–27.1). Estimates of measles vaccine effectiveness in prevention of mortality in children from nine months to thirty-nine months of age ranged from 84.7 percent to 90 percent.

- Senegal: Data from the Khombole study area in Senegal (Garenne and Cantrelle 1986) showed that children six to thirty-six months of age who had been immunized against measles had an overall mortality risk 31 percent lower than nonimmunized controls (*P* = .028).

These data strongly suggest that the survival benefit of measles vaccine is significantly greater than that predicted by measles-specific mortality. Longitudinal data from the Medical Research Council in the Gambia suggest a modest effect on infant mortality but a more marked effect on child mortality when compared with preimmunization data from an adjoining area (Greenwood and others 1987).

The importance of measles in decreasing child survival can also be estimated from retrospective (verbal autopsy) studies of child mortality by cause. Such studies have been used to assess the relative contribution of measles to overall mortality. Using the criteria of age greater than 120 days and rash with fever for at least 3 days, Kalter and others (1990) estimated sensitivity and specificity of a diagnosis of measles as cause of death at 98 percent and 90 percent, respectively. In Sri Lanka, in an analysis of reported deaths among children six months to thirteen years, it was estimated that measles or a measles complication was associated with 53 percent of 122 deaths (WHO/EPI Sri Lanka 1985). In Rangoon, Burma, verbal autopsy follow-up reports of 249 deaths of children age six months to ten years, identified from death certificates, attributed 35 percent of the deaths to measles and its complications (WHO/EPI Burma 1985). Reported causes of mortality attributed to measles included pneumonia, chronic diarrhea, and malnutrition. In a prospective study in Senegal during a period of eight years, measles accounted for 31 percent of deaths of children six months to nine years of age (Pison and Bonneuil 1988).

ALTERNATIVE MEASLES VACCINES. Seroconversion rates to the standard Schwarz strain are low when it is administered prior to nine months of age, and the risk of measles infection is great in high-density areas, where as many as 30 percent of reported measles cases may occur prior to the age of nine months. Because of these factors, improved measles control in areas of high population density requires a vaccine which can be effectively administered before the earliest age of infection, four months to six months. Studies in Mexico by Sabin and others (1983), who used the human diploid Edmonston-Zagreb (EZ) vaccine strain, showed that administration of this vaccine could produce seroconversion in the presence of maternal antibody. Field trials in the Gambia, Guinea-Bissau, Mexico, and Haiti have documented the effectiveness of high-titer EZ vaccine when administered at six months and, in some cases, four months of age (Whittle and others 1984; Aaby and others 1988; Markowitz and others 1990; Job and others 1991). In 1989 the WHO/EPI Global Advisory Group recommended the introduction of high-titer EZ vaccine in areas where measles is a significant cause of mortality in the first year of life (WHO/EPI

1989b). Lack of availability of large quantities of the vaccine has limited the implementation of the WHO recommendation. In Senegal, prospective follow-up of children immunized with high-titer EZ and Schwarz vaccines has shown increased child mortality (Garenne and others 1991). Increased mortality after immunization with high-titer vaccines has also been reported from Guinea-Bissau and Haiti (WHO, personal communication, June 1992). The World Health Organization no longer recommends use of high-titer EZ vaccine (WHO/EPI 1992). Although there is a clear need for an effective measles vaccine for children at six months of age, alternatives to the current EZ vaccine will need to be developed.

Management of Immunization Activities

Many of the obstacles to the reduction of measles morbidity and mortality stem from suboptimal management. Listed below are ten critical areas which determine, in large part, the effectiveness of immunization programs. Each of these areas should be reviewed at least annually at the national and subnational level to assess the appropriateness and effectiveness of policy, strategy, and implementation. Although some factors can be monitored through analyses of routine data (coverage and disease incidence), others require collection of data through supervision, surveys, outbreak investigations, or management audits.

- *Policy.* Is the current immunization policy—for example, schedule—consistent with current technical knowledge (the guidelines of the WHO/EPI Global Advisory Group) and the in-country epidemiology of the EPI diseases? Within-country policy variations may be required to meet different epidemiologic situations (for example, urban slums, rural nomad population).

- *Targets.* Are there national targets for coverage and disease reduction? Are these targets understandable, realistic, and measurable? Do local areas have the responsibility and authority to set local targets, to measure their achievements, and to alter program implementation?

- *Strategies.* Are national and local strategies designed to ensure the achievement of targets? If not, what alterations are needed?

- *Logistics.* Is the national system of vaccine and equipment procurement and distribution adequate to ensure the availability of essential commodities (cold chain, potent vaccines, sterilizers, needles and syringes, vaccination cards) at every immunization delivery point?

- *Training and supervision.* Is there a central authority responsible for ensuring that preservice and inservice education are providing current knowledge on policy, strategy, and practice? Is there a national system of performance assessment, supervision, or surveys which provides data on the quality of immunization delivery (Foster and others 1990; Heiby 1990)?

• *Access.* Do local health jurisdictions have maps of their service areas and a sense of responsibility for the people living within those areas? What percentage of the population has access to immunization services? How can access be increased?

• *Coverage.* What percentage of the at-risk population has been immunized with measles vaccine by twelve months of age? Two methods are used to assess immunization coverage: (a) dividing the number of immunizations reportedly administered under one year of age by the number of surviving infants and (b) completing coverage surveys as recommended by WHO (1988). If local or national targets have not been achieved, what can be done to achieve these targets?

• *Morbidity and mortality reduction.* Is there a routine or sentinel reporting system to monitor trends in measles incidence? Are morbidity reduction targets being achieved? If not, what changes in policy or strategy are needed?

• *High-risk strategy.* Are epidemiologic data available to identify populations at increased risk of dying when infected with measles (high case-fatality rates)? If so, how can strategies be altered to ensure high coverage in those populations?

• *Community participation.* Does the local community participate in immunization through identification of individuals in need of vaccination, publicity of time and place for vaccine delivery, and in disease surveillance?

Surveillance

Achievement of the 1995 morbidity and mortality reduction targets will require improvements in measles surveillance in the following areas:

• Documentation of morbidity and mortality associated with measles infection

• Identification of population groups at high risk of mortality

• The monitoring of trends in measles incidence

• Assessment of the effectiveness of program interventions

• Identification and targeting of program failures in order to reformulate, where necessary, policies and strategies and to define research priorities.

Traditionally, disease surveillance is understood as the routine reporting of morbidity and mortality from health facilities, through intermediary levels, for collation, analysis, and reporting at the national level. This traditional approach to surveillance is flawed on two accounts: (a) measles surveillance data are most useful at the level of collection and (b) achievement of the surveillance objectives listed above requires the use of multiple surveillance methodologies. In table 8-2 we summarize types of surveillance methods useful in effectively managing measles immunization programs.

Table 8-2. Surveillance Methods Used in Measles Control

Surveillance method	Use of data
Routine reporting[a]	Monitor trends in incidence over time Identify foci of measles for case investigation
Sentinel surveillance	Monitor trends in incidence over time Monitor demographic and epidemiologic characteristics of cases Identify high-risk populations
Outbreak investigations[b]	Assess community-level morbidity, mortality, and disability Estimate vaccine efficacy Identify populations at high risk Identify risk factors for vaccine failure
Special studies	Assess susceptibility to infection and vaccine seroconversion by serologic surveys Test alternative vaccine strains and delivery schedules Evaluate impact of measles immunization on survival

a. Useful only if reporting is constant over time.
b. Includes cohort, case-control, and cross-sectional studies.
Source: Authors.

Effective surveillance requires timely and effective use of data at each level of the health system: local, district, national. At the local level, every measles case should be considered for its epidemiologic and management relevance. Each case should be assessed as preventable or nonpreventable. Identification of preventability is not a method of faultfinding but a source of information for problem identification and problem solution. Early identification of cases is the necessary first step in effective outbreak control. Case data, together with locally available coverage data, can also be used to assess vaccine efficacy (Orenstein and others 1985). At district and national levels, subunit coverage and incidence data can be used to assess individual area performance and to identify high-risk areas for supervisory attention. Epidemiologic analyses of national data provide important programmatic data for assessing program status, establishing targets, monitoring performance, and providing information for feedback.

Measles Strategies for the 1990s

Countries, regions and WHO are currently in dialogues on the appropriate goal for measles to be achieved over the next decade.

Control, Elimination, Eradication

At the global level, there is considerable debate as to the appropriate long-term measles objective: control, elimination, or eradication. Understanding of the terminology is essential to this dialogue. *Control* means the reduction of measles morbidity and morality to a level that it is no longer a public health problem. *Elimination* implies the interruption of measles transmission in a geographically defined area, island, nation, or continent. *Eradication* is the interruption of person-to-person transmission, the elimination of the virus reservoir, and the termination of prevention procedures. The current WHO/UNICEF goals of 90 percent reduction in morbidity and 95 percent reduction in mortality by 1995 are consistent with measles control.

Measles elimination has been targeted for the United States, Europe, and the Caribbean (PAHO 1990). Although measles elimination has been achieved in certain populations (the Gambia; São Paulo, Brazil; and Cuba), the goal of sustained measles elimination has been more difficult. In the United States, the measles elimination target of October 1, 1982, was not achieved. Although the program was successful in achieving a remarkable 98 percent reduction in measles incidence, persistent transmission has continued primarily in two population groups: urban infants, and older high school and college-age students. In urban areas, the problem has been one of program implementation, the failure to achieve high coverage in infants from poor families. Intensified efforts are being carried out to increase timely immunization of infants in urban communities. Infection in the older age group reflects the accumulation of susceptibles caused by nonimmunization and vaccine failures, many of which relate to immunizations given prior to the currently recommended age of fifteen months. The addition of a second dose of measles vaccine will, in time, eliminate most of the susceptibles among the older age group.

The high cost of achieving and sustaining measles control has prompted some individuals to propose the global eradication of measles (Hopkins and others 1982; Foege 1984). Much of the advocacy for eradication arises out of the successful smallpox eradication program. Hopkins and colleagues have identified similarities and dissimilarities of measles to smallpox: "Both viruses cause infections which are accompanied by typical rashes and which confer life-long immunity; and both viruses have no animal reservoir and do not produce a chronic carrier state in man" (Hopkins and others 1982, p. 1396). Dissimilarities, they report, include "the highly contagious nature of measles" (70 percent attack rate for measles compared with 33 percent for smallpox), the average age of infection (twelve months to eighteen months for measles as opposed to four to five years for smallpox), the age at which a vaccine is effective (six months to nine months for measles as opposed to at birth for smallpox), and the difficulty in diagnosing mild measles as opposed to the ease of diagnosis of both the acute and the recovered case of smallpox (diagnostic pox and scars for smallpox) (Hopkins and others 1982, p. 1396). Other differences include vaccine effectiveness (99 percent for smallpox as against 80 to 90 percent for measles), the stability of vaccine (one year at ambient temperature for smallpox vaccine as opposed to the cold chain required for measles vaccine), and the effectiveness of outbreak control (achievable within one incubation period for smallpox but difficult beyond the first generation for measles). It should also be noted that smallpox eradication required activities in thirty countries for twelve years (the risk of importation was small); conversely, measles eradication, because of the ease of importations, would require work on a global scale.

The mathematical models of measles transmission for industrial and developing countries both predict that if more than 98 percent of young, susceptible children are protected against measles, the disease can be eradicated in large populations. It is important to note, however, that this prediction is based on the assumptions that the population is homogeneous (there are no isolated subpopulations and everyone is equally likely to mix with infected individuals and be vaccinated) and that vaccination failures are rare. These assumptions clearly do not hold in large urban populations. When these assumptions are relaxed, allowing, for example, for variations in susceptibility to infection, in-home exposure, and access to vaccination, the critical level of protection necessary for eradication rises to nearly 100 percent.

These differences and the data presented in this chapter on disease epidemiology and vaccine efficacy would seem to indicate that measles eradication is not achievable with the current vaccine and the current or projected levels of coverage. This is not to say that measles eradication is not a desirable long-term objective. New, improved vaccines and possibly alternative strategies are needed. However, in a world of limited health resources, careful attention must be given to the opportunity cost of allocating funds to measles eradication instead of to other priority health and development needs.

Mathematical Models

In the past sixty years, many mathematical models of measles transmission and of measles control by vaccination have been developed (for example, Kermack and McKendrick 1927; Dietz 1976; Hethcote 1976; Fine and Clarkson 1982a, 1982b; Schenzle 1989; Anderson and May 1985). These models are based upon the demography and epidemiology of industrial countries and thus describe fairly well the measles patterns in these settings. They do not, however, always accurately describe measles transmission patterns typical of developing countries.

TRANSMISSION. The simplified characteristics of measles transmission at the population level are the same in both industrial and developing countries: infants born to mothers who are immune to measles are protected from infection for several months by transplacental maternal antibodies; the infectivity of measles is high; an individual is both infected and infectious at roughly the same time; case-fatality rates are higher in infancy than in childhood; and recovery from measles results in subsequent long-lasting immunity. Thus, in the simplest model, there are four epidemiologic classes of people: (a) those protected by maternally derived antibodies, (b) those susceptible to infection, (c) those who are infected and infectious, and (d) those who have recovered from measles and are therefore immune. Figure 8-6 traces the progression of individuals among the epidemiologic classes.

Figure 8-6. *Stages in the Measles Infection Cycle of an Individual from Birth through Sequence of Epidemiologic Classes to Death*

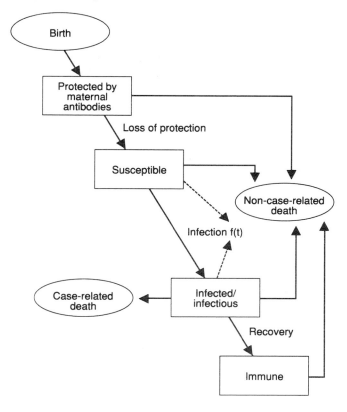

Source: Authors.

Initially, the population consists of infants protected by maternal antibodies and of susceptible individuals who mix randomly. A measles outbreak begins when infected and infectious individuals have contact with a sufficient density of susceptibles. Each time a susceptible individual is encountered, the latter may be infected with a probability proportional to the intensity of exposure. At the earliest stage of the outbreak, most encounters by infectious individuals are with susceptible individuals; therefore, measles spreads quickly. When the illness runs its course in the infected individual, he or she is then immune. As measles transmission progresses through the population, the number of susceptibles decreases whereas the number of immune individuals increases; therefore, it becomes less likely that an infected individual will encounter susceptible individuals and create new infections. If the number of immune individuals is high enough, measles will die out, even though there are still some susceptible individuals in the population: this is the phenomenon of "herd immunity." If, however, susceptibles enter the population (by birth or migration) at a sufficiently high rate, measles may not die out but may instead become endemic.

Immunization programs thus exert their effect at both the individual and the population level: vaccination changes the immune status of the individual and, within the population, it

decreases the probability that a susceptible individual will be exposed to measles.

TRANSMISSION MODELS FOR INDUSTRIAL COUNTRIES. In the models of measles transmission and control for industrial countries, the principal epidemiologic assumption is that the rate of measles spread is independent of the spatial density of the host population; the principal demographic assumption is that the host population is not growing. It is generally assumed that vaccination takes place at a precisely targeted age and that all vaccinations are effective. The measles transmission model for industrial countries yields several predictions:

- The number of susceptibles in the population remains the same in the presence and absence of immunization.
- The median age at infection in the population increases after vaccination.
- In the presence of even modest levels of vaccination, the period between epidemic peaks (interepidemic period) will lengthen.
- At any given level of vaccination coverage, the percentage drop in the incidence of measles should be greater than the level of vaccination coverage.
- The proportion of each cohort that must be immunized to interrupt measles transmission is less than 1.0.

The predictions of this model correspond well to observed pre- and postvaccination measles transmission patterns in the United States and in many European countries.

TRANSMISSION MODELS FOR DEVELOPING COUNTRIES. In contrast, measles transmission models for developing countries explicitly account for the demographic and epidemiologic structure typical of the populations of such countries (John 1990a, 1990b; John and Tuljapurkar 1990; Tuljapurkar and John 1990; Nokes and others 1990), particularly the high rates of population growth. In these models the demographic structure of the host population is determined by the population's fertility and mortality. The distribution of individuals among the four epidemiologic classes at each age is governed by epidemiologic parameters: age pattern of loss of maternal antibodies, age-specific immunization coverage, age-specific infection rate, duration of infectivity, and age-specific case-fatality rate. The demographic structure of the population and the epidemiologic behavior of the infectious disease are linked by the infection rate, which depends on the population's demographic and epidemiologic structure and on the spatial density of the population. More complex developing-country models allow for spatial heterogeneity in infection rates, urban-rural migration, and seasonality in births, deaths, and migration.

The predictions of even the simplest model for developing countries are strikingly different from those of the model for industrial countries:

- The equilibrium proportion of infected individuals in the population (the equilibrium measles prevalence) in-

Figure 8-7. *Interepidemic Interval as Function of Population Growth Rate at Different Levels of Immunization Coverage*

Interepidemic period (years)

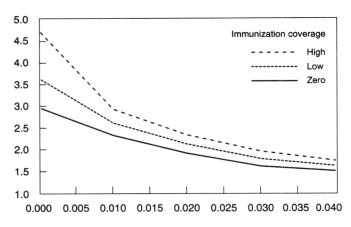

Annual population growth rate

Note: Interepidemic interval (years) plotted as a function of population growth rate, r, for different levels of immunization coverage (low and high) and for no immunization (i=0.0). In the absence of immunization, the inter-epidemic interval shortens as r increases (3.0 years at r=0.0 to 1.5 years at r=4). At r=0.0, immunization sharply increases the periods between epidemics from 3.0 to 4.6 years, while at r=4.0, immunization increases the inter-epidemic period by only 0.4 years.
Source: Authors.

creases as the growth rate of the population increases, both when there is no vaccination in the population and when there is an ongoing vaccination program.

- The mean age at infection in the population need not increase after vaccination, because the remaining post-vaccination cases may be concentrated at the extremes in the youngest and the oldest children; however, the age distribution of cases may change substantially.

- The interepidemic period does not necessarily increase after implementation of a vaccination program in a growing population: when the level of vaccination is a small fraction of the critical level of vaccination required to stop transmission, changes in the interepidemic period are quite small, but when the level of vaccination nears the critical level, the interepidemic period shows a substantial increase (figures 8-7 and 8-8).

- The percentage drop in the incidence of measles, for any given level of vaccination, will be smaller in a growing population than in a nongrowing population: for example, vaccination of 50 percent of the children might induce a drop in measles incidence of 60 percent in an industrial country but of only 52 percent in a rapidly growing population in a developing country.

In contrast to the model for industrial countries, the predictions of the model for developing countries are consistent with the observed effects of immunization programs

in Zaire and Cameroon. Between 1980 and 1985 an intensive measles vaccination program in Kinshasa, Zaire, resulted in the vaccination of almost 60 percent of the children who were twelve months through twenty-three months old, yet "two results expected from [measles transmission models]—a reduction in measles incidence greater than the level of vaccination coverage and a shift in the age distribution of measles to older children—have not occurred in this African urban population" (Taylor and others 1988, p. 792). In addition, the predicted increase in the interval between epidemic outbreaks of measles was not observed: epidemics continued to occur biennially. In Yaoundé, Cameroon, the results of a measles vaccination program showed a slight shift upward in the mean age of infection but no corresponding lengthening of the interepidemic interval (Guyer and McBean 1981). In both cases, the observed results are consistent with the prediction of the simplest transmission model for developing countries.

APPLICATION OF MEASLES MODELS: MEASLES INCIDENCE DYNAMICS. When designing vaccination programs for developing countries, one is rarely faced with the task of fine-tuning the details of vaccination delivery, such as deciding whether the optimum age for vaccination is eight months or nine months. Rather, one weighs the merits of substantial program modifications: decreasing missed opportunities,[2] starting vaccination at six months rather than nine months, instituting annual or semi-annual vaccination days, or changing to two-dose schedules. Mathematical models of measles transmission and control are useful tools for vaccination program design and evaluation.

Figure 8-8. *Combined Effect of Population Growth Rate and Immunization Coverage on Interepidemic Level*

Interepidemic period (years)

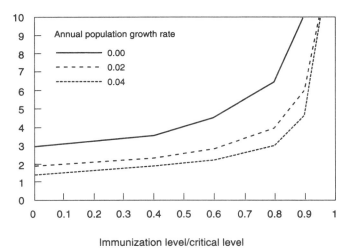

Immunization level/critical level

Note: Horizontal axis shows the ratio of achieved level of immunization and the critical level of immunization required to stop measles transmission.
Source: Authors.

Figure 8-9. *Simulation Model of Measles Incidence after Immunization*

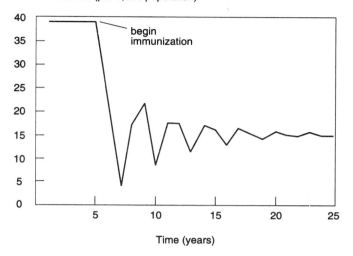

Annual incidence (per 1,000 population)

Source: Authors.

during the twenty-five years projected. Thus, ascertaining whether or not an immunization program has achieved its goals, in the short run, is in fact quite difficult; the "success" of the program depends very much on the relative timing of intervention and evaluation.

DISEASE REDUCTION. We have used a simple measles model for developing countries to estimate measles cases and deaths that would occur under the following five different levels of vaccinations in two settings–high-density urban and low-density rural: no vaccination, measles vaccination at nine months, measles vaccination at nine months and decreased missed opportunities, high-titer Edmonston-Zagreb (EZ) or equivalent measles vaccine at six months, high-titer Edmonston-Zagreb or equivalent measles vaccine at six and twelve months. Because an increase in mortality has recently been observed in populations receiving high-titer vaccine (Garenne and others 1991), development of an alternative safe effective vaccine providing 85 percent or higher seroconversion at six months will be needed. To facilitate a comparison among the two populations, a standard population was used with the following characteristics: a birth rate of 48 per 1,000, an infant mortality rate of 100 per 1,000 live births, a population growth rate of 3.5 percent, and a population under ten years of age of 34 percent. The age distribution of cases and age-specific case-fatality rates for each of the two scenarios are listed in table 8-3. For each scenario, estimates were also made of cases occurring prior to vaccination, of vaccine coverage, and of vaccine efficacy, as shown in table 8-4.

Using the measles model for developing countries and the assumptions listed above, we summarize in table 8-5, for both urban and rural settings, the estimates of the number of cases, the number and percentage of cases prevented, and the number and percentage of deaths prevented.

Several important observations can be made from the simulation model: measles mortality is higher in urban areas than in rural areas because of the younger age of infection, an age at which case-fatality rates are higher; at equivalent

Even though one must recognize the importance of parameter assumptions, the models represent powerful tools for evaluating the potential mortality and morbidity effects of different vaccination programs, for anticipating the dynamic behavior of measles in the population, and for examining the influence of demographic variation on measles transmission patterns. For example, for any given specification of the demographic and epidemiologic parameters, the potential effect of a vaccination program can be estimated and alternative vaccination delivery strategies compared; the effects of changes in the host population due to child survival programs, family planning programs, and urbanization can be studied; and the short-run fluctuations in measles incidence can be predicted.

The nature of the short-run fluctuations in measles incidence following an immunization program is crucial in ascertaining whether the WHO goal of a 90 percent reduction of measles incidence can be achieved by 1995. The introduction of any vaccination program reduces the long-run (equilibrium) incidence of measles in the population. The short-run effect on measles incidence is, however, dominated by the fluctuations in annual incidence (figure 8-9). In the simulation model presented here, immunization results in the desired 90 percent reduction in measles incidence within two years (that is, by year seven), but by year nine, the annual incidence is half of the preimmunization level, which would suggest that this immunization program had not achieved the desired goals, despite the evidence from two years earlier. Yet in year ten, there appears to have been an 80 percent reduction from preimmunization levels. In this model, with this set of parameters, the steady estimate of reduction of disease incidence is from 38 to 14 cases per 1,000 population, a reduction of 63 percent. This model, so configured, assumes that fertility, mortality, and immunization parameters remain unchanged

Table 8-3. *Mathematical Model Assumptions for Unvaccinated Urban and Rural Scenarios: Age-Specific Case-Fatality Rates and Age Distribution of Cases*
(Age distribution in 1990)

Age (months)	Case-fatality rate	Age distribution Urban	Age distribution Rural
<6	—	0	0
6–8	4	18	3
9–11	4	19	6
12–23	5	40	14
24–35	3	10	16
36–47	2	8	18
48–59	1	5	20
60–119	.05	0	23

Source: Authors.

Table 8-4. Mathematical Model Assumptions for Measles: Subjects Immune from Infection at Time of Vaccination, Coverage, and Efficacy of Vaccine

Scenario	Urban			Rural		
	Immune	Cover-age	Efficacy	Immune	Cover-age	Efficacy
Measles vaccine at 9 months	30	60	85	10	60	85
Eliminate missed opportunities	30	80	85	10	80	85
EZ[a] at 6 months	10	80	85	2	80	85
EZ[a] at 6 months and 12 months	10	80	85	2	80	85
	10	60	95	2	60	95

a. Edmonston-Zagreb or equivalent measles vaccine providing 85 percent seroconversion and protection when given at six months of age.
Source: Authors.

levels of coverage, rural strategies are more effective in reducing morbidity and mortality; use of an effective vaccine at six months significantly increases the effectiveness of urban immunization; and two-dose schedules further increase program effectiveness. For simplicity, these calculations do not take into account herd immunity; they do, however, provide an estimate of the long-term effect of alternative strategies for the delivery of measles vaccine. Maximum reductions in morbidity and mortality are obtained with the two-dose vaccine schedule in which a vaccine is used that is effective when administered at six months of age. Coverage levels used in these models represent those currently being achieved by well-managed immunization programs in developing countries. Few countries have been able to achieve and maintain the 95 percent levels achieved in industrial countries.

Simulations are only as accurate as the assumptions and the model used. The assumptions used above reflect data collected from the city of Lagos, Nigeria, Kinshasa, Zaire, and the rural areas of Matlab, Bangladesh. It is our expectation that these data will contribute to the dialogue on alternative measles strategies. The model, reflecting the

currently achieved levels of coverage and vaccine efficacy, projected reductions in morbidity and mortality significantly below the 90 percent morbidity and 95 percent mortality reduction targets established by WHO and affirmed at the 1990 World Summit for Children. According to the model, a two-dose schedule with a vaccine effective at six months of age has the greatest potential for moving operational programs toward the global targets. Further improvements in vaccine coverage and effectiveness will be required to ensure the elimination of measles as a significant cause of childhood morbidity and mortality.

COST-EFFECTIVENESS OF ALTERNATIVE STRATEGIES. Given the above results, we can now consider the costs of the alternative strategies. Costs are predicated on an average cost of $15 per fully immunized child with 40 percent of the cost, or $6, allocated to measles. The cost profile (the contribution of each cost component to total cost) is based on the delivery modality for immunizations in fixed sites (Brenzel 1990). For each alternative strategy, assumptions were made which would change original cost estimates, that is, the incremental costs attributable to each strategy. These assumptions are enumerated below. Costs are assumed to be the same in both urban and rural settings with the exceptions noted.

- Measles immunization at nine months.
- Measles immunization at nine months but a 50 percent increase in vaccine use so that vaccines represent 10 percent of total costs and a 10 percent increase in supervision costs.
- Edmonston-Zagreb or equivalent vaccine given at six months are $6 (the same as measles immunization at nine months). Cost of vaccine is same as currently used measles vaccine. Delivery pattern and sites remain the same. Although one might expect declining average costs because of increasing volume, the effect is probably quite small and thus negligible to average cost.
- Edmonston-Zagreb or equivalent vaccine given at six months and twelve months: cost for second dose is the same

Table 8-5. Simulation Estimates of Measles Cases and Deaths in High-Density Urban and Low-Density Rural Scenarios: Developing Country Model

Scenario	Urban						Rural					
	Cases	Cases prevented	Cases prevented (percent)	Deaths	Deaths prevented	Deaths prevented (percent)	Cases	Cases prevented	Cases prevented (percent)	Deaths	Deaths prevented	Deaths prevented (percent)
No vaccination	36,400	n.a.	n.a.	1,452	n.a.	n.a.	36,400	n.a.	n.a.	806	n.a.	n.a.
Measles vaccine at 9 months	25,744	10,656	29	1,025	425	29	20,193	16,207	45	456	350	45
Vaccine at 9 months and eliminates missed opportunities	22,192	14,208	39	885	567	39	14,791	21,609	59	339	467	58
EZ[a] at 6 months	14,123	22,277	61	563	889	61	12,165	24,235	67	269	537	67
EZ[a] at 6 and 12 months	9,051	27,349	75	361	1,091	75	5,844	30,556	84	140	660	83

n.a. Not applicable.
a. Edmonston-Zagreb or other vaccine that achieves 85 percent seroconversion and protection when administered at six months of age.
Source: Authors' calculations.

Table 8-6. Efficacy and Cost of Alternative Strategies to Increase Measles Coverage in Urban Areas

Strategy	Cases prevented	Deaths prevented	Unit cost $	Coverage (percent)	Doses administered	Total annual cost	Total incremental cost	Total cost per case prevented	Total cost per death prevented	Incremental cost per case prevented	Incremental cost per death prevented	Total cost per DALY	Incremental cost per DALY
Measles vaccine at 9 months (baseline)	10,656	425	6.00	60	30,600	183,600	n.a.	17.23	432.00	n.a.	n.a.	14.90	n.a.
Vaccine at 9 months and missed opportunities	14,208	567	6.42	80	40,800	261,936	78,336	18.44	461.97	22.05	551.66	15.93	19.02
EZ[a] at 6 months	22,277	889	6.00	80	40,800	244,800	61,200	10.99	275.37	5.27	131.90	9.50	4.55
EZ[a] at 6 months and 12 months			6.00	80	40,800								
	27,349	1,091	6.00	60	27,000	406,800	223,200	14.87	372.87	13.37	335.14	12.86	11.56

n.a. Not applicable; increment is determined in relation to this baseline.

a. Edmonston-Zagreb or equivalent vaccine providing 80 percent seroconversion when given at six months of age.

Source: Authors' calculations.

as first dose at six months. Assume that second dose is administered at routine vaccination session or child health visit and therefore does not require additional personnel or outreach. A decrease in volume may predictably increase the average cost of the second dose only if the average cost curve is quite steep.

Using the measles model for developing countries presented earlier, the annual number of cases and deaths in children under ten that would be prevented by each alternative strategy in each scenario was tabulated for use in the cost-effectiveness calculations (tables 8-6 and 8-7). In these calculations, cases and deaths prevented represent the annual number of cases and deaths prevented for the entire cohort of children under ten in any given year. Total annual costs, however, only reflect costs incurred in a single year to immunize the currently eligible children (those under twelve months of age). Costs are expressed in 1990 dollars. In order to compare these results with previous studies, the costs must be converted to the relevant year for which the study data were reported.

The cost per disability-adjusted life-year was calculated under the assumption that a death averted "buys" about sixty years of life or, if one discounts future life-years gained at 3 percent, the annuity stream reveals that a prevented death of a child from measles buys about 29 disability-adjusted life-years. The calculation does not account for DALYs lost to disability caused by measles, because it is estimated that more than 95 percent of years of life lost from measles are due to premature mortality and not to disability (Duflo and others 1986). More refined estimates of DALYs would need to take into account disability caused by measles complications and the concomitant cost in healthy life-years lost. Results of the cost-effectiveness studies are summarized in tables 8-6 and 8-7.

The tables give relative estimates of the cost-effectiveness of alternative strategies to increase measles coverage, notwithstanding all the caveats and assumptions built into the analysis. For urban populations, the most cost-effective strategy appears to be administering Edmonston-Zagreb or equivalent vaccine to children at six months of age. This strategy is also the most cost-effective for rural populations, although use of the current

Table 8-7. Efficacy and Cost of Alternative Strategies to Increase Measles Coverage in Rural Areas

Strategy	Cases prevented	Deaths prevented	Unit cost $	Coverage (percent)	Doses administered	Total annual cost	Total incremental cost	Total cost per case prevented	Total cost per death prevented	Incremental cost per case prevented	Incremental cost per death prevented	Total cost per DALY	Incremental cost per DALY
Measles vaccine at 9 months (baseline)	16,207	350	6.00	60	30,600	183,600	n.a.	77.33	524.57	n.a.	n.a.	18.09	n.a.
Vaccine at 9 months and missed opportunities	21,609	467	6.42	80	40,800	261,936	78,336	12.12	560.89	14.50	669.54	19.34	23.09
EZa at 6 months	24,235	537	6.00	80	40,800	244,800	61,200	10.10	455.87	7.62	327.27	15.72	11.29
EZ[a] at 6 months and 12 months			6.00	80	40,800								
	30,556	666	6.00	60	27,000	406,800	223,200	13.31	10.81	15.56	706.33	21.06	24.36

n.a. Not applicable; increment is determined in relation to this baseline.

a. Edmonston-Zagreb or equivalent vaccine providing 80 percent seroconversion when given at six months of age.

Source: Authors' calculations.

measles vaccine at nine months and use of every missed opportunity along with the current measles vaccine appear to be almost as effective. At least for rural populations, there is no significant difference in the cost-effectiveness of the first three strategies, given the limits of the analysis.

Achieving the 1995 Measles Targets

In 1989, WHO established global EPI targets for the decade of the 1990s: that coverage levels will surpass 80 percent in all countries or areas by the end of 1990 and that levels of 90 percent, in the context of comprehensive maternal and child health services, can be achieved by the year 2000. At the September 1990 World Summit for Children, the WHO 1995 targets for morbidity and mortality reduction were affirmed, 90 percent and 95 percent, respectively. Although global levels of immunization coverage have increased dramatically during the last decade, representing a major achievement of national governments and their collaborating partners, there is still a significant gap between the current levels of coverage and disease reduction and the 1990 targets, as shown in table 8-8.

Achievement of the 1995 and 2000 targets will require increases in both coverage and vaccine efficacy. Eleven strategies, some already a part of the EPI program, hold the potential to increase levels of coverage, increase vaccine efficacy, decrease measles incidence, and decrease measles mortality: (a) vaccination in the first year of life, (b) reduction of missed opportunities, (c) increase in community partnership, (d) registration and follow-up of newborns, (e) use of accelerated immunization strategies, (f) vaccination of high-risk groups, (g) adoption of two-dose measles vaccine schedules, (h) provision of vitamin A supplementation in vitamin A–deficient areas, (i) treatment of severe cases of measles with vitamin A, (j) effective treatment of measles complications, and (k) expansion of the infrastructure. The first six of these strategies, in part developed from experience in the developing world, are important components of the current United States initiative to achieve measles control (United States, National Vaccine Advisory Committee 1991).

Table 8-8. *Measles Coverage and Estimated Disease Reduction, by* WHO *Region, 1989*
(percent)

Region	Measles coverage	Estimated reduction in morbidity[a]
Africa	47	40
Americas	73	62
Mediterranean	70	60
Europe	85	72
Southeast Asia	58	49
Western Pacific	90	77

Note: 1995 target is 90 percent for both measles coverage and morbidity reduction.

a. Coverage times vaccine efficacy (85 percent).

Source: WHO internal data.

Figure 8-10. *Age of Measles Vaccination of 48–59-Month-Old Children in Six Countries*

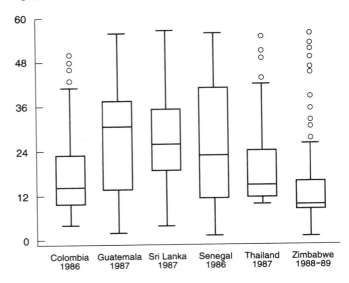

Note: For each population, the median age at immunization is indicated by line inside box. The median age of immunizations administered at ages greater than the median age (approximately the 75th percentile) are graphed as the upper bar of the box. The line extended from the top of the box ends at upper boundary: the observation closest to but less than the sum of the 75th percentile plus 1.5 times the difference between the 25th and 75th percentile. Any observations greater than the boundary were deemed outliers and are plotted individually. The lower boundary was constructed in an analogous manner.
Source: Authors.

VACCINATION IN THE FIRST YEAR OF LIFE. Measles vaccine is effective when administered to a susceptible individual prior to or at the time of exposure to measles. The World Health Organization and UNICEF have emphasized the importance of vaccination in the first year of life in developing countries. Vaccination of older children is less effective in developing countries, because many children (the number increasing with age) may have already become immune through infection with wild virus. Using data from demographic and health surveys (Boerma and others 1990), we provide in figure 8-10 a boxplot of the age distributions of card-documented immunizations from six countries. Except for Zimbabwe, the boxplots show a pattern of delayed measles vaccination.

Increased attention to vaccination in the first year of life, at nine months for the Schwarz strain and six months for alternative vaccines that provide high rates of seroconversion and protection, will increase the probability that a dose of vaccine will be administered to a susceptible infant and thus, depending on age-specific rates of vaccine efficacy, increase program effectiveness in achieving disease reduction.

REDUCTION OF MISSED OPPORTUNITIES. The term "missed opportunities" is defined as contacts of a target-age individual (infant, child, or reproductive-age woman) in need of one or more vaccines with a health facility capable of providing that vaccine and a failure of that contact to provide the needed vaccine(s). There are two types of missed opportunities for immunization: missed vaccination opportunities and missed health facility opportunities.

Missed vaccination opportunities occur when an individual attending a vaccination session fails to receive a needed vaccine or receives one inappropriately timed by age or intervaccination interval. A review of fifteen published articles has documented missed vaccination rates ranging from 8 percent in Mozambique to 76 percent in Indonesia; the median for the fifteen countries was 49 percent (Hirschorn 1990; Grabowsky 1991).

Missed opportunities are also being identified in industrial countries. Investigation of an urban outbreak of measles in the United States identified missed opportunities for measles immunization in fifteen of twenty-six measles cases in an urban outbreak among preschool children (Hutchins and others 1989). Missed opportunities were also documented as a significant factor in the 1990 measles epidemic in the United States (United States, National Vaccine Advisory Committee 1991).

Four methods have been used to assess the rate of missed opportunities:

- *Record reviews.* Facility-held records, vaccination registers, or individual patient immunization cards are reviewed to assess whether all indicated antigens were administered on recorded dates of vaccination contact.
- *Exit interviews.* Child caretakers and reproductive-age women leaving a clinic during a time at which immunizations are being administered are interviewed by health staff. Immunization records are examined for missed or inappropriately timed immunizations (early for age or too short an interval between doses).
- *Clinic observation.* Supervisory staff observe immunization sessions to identify errors in screening, referral, or immunization.
- *Coverage surveys.* As part of surveys to assess immunization coverage, data from individual client-held record cards are reviewed for missed opportunities for immunization on days of recorded attendance at an immunization session and for inappropriately timed immunizations (Cutts, Glik, Gordon, and others 1990). Analyses of these data are facilitated by use of COSAS, a software package which analyzes coverage survey data for coverage, age, intervals between immunizations, and missed opportunities (Boyd 1991).

Ten major causes for missed opportunities for immunization have been identified (Hirschorn 1990).

- Coexistent illness as determined by health worker or child caretaker. In contrast, note that WHO policy calls for immunization at every opportunity. "It is particularly important to immunize children suffering from malnutrition. Low-grade fever, mild respiratory infections or diarrhea, and other mild illnesses should not be considered contraindications to immunization. The decision to withhold immunization should be taken only after serious consideration of the individual child and community. Immunization of children

too ill to require hospitalization should be deferred for decision of hospital authorities" (WHO/EPI 1984, p. 15).

Although recent data suggest decreased rates of seroconversion in children with respiratory infection (Krober 1991), an overall assessment of risks and benefits mandates vaccination of both sick and well children. Because of the risk of nosocomial spread of measles, all children from six months through five years of age who are admitted to a hospital should receive measles vaccine on admission if there is no documentation of age-appropriate measles immunization.

- Incorrect screening by the health worker. (Screening errors relate to a lack of understanding of national vaccination schedule, difficulties in calculating the interval between recorded date of birth and current date, failure to check all antigens, clerical error because of fatigue, or lack of motivation.)
- Vaccine not available.
- Clinic too crowded or disorganized to handle the demand.
- Absence of staff, vaccine, or transport resulting in the cancellation of a scheduled immunization session.
- Mothers too busy to wait, not informed that they should wait, or dissatisfied.
- Health workers' fear of wasting measles vaccine, resulting in refusal to open a multidose vial for one child (WHO and UNICEF recommend opening a vial of vaccine even for one child).
- Acceptance by health worker of an oral history of measles or measles vaccination as a reason for nonimmunization. (Serologic studies have documented the unreliability of histories of measles and measles immunization; all eligible children without written proof of measles vaccination should be immunized with measles vaccine.) The failure of child caretakers to bring the immunization cards to clinic also contributes to this problem.
- Unwillingness of health workers to administer more than one antigen at a time. (Studies have documented the safety and efficacy of simultaneous separate multiple antigen vaccine administration [Foege and Foster 1974]).
- Nonimmunization of individual identified for immunization. This occurs when immunization cards are returned to parents prior to the completion of all immunizations. Such situations may arise when children have been referred for multiple immunizations, for example, DPT, OPV, and measles. Delaying the return of the vaccination card until all antigens required for that vaccination session are administered can eliminate this problem.

When persons eligible for immunizations visit health facilities that are capable of delivering vaccine and vaccines are not given, a missed health facility contact has occurred. Such missed contacts happen in clinics in which administration of vaccines is limited to certain days (infant welfare) or groups (well children). And all too commonly they occur because curative-oriented health workers fail to assess immunization status. Although these missed opportunities may be the most common ones, they are less well documented. Identification of such missed opportunities is facilitated by a unified clinic- or patient-held record system in which immunization and all health contacts are entered on the same record. In the Central African Republic, a comparison of dates of all health facility contacts with opportunities for measles immunization showed that use of all opportunities would have achieved a measles vaccine coverage of 76 percent, rather than the actual 54 percent (Roungou 1991). In Guinea, a community survey estimated that 30 percent of the opportunities for measles immunization had been missed (Cutts, Glik, Gordon and others 1990).

Integrated service delivery in which all health facility contacts are used to screen and immunize all eligible persons can reduce this problem. Although the transition from specialized immunization clinics to routine immunization is initially difficult, the shift to a "comprehensive" approach to vaccine delivery has been effective in reducing the missed health facility opportunity. Pioneered by Shanti Ghosh in Delhi, India, the practice of screening and immunizing all emergency department and outpatient cases prior to their contact with a physician or nurse has been effective in reducing missed opportunities, increasing coverage, and reducing disease morbidity in Zimbabwe and Mozambique (Ekunwe 1984; WHO/EPI Zimbabwe 1989; Hirschorn 1990). Yach and others (1991) estimated 240,000 missed opportunities for measles vaccination per year at two tertiary-level referral hospitals in South Africa. In an investigation of an inner-city measles outbreak in the United States, 38 percent of cases had received DPT or diphtheria-tetanus vaccine at an age when they were eligible to receive measles vaccine (Hutchins and others 1989). In the United States, extension of immunization to contacts with public assistance could significantly increase coverage (United States, National Vaccine Advisory Committee 1991).

INCREASE IN COMMUNITY PARTNERSHIP. Community partnership in immunization is important to the achievement and maintenance of high levels of vaccine coverage. This is well demonstrated in Indonesia, where the PKK, a national organization of women, has become a major partner in childhood immunization. Vaccination coverage provided by outreach vaccinators that had been in the range of 15 to 30 percent increased to 70 to 90 percent in villages where the PKK was active. The PKK organizes the clinics and participates in clinic activities, including the preparation of advance publicity, the weighing of children, the recording of weights, nutrition education, and the distribution of contraceptives. In Liberia and Mozambique, the participation of local chiefs, traditional birth attendants, and village health committees has been effective in increasing coverage (Cutts and others 1988; Bender and Macauley 1990).

Polio eradication is providing many new strategies to increase partnerships. This is best exemplified by the Rotarians around the world, both in the provision of funds (over $200 million) and in the active involvement of local Rotarians in social mobilization and direct assistance in vaccine delivery activities. Prime emphasis is being given to the training of community volunteers to identify and refer eligible children for immunization. In areas where such programs are operational (for example, Ijeru-Ekiti, Nigeria), coverage rates are over 90 percent and drop-out rates are near zero.

REGISTRATION AND FOLLOW-UP OF NEWBORNS. In rural areas where population movement is limited, the enumeration of births and the monitoring of immunization status through the first year of life has proved effective in increasing coverage. In Oman, health facility records of immunization are maintained by month of birth (health facility usage is over 95 percent); a monthly review of immunization records of one-year-old children provides a mechanism for assessing coverage and identifying defaulters for follow-up. Coverage in this population is over 98 percent (Foster 1989). In other places, maintenance of village registers serves the same purpose. Door-to-door visits have also been used to register the at-risk population, identify susceptibles, and refer eligibles for vaccination.

USE OF ACCELERATED IMMUNIZATION STRATEGIES. During the last decade, WHO and UNICEF have promoted accelerated immunization activities as a mechanism to increase coverage (WHO/UNICEF 1985). Historically, immunization days date back to the 1950s, when Sunday vaccination days were instituted to increase polio coverage in the United States. Biennial OPV polio campaigns have been used widely in Latin America, especially in Brazil, and have been credited with the near elimination of that disease from the Western hemisphere (de Quadros, Andrus, and Olive 1991).

Largely through the personal advocacy of the executive director of UNICEF, national immunization days have been established to increase vaccination coverage. Countries using this strategy have included Colombia, Turkey, Senegal, Nigeria, and Côte d'Ivoire. These accelerated strategies have been promoted to achieve several important objectives:

- To elevate the health sector in general, and immunization programs in particular, to the national political agenda. Political leaders have provided leadership in the planning, promotion, and implementation of immunization days.
- To change the public perception of immunization from that of an intermittently available service to that of a basic human right.
- To increase business, voluntary organization, and public support for immunization programs.
- To increase access to immunization services.
- To increase immunization coverage and reduce morbidity and mortality.

Immunization days in many countries, for example, Colombia, Turkey, and Côte d'Ivoire, have been spectacularly successful in achieving their political and coverage targets. Immunization coverage rates have increased to levels in excess of 90 percent; rates of disease incidence have been dramatically reduced.

From the perspective of maintaining high levels of coverage, however, the value of these accelerated strategies has been questioned on four accounts:

- Opportunity cost—the diversion of limited health resources from essential preventive and curative health services to immunization activities.
- Quality and safety—the inability to provide the quantity and quality of supervision required to ensure compliance with basic technical guidelines (Bryce, Cutts, and Saba 1990).
- Cost-effectiveness—the high cost required for a major campaign (vaccine, supplies, cold-chain equipment, personnel, transport, and publicity) and the relative inefficiency of campaigns in providing vaccines to those at greatest risk, children in the first year of life.
- Sustainability—the value of campaigns in promoting and maintaining high rates of vaccine coverage and disease reduction over time.

The expanding experience with accelerated strategies is prompting a shift of policy dialogue from the question of their appropriateness to the question of where, when, and under what conditions accelerated strategies are useful. The poliomyelitis experience in the Americas, especially Brazil, has shown that immunization days are effective in increasing coverage and decreasing disease incidence and can be sustained over time (de Quadros, Andrus, and Olive 1991). For measles, experience in India demonstrated that annual single-day measles campaigns in a village without access to routine vaccine services was effective in achieving and maintaining measles control (John, Ray, and Steinhoff 1984). In Liberia, a country in which only 40 percent of the population had access to health facilities, annual immunization weeks for five consecutive years, epidemiologically timed to precede the measles season, have succeeded in increasing immunization coverage from 15 to 60 percent (CCCD 1990). During 1989, approximately 40 percent of annual immunizations were administered during this vaccination week. Of special importance to the success of these campaigns was the local partnership in the planning, funding of local costs, and implementation of the vaccination weeks. This system, a viable model for many parts of Africa, has unfortunately been destroyed by civil war.

Five conditions are suggested as criteria for the appropriate use of accelerated strategies in achieving local and national EPI targets:

- *Low access* (50 percent access of target population to a facility regularly providing vaccines). In areas of low access to health facilities and where the potential for outreach is limited, accelerated strategies provide an attractive option in achieving coverage and disease reduction targets.

- *Frequency and repeatability*. As needed, accelerated strategies should be conducted annually, as in the Indian example above, or twice a year, as in the polio campaigns in Latin America. For measles, timing the activity to the pre-epidemic season maximizes effect and cost-effectiveness.
- *Decentralization*. As sustainability and effectiveness are very dependent on local participation, responsibility for planning, vaccine delivery, supervision, and evaluation should be decentralized to the level of implementation, for example, district, sector, and so on.
- *Targeting*. Target age groups for immunization, selection of antigens, and timing of accelerated activities need to be based on relevant local data about the availability of the population, physical access to that population, and disease epidemiology.
- *Safety*. Because immunizations (perhaps the most cost-effective of all health interventions) are not totally safe—for example, in the transmission of pathogens through use of nonsterile procedures—systems to ensure quality must be developed and sustained. Systems of training and supervision need to ensure the quality of vaccine delivery as part of accelerated strategies. This includes maintenance of the cold chain and sterilization, appropriate age and intervals for immunization, and instructions to the mother about the need for return visits to complete immunization.

VACCINATION OF HIGH-RISK GROUPS. Four groups of children are particularly at risk from measles and should be vaccinated or, in certain cases, revaccinated. Among refugees, measles has been identified as the main cause of mortality in new refugee populations (Toole and Waldman 1988). Ethiopian refugees in Sudan show a measles CFR of 33 percent (Shears and others 1987). Measles immunization has been identified as a "high priority in emergency relief programs, second only in importance to the provision of adequate food rations" (Toole and others 1989, p. 381).

Hospitalized children, especially those who are severely malnourished, are, if infected, at high risk of measles-associated mortality. Mortality in malnourished children infected with measles in a hospital setting is frequently above 50 percent. Among sixty nosocomial infections requiring admission to a South African hospital, measles and its complications accounted for twenty-eight (47 percent) of readmissions and seven deaths (Cotton and others 1989). All pediatric admissions without written documentation of measles immunization at an appropriate age should be given measles vaccine on admission. Children vaccinated prior to twelve months of age should be reimmunized.

Nosocomial transmission of measles is common in the developing world. In a study in Côte d'Ivoire, 69 percent of measles patients seen at an urban health facility had attended a health facility eight to twenty-one days prior to onset of measles (Foulon and others 1983; Klein-Zabban and others 1987). Nosocomial transmission has also been reported from Taiwan (Gao and Malison 1988); severity of illness was greater in children who had attended the clinic for illness than in those who had attended for well baby care ($P < .01$). Immunization at every opportunity, as advocated by WHO, would have prevented most of these cases.

In urban populations in western and central Africa, measles is primarily a disease of the first two years of life, an age at which CFRs are highest (Taylor and others 1988). Children in urban slums have been identified as at increased risk for high measles mortality (low coverage and low age of infection), and thus such slums are a priority area for targeted immunization (Coetzee, Berry, and Jacobs 1991). Lot quality assessment sampling has been used to identify low coverage areas in Kinshasa, Zaire. Priority attention to these high-risk groups will have maximum effect on measles-associated mortality. Three guides to improve urban immunization have recently been published (UNICEF 1989; Claquin 1991; Cutts 1991). Targeting vaccine to places and groups for which epidemiologic data document increased mortality risk (for example, supplementary feeding centers and girls in poor homes in Bangladesh [Bhuiya and others 1987]), will increase the efficiency of immunization in achieving the mortality reduction goal.

ADOPTION OF TWO-DOSE MEASLES VACCINE SCHEDULES. Ninety percent coverage with a vaccine producing 90 percent efficacy will provide protection to 81 percent of vaccinees, significantly less than the 1995 disease reduction target of 90 percent. Two-dose schedules have the potential to facilitate the achievement of the 90 percent measles reduction target by reducing the number of primary vaccine failures. Two-dose schedules can use the currently available Schwarz vaccine or an improved vaccine providing 85 percent seroconversion for those vaccinated at six months of age. Three two-dose schedules are provided as examples:

- In dense urban areas where risk of infection is highest in the first two years of life, two doses of EZ or equivalent vaccine need to be given as early as possible, for example, at six months and twelve months of age.

- In rural areas with low coverage, immunization at nine and fifteen months of age with Schwarz or equivalent vaccines would be appropriate.

- In countries where high immunization coverage has shifted the age distribution of measles cases to schoolchildren, a second dose of measles vaccine at school entry should be considered. School immunization not only decreases infection in susceptible older children but also decreases the risk of morbidity and mortality in their preschool siblings (measles transmission in schoolchildren has been identified as a source of infection for their high-risk preschool siblings). In Burundi, twenty-five out of twenty-eight cases of measles in school-age children were index cases in their households and the source of infection for thirty-one secondary cases, twenty-eight of whom were younger siblings (Chen 1990). Introduction of two-dose schedules has reduced measles transmission to very low levels in Murmansk and Pskov areas in the former U.S.S.R. and in Czechoslovakia (Davis 1991).

VITAMIN A SUPPLEMENTATION IN DEFICIENT AREAS. The World Health Organization has recommended that vitamin A supplementation become a routine part of immunization programs. Specifically, it recommends the administration of 200,000 international units (IU) to mothers at time of delivery or during the next four weeks, and 25,000 IU at each immunization contact beginning at six weeks of age and with at least four-week intervals (WHO/EPI 1989a, 1992). This recommendation is based on data from Indonesia and India showing that vitamin A supplementation to children in an area of vitamin A deficiency reduced overall mortality (Rahmathullah and others 1990; Sommer 1990). Although Rahmathullah and colleagues (and other researchers) did not show a clear reduction in measles or other specific cause of mortality, there is a growing consensus that vitamin A supplementation in deficient areas will reduce measles case-fatality rates and increase child survival.

TREATMENT OF SEVERE MEASLES WITH VITAMIN A. Therapeutic doses of vitamin A are now recommended for children with severe cases of measles. In a placebo-control double-blind study in South Africa, the risk of death or severe measles complication was reduced by half (RR 0.52 95 percent CI 0.35–0.74) through administration of 400,000 IU of retinyl palmitate (Hussey and Klein 1990).

EFFECTIVE TREATMENT OF MEASLES COMPLICATIONS. Most measles deaths are due to complications, a high proportion of which can be effectively treated through standard treatment practices. Data from Senegal suggest that treatment in the first few days of illness can reduce measles CFRs by 78 percent (Garenne 1992).

EXPANSION OF THE INFRASTRUCTURE. In many areas, at-risk infants have limited access to vaccination services. Development of new vaccine delivery points in such places has to be a long-term priority.

Research Priorities

Improved vaccines and implementation strategy will be required to achieve the 1995 targets. Research is a continuing priority.

OPERATIONAL RESEARCH. The currently available tools (measles vaccines, cold chain, disposable and reusable needles and syringes) have the potential of significantly aiding the effort to reduce measles and measles-associated morbidity and mortality. Operational research is needed to identify the optimal use of these tools to achieve the maximum effect, for example, use of two-dose schedules, targeting of high-risk groups, and accelerated vaccination strategies in urban areas.

VACCINE DEVELOPMENT. Although the current more heat stable vaccine is a highly effective vaccine, further improvements in measles vaccine could significantly increase the effectiveness of efforts to control measles. The ideal criteria for a measles vaccine in the developing world, based on experience acquired in the 1980s and the expected improvements to be gained by the introduction of vaccine capable of providing protection at six months of age, have not yet been met. Listed below are suggested criteria for such a vaccine:

- *Heat stable at 37°C for twelve months.* In the developing world, the areas with highest measles-associated mortality, lack of a reliable cold chain limits many health workers, especially private practitioners, from providing immunization. Resources for fuel and refrigerator maintenance, repair, and replacement are expected to shrink during the next decade.

- *Ability to achieve 95 percent seroconversion and life-long protection when administered at three months of age or earlier.* Access to health facilities is inversely related to age—the younger the age at immunization, the greater the probable contact of that child with health facilities and the opportunity for immunization. An effective vaccine for three-month-old infants would prevent almost all the measles cases that occur before nine months of age. As increasing numbers of infants in the developing world are born to mothers whose antibodies resulted from immunization rather than wild virus infection, infection in the first six months of life may increase in frequency. Immunization in the first few months of life will be needed to address this problem. A major initiative to develop such a vaccine is under way (Bart and Lin 1990).

- *Prepackaged in a single-dose non-reusable syringe.* Single-unit packaging would facilitate expanding vaccine delivery to private practitioners and nurse-midwives operating outside of the health facilities. Use of self-destruct syringes would eliminate sterilization costs and the risks of human immunodeficient virus (HIV) and hepatitis B transmission through reuse of syringes.

- *Affordable.* Vaccine cost should be in the range of the current $0.10 to $0.15 per dose.

Conclusions

Measles immunization is a proven, cost-effective primary health care intervention capable of reducing morbidity and mortality and increasing child survival. The use of current vaccines and strategies will not, however, achieve the targets (90 percent coverage, 90 percent morbidity reduction, and 95 percent mortality reduction) endorsed at the 1990 World Summit for Children. Five priorities have been identified for the 1990s:

- Development of a heat-stable vaccine providing 85 percent or higher protection when administered at six months of age or earlier.

- Operational research to ensure maximum effective use of available technologies within the epidemiologic and resource realities of the local environment.

- Strengthened decentralized management and ownership in the planning, implementation, and evaluation of immunization program.

- Development and use of management and disease information systems to strengthen decisionmaking, implementation, and evaluation.

- Continued awareness and commitment of bilateral and international technical assistance agencies on the need of developing countries for continuing foreign-exchange support for vaccines and cold-chain equipment.

Notes

We appreciate and acknowledge Felicity Cutts, Michael Deming, Michelle Garenne, Mark Grabowsky, Rafe Henderson, Bert Hirschorn, Laurie Markowitz, Walter Orenstein, and Akanne Sorungbe for their thoughtful review of sections of this chapter in manuscript form. The expert clerical support of Pat Jennings, Judith Clark, Quin Long, and Arvis McCormick is also recognized.

1. Except where noted otherwise, all dollar amounts are current U.S. dollars.

2. Missed opportunities: contacts between a child needing vaccination and a health facility with vaccine delivery capability at which needed vaccinations are not provided.

References

Aaby, Peter. 1988. *Malnourished or Overinfected: An Analysis of the Determinants of Acute Measles Mortality.* Copenhagen: Laegeforeningens Forlag.

Aaby, Peter, Jette Bukh, I. M. Lisse, and A. J. Smits. 1981. "Measles Vaccination and Child Mortality." *Lancet* 2:93.

Aaby, Peter, T. G. Jensen, H. L. Hansen, Hans Kristiansen, Jesper Tharup, Anja Poulsen, Morten Sodemann, Marianne Jakobsen, Kim Knudsen, M. C. da Silva, Hilton Whittle. 1988. "Trial of High-Dose Edmonston-Zagreb Measles Vaccine in Guinea-Bissau: Protective Efficacy." *Lancet* 2:809–14.

Aaby, Peter, and J. Leeuwenburg. 1988. "Patterns of Transmission and Severity of Measles Infection: A Reanalysis of Data from the Machakos Area." *Kenya Journal of Infectious Disease* 161:171–74.

Aaby, Peter, I. R. Pederson, Kim Knudsen, M. C. da Silva, C. H. Mordhorst, N. C. Helm-Petersen, B. S. Hansen, Jesper Tharup, Anja Poulsen, Morten Sodemann, Marianne Jakobsen. 1989. "Child Mortality Related to Seroconversion or Lack of Seroconversion after Measles Vaccination." *Pediatric Infectious Disease Journal* 8:197–200.

ACIP. 1989. "Measles Prevention. Recommendations of the Immunization Practices Advisory Committee." *Morbidity and Mortality Weekly Report* 38:1–18.

Anderson, R. M., and R. M. May. 1985. "Age-Related Changes in the Rate of Disease Transmission: Implications for the Design of Vaccination Programs." *Journal of Hygiene* 94:365–436.

Atkinson, W. L., and L. E. Markowitz. 1991. "Measles and Measles Vaccine." *Pediatric Infectious Disease Journal* 2:100–7.

Barclay A. J. G., A. Foster, and A. Sommer. 1987. "Vitamin A Supplements and Mortality Related to Measles: A Randomized Clinical Trail." *British Medical Journal* 294:294–96.

Barnum, H. 1989. "Evaluating Healthy Days of Life Gained from Health Projects." *Social Science and Medicine* 24:833–41.

Bart, K. S., and K. F. Lin. 1990. "Vaccine Preventable Disease and Immunization in the Developing World." *Pediatric Clinics of North America* 37: 735–56.

Bender, D., and R. J. Macauley. 1990. "Immunization Drop-Outs and Maternal Behavior: Evaluation of Reason Given and Strategies for Maintaining Gains Made in the National Vaccination Campaign in Liberia." *International Quarterly of Health Education* 9:283–88.

Bhuiya, Abbas, Bogdan Wojtyniak, Stan D'Souza, Lutfun Nahar, Kashem Skaikh. 1987. "Measles Case Fatality among the Under-Fives: A Multivariate Analysis of Risk Factors in a Rural Area of Bangladesh." *Social Science and Medicine* 24:439–43.

Black, F. L. 1982. "Measles." In Evans, A. S., ed., *Viral Infections of Humans, Epidemiology and Control*, 2d. New York: Plenum Medical Book Company.

———. 1989. "Measles Active and Passive Immunity in a Worldwide Perspective." *Prog Med Virol* 36:1–33.

Bloch, A. B., A. V. K. V. de Silva, R. L. de Sylva. "The Public Health Importance of Measles in Sri Lanka." Typescript. South-East Asia Regional Office, WHO, New Delhi, India.

Bloch, A. B., W. A. Orenstein, W. M. Ewing, W. H. Spain, G. F. Mallison, D. L. Herrmann, A. R. Hinman. 1985. "Measles Outbreak in a Pediatric Practice: Airborne Transmission in an Office Setting." *Pediatrics* 75:676–83.

Boerma, J. T., A. E. Sommerfelt, S. O. Rutsein, and G. Rojas. 1990. "Immunization: Levels, Trends and Differentials." Institute for Resource Development, Columbia, Md.

Borgono, J. M. 1983. "Current Impact on Measles in Latin America." *Review of Infectious Diseases* 5:417–21.

Boyd, D. 1991. "Computerized EPI Information Systems (CEIS)." Resources for Child Health, Arlington, Va.

Brenzel, Logan. 1990. "The Cost of EPI: A Review of Cost and Cost-Effectiveness Studies (1979–1987)." Resources for Child Health, Arlington, Va.

———. 1991. "Cost and Financing of EPI." Resources for Child Health, Arlington, Va.

Brenzel, L., and P. Claquin. 1991. "Immunization Programs and Their Costs." *World Bank Health Sector Priorities Review* HSPR-04. Washington, D.C.

Bryce, J. W., F. T. Cutts, and S. Saba. 1990. "Mass Immunization Campaigns and Quality of Immunization Services." *Lancet* 1:739–40.

Cardenas-Ayala, V. M., C. Sanchez-Vargas. 1989. "Estimation de la razón beneficio/costo de la vacunación contra el sarampión." *Salud Publica México* 31:735–44.

CCCD (Centers for Disease Control). 1990. *African Child Survival Initiative— Combatting Childhood Communicable Diseases, 1989–1990. Annual Report*. Atlanta, Ga.

Chand, Phool, R. N. Rai, Umwa Chawla, K. C. Tripathi, K. K. Datta. 1989. "Epidemiology of Measles—A Thirteen Year Prospective Study in a Village." *Journal of Communicable Disease* 21:190–99.

Chen, R. 1990. "Measles in Muyinga Health Sector, Burundi, 1989–1990." Field report. Centers for Disease Control, Atlanta, Ga.

Claquin, P. 1991. "Urban EPI." Resources for Child Health. Arlington, Va.

Clemens, J. D., Bonita F. Stanton, J. Chakraborty, Shahriar Chowdhury, M. R. Rao, Mohammed Ali, Susan Zimicki, Bogdan Wojtnyiak. 1988. "Measles Vaccination and Childhood Mortality in Rural Bangladesh." *American Journal of Epidemiology* 128:1330–39.

Clements, C. J., J. B. Milstein, Mark Grabowsky, and J. Gibson. 1988. "Research into Alternative Measles Vaccines in the 1990's." Working paper EPI/GEN/88.11. EPI Global Advisory Group. WHO/EPI, Geneva.

Coetzee, N., D. S. Berry, and M. E. Jacobs. 1991. "Measles Control in an Urbanizing Environment." *South African Medical Journal* 79:440–44.

Cotton, M. F., F. E. Berkowitz, Z. Berkowitz, P. J. Becker, and C. Heney. 1989. "Nosocomial Infections in Black South African Children." *Pediatric Infectious Disease Journal* 8:676–83.

Cutts, F. T. 1990. *Measles Control in the 1990s: Principles for the Next Decade*. Geneva: World Health Organization.

———. 1991. "Strategies to Improve Immunization Services in Urban Africa." *Bulletin of the World Health Organization* 69:407–14.

Cutts, F. T., D. C. Glik, A. Gordon, K. A. Parker, S. Diallo, F. Haba, and R. Stone. 1990. "Application of Multiple Methods to Study the Immunization Programme in an Urban Area of Guinea." *Bulletin of the World Health Organization* 68:769–76.

Cutts, F. T., R. H. Henderson, C. J. Clements, R. T. Chen, P. A. Patriarca. 1991. "Principles of Measles Control." *Bulletin of the World Health Organization* 69:1–7.

Cutts, F. T., Kortbeeks, R. Malalane, P. Penicele, K. Gingell. 1988. "The Development of Appropriate Strategies for EPI: A Case Study from Mozambique." *Health Policy and Planning* 3:291–301.

Dabis, F., A. R. Sow, R. J. Waldman, P. Bikakouri, J. Senga, G. Madzou, and T. S. Jones. 1988. "The Epidemiology of Measles in a Partially Vaccinated Population in an African City: Implications for Immunization Programs." *American Journal of Epidemiology* 127:171–78.

Davis, R. M. 1991. "Revised Measles Agenda for the 1990s: From Control to Pre-eradication." *International Child Health II* 3:45–50.

Davis, R. M., E. D. Whitman, W. A. Orenstein, S. R. Preblud, L. E. Markowitz, and A. R. Hinman. 1987. "A Persistent Outbreak of Measles Despite Appropriate Control Measures." *American Journal of Epidemiology* 126:438–49.

Dietz, K. 1976. "The Incidence of Infectious Diseases under the Influence of Seasonal Fluctuations." *Lecture Notes in Biomathematics* 11:1–15.

Dossetor, J., H. C. Whittle, and B. M. Greenwood. 1977. "Persistent Measles Infection in Malnourished Children." *British Medical Journal* 1:1633–35.

Drinkwater, H. 1885. *Remarks upon the Epidemic of Measles Prevalent in Sunderland*. Edinburgh: James Thin.

Duflo, B., H. Balique, P. Ranque, A. N. Diallo, G. Brucker, H. Alavi, and N. Prescott. 1986. "Estimation de l'impact des principales maladies en zone rurale malienne." *Revue d'Epidémiologie et de Santé Publique* 34:405–18.

Edmonson, M. B., D. G. Addiss, J. T. McPherson, J. L. Berg, S. R. Circo, and J. P. Davis. 1990. "Mild Measles and Secondary Vaccine Failure during a Sustained Outbreak in a Highly Vaccinated Population." *JAMA* 263:2467–71.

Ekunwe, E. O. 1984. "Expanding Immunization Coverage through Improved Clinic Procedures." *World Health Forum* 5:361–63.

Ellison, J. B. 1932. "Intensive Vitamin Therapy in Measles." *British Medical Journal* 2:708–11.

Enders, J. F., and T. C. Peebles. 1954. "Propagation in Tissue Cultures of Cytopathogenic Agents from Patients with Measles." *Proceedings of the Society for Experimental Biology* 86:277–86.

Fagbule, D., and F. Orifunmishe. 1988. "Measles and Childhood Mortality in Semi-urban Nigeria." *African Journal of Medical Science* 17:181–85.

Feachem, R. G., and M. A. Koblinsky. 1983. "Interventions for the Control of Diarrhoeal Diseases among Young Children: Measles Immunization." *Bulletin of the World Health Organization* 61:641–52.

Fine, P. E. M., and J. A. Clarkson. 1982a. "Measles in England and Wales—I: An Analysis of Factors Underlying Seasonal Patterns." *International Journal of Epidemiology* 11:5–14.

———. 1982b. "Measles in England and Wales—II: The Impact of Vaccination Programmes on the Distribution of Immunity in the Population." *International Journal of Epidemiology* 11:15–25.

Foege, W. H. 1984. "Banishing Measles from the World." *World Health Forum* 5:63–65.

Foege, W. H., and S. O. Foster. 1974. "Multiple Antigen Vaccine Strategies in Developing Countries." *American Journal of Tropical Medicine and Hygiene* 23:685–89.

Forgy, L., K. McInnes, S. Heinig, and B. Michaels. 1990. *Projected Costs of the Talloires Targets*. Abt and Associates. Washington, D.C.

Foster, A., and G. J. Johnson. 1988. "Measles, Corneal Ulceration, and Childhood Blindness: Prevention and Treatment." *Tropical Doctor* 18:74–78.

Foster, S. O. 1989. UNICEF/EPI consultation, Sultanate of Oman.

Foster, S. O., J. Shepperd, J. H. Davis, and A. N. Agle. 1990. "Working with African Nations to Improve the Health of Their Children." *JAMA* 263: 3303–5.

Foulon, G., M. L. Klein-Zabban, L. Gnansov-Nezzi, and G. Martin-Bouyer. 1983. "Preventing the Spread of Measles in Children's Clinics." *Lancet* 2:1498–99.

Gao, J. P., and M. D. Malison. 1988. "The Epidemiology of a Measles Outbreak on a Remote Offshore Island near Taiwan." *International Journal of Epidemiology* 17:894–98.

Garenne, Michel, and Peter Aaby. 1990. "Pattern of Exposure and Measles Mortality in Senegal." *Journal of Infectious Diseases* 161:1088–94.

Garenne, Michel, and P. Cantrell. "Rougeole et mortalité au Sénégal: étude de l'impact de la vaccination effectuée à Khombole 1965–1968 sur la survie des enfants. Estimation de la mortalité du jeune enfant pour guider les actions de santé des pays en développement." Institut National de Sciences et de Recherche Médicale, Paris. 145:512–32.

Garenne, Michel, Odile Leroy, Jean-Pierre Beau, and Ibrahima Sène. 1991. "Child Mortality after High-Titre Measles Vaccines: Prospective Study in Senegal." *Lancet* 2:903–7.

Ghana Health Assessment Project Team. 1981. "A Quantitative Method of Assessing the Health Impact of Different Diseases in Less Developed Countries." *International Journal of Epidemiology* 10:73–80.

Ginsberg, G. M., and T. H. Tulchinsky. 1990. "Costs and Benefits of a Second Measles Inoculation of Children in Israel, the West Bank, and Gaza." *Journal of Epidemiology and Community Health* 44:274–80.

Gordon, J. E., A. A. Jansen, and W. Ascoli. 1965. "Measles in Rural Guatemala. *Pediatrics* 66:779–86.

Grabowsky, M. 1991. "Missed Opportunities." Resources for Child Health, Arlington, Va.

Greenwood, B. M., A. M. Greenwood, A. K. Bradley, S. Tulloch, R. Hayes, and F. S. Oldfield. 1987. "Deaths in Infancy and Early Childhood in a Well Vaccinated, Rural, West African Population." *Annals of Tropical Pediatrics* 2:91–99.

Guyer, B., and A. M. McBean. 1981. "The Epidemiology and Control of Measles in Yaoundé, Cameroon, 1968–1975." *International Journal of Epidemiology* 10:263–69.

Halsey, N. A., Reginald Boulos, Franz Mode, Jean André, Linda Bowman, R. G. Yaeger, Serge Toureau, Joh Rohde, and Carlo Boulos. 1985. "Response to Measles Vaccine in Haitian Infants 6 to 12 Months Old." *New England Journal of Medicine* 313:544–49.

Heiby, J. R. 1990. *Supervision and the Quality of Care in the Expanded Programme on Immunization*. WHO/EPI/GAG/WP. Geneva.

Hethcote, H. W. 1976. "Qualitative Analysis of Communicable Disease Models." *Mathematical Biosciences* 28:335–56.

Hirschorn, N. 1990. "Missed Opportunities for Immunization." Resources for Child Health, Arlington, Va.

Holt, E. A., Reginald Boulos, N. A. Halsey, L. M. Boulos, C. Boulos. 1990. "Child Survival in Haiti: Protective Effect of Measles Vaccination." *Pédiatrie* 85:188–94.

Hopkins, D. R., J. F. Koplan, A. R. Hinman, and J. M. Lane. 1982. "The Case for Global Measles Eradication." *Lancet* 1:1396–98.

Hussey, G. D., and M. Klein. 1990. "A Randomized Controlled Trial of Vitamin A in Children with Severe Measles." *New England Journal of Medicine* 323:160–64.

Hussey, G. D., and J. Simpson. 1991. "Nosocomial Bacterias in Measles." *Pediatric Infectious Disease Journal* 9:715–17.

Hutchins, S. S., J. Escolan, L. E. Markowitz, C. Hawkins, A. Kimbler, R. A. Morgan, S. R. Preblud, and W. A. Orenstein. 1989. "Measles Outbreaks among Unvaccinated Preschool-Aged Children: Opportunities Missed by Health Care Providers to Administer Measles Vaccine." *Pédiatrie* 83:369–74.

Imperato, P. J., and D. Traore. 1969. "Traditional Beliefs about Measles and Its Treatment among the Bambara of Mali." *Tropical and Geographic Medicine* 21:62–67.

Job, J. S., N. A. Halsey, Reginald Boulos, Elizabeth Holt, Dorothy Farrell, Paul Albrecht, J. R. Brutus, Mario Adrien, Jean André, Edward Chan, Patricia Kissinger, Carlo Boulos, and the Cité Soleil/JHU Project Team. 1991. "Successful Immunization of Infants at 6 Months of Age with High Dose Edmonston-Zagreb Measles Vaccine." *Pediatric Infectious Disease Journal* 10:303–11.

John, A. M. 1990a. "Endemic Disease in Host Populations with Fully Specified Demography." *Population Biology* 37:455–71.

———. 1990b. "Transmission and Control of Childhood Infectious Diseases: Does Demography Matter?" *Population Studies* 44:195–215.

John, A. M., and S. D. Tuljapurkar. 1990. "Childhood Infectious Diseases in LDCs: Immunization Program Design and Evaluation Using Demographic-Epidemiologic Models." Working Paper 22, Research Division, Population Council, New York.

John, T. Jacob, Abraham Joseph, T. I. George, Janaki Radhakrishnan, Rajdayal Singh, Kuryan George. 1980. "Epidemiology and Prevention of Measles in Rural South India." *International Journal of Medical Research* 72:153–58.

John, T. Jacob, M. Ray, and M. C. Steinhoff. 1984. "Control of Measles by Annual Pulse Immunization." *American Journal of Diseases of Children*: 138: 299–300.

Kalter, H. D., R. H. Gray, R. E. Black, and S. A. Gultiano. 1990. "Validation of Postmortem Interviews to Ascertain Selected Causes of Death in Children." *International Journal of Epidemiology* 19:380–86.

Kaschula, R. O., J. Druker, and A. Kipps. 1983. "Late Morphologic Consequences of Measles—A Lethal and Debilitating Lung Disease among the Poor." *Review of Infectious Diseases* 5:395–404.

Kasongo Project Team. 1981. "Influence of Measles Vaccination on Survival Pattern of 7–35 Month Old Children in Kasongo, Zaire." *Lancet* 1:764–67.

Kenyan Ministry of Health and WHO (World Health Organization). 1977. "Measles Immunity in the First Year after Birth and the Optimum Age for Vaccination in Kenyan Children." *Bulletin of the World Health Organization* 55:21–31.

Kermack, W. O., and A. G. McKendrick. 1927. "A Contribution to the Mathematical Theory of Epidemics." *Proceedings of the Royal Society of London*, series A, 115:700–21.

Killewo, Japhet, Cyprian Makwaya, Emmanuel and Rose Munubhi, and Mpembeni. 1991. "The Protective Effect of Measles Vaccine under Routine Vaccination Conditions in Dar Es Salaam, Tanzania: A Case-Control Study." *International Journal of Epidemiology* 20:508–14.

Kipps, A., and R. O. C. Kaschula. 1976. "Virus Pneumonia following Measles." *South African Medical Journal* 50:1083–88.

Klein-Zabban, M. L., G. Foulon, C. Gaudebout, J. Badoual, and J. Assi Adou. 1987. "Fréquence des rougeoles nosocomiales dans un centre de protection maternelle et infantile d'Abidjan." *Bulletin of the World Health Organization* 65:197–201.

Koenig, M. A., M. A. Khan, B. Wojtyniak, J. D. Clements, J. Chakraborty, V. Fauveau, J. F. Phillips, J. Akbar, and U. S. Barua. 1990. "Impact of Measles Vaccination on Childhood Mortality in Rural Bangladesh." *Bulletin of the World Health Organization* 68:441–47.

Koster, F. T., G. C. Curlin, K. M. A. Azia, and Azizul Haque. 1981. "Synergistic Impact of Measles and Diarrhoea on Nutrition and Mortality in Bangladesh." *Bulletin of the World Health Organization* 59:901–8.

Krober, M. S., C. E. Stracener, and J. W. Bass. 1991. "Decreased Measles Response after Measles–Mumps–Rubella Vaccine in Infants with Colds." *JAMA* 265:2095–96.

Lesotho. 1990. Measles control in Lesotho.

Loras-Duclaux, I., L. David, D. Peyramond D. Floret, A. Lachaux, and M. Hermier. 1988. "Etude épidémiologique et évaluation du coût de la rougeole dans les hôpitaux lyonnais durant cinq années." *Pédiatrie* 43:451–54.

McBean, A. M., S. O. Foster, K. L. Herrmann, and C. Gateff. 1976. "Evaluation of a Mass Measles Immunization Campaign in Yaoundé, Cameroon." *Transactions of the Royal Society of Tropical Medicine and Hygiene* 70:206–12.

McFarland, D. A., and D. K. Kraushaar. 1990. "Cost of the EPI and CDD Programmes in Swaziland." Centers for Disease Control, Atlanta, Ga.

Maina-Ahlberg, B. 1979. "Beliefs and Practices Concerning Treatment of Measles and Acute Diarrhea among the Akamba." *Tropical and Geographic Medicine* 31:139–48.

Markowitz, L. 1990. "Measles Control in the 1990s. Immunization before 9 Months of Age." World Health Organization, Geneva.

Markowitz, L. E., and P. Nieburg. 1991. "The Burden of Acute Respiratory Infection Due to Measles in Developing Countries and the Potential Impact of Measles Vaccine." *Review of Infectious Diseases* 13:555–61.

Markowitz, L. E., N. Nzilambi, W. J. Driskell, M. G. Sension, E. Z. Rovira, P. Nieburg, and R. W. Rider. 1989. "Vitamin A Levels and Mortality among Hospitalized Measles Patients, Kinshasa, Zaire." *Journal of Tropical Pediatrics* 35:109–12.

Markowitz, L. E., and W. A. Orenstein. 1990. "Measles Vaccines." *Pediatric Clinics of North America* 37:603–25.

Markowitz, L. E., S. R. Preblud, P. E. M. Fine, and W. A. Orenstein. 1990. "Duration of Live Measles Vaccine—Induced Immunity." *Pediatric Infectious Disease Journal* 8:101–10.

Markowitz, L. E., J. Sepúlveda, J. L. Diaz-Ortega, J. L. Valdespino, P. Albrecht, E. R. Zell, J. Stewart, M. L. Zarate, and R. H. Bernier. 1990. "Immunization of Six-Month-Old Infants with Different Doses of Edmonston-Zagreb and Schwarz Measles Vaccine." *New England Journal of Medicine* 322:580–87.

Mast, Eric, J. L. Berg, L. P. Hanrahan, J. T. Wassell, and J. P. Davis. 1990. "Risk Factors for Measles in a Previously Vaccinated Population and Cost-Effectiveness of Revaccination Strategies." *JAMA* 264:2529–33.

Mathias, R. G., W. G. Meekison, T. A. Arcand, and M. T. Schechter. 1989. "The Role of Secondary Vaccine Failures in Measles Outbreaks." *American Journal of Public Health* 79:475–78.

Morley, D. 1973. "'Severe' Measles." In D. Morley, ed., *Pediatric Priorities in the Developing World*. London: Butterworth.

Mosely, W. H., and L. C. Chen. 1984. "An Analytic Framework for the Study of Child Survival in Developing Countries." In *Child Survival Strategies for Research. Supp. Population and Development Review* 10S:25–45.

Narain, J. P., S. Khare, S. R. S. Rana, and K. B. Banerjee. 1989. "Epidemic Measles in an Isolated, Unvaccinated Population, India." *International Journal of Epidemiology* 18:952–58.

Nokes, D. J., A. R. McLean, R. M. Anderson, and M. Grabowsky. 1990. "Measles Immunization Strategies for Countries with High Transmission Rates: Interim Guidelines Predicted Using a Mathematical Model." *International Journal of Epidemiology* 19:703–10.

Orenstein, W. A., R. H. Bernier, T. J. Dondero, A. R. Hinman, J. S. Marks, K. J. Bart, and B. Sirotkin. 1985. "Field Evaluation of Vaccine Efficacy." *Bulletin of the World Health Organization* 63:1055–68.

Orenstein, W. A., L. Markowitz, S. R. Preblud, A. R. Hinman, A. Tomasi, and K. J. Bart. 1986. "Appropriate Age for Measles Vaccination in the United States." *Developments in Biological Standards* 65:13–21.

PAHO (Pan-American Health Organization). 1990. "Plan to Eliminate Indigenous Transmission of Measles in the English Speaking Caribbean." *Bulletin of the Pan-American Health Organization* 24:240–46.

Panum, P. L. 1939. "Observations Made during the Epidemic of Measles on the Faroe Islands in the Year 1846." *Medical Classics* 3:839–86.

Phillips, M. A., R. G. Feachem, and A. Mills. 1987. *Options for Diarrhoea Control*. EPC Publication 13. London: School of Hygiene and Tropical Medicine.

Pison, G., and N. Bonneuil. 1988. "Increased Risk of Measles Mortality for Children with Siblings among the Fula Bande, Senegal." *Review of Infectious Diseases* 10:468–70.

Ponninghaus, J. M. 1980. "The Cost/Benefit of Measles Immunization: A Study from Southern Zambia." *Journal of Tropical Medicine and Hygiene* 83:141–49.

Preblud, S. R., and S. L. Katz. 1988. "Measles Vaccine." In S. A. Plotkin and E. A. Mortimer, eds., *Vaccines*. Philadelphia: W. B. Saunders.

Prescott, N., A. Prost, and R. Le Berre. 1984. "The Economics of Blindness Prevention in Upper Volta under the Onchocerciasis Control Program." *Social Science and Medicine* 19:1051–55.

de Quadros, C. A., J. K. Andrus, J. M. Olive, C. M. da Silveria, R. E. Eikhof, Peter Carrasco, J. W. Fitzsimmon, and Francisco P. Pinheiro. 1991. "Eradication of Poliomyelitis: Progress in the Americas." *Pediatric Infectious Disease Journal* 10:222–29.

Rahmathullah, Laxmi, B. A. Underwood, R. D. Thulesiraj, R. C. Milton, Kala Ramaswamy, Raheem Rahmathullah, Geneesh Babu, and B. Com. 1990. "Reduced Mortality among Children in Southern India Receiving a Small Weekly Dose of Vitamin A." *New England Journal of Medicine* 323:929–35.

Robertson, R. L. 1985. *Cost of the CCCD Project in Swaziland, 1984–1985*. University Research Corporation.

Robertson, R. L., S. O. Foster, H. F. Hull, and P. J. Williams. 1987. "Cost-Effectiveness of Immunization in The Gambia." *Journal of Tropical Medicine and Hygiene* 88:343–51.

Rosenthal, G. 1990. "Sustainability of EPI." Resources for Child Health, Arlington, Va.

Roungou, J. B. 1991. Coverage Survey, Central African Republic.

Sabin, A. B., A. Flores Arechiga, J. Fernandez de Castro, J. L. Sever, D. L. Madden, I. Shekarchi, P. Albrecht. 1983. "Successful Immunization of Children with and without Maternal Antibody by Aerosolized Measles Vaccine." *JAMA* 249:2651–52.

Sahuguede, P., A. Roisin, I. Sanou, B. Nacro, F. Talls. 1989. "Epidémie de rougeole au Burkina Faso: 714 cas hospitalisés à l'hôspital de Bobo-Dioulasso." *Annals of Pediatrics* 36:244–51.

Schenzle, D. 1989. "An Age-Structured Model of Pre- and Post-vaccination Measles Transmission." *IMA (International Mathematics Association) Journal of Mathematics Applied to Medicine and Biology* 1:16–91.

Shears, P., A. M. Berry, R. Murphy, and M. A. Nabil. 1987. "Epidemiologic Assessment of the Health and Nutrition of Ethiopian Refugees in Emergency Camps in Sudan." *British Medical Journal* 295:314–18.

Shepard, D. S., L. Sanoh, and E. Coffi. 1986. "Cost-Effectiveness of the Expanded Programme on Immunization in the Ivory Coast: A Preliminary Assessment." *Social Science and Medicine* 22:369–77.

Smith, E. A., and S. O. Foster. 1970. "The Effect of the Smallpox Eradication Measles Control Programme on Measles Admissions to the Lagos Infectious Disease Hospital, Yaba, Nigeria." *West African Medical Journal* 19:51–56.

Sommer, A. 1990. "Vitamin A Status, Resistance to Infection, and Childhood Mortality." *Annals of the New York Academy of Science* 587:17–23.

Taylor, W. R., Ruti-Kalisa, Mambu Ma-Disu, and J. M. Weinman. 1988. "Measles Control Efforts in Urban Africa Complicated by High Incidence of Measles in the First Year of Life." *American Journal of Epidemiology* 127:788–94.

Toole, M. J., R. W. Steketee, R. J. Waldman, and P. Nieburg. 1989. "Measles Prevention and Control in Emergency Settings." *Bulletin of the World Health Organization* 67:381–88.

Toole, M. J., and R. J. Waldman. 1988. "An Analysis of Mortality among Refugee Populations in Thailand, Somalia, and Sudan." *Bulletin of the World Health Organization* 66:237–47.

Tuljapurkar, S. D., and A. M. John. 1991. "Disease in Changing Populations: Growth and Disequilibrium." *Population Biology* 40:322-53.

UNICEF. 1990. *Universal Child Immunization Reaching the Urban Poor*. Urban Examples 16. New York.

United States, National Vaccine Advisory Committee. 1991. The Measles Epidemic: The Problems, Barriers, Recommendations.

Verduzco, E., C. Calderon, and E. Velazquez-Franco. 1974. "Repercusiones de la vacunación contra el sarampión en México." *Salud Pública México* 16:707–20.

Voorhoeve, A. M., A. S. Muller, T. W. Schulpen, W. Gemert, H. A. Valkenburg, and H. E. Ensering. 1977. "Agents Affecting Health of Mother and Child in a Rural Area of Kenya. III: The Epidemiology of Measles." *Tropical and Geographic Medicine* 29:428–40.

Walsh, J. A. 1983. "Selective Primary Health Care: Strategies for Control of Disease in the Developing World. IV: Measles." *Review of Infectious Diseases* 5:330–40.

Weierbach, R. 1989. "Rapport de mission au Rwanda du Juillet au 4 Août." Centers for Disease Control, Atlanta, Ga.

White, C. C., J. P. Koplan, and W. A. Orenstein. 1985. "Benefits, Risks, and Costs of Immunization for Measles, Mumps, and Rubella." *American Journal of Public Health* 75:739–44.

Whittle, H. C., A. Bradley-Moore, A. Fleming, and B. M. Greenwood. 1973. "Effects of Measles and the Immune Response of Nigerian Children." *Archives of Diseases of Children* 48:753–56.

Whittle, H. C., M. G. M. Rowland, G. F. Mann, W. H. Lamb, and R. A. Lewis. 1984. "Immunization of 4–6 Month Old Gambian Children with Edmonston-Zagreb Measles Vaccine." *Lancet* 2:834–37.

WHO (World Health Organization). 1988. *Expanded Programme on Immunization Mid-Level Managers Module: Measuring Vaccination Coverage*. Geneva.

———. 1989a. "High Dose EZ Measles Vaccine." EPI/GAG/89/WP13. Geneva.

———. 1989b. "Vitamin A Update." EPI/GAG/89/WP13. Geneva.

———. 1991. "Plan of Action for Global Measles Control." EPI/GAG/91/WP12. Geneva.

———. 1992. "Using Immunization Contacts to Combat Vitamin A Deficiency." EPI/GAG/92.

WHO/EPI (World Health Organization/Expanded Programme on Immunization). 1984. "Expanded Programme on Immunization, Indications and Contraindications for Vaccines Used in the EPI." WHO/WER (*Weekly Epidemological Record*) 59:13–16.

———. 1985. "Expanded Programme on Immunization, Public Health Importance of Measles." WHO/WER 60:103–5. Burma.

———. 1979. "Expanded Programme on Immunization, Measles Immunization." WHO/WER 54:337–39. Kenya.

———. 1986. "Expanded Programme on Immunization, Measles Vaccine Efficacy." WHO/WER 61:356–57. Poland.

———. 1985. "Public Health Importance of Measles." WHO/WER 60:95–97. Sri Lanka.

———. 1989. "Expanded Programme on Immunization, Missed Opportunities for Immunization." WHO/WER 64:32–34. Zimbabwe.

WHO/UNICEF (World Health Organization/United Nations Children's Fund). 1985. *Planning Principles for Accelerated Immunization Strategies. A Joint WHO/UNICEF Statement*. Geneva.

Yach, D., C. Metcalf, P. Lachman, G. Hussey, E. Subotsky, R. Blignaut, A. J. Flisher, H. S. Schaaf, and N. Cameron. 1991. "Missed Opportunities for Measles Immunization in Selected Western Cape Hospitals." *South African Medical Journal* 79:437–39.

9

Tetanus

Robert Steinglass, Logan Brenzel, and Allison Percy

Tetanus is a completely preventable disease caused by contamination of wounds with an anaerobic bacillus, *Clostridium tetani*. The organism is ubiquitous in soil and dust and has the ability to form highly resistant spores. It exists harmlessly in the gut of many animals, including man. If the pathogen is introduced into necrosed tissues, it multiplies and produces a powerful neurotoxin. Tetanus is an endemic environmental hazard, rather than a communicable disease, and consequently does not spread in explosive epidemics (Cvjetanovic, Grab, and Uemura 1978a).

Tetanus in newborns is caused by infection resulting from unsterile methods of cutting the umbilical cord or dressing the stump. The first sign of neonatal tetanus (NNT) is the baby's inability to suck and swallow when a few days old. This inability is due to rigidity of the lips and mouth (lockjaw), which causes a characteristic ironic smile (*risus sardonicus*). Rigidity quickly develops throughout the body, often accompanied by generalized convulsions. Death, usually caused by respiratory failure, occurs between six and ten days of life, two to three days after the onset of symptoms.

In children and adults, tetanus infection follows puncture wounds, cuts, and burns. Cases have been documented that resulted from ear and skin infections, nonsterile injections and surgical procedures, ear-piercing, scarification rituals and tattoos, circumcision, and animal bites or scratches. A relatively common cause of tetanus in adult women is postabortal or postpartum contamination of the uterus, which is associated with a high risk of fatality. Frequently, the portal of entry in non-neonatal tetanus cannot be determined by either the patient or physician.

The World Health Organization (WHO) estimates the case-fatality rate (CFR) of untreated neonatal tetanus to be 85 percent (Stanfield and Galazka 1984; Galazka and Stroh 1986). Marked declines in CFRs in some hospitals are due to control of respiration by medicated relaxation and mechanical ventilation (Simonsen, Bloch, and Heron 1987). Wide variation in CFRs among treated NNT patients has been reported (Bytchenko 1966) and reflects treatment regimens, the vigilance and skill of nursing care, and methods of calculation. In

many instances, significant numbers of terminal patients leave the hospital against medical advice and are recorded as surviving patients. In one series of hospital patients, if all those who left against medical advice are assumed to have subsequently died, which is most probable, the CFR increases from 50.6 percent to 92.6 percent (Al-Mukhtar 1987). If only known outcomes are included in the denominator, the CFR in the above study is 87 percent.

Sharma and Sharma (1982) estimate from several hospital studies that the duration of clinical sickness is nineteen days for newborns who recover and three days for those who die. Recovery in younger persons is usually complete.

On the basis of available evidence, the CFR for non-neonatal tetanus (non-NNT) is estimated to be 40 to 50 percent, and the duration of clinical illness in adults is estimated to be 14 days for those who recover and 4.5 days for those who die (Sharma and Sharma 1982). Rey, Diop-Mar, and Robert (1981) estimate the duration of hospital stay to be between 20 and 40 days. As with NNT, the CFR is largely due to treatment regimens, availability of skilled care, and age distribution of infected patients. The prognosis is poorer in the elderly, who represent a large proportion of all tetanus patients in industrial countries. Some authorities report that survivors do not suffer from incapacitating sequelae (Rey, Diop-Mar, and Robert 1981), whereas others report persisting vertebral changes, ophthalmological changes, limb deformity, and the need for convalescent physiotherapy (Sénécal 1970; Veronesi and Focaccia 1981). Older patients are more likely to suffer sequelae because of exacerbation of preexisting conditions. As tetanus does not confer immunity, reinfection is possible. Given the very high incidence and CFR of neonatal and non-neonatal tetanus in developing countries, the most effective strategy is to prevent the disease from occurring in the first place.

Public Health Significance of Tetanus

A sizeable body of literature exists on the public health significance of tetanus in both industrial and developing countries. Despite this, tetanus remains a neglected disease.

Past and Future Trends in Incidence

Well into the twentieth century, NNT continued to cause high mortality in today's industrial countries. A review of the experience in these countries is instructive.

The decline of NNT in industrial countries to the point of virtual elimination began before the widespread introduction of tetanus toxoid (TT) immunization for children or adults in the 1950s (Heath, Zusman, and Sherman 1964; Bytchenko 1972; Christensen 1972a; Simonsen and others 1987). The decline was due to improved socioeconomic conditions (for example, wearing shoes), sanitation and personal hygiene (for example, cleaner maternal deliveries and immediate treatment of wounds), and advances in wound management (for example, passive immunization with antitetanus serum [ATS] derived from horses). Increasing urbanization, decreasing proportion of the population engaged in agriculture, mechanization of agriculture, increasing use of chemical rather than animal fertilizers, and falling fertility were important factors contributing to the decline. Hygiene associated with childbirth improved (for example, hand washing and cord care) and the proportion of deliveries conducted by trained health workers either at home (as in Holland) or in health facilities increased.

In the United States, NNT incidence declined from 64 per 100,000 live births in 1900 to about 1 per 100,000 live births in the early 1960s (LaForce, Young, and Bennett 1969). In Japan, NNT mortality reached a similar level of 1 per 100,000 live births by 1968, despite a rate of nearly 40 per 100,000 live births only twenty years before. This rapid decline occurred in the absence of a TT immunization program, which was not introduced until the 1970s (Ebisawa 1967, 1972). The control of NNT during the 1970s and 1980s in industrial countries occurred largely because of aseptic obstetric practices. The elimination of NNT owed much to the widespread immunization of children during the 1950s, which led to a cohort of women of childbearing age who could pass maternal antitoxin to their offspring (Christensen 1972a; Simonsen 1989). The fall in non-neonatal tetanus experienced in industrial countries, particularly in children and young adults, was hastened by mass immunization of males and females with TT (Stanfield and Galazka 1984; Simonsen, Bloch, and Heron 1987).

Although instructive, the experience of declining tetanus incidence and improved control in industrial countries is not germane to the situation prevailing in developing countries. With a few notable exceptions, documented levels of NNT today in developing areas are much higher than have ever been reported for today's industrial countries, and few cases are brought to health facilities. In many countries, prospects for rapid improvement in socioeconomic development or in the proportion of births delivered hygienically are not encouraging. Even where birth rates are falling, more babies are being born because of the increased numbers of women of childbearing age. Yet in the second half of this century, TT—an effective and affordable control measure—has become available, along with a structure of national immunization programs through which it can be delivered. Pioneering field trials in developing

countries during the past thirty years have demonstrated dramatically that, despite a contaminated environment, NNT can be rapidly controlled and even eliminated by wide use of TT immunization (Schofield, Tucker, and Westbrook 1961; Newell and others 1966; Berggren and Berggren 1971; Black, Huber, and Curlin 1980).

Unless significant resources are allocated to its rapid reduction, tetanus incidence will decline slowly in developing countries. The pace of decline will be a function of epidemiological risk factors, demographic trends, use of health care, socioeconomic change, political will, resource allocations, and technological advances. The most important factors for the reduction of tetanus cases in developing countries will be increased immunization coverage among children and adults with preparations containing tetanus toxoid, urbanization and urban growth, and declining total fertility rates. The possible development of a high-potency single-dose TT will also hasten the prevention of tetanus.

To accelerate this decline in tetanus, the World Health Assembly of WHO in 1989 set a goal for the Expanded Programme on Immunization (EPI) of global elimination of NNT by 1995. The goal itself has generated increased recognition of the public health importance of NNT. The degree of political will engendered and allocation of required resources will de-

Figure 9-1. *Measles, Neonatal Tetanus, and Pertussis Deaths Prevented and Occurring*

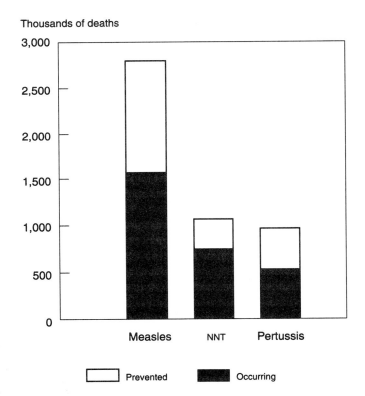

Thousands of deaths

Note: NNT deaths prevented = 325,000; NNT deaths occurring = 754,000.
Source: WHO/EPI 1989b.

termine whether as many as 8 million babies and 2 million children and adults (at current incidence rates) die from tetanus during the 1990s.

Tetanus: A Neglected Disease

With the exception of measles, NNT kills more children than any other vaccine-preventable disease. Called a disease of "peculiar quietness" (Tateno, Suzuki, and Kitamoto 1961), tetanus may be the most underreported lethal infection in the world. If tetanus had the potential to spread in sweeping epidemics or if the disease left lasting disability like polio, or if it occurred primarily in adults like tuberculosis, NNT would probably have attracted the attention of public health authorities long ago.

Instead, NNT kills its victims, who are generally born at home, before they are old enough to be registered or missed by the health system. Routine disease surveillance systems in most developing countries detect only a small fraction of cases, less than 5 percent according to WHO (WHO/EPI 1982). Lacking its own three-digit code in the *International Classification of Diseases* (WHO 1977), NNT is frequently not reported separately from cases of non-NNT, despite epidemiologically significant differences in risk factors and options for prevention. As a result, NNT incidence is often hidden within aggregate figures for "infections specific to the perinatal period" or cannot be disaggregated from tetanus in broader age groupings (for example, from birth to age four).

Neonatal tetanus is there to be found, if one looks for it. A single hospital sometimes admits more patients with NNT than are reported for the entire country (Stanfield and Galazka 1984; Betts 1989). In early global reviews of hospital data, NNT was frequently found to be the leading cause of death in pediatric wards (Bytchenko 1966; Miller 1972). Just as reported smallpox incidence in Ethiopia, India, and elsewhere rose precipitously in the face of stepped-up control and improved surveillance (Fenner and others 1988), so too the number of cases of NNT reported by a hospital in a rural area of Haiti with a successful control program increased even as

incidence per 1,000 live births dropped (Berggren 1974a). In an area of Indonesia with a history of regular reporting through designated sentinel surveillance posts, NNT incidence was five times higher than indicated by the routine surveillance network operating in the same area (WHO 1986).

Neonatal tetanus also is neglected for sociocultural reasons. The family of the baby with NNT is typically, but not exclusively, poor and illiterate and does not view the disease as a biomedical entity amenable to modern medical treatment. From widely scattered parts of the world, it has been reported that the supernatural nature of the signs of NNT suggests some sort of spirit possession (Schofield, Tucker, and Westbrook 1961; Chen 1976; Bastien 1988; Blanchet 1989; Pillsbury 1989). In some areas of presumably lower incidence, NNT is not clearly distinguished from a larger syndrome affecting newborns (Bastien 1988; Nichter 1990). Cases of NNT are likely to be concealed in some cultures, where it is perceived as a punishment from God (Solter, Hasibuan, and Yusuf 1986), possibly because of parental wrongdoing (Bastien 1988). Traditional prohibitions often preclude travel by the mother and newborn in the intimate and secluded period immediately after delivery.

Current Magnitude of Tetanus

The magnitude and preventability of tetanus has been highlighted in several important papers in which the researchers attempted to define the public health agenda for the 1980s. In arguing for selective primary health care, Walsh and Warren (1979) consider NNT to be in the highest priority group for disease control because of its high incidence, high mortality, and cost-effective and feasible means of control. In struggling with problems of scarcity and choice, Evans, Hall, and Warford (1981) conclude that the investment policies of donor agencies should redirect resources to the areas of greatest need with a package of maternal and child health services, including TT to pregnant women. Foege and Henderson (1986) argue that on the basis of cost, feasibility, safety, and effectiveness, the highest priority should be given to immunization against tetanus, measles, pertussis and diphtheria, and polio.

Table 9-1. Estimated Worldwide Morbidity and Mortality from Non-neonatal Tetanus, 1980–1984

Countries	Population[a] (millions)	Average morbidity (per 100,000)	Number of cases (thousands)	Mortality[b] (per 100,000)	Number of deaths (thousands)
Developing countries					
Asia[c]	1,510	15–30	226–528	6–14	90–211
Africa	490	15–35	73–172	6–14	29–69
America	370	3–8	11–30	1–3	3–11
Total	2,290		310–700		122–291
Industrial countries	1,160	0.15	2	0.6	1
Total[c]	3,550		312–702		123–292

a. Figures for 1982. This column does not total correctly in original citation.

b. According to a mean CFR of 40 percent (25 percent to 40 percent in some urban hospitals, 40 percent to 60 percent elsewhere in developing countries). In industrial countries, the CFR is nearly the same, despite intensive care, because most patients are elderly.

c. Excluding China.

Source: Rey and Tikhomirov 1989.

Table 9-2. Age Distribution of Patients with Non-neonatal Tetanus and Case-Fatality Rate in Bombay and Dakar

| | Bombay[a] | | | | Dakar[b] | | | |
| | 1954–68 | | 1977–79 | | 1960–67 | | 1985–86 | |
Age (years)	Percent	CFR	Percent	CFR	Percent	CFR	Percent	CFR
1 month–9 years	47.6	(32.8)	36.1	(6.1)	43.3	(24.9)	39.1	(17.6)
10–19	17.1	(33.7)	14.1	(15.6)	25.0	(24.9)	25.4	(22.5)
20–29	15.1	(61.5)	21.3	(23.5)	12.8	(37.7)	12.6	(45.5)
30–39	11.1	(45.9)	11.3	(38.9)	8.1	(39.2)	6.5	(41.2)
40–49	4.8	(46.8)	8.2	(23.1)	4.9	(36.4)	7.0	(37.8)
50–59	2.9	(49.3)	5.6	(66.7)	n.a.	n.a.	5.3	(46.4)
60+	1.3	(53.3)	3.4	(63.6)	5.8	(63.0)	4.0	(71.4)
Total	99.9	(39.1)	100.0	(21.6)	100.0	(30.0)	99.9	(29.1)

n.a. Data not available.
a. 1954–68 data from Patel and Mehta 1975; 1977–79 data from Vakil and Dalal 1975.
b. 1960–67 data from Rey and others 1968; 1985–86 data from Sow 1989.
Source: Rey and Tikhomirov 1989.

The World Health Organization estimates that tetanus kills 754,000 newborns each year and that another 325,000 deaths are being prevented (WHO/EPI 1989b; see figure 9-1.) Neonatal tetanus typically accounts for one-fourth of infant mortality and half of neonatal mortality in unimmunized populations in developing countries (Galazka, Gasse, and Henderson 1989).

From community surveys, some 270,000 NNT deaths are estimated annually in the Southeast Asia region of WHO and another 200,000 in the African region (WHO/EPI 1987a). Some 130,000 NNT deaths were estimated to occur in seven countries in the Eastern Mediterranean region of WHO in 1981, with 111,000 in Pakistan alone (WHO 1982). Ninety thousand NNT deaths were estimated for the American region in 1984 (Stanfield and Galazka 1984). An additional 60,000 cases, including 40,000 in China alone, are estimated to occur annually in the Western Pacific region (F. Gasse, personal communication, July 3, 1990). These calculations are based on surveys, which will be discussed later.

NON-NEONATAL TETANUS. The magnitude of non-NNT is poorly defined and often overlooked in discussions of tetanus prevention. Stanfield and Galazka (1984) assume that 50 percent of all tetanus cases are non-neonatal. Rey and Tikhomirov (1989) estimate that 300,000 to 700,000 cases of non-NNT, with 120,000 to 300,000 deaths, occurred yearly in the 1980s, excluding those in China (table 9-1). Industrial countries account for less than 2 percent of the total number of non-NNT cases and deaths.

Using age distribution data from four studies conducted from the 1950s to the 1980s in Bombay and Dakar, Rey and Tikhomirov (1989) show that 50 to 60 percent of non-NNT cases and a higher proportion of deaths occur among economically productive individuals from ten to fifty-nine years old (table 9-2).

Following widespread immunization of infants and older children with diphtheria-pertussis-tetanus (DPT) and diphtheria-tetanus (DT) vaccines, an epidemiological shift in the incidence of tetanus toward children and young adults can be expected to occur in developing countries, as it did in industrial countries (Rey, Guillaumont, and Majnoni d'Intignano 1979; Stanfield and Galazka 1984; Cottin 1987; Simonsen, Bloch, and Heron 1987). As recently as the 1950s, NNT in the United States accounted for 25 percent of all tetanus deaths (Heath, Zusman, and Sherman 1964). In Denmark, NNT accounted for more than 50 percent of all tetanus deaths, but since 1970 no NNT deaths have been reported (Simonsen, Bloch, and Heron 1987). In Sri Lanka the proportion of all NNT cases was halved after the first three years (1978–81) of the establishment of the Expanded Programme on Immunization (de Silva 1982). Increased incidence of adult tetanus may occur in some developing countries that are experiencing a demographic transition, where high birth rates in the past outpaced immunization coverage.

Although the proportion of cases which occur at economically productive ages in both developing and industrial countries is likely to increase, the total number of cases at economically productive ages will decline in industrial countries despite aging of the population (figure 9-2). Tetanus will increasingly become a disease of the elderly in industrial countries as a function of poor vaccination coverage and vanishing immunity (WHO/EPI 1981a; WHO/EPI 1983b; Rosmini and others 1987; Simonsen, 1989; Sutter and others 1990).

MATERNAL MORTALITY DUE TO TETANUS. An important though little recognized benefit from immunization of females with TT is the prevention of tetanus mortality in adult women. Mortality is prevented during the period of maternal risk (defined as pregnancy or within six weeks of being pregnant) both from postpartum and postabortal tetanus, as well as from wounds sustained at other times. Tetanus is caused by "inexpert attempts to remove a retained placenta" at delivery and by incomplete abortion (Schofield 1986).

Among 49 women fifteen to fifty years of age admitted with tetanus to one urban hospital in South Africa during a 7.5-year period, tetanus was associated with pregnancy in 20 (40 percent) of these women (Bennett 1976). Seventeen (35 percent) of the total cases were postabortal, two were postpartum, and one occurred during pregnancy. In another review, the genital tract was the portal of entry in 19 percent of more than 500 women with tetanus (Adeuja and Osuntokun 1971). In the United States, LaForce, Young, and Bennett (1969) reported that 6 of 507 tetanus cases were associated with abortion (4) or parturition (2). In the state of Rio de Janeiro from 1966 to 1968, postabortal tetanus constituted 7 (4.8 percent) of the 146 cases with known portal of entry (Ecuador: Ministerio de Salud Pública and UNICEF 1987).

Citing seven studies conducted in India and one each in Japan, Singapore, and Viet Nam, all published from 1960 to 1962, Bytchenko (1966) notes that postpartum and postabortal tetanus (3 to 113 cases, median 17) accounted for 3 to 22 percent (median 8.2 percent) of all cases of tetanus, with CFRs ranging from 64 to 72 percent. A review of 981 tetanus patients admitted to one hospital in New Delhi from 1963 to 1965 found that postabortal and postpartum tetanus caused 47 percent (71) of the 150 cases occurring among women of fifteen to fifty years of age, 25 percent of the 280 female non-neonatal cases, and 7 percent of all tetanus cases (Suri 1967).

In two prospective investigations of maternal mortality in a rural Bangladesh population having a vital registration system, Chen and others (1974) found that maternal deaths (defined as occurring during pregnancy or within ninety days of its termination) accounted for 27 to 30 percent of all adult female deaths. Where cause of death was reported, 3 (7.3 percent) of the 41 maternal deaths were due to postpartum tetanus. Thus, 2 percent of all adult female deaths were due solely to postpartum tetanus. Postabortal tetanus deaths and tetanus not related to pregnancy would further increase the percentage of adult female deaths attributable to tetanus. The tetanus-attributable maternal mortality rate was 56 per 100,000 live births.

Rosenfield and Maine (1985) cite a 1979 WHO estimate that 500,000 females in developing countries die annually from complications of pregnancy, abortion attempts, and childbirth. Maine and others (1987) construct a model for a hypothetical population of 1 million with a crude birth rate of 46 per 1,000 and a maternal mortality rate of 800 per 100,000 births, but they assume a low proportion (2 percent) of maternal mortality to be due to tetanus. The tetanus-attributable maternal mortality rate in this case would be 13 per 100,000 live births.

Tetanus represents an important cause of preventable maternal mortality, although it is sometimes only mentioned in passing in references on safe motherhood (Herz and Measham 1987; Royston and Armstrong 1989). A global review of existing data to determine the magnitude of maternal mortality due to tetanus has recently appeared (Fauveau, Mamdani Steinglass and Koblinsky 1993). From 15,000 to 30,000 deaths due to postpartum and postabortal tetanus are estimated to occur annually.

NEONATAL TETANUS. Much more is known about NNT than about non-NNT or maternal tetanus. Retrospective community surveys using a cluster sampling methodology have been conducted widely since the late 1970s to determine mortality from NNT and to elucidate its epidemiological features (Galazka and Stroh 1986). The surveys generally use a short recall period of four to thirteen months and rely upon a "verbal autopsy" method based on the classic symptoms of NNT (ability to suck during first two days of life, followed by cessation of sucking, stiffness, spasms, and death within the first month of life). As of 1989, forty-two countries had conducted more than seventy-five of these surveys (WHO 1982; Gasse 1990; see table 9-3).

Mortality from NNT ranges from as low as 0 to 2 per 1,000 live births (in Tanzania, Congo, Lesotho, Jordon, Tunisia, and Sri Lanka) to 30 to 67 per 1,000 live births (in Pakistan, Bangladesh, and India). Among surveys which detected NNT and reported the proportion of neonatal deaths due to tetanus, 6 percent (in urban areas in West Bengal, India) to 72 percent (in rural areas in Uttar Pradesh, India) of neonatal mortality was attributable to tetanus (WHO 1982).

The surveys have shown that whenever neonatal mortality exceeds 30 per 1,000 live births, tetanus is invariably a substantial contributor (REACH 1989; see figure 9-3). In some developing countries where measles immunization coverage has rapidly increased, NNT could soon overtake measles as the leading cause of mortality among the vaccine-preventable diseases (WHO/EPI 1987a). These surveys have succeeded in alerting many national decisionmakers about the magnitude of NNT as a public health problem. On the basis of the surveys, WHO estimates that only 2 percent and 5 percent of NNT cases have been reported in the Eastern Mediterranean and Southeast Asian regions of WHO, respectively (WHO/EPI 1982).

Figure 9-2. Reported Tetanus Cases in Poland, by Age, 1965, 1975, 1985

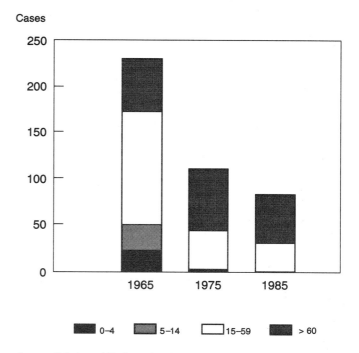

Source: Galazka and Kardymowicz 1989b.

Table 9-3. Estimated Neonatal Mortality and Neonatal Tetanus Mortality Rates Based on Special Community Surveys, 1978–1989
(per 1,000 live births)

WHO region	Country	Year	Number of live births surveyed	Mortality rates		Percent of neonatal deaths due to tetanus
				Neonatal	NNT	
Africa	The Gambia	1980	4,976	—	11	—
	Cameroon	1982	2,102	—	7	—
	Côte d'Ivoire	1982	2,324	34	18	51
	Malawi	1982	2,081	29	12	41
	Ethiopia	1983	2,010	8	5	53
	Zimbabwe	1983	4,103	10	4	39
	Zaire	1983	4,106	—	9	—
	Senegal	1983–86	4,164	51	16	31
	Cameroon	1984	2,118	—	8	—
	Uganda	1984	525	38	15	40
	Togo	1984	4,966	11	6	52
	Burundi	1984	3,099	—	8	—
	Kenya	1984–85	6,566	16	11	67
	Lesotho	1986	—	—	4	—
	Zambia	1986	3,741	14	4	30
	Tanzania (Zanzibar)	1988	2,269	9	2	25
	Congo	1988	3,524	15	2	15
	Ghana	1989	2,694	26	7	29
	Kenya	1989	2,556	21	3	15
	Lesotho	1989	2,467	4	0	0
	Madagascar					
	Urban	1989	3,133	7	0.1	2
	Rural	1989	2,772	2	0.8	38
	Niger	1989	2,550	26	9	33
	Tanzania					
	Kagera	1989	2,118	—	3	—
	Morogoro	1989	2,129	—	3	—
Eastern Mediterranean	Dem. Yemen	1981	6,224	19	4	20
	Egypt (urban)	1981	—	—	3	—
	Pakistan	1981	13,858	52	31	60
	Somalia	1981	5,781	91	21	23
	Sudan	1981	9,632	29	9	32
	Syrian Arab Republic	1981	6,762	—	5	—
	Yemen Arab Republic	1981	5,191	31	3	8
	Jordan	1983	2,850	7	2	13
	Pakistan	1984	9,925	—	28	—
	Iran, Islamic Rep. of	1985	144,000	21	5	24
	Egypt	1986	8,286	12	7	58
	Pakistan	1987	5,859	14	4	29
	Tunisia	1988	9,478	15	2	9
Southeast Asia	Bangladesh	1978	2,432	48	27	56
	Indonesia	1979	1,570	49	23	46
	Indonesia	1980	3,933	—	12	—
	Nepal	1980	3,346	37	15	39
	Thailand	1980	13,659	21	5	23
	India					
	Rural	1980–81	23,482	19–93	5–67	16–72
	Urban	1980–81	25,843	5–26	0–15	0–59
	Bhutan	1982	952	19	13	67
	Indonesia					
	Rural	1982	4,971	21	11	51
	Urban	1982	2,310	17	7	40
	Nepal	1982	1,997	44	24	55
	Indonesia	1983	4,779	—	17	—

WHO region	Country	Year	Number of live births surveyed	Mortality rates		Percent of neonatal deaths due to tetanus
				Neonatal	NNT	
Southeast Asia (continued)	Indonesia	1984	4,836	—	21	35
	Indonesia	1984	4,769	—	9	—
	Sri Lanka	1984	2,841	15	1	7
	Burma	1985	6,000	18	6	33
	Bangladesh	1986	2,077	82	41	50
	India	1986	2,386	37	5	14
	Indonesia	1986	4,707	—	3	—
	Nepal	1988	728	19	4	23
Western Pacific	Philippines	1982	8,754	13	6	48
	Viet Nam	1985	8,270	12	2	16
	Lao PDR	1985	4,996	16	4	25
	Viet Nam	1989	9,199	8	3	40

Source: Gasse 1990.

Although the NNT mortality figures are so high, some epidemiologists consider them to be lower than the true rates, as early neonatal deaths are often missed on retrospective surveys (Foster 1984). Mortality rates for NNT are underestimated for other reasons as well. In Côte d'Ivoire, the longer the recall period (for example, more than seven months), the more likely mothers forget or are unwilling to report NNT in relation to other causes of neonatal mortality (Sokal and others 1988).

Cultural factors also influence underreporting. For example, female neonatal deaths may be undercounted in some cultures (Galazka and Cook 1985). In Indonesia, Arnold, Soewarso, and Karyadi (1986) found a reluctance to discuss infant deaths. In Senegal, self-reports by families resulted in twenty of twenty-six NNT deaths being ascribed to fevers (one), prematurity or low birth weight (three), other causes (five), and unknown causes (eleven) because of variability in diagnosis through verbal autopsy (Garenne and Fontaine 1986).

Biases also may lead to overestimation of NNT mortality. Gray, Smith, and Barss (1990) question whether the differential diagnoses used in community surveys may lack specificity, so that nontetanus deaths are included in estimations. Furthermore, surveys are conducted in expected high-incidence areas, because the intent is to publicize the magnitude of the NNT problem; generalization of survey results is then likely to overestimate NNT mortality for the country as a whole.

No global review of results of prospective as opposed to retrospective community NNT studies in the same geographical area and time period has been published. In general, very few prospective studies have been conducted, but these too demonstrate the enormity of NNT mortality and approximate the rates found on retrospective surveys. In one of the few community surveys for NNT ever conducted in Latin America, Newell and others (1966) demonstrated that tetanus killed 110 per 1,000 newborns. Like other prospective NNT studies, this double-blind controlled trial relied on

registration of all women, establishment and updating of a pregnancy registry during regular home visits by survey staff, and recording of births and deaths. Identifying pregnancies and tracking outcomes eliminates many of the potential biases of the retrospective survey design concerning recall, concealment, and uncertain recording of either live births or deaths.

Longitudinal surveillance by the International Center for Diarrheal Disease Research (ICDDR) in Matlab, Bangladesh, from 1975 to 1977 among a rural population of 260,000 established a NNT mortality rate of 37.4 per 1,000 live births with tetanus responsible for 26 percent of all infant deaths (Chen, Rahman, and Sarder 1980). A prospective survey conducted

Figure 9-3. *Total Neonatal Mortality and Neonatal Tetanus Mortality Rates*

Neonatal tetanus mortality rate
(per 1,000 live births)

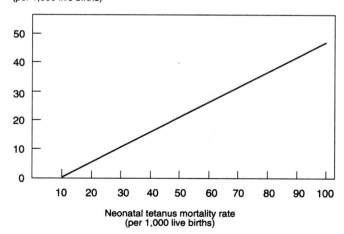

Neonatal tetanus mortality rate
(per 1,000 live births)

Note: If the neonatal mortality rate exceeds 30 per 1,000, neonatal tetanus is invariably a substantial contributor.
Source: REACH 1989; data from WHO/EPI 1987a.

by ICDDR in Teknaf, Bangladesh, determined a NNT mortality rate of 27.4 per 1,000 live births with tetanus responsible for 30.8 percent of neonatal and 21.3 percent of infant deaths (Islam and others 1982). These two prospective survey results are within the range reported in the retrospective studies in Bangladesh (table 9-3).

In the Indonesian province of West Java, a prospective study (Budiarso 1984) gave a NNT mortality rate of 14.7 per 1,000 live births, which also falls within the range of retrospective rates already reported. Finally, in a prospective case-control study in a rural area of thirty villages in Senegal, with a total population of 24,000, all births and deaths were systematically recorded for 43 months; the researchers found a NNT mortality rate of 15.9 per 1,000 live births with tetanus accounting for 31 percent of all neonatal deaths (Leroy and Garenne 1991).

This collective body of research has provided important insights into the epidemiological characteristics of NNT. Data are available on seasonality, age at onset of symptoms and death, age and parity of mothers, and circumstances of delivery and cord cutting. The preponderance of male over female deaths has been observed in many, but not all, studies and has been ascribed to real differences in risk of dying; greater likelihood of males being brought to the hospital, where their deaths would be recorded; differences in cord cutting and handling of males and females; and selectivity in recall (Stanfield and Galazka 1984). As analyzed by week-specific mortality ratios by sex, the practice of male circumcision surprisingly does not appear to explain the larger number of male than female NNT deaths.

In cattle- and horse-raising areas of Punjab, Pakistan, NNT mortality was significantly higher than in nearby farming and urban areas, presumably because of a greater risk of exposure (Suleiman 1982). In Uttar Pradesh, India, exposure-related variables (for example, a previous NNT death in the family, presence of large animals in the home, assistance by an untrained birth attendant) were better predictors of NNT than socioeconomic variables, such as education, income, land ownership, and caste (Smucker and others 1980). The significance of epidemiological factors for NNT, as opposed to the role of socioeconomic factors, was noted also in Senegal (Leroy and Garenne 1991).

Surveys in urban areas have shown consistently lower NNT mortality rates than in neighboring rural areas in Egypt, Iran, and India (Galazka and Stroh 1986; WHO/EPI 1987b, 1987c). Nevertheless, urban rates are high in some cities, such as Jakarta, Indonesia, which has a NNT mortality rate of 6.9 per 1,000 live births (Arnold, Soewarso, and Karyadi 1986).

In most studies, NNT was more likely to occur if the child was delivered at home or by an untrained attendant. Hospital delivery, however, does not guarantee protection from NNT, because infection may still occur as a result of unclean delivery or of unhygienic cord dressing after discharge. In Sri Lanka, from 1975 to 1980, nearly half of NNT deaths (206 of 423) and 75 percent of all births occurred in health facilities (de Silva 1982). Nevertheless, the relative risk of NNT in home delivery

compared with that in delivery in a health facility was still three to one in Sri Lanka (Foster 1984).

In one Indonesian survey, a NNT mortality rate of 23 per 1,000 live births was recorded for babies whose mothers had no prenatal contact with health facilities, as opposed to only 4 per 1,000 for those whose mothers had at least two contacts (WHO/EPI 1983c). In another study in Indonesia, however, NNT mortality rates were similar regardless of the number of prenatal contacts, because TT was not being systematically given (Solter, Hasibuan, and Yusuf 1986). In a prospective study in Senegal, it was found that washing hands with soap on the part of the birth attendant had a significant effect on the occurrence of NNT (odds ratio 5.19, $p = .0001$) when other factors were held constant (Leroy and Garenne 1991).

Prevention of Tetanus

Tetanus can be prevented by a variety of approaches at a cost which is affordable by most countries.

Prevention Strategies

Tetanus can be prevented by immunization, clean cutting and dressing of the umbilical cord, and hygienic wound management. In this section we will concentrate on prevention of NNT through immunization, because data from developing countries on the effect of interventions designed to ensure aseptic cord care are limited (Ross 1986a, 1986b) and information on associated costs is practically nonexistent. Likewise, data on the effect and cost of wound management are rare in developing countries.

Immunization against tetanus is achieved by vaccinating different target groups with vaccines such as DPT, DT, TT and Td (tetanus-diphtheria with a reduced component of diphtheria antigen)—all of which contain tetanus toxoid. Tetanus toxoid and Td are suitable for adults, whereas DPT vaccine is given to

Table 9-4. TT Immunization Schedule for Women

Dose	Time to immunize	Percent protected	Duration of protection
TT–1	At first contact or as early as possible in pregnancy	Nil	None
TT–2	At least four weeks after TT+1	80	Three years
TT–3	At least six months after TT+2 or during subsequent pregnancy	95	Five years
TT–4	At least one year after TT+3 or during subsequent pregnancy	99	Ten years
TT–5	At least one year after TT+4 or during subsequent pregnancy	99	Throughout childbearing years[a]

a. Original document states "for life."
Source: WHO/EPI *Programme on Immunization*, 1988b.

children less than five years old and preferably during infancy. The DT vaccine is used for young children unable to receive DPT and is mainly administered in schools. The schedule recommended by the World Health Organization requires five doses of TT for protection throughout the childbearing years (WHO/EPI 1988b; see table 9-4.)

Protective levels of antibody in the woman ensure protection for the newborn (as well as for the mother herself), since antibody crosses the placenta from mother to baby. Studies on the immunological response to TT have been reviewed by Rey (1982) and Galazka (1982, 1983). The standard series of three DPT injections given at monthly intervals during infancy counts as the first two of the five TT injections required for protection throughout the childbearing years.

Tetanus toxoid costs about $0.02 per dose in multidose vials, can withstand temperatures of 37°C for at least six weeks (WHO/EPI 1990), has more than 95 percent efficacy when used according to the correct schedule, and is extremely safe. Nevertheless, less than half the babies in developing countries have immunity at birth against NNT.

Reactions to TT are minor and local, usually lasting less than one day. Severe systemic reactions are rare, occurring in 1 per 50,000 to 250,000 injections (Christensen 1972b; White and others 1973). In the German Democratic Republic, severe residual damage was virtually unknown (WHO/EPI 1983a). Tetanus toxoid can be given at any stage of pregnancy without increased risk of abortion or congenital abnormality (Heinonen, Shapiro, and Slone 1977). Contraindications to TT immunization are virtually nonexistent (Rey and Tikhomirov 1989).

Researchers have documented the effect of TT immunization on reducing NNT mortality and lowering overall neonatal mortality in developing countries using a variety of control strategies. Immunization of pregnant women in Sri Lanka and Burma resulted in rapid declines in NNT (Stroh and others 1987; Galazka, Gasse, and Henderson 1989). In Sri Lanka after the introduction of EPI in 1978, NNT dropped from 2.16 to 0.06 per 1,000 live births by 1986. In Burma, a community survey found that the NNT mortality rate (3 per 1,000 live births) in EPI operational areas was only one-third the rate in other areas (Stroh and others 1987). The effect of three interventions in Burma was calculated to determine their proportional contribution to the reduction in neonatal tetanus mortality (Stroh and others 1987; see table 9-5). Hospital delivery, although highly efficacious (85 percent), contributed to only 17 percent of the reduction in NNT mortality because coverage with this intervention was only 14 percent. The programmatic efficacy, which is a product of the efficacy and coverage of the intervention, was slightly higher for deliveries by traditional birth attendants (TBAs) and much higher when two doses of TT immunization were given to the pregnant woman.

Mass immunization of 95 percent of women of childbearing age with one dose of TT from 1978 to 1979 in Maputo, Mozambique, followed by routine immunization of pregnant women, resulted in an eightfold drop in reported NNT cases in one hospital (Cliff 1985; WHO/EPI 1988b; Cutts and others 1990).

In Haiti, mass immunization of the entire population of a rural area eliminated NNT and reduced non-NNT to a negligible level (Berggren 1974a). A two-round mass TT campaign in 1985 in Pidie District, Indonesia, achieved 84 percent immunization coverage of all women of childbearing age with two doses of TT. Pre- and postcampaign NNT mortality surveys indicated an 85 percent reduction in NNT mortality. This reduction was likely due to the mass TT campaign, because neonatal mortality attributable to causes other than tetanus remained unchanged (WHO/EPI 1988a). Despite some disruption to routine programs, the Pidie campaign covered a high proportion of the unimmunized backlog, resulting in a dramatic reduction in NNT mortality.

Immunization was shown to be dramatically effective in reducing NNT in Colombia (Newell and others 1966), New Guinea (Schofield, Tucker, and Westbrook 1961), Bangladesh (Black, Huber, and Curlin 1980; Rahman, Chen Chakraborty, Yunus, Chowdhury, Sarder, Bhatia, and Curlin 1982), and many other countries. In Bangladesh, varying NNT mortality between the fourth and fourteenth days explained most of the difference in neonatal and infant mortality rates between the Maternal and Child Health (MCH) and Family Planning intervention area and the control area in a population of 260,000 (Bhatia 1989).

Mosley (1989) has argued that, unique among vaccines, TT is highly effective because NNT incidence is high and the disease has high fatality among otherwise healthy persons. For that reason, a disease-specific intervention against tetanus is able to have a large demographic effect. Unlike measles or pertussis-related deaths, which come at the end of a cycle of synergistic insults (infection, growth retardation, and reduced resistance), NNT has a discrete cause and a specific intervention—TT. Consequently, the so-called replacement mortality phenomenon probably does not occur in the case of NNT. Henry, Briend, and Fauveau (1990) state that given the con-

Table 9-5. Effect of Three Different Interventions on Mortality from Neonatal Tetanus, Burma, 1985

	Intervention		
Characteristics	*Immunization with two doses of tetanus toxoid*	*Hospital delivery*	*Trained birth attendant*
Efficacy[a]	0.91	0.85	0.33
Coverage	0.44	0.14	0.51
Efficacy x coverage	0.40	0.12	0.17
Contribution to reduced neonatal mortality (percent)[b]	58	17	25

a. Defined as:

$$\frac{\text{attack rate without intervention} - \text{attack rate with intervention}}{\text{attack rate without intervention}}$$

b. Defined as:

$$\frac{(\text{efficacy } i \text{ x coverage } i) \text{ x } 100}{\text{sum of (efficacy } i \text{ x coverage } i)}$$

where i is intervention.

Source: Galazka, Gasse, and Henderson 1989; based on data in Stroh and others 1987.

straints in Bangladesh on implementing the full EPI, TT (along with measles vaccination) is the most cost-effective immunization strategy for child survival.

Active and permanent immunization of the entire population and of successive cohorts will be required first to control tetanus and then, because of continuous environmental risks of contamination, to sustain its elimination as a public health problem. Each individual will require five doses of the current tetanus toxoid preparation at appropriate intervals for full lifetime protection. Rey and Tikhomirov (1989) propose a three-stage approach for tetanus control: universal immunization of infants, children, and women of childbearing age, including pregnant women; extension of immunization to schoolchildren and high-risk, easy-to-reach adults (for example, military recruits), as well as more systematic prophylaxis of wounds; and extension of immunization to all other adults, including such neglected groups as the elderly and immigrants.

The relative emphasis and timing of each of these control stages is a decision best made at national and subnational levels based on disease epidemiology, organization of health service delivery, operational and behavioral considerations, availability of resources, and the tradeoffs between costs and benefits of early and late control. The appropriate choice and degree of implementation of strategies will depend on whether the goal is total elimination of all tetanus, the total elimination of NNT, or the elimination (that is, control) of both as public health problems.

The advantages and disadvantages of using various immunization strategies and target groups can be delineated (WHO/EPI 1986) on the basis of discussions by Rey (1982), Cvjetanovic and others (1972), and Schofield (1986). (See table 9-6.) There is a long window of opportunity during which it is possible to immunize women to prevent NNT. Ideally, women entering their childbearing years already should have received five doses of tetanus toxoid, which can be in the form of properly spaced doses of DPT or DT (in childhood) and TT. The prevailing belief in many countries that two doses of TT are sufficient must be changed (Steinglass 1989). The earlier the protection, the greater the reduction of non-NNT, as well. This is important, given that the highest age-specific incidence of tetanus after the neonatal period in developing countries is among children.

There is no global blueprint for NNT control. Strategies need to be determined locally and may differ from one area to another within the same country. In Kilifi District, Kenya, a NNT mortality survey conducted in 1989 by the Resources for Child Health (REACH) project found low levels of NNT mortality (3 per 1,000 live births) as a result of high TT coverage through well-attended prenatal care services (Bjerregaard, Steinglass, Mutie, Kimani, Mjomba, Orinda 1993). Targeting TT to pregnant women was an appropriate strategy in this district because prenatal care coverage is high, although mothers with one child were significantly less well protected with TT than were multiparous women.

Elsewhere in Kenya, however, where prenatal care services are unavailable or not used, girls need immunization during early school grades before attrition. School enrollment levels of boys and girls are greater than 95 percent in some of the same districts where TT coverage among pregnant women is lowest. Approximately 90 percent of women in Kenya deliver their babies at home, despite high levels of prenatal care, so a strategy aimed at schoolchildren will help solve the problem of NNT in the medium term while having a marked, immediate effect on non-NNT.

Through high coverage with DPT in infancy and DT in school, some of the Gulf States in the Middle East have virtually eliminated NNT—despite a TT coverage rate in pregnant women of less than 20 percent. Most girls attend school and women deliver their babies in hygienic conditions. Consequently, no systematic attempt to immunize all women to eliminate NNT is indicated. In Denmark, a vaccination program consisting of three high-potency DT injections in infancy and a single revaccination five years later resulted in continuous protection to about the age of twenty-five (Simonsen and others 1987).

A strategy which relies exclusively on the identification and immunization of women during pregnancy is unlikely to succeed in many areas for operational and cultural reasons. Use of prenatal services at fixed facilities is low or frequently occurs very late in pregnancy, leaving insufficient time to administer two doses to the previously unimmunized woman. With periodic outreach or mobile strategies, trying to identify only pregnant women is like trying to hit a moving target when the marksman, or health worker, is also on the move. A campaign in Bangladesh in which health workers went door-to-door to identify pregnant women was not very successful, given shyness to declare pregnancy, outright resistance to vaccination during pregnancy, and the health workers' failure to refer the women for vaccination sufficiently early in pregnancy (Rahman, Chen, Chakraborty, Yunus, Faruque, and Chowdhury 1982).

Historically, the exclusive focus on pregnant women as a target group for TT has been well intended but operationally impractical in many developing countries. Administration of TT to individuals in this high-risk group is known to have an immediate effect on protecting the newborn. But unless the health services are well developed and appropriately used, a target group focusing on pregnant women exclusively will have low programmatic efficacy and will not achieve a rapid reduction of NNT or non-NNT. Thus a population-wide strategy is required because susceptibility to tetanus is general.

For this reason, WHO recommends continuous immunization of women of childbearing age, including pregnant women. Every contact with the health services is an opportunity to screen a woman's TT status and provide immunization. This strategy is less immediate in protecting individual births than one that focuses on women already pregnant, but its effect on the population will be more rapid. For this strategy to work, a change in attitude of health workers, particularly curative staff, may be needed. Because this target group is less specifically at risk than women already pregnant, more doses of TT will be needed per NNT case

Table 9-6. *Advantages and Disadvantages of Different Immunization Strategies in the Prevention of Neonatal Tetanus*

Approach	Advantages	Disadvantages	When to use
Immunization of pregnant women attending antenatal services	Few additional resources needed Potentially rapid impact on disease incidence	Hesitation about injections during pregnancy Women at highest risk rarely come for antenatal care Only very short periods to immunize women and to maintain immune status	When over 80 percent of pregnant women attend at least twice in antenatal period As part of overall effort to immunize women
Immunization of women of child-bearing age through regular health services	Any contact of women with health worker can be used Better chance of reaching high-risk women (who may not come for preventive care, but would come for curative care for their child)	Cooperation of health staff needed More complex logistics Accessibility of health services may be limited	Preferred when coverage for antenatal care is less than complete and there is reasonable degree of access to general health services May need to be supplemented with (limited) mass campaigns
Immunization of women coming with children to immunization session	Few additional resources needed Women with children are likely to become pregnant again	Women are not reached for first pregnancy Coverage cannot exceed maximum coverage of children	Should be part of any approach If used as only approach, needs periodic supplementation with mass campaigns
Immunization of women coming with or without children to immunization session	Few additional resources needed Women reached for first pregnancy	Accessibility may be limited	Should be part of any approach and may eliminate need for mass campaign if coverage is high
Special outreach clinics (markets, meetings)	Increases accessibility considerably	Needs organization and some extra resources	In places with regular, well-attended markets or other special events and limited access to regular health services
Immunization of school-children	Few additional resources needed Can be incorporated into ongoing school health programs School immunization programs may provide good stimulus for improving health education on immunization	Impact on disease incidence delayed (ten to twenty years) High-risk groups have low school attendance No school health program in most rural areas	Wherever a school health program can be activated without distracting resources from MCH care
Mass campaign	Rapid impact High visibility has good promotional value Men as well as women can be included	Resource intensive Might distract resources from development of regular MCH care May need repetition	Wherever incidence is 10 per 1,000 live births or more When special high-risk areas or groups are not reached otherwise As part of any accelerated immunization activity

Source: WHO/EPI 1986.

averted because many doses will be given to older, less fertile age groups. The World Health Organization recommends the use of long-lasting cards for appropriate screening, immunization, and documentation of protection.

A promising strategy being introduced by the Pan-American Health Organization in Latin America makes use of existing incidence data from routine reporting systems to identify areas at higher-than-average risk for NNT. This strategy permits health staff to target immunization efforts (Cvjetanovic 1972; de Quadros 1990). Another novel strategy is being tried in Indonesia, where prospective brides are required to show proof of TT immunization for marriage registration (Lanasari and Rosenberg 1989).

Economic and Financial Considerations of Prevention

Tetanus has important economic consequences for the developing world. Mortality rates for neonatal tetanus are generally highest in the poorest countries, which have inadequate preventive services.

For infected babies in the poorer countries, tetanus is almost always fatal. Children and adults not adequately protected by TT immunization experience a continuous risk of tetanus from wounds throughout their productive years. Deaths from tetanus, in 40 percent of adult cases and 85 percent of neonatal cases, affect the productive capacity of the population and represent an economic loss to society. Further, hospital treatment of tetanus is expensive for families and society. In countries with limited public health resources, provision of adequate treatment for tetanus constitutes a high opportunity cost compared with health services for other diseases. Given the high cost and poor outcome of treatment, and the fact that most tetanus patients are never brought to health facilities in the first place, the most cost-effective strategy is to prevent this common disease.

The cost to society of tetanus includes economic loss due to death and disability, the cost of treating individuals, and the cost of preventing disease. Although there is a growing body of empirical and theoretical evidence on the cost of preventing tetanus, little work has been done on the loss of productivity because of the disease. In this section we review and discuss cost-benefit and cost-effectiveness analyses of the prevention of NNT and non-NNT through immunization. Other methods of preventing tetanus—such as training TBAs to provide improved obstetrical care—have not been included in the following cost analyses because there is a near total absence of data on costs and the effect of alternative interventions.

Fifteen studies and four simulation models are reviewed (see appendix tables 9A-1–9A-4). The studies, which include six from Africa, six from Asia, and three from the Latin American and Caribbean region, were conducted by a variety of researchers during a twenty-year period, from 1970 to 1990. Examination of TT costs was not the purpose of eight of the studies. In these instances, available cost and coverage data have been used to estimate the cost-effectiveness of immunization strategies.

COST-EFFECTIVENESS STUDIES. The results from cost-effectiveness studies of immunization against tetanus are difficult to compare because of the variability in methods used to determine program costs and outcomes (see appendix tables 9A-1 and 9A-2). Some researchers use actual cost and incidence data, whereas others rely on estimates based on various assumptions. The methods used to estimate program costs vary in four principal ways: (a) type of costs measured, (b) method of allocating shared resources, (c) time frame of analysis, and (d) the strategy and scale of tetanus control.

Researchers measured either the expenditure for the immunization program (Berggren 1974a; Kielmann and Vohra 1977; Rey, Guillaumont, and Majnoni d'Intignano 1970; UNICEF/Jakarta 1985) or the economic costs (Barnum 1980; WHO/EPI 1981b; Robertson and others 1985; Brenzel 1987; Brenzel and others 1987; Shepard and others 1987; de Champeaux and Martin, 1989; Narcisse 1989; Phonboon and others 1989; Brenzel and others 1990; Berman and others 1991).[1] Rey, Guillaumont, and Majnoni d'Intignano (1979) include only vaccine costs in the cost calculations for Dakar, Senegal. In Deschapelles, Haiti, Berggren (1974a) estimated the value of the time spent by health workers to administer tetanus toxoid vaccine during visits to marketplaces, though he used the total expenditure for the five-year program for the cost-benefit calculation of the program. The costs of the Indonesian campaign in Central Lombok reflected UNICEF expenditure and

vaccinators' salaries but did not include costs at the national level or a portion of the routine salaries of health officials (UNICEF/Jakarta 1985). Kielmann and Vohra (1977) predicted the cost in Punjab, India, of importing, storing, and transporting vaccine, as well as managing and administering a hypothetical program.

Among the studies in which economic costs were calculated, the identification and calculation of program costs varied. In several studies the researchers adapted methodologies developed for costing EPI (Brenzel 1987; Brenzel and others 1987; de Champeaux and Martin 1989; Narcisse 1989; Phonboon and others 1989; Brenzel and others 1990; Berman and others 1991). The authors of one study measured the incremental cost of adding different vaccines, like DPT, to EPI in Indonesia on the basis of additional inputs and resources required for each (Barnum, Tarantola, and Setiady 1980). Berman and colleagues (1991) were the only researchers who distinctly evaluated the economic cost of a tetanus immunization campaign. The diversity of underlying assumptions, not always explicit in each study, makes comparing results risky.

Cost-effectiveness studies differed in how shared health resources were allocated to tetanus prevention. For instance, the cost of the tetanus component of EPI was estimated to be 37.5 percent of the total cost in the Gambia (Robertson and others 1985). This proportion was based on the number of contacts for tetanus toxoid (three) compared with total contacts for all doses for full immunization (eight). In many studies, the cost of immunizing women with TT was based on the proportion of annual doses administered to women compared with total annual doses given by EPI (Brenzel 1987; Brenzel and others 1987; Shepard and others 1987; de Champeaux and Martin 1989; Narcisse 1989; Phonboon and others 1989; Brenzel and others 1990).

The time frame used in the cost studies affects the results. Although annual costs of a tetanus control program were calculated in most of the cost-effectiveness studies included in this review, there was no uniform time period across all studies. The researchers in several studies evaluated the cost of an immunization program over a period of several years but did not discount costs to a present value estimate (Berggren 1974a; Barnum, Tarantola, and Setiady 1980). Others measured costs for less than one year, for mass campaigns, for example, which last for a period of months (UNICEF/Jakarta 1985; Narcisse 1989; Berman and others 1991). Further, the point at which a cost-effectiveness study is conducted in the life of an immunization program affects the generalizability of the results. Estimates are likely to be located on different average cost curves at different times during the immunization program, making comparisons of efficiency suspect.

The studies focused on routine immunization of pregnant women, or mass immunization of pregnant women or women of childbearing age. The target population, delivery strategy used, and the scale of the intervention differed. Most studies focused on immunization of women with TT. The required number of doses, and therefore contacts, per woman for full protection was two in most studies, although it ranged from one (Kielmann and Vohra 1977) to three doses (Berggren 1974a; Robertson and others 1985). Pregnant women were the target group in seven of the studies, whereas women of reproductive age were the focus in another seven studies. The cost of vaccinating the entire population with TT was calculated in one study (Rey and others 1979). In another, the researchers examined the cost of the tetanus component of DPT for infants in addition to the cost of TT for women (Barnum, Tarantola, and Setiady 1980).

Mass campaign and routine strategies could be compared in only two studies. In Haiti, the cost-effectiveness of mobile teams, rally posts, and national campaign and fixed centers were evaluated (Narcisse 1989). In Indonesia, a provincial-level campaign was compared with routine services (Berman and others 1991). Berggren (1974a) evaluated the cost of the marketplace strategy in Haiti, as well as that of a comprehensive intervention that included TBA training. Some researchers included the cost of providing routine immunization services to women in a sample of health facilities (WHO/EPI 1981b; Robertson and others 1985; Shepard and others 1987; Berman and others 1991; Brenzel and others 1990). Others examined the total cost of a tetanus control strategy at regional, provincial, or national levels.

Because tetanus incidence is influenced by general social and economic factors, attributing the reduction in incidence exclusively to a specific immunization intervention oversimplifies the situation. In Haiti, the incidence of tetanus declined prior to the onset of the immunization program (Berggren 1974a). The training program for TBAs may have contributed to the eventual decline in cases, although the benefit of training TBAs in Haiti is difficult to measure because training overlapped with provision of ATS at delivery and in treatment of tetanus. In few of the studies was immunization other than TT to women considered. Yet DPT and DT administered in childhood primes the immune system so that even a single future dose of TT before a woman delivers could be protective. None of the researchers, with the exception of Rey, Guillaumont, and Majnoni d'Intignano (1979), addressed the cost of reducing both non-NNT mortality and NNT mortality, and none of them examined the costs or benefits of reaching the target population of school-age children.

The comparability of studies is also limited by variability in methods used to assess outcome. Berman and others (1991) were the only researchers who used NNT mortality data derived from community surveys before and after the intervention. Community survey data on NNT mortality were available before the intervention in Deschapelles, Haiti, although comparison of pre- and postintervention rates had to be based on hospital admissions data (Berggren 1974a). The report on the study done in Central Lombok, Indonesia, had data only from a preintervention community survey (UNICEF/Jakarta 1985). Robertson and others (1985) and Kielmann and Vohra (1977) relied on estimates of NNT mortality from community surveys conducted in notably earlier time periods. In some of the above cases, survey

results were used even though they represented a wider or different geographic area within the country.

The assumed duration of protection from TT also differed among studies. Kielmann and Vohra (1977) assumed that a single, high-potency dose of TT gave lifelong immunity, but NNT deaths averted were calculated only for the year of the campaign. For the mass campaign in Pidie, Indonesia, Berman and others (1991) considered the duration of protection from two doses of TT to be four years for women of childbearing age but only one year for women immunized through routine prenatal care. Berggren (1974a) assumed that three doses of TT provided protection for a minimum of five years.

None of the studies considered the cumulative benefits from priming the immune system with previous tetanus doses. Assumptions that benefits from TT immunization begin at the start of a campaign or the beginning of a year for a routine program are made in order to reduce the complexity of assessing the cost and effectiveness of immunization.

We conclude, then, that the total costs of NNT reduction are likely to be underestimated in this sample of cost-effectiveness studies, whereas the benefits are overestimated or underestimated among studies and even within studies because of varying assumptions.

COMPARISON OF STUDIES BY PROGRAM STRATEGY. Most of the studies in appendix tables 9A-1 and 9A-2 provide analyses of the two broad categories of strategies for TT immunization: routine programs and mass campaigns. Routine programs may include fixed-facility services, mobile teams, outreach, and other strategies; but separate data are rarely available regarding the cost and cost-effectiveness of each of these types of strategies. As a result, we considered all routine programs as a group and compared them with campaigns. For both campaigns and routine programs, target groups may include all women of childbearing age, pregnant women, schoolgirls, infants, and males as well as females. In table 9-7 we compare the unit costs and cost-effectiveness of the routine programs and campaigns in the review. Included in the table are the median values and ranges summarized by strategy.

We were able to compare the cost of routine TT immunization programs in eight studies (see table 9-7). Several of the studies included estimates for different districts, regions, or types of facilities, yielding a total of seventeen observations for the cost per TT dose, per TT second dose (TT2), per case prevented, or per death averted; the study done in the Gambia was the only one to include estimates under all four categories. The outcome measure most frequently available was cost per TT2.

As shown in table 9-7, the cost per TT dose found in the eight studies ranged from $0.40 to $1.76, with a median of $1.14 (all costs are given in 1989 U.S. dollars). The cost per TT2 ranged from $0.66 to $11.87, with a median of $3.38. The wide range in cost per TT2 may reflect different methods for estimating costs as well as varying levels of efficiency and effectiveness of the programs studied. In only two studies, in the Gambia and Indonesia (Aceh), was the cost per case prevented and the cost

Table 9-7. *Unit Costs and Cost-Effectiveness of Tetanus Immunization Programs*
(1989 U.S. dollars)

Source	Location	Subdivision	Cost per TT dose	Cost per TT2	Cost per case prevented	Cost per death averted
Routine Programs						
de Champeaux and Martin 1989	Burkino Faso	Yako	1.01	4.15	—	—
		Gourcy	0.64	2.13	—	—
Shepard and others 1987	Ecuador	n.a.	0.40	—	—	—
Robertson and others 1985	The Gambia	n.a.	1.58	5.23	205	228
Narcisse 1989	Haiti	Fixed centers	0.91	—	—	—
		Horse teams	1.14	—	—	—
WHO/EPI 1981b	Indonesia (Central Java)	n.a.	1.18	3.92	—	—
Berman and others 1991	Indonesia (Aceh)[a]	Tanah Pasir	—	2.20	89	105
		Samudera	—	2.76	113	133
		Matangkuli	—	1.47	60	70
		Jeumpa	—	0.66	27	32
Brenzel and others 1990	Sudan	Darfur	1.76	4.80	—	—
		Kordofan	0.86	2.16	—	—
		Capital	1.33	2.84	—	—
		Nationwide	1.73	4.20	—	—
Phonboon and others 1989	Thailand	Hospitals	—	10.25	—	—
		Health centers	—	11.87	—	—
Minimum	n.a.	n.a.	0.40	0.66	27	32
Maximum	n.a.	n.a.	1.76	11.87	205	228
Median	n.a.	n.a.	1.14	3.38	89	105
Campaigns						
Brenzel 1987	Cameroon	n.a.	1.34	4.16	—	—
Berggren 1974[a,b]	Haiti (Deschapelles)	n.a.	0.34	1.05[b]	98[b,c]	115[b,c]
Narcisse, 1989	Haiti	Mass campaign	1.71	—	—	—
		Rally posts	0.21	—	—	—
Kielmann and Vohra 1977	India (Narangwa)[d]	Initial	0.29	—	—	97
		Maintenance	n.a.	—	—	0.34
UNICEF 1985	Indonesia (Central Lombok)	n.a.	0.23	0.46	44[e]	52[e]
WHO/EPI 1988a	Indonesia (Pidie)	n.a.	0.82	1.84	122	144
Berman and others 1991						
Rey, Guillaumont and Majnoni d'Intignano 1979	Senegal (Dakar)	Mass campaign	—	—	825[f]	2,750[f]
Brenzel and others 1987	Senegal	n.a.	0.76	—	—	—
Minimum	n.a.	n.a.	0.21	0.46	44	52[g]
Maximum	n.a.	n.a.	1.71	4.16	825	2,750
Median	n.a.	n.a.	0.55	1.45	110	115
Total (routine programs and campaigns)						
Minimum	n.a.	n.a.	0.21	0.46	27	32[g]
Maximum	n.a.	n.a.	1.76	11.87	825	2,750[g]
Median	n.a.	n.a.	0.91	2.80	98	110[g]

— Data not available.
n.a. Not applicable.
a. Protective effect of TT2 on all deliveries within three years not considered; hypothetical incidence data.
b. Derived from information reported in cited document. Schedule included three doses of TT.
c. Excludes an additional 630 non-NNT cases prevented.
d. Study was for one high-potency dose of TT with assumed 80 percent efficacy and lifelong immunity; cost data are hypothetical.
e. Assumed NNT mortality rate equals 28.0 (level for seven clusters in Central Lombok district in a thirty-cluster survey).
f. Includes cost per NNT and non-NNT case and death prevented.
g. Excludes India/Narangwal maintenance level estimate.
Source: See first column of this table and tables 9A-2 and 9A-4.

per death averted estimated.[2] The median cost per case prevented was $89, with a range from $27 to $205. The cost per death averted ranged from $32 to $228, whereas the median was $105. The cost per death averted does not differ greatly from the cost per case prevented because of the high case-fatality rate of neonatal tetanus.

Eight studies listed in table 9-7 also included unit costs and cost-effectiveness for TT programs employing campaign strategies. All but one included estimates of the cost per TT dose delivered. As shown in table 9-7, these estimates ranged from $0.21 to $1.71, with a median of $0.55. One of the lowest estimates ($0.29) was from Kielmann and Vohra's study in Narangwal, India, where a single dose of high-titer (30 Lf per milliliter) calcium phosphate-adsorbed vaccine was used. Kielmann and Vohra (1977) found that this single dose was more effective than three doses of aluminum phosphate-adsorbed TT (10 LF per milliliter) given at one-month intervals. If this assertion is true, it may be more appropriate to compare this cost ($0.29) with the cost per TT2 found in Cameroon ($4.16), Deschapelles in Haiti ($1.05), and Central Lombok ($0.46) and Pidie ($1.84) in Indonesia, because these costs represent the nearest estimates of the cost to protect a woman fully against tetanus for several years. The median cost per TT2 was $1.45.

Estimates of the cost per NNT case prevented are available for four studies, and range from $44 to $825, with a median of $110. The wide range in these estimates may be due in large part to different methods of estimating costs and morbidity reductions.

The median cost per NNT death averted in the studies which examined campaign strategies was $115, reflecting a range from $52 to $2,750. The study in Narangwal, India, includes two estimates for the cost per death averted: one for the initial phase, during which 87 percent of all women from fifteen to forty-four years of age were immunized; the other, a much lower estimate ($0.34), for maintenance of the program, in which only the girls fifteen years of age who enter the eligible cohort each year were immunized. This lower estimate has been left out of the calculation of the median cost per death averted ($115) because of its extremely low and hypothetical nature. Because Kielmann and Vohra (1977) assume lifelong immunity from one dose of high-titer vaccine, they claim that only those women who are entering childbearing age will need to be vaccinated during the maintenance phase of the program. Nevertheless, despite the assertion of lifelong immunity, they include in their cost-effectiveness calculations only those deaths prevented in a single year. This results in an underestimate of the cost-effectiveness, if indeed one agrees with the assumption of lifelong protection.

The extremely high estimate of cost per death averted (NNT plus non-NNT) found in Dakar, Senegal, may have resulted from the high-intensity program used in that instance: seven semestral mass vaccination campaigns were undertaken against tetanus (Rey, Guillaumont, and Majnoni d'Intignano 1979). Moreover, the case-fatality rate was only approximately 30 percent because of the high number of cases in those older

than one year, resulting in a large difference between the cost per case prevented and the cost per death averted.

Berggren (1974a, 1974b) estimated that in Haiti an additional 630 cases of non-NNT were prevented. This estimate has not been incorporated into the cost per case or death averted in appendix table 9A-2 or in table 9-7.

In general, this review shows a relatively small range in unit costs and cost-effectiveness. This is surprising given the different methods used in the 15 studies for analyzing the cost and effect of diverse interventions. Little disparity was found between the median values for routine strategies as opposed to campaign strategies, which implies that each strategy may be cost-effective in different circumstances. Whereas median costs per TT and TT2 doses are lower in campaigns, routine strategies were more cost-effective in cases and deaths averted. The choice of strategy must take into account its likely programmatic efficacy—that is, the efficacy of the technology and its expected coverage within the population. In other words, it makes little sense to base a delivery strategy solely on pregnant women attending fixed facilities for prenatal check-ups when, in many countries, only a small minority of women seek prenatal care.

SIMULATION MODELS. We review four hypothetical models which were used to simulate the costs and benefits of alternative tetanus immunization strategies (Cvjetanovic and others 1972; Kessel 1984; Sharma and Sharma, 1984a, 1984b; and Smucker, Swint, and Simmons 1984; see appendix tables 9A-3 and 9A-4). Given the complicated immunologic aspects of tetanus immunization, modeling exercises provide valuable insights from an epidemiologic perspective into the effectiveness of alternative strategies. The greatest weakness of each model is the lack of empirical basis for cost estimates. Kessel (1984) uses an arbitrary system of financial units (from 1 to 100), which ranks the difficulty of implementing alternative immunization strategies with regard to their effect on unit cost per dose (unit costs are expected to rise as the most remote population groups are reached, usually through outreach and mobile services). The results of Kessel's simulations, however, are heavily influenced by the order of magnitude and ranking of these delivery strategies. Cvjetanovic and others (1972) do not consider economic costs of implementing an immunization program but include only vaccine and treatment costs in their model. Sharma and Sharma (1984a, 1984b) base their model on vaccine costs as well, including (unlike the other models) costs of three DPT and three DT shots to young children and schoolchildren, respectively. Only Smucker, Swint, and Simmons (1984) estimate the economic cost of an immunization strategy aimed at TT vaccination of women. Yet they do not consider the integration of TT vaccination (through MCH services) with EPI in India. Joint implementation of immunization of women and children would substantially alter their assumptions about frequency of contact by women with the health system and productivity of health workers (for example, the number of women who could be immunized per day).

Cvjetanovic and colleagues (1972) assume high immunization coverage (90 percent) of pregnant women through routine services and medium coverage (50 percent) of the total population through mass strategies. Empirically, however, these assumptions are reversed. Mass campaigns in Central Lombok and Pidie District, Indonesia; Narangwal, India; and Deschapelles, Haiti, resulted in greater than 80 percent coverage, whereas coverage from routine fixed-facility services was less than 50 percent of the target population of pregnant women. The cost-effectiveness of TT immunization in Kessel's (1984) model is not dependent on coverage levels, which appears counterintuitive from economic theory: average costs change as coverage increases. There is no simulation in any model of the costs and benefits of continuous immunization of women of childbearing age, the strategy recommended by WHO.

As in the empirical studies, varying assumptions were made in the hypothetical models regarding the efficacy of tetanus immunization. The duration of immunity differed among these models from five years (Sharma and Sharma 1984a, 1984b; Smucker, Swint, and Simmons 1984) to ten years (Cvjetanovic and others 1972). The primary series of TT for full protection ranged from two doses (Smucker, Swint, and Simmons 1984 and Sharma and Sharma, 1984a, 1984b) to three doses (Cvjetanovic and others 1972). Sharma and Sharma (1984a, 1984b) include the costs and benefits of three doses of DPT and two doses of DT, whereas Kessel (1984) includes four doses of DPT for preschool children. Cvjetanovic and others (1972) and Sharma and Sharma (1984a, 1984b) include the effect on NNT and non-NNT. Only one model discounts the future costs of the immunization program—at a rate of 12 percent per year (Smucker, Swint, and Simmons 1984). The benefits of the program (for example, deaths averted) are not discounted. Kessel (1984) estimates the effectiveness of tetanus immunization programs by calculating the residual protected fertility achieved by directing efforts at preschool girls, school-age girls, and adult women seeking prenatal care.

As with cost-effectiveness studies, the modeling exercises probably underestimate the costs of delivering immunization services to women and children, whereas benefits are sometimes underestimated and sometimes overestimated. Costs of complementary programs, such as immunization of schoolchildren with DT and infants with DPT and training of traditional birth attendants, are not factored into all the simulations. Similarly, the benefits from NNT reduction are assumed to accrue solely from TT immunization, without regard for active-passive immunization for wound management (including ATS for newborns) and safe deliveries. Thus, the cost per dose and cost per death averted are also underestimated, although, compared with other interventions described in this collection, efforts to control NNT by immunization are likely to be highly cost-effective.

COMPARISON OF RESULTS OF SIMULATION MODELS. Only two of the four models produced usable cost-effectiveness estimates for our present purposes. Although the results of these simulations are not directly comparable to those of the studies, they provide useful insights into the effect of programmatic changes on both the costs and outcomes of tetanus control programs.

Cvjetanovic and others (1972) estimate a range of costs per case prevented from $245 to $595 (all costs are in 1989 U.S. dollars), depending on delivery strategy and target population assumed. Smucker, Swint, and Simmons (1984) vary their coverage assumptions and cost estimates to compare a routine program with a campaign using teams of vaccinators. For the campaign approach, costs per TT dose range from $1.34 to $2.33, whereas the cost per TT2 varies from $2.74 to $5.25. The cost per death averted for this strategy ranges from a low of $6.75 to a high of $11.86. The routine program shows somewhat better results: the cost per TT dose ranges from $0.50 to $0.98; costs per TT2, from $1.03 to $2.20; and the cost per death averted, from $2.59 to $4.87. It should be noted that these costs per death averted are far less than the estimates found in all the empirical studies, which may indicate that the cost estimates were too low or that effectiveness assumptions were overly optimistic.

Kessel (1984), using theoretical financial units as a means of comparing the resource requirements of different strategies, concludes that school-based programs are the most economical in the long run because all the residual fertility of the girls is protected. Sharma and Sharma (1984a, 1984b) favor continuous immunization of pregnant women, because mass immunization programs are projected to lead to only short-term declines in tetanus incidence.

REVIEW OF STUDIES AND SIMULATION MODELS: CONCLUSIONS. This review of empirical work and simulation models has shown that immunization of women with TT is a cost-effective means of controlling NNT. The median cost per NNT case averted is $98 and the median cost per NNT death averted is $110. These estimates are similar for both routine delivery of TT and campaigns. Although cost-effectiveness is but one criterion for choosing among alternative health interventions, these figures compare favorably with those of other interventions presented in the rest of this collection.

For three reasons, however, the results of this review can be generalized only in a limited fashion. First and most important, the cost of controlling tetanus depends on country-specific characteristics, such as the health infrastructure, delivery strategies used, incidence rates of the disease and coverage rates achieved, and the degree of integration of tetanus control within routine EPI, MCH, and school health services. A country with a well-developed health system and universal access to services is more likely to have lower average costs for a TT immunization program than a country which is still extending basic health services to its population. Integration of tetanus control with basic health services will also tend to reduce average costs.

The empirical studies included in this review reflect the cost of providing services at particular coverage levels through specific strategies. The cost of providing routine services at low coverage levels will not be representative of average costs at higher levels, because economic theory predicts that average costs change as volume increases. All the studies were conducted in countries with high NNT incidence, so results cannot be generalized to countries where tetanus incidence is low, and marginal costs of averting cases will consequently be much higher. In no study or simulation did researchers examine the costs and benefits associated with the continuous immunization of women of childbearing age, the current strategy recommended by WHO for the worldwide elimination of tetanus.

The second reason generalization from country-specific results is difficult is because the opportunity cost of health resources is not consistent among countries. A cost per death averted of $144 in Indonesia (Berman and others 1991) may not represent a different set of tradeoffs for resource allocation from a cost of $228 in the Gambia (Robertson and others 1985), and the situation in Indonesia may differ greatly from that in Haiti ($115 per death averted; Berggren 1974a, 1974b). The decision to invest public resources in tetanus control through immunization must be made within the context of the marginal product resulting from competing country-specific use of those same resources.

Finally, variations in the methods used in the empirical studies and simulations hamper casual generalizations of these results. Still, the convergence of many study results around a figure of $110 per death averted suggests that this median estimate can be used as a starting point for determining resource allocations for tetanus control (see table 9-7). Tetanus control through immunization is a highly cost-effective and inexpensive means of reducing infant mortality in the developing world.

ADDITIONAL ECONOMIC ISSUES. In addition to immunization of women and children, other strategies exist which can potentially affect the incidence of NNT. Among these are training of TBAs in more hygienic delivery practices. Several studies allude to the effectiveness of TBA training in reducing NNT, though controlled community studies with pre- and post-intervention evaluation have been rare (Berggren 1974a; Allman 1986). Allman (1986) estimated TBA training to cost $10 per worker between 1977 and 1982. James Heiby reports a figure of $92.50 per worker in Nicaragua during the late 1970s (cited in Allman 1986).

By contrast, many observers conclude that TBA training is not as effective in preventing NNT as vaccination of women (Ross, 1986a, 1986b; Solter, Hasibuan, and Yusuf 1986; Bhatia 1989; Jordan 1989). The expense of training, supervising, and supporting workers to cover the population would also be prohibitive for most developing countries, particularly if case loads per birth attendant are low. Although some evidence suggests that TBA training programs are relatively effective in reducing nontetanus neonatal mortality (Rahman 1982), large-scale efforts are unlikely to be as cost-effective as targeted immunization strategies for NNT reduction.

Immunization of schoolchildren either with a primary series of DT or with additional reinforcing doses of DT after three doses of DPT has been an underused strategy. Besides a simulation exercise (Kessel 1984) which evaluates the costs and benefits of school immunization against tetanus, little empirical data are available about the potential costs (in relation to benefits) of a nationwide school program in a developing country.

The Kessel (1984) model predicts that school immunization is the most cost-effective strategy for reducing NNT deaths, compared with a preschool program, prenatal clinic, and outreach immunization of pregnant women. This model, however, assumes universal access to education and a well-developed institutional base from which to deliver immunizations. The actual situation in most developing countries differs from these assumptions: access is often not universal and attrition rates are high, particularly among young girls—the target population for immunization. Similar to the health sector, the education sector is weak institutionally and financially in most developing countries. Therefore, the applicability of these simulation results for decisionmaking in many developing countries is limited. Still, in countries with high enrollment of female primary school children, DT immunization may prove to be highly cost-effective for tetanus prevention, especially when it is an incremental measure in an integrated primary health care strategy (which may at the same time include vitamin A distribution, administration of anthelmintics, and screening for trachoma).

Single-dose tetanus toxoid vaccine which would confer lifelong immunity is likely to become available for human use within five to ten years. Testing in animals has already begun, with testing in humans expected soon. Funds may be needed in the future to support trials in humans. The vaccine would contain biodegradable microcapsules of different thicknesses which would slowly release tetanus toxoid over a prolonged period. Administered early in life, the vaccine would provide protection for the individual and for future pregnancies. Although unit costs per dose of this vaccine cannot be predicted, it is unlikely to be expensive. The single-dose vaccine would also significantly reduce the number of required immunization contacts, resulting in significant cost savings. This same biotechnology relying on impregnated microcarriers may be useful for delivering other inactivated vaccines.

Pregnant women and those of childbearing age are frequently not screened and immunized with tetanus toxoid when they come into contact with the health system for whatever reason. The World Health Organization recommends immunization of eligible women and infants at every encounter with the health system in order to reduce missed opportunities. Immunization of pregnant women during routine prenatal care visits as early as possible during pregnancy and immunization of women of childbearing age at childhood immunization sessions should lead to reduced costs of the immunization program by substantially increasing efficiency (WHO/EPI 1988b).

Routine immunization of women either is conducted through antenatal clinics and MCH services or is the responsibility of EPI. Where possible, routine TT immunization (and mass immunization strategies) should be designed as integrated efforts with MCH services. If TT immunization is given as part of an integrated package with childhood immunization and prenatal care services, the cost is likely to be reduced.

The World Health Organization has recommended expanding the target population for tetanus toxoid immunization from pregnant women to all women of childbearing age (WHO/EPI 1986). Initially, there was concern that enlarging the population would not be an affordable strategy for developing countries. Gérard Foulon investigated the incremental cost of implementing a five-dose schedule for all women of childbearing age (personal communication, July 12, 1990). He found that total costs would increase within the first five years of adopting this strategy but would then revert to preexpansion costs. If the incremental costs of additional vaccine, storage, training, and monitoring could be financed through donor resources, this policy would not represent an economic burden to developing countries in the short run.

To the extent that parents will quickly replace their lost baby, a death from NNT will continue to exact incalculable costs within the family. In the absence of lactational amenorrhea following a baby's death from NNT, the mother may well become pregnant sooner. Shorter pregnancy intervals are associated with higher infant and child mortality. Even if the older child dies in infancy, too short a birth interval still places the younger child at very high risk. Another pregnancy so soon also jeopardizes the health of the mother.

The REACH project determined that half of immunization costs (capital and recurrent) in developing countries are currently financed by external resources from donor organizations (Brenzel 1989). Tools for making resource allocation decisions, such as cost-effectiveness analyses, have not been used often in cases where resources are abundant. Sustaining immunization coverage gains, however, is becoming a greater priority for program managers, and this translates into selecting the most affordable and effective strategies for tetanus prevention. The estimates calculated in this chapter underscore the need for continued donor assistance in the financing of TT immunization programs, given the economic declines and growing populations faced by most developing countries.

Case Management of Tetanus

This section discusses strategies for the treatment of tetanus and their costs and benefits.

Case Management Strategies

Much of the following discussion on case management of NNT and non-NNT is based on an authoritative essay entitled "Treatment of Tetanus" (Rey, Diop-Mar, and Robert 1981), to which the reader is referred. Death from tetanus commonly occurs in association with spasms, which lead to acute asphyxia. Treatment is largely symptomatic and attempts to prevent and counteract the effects of spasticity and spasms on respiration. Improvements over the past few decades in methods of neu-

rorespiratory resuscitation and use of specialized intensive care units have led to improved outcomes. Nevertheless, even treated tetanus remains extremely serious with the course and prognosis dependent on age, preexisting conditions, superimposed infections and complications of treatment, and availability of medical facilities with advanced equipment and expert staff (Veronesi and Focaccia 1981).

Expert use and timing of sedatives, muscle relaxants, and respiratory assistance (including tracheotomy and artificial ventilation, if indicated) are typically required, but these procedures carry their own iatrogenic risk. Inaccessibility of specialized treatment facilities in much of the world results in delayed admission, a factor associated with increased mortality.

Treatment of NNT and non-NNT patients consists of excising, cleansing, and disinfecting the wound; antibiotic therapy; use of benzodiazepines for their sedating, anticonvulsant, and muscle-relaxing properties; maintenance of effective ventilation, particularly by tracheotomy; parenteral administration of human tetanus immune globulin or antitetanus serum of equine origin, which is less desirable because of frequent adverse side effects; maintenance of water, electrolyte, and nutritional balance; and intensive nursing care. (Neonates in particular require assisted respiration in specialized neonatal intensive care units.) The effectiveness of this symptomatic treatment depends on financial and human resources rarely available where tetanus most frequently occurs.

Following the treatment outline above, hospitals in France and Japan have recorded impressive reductions in fatality of non-NNT patients to a rate of approximately 10 percent despite the increasing age of patients in recent years (Rey, Diop-Mar, and Robert 1981; Ebisawa and Homma 1986). The principal determinant of survival in Japan was admission to an intensive care unit where staff, including anesthesiologists, were trained in treatment of tetanus. After 1974, gastrointestinal and cardiac complications overtook respiratory insufficiency with or without pulmonary infection as the leading cause of death for Japanese tetanus patients. Rey, Diop-Mar, and Robert (1981) report that intensive care of newborns has in a few instances even reduced neonatal fatality to 10–20 percent from 90 percent, although the risk of incapacitating sequelae has increased owing to survival after intensive care.

Rey, Diop-Mar, and Robert (1981) suggest that in developing countries a compromise between modern medical advances and available resources is needed. They advocate establishment of special care units in facilities admitting more than 100 cases per year. Such a unit would admit other patients also requiring continuous monitoring.

Practically, the financial and human resources which they recommend for tetanus patients may still be out of reach for most developing countries: one doctor continuously available; two daytime nurses and one nighttime nurse, which would require a team of six to eight trained nurses; several orderlies; oxygen; apparatus for aspiration, intravenous infusion, catheterization of veins or bladder, and tracheotomy; nasogastric tubes; and appropriate sedatives, antibiotics, and serum. Laboratory tests, bacteriological examinations, and air condition-ing are desirable but may have to be omitted.

Even with relatively simple and inexpensive treatment, it is in the newborn that the most noticeable improvement in survival rate is found (Rey, Diop-Mar, and Robert 1981). Schofield (1986) observes, however, that with routine treat-ment an overall fatality reduction of only 10 percent can be expected. Even in the United States as recently as 1953–61, the case-fatality rate for all tetanus remained as high as 63 percent (Bytchenko 1966). In the absence of sophisticated equipment and the most advanced drugs, the quality and continuity of nursing care, which allows early recognition and treatment of potentially life-threatening complications, is probably the most important factor when case fatality varies greatly from place to place (Barten 1969).

Cost and Benefits of Treatment

There have been some attempts to examine the costs and benefits of treatment of tetanus compared with prevention though immunization. Treatment costs are more relevant for non-NNT, since NNT cases are rarely brought to the hos-pital and the case-fatality rate of NNT approaches 100 per-cent. Cvjetanovic and others (1972) state that treatment costs may vary from $50 to $900 ($148 to $2,665), with an average of $200 per case ($592) in developing countries.[3] Rey, Guillaumont, and Majnoni d'Intignano (1979) esti-mate treatment costs from $15,000 to $20,000 ($28,500 to $38,000) per case in the United States and $10,000 to $16,000 ($19,000 to $30,500) in France. Berggren (1974a) estimates treatment costs of $12 ($30) per day at Albert Schweitzer Hospital in Haiti, with an average of seventeen days of treatment. Rey and Tikhomirov (1989) report a mean hospital stay for non-NNT patients of sixteen days, though a significant proportion of cases die within the first two or three days. Griffith and Sachs (1974) report a mean hospital stay in Ludhiana, India, of eighteen and one-half days and a direct daily cost of 991 rupees ($226). When only surviving patients are considered, a total of 1,857 rupees ($423) were spent to treat each infant.

Table 9-8 provides treatment costs per case of tetanus (NNT and non-NNT) in various locales. It must be emphasized that treatment protocols (use of drugs, ATS, tetanus immune globu-lin, ventilation, and so on) are not uniform and that cost methodologies vary; therefore, comparison of these estimates is not straightforward. Nevertheless, with a median cost per NNT death averted of $110 by means of TT immunization (table 9-7), prevention of tetanus is by far more cost-effective than treatment. Cvjetanovic and others (1972) estimated that cu-mulative savings in treatment costs over the course of thirty years would exceed by a factor of more than 2.5 to 1 the cost of continuous immunization of pregnant women. Costs associ-ated with passive immunization as part of wound management would also decrease as the population becomes protected by TT. Berggren (1974a) calculated that more than 50,000 hospi-tal days were saved over a four-year period by Haiti's vigorous

Table 9-8. Costs Per Capita of Tetanus Treatment and Immunization in Selected Areas
(1989 U.S. dollars)

Location	Type of case	Cost of treatment	Cost of vaccination
Argentina	Average	160–2,553	0.80
India (Delhi, Safdar-jang Hospital)	Average	319	—
Iran, Islamic Rep. of	Government hospital	319–807	1.00
	Private hospital	957–2,042	6.40–10.50
Senegal (Dakar)	Fatal	255–511	} 0.90–1.80
	Surviving	460–2,374	
	Average	638–766	
Yugoslavia	Simple	287	} 0.30–1.60
	Artificial respiration required	2,872	
Developing countries	Average	319–957	1.00–1.60

— Data not available.
Note: All costs have been converted into 1989 U.S. dollars, assuming costs in original studies were in 1970 dollars.
Source: Cvjetanovic, Grab, and Uemura 1978.

tetanus immunization program, which allowed a redistribution of $600,000 worth of care from tetanus to other priorities. He estimated a benefit-to-cost ratio of 9 to 1.

Rey, Guillaumont, and Majnoni d'Intignano (1979) esti-mate the costs of alternative immunization strategies and benefits in treatment costs saved over a thirty-year period (see table 9-9) based on the model developed by Cvjetanovic and others (1972). Assuming that the cost per vaccination is $1.18 (all costs have been converted to 1989 U.S. dollars) and the treatment cost for one case is $592, they calculate that contin-uous vaccination of pregnant women would result in the lowest cost per case averted ($245), compared with one mass vacci-nation campaign ($463 per case averted), repeated mass cam-paigns ($595), and a combination of repeated mass campaigns and continuous vaccination ($468). This model does not, however, examine costs of continuous (routine) immunization of all women of childbearing age.

This information on the costs of treatment of non-neonatal tetanus can be used to estimate the cost-effectiveness of case management.[4] The range of treatment costs for developing countries cited in table 9-8 is from $319 to $957. Footnote b of table 9-1 indicates that treatment in hospitals of non-neonatal tetanus cases may reduce the case-fatality rate by 15 to 20 percentage points. Dividing the cost of treatment by this change in CFR gives a range in estimated cost per death averted of $1,595 to $6,380. As mentioned above, Cvjetanovic and others (1972) estimate an average cost of $592 per case treated in developing countries, resulting in a cost per death averted of $2,960 to $3,947, depending on the assumed reduction of 15 to 20 percentage points in the CFR. Thus, treatment of non-neonatal tetanus appears to be substantially less cost-

Table 9-9. Cost-Benefit and Cost-Effectiveness of Various Immunization Programs in Developing Countries over a Thirty-year Period
(1989 U.S. dollars)

Immunization program	Cumulative cost	Number of cases averted	Treatment cost saved	Cost per case averted
None[a]	n.a.	n.a.	n.a.	n.a.
One mass campaign[b]	592,288	1,278	756,944	463
Repeated mass campaigns at ten-year intervals[b]	2,194,391	3,686	2,183,173	595
Continuous vaccination of pregnant women[c]	1,513,761	6,184	3,662,708	245
Combination of repeated mass campaigns and continuous vaccination of pregnant women	3,708,152	7,922	4,692,105	468

n.a. Not applicable.

Note: Assumes population of one million at beginning of the period; thereafter, annual growth rate is 2 percent. Cost of one vaccination is $1.18; treatment cost for one case is $592.

a. Without immunization program, incidence would be 400 per 100,000 newborns and 18 per 100,000 population.

b. Assumes coverage of 50 percent, vaccine effectiveness of 95 percent.

c. Assumes coverage of 90 percent, vaccine effectiveness of 95 percent.

Source: Rey, Guillaumont, and Majnoni d'Intignano 1979, based on Cvjetanovic and others (1972).

effective than prevention. Prevention should therefore remain the intervention of top priority.

Non-NNT is important from an economic perspective in that treatment costs are high, death is common, long-term disability may ensue, and prolonged illness may result in lost productivity for the family and society (Rey, Guillaumont, and Majnoni d'Intignano 1979). Age-distribution data from studies conducted in Bombay (1954–79) and Dakar (1960–86) indicate that a high proportion of deaths and between 50 and 60 percent of non-NNT cases occur among the economically productive groups age ten to fifty-nine years (Rey, Guillaumont, and Majnoni d'Intignano 1979).

With increasing immunization of infants and older children with DPT and DT, an epidemiological shift in incidence to older age groups is expected to continue. These epidemiological shifts will have an effect on the economic productivity of developing societies.

The annual cost fully to protect the entire adult population of the developing world is difficult to estimate because vaccinations administered in past years may still be protective. Unlike infants (a cohort which renews itself annually and is consequently easily calculated), women receive multiple doses of TT at varying intervals over a thirty-year reproductive span; and women enter and leave the eligible age range continuously (Steinglass 1990). Still, assuming a cost of $0.91 per dose of TT (table 9-7), a five-dose schedule for lifelong protection, and a total adult population of 2.4 billion, we arrive at a cost of approximately $10.9 billion to

protect this population for life against tetanus and their offspring against NNT. This figure is less than the total potential savings resulting from avoided economic loss, avoided treatment, and prevention of disability. The cost to protect all unimmunized women of childbearing age would be less than half this amount and would eliminate NNT and reduce adult tetanus by half.

The estimates of tetanus deaths can be used to project crude cost-effectiveness figures for prevention of adult tetanus cases.[5] Murray, Yang, and Qiao (1992) estimate that 10.6 million deaths occur annually in developing countries in the adult age group (fifteen to fifty-nine years of age). From tables 9-1 and 9-2 earlier in this chapter, we can estimate that 132,500 (1.25 percent) of these deaths are due to tetanus. An individual in a developing country has approximately a 24 percent chance of dying of any cause between the ages of fifteen and fifty-nine (Murray, Yang, and Qiao 1992). By derivation, an adult in a developing country has approximately a 0.3 percent chance of dying of tetanus between those ages.

Full immunization by the age of fifteen (through a combination of DPT, DT, Td, and TT during infancy, at school, and during other contacts with the health system) would require five properly spaced shots and would most likely fully protect an individual from the risk of tetanus for life.

Unfortunately, few of the studies reviewed earlier included examinations of the cost of providing tetanus as a part of infant and school immunization programs. For the most part, they focused on reaching adult women in order to prevent neonatal tetanus deaths. The marginal cost of providing the "T" in DPT is likely to be very small, and the costs of providing DT or Td to schoolchildren might be substantially different from the costs of providing TT to pregnant women. Nevertheless, the median cost per TT dose of $0.91 (table 9-7) is the most reasonable estimate we have available of the unit cost of delivering tetanus immunization. If five doses were provided at a median cost of $0.91 per dose, full protection could be bought for $4.55.

If this cost is divided by the individual risk of an adult dying of tetanus between the ages of fifteen and fifty-nine (0.3 percent), we can derive a cost per death averted of $1,517. This cost of preventing adult tetanus is nearly fourteen times higher than the median cost per NNT death averted ($110) found in table 9-7, but it compares well with other adult interventions discussed elsewhere in this collection.

Research Agenda for the 1990s

A review of the recent literature has identified a research agenda for the 1990s. Such a lengthy list is not meant to suggest that current control efforts should await research findings. Enough is already known about the benefits of NNT control efforts to justify vigorous implementation at country level. The research agenda includes topics in vaccinology, epidemiology, programmatic concerns, and behavioral science.

Vaccinology

• Determine the nature, action, and duration of immunity from primary and reinforcing doses of TT with varying potencies and intervals in different settings (Jones 1983).

• Define the effect of the varying levels of maternal tetanus antitoxin on the level and duration of infant tetanus antitoxin following varying doses of DPT (WHO/EPI 1989b).

• Develop and test a TT vaccine which is more immunogenic with fewer doses, such as a single-dose high-potency TT with pulsed or continuous release of toxoid, with or without adjuvants, that uses alternative polymers as the vehicle (Galazka 1983; WHO/EPI 1989a).

Operational Strategies

• Identify and implement alternative cost-effective NNT prevention strategies in a variety of settings (including hard-to-reach areas), identify costs and operational constraints, and document the effect on immunological status and NNT incidence. Such strategies include expanding the TT schedule to five doses and the target groups to all women of childbearing age, immunizing at every contact with the health services, offering immunization at markets, immunizing schoolchildren in the early grades, launching mass campaigns every five or ten years, incorporating TT in national vaccination days, enforcing compulsory TT before marriage certificates are issued, scheduling a routine dose of TT at the start of every decade of life—at ages ten, twenty, thirty, and forty.

• Determine practical methods of screening and immunizing all women of childbearing age on every contact with the health services.

• Determine methods of identifying and routinely immunizing women entering the childbearing age.

• Explore potential use of TT outside the cold chain, including the possibility of administration by prefilled single-use injection devices which can be used by peripheral workers—for example, TBAs or village health workers (WHO/EPI 1989a; WHO/EPI 1989b).

• Study use, distribution, and effect of disposable delivery kits in a variety of settings.

Monitoring

• Develop and apply valid criteria, guidelines, operational indicators, and methodologies to monitor levels of TT coverage and protection, clean delivery, and cord care (Steinglass 1988; WHO/EPI 1989b).

• Review experience using lifetime home-based records and develop several record-keeping options for TT protection in areas employing different NNT prevention strategies. Study factors for promoting retention of records by the public.

• Include in the standard thirty cluster community surveys of immunization coverage questions on maternal TT status, age and parity of mother and protection status of delivery, number of prenatal care visits, place of delivery and attendant, and circumstances of delivery.

• Include TT in surveys on missed opportunities for immunization to determine magnitude and correction of problem.

• Conduct serological (gold-standard) assessments of immunologic and immunization status in the community as part of NNT mortality and thirty cluster coverage surveys (Schofield 1986).

Surveillance

• Develop various methods of identifying high-risk population subgroups and areas for focused interventions.

• Determine the magnitude of maternal mortality due to tetanus.

• Determine the feasibility of community-based surveillance and reporting of NNT cases and the utility of case investigations.

• Determine methods of documenting the absence of NNT as part of the elimination effort.

• Determine in selected areas the relationship of altitude to NNT incidence to concentrate control activities in high-risk areas.

Impact Evaluation

• Assess sustained effect of TBA training on changing delivery and cord care practices and on NNT and neonatal mortality in "before" and "after" control and experimental areas (Ross 1986a).

• Conduct retrospective case-control studies of the effect of TBA training (and TT immunization) on neonatal mortality and NNT in areas where some TBAs have been trained and others have not (Ross 1986b).

• Conduct studies on the incremental effect of TBA training, above that achieved by TT immunization alone, on NNT and neonatal mortality (Ross 1986b).

Social Factors

• Review experiences of the use of techniques of social marketing and social mobilization directed at the problem of NNT.

• Conduct market research and practical behavioral research on immunization acceptability, intrapartum and postpartum care, and cultural perceptions of NNT to identify and overcome resistance on the part of the public and providers and to promote TT immunization and clean delivery practices (Bastien 1988; Pillsbury 1989).

- Study methods of community involvement for routine identification and referral of females for TT, including use of TBAS, women's groups, political structure, and religious leaders.

Cost-Effectiveness

- Study the cost and cost-effectiveness of alternative NNT control strategies, especially TT immunization of all women of childbearing age and TBA training. Study the logistical implications and resource requirements for widened immunization target groups, so as to influence local decisions on resource allocation.
- Refine simple costing guidelines on alternative NNT prevention strategies for use by program managers for decisions on resource allocation.

Conclusions

Tetanus kills 750,000 babies annually, and non-NNT kills an additional 120,000 to 300,000 persons. Neonatal tetanus is completely preventable by means of maternal immunization with tetanus toxoid or aseptic care of the umbilical cord. Prevention of NNT will reduce neonatal mortality by up to half and infant mortality by up to one-quarter in unimmunized populations. Increasingly, the level of NNT is being recognized as a barometer of the health status and well-being of mothers and newborns, with each case attesting to multiple failures of the health system (Galazka and Cook 1985).

Prevention of NNT should be a priority for resource allocation in many developing countries, given the magnitude of the disease (high incidence rates in poorer countries), the severity of the disease (high case-fatality rates even with treatment), the high cost of treatment, and the availability of a safe, highly efficacious, and cost-effective vaccine.

The strategies chosen for immunization, as well as the target groups, should be defined locally and will depend on a number of different factors, including:

- Level of incidence
- Level of resources available (nationally and from donors)
- Organization and utilization of health services (particularly preventive and MCH services)
- Existence of other channels for contact (schools, bride registration, TBAS, and so on)
- Immediacy of desired effect (use of campaigns or routine immunization)

- Cost-effectiveness and opportunity cost of other health interventions and strategies
- Incremental cost of different TT strategies
- Operational and behavioral considerations

As was demonstrated by the studies in Deschapelles, Haiti (Berggren, 1974a), and Pidie District, Indonesia (Berman and others 1991; WHO/EPI 1988a), mass campaigns can be effective in rapidly reducing the backlog of unimmunized individuals in the target population. Continuous immunization through routine services is a more common approach and will be necessary in most cases to ensure continued protection of the population over time. In the cost studies reviewed, the median cost per NNT death averted was $110.

As Berman and others (1991) noted: "The appropriate agenda for planning is not an absolute choice amongst different strategies, but a flexible schedule for how different approaches can be combined over time to maximize results at an affordable cost. This approach was suggested by Cvjetanovic et al. (1972) and still remains valid."

The World Health Organization now recommends efforts to eliminate NNT worldwide by 1995. Achievement of this global target will require a global commitment of resources and mobilization of political will at all levels. Unlike other eradication and elimination efforts (for example, smallpox and polio), there can be no cessation of vaccination and revaccination efforts once NNT elimination is achieved, because the infective agent exists in the environment and cannot be eradicated. Elimination itself will need to be sustained forever by means of active immunization. Neonatal tetanus is easily preventable and can be eliminated as a public health problem in most countries at a reasonable cost. This cost would be affordable for most countries, although many of the poorer countries (which also tend to have the largest tetanus problem) will require donor assistance for years into the future.

Appendix 9A. Cost-Effectiveness of Tetanus Immunization Programs

Two of the following four tables examine the cost-effectiveness of tetanus immunization programs from the standpoint of epidemiologic data, cost, and effectiveness data. The other two tables use the same data to examine simulation models of cost-effectiveness.

Table 9A-1. Studies of Cost-Effectiveness of Tetanus Immunization Programs: Epidemiologic Data

Location (source)	Intervention year	Strategy	Target group	Population total	Population Target	Number of TT immunizations given				NNT incidence rate[a]	NNT mortality rate[a]	Case-fatality rate
						One	Two	Three or more	Total			
Burkina Faso (de Champeaux and Martin 1989)[b]	1987	Fixed centers	Women 15–44	—	—	6,043 / 13,832	1,957 / 5,928	0 / 0	8,000 / 19,760	—	—	—
Cameroon (Brenzel 1987)	1987	Mass campaign	Women 15–49	—	—	—	—	—	151,415	—	—	—
Ecuador (Shepard and others 1987)	1974–85	Fixed centers	Pregnant women	—	—	—	—	—	179,765	—	—	—
The Gambia (Robertson and others 1985)	1980–81	Fixed centers and outreach	Pregnant women nationwide	—	—	—	84 percent	—	—	—	40 in unimmunized (1965)	90 percent (1982)
Haiti/ Deschappelles (Berggren 1974a,b)[c]	1967–71	Mass	Females ten and older	94,000	—	247,677	213,002	178,327	639,006	64 (1967)	60 (1966)	85 percent[d]
		Marketplace	All people ten and older	—	—	—	—	—	—	9 (1972)	—	—
		Rally posts	Children	—	—	—	—	—	—	—	—	—
Haiti (Narcisse 1989)	1988	Fixed centers	Women 15–44	—	—	—	—	—	165,713	—	—	—
		Mass campaign	Women 15–44	—	—	—	—	—	542,461	—	—	—
		Rally posts	Women 15–44	—	—	—	—	—	165,713	—	—	—
		Horse teams	Women 15–44	—	—	—	—	—	127,496	—	—	—
India/Narangwal (Kielmann and Vohra 1977)[e]	1972–73	Campaign	Women 15–44	13,000,000	1,820	1,583 (87 percent)	0	0	1,583	—	25	—
Indonesia/Central Java (WHO/EPI 1981b)[f]	1979–80	Fixed centers and outreach	Pregnant women	1,400,000 two rural sites	—	—	—	—	—	—	—	—
Indonesia/Central Java (Barnum, Tarantola, and Setiady 1980)[f]	1979–84	Fixed centers and outreach	Children Pregnant women	—	—	—	—	—	—	—	—	—
Indonesia/Pidie (WHO/EPI 1988; 1988a; Berman and others 1991)[g]	1985	Mass campaign	Women 10–45	380,000	95,300	83,642 (88 percent)	67,962 (71 percent)	—	151,604	—	Provincial: 20.9 (1984)[d] Pidie (5 clusters): 32.1 ± 15 (1984) Pidie (30 clusters): 4.9 ± 2.6 (1987)	85 percent[d]

(Table continues on the following page.)

Location (source)	Intervention year	Strategy	Target group	Population total	Population Target	Number of TT immunizations given — One	Two	Three or more	Total	NNT incidence rate[a]	NNT mortality rate[a]	Case-fatality rate
Indonesia/Aceh (Berman and others 1991)[h]	1985	Fixed centers	Pregnant women in four sub-districts	— — — —	358 462 732 2,435	— — — —	43 97 205 1,948	— — — —	— — — —	— — — —	— — — —	85[d] pecent
Indonesia/Central Lombok (UNICEF 1985)[i]	1985	Campaign	All women of reproductive age	577,000	140,000	129,728 (93 percent)	125,982 (90 percent)	—	255,710	—	Seven clusters: 28 ± 9.7 (1983) Provincial level: 16.7	85[d] percent
Senegal/Dakar (Rey and others 1979)[j]	1970	Mass campaign (two times) (hypothetical)	Total population	650,000	650,000	—	—	—	—	300/650,000	100/650,000	30–40 percent
	1970–73	Mass campaign (seven times) (real data)	Total population	650,000	650,000	—	—	—	—	—	—	—
Senegal (Brenzel and others 1987)	1987	Mass campaign	Pregnant women	—	—	—	—	—	71,546	—	—	—
Sudan (Brenzel and others (1987)	1988	Fixed centers and mobile teams	Pregnant women Pregnant women Pregnant women Pregnant women	— — — —	190,120 180,177 119,556 920,030	40,686 69,548 68,864 332,131	23,575 45,405 60,854 231,848	— — — —	64,261 114,953 129,718 563,979	— — — —	— — — —	— — — —
Thailand (Phonboon and others 1989)[k]	1987	Fixed centers and outreach	Pregnant women	3,025,000	—	—	42–70 percent	—	—	—	—	—

— Not available.

a. Per 1,000 live births unless otherwise noted.

b. In Yako, EPI used oral polio vaccine and DPT. In Gourcy, EPI used DPTP (DPT with injectable polio).

c. Three doses of TT one month apart; minimum five years protection. Numbers of TT immunizations derived from information in cited document. Incidence based on hospital admissions. Mortality estimate rom retrospective community survey. Calculations use actual program intervention data.

d. WHO estimate of case-fatality rate.

e. Assumes lifelong immunity from one dose of high-potency (30Lf/ml) calcium phosphate-adsorbed TT with 80 percent efficacy.

f. Uses hypothetical model of incidence.

g. Two doses of TT. Coverage figures differ slightly by source.

h. Two doses of TT. Targets derived from information reported in document.

i. Hypothetical incidence data. Targets derived from information reported in document.

j. Two doses of TT. Previous vaccination history ignored.

k. Hypothetical study of ten-year program of TT2. Low CFR due to high proportion of cases in people over one year of age.

k. Two doses of TT.

Source: See first column of this table.

Table 9A-2. Studies of Cost-Effectiveness of Tetanus Immunization Programs: Cost and Cost-Effectiveness Data

Location (source)	Subdivision	Year	Total Cost		Cost per TT dose		Cost per TT2		Cost per case prevented[a]		Cost per death averted[a]	
			Current dollars	1989 dollars	Current dollars	1989 dollars	Current dollars	1989 dollars	Current dollars	1989 dollars	Current dollars	1989 dollars
Burkina Faso (de Champeaux and Martin 1989)[b]	Gourcy	1987	11,568	12,607	0.59	0.64	1.95	2.13	—	—	—	—
	Yako		7,447	8,116	0.93	1.01	3.81	4.15	—	—	—	—
Cameroon (Brenzel 1987)[b]	n.a.	1987	186,218	202,955	1.23	1.34	3.82	4.16	—	—	—	—
Ecuador (Shepard and others 1987)[b]	n.a.	1985	62,918	72,482	0.35	0.40	—	—	—	—	—	—
The Gambia (Robertson and others 1985)[c]	n.a.	1980	125,315	188,463	1.05	1.58	3.48	5.23	136.36	205.07	151.53	227.89
Haiti/Deschapelles (Berggren 1974a,b)[d]	n.a.	1969	67,000	226,346	0.10	0.34	0.31	1.05	28.88	97.57	33.98	114.79
Haiti (Narcisse 1989)[b]	n.a.	1988	143,926	150,867	0.87	0.91	—	—	—	—	—	—
			888,990	931,862	1.63	1.71	—	—	—	—	—	—
			32,846	34,430	0.20	0.21	—	—	—	—	—	—
			138,890	145,588	1.09	1.14	—	—	—	—	—	—
India/Narangwal (Kielmann and Vohra 1977)[e]	Initial period	1972	253,846	751,750	0.10	0.29	—	—	—	—	32.85	97.27
	Maintenance phase		n.a.	n.a.	n.a.	n.a.	n.a.	n.a.	n.a.	n.a.	0.12	0.34
Indonesia/Central Java (WHO/EPI 1981b)[f]	n.a.	1980	—	—	0.62	1.18	2.06	3.92	—	—	—	—
Indonesia/Central Java (Barnum and others 1980)[f]	n.a.	1978	32,800,000	62,352,475	—	—	—	—	8.70	16.54	135.00	256.63
Indonesia/Pidie (WHO/EPI 1988a; Berman and others 1991)[g]	n.a.	1985	108,355	124,825	0.71	0.82	1.59	1.84	106.25 (92–127)	122.40 (106–146)	125.00 (108–147)	144.00 (124–179)
Indonesia/Aceh (Berman and others 1991)[h]	Tanah Pasir	1985	82	94	—	—	1.91	2.20	77.38	89.15	91.04	104.88
	Samudera		233	268	—	—	2.40	2.76	97.90	112.78	115.18	132.69
	Matangkuli		261	301	—	—	1.27	1.47	51.98	59.88	61.15	70.45
	Jeumpa		1,114	1,284	—	—	0.57	0.66	23.34	26.89	27.46	31.64
Indonesia/Central Lombok (UNICEF 1985)[i]	NNT mortality, 28.0	1985	50,000	57,600	0.20	0.23	0.40	0.46	38.43	44.27	45.21	52.09
	NNT mortality, 18.3	—	—	—	—	—	—	—	58.80	67.74	69.18	79.69
	NNT mortality, 37.7	—	—	—	—	—	—	—	28.54	32.88	33.58	38.68
	NNT mortality, 16.7	—	—	—	—	—	—	—	64.44	74.23	75.81	87.33

(Table continues on the following page.)

Table 9A-2 (continued)

Location (source)	Subdivision	Year	Total Cost Current dollars	Total Cost 1989 dollars	Cost per TT dose Current dollars	Cost per TT dose 1989 dollars	Cost per TT2 Current dollars	Cost per TT2 1989 dollars	Cost per case prevented[a] Current dollars	Cost per case prevented[a] 1989 dollars	Cost per death averted[a] Current dollars	Cost per death averted[a] 1989 dollars
Senegal/Dakar (Rey and others 1979)[j]	Hypothetical	1970	—	—	—	—	—	—	175.00	558.45	528.00	1,684.92
	Real data	1971	70,000	214,468	—	—	—	—	269.23	824.88	897.44	2,749.59
Senegal (Brenzel and others 1987)[b]	n.a.	1987	49,786	54,261	0.70	0.76	—	—	—	—	—	—
Sudan (Brenzel and others 1990)[b]	Darfur	1988	108,065	113,277	1.68	1.76	4.58	4.80	—	—	—	—
	Kordofan		93,776	98,298	0.82	0.86	2.07	2.16	—	—	—	—
	Capital		164,819	172,768	1.27	1.33	2.71	2.84	—	—	—	—
	National level		929,577	974,406	1.65	1.73	4.01	4.20	—	—	—	—
Thailand (Phonboon and others 1989)[b]	Hospitals	1985–	—	—	—	—	8.90	10.25	—	—	—	—
	Health centers	86	—	—	—	—	10.30	11.87	—	—	—	—

— Not available.

n.a. Not applicable.

a. NNT only, unless otherwise specified.

b. Calculated from cost-effectiveness study of entire EPI.

c. Cost of expatriate personnel excluded. Costs based on three contacts required to receive TT3 (three of eight contacts = 37.5 percent of total costs).

d. Total cost is expenditures only. Cost per case and death averted excludes another 630 non-NNT cases prevented. If these were included, the cost per case prevented would fall to $23 ($77 in 1989 dollars), and the cost per death averted would drop to $29 ($99 in 1989 dollars).

e. Hypothetical cost data for 2.6 million women age fifteen to forty-four.

f. Range in cost per TT = $0.56–$0.76; range in cost per TT2 = $1.43–2.61. Cost data include five years' cost of DPT and TT and cases and deaths from diphtheria, pertussis, and tetanus.

g. Cost per TT dose and case prevented derived from information reported in cited documents. Applying upper and lower confidence intervals (17–47) around 32.1/1,000 in five clusters of 1984 survey in Pidie and 2.3–7.5/1,000 in thirty-cluster survey in 1987, cost per death averted ranges from $45–$211 ($52–$243) in 1989 U.S. dollars.

h. Cost per case and death prevented does not take into account the protective effect of TT2 on all deliveries within three years. Cost per case prevented data derived from information reported in cited document.

i. Cost excludes administrative salaries at national level. Cases and deaths averted estimated from data reported in cited document, assuming vaccine efficacy of 95 percent; general fertility rate of 110/1,000; average duration of protection of three years.

j. Total costs include only vaccine costs. Costs for second study, using real data, were likely incurred over entire four-year period. Authors assume cost year is 1971.

Source: See first column of this table.

214

Table 9A-3. Simulation Models of Cost-Effectiveness of Tetanus Immunization Programs: Epidemiologic Data

Source	Location	Strategy	Target group	Population		TT coverage		NNT incidence[a]	NNT mortality[a]	Case-fatality rate
				Total	Target	TT1	TT2			
Cvjetanovic and others 1972[b]	—	Mass campaign	Total population	1,000,000	1,000,000	—	—	4 Neonatal	—	With treatment: 80 percent general
		Repeated mass campaign (3x)	Total population	1,000,000	1,000,000	—	—	18/100,000 (adult)	—	30 percent newborn
		Continuous pregnant	Pregnant women	1,000,000	1,000,000	—	—	—	—	Without treatment: 90 percent general
		Continuous pregnant and repeated mass (3x)	Pregnant women and total population	1,000,000	1,000,000	—	—	—	—	40 percent newborn
Kessel 1984[c]	—	Preschool	Children	—	—	—	—	—	10–30	—
		Primary school	Children	—	—	—	—	—	—	—
		Antenatal TT	Pregnant women	—	—	—	—	—	—	—
		Antenatal outreach	Pregnant women	—	—	—	—	—	—	—
Sharma and Sharma 1984a,b[d]	India/rural Uttar Pradesh	Continuous (50–80 percent)	Pregnant women	—	—	—	—	Adult: 185/100,000	—	Adult: 50 percent
			Children 5–10 Children 10–15 Children < 5	—	—	—	—	Neonatal: 68.8	66.7	Rural: 97 percent
		Mass—repeated every five years (50 percent coverage)	Women 15–44 All adults							
Smucker and others 1984[e]	India/Uttar Pradesh (2 districts)	Campaign (teams) every 5 years	Women 10–44	3,529,048	882,262	75–95 percent	60–90 percent	—	53	—
		Outreach (continuous)	Women 10–44	3,529,048	882,262	75–95 percent	60–90 percent	—	53	—

— Not available.

a. Per 1,000 live births unless otherwise indicated.

b. Includes NNT and not NNT. Assumes 50 percent coverage for campaign and 90 percent coverage for continuous strategy. Booster given one year after TT2. Thirty-year time horizon.

c. Excludes cases and deaths from non-NNT.

d. Vaccine efficacy is 90 percent, twenty-five year time horizon, two TT per woman. Boosters given every five years. NNT mortality from sample of 3,267 births. Excludes cases and deaths from non-NNT. Intervention year 1978.

Table 9A-4. *Simulation Models of Cost-Effectiveness of Tetanus Immunization Programs: Cost and Cost-Effectiveness Data*

Source	Location	Cost year	Total cost		Cost per TT dose		Cost per TT2 dose		Cost per case prevented[a]		Cost per death averted[a]	
			Current dollars	1989 dollars	Current dollars	1989 dollars	Current dollars	1989 dollars	Current dollars	1989 dollars	Current dollars	1989 dollars
Cvjetanovic and others 1972[b]	—	1972	—	—	—	—	—	—	156.50	463.47	—	—
									201.00	595.25	—	—
									82.70	244.91	—	—
									158.10	468.20	—	—
Kessel, 1984[c]	—	—	—	—	—	—	—	—	Uses hypothetical financial units, not actual dollars. Concludes that school-based immunization is most economical for long term complementary strategy.			
Sharma and Sharma 1984[a,b]	India/rural Uttar Pradesh[c]	—	—	—	—	—	—	—	Favors continuous immunization of pregnant women. Mass immunization leads to short-lived declines in cases and deaths.			
Smucker and others 1984[d]	India/Uttar Pradesh (2 districts)	1978 (?)	1,147,795	2,181,947	0.70	1.34	1.44	2.74	—	—	3.55	6.75
			1,461,477	2,778,443	1.23	2.33	2.76	5.25	—	—	6.24	11.86
			431,222	819,749	0.26	0.50	0.54	1.03	—	—	1.36	2.59
			613,517	1,166,290	0.52	0.98	1.16	2.20	—	—	2.56	4.87

a. Cost per case and death averted is for NNT only, unless otherwise specified.
b. No discounting of costs and benefits.
c. Gives rankings of cost per prevented death at different NNT mortality rates. Makes assumptions regarding ranking of financial units and strategies.
d. First line for each strategy: most cost-effective scenario. Second line for each strategy: least cost-effective scenario costs for twenty-five year period discounted at 12 percent per year; deaths not discounted.

Notes

The authors wish to acknowledge their gratitude to Mary Carnell, Pierre Claquin, Nancy Cylke, Michael Favin, Rebecca Fields, Stanley Foster, Artur Galazka, François Gasse, Mary Harvey, Diane Hedgecock, Norbert Hirschhorn, and Dean Jamison for their assistance and comments on earlier drafts of this chapter and to the Resources for Child Health Project (John Snow, Inc.) under a contract (DPE-5982-Z-00-9034-00) with the U.S. Agency for International Development for their support and encouragement.

1. The term "economic costs" refers to the value of all resources used, including those which were donated and those for which there was no additional expenditure (for example, personnel time and amortization of vehicles and equipment).

2. In the case of Indonesia (Aceh), as well as Indonesia (Pidie), only the cost per death averted was given in the source cited. The World Bank authors have calculated the cost per case averted from this information using the WHO estimate of 85 percent case fatality for NNT.

3. All dollar amounts in parentheses in this section are 1989 U.S. dollars.

4. The authors would like to thank Dean Jamison for his assistance with the calculations in this paragraph.

5. The authors would like to thank Dean Jamison for his assistance with the calculations in this paragraph.

References

Adeuja, A. O. G., and B. O. Osuntokun. 1971. "Tetanus in the Adult Nigerians. A Review of 503 Patients." *East African Medical Journal* 48:683–91.

Allman, Suzanne. 1986. "Childbearing and the Training of Traditional Birth Attendants in Rural Haiti." *Medical Anthropology Quarterly* 17:40–43.

Al-Mukhtar, M. Y. 1987. "Birth Care Practice and Tetanus Neonatorum: A Hospital-Based Study in Mosul." *Public Health* 101:453–56.

Arnold, R. B., T. I. Soewarso, and Albertus Karyadi. 1986. "Mortality from Neonatal Tetanus in Indonesia: Results of Two Surveys." *Bulletin of the World Health Organization* 64:259–62.

Barnum, H. N., Daniel Tarantola, and I. F. Setiady. 1980. "Cost-Effectiveness of an Immunization Programme in Indonesia." *Bulletin of the World Health Organization* 58:499–503.

Barten, J. J. C. 1969. "Neonatal Tetanus: A Review of 134 Cases." *Tropical and Geographical Medicine* 21:383–88.

Bastien, J. W. 1988. *Cultural Perceptions of Neonatal Tetanus and Programming Implications, Bolivia.* Arlington, Va.: John Snow, REACH.

Bennett, M. J. 1976. "Postabortal and Postpartum Tetanus: A Review of 19 Cases." *South African Medical Journal* 50:513–16.

Berggren, G. G., Adeline Verly, Nicolle Garnier, Walbourg Peterson, Douglas Ewbank, and Wooly Dieudonné. 1983. "Traditional Midwives, Tetanus Immunization, and Infant Mortality in Rural Haiti." *Tropical Doctor* 13:79–87.

Berggren, W. L. 1974a. "Administration and Evaluation of Rural Health Services. I. A Tetanus Control Program in Haiti." *American Journal of Tropical Medicine and Hygiene* 23:936–49.

———. 1974b. "Control of Neonatal Tetanus in Rural Haiti through the Utilization of Medical Auxiliaries." *Bulletin of the Pan-American Health Organization* 8:24–29.

Berggren, W. L., and G. G. Berggren. 1971. "Changing Incidence of Fatal Tetanus of the Newborn: A Retrospective Study in a Defined Rural Haitian Population." *American Journal of Tropical Medicine and Hygiene* 20:491–94.

Berman, Peter, John Quinley, Burhannudin Yusuf, Syaifuddin Anwar, Udin Mustaini, A. Azof, and Iskander. 1991. "Maternal Tetanus Immunization in Aceh Province, Sumatra: The Cost-Effectiveness of Alternative Strategies." *Social Science and Medicine* 33:185–92.

Betts, C. D. 1989. *Assessment of Neonatal Tetanus and Its Control in Bolivia.* Arlington, Va.: John Snow, REACH.

Bhatia, Shushum. 1989. "Patterns and Causes of Neonatal and Postneonatal Mortality in Rural Bangladesh." *Studies in Family Planning* 20:136–46.

Bjerregaard, P., R. Steinglass, D. M. Mutie, G. Kimani, M. Mjomba, and V. Orinda. 1993. "Neonatal Tetanus Mortality in Coastal Kenya: A Community Survey." *International Journal of Epidemiology* 22(1).

Black, R. E., D. H. Huber, and G. T. Curlin. 1980. "Reduction of Neonatal Tetanus by Mass Immunization of Non-pregnant Women: Duration of Protection Provided by One or Two Doses of Aluminum-Adsorbed Tetanus Toxoid." *Bulletin of the World Health Organization* 58:927–30.

Blanchet, Thérèse. 1989. *Perceptions of Childhood Diseases and Attitudes towards Immunization among Slum Dwellers, Dhaka, Bangladesh.* Arlington, Va.: John Snow, REACH.

Brenzel, L. E. 1987. *Cost-Effectiveness of Immunization Strategies in the Republic of Cameroon.* Arlington, Va.: John Snow, REACH.

———. 1989. *The Cost of EPI: A Review of Cost and Cost-Effectiveness Studies (1979–1987).* Arlington, Va.: John Snow, REACH.

Brenzel, L. E., Pierre Claquin, Ian McLellan, and Sally Stansfield. 1987. *Rapid Assessment of Senegal's Acceleration Phase.* Evaluation Publication 5. New York: UNICEF.

Brenzel, L. E., Michael Enright, Rachel Feilden, K. S. Lwin, Siraj Mustafa, A. H. Omer, Atahir Osman, Ahmed Babiker, and Allison Percy. 1990. *Report on the Cost-Effectiveness of the Expanded Program of Immunization in the Republic of Sudan,* vols. 1–5. Arlington, Va.: John Snow, REACH.

Budiarso, L. R. 1984. *Prospective Study on Infant and Childhood Mortality in Sukabumi, 1982–83.* Jakarta: Government of Indonesia, Department of Health.

Bytchenko, Boris. 1966. "Geographical Distribution of Tetanus in the World, 1951–60: A Review of the Problem." *Bulletin of the World Health Organization* 34:71–104.

———. 1972. "Recent Trends of Tetanus Mortality in the World." In Geoffrey Edsall, ed., *Proceedings of the Third International Conference on Tetanus.* Pan-American Health Organization Scientific Publication 253. Washington, D.C.

Chen, L. C., M. C. Gesche, Shamsa Ahmed, A. I. Chowdhury, and W. H. Mosley. 1974. "Maternal Mortality in Rural Bangladesh." *Studies in Family Planning* 5:334–41.

Chen, L. C., Mizanur Rahman, and A. M. Sarder. 1980. "Epidemiology and Causes of Death among Children in a Rural Area of Bangladesh." *International Journal of Epidemiology* 9:25–33.

Chen, P. C. Y. 1976. "The Traditional Birth Attendant and Neonatal Tetanus: The Malaysian Experience." *Journal of Tropical Pediatrics and Environmental Child Health* 22:263–64.

Christensen, P. E. 1972a. "Comments on Epidemiology and Immunology of Tetanus in Denmark." In Geoffrey Edsall, ed., *Proceedings of the Third International Conference on Tetanus.* Pan-American Health Organization Scientific Publication 253. Washington, D.C.

———. 1972b. "Side Reactions to Tetanus Toxoid." In Geoffrey Edsall, ed., *Proceedings of the Third International Conference on Tetanus.* Pan-American Health Organization Scientific Publication 253. Washington, D.C.

Cliff, J. 1985. "Neonatal Tetanus in Maputo, Mozambique. Part II: Preventative Measures." *The Central African Journal of Medicine* 31:27–32.

Cottin, J. F. 1987. "Le tétanos en France 1984–85." *Bulletin Epidémiologique Hebdomadaire* 10:37–39.

Cutts, F. T., A. Soares, A. V. Jecque, J. Cliff, S. Kortbeek, and S. Colombo. 1990. "The Use of Evaluation to Improve the Expanded Programme on Immunization in Mozambique." *Bulletin of the World Health Organization* 68:199–208.

Cvjetanovic, B. 1972. "Epidemiology of Tetanus Viewed from a Practical Public Health Angle." In Geoffrey Edsall, ed., *Proceedings of the Third International Conference on Tetanus.* Pan-American Health Organization Scientific Publication 253. Washington, D.C.

Cvjetanovic, B., B. Grab, and K. Uemura. 1978a. "Epidemiological Models of Acute Bacterial Diseases." *Bulletin of the World Health Organization* 56 (Supplement 1):11–28.

———. 1978b. "Tetanus: An Endemic Disease without Interhuman Transmission." *Bulletin of the World Health Organization* 56 (Supplement 1):29–45.

Cvjetanovic, B., B. Grab, K. Uemura, and Boris Bytchenko. 1972. "Epidemiological Model of Tetanus and Its Use in the Planning of Immunization Programmes." *International Journal of Epidemiology* 1:125–37.

de Champeaux, Antoine, and Bruno-Jacques Martin. 1989. *Evaluation du Programme Elargi de Vaccination, Province de la Sissili.* Centre Muraz, Burkina Faso: Organisation de Coordination et de Coopération pour la Lutte contre les Grandes Endémies (OCCGE), Unité de Vaccinologie.

de Quadros, C. A. 1990. "Defining High Risk Areas and Groups." In *Neonatal Tetanus Elimination: Issues, and Future Directions.* Arlington, Va.: John Snow, REACH/MotherCare.

de Silva, A. V. K. V. 1982. "Neonatal Tetanus Problem in Sri Lanka." *Pakistan Pediatric Journal* 6:214–27.

Ebisawa, Isao. 1967. "Mortality of Tetanus in Japan: An Unintentional Control Observation." In Leo Eckmann, ed., *Principles on Tetanus: Proceedings of the Second International Conference on Tetanus.* Bern, Switzerland: Hans Huber.

———. 1972. "Mortality and Sex Ratio of Tetanus in Japan." In Geoffrey Edsall, ed., *Principles on Tetanus: Proceedings of the Third International Conference on Tetanus.* Pan-American Health Organization Scientific Publication 253. Washington, D.C.

Ebisawa, Isao, and Reiko Homma. 1986. "Tetanus in Japan: Trends of Mortality, Case Fatality, and Causes of Death." *Japanese Journal of Experimental Medicine* 56:155–61.

Ecuador: Ministerio de Salud Pública and UNICEF. 1987. *Curso Basico de Vigilancia Epidemiológica de Enfermedades Immunoprevenibles.* Modulo 4 p. 40: Quito.

Evans, J. R., K. L. Hall, and Jeremy Warford. 1981. "Shattuck Lecture—Health Care in the Developing World: Problems of Scarcity and Choice." *New England Journal of Medicine* 305:1117–27.

Fauveau, Vincent, M. Mamdani, Robert Steinglass, and Marjorie Koblinsky. 1993. "Maternal Tetanus: Magnitude Epidemiology and Potential Control Measures." *International Journal of Gynecology and Obstetrics* 40(1):3–12.

Fenner, Frank, D. A. Henderson, Isao Arita, Zdenek Jezek, and I. D. Ladnyi. 1988. *Smallpox and Its Eradication.* Geneva: World Health Organization.

Foege, W. H., and D. A. Henderson. 1986. "Management Priorities in Primary Health Care." *Reviews of Infectious Diseases* 8:313–21.

Foster, S. O. 1984. "Immunizable and Respiratory Diseases and Child Mortality." In W. H. Mosley and L. C. Chen, eds., *Child Survival: Strategies for Research,* special supplement, *Population and Development Review* 10:119–40.

Galazka, Artur. 1982. "Tetanus Toxoid—Nature and Action." *Pakistan Pediatric Journal* 6:120–43.

———. 1983. *Immunization of Pregnant Women against Tetanus.* EPI/GEN/83/5. Geneva: World Health Organization.

Galazka, Artur, and Robert Cook. 1985. "Neonatal Tetanus Today and Tomorrow." In Guiseppe Nistico, P. Mastroeni, and M. Pitzurra, eds., *Proceedings of the Seventh International Conference on Tetanus.* Rome: Gangemi.

Galazka, Artur, François Gasse, and R. H. Henderson. 1989. "Neonatal Tetanus and the Global Expanded Programme on Immunization." In Elton Kessel and A. K. Awan, eds., *Maternal and Child Care in Developing Countries: Assessment, Promotion, Implementation. Proceedings of the Third International Congress for Maternal and Neonatal Health.* Thun, Switzerland: Ott.

Galazka, Artur, and B. Kardymowicz. 1989. "Tetanus Incidence and Immunity in Poland." *European Journal of Epidemiology* 5:474–79.

Galazka, Artur, and George Stroh. 1986. *Neonatal Tetanus: Guidelines on the Community-Based Survey on Neonatal Tetanus Mortality.* WHO/EPI/GEN/86/8. Geneva: World Health Organization.

Garenne, Michel, and Olivier Fontaine. 1986. "Assessing Probable Causes of Death Using a Standardized Questionnaire: A Study in Rural Senegal." Paper presented at the Seminar on Comparative Studies of Mortality and Morbidity: Old and New Approaches to Measurement and Analysis, University of Siena, International Union for the Scientific Study of Population and Institute of Statistics, July 7–12, Siena, Italy.

Gasse, François. 1990. *Neonatal Tetanus Elimination Initiative: Progress Report and Recommendation.* EPI/MCH/NNT/GEN/90.1. Geneva: World Health Organization.

Gray, R. H., G. S. Smith, and P. G. Barss. 1990. *The Use of Verbal Autopsy Methods to Determine Selected Causes of Death in Children.* Baltimore: Johns Hopkins University, Institute for International Programs.

Griffith, J. A., and D. L. Sachs. 1974. "Tetanus Neonatorum: Social and Economic Dimensions for Teaching and Program Planning." *Indian Pediatrics* 11:409–15.

Haaga, J. G. 1986. "Cost-Effectiveness and Cost-Benefit Analyses of Immunization Programmes in Developing Countries." In D. Jelliffe and E. F. P. Jelliffe, eds., *Advances in International Maternal and Child Health,* vol. 6. Oxford: Clarendon Press.

Heath, C. W., Jack Zusman, and I. L. Sherman. 1964. "Tetanus in the United States, 1950–1960." *American Journal of Public Health* 54:769–79.

Heinonen, O. P., Samuel Shapiro, and Dennis Slone. 1977. "Immunizing Agents." In *Birth Defects and Drugs in Pregnancy.* Littleton, Mass.: Publishing Sciences Group.

Henry, Fitzroy, André Briend, and Vincent Fauveau. 1990. "Child Survival: Should the Strategy be Redesigned? Experience from Bangladesh." *Health Policy and Planning* 5:226–34.

Herz, B. K., and A. R. Measham. 1987. *The Safe Motherhood Initiative: Proposals for Action.* World Bank Discussion Papers 9. Washington, D.C.

Islam, M. S., M. M. Rahaman, K. M. S. Aziz, Mizanur Rahman, M. H. Munshi, and Yakub Patwari. 1982. "Infant Mortality in Rural Bangladesh: An Analysis of Causes During Neonatal and Post-neonatal Periods." *Journal of Tropical Pediatrics* 28:294–98.

Jones, T. S. 1983. "The Use of Tetanus Toxoid for the Prevention of Neonatal Tetanus in Developing Countries." In N. A. Halsey and C. A. de Quadros, eds., *Recent Advances in Immunization: A Bibliographic Review.* PAHO (Pan-American Health Organization) Scientific Publication 451. Washington, D.C.

Jordan, Brigitte. 1989. "Cosmopolitical Obstetrics: Some Insights from the Training of Traditional Midwives." *Social Science and Medicine* 28:925–44.

Kessel, Elton. 1984. "Strategies for the Control of Neonatal Tetanus." *Journal of Tropical Pediatrics* 30:145–49.

Kielmann, A. A., and S. R. Vohra. 1977. "Control of Tetanus Neonatorum in Rural Communities—Immunization Effects of High-Dose Calcium Phosphate-Adsorbed Tetanus Toxoid." *Indian Journal of Medical Research* 66:909–16.

LaForce, F. M., L. S. Young, and J. V. Bennett. 1969. "Tetanus in the United States (1965–1966): Epidemiologic and Clinical Features." *New England Journal of Medicine* 280:569–74.

Lanasari, Rosaline, and Zeil Rosenberg. 1989. "Tetanus Toxoid Immunization of Prospective Brides in Central Java, Indonesia." *Health Policy and Planning* 4:235–38.

Leroy, Odile, and Michel Garenne. 1991. "Risk Factors of Neonatal Tetanus in Senegal." *International Journal of Epidemiology* 20:521–26.

Maine, Deborah, Allan Rosenfield, Marilyn Wallace, A. M. Kimball, B. E. Kwast, Emile Papiernik, and Sharon White. 1987. "Prevention of Maternal Deaths in Developing Countries: Program Options and Practical Considerations." Paper presented at International Safe Motherhood Conference, 10–13 February, Nairobi, Kenya.

Miller, J. K. 1972. "The Prevention of Neonatal Tetanus by Maternal Immunization." *Environmental Child Health* 18:160–67.

Mosley, W. H. 1984. "Will Primary Health Care Reduce Infant and Child Mortality? A Critique of Some Current Strategies, with Special Reference to Africa and Asia." In J. C. Caldwell and Gigi Santowi, eds., *Selected Readings in the Cultural, Social, and Behavioral Determinants of Health*. Health Transition Series no. 1. Canberra: Highland Press for Health Transition Center of the Australian National University.

Murray, C. J. L., Gonghaan Yang, and Xinjian Qiao. 1992. "Adult Mortality: Levels, Patterns, and Causes." In R. G. A. Feachem, Tord Kjellstrom, C. J. L. Murray, Mead Over, and M. A. Phillips, eds., *The Health of Adults in the Developing World*. Oxford: Oxford University Press.

Narcisse, Maryse. 1989. *Analyse du coût, coût-efficacité des stratégies du Programme Elargi de Vaccination en Haiti*. Port-au-Prince, Haiti: Ministère de la Santé Publique et de la Population, Bureau de Coordination du Programme Elargi de Vaccination.

Newell, K. W., A. D. Lehmann, D. R. Leblanc, and N. G. Osorio. 1966. "The Use of Toxoid for the Prevention of Tetanus Neonatorum: Final Report of a Double-Blind Controlled Field Trial." *Bulletin of the World Health Organization* 35:863–71.

Nichter, Mark. 1990. "Vaccinations in South Asia: False Expectations and Commanding Metaphors." In Jeannine Coreil and J. D. Mull, eds., *Anthropology and Primary Health Care*. Boulder, Colo.: Westview Press.

Patel, J. C., and B. C. Mehta. 1975. "Tetanus: A Study of 8,697 Cases." In *Proceedings of the Fourth International Conference on Tetanus*. Lyons: Fondation Mérieux.

Phonboon, K., D. S. Shepard, S. Ramaboot, P. Kunasol, and S. Preuksaraj. 1989. "The Thai Expanded Programme on Immunization: Role of Immunization Sessions and Their Effectiveness." *Bulletin of the World Health Organization* 67:181–88.

Pillsbury, Barbara. 1989. *Immunization: The Behavioral Issues: Behavioral Issues in Child Survival Programs: A Synthesis of the Literature with Recommendations for Project Design and Implementation*. Monograph 3. Washington, D.C.: International Health and Development Associates.

Rahman, Makhlisur, L. C. Chen, J. Chakraborty, M. Yunus, A. I. Chowdhury, A. M. Sarder, Shushum Bhatia, and G. T. Curlin. 1982. "Use of Tetanus Toxoid for the Prevention of Neonatal Tetanus. 1. Reduction of Neonatal Mortality by Immunization of Non-pregnant and Pregnant Women in Rural Bangladesh." *Bulletin of the World Health Organization* 60: 261–67.

Rahman, Makhlisur, L. C. Chen, J. Chakraborty, M. Yunus, A. S. G. Faruque, and A. I. Chowdhury. 1982. "Use of Tetanus Toxoid for the Prevention of Neonatal Tetanus. 2. Immunization Acceptance among Pregnant Women in Rural Bangladesh." *Bulletin of the World Health Organization* 60:269–77.

Rahman, Shafiqur. 1982. "The Effect of Traditional Birth Attendants and Tetanus Toxoid in Reduction of Neonatal Mortality." *Journal of Tropical Pediatrics* 28:163–65.

REACH (Resources for Child Health Project). 1989. *EPI Essentials: A Guide for Program Officers*. Arlington, Va.: John Snow.

Rey, Michel. 1982. "Prevention of Neonatal Tetanus by Immunization." *Pakistan Pediatric Journal* 6:103–19.

Rey, Michel, I. Diop-Mar, C. Lafaix, M. Guérin, and B. Schaff. 1968. "Le tétanos à Dakar, problème de santé publique." *Bulletin et Mémoires de Faculté des Médicins Pharmocologiques* 16:77–87.

Rey, Michel, I. Diop-Mar, and D. Robert. 1981. "Treatment of Tetanus." In Ricardo Veronesi, ed., *Tetanus: Important New Concepts*. Amsterdam: Excerpta Medica.

Rey, Michel, P. Guillaumont, and B. Majnoni d'Intignano. 1979. "Benefits versus Risk Factors in Tetanus." *Developments in Biological Standardization* 43:15–23.

Rey, Michel, and E. Tikhomirov. 1989. "Non-neonatal Tetanus over the World." In Giuseppe Nistico, Bernard Bizzini, Boris Bytchenko, and René Triau, eds., *Proceedings of the Eighth International Conference on Tetanus*. Rome: Pythagora Press.

Robertson, R. L., S. O. Foster, H. F. Hull, and P. J. Williams. 1985. "Cost-Effectiveness of Immunization in The Gambia." *Journal of Tropical Medicine and Hygiene* 88:343–51.

Rosenfield, Allan, and Deborah Maine. 1985. "Maternal Mortality—A Neglected Tragedy: Where is the M in MCH?" *Lancet* 2:83–85.

Rosmini, F., M. Wirz, G. Gentili, C. Colotti, M. Rossini Ricci, E. Franco, I. Terzi, and P. Pasquini. 1987. "Year of Birth, Sex, and Residence as 'Determinants' of Tetanus Incidence and Immunity in Italy." *European Journal of Epidemiology* 3:377–80.

Ross, D. A. 1986a. "Does Training TBAs Prevent Neonatal Tetanus?" *Health Policy and Planning* 1:89–98.

———. 1986b. "The Trained Traditional Birth Attendant and Neonatal Tetanus." In Amelia Mangay-Maglacas and John Simons, eds., *The Potential of the Traditional Birth Attendant*. Geneva: World Health Organization.

Royston, Erica, and Sue Armstrong, eds. 1989. *Preventing Maternal Deaths*. Geneva: World Health Organization.

Schofield, Frank. 1986. "Selective Primary Health Care: Strategies for Control of Disease in the Developing World. XXII. Tetanus: A Preventable Problem." *Reviews of Infectious Diseases* 8:144–56.

Schofield, F. D., V. M. Tucker, and G. R. Westbrook. 1961. "Neonatal Tetanus in New Guinea: Effect of Active Immunization in Pregnancy." *British Medical Journal* 2:785–89.

Sénécal, J. 1970. "Tetanus." In D. B. Jelliffe and H. C. Trowell, eds., *Diseases of Children in the Subtropics and Tropics*, 2d ed. London: Edward Arnold.

Sharma, Monica, and P. D. Sharma. 1984. "The Dynamics of Tetanus Epidemiology and Control in Rural Uttar Pradesh Studied through Computer Simulation." *Social Science and Medicine* 18:303–13.

Sharma, P. D., and Monica Sharma. 1982. "An Approach to Health Planning in India via Computer Simulation of Epidemiological Models: A Case Study of Tetanus." *Health and Population: Perspectives and Issues* 5:139–67.

———. 1984. "Impact of Alternate Immunisation Strategies on Tetanus Neonatorum in India." *Indian Pediatrics* 21:839–52.

Shepard, D. S., R. L. Robertson, C. S. M. Cameron, Pedro Saturno, Marjorie Pollack, and Jacques Manceau. 1987. *The Cost-Effectiveness of Immunization Strategies in Ecuador*. Arlington, Va.: John Snow, REACH.

Simonsen, Ole. 1989. "Vaccination against Tetanus and Diphtheria: Evaluation of Immunity in the Danish Population, Guidelines for Revaccinations, and Methods for Control of Vaccination Programs." *Danish Medical Bulletin* 36:24–47.

Simonsen, Ole, M. W. Bentzon, Keld Kjeldsen, H. A. Venborg, and Iver Heron. 1987. "Evaluation of Vaccination Requirements to Secure Continuous Antitoxin Immunity to Tetanus." *Vaccine* 2:115–22.

Simonsen, Ole, A. V. Bloch, and Iver Heron. 1987. "Epidemiology of Tetanus in Denmark 1920–1962." *Scandinavian Journal of Infectious Diseases* 9: 437–44.

Smucker, C. M., G. B. Simmons, Stan Bernstein, and B. D. Misra. 1980. "Neo-natal Mortality in South Asia: The Special Role of Tetanus." *Population Studies* 34:321–35.

Smucker, C. M., J. M. Swint, and G. B. Simmons. 1984. "Prevention of Neonatal Tetanus in India: A Prospective Cost-Effectiveness Analysis." *Journal of Tropical Pediatrics* 30:227–36.

Sokal, D. C., G. Imboua-Bogui, G. Soga, C. Emmou, and T. S. Jones. 1988. "Mortality from Neonatal Tetanus in Rural Côte d'Ivoire." *Bulletin of the World Health Organization* 66:69–76.

Solter, S. L., A. A. Hasibuan, and Burhanuddin Yusuf. 1986. "An Epidemiological Approach to Health Planning and Problem-Solving in Indonesia." *Health Policy and Planning* 1:99–108.

Sow, Abdourahmane. 1989. "Tetanus in Dakar, Senegal 1985–1986." Personal communication. Cited in Rey and Tikhomirov 1989.

Stanfield, J. P., and Artur Galazka. 1984. "Neonatal Tetanus in the World Today." *Bulletin of the World Health Organization* 62:647–69.

Steinglass, Robert. 1988. *Monitoring Tetanus Toxoid Coverage through Routine Reporting: Present and Proposed Methods.* Arlington, Va.: John Snow, REACH.

———. 1989. "The Control of Neonatal Tetanus." *Mothers and Children, Bulletin on Infant Feeding and Maternal Nutrition* 9:4–5.

———. 1990. *Monitoring Tetanus Toxoid Coverage and Activity Using Service Statistics.* In *Neonatal Tetanus Elimination: Issues and Future Directions.* Arlington, Va.: John Snow, REACH/MotherCare.

Steinglass, Robert, D. M. Mutie, Geoffrey Kimani, Mary Mjomba, Vincent Orinda, and Peter Bjerregaard. 1989. "Neonatal Tetanus Mortality in Kilifi District, Kenya: Results of a Community Survey, 1989." Forthcoming in *International Journal of Epidemiology.*

Stroh, George, U Aye Kyu, U Thaung, and U Kyaw Lwin. 1987. "Measurement of Mortality from Neonatal Tetanus in Burma." *Bulletin of the World Health Organization* 65:309–16.

Suleiman, Omar. 1982. "Mortality from Tetanus Neonatorum in Punjab (Pakistan)." *Pakistan Pediatric Journal* 6:152–83.

Suri, J. C. 1967. "The Problem of Tetanus in India." In Leo Eckmann, ed., *Principles on Tetanus: Proceedings of an International Conference on Tetanus.* Bern, Switzerland: Huber.

Sutter, R. W., S. L. Cochi, E. W. Brink, and B. I. Sirotkin. 1990. "Assessment of Vital Statistics and Surveillance Data for Monitoring Tetanus Mortality, United States, 1979–1984." *American Journal of Epidemiology* 131:132–42.

Tateno, Isao, Shigeto Suzuki, and Osama Kitamoto. 1961. "Epidemiology of Tetanus in Japan." *Japanese Journal of Experimental Medicine* 31:365–80.

UNICEF (United Nations Children's Fund)/Jakarta. 1985. "Tetanus Toxoid Campaign in West Nusa Tenggara, Indonesia." *Assignment Children* 69/72: 369–80.

Vakil, B. J., and N. J. Dalal. 1975. "Ways of Inoculation, Portals of Entry of Tetanus, and Risk Evaluation of a Wound." In *Fourth International Conference on Tetanus.* Lyons: Fondation Mérieux.

Veronesi, Ricardo, and R. Focaccia. 1981. "The Clinical Picture." In Ricardo Veronesi, ed., *Tetanus: Important New Concepts.* Amsterdam: Excerpta Medica.

Walsh, J. A., and K. S. Warren. 1979. "Selective Primary Health Care: An Interim Strategy for Disease Control in Developing Countries." *New England Journal of Medicine* 301:967–74.

White, W. G., G. M. Barnes, E. Barker, D. Gall, P. A. Knight, A. H. Griffith, R. M. Morris-Owen, and J. W. G. Smith. 1973. "Reactions to Tetanus Toxoid." *Journal of Hygiene* 71:283–97.

WHO (World Health Organization). 1977. *International Classification of Diseases. Manual of the International Statistical Classification of Diseases, Injuries, and Causes of Death.* Vols. 1 and 2. Ninth revision. Geneva.

———. 1982. *Prevention of Neonatal Tetanus.* Eastern Mediterranean Regional Office Technical Publication 7. Alexandria, Egypt.

———. 1986. *The Expanded Programme on Immunization in South-East Asia.* Regional Health Papers 12. New Delhi: South-East Asia Regional Office.

WHO/EPI (World Health Organization/Expanded Programme on Immunization). 1981a. "Disease Incidence and Immunization Coverage, Poland 1950–1980." *Weekly Epidemiological Record* 56:281–84.

———. 1981b. "An Economic Appraisal: Indonesia." *Weekly Epidemiological Record* 56:99–101.

———. 1982. "The Use of Survey Data to Supplement Disease Surveillance." *Weekly Epidemiological Record* 57:361–62.

———. 1983a. "Adverse Reactions to Immunization, German Democratic Republic." *Weekly Epidemiological Record* 58:62–64.

———. 1983b. "Disease Incidence and Immunization Coverage, Hungary." *Weekly Epidemiological Record* 58:77–80.

———. 1983c. "Neonatal Tetanus Mortality Surveys, Indonesia." *Weekly Epidemiological Record* 58:56–57.

———. 1986. *Prevention of Neonatal Tetanus through Immunization.* WHO/EPI/GEN/86.9. Geneva.

———. 1987a. *Issues in Neonatal Tetanus Control.* EPI/GAG/87/WP.11. Geneva.

———. 1987b. "Neonatal Tetanus Mortality Surveys, Egypt." *Weekly Epidemiological Record* 62:332–35.

———. 1987c. "Neonatal Tetanus Mortality Surveys, Iran." *Weekly Epidemiological Record* 62:38–40.

———. 1988a. "Impact of Tetanus Toxoid Immunization, Indonesia." *Weekly Epidemiological Record* 63:301–2.

———. 1988b. *Neonatal Tetanus: Immunize All Women of Childbearing Age.* Geneva.

———. 1989a. *Progress report: March 1989–October 1989. Research and Development Group Meeting.* EPI/RD/89 WP. 4. Oct. Geneva.

———. 1989b. *A Vision for the World: Global Elimination of Neonatal Tetanus by the Year 1995: Plan of Action.* EPI/GAG/89/WP.9. Geneva.

———. 1990. "Stability of Vaccines." *Weekly Epidemiological Record* 65:233–35.

10

Rheumatic Heart Disease

Catherine Michaud, Jorge Trejo-Gutierrez, Carlos Cruz, and Thomas A. Pearson

Rheumatic heart disease (RHD) is the most common form of heart disease among children and young adults in many developing countries. It affects more than 4 million people worldwide and causes approximately 90,000 deaths each year. This heavy toll could be reduced, because RHD is always triggered by a controllable infectious agent: group A streptococci.

The chain of events leading to RHD is complex and evolves over several years. It starts with acute group A streptococcal pharyngitis (GASP), or strep throat, which is extremely common among school-age children. If they are not treated effectively, 3 percent of GASP episodes lead to rheumatic fever (RF), a disease that damages the heart, particularly the heart valves. Heart valve injuries occur because group A streptococci precipitate an immunological assault against the body's own heart valves and some other tissues.

Rheumatic fever lasts for only several weeks but often leaves permanent scars which cause rheumatic heart disease. Damaged valves no longer open or close properly, thus disrupting normal blood flow. These hemodynamic changes overload the heart and lead to progressive cardiac insufficiency and often to premature death. Finally, the severity of valve injuries tends to increase over time, because RF recurs in 75 percent of children who had a first attack of RF when they suffer new episodes of streptococcal pharyngitis (figure 10-1). In the absence of any intervention, among 1,000 children with pharyngitis, 200 would have pharyngitis caused by group A streptococci, 6 would suffer an initial RF attack, 5 would later have recurrences of RF, and 2 would die from intractable cardiac failure.

Interventions to prevent RHD can be directed at different points in the chain of events leading from GASP to intractable cardiac failure. Primary prevention targets cases of pharyngitis and consists of a single injection of benzathine penicillin, which effectively treats GASP and prevents the occurrence of RF. Secondary prevention targets RF cases and consists in monthly injections of benzathine penicillin for several years to prevent recurrences of GASP that might trigger new bouts of RF. Tertiary prophylaxis targets severe cases of RHD. It interrupts the progression to intractable cardiac failure by means of surgical repair or replacement of damaged heart valves. A vaccine that could prevent the occurrence of GASP is not yet available.

The cost-effectiveness of various strategies is determined by the number of total cases that have to be treated to prevent one death and is limited by difficulties in finding the cases. Primary prevention in developing countries is impractical when the diagnosis of GASP cannot be confirmed. Secondary prevention therefore remains the cornerstone of RHD prevention. Tertiary prophylaxis is a cost-effective alternative in spite of the high cost of surgery because it can be very specifically directed to a small number of cases.

In industrial countries the incidence of RF and prevalence of RHD decreased during the past decades as socioeconomic conditions improved and penicillin treatment became available. Fewer than 1,000 cases of RHD, and almost no deaths, now occur each year in industrial countries. The challenge is to achieve a similar reduction in developing countries, despite

Figure 10-1. Chain of Events Leading to Rheumatic Heart Disease Showing Percentage That Will Develop the Next Stage

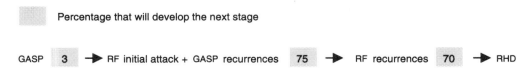

Percentage that will develop the next stage

GASP   3 ➜ RF initial attack + GASP recurrences   75 ➜ RF recurrences   70 ➜ RHD

Source: Authors, from epidemiologic data.

scarce resources, slow socioeconomic growth, and limited access to health care.

In this chapter we review the epidemiology, pathogenesis, and clinical manifestations of RF and RHD; discuss possible interventions and analyze their cost-effectiveness; and, finally, outline areas which require further research.

Background

The distribution of RF and RHD is quite different in industrial and developing countries, and has evolved over time. The distribution of the disease also varies within each country between rural and urban areas and among different population groups. The major determinants of the disease are socioeconomic conditions, access to medical care, and the changing virulence of group A streptococci.

In Industrial Countries

Rheumatic fever and rheumatic heart disease have virtually disappeared in industrial countries. The average annual RF incidence is now below 0.5 per 100,000, and RHD prevalence is less than 0.05 per 1000.

The progressive decline in RF and RHD started simultaneously in several Western countries at the beginning of the twentieth century, several decades before penicillin treatment became available. With the introduction of penicillin, at the end of World War II, the decline accelerated rapidly among higher socioeconomic groups but lagged behind among the poor. Inadequate housing and overcrowding favor the spread of streptococcal infection from person to person, undernutrition impairs the immune response, and streptococci remain longer in the throat in the absence of penicillin treatment. The number of rheumatic fever and rheumatic heart disease cases have nevertheless slowly decreased even in communities in which the use of penicillin was not widespread, perhaps as a consequence of lower virulence of group A streptococci. These observations indicate that penicillin treatment was only one among several factors that prompted the decline of RF and RHD (Gordis 1985; Gordis, Lilienfeld, and Rodriguez 1969a and 1969b; Massell and others 1988).

The frequency of occurrence of pharyngitis has also decreased in industrial countries, but not the proportion of pharyngitis caused by group A streptococci. Streptococci cause 15 to 30 percent of all pharyngitis, and this proportion does not vary significantly within and between nations worldwide (Markowitz 1985). The potential to develop RF and RHD therefore persists in industrial countries, as was evidenced by outbreaks of RF that have occurred in several small communities since 1986 in the United States and northern Italy. In each instance, RF followed a similar new epidemiologic pattern: RF cases were concentrated among middle-class families with ready access to medical care. The resurgence of RF, following this new pattern, has raised great concern and requires close monitoring (Hosier and others 1987; Kaplan and Markowitz 1988; Veasy and others 1987; Wald and others 1987).

In the Developing World

In sharp contrast to the situation prevailing in industrial countries, RF and RHD are quite common in developing countries, where the incidence of RF ranges from 6.9 to 100 cases per 100,000 people (table 10-1), and the prevalence of RHD ranges from 1.0 to 18.6 cases per 1,000 (table 10-2). These rates are similar to rates that were common in Western countries at the beginning of this century (WHO 1988). Their broad range illustrates disparities existing among different geographic regions, among various ethnic and socioeconomic groups, and between urban and rural populations. For instance, several minority groups in the Pacific Islands still suffer from a very high prevalence of RHD, ranging between 7.6 and 18.6 cases per 1,000 persons, even though the prevalence of RHD is quite low in the general population. In New Zealand, most cases of RHD were reported from the northern part of North Island, where Maori and Polynesian populations are concentrated (Neutze 1988a). In Australia, RF and RHD persist only among aboriginal communities living in the Northern Territory (MacDonald and Walker 1989). The differences observed between various ethnic groups are probably attributable to their lower socioeconomic conditions, rather than to a particular genetic susceptibility to the disease.

The prevalence of RHD is determined worldwide by the level of socioeconomic development and by access to health care, but in addition, it differs strikingly between urban and rural settings. The prevalence of RHD tends to be higher among the urban poor than among rural poor. It ranges from 8.5 to 11 cases per 1,000 individuals in the largest cities of Africa, Asia, and Latin America, whereas in rural areas, RHD prevalence does not exceed 3.5 per 1,000 on average (Strasser 1985).

Table 10-1. Annual Incidence of Rheumatic Fever in Selected Areas

Location	Year	Incidence (per 100,000)	Age group (years)
England and Wales	1963	4.7	1–14
Baltimore (United States)	1964	15.3	5–19
Denmark	1970	10.7	All
Singapore	1971	92	All
Cyprus	1972	27–43	All
Hong Kong	1972	23	All
Czechoslovakia	1972	8.5	<15
Iran, Islamic Rep. of	1973	59–100	All
Kuwait	1983	19.6	<14
Auckland (New Zealand)[a]	1984	70.7	<15
Hawaii (United States)[b]	1976–80	14.4	4–18
Salt Lake County (United States)	1985	18.1	5–17

a. Maori population.
b. Incidence (per 100,000) by ethnic group was Samoan, 96.5; Hawaiian, 27.2; Filipino, 9.0; and Chinese, 6.9.
Source: Adapted from Majeed and others 1987.

Table 10-2. Prevalence of Rheumatic Heart Disease in School-age Children in Different Areas

Location	Year	Prevalence (per 1,000)
Africa		
Algeria	1970	15.0
Nigeria	1970	0.–3.0
Egypt	1973	10.0
Morocco	1973	9.9
Soweto, South Africa	1975	6.9
Côte d'Ivoire	1985	1.9
Latin America		
Brazil	1968–70s	1.6–6.8
Montevideo, Uruguay	1970	1.0
	1985	10.0
La Paz, Bolivia	1973	17.0
Mexico City, Mexico	1977	8.5
San Juan, Puerto Rico	1980	1.6
Caracas, Venezuela	1985	10.0
Porto Allegre, Brazil	1985	10.0
São Paulo, Brazil	1985	10.0
Asia		
Tokyo, Japan	1966	0.3
Taiwan, Republic of China	1970	1.4
India	1970s	6.0–11
Pakistan	1970s	1.8–11
Thailand	1974	1.2–2.1
China	1979	0.4–2.7
Mongolia	n.d.	3.5
New Delhi, India	1985	11.0
Pacific		
Torres Strait Islands, Australia	1978	4.7–12.5
Rarotonga, Cook Islands	1982	18.6
French Polynesia	1988	11.2
Waikito, New Zealand[a]	n.d.	7.6 (Maori)
		1.0 (non-Maori)

n.d. No date available.

a. Subjects in this study were age five to twenty-nine years.

Source: Adapted from WHO, 1988.

Trends observed during the past several decades in developing countries vary. The prevalence of RHD is increasing in the largest cities undergoing rapid growth, particularly in slum areas. In India the prevalence of RHD has increased with rapid urbanization, and now reaches 6 cases per 1,000 people on average for the whole country (WHO 1980a). The prevalence of RHD seems to be much lower in China than it is in India. Richard Bumgarner estimated in 1990 that there were 410,000 cases of RHD in China, which corresponds to an average RHD prevalence of 1.4 per 1,000 for the whole country (Bumgarner, personal communication). In middle-income economies—for example, Thailand—the prevalence of RHD is decreasing.

Pathogenesis

Group A streptococci are very common human pathogens. Between 20 and 30 million cases of group A streptococcal infections occur each year in the United States alone. These cases include infections of the skin and throat (GASP), forms of pneumonia, and a recently identified disease resembling toxic shock. Scarlet fever is the result of infection by streptococci that elaborate an erythrogenic toxin against which the host has no antibodies.

The exact nature of the interaction between group A streptococci and the human host leading to RF is not fully understood. Several hypotheses were developed to explain how streptococci might damage the heart:

- Direct tissue invasion by group A streptococci
- Toxic effects of streptococcal products, particularly streptolysins S or O, which are known to be capable of inducing tissue injury
- Reactions like serum sickness, mediated by antigen-antibody complexes
- Autoimmune phenomena induced by similarity or identity between certain streptococcal antigens and human tissue components

Even though direct tissue invasion and toxic effects of streptolysins may play a role, most attention has recently been directed to the immunological process involved. Almost every part in the immune system, cellular and humoral, is involved in RF. Group A streptococci selectively amplify or downregulate various immune pathways which are likely to be critical in the subsequent development of RF after an episode of streptococcal pharyngitis (Cairns 1988; Goldstein 1967).

Recent research has unraveled the key role played by M proteins in the immunological process (Fischetti 1991). M proteins cover the surface of the bacterial cell wall and appear as hairlike projections. They give a streptococcus the ability to resist ingestion by white blood cells. To overcome the effect of M proteins, the human host produces antibodies directed against M proteins. These antibodies neutralize the protective capacity of the M protein and allow the streptococcus to be engulfed and destroyed by white blood cells. Group A streptococci have further increased their ability to evade the immune system through antigenic variation. There are more than eighty different serotypes, or varieties of M proteins, and laboratory tests suggest that antibodies against one serotype do not offer protection against others. The low incidence of GASP observed in adulthood may be due either to an undefined, age-related factor or to a broad immunity that individuals acquire through contact with streptococci as children.

Different serotypes of group A streptococci cause the two major nonsuppurative sequelae of GASP: RF and glomerulonephritis. Serotypes of group A streptococci isolated from children with RF and their families differ from those isolated from children with poststreptococcal nephritis and their families (Majeed and others 1987). This chapter deals only with RF.

Rheumatic fever occurs when antibodies developed against M proteins cross-react with the host's own heart tissues because some fragments (epitopes) of the M protein closely resemble fragments of valve glycoproteins and valve fibroblasts, leading

Table 10-3. Frequency of Major Manifestations in Initial Attacks of Rheumatic Fever in Prospective Studies
(percent)

Manifestation	Kuwait	India	United Kingdom	United States
Carditis	46	34	55	42
Polyarthritis	79	67	85	76
Chorea	8	20	13	8
Nodules	0.5	3	**	1
Erythema marginatum	0.5	2	**	4

** Negligible amount.
Source: Adapted from Markowitz 1988.

to permanent valvular damage. The exact role of such cross-reactive antibodies in the genesis of RHD, however, is not yet understood (Fischetti 1991).

Other researchers have identified genetic markers—B lymphocyte alloantigens—which might determine greater susceptibility to RF (Patarroyo and others 1979). For instance, RF happened more often in monozygotic than dizygotic twins, but the numbers studied were very small (Taranta and others 1959). These findings still require confirmation in various ethnic groups.

There is no single determinant for RF. Several risk factors pertaining to the environment, the host, and the agent interact and ultimately cause RF. Only a few of the mechanisms involved are fully understood. For instance, the observation that the sera of patients contained antibodies against heart tissues dates back half a century, but the exact amino-acid sequence of heart cross-reactive epitopes was identified in M proteins only recently.

Clinical Aspects

Rheumatic fever occurs in 3 percent of all GASP episodes (Denny 1987). No direct relationship exists between the severity of GASP symptoms—fever, sore throat—and the development of RF ten to thirty-five days later. Furthermore, GASP causes no symptoms in 30 to 50 percent of all children who later develop RF (Maharaj and others 1987).

The clinical findings vary greatly and are determined by the site of involvement, the severity of the attack, and the stage at which the patient is first examined. The most common symptoms of RF are redness and pain of the joints (arthritis) and a typical heart murmur (carditis). The clinical diagnosis of RF may be difficult because the severity and the combination of RF symptoms vary among different individuals. The onset is usually acute when arthritis is the presenting manifestation and more gradual when carditis is the initial clinical feature. When carditis is the sole clinical manifestation, it can be difficult to determine when the attack began.

Arthritis and carditis are sometimes accompanied by chorea, subcutaneous nodules, or erythema marginatum. Chorea occurs in 10 to 15 percent of patients and is self-limited. The

rapid random, nonrhythmic movements of chorea most often affect the muscles of the face and arms. Subcutaneous nodules are round, hard, painless swellings, which occur in 5 to 10 percent of rheumatic patients. Erythema marginatum is the characteristic skin rash of RF and occurs in fewer than 5 percent of patients. Symptoms observed during the initial attack of RF tend to be different from those observed during subsequent episodes of RF (Nelson 1983).

Initial Rheumatic Fever Attack

During the initial attack of RF it is common to observe migrating arthritis with painful, red, hot swellings of one or several large joints—knees, elbows, wrists, and ankles. Arthritis may last up to three months; it causes significant morbidity but ultimately leaves no sequelae (WHO 1988). Arthritis tends to be less frequent in subsequent episodes of RF. The frequency of carditis, on the contrary, tends to increase with recurrent episodes of RF.

Carditis often causes few symptoms, and it is rarely life threatening. The onset of carditis may be asymptomatic—so-called silent carditis—or insidious, with only a few vague symptoms such as lethargy, poor appetite, and chronic respiratory infections. In this instance, patients seek health care only much later, when they suffer from shortness of breath (Markowitz 1988).

Recurrent RF Episodes

After the initial attack, RF is characterized by frequent recurrences of the disease after a varying number of intercurrent years of freedom from symptoms. The risk for RF recurrence, following subsequent GASP, increases dramatically from 3 percent to 75 percent (Denny 1987). Recurrent bouts of carditis often cause long-term sequelae because when the inflammatory process heals in the heart, it leaves scars on the valves, which impair their normal opening or closure.

Table 10-4. Outcomes of 10,000 Hypothetical Cases of Rheumatic Fever without Treatment

Outcome	Initial attack without recurrence		Initial attack with recurrence		Total	
	Number	Percent	Number	Percent	Number	Percent
Total cases	2,500	25	7,500	75	10,000	100
Recover	1,475	59	1,500	20	2,975	30
Carditis	1,025	41	6,000	80	7,025	70
Mild	369	15	840	11	1,209	12
Moderate/ severe cardiomegaly	431	17	1,920	26	2,351	24
Congestive heart failure leading to death	22	9	3,240	43	3,465	35

Source: Authors, from epidemiologic data.

Table 10-5. Age Distribution at First Attack of Rheumatic Fever and Death in 10,000 Hypothetical Cases without Treatment

Ages (years)	Number	Percent
At first attack		
< 5	800	8
6–8	2,000	20
9–11	3,600	36
12–15	2,600	26
> 15	1,000	10
Total	10,000	100
At death		
< 5	87	2.5
5–14	485	14
15–44	1,975	57
45–64	814	23.5
>65	104	3
Total	3,465	100

Source: Authors, from epidemiologic data.

In developing countries, the initial episode of RF is often unnoticed, and arthritis tends to be reported less often than in Western countries. Because of these differences, RF seemed to follow a different clinical course in developing countries. Careful longitudinal studies have not substantiated such differences. Carditis occurs in 34 to 55 percent of children during the initial RF attack and in 65 to 85 percent of subsequent RF episodes in different parts of the world (Majeed and others 1981; Padmavati and Gupta 1988; Potter and others 1978; Sanyal and others 1974; see table 10-3). Carditis, nevertheless, runs a more severe course in developing countries because the initial attack of RF occurs at a much younger age, and RF recurs more often.

Rheumatic Heart Disease

Approximately 90 percent of children who have carditis during RF episodes will develop RHD. This disease is a chronic and progressive condition resulting from permanent scarring of heart valves, following RF. It often causes little morbidity in its early stages. Children attend school, run, and play (McLaren and others 1978). A few, however, suffer from exhaustion when they exercise. As RHD becomes more severe with recurrent bouts of RF, children and young adults can no longer attend school or work, and they withdraw from play and other social activities. Finally, severe congestive cardiac failure occurs, and medical treatment often fails. Heart surgery then remains the only possible intervention.

Disease Outcome

The age at which the first RF attack occurs and the frequency and severity of RF recurrences determine the outcome of RHD. Young children six to thirteen years old are at highest risk for recurrences, and they suffer a more fulminant course of the disease. Table 10-4 illustrates the outcome of 10,000 RF hypothetical episodes based on different epidemiologic studies. These studies have shown that initial episodes of RF occurred before age fifteen in 90 percent of cases (table 10-5). Thirty percent of all children having one or more RF episodes recover completely even in the absence of treatment; 12 percent develop mild carditis; 23 percent develop cardiomegaly but no congestive heart failure. Among the remaining 35 percent, the damage to the heart valve is so severe that it causes progressive heart failure and early death.

Diagnosis

The diagnosis of RF requires a combination of clinical and laboratory criteria because no single symptom or laboratory test is pathognomonic of the disease. Rheumatic carditis, or permanent valvular lesions of RHD are suspected when a heart murmur is audible at auscultation. The initial detection of heart murmurs can be successfully done by health workers (Irwig and others 1985). To confirm the diagnosis and to determine the extent of underlying heart damage, however, chest x-ray, electrocardiogram, and, if possible, echocardiography or cardiac catheterization are required.

Jones Criteria

Dr. T. Duckett Jones systematized clinical diagnosis of RF in 1944 and classified the observed symptoms into major and minor manifestations. Jones criteria have been only slightly modified by subsequent revisions and remain the mainstay for the diagnosis of rheumatic fever today (tables 10-6 and 10-7; figure 10-2). Standardized diagnostic criteria are important to ensure comparability of epidemiological data, for the evaluation of prevention and care programs, and to guide therapeutic decisions. Underdiagnosis will prevent affected children from

Table 10-6. Changes in the Original Jones Criteria for the Diagnosis of Acute Rheumatic Fever

Manifestation	Year			
	1944	1951	1956	1965/1984
Carditis	M	M	M	M
Polyarthritis	—	M	M	M
Chorea	M	M	M	M
Subcutaneous nodules	M	M	M	M
Erythema marginatum	m	—	m	m
Arthralgia	M	—	m	m
Fever	m	m	m	m
Erythrocyte sedimentation rate	m	m	m	m
History of acute rheumatic fever or rheumatic heart disease	M	m	m	m
Evidence of prior streptococcal infection	—	m	m	R

— Not available.

Note: M = Major manifestation; m = minor manifestation; R = required manifestation.

Source: WHO 1988.

Table 10-7. Cases of Rheumatic Heart Disease in the Developing World, 1985

Location	Population age 6–16 years (thousands)	Total cases[a] (thousands)	Deaths[b] per year (thousands)
Asia			
Urban	189,000	1,510	—
Rural	485,000	971	—
Total	674,000	2,481	56
Latin America			
Urban	73,000	584	—
Rural	33,000	66	—
Total	106,000	650	15
Middle East/ North Africa			
Urban	32,000	253	—
Rural	81,000	162	—
Total	113,000	415	9
Sub-Saharan Africa			
Urban	40,000	319	—
Rural	100,000	200	—
Total	140,000	519	12
Total		4,065	92

— Not available.

a. These are conservative estimates, based on the following assumptions: (a) mean urban prevalence 8/1,000; (b) mean rural prevalence 2/1,000. Those severely affected will die within twenty years of the initial attack of RF.

b. Assumes 45 percent of cases each year result in death within 20 years. Calculation for number of deaths per year is as follows: Total number of cases in the region/20∞0∞45.

Source: Authors, from epidemologic data.

receiving proper treatment, whereas overdiagnosis may create unnecessary emotional and psychological suffering among patients and parents (Jones 1944).

GASP: *Laboratory Diagnosis*

Laboratory tests can provide direct identification of group A streptococci or retrospective evidence of infection with group A streptococci. Direct identification of group A streptococci from the throats of children suffering from pharyngitis is required to diagnose GASP. This can be done through cultures, or by means of rapid antigen detection tests. Cultures on blood agar plates are exceptionally effective as a diagnostic tool. However, they require laboratory facilities, and bacteriologic identification takes eighteen to twenty-four hours. Rapid antigen detection tests provide an immediate diagnosis. They have a good specificity of 98 percent, but their sensitivity varies with the amount of antigen present between 44 percent and 100 percent. Negative results, therefore, must be confirmed by a culture (Kaplan and Markowitz 1988). The sensitivity of rapid antigen detection tests needs to be increased to ensure reliable diagnosis and improved clinical management.

Retrospective evidence is important to confirm the diagnosis of RF. Titers of antistreptolysin O (ASO), which is an anti-

body developed against extracellular products of group A streptococci, peak within three weeks following GASP and provide retrospective evidence of infection with group A streptococci. A single ASO titer does not provide a reliable measure of the time elapsed since infection because the rate of decrease of ASO titers is highly variable (Denny 1987).

The Public Health Significance

Children bear the major burden of disease resulting from RF and RHD. This burden is likely to increase with continuing population growth in developing countries. RF and RHD have high economic costs which could be reduced through effective prophylaxis of RF and RHD.

Current levels in the Developing Countries

The first African case of RHD was reported by Procter and Hargreaves in eastern Africa in 1932, but the importance of RF and RHD in developing countries was not recognized until the 1950s (Anabwani, Amoa, and Muita 1989). Rheumatic heart disease is the most common form of heart disease among children and one of the most common cardiovascular diseases

Figure 10-2. Jones Criteria (Revised) for Guidance in the Diagnosis of Rheumatic Fever

Major Manifestations

Carditis

Polyarthritis

Chorea

Erythema Marginatum

Subcutaneous Nodules

Minor Manifestations

Clinical

- Previous rheumatic fever or rheumatic heart disease

- Arthralgia

- Fever

Laboratory

- Acute phase reactants Erythrocyte sedimentation rate, C-reactive protein, leukocytosis

- Prolonged P-R interval

Supporting evidence of streptococcal infection

- Increased Titer of Anti-Streptococcal Antibodies ASO (anti-streptolysin O), others

- Positive Throat Culture for Group A Streptococcus

- Recent Scarlet Fever

Note: Two major or one major and two minor manifestations plus evidence of preceding streptococcal infection indicates a high probability of acute rheumatic fever.

This figure shows the recommendation of the American Heart Association (Circulation 1984). It has been approved by the WHO Study Group (1988) with the provision that the following be dealt with separately and be exempted from fulfilling the Jones criteria: "pure"chorea, late on-set carditis, and rheumatic recurrence.

Source: WHO 1988.

Table 10-8. Hospital Admissions for Rheumatic Heart Disease
(percent)

Country	Admissions as percentage of all cardiac admissions
Asia	
Bangladesh	34.0
Burma	30.0
Mongolia	30.0
Pakistan	23.0
Thailand	34.0
Africa	
Ethiopia	34.8
Ghana	20.6
Malawi	23.0
Nigeria (Ibadan)	18.1
Nigeria (Kano)	23.0
South Africa	25.0
Tanzania	9.7
Uganda	24.7
Zambia	18.2

Source: WHO 1980a; Hutt 1991.

among young adults in tropical and subtropical countries (Sharper 1972). In 1985 an estimated 4.2 million people—mostly children and young adults—were suffering from RHD; 500,000 of these people had at least one episode of RF, and approximately 90,000 of those affected died (table 10-8).

The outstanding features of RF and RHD in tropical and subtropical regions are the young age at which the initial attack of RF occurs, the high recurrence rate, and the more fulminant course of RHD. In Thailand, peak RF incidence occurred between ages nine and eleven, and peak RHD prevalence between twelve and sixteen (Vongprateep, Dharmasakti, and Sindhavanonda 1988). A similar age distribution was observed in other developing countries.

Rheumatic fever and rheumatic heart disease cause severe disability and are a frequent cause for hospitalization. About 10 to 35 percent of all clinical cardiac patients in hospitals in Sub-Saharan Africa and Asia were suffering from RHD (Hutt 1991; see table 10-9). In Barangwanath Hospital, Soweto, in the Republic of South Africa, RF and RHD accounted for 11 per 1,000 of all pediatric patients under age ten (Edington and Gear 1982). The average length of hospital stay of three to four weeks, for both RF and RHD, meant prolonged absence from school or work.

In the 1960s, cardiac valvular surgery became available. The high number of children and young adults referred for surgery confirmed the young age of occurrence and the severity of RHD in developing countries. In Nairobi, Kenya, 33 percent of all valvotomies were done in children under age sixteen; in Johannesburg, South Africa, 44 percent of patients that underwent valvuloplasty were fifteen or younger, and 26 percent were under twelve (Anabwani, Amoa, and Muita 1989; Antunes and others 1987). Heart surgery was not available, however, in many developing countries,

and children were sometimes referred abroad at high cost. For instance, by mid-1985, 238 RHD cases from French Polynesia had been evacuated to France to undergo heart surgery (Vigneron 1989).

Women of childbearing age are at the highest risk of suffering complications from RHD during pregnancy. The important hemodynamic changes occurring during pregnancy may precipitate cardiac failure in women with RHD. Rheumatic heart disease is an important obstetric complication in Africa, making up 75 to 90 percent of all symptomatic heart disease cases during pregnancy. In Cape Town, South Africa, closed mitral valvotomies were performed in 41 women age eighteen to forty-one between 1965 and 1985 (Vasloo and Reichart 1987).

Approximately 90,000 deaths due to RHD occur each year among all those affected. Peak mortality reported from autopsy studies in Mulago Hospital, Kampala, Uganda, occurred between ages twenty-four and thirty-four (Shaper 1972; see figure 10-3). Adults living beyond age thirty-five tend to suffer from less severe cardiac damage and, therefore, have lower mortality rates. The death rate from RHD is highest among young adults. In Sub-Saharan Africa, up to 20 percent of all deaths confirmed at autopsy were due to RHD (Hutt 1991). Rheumatic heart disease causes approximately 1 out of 150 deaths occurring between the ages of sixteen and forty-nine in developing countries.

Table 10-9. Cost-Effectiveness of Different Prophylactic Strategies

Treatment	Unit cost (dollars)	Cases treated to prevent one death[a]	Cost per death averted (dollars)	DALYs gained[b]	Cost per DALY (dollars)
Prevention of pharyngitis[c]	60	682	40,920	39	1,049
Prevention of RF[d]	1,380	4	5,520	39	142
Prophylaxis of RHD[e]	8,500	1.5	12,750	30	425

a. Assuming 100 percent efficacy of each treatment, approximately 500 pharyngitis cases, 100 GASP, three RF, or one severe RHD case would have to be treated to prevent one death.
b. Twenty DALYs per death averted. DALYs per disability reduction: three for mild carditis (10 percent for thirty years); six for moderate carditis (20 percent for thirty years); ten for severe carditis (50 percent for twenty years). The first two prevention strategies provide a gain of thirty-nine DALYs because these interventions reduce the disability from mild and moderate carditis in addition to reducing disability and death from severe carditis; the last strategy does not reduce disability from mild or moderate carditis.
c. Primary prevention entails one benzathine-penicillin injection each year for ten years. Efficacy of intervention is 70 percent.
d. Secondary prevention entails one benzathine-penicillin injection per month for five years and assumes one hospitalization of twenty-four days. Efficacy of intervention is 80 percent.
e. Tertiary prophylaxis entails valvuloplasty or valve replacement and includes hospitalization. Efficacy of intervention is 70 percent. Unit costs range from $5,000 to $12,000; costs per death averted from $7,500 to $18,000; and costs per DALY from $250 to $600.
Source: Authors, from epidemiologic data.

Figure 10-3. Ages of Subjects with Rheumatic Heart Disease at Autopsy in Mulago Hospital, Kampala, Uganda, 1960–65

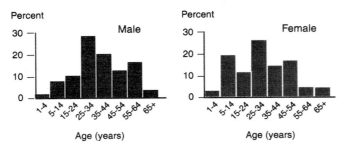

Source: Sharper 1972.

Possible Patterns of Morbidity and Mortality by 2015

Total morbidity and mortality attributable to RF and RHD is likely to increase during the next twenty-five years because the total population at highest risk for RF, those between the ages of five and fifteen, will increase and reach 1.2 billion by the year 2015. Half of them will live in urban areas (United Nations 1988). Assuming no changes in the incidence or in the prevention of RHD by the year 2015, approximately 6 million school-age children will suffer from RHD. The level of socioeconomic development, access to health care, and progress toward better preventive strategies (that is, a vaccine) will ultimately determine the disease burden resulting from RF and RHD.

Economic Costs

Rheumatic fever and rheumatic heart disease incur direct as well as indirect costs. Estimates of direct costs of RHD are not available in most developing countries. Neutze estimated the financial cost incurred to the state in New Zealand in 1985 and showed that the country spent $2 million to treat 5,625 RF and RHD patients.[1] This represents an average cost of $355 per case per year. Hospital care, including heart surgery, represented 87 percent and ambulatory treatment 13 percent of the total expenditure. The average hospital stay was twenty-four days for RF, twenty-one days for RHD, and twenty-seven days for surgery (Neutze 1988b).

The indirect costs of RHD are quite high because it is primarily adolescents and young adults who are disabled or die during their most productive years. Mild carditis results in 10 percent disability and moderate carditis 25 percent disability for thirty years. Deaths from RHD are due to progressive heart failure and occur most often between the ages of twenty-five and thirty-four, on average twenty years after the initial RF attack. In addition, RHD causes approximately 50 percent disability during the twenty years preceding death. Thus, one can estimate the disability resulting from mild carditis to be three disability-adjusted life-years (DALYs) and the disability from moderate carditis to be six DALYs. Severe carditis causes the loss of twenty DALYs as a result of premature death and the loss of an addi-

tional ten DALYs, assuming that RHD causes 50 percent disability during the twenty years preceding death. The total indirect cost per RHD death, therefore, was estimated to be thirty DALYs.

Elements of Preventive Strategy

Interventions to prevent RHD can be targeted at different points in the chain of events leading from GASP to intractable cardiac failure. Two different intervention strategies—mass penicillin prophylaxis or a vaccine—could prevent GASP. Mass chemoprophylaxis is not practical, however, unless the population at risk can be precisely targeted (for example, military recruits), and a vaccine is not yet available. Primary and secondary prevention therefore aim at reducing the occurrence of RF. Primary prevention averts the first attack of RF with a single injection of benzathine penicillin, and secondary prevention hinders recurrences of RF by providing monthly injections of benzathine penicillin. Finally, rehabilitation through cardiac surgery corrects damage to the valves and interrupts the progression to cardiac failure (figure 10-4).

Mass Chemoprophylaxis

Routine administration of benzathine penicillin injections was introduced among all U.S. military recruits after World War II because more than 20,000 cases of RF had occurred in navy and marine recruits between 1942 and 1945. The strategy was carried out effectively, and it prevented further epidemics of RF. Routine administration was discontinued in the early 1980s but was resumed after two outbreaks of RF occurred in 1986–87 at the naval training center in San Diego, California, and at the Fort Leonard Wood Army Training Base in Missouri. Both military epidemics were effectively terminated by the reintroduction of mass benzathine penicillin prophylaxis to all military recruits who were not allergic to penicillin (Bisno 1991).

Figure 10-4. Prevention of Rheumatic Fever and Rheumatic Heart Disease

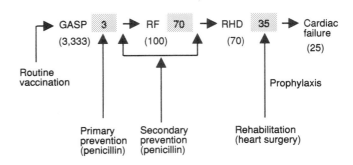

Source: Authors, from epidemiological data.

Vaccine Development

A vaccine could prevent GASP, but vaccine development has been slow because initial vaccine candidates induced the production of antibodies that cross-reacted with the heart valves. A vaccine is unlikely to become available for several more years.

Recombinant DNA technology now provides the means to develop synthetic vaccines. An important first step toward the development of a synthetic vaccine was to discover the structure of M proteins and to learn the sequence of amino acids of different M proteins. M proteins encompass hypervariable and conserved regions. Hypervariable regions differ among different serotypes, but conserved regions are common to all serotypes. Protection against group A streptococci could be induced by antibodies directed to some conserved regions common to all M proteins (Fischetti 1991).

Primary Prevention

Primary prevention consists of a single injection of benzathine penicillin (or oral penicillin) each day for ten days to treat GASP effectively and prevent the occurrence of RF. Difficulties in finding cases and in establishing the diagnosis of GASP limit the effectiveness of this strategy. Primary prevention has been successful in industrial countries where GASP can be readily diagnosed. In many developing countries, however, GASP cannot be diagnosed because laboratory facilities required to identify group A streptococci are not available, and rapid antigen detection tests do not yet have the sensitivity required for a reliable diagnosis. Even where GASP can be diagnosed, the finding of cases is limited by biological factors, because GASP causes no symptoms in 30 to 50 percent of those who later develop RF. Children at greatest risk live in poor, overcrowded conditions and often have only limited access to health services.

In the absence of proper GASP diagnosis, the targeting required for effective primary prevention is impractical. Several hundred episodes of pharyngitis would have to be treated to prevent a single death from intractable cardiac failure (table 10-4). Twenty percent of all pharyngitis episodes are due to group A streptococci. Thus 333 out of 1,000 episodes of pharyngitis would be GASP and would lead to 10 cases of RF (3 percent), 7 cases of RHD (70 percent), and 2 or 3 deaths from intractable cardiac failure (35 percent). Because children remain at high risk between the ages of five and fifteen and commonly have pharyngitis at least twice a year, penicillin treatment would be required approximately twice a year for ten years to prevent RF effectively. Therefore, even though a single injection of benzathine penicillin costs only $3, averting one death would cost $40,920, or $1,049 per DALY (table 10-9).

Secondary Prevention

Long-term penicillin prophylaxis is the cornerstone of RF prevention in developing countries in which GASP cannot be diagnosed. It targets children who have had an initial attack of RF and consists of monthly injections of benzathine penicillin to prevent recurrences of GASP that might trigger new bouts of RF. Secondary prophylaxis should be given to those under the age of twenty-four for at least five years.

The advantage of secondary prophylaxis is that it targets a much smaller population, because only 3 percent of GASP episodes are followed by an initial attack of RF. Rheumatic fever cases are usually diagnosed when the patients seek treatment. In some instances, rheumatic carditis has been actively searched for among schoolchildren. Health care workers can be trained to note heart murmurs and to refer these children for further investigation.

The greatest challenge of secondary prevention is to ensure long-term compliance with monthly injections of benzathine penicillin for several years (Gordis, Lilienfeld, and Rodriguez 1969b; WHO Study Group 1988). In Hamilton, Australia, for instance, hospital contact was maintained by less than half of a group of RF patients during a ten-year period. Secondary prevention programs therefore require the establishment of a registry of RF/RHD patients and good coordination at various levels of the health system to ensure the proper follow-up of all RF patients.

Substantial experience now exists in many developing countries. The World Health Organization implemented secondary RF prevention programs in Barbados, Cyprus, Egypt, India, Iran, Mongolia, and Nigeria, as well as in several Latin American countries. In 1970 the cost of the program was estimated to be $325 per month, which was considerably less than the cost of maintaining pediatric beds at $1,260 per month (Hassell and Stuart 1974). The success of the programs nevertheless differed among countries. Compliance was considered adequate if fewer than 30 percent of benzathine penicillin injections were missed. In Barbados the introduction of RF identification cards and vigorous follow-up ensured compliance by 89 percent of all patients. In other countries, prophylaxis was effective in only 80 percent of the cases. The WHO study also demonstrated that patients who had only occasional or no penicillin prophylaxis at all spent on average six times as much hospitalization time as those on full prophylaxis (Strasser 1985). The importance of community participation was further demonstrated in Soweto, South Africa, where regular attendance to clinic-based prophylaxis increased from 17 percent to 38 percent seven months after a community outreach program was established (Edington and Gear 1982). In Thailand the National Control Program for RF/RHD was developed by an initial working group and was effectively implemented once it had been approved by the government. Ongoing evaluation provides the information required to make the necessary changes (Vongprateep, Dharmasakti, and Sindhavanonda 1988).

Cost estimates were based on the following assumptions: a benzathine penicillin prophylaxis once each month for five years and one hospitalization of twenty-four days for each initial RF attack to avert death among 34 percent of patients.

Under these assumptions, the cost of secondary prophylaxis to avert one death is $5,520, or $142 per DALY.

Tertiary Prophylaxis

Tertiary prophylaxis can reverse the progression of intractable cardiac insufficiency by means of surgical repair or replacement of damaged heart valves. Surgical interventions are important in developing countries because children and young adults often seek treatment when they already suffer from severe cardiac failure. The natural history of the disease demonstrates that surgical treatment is the only effective method in those instances (Antunes and others 1987).

Different types of surgical interventions exist to repair damaged heart valves: a mechanical valve prosthesis or biological valves are inserted in the heart to replace damaged heart valves; valvuloplasty conserves and repairs damaged valves rather than replacing them. Mechanical prostheses cause a high incidence of thromboembolic events which are potentially lethal, and anticoagulant therapy is required to avoid them; many biological valves degenerate early as a result of fibrosis and calcification, leading to early cardiac failure in young patients (Abid and others 1989). Thus despite immense strides in the perfection of materials and design, the ideal valve remains elusive. Consequently, the desirability of preservation of heart valves has become more appreciated. Valvuloplasty causes very few thromboembolic events. Monthly benzathine penicillin prophylaxis is required after surgery to prevent GASP and to avoid damage to the new cardiac valves (Antunes and others 1987).

The cost-effectiveness of those procedures needs careful evaluation because so many children and young adults suffer today from debilitating or intractable cardiac failure. Richard Bumgarner found that in China, out of 410,000 children suffering from RHD, 80,000 need valvular replacement (Bumgarner, personal communication). The mean cost of tertiary prophylaxis to avert one death is $12,750, or $425 per DALY (table 10-9). Tertiary prophylaxis is an attractive option despite high intervention costs.

Elements of Case Management Strategy

The experience gained thus far has led to the formulation of clear guidelines for the clinical management of cases of RF and RHD.

Acute Rheumatic Fever

The patient who has even a suspicion of RF should be hospitalized for diagnosis and initial treatment. In most secondary-level hospitals the diagnosis can be established according to Jones criteria. Other diagnostic procedures usually include chest x-ray, blood cell count, erythrocyte sedimentation rate, C-reactive protein, and ASO titer. A limitation in developing countries is the availability of a microbiological laboratory for throat culture and exclusion of infective endocarditis.

Once the diagnosis has been established, the management is straightforward:

- Eradication of group A streptococci from the throat by a course of penicillin.

- Acetylsalicylic acid (aspirin) or, in serious cases of carditis, corticosteroid treatment to suppress the accompanying inflammatory response. Response to acetylsalicylic acid and corticosteroid is so good that it should not be administered until the diagnosis is confirmed.

- Bed-chair rest in the hospital until cardiac manifestations subside, and mobilization when the acute phase reactants have returned to normal.

- In rare instances of severe carditis, cardiac valve replacement or valvuloplasty might be considered.

- Long-term penicillin prophylaxis.

Chronic Rheumatic Heart Disease

The initial management of the patient with RHD is directed at the control of heart failure. Cardiac arrhythmias are rare in young patients but increase with age. Cardiotonic (usually digitalis) is the appropriate drug to control arrhythmias and increase myocardial contractility. Diuretics are usually given to control fluid retention associated with heart failure. The most important therapeutic decision in RHD is the timing of surgical intervention, a costly tertiary prophylaxis requiring tertiary-care centers.

In all cases, with or without surgery, long-term penicillin prophylaxis and prophylaxis of bacterial endocarditis before other surgical procedures must be ensured.

Priorities

Secondary prophylaxis is the most cost-effective approach to prevent RF and RHD in developing countries. It is important to take into account the level of training of health care providers and the coverage of the health system while planning and implementing secondary prophylaxis in each country.

Priorities for Resource Allocation

Recent experiences in several developing countries have demonstrated that secondary prophylaxis is a cost-effective approach. In addition to providing penicillin, it is important to provide careful training of health care personnel in diagnosing heart murmurs and to ensure close follow-up of patients with RF and RHD by sensitizing health care providers and communities to the need for monthly penicillin injections. Where a good health care infrastructure is already in place, prevention of RHD can be included in national health plans with little added cost. In areas with little health coverage, populations at highest risk—school-age children of low socioeconomic groups enrolled in school in large urban areas—could receive special attention and secondary prophylaxis through the school system.

Priorities for Research

Further research is crucial to reduce the present burden of disease due to RF and RHD. New tools are needed to diagnose pharyngitis due to group A streptococci in developing countries and to produce a vaccine. Research is also important to monitor changes in the epidemiology of RF and RHD and to assess the effectiveness of interventions.

- Biomedical research is necessary to unravel fully the pathogenesis of RHD and to develop a simple diagnostic test and a vaccine.

- Epidemiologic research is important to assess the magnitude of the problem in different geographic areas and to monitor trends.

- Finally, operations research is essential to evaluate the effect of interventions.

References

Abid, F., N. Mzah, F. El Euch, and M. Ben Ismail. 1989. "Valve Replacement in Children under 15 Years with Rheumatic Heart Disease." *Pediatric Cardiology* 10:199–204.

Anabwani, G. M., A. B. Amoa, and A. K. Muita. 1989. "Epidemiology of Rheumatic Heart Disease among Primary School Children in Western Kenya." *International Journal of Cardiology* 23:249–52.

Antunes, M. J., M. P. Magalhaes, P. R. Colsen, and R. H. Kinsley. 1987. "Valvuloplasty for Rheumatic Mitral Valve Disease, a Surgical Challenge." *Journal of Cardiovascular Surgery* 94:44–56.

Behrman, Richard E., and Victor C. Vaughan, eds. 1983. *Nelson Textbook of Pediatrics*, twelfth edition. Philadelphia: W. B. Saunders Company.

Bisno, A. L. "Group A Streptococcal Infections and Acute Rheumatic Fever." 1991. *New England Journal of Medicine* 325:783–93.

Cairns, L. M. 1988. "The Immunology of Rheumatic Fever." *New Zealand Medical Journal* 101:388–91.

Denny, F. W. 1987. "T. Duckett Jones Memorial Lecture: T. Duckett Jones and Rheumatic Fever in 1986." *Circulation* 76:963–70.

Edington, M. E., and J. S. Gear. 1982. "Rheumatic Heart Disease in Soweto— A Program for Secondary Prevention." *South African Medical Journal* 62: 523–25.

Fischetti, V. A. 1991. "Streptococcal M Protein." *Scientific American*, June, 58–65.

Goldstein, I., P. Rebeyrotte, J. Parlebas. 1968. "Isolation from Heart Valves of Glycopeptides which Share Immunological Properties with Streptococcus hemolyticus Group A Polysaccharides." *Nature* 219:866–8.

Gordis, Leon. 1985. "T. Duckett Jones Memorial Lecture. The Virtual Disappearance of Rheumatic Fever in the United States: Lessons in the Rise and Fall of the Disease." *Circulation* 72:1155–62.

Gordis, Leon, Abraham Lilienfeld, and Romeo Rodriguez. 1969a. "Studies in the Epidemiology and Preventability of Rheumatic Fever—I. Demographic Factors in the Incidence of Acute Attacks." *Journal of Chronic Diseases* 21:645–54.

———. 1969b. "Studies in the Epidemiology and Preventability of Rheumatic Fever—II. Socio-economic Factors and the Incidence of Acute Attacks." *Journal of Chronic Diseases* 21:655–66.

Hassell, T. A., and K. L. Stuart. 1974. "Rheumatic Fever Prophylaxis: A Three Year Study." *British Medical Journal* 2:39–40.

Hosier, D. M., J. M. Craenen, D. W. Teske, and J. J. Wheller. 1987. "Resurgence of Acute Rheumatic Fever." *American Journal of Diseases of Children*. 141:730.

Hutt, Michael S. R.. 1991. "Cancer and Cardiovascular Disease." In R. G. Feachem and D. T. Jamison, eds., *Disease and Mortality in Sub-Saharan Africa*. New York: Oxford University Press.

Irwig, L. M., B. Porter, T. D. Wilson, L. D. Saunders, Lucy A. Wagstaff, N. Liesch, S. G. Reinach, M. S. Makhaya, and J. S. Gear. 1985. "Clinical Competence of Pediatric Primary Health Care Nurses in Soweto." *South African Medical Journal* 67:92–95.

"Jones Criteria (Revised) for Guidance in the Diagnosis of Rheumatic Fever." 1984. *Circulation* 69:203A–208A.

Jones, T. D. 1944. "The Diagnosis of Rheumatic Fever." *JAMA* 126:481–84.

Kaplan, Edward L., and Milton Markowitz. 1988. "Rheumatic Fever in the United States: No Longer a Disease of the Past." *New Zealand Medical Journal* 101:402–4.

MacDonald, K. T., and A. C. Walker. 1989. "Rheumatic Heart Disease in Aboriginal Children in the Northern Territory." *Medical Journal of Australia* 150:503–5.

McLaren, M. J., D. M. Hawkins, H. J. Koornhof, K. R. Bloom, D. M. Bramwell-Jones, E. Cohen, G. E. Gale, K. Kanarek, A. S. Lachman, J. B. Lakier, W. A. Pocock, and J. B. Barlow. 1978. "Epidemiology of Rheumatic Heart Disease in Black School Children of Soweto, Johannesburg." *British Medical Journal* 3:474–78.

Maharaahj, B., R. B. Dyer, W. P. Leary, D. D. Arbukle, T. G. Armstrong, and D. J. Pudifin. 1987. "Correspondence: Screening for Rheumatic Heart Disease amongst Black School Children in Inanda, South Africa." *Journal of Tropical Pediatrics* 33:60–61.

Majeed, H. A., N. N. Khan, M. Dabbagh, and others. 1981. "Acute Rheumatic Fever during Childhood in Kuwait. The Mild Nature of the Attack." *Annals of Tropical Pediatrics* 1:13–20.

Majeed, H. A., F. A. Khuffash, D. C. Sharda, S. S. Farwana, A. F. el Sherbiny, and S. Y. Ghafour. 1987. "Children with Acute Rheumatic Fever and Acute Poststreptococcal Glomerulonephritis and Their Families in a Subtropical Zone: A Three Year Prospective Comparative Epidemiological Study." *International Journal of Epidemiology* 16: 561–67.

Markowitz, Milton. 1970. "Eradication of Rheumatic Fever. An Unfulfilled Hope." *Circulation* 41:1077–84.

———. 1983. "Rheumatic Fever." In Richard E. Behrman, and Victor C. Vaughan, eds., *Nelson Textbook of Pediatrics*, twelfth edition. Philadelphia: W. B. Saunders Company.

———. 1985. "The Decline of Rheumatic Fever: Role of Medical Intervention. Lewis W. Wannaker Memorial Lecture." *Journal of Pediatrics* 106:545–50.

———. 1988. "Evolution and Critique of Changes in the Jones Criteria for the Diagnosis of Rheumatic Fever." *New Zealand Journal of Medicine* 101: 392–94.

Massell, B. F., C. G. Chute, A. M. Walker, and G. S. Kurland. 1988. "Penicillin and the Marked Decrease in Morbidity and Mortality from Rheumatic Fever in the United States." *New England Journal of Medicine* 318:280–86.

Neutze, J. M. 1988a. "Rheumatic Fever and Rheumatic Heart Disease in the Western Pacific Region." *New Zealand Medical Journal* 101:404–6.

———. 1988b. "The Third International Conference on Rheumatic Fever and Rheumatic Heart Disease." *New Zealand Medical Journal* 101:387.

Padmavati, S., and Vijay Gupta. 1988. "Reappraisal of the Jones Criteria: The Indian Experience." *New Zealand Medical Journal* 101:391–92.

Patarroyo, M. E., R. J. Winchester, Alberto Vejerano, Allan Gibofsky, Fernand Chalem, J. B. Zabriskie, and H. G. Kunkel. 1979. "Association of a B-Cell Alloantigen with Susceptibility to Rheumatic Fever." *Nature* 278:173–74.

Potter, E. V., Mauri Svartman, Isahak Mohammed, Reginald Cox, Theo Poon-King, and D. P. Earle. 1978. "Tropical Acute Rheumatic Fever and

Associated Streptococcal Infections Compared with Concurrent Acute Glomerulonephritis." *Journal of Pediatrics* 92:325–33.

Sanyal, Shyamal. K., M. K. Thapar, S. H. Ahmed, Vijaya Hooja, and Promila Tewari. 1974. "The Initial Attack of Acute Rheumatic Fever During Childhood in North India. A Prospective Study of the Clinical Profile." *Circulation* 49:7–12.

Sharper, A. G. 1972. "Cardiovascular Disease in the Tropics—I. Rheumatic Heart." *British Medical Journal* 3:683–86.

Strasser, Toma. 1985. "Cost-Effective Control of Rheumatic Fever in the Community." *Health Policy* 5:159–64.

Taranta, Angelo, Jeta Torosdag, Julius D. Metrakos, Wanda Jegier, and Irene Uchida. 1959. "Rheumatic Fever in Monozygotic and Dizygotic Twins." *Circulation* 20:778.

Vasloo, M. B., and B. Reichart. 1987. "The Feasibility of Closed Mitral Valvotomy in Pregnancy." *Journal of Thoracic and Cardiovascular Surgery* 93:675–79.

Veasy, L. George, S. E. Wiedmeier, G. S. Orsmund, H. D. Ruttenburg, M. M. Boucek, S. J. Roth, V.F. Tait, J. A. Thompson, J. A. Daly, E. L. Kaplan, and H. R. Hill. 1987. "Resurgence of Acute Rheumatic Fever in the Intermountain Area of the United States." *New England Journal of Medicine* 316:421–26.

Vigneron, Emmanuel. 1989. "The Epidemiological Transition in an Overseas Territory: Disease Mapping in French Polynesia." *Social Science and Medicine* 29:913–22.

Vongprateep Choompol, Duangsuda Dharmasakti, and Kamol Sindhava-nonda. 1988. "The National Program and the Control of Rheumatic Heart Disease in Two Project Areas of Thailand." *New Zealand Medical Journal* 101:408–10.

Wald, Ellen R., Barry Dashefsky, Cindy Feidt, Darleen Chiponis, and Carol Byers. 1987. "Acute Rheumatic Fever in Western Pennsylvania and the Tristate Area." *Pediatrics* 80:371–74.

WHO (World Health Organization). 1980a. "Community Control of Rheumatic Fever in Developing Countries: 1. A Major Public Health Problem." *WHO Chronicles* 34:336–45.

———. 1980b. "Community Control of Rheumatic Fever in Developing Countries: 2. Strategies for Prevention and Control." *WHO Chronicles* 34: 389–95.

———. 1988. "Rheumatic Fever and Rheumatic Heart Disease." *Study Group Report.* Technical Report 764.

11

Tuberculosis

Christopher Murray, Karel Styblo, and Annik Rouillon

Tuberculosis is an ancient disease that has long been a significant public health challenge in the world and remains a significant health problem in developing countries. In the last century, tuberculosis was responsible for nearly one in ten deaths in Europe (Preston, Keyfitz, and Schoen 1972). There is reliable evidence that irrespective of its magnitude, the tuberculosis problem in industrial countries has been decreasing for at least the last forty years, since the introduction of antituberculosis chemotherapy. In many industrial countries, a steady decrease in mortality from tuberculosis in the pre-chemotherapy era was observed from the turn of this century if not before (Frost 1937; Styblo 1986). The elimination of tuberculosis in most industrial countries will not be substantially influenced by acquired immunodeficiency syndrome (AIDS) because of the low prevalence of tuberculous infection in subjects age twenty to fifty years in whom infection from the human immunodeficiency virus (HIV) is most frequent (Styblo 1989). In developing countries, however, tuberculosis continues to be an important problem and there appears to have been virtually no tendency for tuberculosis to eliminate itself in the absence of intensive control measures. Unlike in industrial countries, HIV infection will result in a considerable increase of tuberculosis cases in those developing countries where both tuberculous and HIV infections are prevalent. Tuberculosis remains, therefore, one of the top priorities for action in developing countries, because tools exist to diagnose and cure infectious cases of tuberculosis and thus to decrease transmission of tuberculous infection.

The epidemiology of tuberculosis is complex and a certain knowledge of the natural history of tuberculosis is required in order to discuss the policy options. Tuberculosis is caused by the bacillus *Mycobacterium tuberculosis*, which in most cases attacks the lungs. Infection is most commonly transmitted from persons with pulmonary tuberculosis to other persons, in particular when coughing or sneezing. The most important exception to the airborne route of infection is infection of the digestive tract through contaminated milk containing *Mycobacterium bovis* from cows suffering from tuberculosis, which causes a disease clinically similar to tuberculosis.

One or more bacilli reaching the lung tissue can cause a nonspecific inflammatory response, which may result in a primary complex. The primary complex has two components, one in the lung and the other in the corresponding lymph node or nodes. In most cases, both the primary pulmonary lesions and lesions in lymph nodes heal spontaneously, leaving behind a focus of a few "dormant" bacilli that can be reactivated and cause clinical disease at any moment during an individual's lifetime. Before the development of allergy and immunity, some bacilli escape from the primary lesions into the blood stream and set up blood-borne foci in other parts of the body, for example, in the kidneys, ends of long bones, spine, or brain. In newborns and small children the infection progresses either in the primary site or metastatic foci, and serious forms of tuberculosis may develop, in particular, miliary tuberculosis and tuberculous meningitis. These forms of tuberculosis also occur in adolescents and adults but much less frequently than in newborns and small children.

Two to six weeks after the primary infection, the body's immune system develops a certain level of cell-mediated immunity to M. *tuberculosis* antigens. This leads to the formation of granulomas—a type of histological pattern—around the focus of the bacilli. When these areas become calcified, they may be detected on a chest x-ray as a calcified primary complex. (If the calcified lesions of the primary complex in the lung and the lymph node are too small, they may not be seen on an x-ray.) Clinical disease, however, may occur weeks to years after the primary infection with the bacillus, although about 80 percent of all cases occur during the first two years after infection (Sutherland 1968). The probability of progressing from a primary infection to clinical tuberculosis is discussed more fully below. The key aspect of the natural history of tuberculosis is that infection may lead, in a relatively small proportion of infected persons, to clinical disease at a later date. Consequently, the process of elimination of tuberculosis in a community is very slow, because a certain risk of latent infections developing into active tuberculosis (endogenous exacerbation) cannot be completely prevented.

Four important diagnostic strategies are used to detect tuberculous infection and clinical disease. First, a recently or remotely infected person, whether or not he or she has clinical disease, develops a certain degree of cell-mediated immune response to M. *tuberculosis* antigen. An intradermal injection of tuberculin (preferably purified protein derivative) will cause an induration in forty-eight to seventy-two hours. This skin test (Mantoux test) permits a relatively easy detection of the prevalence of tuberculous infection in any population. The tuberculin test does not distinguish, however, between recent and remote infections or between an infection caused by M. *tuberculosis* and one caused by M. *bovis* or by some other mycobacteria. In spite of these limitations, tuberculin sensitivity surveys in a representative sample of a population are one of the mainstays of tuberculosis epidemiology. The tuberculin test, however, has a limited value for the diagnosis of clinical tuberculosis. If the test is positive, it does not distinguish between infection and disease; if it is negative it does not always exclude disease. Studies by Canetti (1939, 1972) indicate that most patients who have been infected and have a positive skin test maintain viable bacilli within their bodies.

Second, detection by microscopy of acid-fast bacilli (nearly always identical with tubercle bacilli) in sputum and other specimens (for example, gastric washings) is the most important tool to detect highly infectious cases of tuberculosis. There is strong evidence (Rouillon, Perdrizet, and Parrot 1976; Styblo 1984) that those patients whose sputa contain sufficient bacilli to be detected by microscopy are highly infectious. These cases are referred to as "smear-positive."

Third, the culture of specimens for mycobacteria detects, in about four to six weeks, tubercle bacilli in sputum containing insufficient bacilli to be detected by microscopy. These cases are then classified as sputum smear-negative but "culture-positive" pulmonary tuberculosis. Patients whose sputum is smear-negative and culture-positive or culture-negative are several times less infectious than smear-positive cases.

Fourth, in smear- and culture-negative patients (particularly in children and young adults) diagnosis of tuberculosis is made on the basis of clinical examination and interpretation of chest x-ray.

Extrapulmonary tuberculosis is diagnosed by, in a number of cases, bacteriology (in patients with tuberculous meningitis, lymphadenitis, genitourinary tuberculosis, and the like) or by histology of biopsy material. Depending on the site of infection, roentgenologic and other special examinations are required to diagnose extrapulmonary tuberculosis. It is important to stress that extrapulmonary tuberculosis is either noninfectious or the degree of infectivity is very low.

The natural history of tuberculosis illustrates that patients suffering from smear-positive pulmonary tuberculosis are the main source of infection. For the rest of this chapter, therefore, tuberculosis will be divided into two categories: (a) sputum smear-positive tuberculosis, which will be referred to as smear-positive tuberculosis; and (b) other tuberculosis, which includes pulmonary tuberculosis, in which the sputum is smear negative, and extrapulmonary tuberculosis. Because children rarely suffer from sputum smear-positive tuberculosis, most cases of tuberculosis in children will be included in the category "other tuberculosis." (If children are smear positive, they are highly infectious sources of infection. If they are smear negative and culture positive or smear negative and culture

negative they are much less infectious.) The above two categories are sometimes labeled infectious or open tuberculosis and noninfectious tuberculosis, respectively (India, Ministry of Health and Family Welfare 1986). The distinction between sputum smear-positive tuberculosis and other tuberculosis is particularly important when considering the policy options for tuberculosis control and prevention.

Tuberculosis without detection and the institution of adequate treatment is highly fatal—specific studies will be reviewed below. Because mycobacteria are able to survive within host lesions as persisters (dormant bacilli), treatment is long and requires, in smear-positive cases, the combination of at least two drugs in the initial intensive phase. Length of treatment ranges from six to eighteen months.

Tuberculosis Incidence and Mortality

In the following section, we outline the empirical and epidemiological basis for estimating tuberculosis incidence and mortality.

Tuberculosis Incidence

To put tuberculosis in the proper perspective we need to know the number and the age distribution in new cases of tuberculosis which develop in a community each year, as well as the number and the age distribution of patients who die from tuberculosis each year. Health information systems in developing countries are too incomplete to provide meaningful information on the incidence or mortality of tuberculosis (Styblo and Rouillon 1981). We are forced to estimate the burden of tuberculosis indirectly by using several epidemiological parameters. These include the average annual risk of tuberculous infection and the incidence of smear-positive pulmonary tuberculosis, the proportion of all cases of tuberculosis that are smear positive, and case-fatality rates for smear-positive tuberculosis and other tuberculosis.

ANNUAL AVERAGE RISK OF TUBERCULOUS INFECTION. Tuberculosis epidemiologists have used skin tests to measure the prevalence of infection in communities. A technique has been developed for converting this information on prevalence of

Table 11-1. Estimated Risks of Tuberculosis Infection in Developing Countries 1985–90
(percent)

Area	Risk of infection	Annual decrease in risk
Sub-Saharan Africa	1.50–2.50	1–2
North Africa and western Asia	0.50–1.50	4–5
Asia	1.00–2.00	1–3
South America	0.50–1.50	2–5
Central America and the Caribbean	0.50–1.50	1–3

Source: Based on Cauthen, Pio, and ten Dam 1988.

Figure 11-1. *Relationship between Annual Risk of Infection and Incidence of Smear-Positive Tuberculosis*

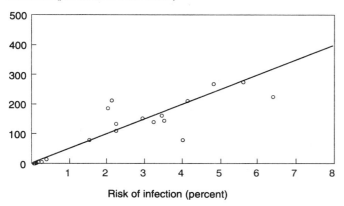

Incidence (per 100,000 U.S. dollars)

tuberculous infection into a series of annual risks of tuberculous infection (Styblo, Meijer, and Sutherland 1969; Sutherland 1976). If several tuberculin surveys of the same population have been made at different times (using similar techniques and testing a representative sample of subjects of the same age not vaccinated with BCG [bacille Calmette-Guérin]), the level of and percentage decrease in the risk of infection can be estimated. Techniques have been developed to estimate, if the pattern of the annual risk of infection by age is assumed, the level and time trend in the annual risk of infection from a single tuberculin survey (Sutherland 1976). The annual risk of infection tells us the probability that any individual will be infected or reinfected with M. *tuberculosis* in one year. This measure has become the standard indicator of the tuberculosis burden in a community (Leowski 1988).

Since the 1950s many different tuberculin sensitivity surveys in developing countries have provided us with an approximate picture of the annual risk of infection in different regions of the developing world. Our best estimates, based on a recent review of survey data on the annual risk of infection, are presented in table 11-1. The annual risk of tuberculous infection is probably highest in Sub-Saharan Africa, followed closely by Asia. For comparison the annual risk of infection in the Netherlands in 1985 was 0.012 percent (Styblo 1989).

INCIDENCE OF SMEAR-POSITIVE TUBERCULOSIS. Incidence of smear-positive pulmonary tuberculosis is one of the two key epidemiological indexes (the other being the average annual risk of tuberculous infection) for evaluation of the overall tuberculosis situation. Lack of data on smear-positive tuberculosis cases in developing countries makes it difficult to convey the enormity of the tuberculosis problem to the public health community. It is not possible readily to obtain reliable information on incidence of smear-positive tuberculosis in developing countries because case-

detection rates can be only a fraction of the respective true incidence rates.

Prevalence of smear-positive cases is of limited value as an epidemiological index because it largely depends on the quality of chemotherapy of smear-positive cases and the extent and quality of case finding. (In industrial countries, prevalence may be substantially lower than incidence, especially in countries where a six-month course of treatment is given to patients. In developing countries, prevalence may be several times higher than incidence if treatment results are poor and the case-detection rate is low.) For these very same reasons, prevalence may be an important indicator for management of a national tuberculosis control program, but estimates of prevalence depend on too many locally specific parameters to be made here for regions or for the developing world as a whole.

The relationship between the annual risk of infection and the incidence of smear-positive tuberculosis can provide one of the only means of estimating the incidence of smear-positive tuberculosis (Styblo 1985). Styblo examined the relationship between the annual risk of infection and incidence of smear-positive pulmonary tuberculosis using a variety of data sources from the developing and industrial world. We have recomputed this relationship using only the results of a series of surveys sponsored by the World Health Organization in developing countries and data from the Netherlands before chemotherapy was widely available. We must note that for some of these surveys data are available on the prevalence of smear-positive tuberculosis, not the incidence. In such cases, we derived the incidence rates by using the historical observation that the prevalence of smear-positive tuberculosis was usually twice the incidence in the communities without widespread institution of chemotherapy (Holm 1970). In these developing countries, the relationship between the annual risk of infection and incidence of pulmonary smear-positive tuberculosis was linear. A least squares regression line (figure 11-1) gives an

Table 11-2. *Estimated Incidence of Smear-Positive Tuberculosis in Developing Countries, 1985–90*

Area	Cases			Incidence (per 100,000)
	Low	Midpoint	High	
Sub-Saharan Africa[a]	342,921	591,445	839,970	117
North Africa and western Asia	52,592	145,640	238,687	54
Asia	1,141,877	2,298,393	3,454,909	79
South America	57,937	160,440	262,943	54
Central America and the Caribbean	30,022	83,138	136,266	54
Total	1,625,349	3,279,056	4,932,775	79

Note: Based on annual risk of infection for each region presented in table 11-1, 1990 population, and incidence of thirty-nine to fifty-nine cases per 100,000 population for each 1 percent annual risk of infection.

a. Includes cases attributable to dual HIV/tuberculosis infections.

Source: Authors.

Figure 11-2. Age Distribution of Smear-Positive Tuberculosis in Four Sub-Saharan Tuberculosis Programs

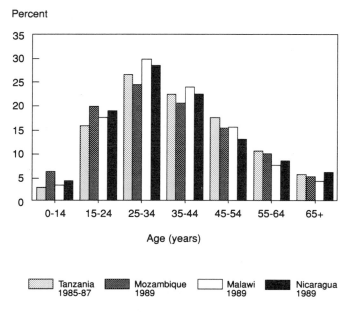

Source: Tanzania: Chum and others 1988; other countries: government registry data.

estimate of 49 cases of smear-positive tuberculosis per 100,000 for every 1 percent annual risk of infection. The 95 percent confidence interval for the coefficient is 39 to 59.[1]

Using the estimates of the risk of infection for different regions in table 11-1 and the confidence interval for the relationship between incidence of pulmonary smear-positive tuberculosis and the risk of infection, we have calculated the low and high estimates of the incidence of smear-positive tuberculosis for different regions (table 11-2). The midpoint of the confidence interval of the estimates of smear-positive incidence is 3,208,000 cases, or an incidence of 77 per 100,000 in the developing world. These must be viewed as only crude estimates, which nevertheless illustrate the continuing magnitude of the tuberculosis problem.

AGE DISTRIBUTION OF SMEAR-POSITIVE TUBERCULOSIS. The age distribution of incidence is important in determining the effect on public health of smear-positive tuberculosis and the most appropriate means of preventing or controlling tuberculosis. From the historical record of industrial countries and epidemiological models, the age and sex distribution of incidence appears to change as the annual risk of infection declines. Because most developing countries have annual risks of tuberculous infection between 1 and 2 percent, we propose to use the age distribution of the incidence of smear-positive tuberculosis from a developing country with an annual risk of infection in this range. There is no reason to believe that the epidemiology and thus the age distribution of incidence for a

given annual risk of infection will vary substantially between communities. Because the tuberculosis control program in Tanzania is well organized and captures most of the tuberculosis cases, the age distribution from Tanzania will be used as representative of the developing world. In figure 11-2 we show the age distribution of smear-positive tuberculosis in Tanzania for 1985–87 (Chum and others 1988), Malawi for 1989, Mozambique for 1989, and Benin for 1989. The pattern is remarkably similar in these four countries, all of which have good programs and case registration. It is important to note that BCG coverage in Tanzania was roughly 50 percent in 1983–87 (Bleiker and others 1987), based on scar examination in the National Tuberculin Survey in Tanzania carried out on 80,000 schoolchildren from twenty regions selected at random from 1983 to 1987, which is below the officially reported average for the developing world (UNICEF 1988). Thus any effect such BCG coverage may have on preventing tuberculosis in children is partially represented in the age distribution; because world coverage is probably higher than in Tanzania, the estimate for the incidence of smear-positive tuberculosis in children based on this age distribution may be slightly high. Clearly, smear-positive cases are relatively rare in children; smear-positive tuberculosis is concentrated in adults—more than 80 percent of cases occur between the ages of fifteen and fifty-four, according to the data from these four countries.

INCIDENCE OF OTHER FORMS OF TUBERCULOSIS. Estimates of the incidence of smear-negative pulmonary and extrapulmonary

Figure 11-3. Smear-Positive Tuberculosis as a Proportion of All Cases of Tuberculosis, by Age, United States (1985–87) and Norway (1951–72)

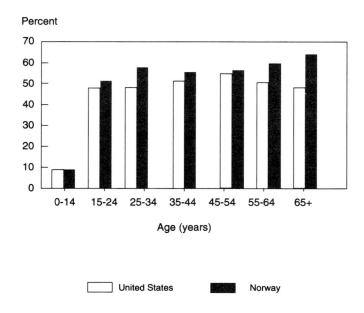

Source: United States: CDC (unpublished data); Norway: Tuberculosis Surveillance Research Unit (TSRU; unpublished data).

Figure 11-4. Estimated Age Distribution of Tuberculosis in the Developing World, 1990

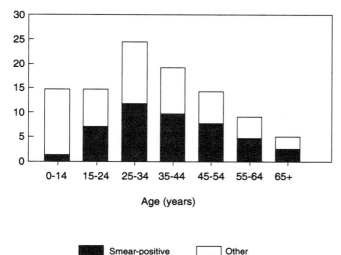

Percent

Age (years)

■ Smear-positive   □ Other

Source: Authors.

tuberculosis are also needed. These forms of tuberculosis are particularly difficult to quantify because the main diagnostic tool used in developing countries, sputum microscopy, does not detect these cases. Because the diagnosis of extrapulmonary tuberculosis is often based on clinical criteria, no survey data are available to estimate the relation between the risk of infection and other tuberculosis. In the past, estimates of smear-positive tuberculosis have simply been doubled to provide a figure for other tuberculosis (Styblo and Rouillon 1981; Leowski 1988). The distribution of total cases between the categories sputum smear-positive and other tuberculosis cannot be accurately established. Whereas smear-positive tuberculosis and tuberculosis positive by culture can be objectively determined, the number of culture-negative cases detected depends on various factors, such as whether or not mass miniature radiography is used to find cases (this method was extensively employed in Europe in the 1950s, 1960s, and 1970s), the criteria used for activity in asymptomatic cases, age group, and so on. We will assume that within each age group, using the same diagnostic approach, the percentage of cases that are sputum smear-positive and the percentage of other cases should be the same independently of the overall annual risk of infection. The proportion of all tuberculosis cases in the United States and Norway that are smear-positive by age is shown in figure 11-3 (Galtung Hansen 1955; and personal communication from the Centers for Disease Control in Atlanta (CDC) in 1989). Because the data set for the United States is larger and no mass miniature radiography was used on a large scale, we will use the ratio of cases of other tuberculosis to smear-positive tuberculosis within each age group in the United States. Using the age distribution of the incidence of

smear-positive tuberculosis in Tanzania and the age-specific ratios of other to smear-positive in the United States, we have derived the rough estimate of the age distribution of other tuberculosis shown in figure 11-4. Although the assumptions underlying these estimates of other tuberculosis may be challenged on many grounds, we believe it is preferable to make some objective attempt to estimate the age distribution of smear-negative and extrapulmonary tuberculosis in developing countries because it is an important input to policy decisions.

Our estimations imply that there are 1.22 cases of smear-negative and extrapulmonary tuberculosis for every case of smear-positive tuberculosis in developing countries with an annual risk of infection between 1 and 2 percent and an overall age distribution similar to Tanzania. Low and high estimates of the number of new cases of smear-negative and extrapulmonary tuberculosis for each region in the developing world are provided in table 11-3. For all types of tuberculosis combined, the data in table 11-4 indicate that the incidence of tuberculosis exceeds 260 per 100,000 in Sub-Saharan Africa.

HIV-ASSOCIATED TUBERCULOSIS INCIDENCE. The close relationship between HIV infection and clinical tuberculosis that has been widely observed will substantially affect the predicted incidence of clinical tuberculosis in regions with high levels of HIV seropositivity. Using the most recent estimates of country-specific seroprevalence provided by the World Health Organization, we estimate that there are approximately 4.9 million HIV-seropositive patients in Sub-Saharan Africa. Using estimates of the prevalence of tuberculosis infection in the region, we arrive at the approximate figure of 2.1 million cases of dual HIV and tuberculosis infections. Individuals with dual infections have much higher rates of breakdown from infection to clinical disease (Selwyn and others 1989). A range for the annual breakdown rate in dually infected individuals of 5 to 10 percent has been used to estimate that an additional 105,000 to 210,000 cases of tuberculosis occur each year in Sub-Saharan Africa. These extra cases have been included in tables 11-2 through 11-6. If seroprevalence continues to rise, the tuberculosis burden attributable to the HIV epidemic will also rise. For the estimates in this chapter, we assume the same clinical spectrum between smear-positive and other tuberculosis for HIV-positive patients (Chaisson and Slutkin 1989).

Tuberculosis Mortality

This section discusses death rates of tuberculosis and their age distribution.

CASE-FATALITY RATES. In order to calculate tuberculosis mortality from the estimates of incidence derived above, we need to estimate the case-fatality rate. Without appropriate chemotherapy, tuberculosis is highly fatal. Two types of sources provide information on the relationship between incidence and tuberculosis mortality: data from before chemotherapy was available in industrial countries and survey data from southern India. First, Drolet (1938) investigated the relation between

Table 11-3. Estimated Incidence of Other Forms of Tuberculosis in Developing Countries, 1990

Area	Cases			Incidence (per 100,000)
	Low	Midpoint	High	
Sub-Saharan Africa[a]	418,363	721,563	1,024,763	143
North Africa and western Asia	64,162	177,680	291,198	66
Asia	1,393,090	2,804,039	4,214,989	96
South America	70,683	195,737	320,791	66
Central America and the Caribbean	36,627	101,429	166,231	66
Total	1,982,925	4,000,448	6,017,972	96

Note: Based on the relationship between smear-positive tuberculosis and other forms of tuberculosis in the United States by age, combined with the age distribution of smear-positive tuberculosis in Tanzania.

a. Includes cases attributable to dual HIV/tuberculosis infections.

Source: Authors.

Table 11-5. Estimated Cases of Tuberculosis Detected and Case-Fatality Rates in Developing Countries, 1990

Area	Cases detected	Percentage of total cases actually detected	Case-fatality rates[a] (percent)	
			Low	High
Sub-Saharan Africa	325,132	25	39	47
North Africa and western Asia	222,686	69	26	29
Asia	2,572,809	50	32	37
South America	221,856	62	28	32
Central America and the Caribbean	62,054	34	38	45
Total	3,404,537	47	33	38

Note: Based on assumption that 15 percent of patients receiving standard chemotherapy die; this is a conservative assumption.

Source: Authors.

the tuberculosis mortality rate and reported incidence in selected American cities from 1915 to 1935. He found that the estimated case-fatality rate for all types of tuberculosis in Detroit and New Jersey was 58.8 percent and 54.9 percent, respectively. The calculated case-fatality rate varied little during that twenty-year period. Similar case-fatality rates for all forms of tuberculosis were recorded in European countries—Denmark, 1925–34: 51.2 percent (Lindhart 1939); Norway, 1925–44: 50.6 percent (Galtung Hansen 1955); and England and Wales, 1933–35: 49.1 percent (Drolet 1938). The most detailed study is from Berg (1939), who followed 6,162 smear-positive patients for periods of up to twenty years. After two years, 40.1 percent had died; deaths increased to 60.7 percent

Table 11-4. Estimated Incidence of All Forms of Tuberculosis in Developing Countries, 1990

Area	Cases			Incidence (per 100,000)
	Low	Midpoint	High	
Sub-Saharan Africa[a]	761,284	1,313,008	1,864,733	260
North Africa and western Asia	116,754	323,320	529,885	120
Asia	2,534,966	5,102,432	7,669,898	174
South America	128,619	356,177	583,734	120
Central America and the Caribbean	66,649	184,567	392,485	120
Total	3,608,272	7,279,504	10,950,735	175

Note: Based on annual risk of infection for each region presented in table 11-1, 1990 population, and incidence of thirty-nine to fifty-nine cases per 100,000 population for each 1 percent annual risk of infection and also the relationship between smear-positive tuberculosis and other forms of tuberculosis in the United States by age, combined with the age distribution of smear-positive tuberculosis in Tanzania.

a. Includes cases attributable to dual HIV/tuberculosis infections.

Source: Authors.

at five years and 73.3 percent at ten years. Berg found that even fifteen to nineteen years after diagnosis, smear-positive patients had mortality rates five times higher than the general population of the same age. Second, a five-year study of the natural history of tuberculosis in Bangalore, India, found that 49 percent of smear-positive and culture-positive patients whose tuberculosis was detected on the first round of the survey were dead within five years (Olakowski 1973; National Tuberculosis Institute, Bangalore 1974). Mortality was concentrated in the first year and a half, during which 30 percent of the patients died. The death rate among new cases dropped in the second and third rounds (32.4 percent over three and one-half years in the first round and 33.9 percent over two years in the second round) because all round 2 patients received isoniazid for one month. Taken together, these data suggest that, without treatment, from 50 to 60 percent of tuberculosis patients will die.

The case-fatality rate for smear-positive patients is thought to be higher than for all forms of tuberculosis combined. Rutledge and Crouch (1919) followed 1,229 patients who had smear-positive tuberculosis and found that 66 percent of them were dead within four years. Lindhart (1939) found in Denmark that 66 percent of patients who were bacteriologically positive died. Berg's results for smear-positive patients provide the most direct evidence on the higher case-fatality rate of smear-positive tuberculosis. A higher mortality of smear-positive patients has also been shown in the study in southern India (Olakowski 1973). Of the 126 bacillary patients detected in round 1, the death rate in the culture-positive and smear-negative group (62 patients) was 45.2 percent at five years and 53.1 percent in the smear-positive group (64 patients) for the same period. Case-fatality rates must also be expected to vary between communities as a result of other factors, such as nutrition and concurrent infections. Still, the above studies provide a rough indication of the likely range in case-fatality rates from tuberculosis. If the case-fatality rate for smear-positive tuberculosis is higher than for all forms of tuberculosis, then the case-fatality rate of other tuberculosis on average must be somewhat lower. In other tuberculosis, however, some forms, such as tuberculous meningitis, will cause 100 percent or very high case-fatality rates if the patients receive no treatment. For the rest of this chapter, we will assume that the case-fatality rate for smear-positive tuberculosis is 60 to 70 percent; for other tuberculosis as a whole, 40 to 50 percent; and for all forms combined, 50 to 60 percent.

TUBERCULOSIS DEATH RATES IN DEVELOPING COUNTRIES. The tuberculosis death rates in developing countries cannot be as high as the incidence rates and a case-fatality rate of 50 to 60 percent imply, because a significant proportion of cases are detected by existing health services and the patients receive treatment. For all those cases that are estimated to be detected and receive treatment, we assume the case-fatality rate is reduced to 15 percent after five years. For example, in the East African and British Medical Research Council survey in Kenya the case-fatality rate for patients receiving standard chemotherapy was 13 percent after twelve months (East African and British Medical Research Council 1977, 1979). In many countries, however, the case-fatality rate may be over 15 percent for those receiving chemotherapy, after five years of follow-up, making the following estimates of mortality conservative.

Estimates of the percentage of new cases that are detected and the patients treated are based on the number of cases of tuberculosis detected that are reported by countries to the World Health Organization (table 11-5; WHO 1988). Because reporting is extremely variable, these estimates are based on the highest number of cases reported by each country for any year in the last decade. This basis is justified by the assumption that year-to-year variation in the number of cases reported, which can be greater than an order of magnitude, is due more to incomplete reporting of health service activities than to changes in the epidemiology of tuberculosis. The number of new cases reported from some programs has been confused with the total number registered at the end of the year, which includes old cases. We have adjusted the country estimates for

specific countries to reflect newly registered cases.[2] In addition, the highest number of cases reported in the last ten years has been adjusted upward by 20 percent for those regions with an active private sector to try to account for those cases that are detected in the private sector but are not reported to the government; in Asia, where data for some large countries may include a large number of retreatment cases, we have not adjusted the figures by 20 percent.

Separate estimates for the percentages of smear-positive and other cases are needed. The primary mode of case detection varies across regions; for example, in Sub-Saharan Africa, sputum microscopy is the main tool, whereas in China, much greater emphasis is placed on chest radiography. We will assume arbitrarily that 50 percent of cases detected are smear positive and 50 percent are other tuberculosis. This mix between smear-positive and other tuberculosis cases is probably an underestimate for Sub-Saharan Africa and an overestimate for Asia. The detection rate of the various forms of tuberculosis and the likely range of case-fatality rates discussed above can be combined to estimate the tuberculosis death rates from smear-positive tuberculosis and other tuberculosis.

In table 11-6 we show estimated deaths each year from all forms of tuberculosis based on the calculations of the tuberculosis death rates discussed above. The wide confidence intervals reflect the cumulative uncertainty in the parameters of the estimation procedure. The midpoints of the confidence intervals give a total number of deaths from tuberculosis in the developing world of almost 2.7 million. Tuberculosis, therefore, accounted for approximately 6.9 percent of all deaths in the developing world in 1990 (United Nations 1986).[3]

AGE DISTRIBUTION OF TUBERCULOSIS DEATHS. To estimate the age distribution of tuberculosis deaths, we must take into

Table 11-6. Estimated Incidence of All Forms of Tuberculosis in Developing Countries, 1990

| Area | Cases | | | Incidence (per 100,000) |
	Low	Midpoint	High	
Sub-Saharan Africa[a]	300,604	585,591	870,578	116
North Africa and western Asia	29,881	90,960	152,039	34
Asia	811,303	1,824,756	2,838,208	62
South America	35,915	110,548	185,180	37
Central America and the Caribbean	25,217	79,966	134,715	52
Total	1,202,920	2,691,820	4,180,720	65

a. Includes deaths attributable to dual HIV/tuberculosis infections.
Source: Authors.

Figure 11-5. *Estimated Distribution of Deaths from Tuberculosis in the Developing World, 1990*

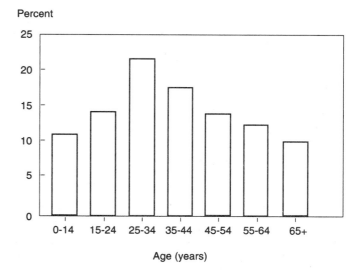

Source: Authors.

Table 11-7. Distribution of Tuberculosis Deaths by Age in Three European Countries before the Availability of Anti-Tuberculosis Chemotherapy
(percent)

Age (years)	Czechoslovakia 1940	Norway 1931	Norway 1941	Norway 1951	Netherlands 1931	Netherlands 1941	Netherlands 1951
0–14	11.7	11.8	10.3	8.0	24.0	19.4	13.6
15–24	22.0	30.6	25.4	10.8	22.4	20.3	12.8
25–34	18.7	25.9	25.4	24.4	20.8	20.7	16.9
35–44	14.0	14.5	9.6	13.2	11.7	13.1	12.8
45–54	12.5	7.7	9.6	13.2	7.7	9.6	11.6
54–64	11.4	5.0	6.6	13.2	6.3	8.2	13.4
65+	9.7	4.5	6.5	13.4	7.1	8.7	18.9
Risk of infection	5.5[a]	—	—	—	3.7	1.8	0.5

— Not available.

Note: Based on age-specific mortality rates for each country and the estimated population age structure for the developing world in 1990.

a. 1938 figure.

Source: Authors.

consideration the age distribution of new cases and the relation between case-fatality rates and age. Clearly, the relation is complex; for example, the death rates may also vary by age because certain age groups or sexes may be more likely to seek treatment and be cured. For example, comparing the distribution of smear-positive patients by age and sex between Malawi and Tanzania, it is evident that women in Tanzania are much less likely to seek care than men. The reduction of female case-detection rates by sex bias in access to care is probably quite widespread, especially in South Asia. Tuberculosis case-fatality rates tend to increase steadily at older ages (Berg 1939; Styblo 1984). We have derived from the Berg data the relation between age-specific case-fatality rates with some data from Styblo (1984) on mortality in the age group zero through fourteen.[4] Figure 11-5 provides the crude estimates of the age pattern of tuberculosis deaths in a country with an annual risk of infection of 1 to 2 percent, where the probability of detection is equal for smear-positive tuberculosis across all age groups and equal for other tuberculosis across all age groups.

This estimated pattern can be compared with the age distribution of tuberculosis deaths in Western countries when the annual risk of infection was similar to that now seen in the developing world. The age distribution of tuberculosis deaths adjusted to the age structure of the developing world in Czechoslovakia, Norway, and the Netherlands (Tuberculosis Surveillance Research Unit 1966) is illustrated in table 11-7. The percentage of deaths in children under fifteen ranged from approximately 10 to 20 percent. However, overall, the tuberculosis death rates in children were considerably lower in the Netherlands than in Czechoslovakia, even at higher risks of infection. Clearly, there are other variables that are significant determinants of the reported age distribution of tuberculosis death rates. One explanation may be the high rates of M. *bovis* infection in the Netherlands at the time. According to our estimates for Tanzania, 11 percent of tuberculosis deaths occur

in children under age fifteen, which is within the lower range for the three industrial countries in table 11-7. The comparatively lower value may be a result of the higher BCG coverage in Tanzania now than in these countries at the time. Variation in the age pattern of tuberculosis deaths highlights the tentative nature of the estimates presented here. The basic conclusion, however, that tuberculosis is concentrated in the adult age groups, appears to be robust.

As implied in this discussion, the age pattern of tuberculosis deaths shifts toward higher ages as the annual risk of infection declines. Using data from the United States which has been adjusted to the 1990 age structure of the developing world, we demonstrate in figure 11-6 how the mean age of death increases as the risk of infection declines. The number of deaths in children declines faster than the annual risk of infection; this relationship will become important when we consider the cost-effectiveness of BCG.

Trends in Incidence and Mortality

We have estimated cases and rates of tuberculosis in the year 2015 using the midpoints of the ranges of the annual risk of infection in table 11-1, population projections, and the rates of decline in the annual risk of infection, also reported in table 11-1 (table 11-8). These estimates are based on the assumption that the rates of decline in the annual risk of infection observed between 1970 and 1985 will continue into the future. In other words, the projections are based on the assumption that the socioeconomic changes and tuberculosis control activities that caused the decline in the risk of infection in the last two decades will continue at the same rate. Such projections suffer

Figure 11-6. Shifting Age Structure of Tuberculosis Deaths in the United States, 1937

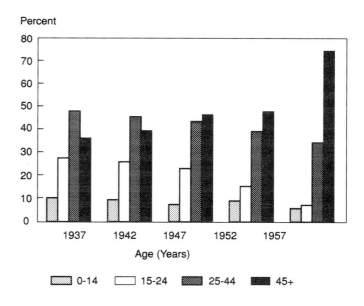

Note: Adjusted for age structure changes.
Source: Authors.

Table 11-8. Projected Cases and Deaths for all Forms of Tuberculosis in 2015

	Cases			
Area	Smear-positive	Other	Total	Deaths
Sub-Saharan Africa[a]	1,270,366	1,549,846	2,820,212	1,257,791
North Africa and western Asia	128,607	156,900	285,507	80,288
Asia	1,873,615	2,285,810	4,159,424	1,487,316
South America	98,667	120,373	219,040	67,965
Central America and the Caribbean	79,980	97,575	177,555	76,919
Total	3,451,235	4,210,504	7,661,738	2,970,279

Note: These projections are based on the following assumptions: (a) the current rate of decline in the annual risk of infection will continue over the next twenty-five years except in Sub-Saharan Africa, where it will not change because of the HIV epidemic; (b) the percentage of cases detected will remain the same in each region; (c) the percentage of patients treated with standard and short-course chemotherapy, and thus the population cure rate, will remain constant.

Source: Authors.

from all the same limitations as any projection of current trends. For Sub-Saharan Africa, we have assumed no net increase in the seroprevalence of HIV and no net decline in the annual risk of infection in making these projections to represent the potential contribution of the HIV epidemic. This is an extremely conservative assumption that probably underestimates the contribution of HIV-associated tuberculosis to the total tuberculosis caseload and the real potential for an increase in the risk of infection in the HIV-negative population, given an increasing number of sputum-positive patients. According to these conservative assumptions, tuberculosis will remain a significant problem in all developing world regions referred to in table 11-8. In Africa, population growth alone will lead to an absolute increase in the number of cases.

Social and Economic Costs

There are few if any studies of the actual costs or consequences of tuberculosis on the family, community, or economy in developing countries. The special burden of ill health and death caused by tuberculosis, however, follows from the age distribution of its incidence. Although morbidity and mortality in any age group have significant social and economic costs, the death of adults in their prime, who are the parents, community leaders, and producers in most societies, cause a particularly onerous burden. The incidence of tuberculosis is concentrated in adults age fifteen through fifty-four. For example, whereas the overall incidence in Africa of tuberculosis in 1985 is estimated to be 260, in adults it is approximately 390 per 100,000.

One of the greatest costs to society and the economy from tuberculosis is mortality. It has been estimated that there are just under 10.6 million deaths in adults age fifteen through fifty-nine in the developing world (Murray and Feachem 1990). Of these, our figures suggest that approximately 18.5 percent are due to tuberculosis. Not all these deaths are preventable.

Of avoidable adult deaths, 26 percent are probably due to tuberculosis.

The consequences of adult death from tuberculosis on children and other dependents can also be great. Studies have shown that, when a mother dies, her children suffer higher rates of mortality (Greenwood and others 1987). One can speculate that similar relationships exist for paternal death. Several studies from industrial countries have shown that tuberculosis is concentrated in lower socioeconomic groups, those households least able to cope with the burden of tuberculosis. Pryer (1989) found that in households in which one parent suffers from a serious debilitating disease, such as tuberculosis, children are two and one-half times more likely to be severely malnourished. Because tuberculosis deaths are concentrated in the segment of the population that is economically most productive, the economic cost of tuberculosis in lost production must be greater than that of a disease that exclusively affects children or the elderly.

Prevention

Before discussing specific measures to prevent or treat tuberculosis in developing countries, we will summarize the rationale for tuberculosis control programs in countries with a low prevalence of HIV infection. The presence of a significant proportion of the population infected with HIV may change the strategy for control.

- Unlike many other infectious diseases seen in developing countries, tuberculosis can be controlled with existing tools because the infectious agent is almost exclusively in the diseased person, who can be quickly rendered noninfectious.

- The detection of infectious, particularly smear-positive, cases of pulmonary tuberculosis and their cure are the key to effective prevention and control of the disease, both in industrial and developing countries. In addition, detection and treatment of cases reduce suffering and if adequately applied, very much lower the death rate of tuberculosis.

- Because a balance exists in developing countries between the tubercle bacillus and people in the absence of human-made interference (that is, case finding and chemotherapy), any reduction in the sources of infection will inevitably improve the epidemiological situation. If all or nearly all smear-positive cases of pulmonary tuberculosis diagnosed at present in any developing country could be rendered noninfectious, the risk of tuberculous infection would immediately start to fall. A decrease in the annual risk of tuberculous infection of 4 percent or more would not only result in a decrease in the incidence rate of the disease but would also outweigh increases in the population; consequently the absolute number of smear-positive cases would fall as well. A 5 percent decrease in the risk of infection each year would ensure that the tuberculosis problem in a given community or country would halve itself about every fourteen years.

• Reliable diagnostic tools that enable detection of the great majority of smear-positive cases of pulmonary tuberculosis and highly efficient chemotherapy regimens that can cure nearly all discovered cases of tuberculosis are available.

There are three main strategies for preventing tuberculosis: BCG vaccination, chemoprophylaxis, and decreasing sources of infection through case treatment. Each will be discussed in turn.

BCG Vaccine

The bacillus of Calmette and Guérin (BCG) was developed in 1921. Since that time it has become one of the most widely used yet controversial vaccines. Although BCG coverage has been up to now quite high on average compared with other immunizations, the effectiveness of BCG in preventing tuberculosis in adults remains controversial. From clinical trials conducted in the United Kingdom and in the United States it was found that BCG was up to 80 percent effective (Aronson, Aronson, and Taylor 1958; Great Britain Medical Research Council 1972). Important vaccine trials in southern India, however, revealed no effectiveness of BCG (Tuberculosis Prevention Trial 1979; Tuberculosis Prevention Trial, Madras 1980). Reports from a variety of prospective trials in the industrial world and more recent case-control studies in developing countries state effectiveness ranging from 0 to 80 percent (Clemens, Chung, and Feinstein 1983; Smith 1987).

Many explanations and theories have been advanced to explain this variance, including differences in strains of BCG, infections with other mycobacteria, and differences in susceptibility resulting from factors such as nutritional status (Fine 1989). Although there is no consensus on the effectiveness of BCG, we will assume that BCG is between 40 and 70 percent effective in preventing tuberculosis in children age zero through fourteen when given at birth. Some would argue that BCG given at birth may protect beyond fifteen years; there is, however, no evidence of this, especially in developing countries.

The BCG vaccine is given as early as possible in life, preferably at birth, in the vast majority of developing countries. Serious consideration might also be given to "indiscriminate (re)vaccination" (that is, without prior tuberculin testing) at older ages, irrespective of vaccination at birth. Depending on the feasibility of coverage, BCG (re)vaccination could be given to children entering and leaving school, pregnant women during prenatal care visits to health facilities, or to the general population during routine contacts with health workers. For example, tetanus toxoid is now considered by many to be an integral component of prenatal care; BCG could be delivered at the same time for only a small increase in the total cost. The actual effect of BCG (re)vaccination at older ages has not been studied; there seems little reason to believe that it would be harmful, however, and it may have some beneficial effect.

Still, we must realize that vaccination of newborns with BCG is a problem in those developing countries where there is a high prevalence of HIV infection among mothers. The WHO Expanded Programme on Immunization, which is responsible for the program of vaccination against six selected childhood diseases in the world, has been continuing BCG vaccination of newborns and small children, including those whose mother is known to be or suspected of being infected with HIV. As of the time of writing, evidence remains inconclusive regarding the rate of adverse reactions after BCG immunization among asymptomatic HIV-infected individuals. The vaccine should be withheld from individuals with symptomatic HIV infection (WHO 1987).

The effect of mass BCG vaccination on the epidemiological situation of tuberculosis was overestimated until the mid-1970s (Styblo and Meijer 1976). As mentioned earlier, tuberculosis is largely transmitted by persons with sputum smear-positive pulmonary tuberculosis. From the age distribution of smear-positive patients, it is clear that even complete BCG coverage can have little effect on the annual risk of infection. Total coverage with BCG, however, will have a significant effect on tuberculosis mortality in children, if BCG is 40 to 70 percent effective, as we have assumed. Based on the assumptions discussed above, complete coverage could reduce total tuberculosis mortality by 4 to 7 percent. The vaccine will most likely have very limited effect on the remaining 90 percent and more of tuberculosis mortality. Evidently, the expansion of BCG coverage alone cannot or should not be the sole means employed to control tuberculosis in any community.

Cost-Effectiveness of BCG

For two principal reasons, generalizable estimates of the cost-effectiveness of BCG cannot be made. First, there may be substantial differences in the computed average and marginal costs of BCG programs, depending on the program considered. Second, the cost-effectiveness of BCG is inversely proportional to the annual risk of infection.

When more than one vaccine is given at the same time, average costs for delivering each particular immunization are often calculated by dividing the cost per client contact by the number of vaccinations received. Thus the difference between marginal costs and average costs for a BCG program will depend on whether BCG is delivered in an independent campaign, in a contact with mother and child, or along with other immunizations such as the first DPT (diphtheria-pertussis-tetanus) vaccination. The Expanded Programme on Immunization has not, unfortunately, collected data on how BCG is delivered in each country. We conclude that the marginal cost-effectiveness of expanding BCG will necessarily depend on the location and timing of vaccination in a particular country.

As the annual risk of infection declines, if all else remains the same, the cost of immunizing all newborns does not change. The benefits of BCG immunization in cases or deaths averted, however, will decline inversely to the risk of infection. For example, as the risk of infection declines from 2 percent to 1 percent, the cost per death averted will more than double. The increase in the cost per death averted is greater than the decline in the risk of infection because the age distribution of deaths also shifts away from children as the risk of infection declines (see figure 11-6). The expected relation between the risk of infection and the cost per death averted by BCG is illustrated in figure 11-7.

In only one study has an attempt been made to cost a BCG program and estimate its effect in a developing country. Barnum, Tarantola, and Setaidy (1980) estimated the cost of operating a BCG program alone and also the marginal cost of adding a BCG program to an existing DPT program. Their estimates of deaths averted were based on local incidence and case-fatality rates of tuberculosis and an assumed effectiveness for BCG of 50 percent. Using their original data, we have recalculated the cost per discounted death averted in U.S. dollars.[5] Deaths prevented by BCG vaccination now occur over the next fourteen years; these are discounted to present value for comparison with interventions that avert deaths in the current time period. The cost in 1986 U.S. dollars per death discounted at 3 per cent was $644 for the BCG program alone and $144 for the marginal BCG program. At the time in Indonesia, survey data suggested that the risk of infection was approximately 3 percent: regional surveys reported annual risks of infection of between 2 and 4 percent (Cauthen, Pio, and ten Dam 1988). It must be stressed that these estimates of cost-effectiveness do not take into consideration the potential benefits of BCG in reducing leprosy (Fine 1989).

With no evidence at all on the efficacy of indiscriminate adult (re)vaccination with BCG, it is difficult to discuss the cost-effectiveness of adult BCG vaccination. Because tuberculosis mortality is concentrated in the young adult ages, revaccination, if it proved to be as effective as the vaccination of infants, would be more cost-effective. This, of course, assumes

that delivery of BCG to adults could be feasible at the same average or marginal costs as its delivery to infants.

Chemoprophylaxis

Secondary prevention of clinical tuberculosis can be accomplished by treating patients with tuberculosis infections. Chemoprophylaxis is applied either to freshly infected so-called tuberculin converters or to those who have been infected with virulent tubercle bacilli in the more distant past. The latter either do or do not have abnormalities in the lungs on x-ray.

Tuberculin converters undoubtedly represent a very rewarding group in terms of chemoprophylaxis results and thus chemoprophylaxis policy has been adopted as a routine procedure in a number of low-prevalence countries. Mass chemoprophylaxis of converters is impossible, however, since their identification depends on repeated tuberculin tests of the population. However, a selective search for converters in high-risk groups, such as close family contacts of smear-positive sources, is a feasible alternative. As discussed later, 6 to 10 percent of recent infections evolve into clinical tuberculosis. In developing countries, where large percentages of the population have been infected, the International Union against Tuberculosis and Lung Disease (IUATLD) recommends chemoprophylaxis only for all non-BCG-vaccinated children age five years or under, with no symptoms of tuberculosis. In children with symptoms, standard treatment should, of course, be given.

Chemoprophylaxis in tuberculin-positive subjects who have not developed clinical tuberculosis would reduce the number of sources of infection, if given for six to twelve months. In most developing countries, this group is very large, and resources would be far better directed to the detection of cases and to treatment. Still, chemoprophylaxis might play a very important role both in industrial and developing countries in subjects with the dual HIV and tuberculous infections but without clinical and bacteriological signs of tuberculosis. Research on HIV chemoprophylaxis is under way in several Sub-Saharan African countries.

Studies in industrial countries have found cost-effectiveness ratios per case averted to be greater than $7,000 for a twenty-four-week regimen (Snider, Caras, and Koplan 1986). Without accurate data to review the cost-effectiveness of chemoprophylaxis in developing countries, we can only make some comparisons with the costs per case treated. Because only 6 to 10 percent of those who have recently become skin-test positive develop clinical diseases, 10 to 16.7 recent tuberculin-positive patients must be given chemoprophylaxis to prevent one case of tuberculosis, assuming prophylaxis is 100 percent effective. In tuberculin-positive patients as opposed to new converters, the ratio would be one or two orders of magnitude higher because the long-term breakdown rate is only 25 to 40 per 100,000 per year. The drug costs for chemoprophylaxis are lower than for treatment, but the costs of administration, screening, transport, delivery, and monitoring would be similar. Thus, chemoprophylaxis is unlikely to be more cost-effective in developing countries than case treatment of

Figure 11-7. Cost-Effectiveness of BCG and Case Treatment as a Function of the Annual Risk of Infection

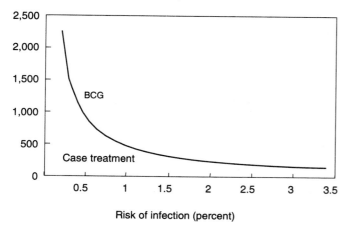

Cost per death averted (U.S. dollars)

patients presenting with symptoms suggestive of tuberculosis as discussed later. One exception may be in children under five exposed to an adult with active smear-positive pulmonary tuberculosis.

Decreasing Sources of Infection

The transmission of tuberculosis appears to take an extremely regular and stable course in comparison with most other infectious diseases such as malaria, schistosomiasis, or cholera. Each infectious or smear-positive person infects many others each year. The number of new infections caused each year by a person with smear-positive tuberculosis can be estimated from survey data on the number of new infections and the prevalence of smear-positive tuberculosis. It has been estimated from data from developing and industrial countries that an undiagnosed and untreated smear-positive source of tuberculous infection would infect on average between ten and fourteen persons per year (Sutherland and Fayers 1975; Styblo 1984). Each smear-positive person continues to excrete the bacillus for an average of two years, thus leading to the well-known 2:1 ratio of prevalence to incidence (Styblo 1984). A person with smear-positive tuberculosis will be responsible for approximately twenty to twenty-eight new infections before either dying or becoming smear negative. Figure 11-8 is an illustration in a schematic form of the nature of tuberculosis transmission.

A certain percentage of these new infections or reinfections caused by a smear-positive person will in turn break down and lead to clinical tuberculosis. Reference is made to three reports of newly infected persons to determine the percentage that developed clinical tuberculosis: the British Medical Research Council study (Sutherland 1976) found that 8.1 percent of converters developed clinical tuberculosis within fifteen years; in Saskatchewan, 6.4 percent of recently infected individuals developed clinical tuberculosis within a few years after primary infection (Barnett, Grzybowski, and Styblo 1971); and a Tuberculosis Surveillance Research Unit study of European data found that 6.0 percent of converters developed bacillary tuberculosis in five years (Sutherland 1968)). For the purposes of modeling transmission, we will assume that from 6 to 10 percent of new infections will eventually develop some form of clinical tuberculosis.[6] In figure 11-8 we show that the new infections could lead to 100 cases of smear-positive tuberculosis and 122 cases of smear-negative or extrapulmonary tuberculosis. The transmission cycle would then repeat itself over and over.

The steady state illustrated in figure 11-8 is a close approximation of reality in most of the developing world. Data on the annual risk of infection summarized in table 11-1 showed that the annual decline in the risk of infection for Africa and Asia was between 1 and 3 percent. Population in these regions is also growing at an annual rate of 1 to 3 percent, so the absolute number of cases of smear-positive tuberculosis remains nearly

Figure 11-8. Tuberculosis Transmission Schematic

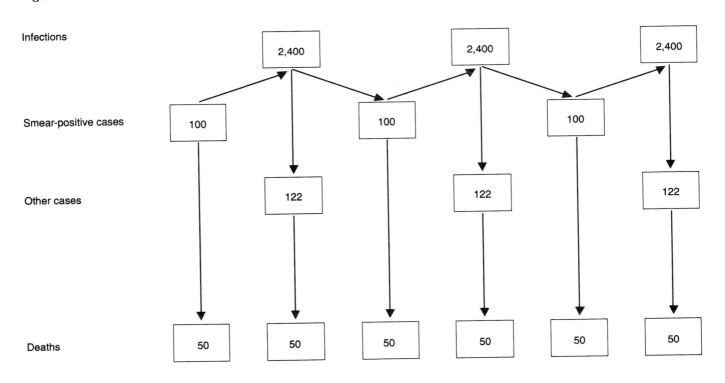

Source: Authors.

constant. In other words, each smear-positive case of tuberculosis must lead on to approximately one more smear-positive case after a round of transmission. The best way to prevent tuberculosis, therefore, is to interrupt the transmission cycle. As early as 1961, Crofton (1962) realized that chemotherapy for smear-positive patients, which rapidly renders them non-infectious, is the best way to reduce the transmission of the disease.

Risk Factors

The history of tuberculosis in industrial countries clearly demonstrates an important role for socioeconomic change in the decline of tuberculosis. In figure 11-9 we show how the age-specific tuberculosis mortality rates in the United States declined from 1900 to 1950, before chemotherapy was available. This decline appears to have been due to a decrease in transmission, because the case-fatality rates remained constant in this period (Drolet 1938). Reduction in transmission may have been a result of improvements in housing, nutritional standards, general health, and perhaps most important the policy, instituted at the turn of the century, of isolating infectious sources of tuberculosis in sanatoriums. During the first four decades of this century the annual risk of infection in most industrial countries was falling about 3 to 5 percent per year (Styblo 1984).

With the introduction of chemotherapy, tuberculosis mortality rates declined at a faster rate, approaching 10 to 12 percent. In some developing countries that have reliable registration of vital statistics, such as Chile, tuberculosis mortality was fluctuating and high before 1945, after which it declined precipitously. The most famous example of the effect of chemotherapy is in the Eskimos. In populations in Canada and Greenland, the risk of infection before 1950 approximated 25 percent per year. After aggressive case detection and treatment were instituted, the annual risk of infection declined by 17 to 20 percent per year. Tuberculosis mortality has followed a similar precipitous decline (Johnson 1973; Grzybowski, Styblo, and Dorken 1976).

The experience of industrial countries, and some disadvantaged groups in these countries, indicates that although socioeconomic changes can reduce the transmission of tuberculosis, widespread use of chemotherapy can greatly accelerate the decline in tuberculosis. In many parts of the developing world tuberculosis is declining at a rate of 1 to 2 percent per year. Improved case detection and case treatment could realistically accelerate that decline to 5 to 10 percent per year.

Three specific risk factors for developing tuberculosis deserve note. First, for the last few years we have been witnessing the strongest risk factor for developing tuberculosis in individuals remotely or recently infected with tubercle bacilli–HIV infection. The mechanism is easy to understand: the decrease in immunity caused by HIV infection results in the flaring up of this virulent agent, the tubercle bacillus.

Tuberculosis is thus one of the diseases in developing countries most influenced by the HIV pandemic. The interactions

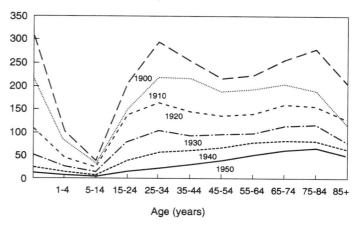

Figure 11-9. Age-Specific Tuberculosis Death Rates in the United States, 1900–50

Deaths (per 100,000 population)

Source: Vital and Health Statistics

between HIV and tuberculosis infections, particularly in countries where both infections are prevalent, appear more and more clearly. In several African countries, a considerable increase in newly discovered cases has already been documented (for example, Tanzania and Malawi). Tuberculosis is a frequent presenting symptom of HIV infection and AIDS in these and other countries.

The WHO Global Programme on AIDS, the WHO tuberculosis unit, and the IUATLD have initiated studies on the study on the various facets of the interactions of these two diseases, particularly, the epidemiological effect of HIV infection on the overall tuberculosis situation. Researchers suspect not only that HIV infection will increase the incidence of tuberculosis in individuals already carrying the tubercle bacillus, as a result of the decrease in immunity, but that the excess sources of infection will result in an increase in the annual risk of tuberculous infection in the country.

The two other specific potential risk factors for developing tuberculosis are mining and associated silicosis and malnutrition. The association between silicosis and tuberculosis has long been noted (Brink, Grzybowski, and Lane 1960). This relationship may explain in part the high incidence of tuberculosis in southern Africa and the Altiplano of South America, where a significant proportion of the adult male population works in mining and where there is an elevated prevalence of silicosis (De Beer 1984). Although the validity of this hypothesis has not been rigorously tested, the association between silicosis and high incidence of tuberculosis is accepted by many authors.

Malnutrition has been associated with increased incidence of and deaths from tuberculosis. During World War II, tuberculosis rates increased in European countries affected by the war, particularly in some special groups, such as in camps (Cochrane 1948) and in the Warsaw Ghetto

(Schechter 1953). There has been, however, no careful, controlled demonstration of this association, because crowding, recirculating air, and poor sanitation seem to be at least as important. Conversely, despite improvements in nutritional intake, the case-fatality rate for tuberculosis remained unchanged in the United States, England, Denmark, and other industrial countries from the turn of the century until the introduction of chemotherapy. Improvement in nutritional status may alter the probability of those who are infected developing clinical tuberculosis, and it may decrease the breakdown rate from infection to disease. As a pragmatic means of preventing tuberculosis, however, improving the general nutritional status of the population holds little promise, unless it is combined with an efficient program of case detection and treatment.

Curative Care

The subject of curative care can naturally be divided into tuberculosis detection and chemotherapy. We will address each of these in turn, highlighting the policy options.

Case Detection

There are two main issues in detecting cases of clinically significant tuberculosis: active as opposed to passive detection strategies and the choice of diagnostic technology. "Active detection" means an attempt to screen the population at large or target populations, such as military recruits, for evidence of tuberculosis. "Passive detection" means screening and diagnosing only those patients who visit a health service provider because of symptoms suggestive of tuberculosis. In the 1950s and 1960s, the choice between active and passive detection in industrial and developing countries was a controversial topic (Styblo and others 1969; Meijer and others 1971; WHO 1974; Toman 1979; Styblo and Meijer 1980). In the last two decades, a consensus for passive case detection of tuberculosis in all countries has developed—both WHO and the IUATLD advocate this policy.

Three assumptions underlie the wide acceptance of passive case detection as the primary strategy in tuberculosis control. First, 90 percent of patients with smear-positive pulmonary tuberculosis have objective symptoms, such as cough, fever, loss of weight, sputum, or hemoptysis. These symptoms develop quite soon after the onset of the disease, prompting the patient to seek medical advice. Second, the great majority of sputum smear-positive tuberculosis cases develop in a shorter period of time than the shortest feasible interval between two mass radiography survey rounds. That is why smear-positive tuberculosis cases were detected outside (and usually earlier than) the periodic case-finding campaigns conducted by the regular health services. Third, appropriate diagnostic and curative care ought to be physically, socially, and economically available. Most infections, before chemotherapy is instituted, would therefore occur within the family. Whereas in industrial countries it is estimated that two to three persons would be infected by a person with smear-positive tuberculosis before its detection, this number may be four or five in developing countries, because of a higher number of close contacts. No contacts will be infected after the start of adequate chemotherapy. The validity of these assumptions depends on local conditions, cultural perception of disease, access to care, and the effectiveness of health services.

Regardless of the technology used, active case detection is more expensive per case detected because the yield of tuberculosis per patient screened is lower. For example, if the incidence of smear-positive tuberculosis is 100 per 100,000 people, then the sputum of more than 1,000 people would have to be screened to detect one case of smear-positive tuberculosis, provided it is the general population that is being screened. If specific high-risk groups were identified, the yield would clearly be higher. For comparison, the use of sputum microscopy to screen patients who present with cough in Tanzania yields one patient in ten with smear-positive tuberculosis. Another argument against active case detection is that persons actively identified as being infected may be less likely to comply with long drug regimens. Clearly, they did not yet consider their health to be impaired enough to seek treatment. Moreover, a proportion of smear-negative persons with few or no clinical symptoms cure spontaneously and in a number of cases the disease is in regression (Styblo and others, 1969; Meijer and others 1971; National Tuberculosis Institute, Bangalore 1974). In developing countries, active case finding was studied by the Kenyan and British Research Councils in the late 1970s and early 1980s. These studies have yielded seven reports, and the conclusion in the last study is that a patient suffering from symptoms suggestive of pulmonary tuberculosis nearly always seeks medical advice from a health unit, usually several times. In many instances, however, health workers at the peripheral level do not think of tuberculosis and do not examine the sputum themselves or do not refer the patient to the nearest microscopy center for sputum examination for tubercle bacilli. In many developing countries, public transportation is rudimentary; even if available, it is not always affordable to poor people. Moreover, the Kenyan studies have shown that active case finding, except in health units, is not feasible.

The second issue in case detection is the choice of technology. At present, the main options are sputum microscopy, sputum culture, and radiology. To illustrate the yield and likely cost of case detection using microscopy (Ziehl-Nielsen stain), we shall examine data from the National Tuberculosis and Leprosy Programme in Tanzania. In that country, one in seven people who are suspected of having tuberculosis and are screened is identified as having smear-positive tuberculosis. Normally, three smears are conducted on each patient. The cost of supplies and reagents alone for these thirty smears is $2.50. A microscopist can examine about twenty sputa per day. The effective cost per case detected using sputum microscopy in Tanzania is $5.46, including the depreciated cost of the microscopes. In Tanzania, three sputa are examined to increase test sensitivity; the increased sensitivity achieved with the third smear is in fact small and could be sacrificed to reduce the cost.

Sputum culture is used to diagnose pulmonary tuberculosis in those patients who produce too few bacilli to be detected on a smear, to confirm sputum microscopy, and to characterize the type of mycobacterium. Because culture takes several weeks to yield results, it is not useful as a primary diagnostic tool in developing countries. For retreatment cases, however, culture and sensitivity may be very important to determine the most cost-effective drug regimen.

There are at least two different roles for chest radiography in the diagnosis and treatment of tuberculosis. First, for diagnosing smear-positive tuberculosis, chest radiography can be used to identify a group with a much higher probability of being smear positive. The resulting yield on sputum microscopy can be increased and many fewer total smear examinations undertaken. In areas where the prevalence of smear-positive tuberculosis is low, the increased yield may be important for maintaining the quality of sputum examinations. Unfortunately, x-rays are not 100 percent sensitive in detecting tuberculosis, so an initial screening with chest radiography will decrease the total yield as compared with sputum culture—for example, in Bangalore, x-ray was 87 percent sensitive. Second, chest radiography is essentially the only available tool for use in the periphery of most developing countries for the diagnosis of smear-negative tuberculosis. Sputum culture, although the gold standard for smear-negative diagnosis, takes too long and is too difficult to implement in the periphery of most developing countries. The role of chest radiography depends on the desirability of detecting and treating smear-negative tuberculosis; this subject will be discussed later in relation to cost effectiveness.

The cost per case of tuberculosis detected by x-ray depends largely on three factors. First is the prevalence among symptomatic patients presenting with x-rays suggestive of tuberculosis at health services. This can reportedly vary from one in two in China to a more realistic rate of one in four or five in Tanzania. The second factor is the cost of x-ray machines, which are expensive capital investments. The depreciated capital cost per patient screened depends on how much the machine is used. A district-level machine used for the diagnosis of many diseases is likely to be less expensive per patient than an underused machine dedicated to the detection of tuberculosis. Considerations of depreciated capital cost will require x-rays to be used at a level in the health services that has an adequate patient load. On the basis of hypothetical cost calculations, the cost per case of tuberculosis detected using chest radiography varies from $6 to $10 in China and Tanzania, assuming a caseload of 5,000 x-rays per year on a machine that costs $50,000 and lasts ten years. More research is needed on defining the true average and marginal costs of deploying chest radiography in various conditions for the diagnosis of smear-negative pulmonary tuberculosis.

New diagnostic technologies based on the enzyme-linked immunoabsorbent assay or DNA probes for mycobacterial DNA or RNA are currently being investigated (Daniel 1989; Bloom 1989). If these technologies yield new tools that can be inexpensively applied in developing countries, passive case detection may be improved, especially for smear-negative and extrapulmonary tuberculosis, which cannot be diagnosed by sputum microscopy. Active case detection in some high-risk groups would perhaps become feasible.

A limited number of interventions are available to improve the effectiveness of passive case detection. The factors that would be most important in improving such effectiveness are a high cure rate of diagnosed cases and a friendly relationship between the treating health staff and the patient. Public education can increase general awareness of the symptoms of tuberculosis and encourage those suspected of having it to seek medical advice. Improved diagnostic skills of primary health care providers, transport of sputum or a patient to a microscopy center, and availability of x-ray facilities can also improve the detection of both smear-positive tuberculosis and other tuberculosis. Finally, if diagnosis and adequate treatment are free, as recommended by WHO and IUATLD, more patients will seek early care.

Treatment

The first antituberculosis drug, streptomycin, became available in the early 1940s. In 1952, three antituberculosis drugs were available (streptomycin; para-aminosalicylic acid, or PAS; and isoniazid) which were able to cure virtually all patients however severe their disease, provided that their bacilli were initially sensitive to the above drugs. Such results were achieved in Edinburgh in 569 cases as far back as 1953 and 1954 and in 2,506 cases treated in 1955–56 (Crofton 1961). Since then a variety of chemotherapeutic agents have been developed. The six drugs recommended by WHO and the IUATLD and most commonly used in developing countries for tuberculosis are isoniazid, streptomycin, thiacetazone, ethambutol, rifampicin, and pyrazinamide. These drugs are used in a host of combinations for different durations (table 11-9).

Despite the availability of powerful and potentially effective antituberculosis drugs, tuberculosis treatment programs in most developing countries have not been very successful. Overall cure rates for most national programs in poor developing countries are below 50 percent. Evidently, the "standard" chemotherapy (isoniazid, streptomycin, and thiacetazone) recommended by the WHO Expert Committee on Tuberculosis (WHO 1974) for use in developing countries is presently, and probably will be in the future, beyond the organizational resources of many of them. This was clear to Canetti more than thirty years ago. As the principal reporter to the Panel on Eradication of Tuberculosis he stated: "On the global level, and among the efforts required to make some headway towards tuberculosis eradication, an absolute priority stands out imperatively: to develop chemotherapeutic methods adapted to the conditions prevailing in underdeveloped countries" (Canetti 1962).

In the 1960s and 1970s, experience showed that Canetti was right. In many poor developing countries in Africa, many parts

Table 11-9. Examples of Anti-tuberculosis Chemotherapy Regimens Used in Developing Countries

Regimen	Duration (months)
New smear-positive standard	
2SH/10TH	12
2SH/10EH	12
2SH/10S$_2$H$_2$	12
Short-course	
2SHRZ/6TH	8
2SHRZ/4HR or 2EHRZ/4HR	6
2HRZ/4HR	6
2RZ/4H$_3$R$_3$	6
New smear-negative	
2STH/10TH	12
2SHRZ/6TH	8
Retreatment	
2SHRZE/1HRZE/5H$_3$R$_3$E$_3$	6
2SHRZE/1HRZE/5TH	8

Note: S = steptomycin 1 gm; H = isoniazid 300 mg; R = rifampicin 450/600 mg; Z = pyrazinamide 1500/200 mg; E = ethambutol 25 mg/kg; T = thiacetazone 150 mg. Subscripts indicate the number of times each week drugs are given during intermittent therapy.

Source: Authors.

of Southeast Asia, and certain parts of Latin America, signs of improvement in the epidemiological situation of tuberculosis were the exception, despite widespread attempts at disease control. The most important reason for the failure of such control programs was the low cure rate. As Canetti postulated, unless a large increase in the cure rate for smear-positive pulmonary tuberculosis can be achieved, there will be no marked improvement in the tuberculosis problem in many developing countries in the foreseeable future.

Although there are many interesting issues in tuberculosis treatment, in this discussion we will stress the choice between WHO standard chemotherapy regimens that last from twelve to eighteen months and use fewer and cheaper drugs (isoniazid, streptomycin, and thiacetazone), and short-course chemotherapy that lasts from six to eight months and uses multiple and more expensive drugs (rifampicin and pyrazinamide). To compare these two strategies with chemotherapy, we must examine the relative effectiveness of each and the relative costs of each. Because of the great diversity in effectiveness and costs between countries, the emphasis will be on the key determinants of the effectiveness and costs of the two regimens. It should be stressed that the regimen with a higher cure rate leads to a more rapid reduction in the risk of tuberculosis infection and the incidence of active tuberculosis.

Effectiveness of Chemotherapy

The effectiveness of standard and short-course chemotherapy depends on three main factors: the cure rate, acquired drug resistance, and the effect on the trend of the risk of tuberculous infection. Without question, the most important of these

factors today in nearly all contexts is the cure rate, which decisively influences the remaining two factors.

One determinant of the cure rate is the biological effectiveness of WHO standard and short-course chemotherapy given under ideal conditions of 100 percent compliance. With short-course chemotherapy, after two months of treatment 80 to 90 percent of smear-positive pulmonary cases will have converted to sputum-negative status. Under WHO standard therapy, after two months 50 percent will remain smear positive. The "permanent" cure rate is a more important aspect of the treatment regimens. In figure 11-10 we show the percentage of patients who will remain or become smear positive, say, two years after the start of the (first) treatment (with no retreatment during the first two years), provided that chemotherapy is discontinued at each point in time. We shall refer to them as "failures.") (Patients who remained or became smear positive and died during the first two years will also be referred to as failures. Under short-course chemotherapy (for example, 2SHRZ/6TH [see table 11-9]), about 40 percent of those who discontinue chemotherapy at two months may be failures compared with approximately 10 percent of those who complete six months of short-course chemotherapy. Under standard chemotherapy (for example, 2STH/10TH), the failure rate in patients who discontinue standard chemotherapy after two months may reach 65 to 70 percent, and in those who complete six months it might be approximately 50 percent. The failure rate begins to drop significantly on WHO standard chemotherapy only after six months. By twelve months, under ideal conditions of 100 percent compliance, approximately 10 percent will become failures if treatment is stopped.

Since standard and short-course chemotherapy both give high cure rates and do not lead to secondary resistance in

Figure 11-10. Patients Failing Therapy after Two Years of Follow-up, as a Function of Months of Chemotherapy

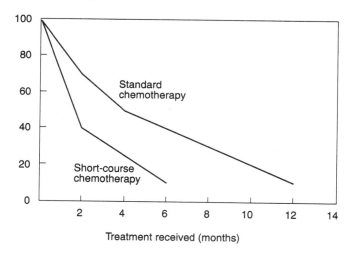

Source: Author.

controlled clinical trials, compliance is the most important determinant of the cure rate in national tuberculosis programs. There is a vast and detailed literature on compliance in general and on tuberculosis in particular (WHO Tuberculosis Chemotherapy Centre 1963; Haynes, Taylor, and Sackett 1979; Fox 1983a, 1983b; Chaulet 1987; Reichman 1987). Many of the factors that one might expect would influence patients' compliance with antituberculosis drug regimens, such as the severity of side effects, have not been empirically observed. There is a clear consensus, however, that the duration of treatment adversely affects compliance (Haynes 1979). Moodie (1967) in unusual circumstances in Hong Kong found that most noncompliers dropped out in the first three weeks; but all other studies have observed a steady dropping out over time (East African and British Medical Research Council 1977, 1979). Improved net compliance in shorter regimens is an important advantage of short-course chemotherapy over standard chemotherapy. Given the relapse rate as a function of months of treatment discussed above, in a situation where patients continue to drop out over time, short-course chemotherapy will have a higher total cure rate.

Another determinant of tuberculosis chemotherapy compliance is the degree of supervision of treatment. A spectrum exists, from giving supplies of drugs for multiple months to patients all the way to hospitalization for the entire duration of treatment. Between these extremes, a wide variety of supervision strategies are possible, including daily patient visits to health centers, health visitors contacting patients in the home, periodic urine tests to monitor compliance, and hospitalization for the first two months of treatment. Although increased supervision increases compliance in most settings (Haynes 1979), increased supervision also means increased cost. The balance of this tradeoff will depend on the specific institutional and cultural characteristics of each community. For example, in Madras, in areas where most of the population has ready access to health centers, entirely ambulatory care has been successful (Tuberculosis Chemotherapy Centre, Madras 1959; Dawson and others 1966). On the other hand, in many parts of rural Sub-Saharan Africa, the only way to guarantee daily supervision of chemotherapy may be to hospitalize patients for the first two months of chemotherapy; this has been the experience in seven African countries (Tanzania, Kenya, Mozambique, Malawi, Benin, Senegal, and Mali) (Styblo and Chum 1987).

The rationale for hospitalizing patients to ensure close supervision of the initial intensive phase is much greater in short-course chemotherapy than in WHO standard chemotherapy. Two months of short-course chemotherapy will convert smear-positive sputum into smear-negative sputum in about 90 percent of patients, and in another two to four weeks, in the remaining 10 percent. Even if they stop taking drugs one or two months after they leave the hospital, many will not relapse. In Tanzania, approximately 50 percent of smear-positive patients enrolled in WHO standard chemotherapy remain smear and culture positive at two months. For standard chemotherapy, it is crucial to continue to take isoniazid and thiacetazone

combined tablets daily for at least another two months to achieve 90 percent sputum conversion.

In all probability, the patient's perception of the effectiveness of treatment and the balance between discounted future costs and benefits of treatment are also important determinants of compliance. In Tanzania and other IUATLD-assisted national tuberculosis programs, it has been observed that both the perceived effectiveness of treatment and individual and group education of patients during the initial intensive phase of short-course chemotherapy positively affected compliance during the continuation phase.

Other possible determinants of compliance include the number of medications taken at each time, the number of doses per week, and the cost of therapy to the patients. Combination tablets of isoniazid and thiacetazone and isoniazid and rifampicin have been in use in national tuberculosis programs of many developing countries for several years. Conversely, intermittent standard chemotherapy (streptomycin and isoniazid) has never been used on a large scale in developing countries. In India, it has been shown that intermittency leads to increased irregularity of compliance (Pamra and Mathur 1973). Also Blackwell (1979) could not validate the expected relationship between reduced number of doses and improved compliance. The advantages and disadvantages of intermittent standard chemotherapy will not be addressed further here. The common sense notion that increasing costs both in time and money will decrease compliance has been confirmed in most studies (Haynes 1979). To maximize compliance, tuberculosis chemotherapy should be free and the spatial and temporal ease of access to treatment should be improved. When alternative treatments are available in the private and public sector, patients may initially prefer to pay for therapy perceived as better, but when funds run out they may switch to the public sector (Uplekar and Shepard 1991). This mixing of different drug regimens will tend to increase the failure rate and the probability of secondary resistance.

The second factor determining the effectiveness is the development of drug resistance. Under ideal conditions, such as in many clinical trials in patients with sensitive bacilli, the cure rates for both standard and short-course chemotherapy are over 95 percent. In patients infected with tubercle bacilli that are isoniazid resistant, the cure rate with total compliance is greatly reduced (Shimao 1987). Isoniazid resistance is already a significant problem in many developing countries (Kleeberg and Boshoff 1980). A systematic application of short-course chemotherapy referred to above (2SHRZ/6TH) in new smear-positive cases makes it virtually impossible to select for a bacillus resistant to all four drugs. Decreased development of resistance means that short-course chemotherapy is a substantially more effective long-term strategy for tuberculosis control than standard chemotherapy. It has to be stressed that acquired (and in contacts of the index cases, primary) resistance to both isoniazid and rifampicin results in incurability of the majority of such cases in developing countries, with serious consequences for elimination of tuberculosis.

Finally, tuberculosis is maintained in the community by the transmission of the bacillus from smear-positive patients to susceptible hosts. Short-course chemotherapy converts most patients to smear negativity faster than standard chemotherapy and more effectively because of higher cure rates and higher compliance. Therefore, fewer patients transmit the bacillus to new hosts. Short-course chemotherapy will thus lead to a more rapid reduction in the risk of infection and incidence of clinical tuberculosis. This transmission effect for the treatment of smear-positive tuberculosis has a significant effect on the choice of chemotherapy.

Costs of Chemotherapy

The cost of any tuberculosis control program is made up of the costs of many components, including drugs, staff, transportation, training, and hospitalization. Although drugs form a considerable portion of the budget, probably from 20 to 40 percent, they are not the only cost. Cost differences between short-course and standard chemotherapy, however, are attributable to the costs of drugs and hospitalization. The choice of suppliers, such as UNIPAC, Chinese pharmaceutical firms, or European companies, will have a substantial bearing on the costs of standard and short-course chemotherapy. Likewise, the size of the drug purchases have a significant influence on cost. Without a single agency or group that can evaluate the routine quality of antituberculosis drugs produced by different manufacturers, it is difficult to choose the most cost-effective supplier or suppliers. In general, the short-course regimen used in IUATLD national tuberculosis programs is approximately $20 to $25 more per patient than standard chemotherapy, depending on the supplier.

Another potential source of cost differences between treatment regimens is the level and intensity of supervision. Both standard and short-course chemotherapy should be given whenever possible on an entirely ambulatory basis. In some rural areas, however, where the population is without ready access to health facilities, daily regimens may have to be delivered in district hospitals to maintain acceptable compliance and cure rates. The experience of the national tuberculosis programs in Tanzania, Malawi, and Mozambique has indicated that hospitalization during the intensive phase of chemotherapy is indeed necessary in many areas. Not only will this improve compliance, but expensive and valuable drugs can be better accounted for in these conditions. Because two months of short-course chemotherapy can permanently cure more than 60 percent of patients as compared with standard chemotherapy, which cures only 30 percent, the higher cost of hospitalization may be more justified for short-course regimens in some circumstances.

This discussion has thus far been implicitly restricted to the treatment of smear-positive tuberculosis. Once other forms of tuberculosis have been identified, treatment costs for other tuberculosis should be similar to standard chemotherapy except for serious forms of smear-negative tuberculosis, such as miliary tuberculosis, tuberculous meningitis, Pott's disease,

Figure 11-11. Tuberculosis Program Costs

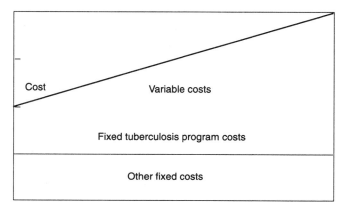

Source: Authors.

and so on. Those with these forms should be enrolled in short-course chemotherapy (patients with tuberculous meningitis should also be given rimactazid in the continuation phase of treatment). For treatment of cases in which the sputum or culture fails to convert in the first round of treatment, the drug costs are particularly high, because these patients harbor tubercle bacilli, frequently resistant, in developing countries, to isoniazid and/or streptomycin. Many of them have to be treated with short-course chemotherapy for retreatment cases, which should ideally contain three drugs to which the bacilli are sensitive. A retreatment regimen includes, as a rule, rifampicin and pyrazinamide. In the IUATLD-assisted national tuberculosis programs the following regimen is used: 2SHRZE/1HRZE/5H3R3E3 for patients resistant to isoniazid or 2SHRZE/1HRZE/5TH for patients sensitive to isoniazid. In programs that are committed to treating all patients that present for care, retreatment must also be considered in examining short-course and standard chemotherapy. Because failure rates are higher for standard chemotherapy, more resources would have to be devoted to retreatment of these patients.

Cost-Effectiveness

The cost-effectiveness of treating smear-positive tuberculosis will be addressed first. In general, the cost per death averted directly and indirectly will be lowest for smear-positive tuberculosis, higher for other tuberculosis, and highest for retreatment cases. Although this statement may run counter to intuitive notions of the clinical costs of treating each type of tuberculosis, the rationale is based on the effect of interrupting transmission, as explained more fully below.

Few studies have examined the cost-effectiveness of tuberculosis treatment in developing countries (Feldstein, Piot, and Sundaresan 1973; Barnum 1986; Joesoef, Remington, and Tjiptoherijanto 1989; Murray, Styblo, and Rouillon 1990). The authors of two of these investigations reported that per case cured short-course chemotherapy was more cost-effective. They did not, however, report figures on the cost per death averted. To fill the gap in information on the cost-effectiveness of short-course and WHO standard chemotherapy, the national tuberculosis programs in Malawi, Mozambique, and Tanzania have been studied by Murray and others (1991) and DeJonghe and others (1992).

Before detailing the costs per case treated, some unit cost definitions are needed. Program costs in these three countries can be divided into three components. The first is variable costs, which are a direct function of the number of patients treated and include costs such as drugs, reagents for diagnosis, and food during hospitalization. The second component is the fixed costs associated with the tuberculosis program itself, such as the salaries of district and regional tuberculosis coordinators, capital costs of vehicles, and administrative costs of the tuberculosis unit. The third component is the fixed costs incurred through use of the primary health care infrastructure, such as clinics and district hospitals. These three types of costs are illustrated in figure 11-11. Three unit costs can also be defined. Marginal costs are here defined as the average variable costs per case; average incremental costs are variable costs plus the fixed tuberculosis program costs per case; and average costs are total costs, including the fixed costs outside the tuberculosis program per case.

Table 11-10. Estimated Costs per Case Treated in Malawi, Mozambique, and Tanzania
(1989 U.S. dollars)

Treatment and type of cost	Malawi	Mozambique	Tanzania
Short-course chemotherapy with hospitalization[a]			
Average cost	160	217	174
Average incremental cost	99	155	127
Marginal cost	69	140	101
Standard chemotherapy with hospitalization			
Average cost	91	73	72
Average incremental cost	71	54	63
Marginal cost	42	40	37
Ambulatory short-course chemotherapy			
Average cost	66[b]	55	50
Average incremental cost	45[b]	36	41
Marginal cost	19[b]	18	15
Retreatment chemotherapy with hospitalization			
Average cost	209	323	252
Average incremental cost	141	232	182
Marginal cost	97	206	146

a. Hospitalization for sixty days during the intensive phase of chemotherapy.
b. Hypothetical estimate based on measured costs; ambulatory therapy is not actually provided.
c. Hospitalization for ninety days.
Source: Authors.

Table 11-11. Estimated Average Incremental Cost per Patient Treated in Low- and Middle-Income Countries
(dollars)

GDP per capita	Short-course hospital[a]	Short-course ambulatory[b]	Standard hospital[c]	Standard ambulatory[d]
150	136	63	113	41
250	181	70	159	48
500	296	87	274	64
750	411	104	389	82
1,000	526	122	504	100
1,250	641	139	619	117
1,500	756	156	734	134

a. Short-course chemotherapy with sixty days of hospitalization during the intensive phase.
b. Short-course chemotherapy with daily supervision during the intensive phase.
c. Standard chemotherapy with sixty days of hospitalization during the intensive phase.
d. Standard chemotherapy with daily supervision during the intensive phase.
Source: Authors.

In table 11-10 we provide the estimated average, average incremental, and marginal costs per case treated under short-course, standard, and retreatment regimens for smear-positive cases with and without hospitalization. These costs cannot easily be generalized to developing countries that have substantially higher incomes per capita than those in Malawi, Mozambique, and Tanzania, whose gross domestic product (GDP) per capita is under $300. Some treatment costs require foreign currency or are internationally traded goods; other costs are local costs that can be paid in local currency and are not traded commodities. By separating the external costs from the domestic costs, we can generate more representative estimates of the cost of treating patients in countries with different incomes per capita. The external component of the cost is assumed to be the same in all countries, whereas the domestic component is assumed to be proportional to GDP per capita. In table 11-11 we give our best estimates of the cost of chemotherapy in countries with different levels of income.[7] Notably, the cost of chemotherapy with hospitalization increases much more rapidly than ambulatory strategies as GDP per capita increases. In other words, chemotherapy with hospitalization is relatively more affordable in low-income countries.

The benefits of chemotherapy can be divided into the direct benefits for the patient of cure and a reduced death rate and the indirect benefit of reduced transmission. A life table for the prognosis of smear-positive pulmonary tuberculosis based on the most detailed study of the prognosis of pulmonary tuberculosis by Berg (1939) is provided in table 11-12. The Bangalore epidemiological study confirms the general case-fatality rates in a developing country (Olakowski 1973; National Tuberculosis Institute, Bangalore 1974). For each program, the cohort results of chemotherapy have been used to construct an alternative life table of the fate of cases treated by the program. Comparison of the treatment life table and natural progression

Table 11-12. Life Table for Untreated, Smear-Positive Pulmonary Tuberculosis

Year after diagnosis	Population alive at beginning of year	Deaths during year	Population excreting bacillus at beginning of year
0	100,000	28,596	100,000
1	71,404	11,564	51,334
2	59,840	9,771	30,928
3	50,070	5,705	18,605
4	44,364	5,055	11,851
5	39,309	3,545	7,549
6	35,764	3,225	4,938
7	32,538	2,074	2,230
8	30,464	1,942	2,174
9	28,522	1,818	1,463
10	26,704	—	985

— Not available.

Note: Based on Berg's study of 6,162 cases. By convention, the radix of the starting population is set at 100,000.

Source: Berg 1939; authors.

life table allows us to quantify the marginal benefits of treatment. A model based on the principle that in an untreated population one case of tuberculosis will lead to one case of smear-positive tuberculosis in the future has been constructed. Transmission benefits have been counted for four transmission cycles, which occur over the next eighteen and one-half years. Deaths averted and years of life saved have been discounted at 3 percent. In the model, it is assumed that passive case detection will lead to diagnosis after three months of symptoms and that during the first three months before diagnosis the rate of transmission is 50 percent higher than normal. This captures the increased rate of transmission to close household contacts during the period before diagnosis. The false positive diagnosis rate has been studied in Tanzania and is less than 5 percent. The study results are based on an assumed false positive rate of 5 percent for all three programs.

The cost-effectiveness ratios for short-course and standard chemotherapy with and without hospitalization during the intensive phase are summarized in table 11-13. Four ratios are provided for each intervention: the cost per case cured; the cost per direct death averted; the cost per total death averted, which includes deaths averted due to decreased transmission over the next eighteen and one-half years; and the cost per year of life saved, including transmission benefits. Three conclusions follow from the cost-effectiveness ratios. First, chemotherapy for smear-positive tuberculosis is extremely cost-effective. The average incremental cost per year of life saved ranges from $1 to $4. Second, short-course chemotherapy is preferable to standard chemotherapy in virtually all situations. The ratios in table 11-13 show that short-course chemotherapy is cheaper than standard chemotherapy for virtually all indicators of cost-effectiveness. The absolute difference in the cost per unit benefit is not large, but the cost-effectiveness ratios do not tell the whole story. The cure rate with short-course chemotherapy in all three countries is approximately 25 percentage points higher than with standard chemotherapy. In

economic terms, the depth of the margin is much greater with short-course chemotherapy than with standard chemotherapy. There are also several other unquantified benefits to short-course chemotherapy. Rates of secondary resistance with short-course chemotherapy are much lower. And the cost of retreating failures has not been built into the comparison. With standard chemotherapy many more patients will require the expensive retreatment regimens. The benefits of short-course and standard chemotherapy are summarized in table 11-14.

We do not arrive at equally robust conclusions concerning the appropriate role of hospitalization with short-course chemotherapy. Clearly, ambulatory chemotherapy is much cheaper per patient treated. Experience in Tanzania and Mozambique has shown that in urban areas with good health service facilities high cure rates can be achieved with ambulatory short-course chemotherapy. In the rural areas, these same programs have not been successful in employing ambulatory

Table 11-13. Estimated Average Incremental Unit Costs per Case Cured and per Death Averted in Malawi, Mozambique, and Tanzania
(1989 U.S. dollars)

Treatment and type of cost	Malawi	Mozambique	Tanzania
Short-course chemotherapy with hospitalization			
Per case cured	165	232	202
Per direct death averted	200	267	236
Per total deaths averted	38	57	47
Per year of life saved	1.7	2.6	2.1
Standard chemotherapy with hospitalization			
Per case cured	215	301	270
Per direct death averted	187	272	227
Per total deaths averted	54	76	68
Per year of life saved	2.4	3.4	3.1
Ambulatory short-course chemotherapy			
Per case cured	107	81	101
Per direct death averted	130	94	117
Per total deaths averted	25	20	23
Per year of life saved	1.1	0.9	1.1
Ambulatory standard chemotherapy			
Per case cured	111	82	107
Per direct death averted	96	74	90
Per total deaths averted	28	21	27
Per year of life saved	1.3	0.9	1.2

Note: For Malawi, the estimates for standard chemotherapy with hospitalization and ambulatory short-course and standard chemotherapy are not based on actual program results. The costs are based on estimates of the likely cost of ambulatory chemotherapy, and the results of treatment are the average results achieved in Tanzania and Mozambique.

The results for ambulatory treatment are based on the overall results of the program for each country, not on specific results of ambulatory chemotherapy. They are applicable only to those urban areas where high compliance can be maintained with daily supervised chemotherapy in the intensive phase.

Source: Authors.

Table 11-14. Costs and Benefits of Short-Course Chemotherapy and Standard Chemotherapy Based on National Tuberculosis Programs of Malawi, Mozambique and Tanzania

Parameter	Standard chemotherapy	Short-course chemotherapy
Average incremental cost per year of life saved with hospitalization (U.S. dollars)	3.00	2.00
Cure rate	60	85
Percent of cases requiring retreatment (percent)	30	10

Source: Authors.

chemotherapy. Because the determinants of compliance are complex and often locally specific, we cannot make general conclusions. We can, however, estimate the marginal cost per patient cured through hospitalization for any given percentage point increase in the cure rate purchased through hospitalization during the intensive phase. In figure 11-12 we show, for Malawi, Mozambique, and Tanzania, the relation between the marginal cost per case cured and the absolute percentage point increase in the cure rate achieved through hospitalization. We show that once the cure rate is increased by as much as 10 to 15 percentage points, hospitalization becomes relatively inexpensive per marginal patient cured. In middle-income countries, where the cost of hospitalization increases much more than ambulatory chemotherapy, the increase in the cure rate would have to be substantially higher to achieve the same marginal cost per patient cured.

In countries with poorly trained microscopists or frequent atypical mycobacteria infections, the predictive value positive of sputum positivity could be lower than 95 percent. The potential of wasting scarce resources on patients without tuberculosis puts a high premium on training health workers and microscopists to diagnose tuberculosis correctly.

Chemotherapy for Smear-Negative Pulmonary Tuberculosis

The cost-effectiveness of chemotherapy for smear-negative pulmonary tuberculosis is much more difficult to assess. The criteria both for diagnosis and effective therapy are less objective. A series of studies (see Toman 1979 for review and discussion) have shown that there is substantial variation in the x-ray diagnosis of active tuberculosis both between observers and by the same observer seeing the same film at different times. Cost-effectiveness can be discussed only in hypothetical terms and using realistic values from a variety of studies for the key parameters. There are four main determinants of the cost-effectiveness of chemotherapy for smear-negative pulmonary tuberculosis: the predictive value positive of x-ray diagnosis; the case-fatality rate of untreated smear-negative cases or cases suggested by x-ray; the effective cure rate of chemotherapy; and, perhaps most important, the percentage of tuber-

culosis cases diagnosed only by x-rays that would, if left untreated, progress to smear-positive tuberculosis.

The Bangalore epidemiological study provides one of the few sources for estimating these parameters (Olakowski 1973). Of 304 persons considered to have active or probably active tuberculosis according to radiological findings but who were smear and culture negative, a total of 13 percent became bacteriologically positive during five years of observation. If half of these were smear positive, that would be only 6.5 percent of those whose x-ray was suggestive of tuberculosis who went on to become infectious smear-positive patients. This percentage is the product of the specificity of the original x-ray diagnosis and the probability of true smear-negative persons progressing on to become smear positive. If diagnosis was only 50 percent specific, then 13 percent of the true smear negatives would have progressed on to become smear positive. This should be taken as the minimum estimate because smear-negative, culture-positive patients were excluded from the analysis. Short-course chemotherapy trials in Hong Kong have shown in a much more medically sophisticated setting that 56 percent of patients whose x-ray was suggestive of tuberculosis went on to develop bacteriologically positive or clinically active disease during a period of sixty months (Hong Kong Chest Service/Tuberculosis Research Centre, Madras/British Medical Research Council 1984).

In the Bangalore study, although the percentage becoming bacteriologically positive was low, the death rate of those whose x-ray was suggestive of tuberculosis was 30.9 percent over five years as compared with approximately 50 percent in bacteriologically confirmed cases. The mortality rate in the former cases was well over twice the baseline death rate in the study population.

Figure 11-12. Marginal Cost per Case Cured with Hospitalization and Short-Course Chemotherapy in Three Countries

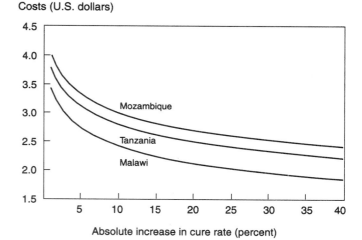

Costs (U.S. dollars)

Note: Costs are drawn on a log scale.
Source: DeJonghe 1993.

Using the average incremental unit cost for ambulatory therapy in Malawi, Mozambique, and Tanzania and a cheap short-course regimen for smear negatives ($16 per course), we will calculate the hypothetical cost-effectiveness. We will assume a predictive value positive of 50 percent for active disease detected on x-ray. The true value will be locally specific and could well range between 25 and 75 percent. For true smear-negative cases, we will assume a case-fatality rate of 40 percent. Because the regimen proposed is ambulatory and the symptoms in smear-negative patients are often less severe, we will assume that the effective cure rate would be on the order of 50 percent. With this set of assumptions, the cost per death averted is $450, or nearly ten times the cost per death averted of short-course chemotherapy with hospitalization for smear-positive patients and twenty times the cost of ambulatory short-course chemotherapy.

If a percentage of smear-negative cases do not progress to become smear-positive cases, then the costs of treating smear-negative patients are nearly an order of magnitude greater than the costs of treating smear-positive patients. On the basis of the Bangalore data, however, we expect that at least 10 to 15 percent would progress to become smear-positive patients. Treating smear-negative patients that go on to become smear positive cuts out the prediagnosis transmission that cannot be affected with chemotherapy for those who are smear positive. This prediagnosis transmission bonus accounts for nearly one-fifth of total transmission. If 15 percent of the cases progress to become smear positive, the cost per death averted by treating smear-negative patients is reduced to $185 and $155 if 20 percent become infectious. This is still three and one-half to eight times more expensive than treating smear-positive patients. In comparison with many other health sector interventions, this is relatively inexpensive per death averted or year of life saved. If the predictive value positive of x-ray diagnosis can be increased to 70 percent, the cure rate increased to 65 percent, and 20 percent of cases go on to be smear negative, the cost per death averted could be as low as $85.

The Ratchet Effect

Investments in chemotherapy for smear-positive tuberculosis are relatively secure as compared with investments in other infectious diseases. An illustration of how chemotherapy programs can ratchet down the incidence of tuberculosis is presented in figure 11-13. The top line shows the slow decline in the annual risk of infection in the absence of an effective program. After twenty-five years the annual risk of infection will only be reduced by 20 percent. A good tuberculosis control program should be able to reduce the annual risk of infection by at least 6 percent per year—for example, since the 1950s, the annual risk of infection in the West has been declining by about 10 percent per year. If after seven years, as shown in figure 11-13, the program collapses, then the annual risk of infection will revert to its baseline rate of 1 percent decline. There is no reason to expect, as with malaria, schistosomiasis, or hookworm, that the risk of infection will increase back to

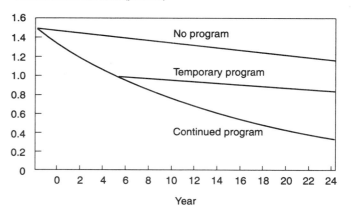

Figure 11-13. The Ratchet Effect

Annual risk of infection (percent)

Source: DeJonghe 1993.

previous levels. The number of people infected by a smear-positive patient is a function of the social patterns of interaction and household structure, not of the overall risk of infection. The last line shows the rapid decline in the risk of infection if investments in chemotherapy are maintained. Each investment, even if only temporary, has a permanent effect of ratcheting down the annual risk of infection and thus incidence.

With the HIV epidemic, it is possible that the baseline decline in the annual risk of infection in Sub-Saharan Africa may not persist and may even be reversed. In this scenario, although the annual risk of infection will not be ratcheted down by investments in chemotherapy, there will be a persisting benefit. The two lines labeled "No program" and "Temporary program" in figure 11-13 would increase slowly at the same rate, maintaining a permanent difference in the ultimate risk of infection, even many years into the future.

BCG and Case Treatment

One would like to compare the two main interventions for tuberculosis control: BCG and case treatment. They are, however, not truly comparable because even complete BCG coverage at birth will affect only 4 to 7 percent of mortality. Case treatment is absolutely necessary to reduce the other 90 percent and more of mortality. How does the cost-effectiveness of expanding BCG coverage compare with expanding case-treatment activities? The cost per death averted can be compared directly using the studies mentioned earlier. Some may object that a death between the ages of 0 and 14 represents a greater loss of years of life than a death at age 35. If we choose to examine discounted years of life lost, however, it will not significantly alter the comparison. A death at age 7, the midpoint for deaths averted by BCG, represents, at a 3 percent discount rate, 29.7 years of life lost, whereas a death at age 34, the average age of a tuberculosis death, represents 23.4 years at a similar discount rate. Therefore, we can examine the cost-effectiveness of the two interventions using the cost per death averted, bearing in mind that discounted years of life lost would change the relationship by less than 20 percent.

The cost per death averted through tuberculosis chemotherapy should change little as the risk of infection in a community declines. If all else remains the same, the only change would be the slight increase in the cost of detection as more cases of cough would have to be screened per case of tuberculosis detected. This does not hold true for any immunization, including BCG. The cost of immunizing all infants will not change as the risk of infection declines, but the benefits in terms of deaths averted will decline proportionately to the risk of infection. In other words, the cost per death averted through BCG must be inversely proportional to the risk of infection. In figure 11-7 we show two hypothetical curves for the cost per death averted as a function of the risk of infection. The curve for the cost-effectiveness of BCG is estimated on the basis of a single data point for Indonesia and the average cost per death averted for short-course chemotherapy with hospitalization during the intensive phase is based on data from Malawi, Mozambique, and Tanzania. Although the data are clearly weak, the principle is clear. At low annual risks of infection, case treatment is a substantially more cost-effective strategy than expanding BCG coverage. At higher risks of infection, the costs of both interventions are of the same order of magnitude. This curve should not be interpreted to mean that countries with low risks of infection should curtail BCG immunization activities. The discussion so far provides no insight into the savings from cutting back an existing activity as opposed to the potential reduction in benefits. This discussion does not imply that the policy choice in tuberculosis control is between BCG and case treatment. Some combination of the two is likely to be desirable in many countries. It does, however, indicate that BCG becomes relatively less attractive as the risk of infection declines.

Research Priorities

This discussion of tuberculosis leads naturally to some general recommendations for tuberculosis research. These can be divided into six areas.

EPIDEMIOLOGY. The wide confidence intervals in the estimates of incidence, prevalence, and mortality highlight the need for epidemiological research. Many countries require basic information on incidence and mortality rates and their distribution by age and socioeconomic status in order to establish the importance of tuberculosis as a health sector priority. For those countries that do not register vital statistics, new survey techniques based on the verbal autopsy may provide the tools with which tuberculosis mortality can be quantified.

PREVENTION. Because of the uncertain and variable effectiveness of BCG, a new effective vaccine would be an important tool, especially if it also prevented tuberculosis in already infected individuals. Fine (1989), however, has pointed out that, for moral and technical reasons, it will be difficult to test appropriately the effectiveness of any new vaccines. Research is also needed to explore the most appropriate role for chemoprophylaxis in developing countries.

DIAGNOSIS. Development of new tools for the rapid diagnosis of tuberculosis would substantially improve case detection. Research into serological or sputum diagnosis that can be deployed in peripheral health facilities in developing countries should be a priority.

CHEMOTHERAPY. Development of new, shorter acting, cheap drugs would help address two important issues in tuberculosis control: compliance and cost. Although opportunities exist for developing new drugs (Sensi 1989), relatively little research is under way. Another possibility that seems worth exploring is the use of depot preparations and four drug combination pills which could solve compliance problems.

PROGRAM DESIGN. There is an urgent need for operational and health economics research on strategies for tuberculosis control. Some key issues have been highlighted in this chapter: what is the tradeoff between the cost of supervision and the improvement in compliance, taking the existing infrastructure into consideration? What is the cost-effectiveness of alternative diagnosis strategies? These and many other issues need to be addressed in an organized fashion.

HIV AND TUBERCULOSIS INTERACTIONS. The interaction between HIV and tuberculosis has not been fully addressed in this chapter. It appears that immune-suppressed patients with HIV have a high probability of developing clinical tuberculosis. In Central and East Africa, tuberculosis programs are already reporting an increase in the number of cases of tuberculosis. The effect of any HIV-tuberculosis interaction on the annual risk of infection for the rest of the population is not known. Epidemiological study of these relationships has just begun and should be considered a priority for research.

Major Operational Conclusions

This review of tuberculosis can be summarized in six main points.

- The magnitude of the tuberculosis problem is simply staggering. Our estimates suggest that 2.7 million people die from tuberculosis each year. This is probably more than from any other single pathogen. The burden of tuberculosis extends beyond morbidity; the annual incidence of new cases of all forms of tuberculosis is over 7.3 million in the developing world. Tuberculosis is unique among the main killers of the developing world in that it afflicts nearly all age groups. Many children die from tuberculous meningitis and miliary tuberculosis. But the greatest burden of tuberculosis incidence and mortality is concentrated in adults age fifteen to fifty-nine. These are the parents, workers, and leaders of society. This heavy toll of the care givers makes tuberculosis a unique problem.

- In at least the last decade and a half, tuberculosis has been ignored by much of the international health community. Shimao (1989) has outlined the decline of the human and institutional capacity to address the tuberculosis problem over the last decades, which is but one symptom of a general lack of priority attached to tuberculosis action and research. Another example is the study done by the Institute of Medicine (1986) of vaccine development priorities for the developing world. The institute classified diseases into three levels of priority for research on vaccines. Whereas leprosy received significant attention, tuberculosis was not even mentioned in the lowest priority group. Clearly, focusing international attention on tuberculosis is the necessary first step if more resources are to be directed to combatting the disease.

- Existing diagnostic technology and chemotherapeutic agents can be used effectively in developing countries to cure tuberculosis. The IUATLD-assisted national tuberculosis programs (for example, those in Malawi, Mozambique, and Tanzania) have shown that short-course chemotherapy can be applied on a national scale with excellent results. Cure rates approaching 90 percent, even taking into consideration problems with compliance, can be achieved in the most difficult circumstances.

- Short-course chemotherapy and BCG immunization (in countries with high risks of infection) are some of the most cost-effective health interventions available in the health armamentarium. The analysis of the programs in Malawi, Mozambique, and Tanzania has shown that treating smear-positive tuberculosis costs $20 to $57 per death averted. The cost per discounted year of life saved is therefore $1 to $3. There are few interventions that are as cost-effective as tuberculosis case treatment.

- On the basis of country-by-country estimates, taking into consideration the estimated incidence and current levels of case detection and treatment, we estimate that $150 million in extra resources is needed to treat 65 percent of smear-positive patients in low-income countries and 85 percent of smear-positive cases in middle-income developing countries with short-course chemotherapy. Of this $150 million, approximately $70 million in foreign currency is required to address the problem of smear-positive tuberculosis.

- Evidence has accumulated that the interaction between HIV and tuberculosis may significantly exacerbate the epidemiological situation of tuberculosis. The potential rise, as a result of this interaction, in the risk of infection in Africa and other regions, depending on the spread of HIV, makes our operational conclusions about tuberculosis all the more pressing.

The combination of the enormous burden of the disease, years of neglect, the existence of effective interventions, and the availability of one of the most cost-effective interventions must make tuberculosis one of the highest priorities for action and research in international health.

Notes

1. The linear relationship between the annual risk of infection and the incidence of smear-positive tuberculosis will not hold at low annual risks of infection. As the annual risk of infection declines, the percentage of cases resulting from endogenous reactivation that are related to past levels of the annual risk of infection (during the last fifty to ninety years) rather than to current levels will increase.

2. There are two other problems with the interpretation of reported newly registered cases. For most countries, no distinction is provided between smear-positive cases and other cases. For countries in Latin America, the Middle East, and China, where a substantial portion of diagnosis is through x-ray, the numbers detected can be misleading. For example, in China, the widespread use of x-ray for diagnosis and the poor quality of microscopy means that only 10 to 20 percent of cases detected are smear positive. Many of the undetected smear-positive cases are probably diagnosed as smear negative with tuberculosis suggested by the x-ray. Many of the putative smear-negative cases, however, are probably misdiagnosed or overdiagnosed. Thus, if the total number of cases detected is divided by the estimated incidence, we will substantially overestimate case-detection rates. On the basis of discussions with national programs, we have adjusted the cases reported by China to reflect the likely overdiagnosis of smear-negative cases; data presented in Fox (1990) have been used to adjust the Indian data.

3. The midpoint of the confidence interval estimates is not equal to the expectation of the interval. When two 95 percent confidence intervals are multiplied, the resulting interval is actually much larger. In addition, the expectation is slightly lower than the interval midpoint.

4. If the age-specific case-fatality rate for ages twenty-five through twenty-four is assumed to be indexed at 1, then the other rates are: zero through fourteen, 0.9; fifteen through twenty-four, 1.15; twenty-five through thirty-four, 1.0; thirty-five through forty-four, 1.07; forty-five through fifty-four, 1.15; fifty-five through sixty-four, 1.65; and sixty-five and over, 2.5. The ratios for ages fifteen through sixty-five and over are based on Berg (1939); the ratio for ages zero through fourteen is based on case registration and tuberculosis mortality data for London during 1933–34 in Styblo (1984).

5. All dollar amounts are 1986 U.S. dollars.

6. The studies cited refer to the risk of developing clinical tuberculosis soon after primary infection. What about the risk of persons infected with tubercle bacilli developing clinical tuberculosis, with or without a fresh reinfection? Because it is not possible to detect reinfection with tubercle bacilli by tuberculin testing, it cannot be discovered directly whether or not exogenous reinfection is important in the development of tuberculosis in an adult. It is evident that in countries with low annual risks of infection, tuberculosis in elderly and old persons is predominantly a result of endogenous exacerbation among those remotely infected with tubercle bacilli. In developing countries, exogenous reinfection seems to play an important role in developing active tuberculosis in the adult population, because 0.5 to 2.5 percent or more of previously infected individuals are annually reinfected with tubercle bacilli, as was the case in industrial countries some two to four decades ago (Canetti 1972; Jancik and Styblo 1976). Strong evidence for the latter is the rapid decline in tuberculosis incidence in Eskimos over the space of twenty years, not only in children and young adults but also in elderly and old people, when aggressive case detection and adequate chemotherapy was introduced (Grzybowski, Styblo, and Dorken 1976).

7. This method is a modification of that of Barnum and Greenberg in chapter 21, this collection, who have calculated unit costs by the percentage of GDP per capita. External costs or the costs of internationally traded goods

whether they are domestically produced or not will not vary in proportion to GDP per capita. Local costs of nontraded goods, most notably labor, will in all probability change in proportion to GDP per capita. The distinction between external and domestic costs not only leads to different estimates of unit costs but can alter the relative cost of different interventions. As discussed in the text, the cost of an intervention with a higher domestic percentage of total cost will rise at a faster rate than the cost of an intervention with a higher percentage of external costs. Thus in a low-income country one intervention with a large domestic component may be cheaper than an alternative with a large external component. The relative cost-effectiveness rank could, however, reverse as income per capita rises.

References

Aronson, J., C. Aronson, and H. Taylor. 1958. "A 20-Year Appraisal of BCG Vaccination in the Control of Tuberculosis." *Archives of Internal Medicine* 101:881–93.

Barnett, G. D., S. Grzybowski, and K. Styblo. 1971. "Present Risk of Developing Active Tuberculosis in Saskatchewan According to Previous Tuberculin and X-Ray Status." *Bulletin of the International Union against Tuberculosis* 45:51–74.

Barnum, H. N. 1986. "Cost Savings from Alternative Treatments for Tuberculosis." *Social Science and Medicine* 23:847–50.

Barnum, H. N., D. Tarantola, and I. F. Setaidy. 1980. "Cost-Effectiveness of an Immunization Programme in Indonesia." *Bulletin of the World Health Organization* 58:499–503.

Berg, G. 1939. "The Prognosis of Open Pulmonary Tuberculosis. A Clinical-Statistical Analysis." *Acta Tuberculosea Scandinavica*, supplementum IV:vii–viii, 1–207.

Blackwell, B. 1979. "The Drug Regimen and Treatment Compliance." In R. B. Haynes, D. W. Taylor, and D. L. Sackett, eds., *Compliance in Health Care*. Baltimore: Johns Hopkins University Press, 1979.

Bleiker, M. A., H. J. Chum, S. J. Nkinda, and K. Styblo. 1987. "Tanzania National Tuberculin Survey, 1983–1986." In *Tuberculosis and Respiratory Diseases. Proceedings of the 26th IUAT (International Union against Tuberculosis) World Conference on Tuberculosis and Respiratory Diseases*. Tokyo: Professional Post-Graduate Services.

Bloom, B. 1989. "An Ordinary Mortal's Guide to the Molecular Biology of Tuberculosis." *Bulletin of the International Union against Tuberculosis and Lung Disease*. 64:50–58.

Brink, G. C., S. Grzybowski, and G. B. Lane. 1960. "Silicotuberculosis." *Canadian Medical Association Journal* 94:999.

Canetti, G. 1939. *Les réinfections tuberculeuses latentes du poumon*. Paris: Vigot Editions.

———. 1962. "L'éradication de la tuberculose dans les differents pays, compte tenu des conditions existantes (problèmes théoriques et solutions pratiques)." *Bulletin of the International Union against Tuberculosis* 2:608–42.

———. 1972. "Endogenous Reactivation and Exogenous Reinfection. Their Relative Importance with Regard to Development of Nonprimary Tuberculosis." *Bulletin of the International Union against Tuberculosis* 47:116–22.

Cauthen, G. M., A. Pio, and H. G. ten Dam. 1988. *Annual Risk of Tuberculous Infection*. WHO/TB/88.154. Geneva: World Health Organization.

Chaisson, R. E. and G. Slutkin. 1989. "Tuberculosis and Human Immunodeficiency Virus Infection." *Journal of Infectious Diseases* 159: 96–100.

Chaulet, P. 1987. "Compliance with Anti-tuberculosis Chemotherapy in Developing Countries." *Tubercle* 68:19–24.

Chum, H. J., K. Styblo, M. R. A. van Cleef, and M. Gunzareth. 1988. "Further Development in Tanzania National Tuberculosis and Leprosy Programme." Paper presented at the IUATLD (International Union against Tuberculosis and Lung Disease) Conference, Dubrovnik.

Clemens, J. D., J. J. H. Chung, and A. R. Feinstein. 1983. "The BCG Controversy. A Methodological and Statistical Reappraisal." *JAMA* 249(17): 2362–69.

Cochrane, A. L. 1948. "Tuberculosis among Prisoners of War in Germany." *British Medical Journal* 2:656.

Crofton, J. 1962. "The Contribution of Treatment to the Prevention of Tuberculosis." *Bulletin of the International Union against Tuberculosis* 32:643–53.

Daniel, T. M. 1989. "Rapid Diagnosis of Tuberculosis: Laboratory Techniques Applicable in Developing Countries." *Reviews of Infectious Diseases* 2(supplement 2):S471–S478.

Dawson, J. J. Y., S. Devadatta, Wallace Fox, S. Radakrishna, C. V. Ramakrishnan, P. R. Somasundavam, H. Stott, S. P. Tripathy, S. Vehi. 1966. "A 5 Year Study of Patients with Pulmonary Tuberculosis in a Concurrent Comparison of Home and Sanatorium Treatment for One Year with Isoniazid plus PAS." *Bulletin of the World Health Organization* 34:533–51.

DeJonghe, E., C. J. L. Murray, H. G. Chum, D. S. Nyangulu, A. Salamao, and K. Styblo. 1991. "Cost-Effectiveness of Chemotherapy for Sputum Smear-Positive Pulmonary Tuberculosis in Malawi, Mozambique, and Tanzania." WHO, Tuberculosis Unit, Geneva. Forthcoming 1993 in *International Journal of Health Management* 8.

Drolet, G. J. 1938. "Present Trend of Case Fatality Rates in Tuberculosis." *American Review of Tuberculosis* 37:125–51.

East African and British Medical Research Council. 1977. "Tuberculosis in Tanzania: A Follow-Up of a National Sampling Survey of a Drug Resistance and Other Factors." *Tubercle* 58:55–78.

———. 1979. "Tuberculosis in Kenya: Follow-Up of the Second National Sampling Survey and a Comparison with the Follow-Up Data from the First (1964) National Sampling Survey." *Tubercle* 60:125–49.

Feldstein, M. S., M. A. Piot, and T. K. Sundaresan. 1973. "Resource Allocation Model for Public Health Planning. A Case Study of Tuberculosis Control." *Bulletin of the World Health Organization* 48 (supplement):1–110.

Fine, P. E. M. 1989. "The BCG Story: Lessons from the Past and Implications for the Future." *Reviews of Infectious Diseases* 2(supplement 2):S353–S359.

Fox, W. 1983a. "Compliance of Patients and Physicians: Experience and Lessons from Tuberculosis." Part 1. *British Medical Journal* 287:33–35.

———. 1983b. "Compliance of Patients and Physicians: Experience and Lessons from Tuberculosis." Part 2. *British Medical Journal* 287:101–5.

———. 1990. "Tuberculosis in India: Past, Present, and Future." *Indian Journal of Tuberculosis* 37:175–213.

Frost, W. H. 1937. "How Much Control of Tuberculosis?" *American Journal of Public Health* 27:759–66.

Galtung Hansen, O. 1955. *Tuberculosis Mortality and Morbidity and Tuberculin Sensitivity in Norway*. WHO EURO-84/15. Copenhagen: World Health Organization.

Great Britain Medical Research Council. 1972. "BCG and Vole Bacillus Vaccines in the Prevention of Tuberculosis in Adolescence and Early Life." *Bulletin of the World Health Organization* 46:371–85.

Greenwood, A., B. M. Greenwood, A. K. Bradley, K. Williams, F. Shenton, S. Tulloch, P. Byass, and F. S. J. Oldfield. 1987. "A Prospective Survey of the Outcome of Pregnancy in a Rural Area of The Gambia, West Africa." *Bulletin of the World Health Organization* 65:636–43.

Grzybowski, S., K. Styblo, and E. Dorken. 1976. "Tuberculosis in Eskimos." *Tubercle* 57(supplement 4):1–58.

Haynes, R. B. 1979. "Determinants of Compliance: The Disease and Mechanics of Treatment." In R. B. Haynes, D. W. Taylor, and D. L. Sackett, eds., *Compliance in Health Care*. Baltimore: Johns Hopkins University Press, 1979.

Haynes, R. B., D. W. Taylor, and D. L. Sackett. 1979. *Compliance in Health Care*. Baltimore: Johns Hopkins University Press.

Holm, J. 1970. "Our Enemy: The Tubercle Bacillus." *International Tuberculosis Digest* 5 (IUATLD special publication.)

Hong Kong Chest Service/Tuberculosis Research Centre, Madras/British Medical Research Council. 1984. "A Controlled Trial of 2-month, 3-month, and 12-month Regimens of Chemotherapy for Sputum Smear-Negative Pulmonary Tuberculosis." *American Review of Respiratory Diseases* 130:23–28.

India, Ministry of Health and Family Welfare. 1986. *Health Atlas of India.* Directorate General of Health Services, New Delhi.

Institute of Medicine. 1986. *New Vaccine Development Establishing Priorities.* Vol. 2. *Diseases of Importance in Developing Countries.* Washington D.C.: National Academy Press.

Jancik, E. H., and K. Styblo. 1976. "Die Problematik der postprimaren mykobakteriellen Superinfektion-Versuch einer epidemiologisch-klinischer Sicht." In *Brecke: Fortbildung in Thoraxkrankheiten*, vol. 7. Stuttgart: Hipokrates Verlag.

Joesoef, M. R., P. L. Remington, and P. Tjiptoherijanto. 1989. "Epidemiological Model and Cost-Effectiveness Analysis of Tuberculosis Treatment Programmes in Indonesia." *International Journal of Epidemiology* 18:174–79.

Johnson, M. W. 1973. "Results of Twenty Years of Tuberculosis Control in Alaska." *Health Services Reports* 88:247–54.

Kleeberg, H. H., and M. S. Boshoff. 1980. "A World Atlas of Initial Drug Resistance." Report to the Scientific Committee on Bacteriology and Immunology of the International Union against Tuberculosis.

Leowski, J. 1988. *Global Status of Tuberculosis Control and Its Prospects.* WHO/TB/88.156. Geneva: World Health Organization.

Lindhart, M. 1939. *The Statistics of Pulmonary Tuberculosis in Denmark, 1925–1934. A Statistical Investigation on the Occurrence of Pulmonary Tuberculosis in the period 1925–1934, Worked Out on the Basis of the Danish National Health Service File of Notified Cases and of Deaths.* Copenhagen: Ejnar Munksgaard.

Meijer, J., G. D. Barnett, A. Kubik, and K. Styblo. 1971. "Identification of Sources of Infection." *Bulletin of the International Union against Tuberculosis* 45:5–50.

Moodie, A. S. 1967. "Mass Ambulatory Chemotherapy in the Treatment of Tuberculosis in a Predominantly Urban Community." *American Review of Respiratory Diseases* 95:384–97.

Murray, C. J. L., E. DeJonghe, H. G. Chum, D. S. Nyangulu, A. Salamao, and K. Styblo. 1991. "Cost-Effectiveness of Chemotherapy for Pulmonary Tuberculosis in Three Sub-Saharan Countries." *Lancet* 338:1305–8.

Murray, C. J. L., and R. G. Feachem. 1990. "Adult Mortality in the Developing World." *Transactions of the Royal Society of Tropical Medicine.*

National Tuberculosis Institute, Bangalore. 1974. "Tuberculosis in a Rural Population of India: A Five-Year Epidemiological Study." *Bulletin of the World Health Organization* 51:473–88.

Olakowski, T. 1973. *Assignment Report on a Tuberculosis Longitudinal Survey, National Tuberculosis Institute, Bangalore* WHO Project: India 0103. Published in Geneva. SEA/TB/129. World Health Organization, Regional Office for South East Asia.

Pamra, S. P., and G. P. Mathur. 1973. *Indian Journal of Tuberculosis* 20:108.

Preston, S. H., N. Keyfitz, and R. Schoen. 1972. *Causes of Death; Life Tables for National Populations.* New York: Seminar Press.

Pryer, J. 1989. "When Breadwinners Fall Ill: Preliminary Findings from a Case Study in Bangladesh." *IDS Bulletin* 20(2):49–57.

Reichman, L. B. 1987. "Compliance in Developed Nations." *Tubercle* 68:25–29.

Rouillon, A., S. Perdrizet, and R. Parrot. 1976. "Transmission of Tubercelle Bacilli: The Effects of Chemotherapy." *Tubercle* 57:275–99.

Rutledge, C. J. A., and J. B. Crouch. 1919. "The Ultimate Results in 1,694 Cases of Tuberculosis Treated at the Modern Woodmen of America Sanatorium." *American Review of Tuberculosis* 2:755–63.

Schechter, M. 1953. "Health and Sickness in Times of Starvation and Food Shortage." *Harofe Haivri* 2:191.

Selwyn, Peter A., Diana Harterl, Victor A. Lewis, Ellie E. Schoenbaum, Sten H. Vermund, Robert S. Klein, Angela T. Walker, Gerald H. Friedland.

1989. "A Prospective Study of the Risk of Tuberculosis among Intravenous Drug Users with Human Immunodeficiency Virus Infection." *New England Journal of Medicine* 320:545–50.

Sensi, P. 1989. "Approaches to the Development of New Antituberculosis Drugs." *Reviews of Infectious Diseases* 2(supplement 2):S471–S478.

Shimao, T. 1987. "Drug Resistance in Tuberculosis Control." *Tubercle* 68(supplement 2):5–15.

———. 1989. "Institutional Capacity for Disease Research and Control: Tuberculosis." In M. Reich and E. Marui, eds., *International Cooperation for Health; Problems, Prospects, and Priorities.* Dover, Mass.: Auburn House.

Smith, P. G. 1987. "Case-Control Studies of the Efficacy of BCG against Tuberculosis." In *Tuberculosis and Respiratory Diseases. Proceedings of the 26th IUAT (International Union against Tuberculosis) World Conference on Tuberculosis and Respiratory Diseases.* Tokyo: Professional Postgraduate Services.

Snider, D. E., G. J. Caras, and J. P. Koplan. 1986. "Preventive Therapy with Isoniazid. Cost-Effectiveness of Different Durations of Therapy." *JAMA* 255(12):1579–83.

Stilwell, J. A. 1976. "Benefits and Costs of the Schools BCG Vaccination Programme." *British Medical Journal* 1:1002–4.

Styblo, K. 1980. "Recent Advances in Epidemiological Research in Tuberculosis." *Advances in Tuberculosis Research* 20:1–63.

———. 1984. "Epidemiology of Tuberculosis." In G. Meissner and others, eds., *Infektionskrankheiten und ihre Erreger: Mykobakteria und mykobakteriellen Krankheiten*, vol. 4. Jena: Gustav Fischer Verlag.

———. 1985. "The Relationship between the Risk of Tuberculosis Infection and the Risk of Developing Infectious Tuberculosis." *Bulletin of the International Union against Tuberculosis* 60:117–19.

———. 1986. "Tuberculosis Control and Surveillance." In D. C. Flenley and T. L. Petty, eds., *Recent Advances in Respiratory Medicine*, vol. 4. Edinburgh: Churchill Livingstone.

———. 1988. "The Relationship between the Annual Risk of Tuberculosis Infection and the Incidence of Smear-Positive Pulmonary Tuberculosis." Unpublished.

———. 1989. "Overview and Epidemiologic Assessment of the Current Global Tuberculosis Situation with an Emphasis on Control in Developing Countries." *Reviews of Infectious Diseases*, 11(Supplement 2):S339–46.

Styblo, K., and H. J. Chum. 1987. "Treatment Results of Smear-Positive Tuberculosis in the Tanzania National Tuberculosis and Leprosy Programme: Standard and Short-Course Chemotherapy." In *Tuberculosis and Respiratory Diseases. Proceedings of the 26th IUAT (International Union against Tuberculosis) World Conference on Tuberculosis and Respiratory Diseases.* Tokyo: Professional Postgraduate Services.

Styblo, K., D. Dankova, J. Drapela, J. Galliova, Z. Jezek, J. Krivanek, Kubik, M. Langerova, and J. Radkovsky. 1969. "Epidemiological and Clinical Study of Tuberculosis in the District of Kolin, Czechoslovakia." *Bulletin of the World Health Organization* 37:819–74.

Styblo, K., and J. Meijer. 1976. "Impact of BCG Vaccination Programmes in Children and Young Adults on the Tuberculosis Problem." *Tubercle* 57:17–43.

———. 1980. "The Quantified Increase of the Tuberculous Infection Rate in a Low Prevalence Country to be Expected if the Existing MMR Programme were Discontinued." *Bulletin of the International Union against Tuberculosis* 55:3–8.

Styblo, K., J. Meijer, and I. Sutherland. 1969. "The Transmission of Tubercle Bacilli: Its Trend in a Human Population, Tuberculosis Surveillance Research Unit (TSRU)" *Bulletin of the International Union against Tuberculosis* 42.

Styblo, K., and A. Rouillon. 1981. "Estimated Global Incidence of Smear Positive Pulmonary Tuberculosis. Unreliability of Officially Reported Figures on Tuberculosis." *Bulletin of the International Union against Tuberculosis* 56:118–26.

Sutherland, I. 1968. *The Ten-Year Incidence of Clinical Tuberculosis Following 'Conversion' in 2,550 Individuals Aged 14 to 19 Years*. Tuberculosis Surveillance Research Unit (TSRU) Progress Report. The Hague.

————. 1976. "Recent Studies in the Epidemiology of Tuberculosis Based on the Risk of Being Infected with Tubercle Bacilli." *Advances in Tuberculosis Research* 19:1–63.

Sutherland, I., and P. M. Fayers. 1975. "The Association of the Risk of Tuberculosis Infection with Age." *Bulletin of the International Union against Tuberculosis* 50:70–81.

Toman, K. 1979. *Tuberculosis Case-Finding and Chemotherapy*. Geneva: World Health Organization.

Tuberculosis Chemotherapy Centre, Madras. 1959. "A Current Comparison of Home and Sanatorium Treatment of Pulmonary Tuberculosis in South India." *Bulletin of the World Health Organization* 21:44–51.

Tuberculosis Prevention Trial, Madras. 1979. "Trial of Vaccines in South India for Tuberculosis Prevention: First Report." *Bulletin of the World Health Organization* 57:819–27.

————. 1980. "Trial of BCG Vaccines in South India for Tuberculosis Prevention." *Indian Journal of Medical Research* 72(supplement):1–74.

Tuberculosis Surveillance Research Unit. 1966. *Progress Report*. The Hague.

UNICEF (United Nations Children's Fund). 1988. *State of the World's Children*. Oxford: Oxford University Press.

United Nations. 1986. *World Population Prospects. Estimates and Projections as Assessed in 1984*. New York.

WHO (World Health Organization). 1974. *Expert Committee on Tuberculosis, Ninth Report*. Technical Report Series 552. Geneva.

————. 1987. "Statement from Consultation on Human Immunodeficiency Virus (HIV) and Routine Childhood Immunization." *Weekly Epidemiological Record* 62:297–99.

————. 1988. "Reported Annual Incidence of Tuberculosis 1974–1987." Geneva. Mimeo.

WHO (World Health Organization)/Tuberculosis Chemotherapy Centre. 1963. "Drug Acceptability in Domiciliary Tuberculosis Control Programmes." *Bulletin of the World Health Organization* 29:627–39.

12

Leprosy

Myo Thet Htoon, Jeanne Bertolli, and Lies D. Kosasih

Leprosy has been referred to as one of the oldest diseases known to humankind. The earliest written records describing true leprosy come from India and there it was known as *kushta*. It is believed that from India it spread eastward to China and Japan and then westward to the lands bordering the Mediterranean. During the fourteenth century, the leprosy epidemic reached its peak in Europe. During the height of the epidemic there may have been as many as 2,000 hospices in France alone to care for the victims of leprosy (Browne 1985). The influence of the Crusades on the spread of leprosy in Europe and the effect of the "Black Death" (which wiped out a third of the population of that continent in 1349) on the decline of the leprosy epidemic has long been debated. For reasons still unknown, Europe was rid of the disease by the early nineteenth century. The last known indigenously contracted leprosy case in Britain was diagnosed in 1798 (Browne 1985). This decline of leprosy prevalence in Europe even before the advent of effective treatment and a century before the discovery of sulfone drugs has been mainly attributed to the changing socioeconomic environment brought about by the industrial revolution.

Leprosy is an infectious disease caused by *Mycobacterium leprae*. The host response to this infectious agent depends on the cellular immune mechanism. A person with a good cellular immune response who develops leprosy is more likely to have the milder tuberculoid type, whereas those with weak or lacking cellular immunity are likely to develop the lepromatous type (Bloom and Godal 1983).

The clinical spectrum of leprosy varies from a single benign hypopigmented skin patch that may heal spontaneously to widespread damage to nerves, bones, eyes, muscles, and kidneys. Long-standing disease may produce severe mutilation of the face and extremities, making the psychological trauma of leprosy victims at least as important as the physical suffering. The Ridley and Jopling classification system (Ridley 1974) defines the immunological spectrum of leprosy in clinical and histological terms, dividing it into indeterminate (I), tuberculoid (TT), borderline tuberculoid (BT), borderline (BB), borderline lepromatous (BL), and lepromatous (LL) types. The multibacillary form of the disease (BB, BL, and LL) is highly infectious and strongly positive on bacterial examination,

whereas the paucibacillary form (I, TT, and BT) is generally less infectious and is bacteriologically negative.

Onset of leprosy is usually gradual, and the first signs may not be apparent for quite some time after infection. The insidious onset and uncertain time of exposure make it difficult to calculate the exact incubation period. The average incubation period of leprosy is estimated to be two to four years, though it may vary from nine months to twelve years (WHO 1985b).

Before the days of modern chemotherapy for leprosy, the duration of illness was lifelong for some cases. Even with the discovery of dapsone, lepromatous cases were treated for life. With the recent discovery of newer drugs, the duration of illness has been drastically reduced. The World Health Organization now recommends that duration of treatment for a paucibacillary case be six months and for a multibacillary case, two years or until the skin smear becomes negative (WHO 1982), which may be on average three and one-half years. Even though the present therapy still takes months and sometimes years to cure a patient, when compared with previous treatments, it has greatly improved the prospects for a quick cure.

Since patients rarely die of leprosy, the case-fatality rate is negligible (Walsh [1988] estimates it is 0.1 percent). A few may die from complications of septic wounds or from severe reactions. This low case-fatality rate has made the disease appear to be less serious, especially when priorities are being set for health care by politicians and health administrators according to mortality rates and public outcry. Leprosy tends to be given a low priority, but the disability and economic loss it causes, along with the social and psychological problems the patient and his or her family suffer, make it more than an insignificant disease.

The disability suffered by leprosy patients is a secondary consequence of nerve damage caused by infection with *M. leprae*. The resulting anesthesia makes leprosy patients vulnerable to accidental injury of anesthetic tissue. In 1970 WHO formulated a disability grading system which categorized disability from such injury into three grades. The system has since been simplified. It is still a three-grade system (grades 0, 1, and 2 rather than grades 1, 2, and 3) with two separate sets of criteria, one for the hands and feet, and one for the eyes. The new grade 2, however, includes the previous grades 2 and 3.

The current grading system is as follows. For the hands and feet, the criteria for grade 0 are no anesthesia and no visible deformity or damage. A grade 1 condition is indicated by the presence of anesthesia, but no visible deformity or damage, whereas grade 2 is indicated by the presence of visible deformity or damage. Each hand and foot is to be assessed and graded separately. "Damage" in this context includes ulceration, shortening, disorganization, stiffness, and loss of part or all of the hand or foot. For the eyes, criteria for grade 0 are no eye problems due to leprosy and no evidence of visual loss. Grade 1 is indicated by the presence of eye problems due to leprosy but with vision remaining at six-sixty or better or the ability to see well enough to count fingers at 6 meters. Visual impairment is classified as grade 2 when vision is worse than six-sixty or the patient is unable to count fingers at 6 meters. "Eye problems due to leprosy" include corneal anesthesia, lagophthalmos, and iridocyclitis. Each eye is to be assessed and classified separately (WHO, Regional Office of the Western Pacific 1988).

The percentage of untreated patients who are disabled may reach 50 percent if the less serious forms (grade 1) of anesthesia arising from peripheral nerve trunk involvement are considered. If only the more serious forms (currently grade 2) of disability are considered, the percentage is about 32 percent (WHO 1980). Among the newly diagnosed patients, the percentage who are disabled (all grades) ranges from 2.7 percent in India (Mittal 1991) to 16 percent in some areas of Myanmar (formerly Burma) (Myint, Htoon, and Shwe 1992). Although multidrug therapy has reduced the occurrence of disability, the proportion of treated patients who are disabled remains high in some areas because many patients are diagnosed after irreversible nerve damage has occurred. Early diagnosis and treatment are thus important in reducing the proportion of disabled patients. Another reason that disability may remain common is the failure of leprosy control programs to incorporate the use of simple technologies for disability prevention as well as patient education. It must be noted, however, that despite rigorous efforts, even regarding early diagnosis and treatment, some patients will develop disability.

The World Health Organization has estimated that two-thirds of the leprosy cases in the world are still unregistered, so there may be as many as 2 million undetected, partially disabled patients (grade 2) in addition to the registered cases. It is estimated that 250,000 of those with leprosy are blind (vision three-sixty). This figure increases if a visual acuity of less than six-sixty is considered (Courtwright and Johnson 1988).

The clinical entity of leprosy represents a spectrum of immunological reactions to infection by M. *leprae*. Some patients have skin patches only (uncomplicated leprosy), and others have skin lesions complicated by immunological reactions ranging from mild to serious, producing such conditions as neuritis, iritis, and increased inflammatory response in the skin lesions. Very little is known about the incidence of reactions in leprosy patients because of the problems in defining the appropriate denominator, the total number of cases of the disease. Data on reaction incidence are usually from clinic sources, but many undetected cases exist which are not counted in clinic data.

There was initial concern that with the introduction of new bacteriocidal drugs in multidrug therapy, more patients might have reactions due to the release of antigens from the killed bacilli. But the results of studies of reaction incidence are encouraging. In a study by Boerrigter, Ponnighaus, and Fine (1988), the rates of the more serious type I reactions range from 76.9 per 1,000 person-years to 43.6 per 1,000 person-years in paucibacillary cases treated with the WHO multidrug therapy regimen. (Reactions are discussed later in this chapter.) Other secondary complications of leprosy infections include tissue necrosis, plantar ulceration, secondary bacterial cellulitis and osteomyelitis, and progressive absorption of the digits of the hands and feet.

Distribution and Risk Factors

Although leprosy is one of the oldest diseases known to humankind, very little is known about its natural history. The mode of transmission is still not known with certainty. The isolation of bacilli from loosened squamous epithelium of intact skin and from nasal washings of untreated lepromatous cases has led to the hypothesis that the portals of exit are ulcers on the skin and the respiratory tract (WHO 1985b). The two widely accepted modes of transmission are direct skin-to-skin contact and droplet dispersion, but there is still no clear-cut evidence to support their role in the spread of infection.

Age Distribution

The incidence of leprosy is bimodal. The first peak occurs between the ages of ten and twenty years and the second peak between the ages of thirty and fifty (Dominguez and others 1980). Clinical leprosy may occur in infants, but it does so rarely and only in children of those with the disease.

Sex Distribution

In most endemic countries both the prevalence and the incidence of leprosy is higher in males than in females. The higher occurrence in males has been attributed to the greater mobility of males, which provides greater opportunity for exposure and contact with infectious cases. It may also be attributable to failure to detect disease in females because of social attitudes, which result in less thorough examination of females by health workers. In a cohort study conducted in Myanmar from 1964 to 1976 in a population of 61,000 people living in highly endemic areas, the prevalence of leprosy for males was 42.2 per 1,000 and that of females was 32.6 per 1,000. The incidence rate for males and females was 7.0 per 1,000 per year and 4.9 per 1,000 per year, respectively (Dominguez and others 1980).

Host Factors

Until recently, humans were considered to be the only hosts and sources of M. *leprae* (Walsh and others 1977), but now there is evidence that armadillos are naturally infected with an organism which is indistinguishable from M. *leprae*. There is little evidence that these animals transmit the infection to humans, because armadillos are not found in areas of the world in which leprosy is hyperendemic.

That genetic factors as well as environmental factors have a role in the pathogenesis of leprosy is demonstrated by both twin and family studies which indicate that host genetics influence the type of disease that develops after infection (WHO 1985b).

Contact Status

The household contacts of persons with leprosy are at a greater risk of infection than nonhousehold contacts. And household contacts of those with lepromatous leprosy have a higher risk of infection than household contacts of those with non-lepromatous leprosy. A study conducted in the Philippines found that the attack rate in nonhousehold contacts was 0.83 per 1,000 person-years of observation. In contrast, incidence rates in household contacts of nonlepromatous and lepromatous cases were 1.6 and 6.23 per 1,000 person-years of observation (WHO 1985b). A similar study in Myanmar found that the cumulative incidence among nonhousehold contacts was 5.9 per 1,000 population per year and 21.9 per 1,000 per year among household contacts of lepromatous cases. For border-line cases it was 10 per 1,000 per year and for indeterminate and tuberculoid cases it was 7.6 per 1,000 per year (Lwin and others 1985).

Leprosy has been generally associated with poverty, and crowding may facilitate transmission (Noordeen 1985). Economic development has been proposed as a reason for the decline of leprosy prevalence in Europe and Japan. Consistent with this hypothesis is the twenty-year lag in the decline of leprosy (relative to the rest of the country) that was observed in the Okinawa prefecture in Japan, which had the slowest rate of economic development in the country. These shifts in risk factors appear to occur independently of any leprosy control activity, because they have been observed in countries with strict or relaxed isolation policies and in the absence of any other control measures. Once the situation is reached in which each new lepromatous case fails to produce, on average, one new secondary lepromatous case, the capacity for endemic persistence is broken, and disease incidence will gradually decline and ultimately reach zero (WHO 1985b). This process has important implications for leprosy intervention programs in endemic areas.

Physiological Factors

Claims have been made that puberty, menopause, pregnancy, lactation, stress due to infections, and malnutrition favor the onset of leprosy or lead to deterioration of a patient's clinical condition. These factors need to be studied in more detail to gain further information. Recent studies in Ethiopia suggest that there is a relationship between pregnancy and the onset or reactivation of the disease (WHO 1985b).

Current Prevalence and Trends

Estimating the number of leprosy cases in the world is a difficult task because the projections have to be based on the registered cases. These data may not be kept up to date, may contain misdiagnosed cases, and may be affected by incomplete reporting. With consideration of these potential inaccuracies, it has been estimated that the prevalence of leprosy in the world is 5.5 million cases. The geographic distribution of cases in the six WHO regions is shown in appendix 12A, table 12A-1. Of the 3.7 million registered cases in all the WHO regional areas, Southeast Asia has the largest estimated number of patients, 2.7 million. In this region, the majority of the cases (2.5 million) are in India.

There is no uniform distribution of either the disease itself or the various clinical forms. At the subcontinental level, the following patterns are recognized (WHO 1985b; see table 12A-1)

- *Tropical and subtropical belt of Africa and southern Asia.* This is considered to be the original source of leprosy; in these areas the disease can be traced back at least 2,500 years and remains endemic today.

- *Mediterranean basin.* Leprosy has probably been present in this region for 2,000 years, and still persists today, although prevalence of the disease is low and declining.

- *Northern Europe.* Leprosy was widespread in this area 1,000 years ago, reaching as far north as the Arctic Circle; however, from the thirteenth century, the prevalence of the disease has declined progressively. The decline observed in some populations of North America is in some ways comparable to the decline that occurred in northern Europe.

- *South and Central America.* Leprosy was introduced into this region from Europe and Africa, and the disease remains endemic today, although the incidence is declining in Venezuela.

- *Pacific Islands and Australia.* Leprosy has been introduced into several island populations during the last 200 years, and in some instances epidemics have occurred that have lasted for several decades.

The lepromatous proportion of cases (as estimated from case registries) also differs from region to region. In Europe this proportion is 20 percent, whereas in Sub-Saharan Africa it is 5 percent. In northern Asia it is between 5 and 20 percent (WHO 1985b). These differences may be the reflection of genetic, environmental, and cultural differences in the host populations. Diagnostic and reporting practices may also help explain the variation in the lepromatous proportion. The immunoepidemiologic studies conducted in Sri Lanka show that 5 percent of the total household contacts studied had antibodies to phenolic glycolipid antigen, which is produced by *M. leprae*. In the hyperendemic community of Micronesia, approximately 10 percent of the population have been found to have this antibody (WHO 1985b).

In endemic areas, the prevalence of leprosy is maintained at a relatively constant level. During the past century, however, increases in the prevalence of leprosy have occurred in some areas of the world according to a distinct temporal pattern.

In Nauru, Ponape, and Truk, Hawaii, Irian Jaya, and eastern Nigeria, leprosy epidemics have been reported with prevalence proportions of 10 to 30 percent. These epidemics have appeared in communities in which leprosy has been introduced only recently and where environmental factors favor the rapid spread of infection. The epidemics are characterized by a rapid increase in the incidence of paucibacillary disease and a very low initial incidence of multibacillary leprosy, little clustering among household contacts, and fairly equal distribution of cases by age. Incidence reaches a peak and is followed by a fairly rapid spontaneous decline (perhaps attributable to the infection of all susceptible individuals). During this decline the proportion of multibacillary forms of the disease increases, a shift is seen toward a higher incidence in children, and there is increased disease clustering among household contacts. Gradually the conventional pattern of endemic leprosy emerges (WHO 1985b).

Irgens and Skjaerven (1985) report that epidemiologic surveillance in Norway, the United States, Nigeria, Japan, Venezuela, India, and China, covering periods from 1851 to 1981, has indicated a consistent decline in incidence rates of leprosy. At the same time, the age at onset, the ratio of male cases to female cases, and the proportion of multibacillary cases have been increasing. The increasing age at onset may be attributable to postponement of infection to a later age or an increasing fraction of patients with long incubation periods or both. The increasing importance of long incubation periods is consistent with the shift toward multibacillary cases, in which the incubation period is longer than that in paucibacillary cases.

This mechanism was also reported during the decline of tuberculosis. Irgens and Skjaerven (1985) propose the general principle that an increasing fraction of new patients with long incubation periods, resulting in an increasing age at onset, should be expected in any disease in rapid decline which also has a long and varying incubation period. This theory offers a basis for assessment of secular trends.

Economic Costs

The indirect costs of an illness are all costs other than those for health care. As mentioned earlier, leprosy affects people in the prime of life, with peak incidence between ten and twenty years of age and again between thirty and fifty. As many as 16 percent (Myint, Htoon, and Shwe 1992) of those with the disease may have serious (currently grade 2) disability with concomitant loss of productivity. Thus, the indirect costs from loss of productivity might be expected to be significant.

The productivity loss due to deformity from leprosy in India was evaluated in a survey by Max and Shepherd (1989) of 550 leprosy patients randomly sampled from a rural and an urban area in the state of Tamil Nadu, India. Their analysis showed that elimination of deformity would raise the probability of gainful employment from 42.2 to 77.6 percent. The authors' extrapolation to all of India's estimated 645,000 leprosy patients with deformity suggested that elimination of deformity would raise productivity by $130 million per year. This amount is one-eleventh of India's entire official development assistance for all purposes from all sources in 1985 ($1,470 million).

In addition to the cost of loss of productivity, there are social costs associated with the loss of healthy life brought about by leprosy. These include (but are not limited to) the burden on family members of living with and caring for a disabled relative. The cost of these social consequences should be considered as part of the indirect costs of leprosy. Though they are not insignificant, these social costs are not readily calculable. They will vary from community to community and will be associated with the social and cultural values each society attaches to an individual's life.

The direct cost of an illness refers to the costs of medical care (paid by patients or society) to control or treat the illness. The direct costs of leprosy include the costs of drugs, drug delivery, supervision of drug delivery, laboratory facilities for diagnosis and for monitoring response to treatment, and reconstructive surgery and rehabilitation. The effectiveness of a control program depends greatly on adequacy of case detection, which in turn depends on the level of knowledge of health workers and members of the community. Therefore, the costs of case detection or screening efforts as well as training of health workers and education of the community must be included along with the direct costs.

Direct costs of leprosy have not been assessed systematically. Lechat and others (1978) tested the relative cost-effectiveness of current or potential control methods using a computer simulation model. The model has potentially serious limitations, however (Lechat 1981), and so will not be discussed further here. Wardekar (1968) found that the development of deformity results in increased use of medical care. Deformity thus adds to direct costs as well as indirect costs. In addition to the cost of medical care borne by the leprosy patient, wages lost while seeking care must also be considered as part of the direct cost. A more detailed discussion of costs and effectiveness of various control programs is presented in appendixes 12B–12G. The total cost of a leprosy control program is estimated in appendix 12H.

Prevention Strategy

Though leprosy has plagued humankind for centuries, gaps in knowledge about the disease still exist, especially with regard to the natural history of disease and transmission. Even though great advances have been made in the microbiology, immunology, epidemiology, and treatment of leprosy during the past two decades, from 1966 to 1985 there was a 90 percent increase in the number of registered cases. But more recently, from 1985 to 1990, the number of registered cases has declined by more than 30 percent. This decline has been attributed to the implementation of multidrug therapy and the consequent release of large numbers of patients from treatment. Multidrug therapy is also thought to increase the proportion of patients who present at an early stage of the disease, and thus it has a role in preventing and reducing the number and degree of deformity among new cases (Noordeen, Bravo, and Daumerie 1991) The risk factors and the primary prevention measures employed in leprosy control are presented in table 12A-2.

Leprosy is a disease with high infectivity but low pathogenicity and virulence. At present no specific primary preventive measure has been devised, and until this occurs, the main strategy for the prevention of leprosy must be early diagnosis and adequate and regular treatment.

Behavior

Many studies on social factors influencing leprosy have shown that it is a disease affecting the lower socioeconomic classes and that poor nutrition, sanitation, and personal hygiene, as well as overcrowding, are some of the factors which interact to influence persistence of the disease (Noordeen 1985). Improvement of economic conditions is beyond the scope of efforts to prevent leprosy. Still, any improvement of nutrition, sanitation, and personal hygiene through more broadly based health and education efforts should reduce the incidence of leprosy as well as that of a number of other diseases.

Environment

Lack of an adequate supply of clean water can lead to poor personal hygiene, which in turn may promote the transmission of leprosy, especially the skin contact mode of transmission. Though no supportive evidence has been presented for this theory, it is conceivable that the improvement in domestic water supplies in communities in which leprosy is highly endemic may disrupt the chain of transmission.

The high incidence rate among household contacts of leprosy cases may be attributable to overcrowding (Noordeen 1985). If droplet spread of infection does, in fact, occur in leprosy transmission, it is feasible that it might be facilitated in close quarters. Dealing with overcrowding is best done through a multisectoral approach involving population control, economic development, education, and health care services. Leprosy control would be only one of the many benefits of such a strategy.

Immunization

Several follow-up studies of the efficacy of BCG (bacille Calmette-Guérin) vaccine for the prevention of leprosy have been conducted. These studies have consistently found a protective effect of BCG against leprosy, but the vaccine effectiveness ranges from 80 percent in Uganda (Stanley and others 1981)

to 20 percent in Myanmar (Lwin and others 1985; see table 12A-3). In a recent case-control study conducted in Tamil Nadu, India, researchers found that BCG vaccine appears to increase the risk of indeterminate leprosy while offering 61 percent protection against borderline disease (Muliyil, Nelson, and Diamond 1991).

The wide range of effectiveness has been attributed to different vaccine strains, regional and racial differences, and the prevalence of environmental mycobacteria. Despite the large number of studies of the subject, however, the effectiveness of BCG vaccine for leprosy control is still not well understood. The cost per dose of BCG is approximately $0.05 (UNICEF 1991).

A combination of killed M. leprae and BCG vaccine was used for the treatment of borderline lepromatous and lepromatous patients in Venezuela (Convit and others 1982) with promising results. Recently Talwar and others (1990) have found that lepromatous patients given a combination of multidrug therapy and a candidate antileprosy vaccine based on Mycobacterium w show distinctly better clinical improvement. Such observations that vaccines may be effective even when given after infection has occurred may revolutionize control efforts in many endemic communities.

Even if BCG is only 30 percent effective in preventing leprosy, as was reported from southern India and Myanmar (Noordeen 1983; Lwin and others 1985), this is good news for leprosy control, because the 30 percent reduction would be a spillover benefit from tuberculosis control programs already in place. This spillover benefit is another reason to support BCG vaccination in childhood immunization programs. Further studies must be conducted to determine the optimal age for vaccine administration for protection against both tuberculosis and leprosy. Because these two diseases have different incubation and exposure periods, a single dose of vaccine, which is sufficient to prevent tuberculosis, may not be sufficient to prevent leprosy. (See appendix 12E for discussion of the cost issues involved in immunization.)

With use of recombinant DNA techniques, it may be possible in the near future to develop a multivaccine which is effective against both leprosy and tuberculosis. It will be necessary, however, to learn more about the antigens relevant to protective immunity. Katoch and others (1990) review recent progress in applying advances in molecular biology of M. leprae to the problem of vaccine development. Several trials of vaccines against leprosy are currently planned or under way.

Health Education

Education regarding leprosy should be directed toward two different groups: first, leprosy patients and their immediate family, and second, the community. The nature of the educational material should also be different for these two groups because the message or aim of the education program in each case is different. Leprosy patients should be thoroughly educated about the nature and natural history of the disease. Certain age-old beliefs should be delicately handled, as they may not be easily dispelled. The importance of regular compliance with prescribed therapy should also be stressed. Education of leprosy patients should be an ongoing process, and although it is time consuming, it should not be neglected. Failures in treatment with dapsone in the past have been attributed to neglect of patient education, although it is hard to pinpoint the number of relapses attributable to lack of health education.

Education to prevent injury in patients with nerve damage may reduce the loss of productivity which is so costly in leprosy. The patient's role in preventing permanent injury to hands and feet can be significant if he or she is taught to avoid activities that may potentially cause injury, to inspect anesthetic tissue regularly, and to practice early and correct wound care. Similarly, patients should be taught to prevent the opthalmologic complications of leprosy by avoiding eye dryness and protecting the eyes from injury (Watson 1988).

Educating the immediate family and the community is also necessary, especially in highly endemic areas. This will promote the early diagnosis of cases by making the community more aware and accepting of the disease. The goal of the program would be to encourage patients to come forward and obtain treatment rather than being ashamed of and concealing their disease. This is important because through early diagnosis a significant reduction in permanent disability can be achieved (Lechat 1985). Another goal of the health education effort is to dispel social stigmas through promotion of understanding of the disease. This will encourage a social environment in which the leprosy patient is treated in the same way as a person with any other disease. This social support is necessary if the leprosy patient is to lead the socially and economically productive life to which he or she is entitled according to World Health Assembly resolution WHA30.43.

Education of the community should be conducted as part of a general health education program. Education of persons with leprosy and their families should be a regular part of treatment. Although including education in treatment programs will add to their cost, the costs of neglecting education must also be considered. In the past, leprosy control programs which neglected education had limited effectiveness because of social discrimination, poor drug compliance, and lack of openness in dealing with the disease (Lechat 1985).

Treatment

If modern chemotherapy is to be of any help to leprosy patients, early diagnosis is crucial. It is important that cases be diagnosed before deformity has occurred so that they may be cured without leaving behind residual signs of this stigmatizing disease. Early case-finding activity must be promoted by leprosy control programs. Case finding may be passive or active. Passive case finding happens when patients come on their own to obtain treatment. It is greatly improved by increasing the accessibility of health care and also by promoting health education. A drawback of relying on passive case finding is that persons who are motivated to seek treatment on their own

usually have advanced disease and are already disabled. Such advanced cases have also acted for some years as a source of infection in the community. Active case finding usually involves screening of schoolchildren, contact surveillance, and mass population screening activities (Lechat 1985). Pre-employment screening of workers and military recruits may also be done but is usually not of much significance in leprosy control.

At present there is no specific screening test for leprosy which can discriminate an active from an inactive case with certainty (the current status of serological techniques in the epidemiology of leprosy is reviewed in Bharadwaj and Katoch 1990). Screening is based on clinical examination. This requires special training of health workers and is an expensive, time-consuming activity. The advantage of a well-conducted screening program is that cases are usually detected in their early stages. Because screening is costly, WHO has laid down guidelines for countries in which prevalence of leprosy is low (less than 1 per 1,000 population) and resources and personnel are lacking. In these countries, WHO recommends focusing only on surveillance of household contacts of lepromatous cases for a minimum of ten years after the index case is bacteriologically negative and on surveillance of household contacts of non-lepromatous cases for five years from the time of diagnosis of the index case. If these tasks prove impossible, it is recommended that contacts be examined at least once (WHO 1977).

Mass population screening programs are cost-efficient only in highly endemic communities and require careful planning and teamwork so that at least 95 percent of the population is covered. Without such high coverage the program may be unsuccessful, because those who are unwilling to come forward to be treated will continue to act as reservoirs of infection (WHO 1980; see appendix 12E for further discussion of the cost issues involved in screening).

Because most of the control programs in developing countries employ paramedical health workers for leprosy diagnosis at the village level, diagnostic criteria are needed which are simple and easily taught. The World Health Organization's four cardinal signs are useful for this purpose, although they may not be highly sensitive or specific. These four criteria are (a) a hypopigmented or hyperpigmented patch or macule, (b) an enlarged hard or tender nerve, (c) anesthesia in the area of the skin lesion, and (d) a positive skin smear. At least two of the first three criteria must be present.

With the introduction of more effective multidrug therapy, the cost of treatment per case has increased. Outlay of funds for drugs in specific control areas will also depend on the specificity of the health workers' diagnosis. Training of health workers thus improves the cost-effectiveness of treatment.

In the future, if diagnostic tools such as the polymerase chain reaction (PCR) technique are perfected, earlier and more rapid diagnosis of leprosy may be possible. At present, however, PCR is not easy to adapt to field conditions for several reasons, including the required use of radioisotopes and the expense of setting up the technique (Bloom 1990). Gillis and Williams

(1991) review possible uses of the PCR technique for studying leprosy.

Good Practice and Actual Practice

Treatment of leprosy is designed to render infectious patients noninfectious. Because there is no known animal reservoir for the disease, the chain of transmission could be interrupted if infectious cases in the community were made noninfectious through adequate and regular treatment. The chances of achieving control are greatly increased when at least 90 percent of the estimated multibacillary (infectious) cases are registered and treated regularly (WHO 1980). Historically, failure of many control programs in hyperendemic countries has been attributed to poor coverage and inadequate and irregular treatment of multibacillary cases. The number of new unregistered multibacillary cases is thus a useful indicator of continued transmission (WHO 1980).

As mentioned previously, a decline in the prevalence of leprosy has followed the introduction of MDT. Although MDT is thought to have led to a reduction in the number and degree of deformities among new cases, it does not completely prevent the reactions which lead to deformity (Noordeen, Bravo, and Daumerie 1991; Cellona and others 1990). The increasing acceptance of MDT among national health services and leprosy patients themselves is due to the fixed and relatively short duration of treatment; the low levels of toxicity and side effects; low relapse rates following completion of treatment; and the reduction in frequency and severity of erythema nodosum leprosum reactions (Noordeen, Bravo, and Daumerie 1991). Effective coverage of patients with MDT differs widely from country to country (Declercq and Gelin 1991), although on average it had reached 56 percent by October 1990 (Noordeen, Bravo, and Daumerie 1991).

The mode of delivery of treatment depends on the available resources, caseload, communication, manpower, and the type of drug schedule used. Two types of delivery used in hyperendemic countries are domiciliary treatment and stationary clinic treatment. Domiciliary treatment results in high coverage but is very costly, especially when supervised, because treatment with rifampicin and clofazimine must be given at least once a month. With domiciliary treatment, the delivery cost may outstrip available resources. In the latter case, the service area of the treatment program may have to be reduced, with rotation to a new area after completion of a minimum of two years treatment, or the program may have to be operated through a stationary clinic open at fixed times on fixed days of the week.

Treatment of locally endemic disease was one of the goals set for primary health care by the World Health Organization at the 1978 conference at Alma Ata. As a result of this recommendation, vertical leprosy control programs were dismantled in favor of integration of leprosy control into primary health care programs. The expectation was that with more personnel working in leprosy control, case finding would improve. In practice, however, because of the social stigma attached to leprosy, primary health care workers are often not highly motivated to work with leprosy patients, and case finding and management have suffered. This experience shows that training of primary health care workers should include education about leprosy and encouragement of the workers to take a more active role in case finding and management.

Because primary health care workers are not specifically trained to diagnose leprosy patients, they may be inaccurate diagnosticians. In particular, if their diagnoses are not highly specific, drugs and other resources will be wasted on patients who are false positives. In addition, patients who are falsely diagnosed will undergo unnecessary psychological stress. Therefore, it is important that primary health care workers be trained to improve their diagnostic skills and that the training be repeated at regular intervals to maintain a high level of diagnostic accuracy.

With the integration of leprosy control activities into primary health care programs, other activities such as WHO's Expanded Programme on Immunization compete with leprosy control for health care workers' time. In countries where leprosy is hyperendemic and resources are limited, the role of leprosy control may be reduced to drug delivery activities alone. Active case finding may have to be neglected, which will in turn result in a greater number of new cases with disability. The cycle of disability, social stigma, economic losses, poor treatment compliance, and further development of disability would then be perpetuated as in the days of dapsone monotherapy. Another danger is that poor compliance may lead to resistance to the newer drugs, as it did for dapsone monotherapy (WHO 1982).

Case Management

Treatment of leprosy is simple in the sense that there are very few alternative choices of drugs, but successful treatment is actually difficult. Often, case management has been simply equated with issuing patients the necessary drugs. But the psychological and social aspects of the disease must not be overlooked by health care workers, though this kind of comprehensive care can be difficult when caseloads are high. Health workers are often not trained to tackle the complexity of the problems leprosy presents. Failure to treat the leprosy patient as an individual in a comprehensive manner has often resulted in high treatment failure rates in countries in which leprosy is a significant problem. This high failure rate has also been attributed to the long duration of therapy. In the days of monotherapy with dapsone, paucibacillary patients were usually on a daily dapsone dose for five to seven years, and multibacillary patients were frequently on a daily dose for their lifetime. Lapses in compliance were common with such a long course of treatment, especially when unsupervised. This problem was further compounded by the irregular distribution of drugs by health care workers.

In the past, despite uneven patient compliance, treatment was often continued indefinitely because of the possibility of relapse. This resulted in great demand on leprosy clinics and control workers and precipitated a decline in the quality of treatment (WHO 1982).

Many control programs continue to have high dropout rates. A number of investigations have indicated that even the patients who collect the drugs regularly from leprosy clinics do not necessarily ingest them. Researchers of earlier studies in Malawi (Ellard and others 1974) and Myanmar (Hagan and Smith 1979) used urinary analysis to monitor the regularity of dapsone self-administration. They found that not more than 50 percent of the outpatients had taken the prescribed dose in the three days prior to attendance.

This irregular treatment is suspected of having been the main reason for the development of dapsone resistance. In 1981 it was estimated that the prevalence of dapsone resistance for all of Malaysia was as high as 10 percent of all treated multibacillary patients (WHO 1988b). The secondary dapsone resistance in India was estimated at 23 per 1,000 multibacillary cases in 1978 and in Jiengsin Province, China, it was 51 per 1,000, compared with 35 to 40 per 1,000 multibacillary cases in Shanghai (WHO 1982). Pearson and his colleagues (1977) reported an even more disturbing situation in Ethiopia. The resistance proportion was found to be 190 per 1,000. Along with reports of secondary dapsone resistance from all over the world, primary dapsone resistance has been reported in Ethiopia, India, the Philippines, and Malaysia (WHO 1982).

Fortunately, the effectiveness of the multidrug alternative to dapsone monotherapy has been quite encouraging. Boerrigter, Ponnighaus, and Fine (1988) found a relapse rate of 4.17 per 1,000 person-years among paucibacillary cases treated with the multidrug regimen recommended by WHO, as compared with 12.9 per 1,000 person-years observed by Jesudasan, Christian, and Bradley (1984) among cases treated with dapsone alone. The World Health Organization (Noordeen, Bravo, and Daumerie 1991) has recently reported a relapse rate of 0.10 percent per year for paucibacillary patients and 0.06 percent per year for multibacillary patients.

In a three-year assessment of multidrug therapy in India by Ganapati, Revankar, and Pai (1987), it was observed that out of an initial 253 persons with multibacillary leprosy who were treated, 67 percent were smear negative after twenty-four doses (two-year standard WHO regimen) and 75 percent were smear negative after thirty-six doses. In the same study, 18 patients who were smear positive at the end of the two-year multidrug treatment were observed without further treatment; it was found that 17 of them went on to become smear negative within two years. This study showed that multidrug therapy has a distinct advantage over dapsone monotherapy and is an effective regimen for both individual treatment and public health intervention.

In a follow-up study of 129 persons with paucibacillary leprosy who were treated for one year with the multidrug regimen recommended by WHO, Ramanan and others (1987) found that 83.7 percent had clinically active leprosy at the end of the year of treatment. Further studies are necessary to determine whether it is advisable to continue treatment of those with paucibacillary leprosy beyond the recommended six

months. A study by Neik and others (1988) found that 53 percent of those with multibacillary leprosy who were treated with the multidrug regimen recommended by WHO were rendered smear negative within two years and 94 percent within four and one-half years.

Unless new developments in vaccine production occur within a few years, there is little reason to expect that there will be a change in case management in the next decade. Any uncontrolled trial of a vaccine, of chemotherapy, or of a chemoprophylaxis program in a population that is beginning to undergo a "natural" shift in risk factors is bound to appear a success, although slowly. Even a controlled trial that alters environmental or host factors may not show rapid changes in subsequent incidence rates for the population because of the additional effects accompanying the natural decline described above. There is a minimum incubation period for leprosy, but the maximum interval from primary infection to disease onset may be as long as a lifetime. Thus cases may continue to appear for many years after the effective cessation of transmission, unless it becomes possible to eradicate the residual bacilli in all infected persons (Dharmendra 1986).

The case management strategy for leprosy can be divided into four categories.

- Treatment of leprosy
- Treatment of complications of leprosy
- Reconstructive surgery
- Psychological therapy and rehabilitation

Each category presents a unique treatment problem and must be tackled at different stages of the disease process. Case management interventions for leprosy are summarized in table 12A-4.

The primary and secondary level of management facilities should be general health care facilities that are already established in the community. This is important not only from the economic and feasibility aspect but also from a psychological standpoint. Separate facilities for the treatment of leprosy add to the isolation and stigmatization of patients with this disease.

Treatment of Leprosy

The treatment of leprosy with multidrug regimens serves four purposes. First, it interrupts the chain of transmission in the community by rendering infectious cases noninfectious. Though multibacillary cases may have infected others prior to treatment, one can assume that once they are treated, their role in the transmission of the disease has been diminished. Second, it cures patients of the disease. Third, it prevents the emergence of drug-resistant strains in the future. Last, it halts the disease process, and if the disease is treated in its early stage, it will prevent further development of deformity.

Treatment regimens for leprosy are considered separately for paucibacillary and multibacillary cases. Paucibacillary leprosy includes indeterminate and tuberculoid cases in the Madrid classification (WHO 1980) and I, TT, and BT leprosy in the Ridley and Jopling classification (Ridley 1977), whether diagnosed clinically or histopathologically. The bacteriological index must be less than two at any site (according to the Ridley scale [WHO 1982]). The World Health Organization has recommended a short course of therapy for paucibacillary cases with 600 milligrams of rifampicin once a month for six months to be given under supervision along with 100 milligrams of dapsone (1–2 milligrams per kilogram of body weight) daily for six months. The cost of drugs for the six-month course of treatment for a paucibacillary case is $2.15. It is estimated that the cost of delivery of the drugs is $4.50 and the cost of supervision of drug delivery an additional $1.35, bringing the total cost to $8.00 (see appendix 12C for details).

It is recommended that if treatment is interrupted, the regimen should be started again where it was left off and the full course completed. If relapse occurs after termination of treatment (release from control or discharge), the same treatment is to be restarted (WHO 1980).

Multibacillary leprosy includes both lepromatous and borderline leprosy in the Madrid classification (WHO 1980) and LL, BL, and BB leprosy in the Ridley and Jopling classification (Ridley 1977). The regimen recommended by WHO for a multibacillary case is 600 milligrams of rifampicin and 300 milligrams of clofazimine in a single dose once a month to be given under supervision along with 100 milligrams of dapsone and 50 milligrams of clofazimine daily to be self-administered. This treatment is to be followed for at least two years and is to be continued wherever possible until the patient achieves skin smear negativity (WHO 1988). The average duration of treatment for multibacillary cases should be about three and one-half years (S. K. Noordeen, Chief Medical Officer, Leprosy, Division of Communicable Diseases, WHO, personal communication August 30, 1989). The cost of drugs for a course of treatment of three and one-half years for a multibacillary case is $81.66. The cost of delivery is estimated at $31.50, and supervision of delivery is an additional $9.45, bringing the total cost of treatment to $122.61 per case. Considering that approximately 20 percent of cases are multibacillary and 80 percent are paucibacillary, the average cost per case is $30.92, a weighted average (see appendix 12C for further discussion).

The case management strategy outlined above should be implemented at all the four levels of management, namely household, primary, secondary, and tertiary. Apart from surgical care, both diagnostic and medical care should be provided at these four levels but at different levels of sophistication.

At the household level, simple diagnostic procedures should be performed by primary health care workers and the necessary drugs should be distributed if resources are available. At the primary management level, both diagnostic and medical treatment should be made available, especially when lack of resources prevents delivery of services at the household level. Even in instances in which household care could be provided, care at the primary level is still necessary for supervision and monitoring of therapeutic response and also in circumstances

in which second-line drugs, such as ethionamide or protionamide, must be introduced.

The role of the secondary level of management in the treatment of leprosy is limited and should be mainly concerned with treatment and diagnosis of the side effects of the multiple drug regimens (such as sulfone allergy to dapsone and liver toxicity from rifampicin) which are being prescribed in the catchment area of that facility. The tertiary level of management should be concerned with research and development of new drugs and treatment procedures and monitoring of drug resistance and side effects.

Treatment of Complications

Two types of reactions occur in leprosy patients. Type I reaction, which is seen commonly in cases of the tuberculoid spectrum, is the most serious type of the two because the patient may suffer from severe nerve damage within days and needs immediate referral, prompt care, and in some cases even hospitalization. Type II reaction, which is also known as erythema nodosa leprosum (ENL), is seen in the lepromatous spectrum of cases. Although it does not give rise to nerve damage immediately, ENL is an important clinical problem because patients may suffer from repeated episodes, which may cause a loss of confidence in the treatment regimen.

Reactions are only occasionally medical emergencies, although type I reactions require urgent action because of the potential for nerve damage and deformities. The most effective treatment at present for both types of reactions is prednisolone, which should be given in a very high dose, as much as 20 to 80 milligrams per day, to be slowly reduced, depending on the clinical response, to a daily maintenance dose of 5 to 10 milligrams. The duration of treatment varies from patient to patient. The daily prednisolone requirement may be discontinued within two to three months or continued for more than two years. Other general supportive therapy such as analgesics and sedatives, along with adequate rest and nutrition, is also important (WHO 1980).

Thalidomide has proven effective for ENL cases, with few toxic effects. But its known teratogenic effect prevents widespread use in the field from being a feasible option even though the drug is relatively inexpensive (WHO 1980). Clofazimine in a 200 to 300 milligram daily dose has an anti-inflammatory effect, but it takes four to six weeks to exert its effect and is toxic if used for long periods (Jacobson 1985). Its use in the treatment of reactions is limited to severe cases, but if used together with prednisolone it may lower the daily requirement of the latter.

Ulcers, another complication in leprosy, are a consequence of anesthesia occurring in the extremities due to peripheral nerve damage. Once the peripheral nerves have been damaged, nothing can be done to reverse the damage. Care of the anesthetic extremity becomes extremely important for the prevention of ulcers. The precipitating cause of ulcers are burns, mechanical pressure, and accidental injury to the hands and feet. The most effective way to treat ulcers is to immobilize or rest the affected part of the extremity. Antibiotics, along with surgical dressing, will also shorten the course of the ulcer.

Treatment of mild nerve damage and ulcers may be undertaken at the household level with frequent visits to the health care facility for necessary drugs and supervision. If a reaction is severe, with signs of nerve compression, the patient should be referred to a secondary facility. Ulcers complicated by osteomyelitis will require surgical intervention, which may be obtained by referral to a secondary-care facility. Tertiary care may be needed in some few cases in which reactions cannot be controlled or if osteomyelitis and osteoarthritis have become so advanced that amputation is necessary.

Reconstructive Surgery

Because reconstructive surgery is expensive and is not important for control of leprosy, it has been neglected by many control programs. But reconstructive surgery is very important for the social and psychological well-being of the patient. Correction of various deformities will also increase the economic productivity of leprosy patients. A further consequence is the promotion of trust in the health care system, and along with it, drug compliance.

Reconstructive surgery must be obtained in highly specialized tertiary-care facilities with a staff of reconstructive surgeons. The direct benefits in dollars are hard to estimate, especially when self-esteem and happiness are the greatest benefits of these procedures. Reconstructive surgery is required in 2 to 5 percent of all cases (Myanmar, Ministry of Health 1985).

Psychological Therapy and Rehabilitation

It is well known that many leprosy patients suffer from psychological and social problems. Many control programs focus their efforts on drug distribution and treatment of complications and pay little attention to the psychological and social problems of the patients. This lack of attention may be contributing to high dropout rates. Primary health care workers are normally not trained to provide psychological or rehabilitation services, but they should at least be trained to identify problem cases and refer them to secondary referral facilities.

Rehabilitation in leprosy involves the combined and coordinated use of medical, social, educational, and vocational measures for training or retraining the individual to the highest possible level of functional ability. The surest and least expensive rehabilitation is to prevent physical disability, which is done through patient education about self-care and through early diagnosis and treatment by clinicians. Rehabilitation must begin as soon as the disease is diagnosed (WHO 1980). Rehabilitation activities include:

- Health education of the public so as to reduce prejudice against the disease.

- Vocational training, which may be given in an institutional setting or on a part-time basis. Such training should not disrupt the patient's life.

- Prevention of disabilities by simple methods that can be applied in the field, such as simple forms of physiotherapy, provision of special footwear and crutches, and the teaching of patients to avoid injury and, when it occurs, to attend to it early (Watson 1988).

Priorities for Operations Research

As mentioned in the section on prevention, more research is necessary to understand the variability in the efficacy of BCG vaccine for the prevention of leprosy and to develop a more effective vaccine. Preliminary research has indicated that certain vaccines against leprosy used in combination with MDT as immunotherapeutic agents appear to be effective in the treatment of leprosy patients. More studies are needed to evaluate these findings. In addition, the sensitivity analyses presented in appendix 12D indicate that further efforts are necessary to determine more precisely the reduction in permanent disablement brought about by treatment of complications. Additional research that should be done includes study of the mechanism of transmission, incubation period, sensitivity and specificity of diagnosis by various methods, and the morbidity risks associated with early lesions of different types. Development of drugs that act faster than the current ones should also be investigated and the effectiveness of intervention programs determined.

Priorities for Resource Allocation

The application of basic concepts and principles of economic analysis and management science suggests that early diagnosis and adequate and appropriate treatment should be given the highest priority in leprosy control. Current projections indicate that a 60 to 80 percent reduction in the prevalence of leprosy may be achieved within five to seven years with widespread use of MDT (Noordeen, Bravo, and Daumerie 1991). Even if such a reduction in prevalence can be realized, disability in cured patients will still be a problem for many years. In addition, a continuing slow trickle of new cases (infected many years earlier) can be expected because of leprosy's long incubation period. The second priority for resource allocation should thus be research, with emphasis on development of a vaccine effective in preventing transmission and development of drugs with quicker action. Finally, resources should be allocated to prevention and treatment of disability in patients with nerve damage.

Conclusion

It is our conclusion that the benefits of leprosy control programs have been underestimated in the past and that the effect of the disease is significant in many developing countries. Studies of the currently recommended multidrug therapy program have found that it is effective in controlling leprosy. Furthermore, the cost-effectiveness analysis presented in this chapter indicates that the cost per year of healthy life gained (YHLG) from implementation of this regimen is quite low. Ranking leprosy control on a list of health care priorities will, of course, depend on its comparison with intervention programs for other diseases. Still, we urge the priority setters to consider the significant intangible benefits of a leprosy control program as well as the cost per YHLG presented here.

Appendix 12A. Tables

The tables below summarize incidence and risks of leprosy and its prevention and management.

Table 12A-1. Registered Leprosy Cases, by WHO Region

WHO region	Prevalence (per 10,000)	Incidence (per 10,000)
Africa	9.2	0.71
Americas	4.2	0.42
Southeast Asia	20.5	3.72
Europe	0.1	0.00
Eastern Mediterranean	2.6	0.15
Western Pacific	1.0	0.09
Total	7.1	1.09

Source: Noordeen, Bravo, and Daumerie 1991.

Table 12A-2. Risk Factor and Points of Prevention for Leprosy

Risk factor/point of prevention	Mechanism	Relevance to leprosy
Behavior		
Personal hygiene	Transmission	Low
Environmental		
Domestic water	Transmission	High
Public health		
Immunization with BCG vaccine	Resistance to infections	Medium
Health education	Transmission	Medium
Treatment		
Early diagnosis	Transmission	High
Adequate and regular treatment	Transmission	High

Source: Authors.

Table 12A-3. BCG Vaccine Efficacy in Control of Leprosy

Area	Subjects	First year	Age at vaccination (years)	Vaccine used	Follow-up (years)	Vaccine efficacy (percent)	Source
Uganda	16,150	1960	0–10	Glaxo	8	80	Stanley and others 1981
New Guinea	5,000	1962	All	Japan	14	48	Bagshawe and others 1989
South India	210,337	1968	All	Paris and Copenhagen	5–10	23	Noordeen 1986
Burma	28,220	1964	0–14	Glaxo	11–14	20	Lwin and others 1985
Malawi	80,622	1979	0–15	Glaxo	Less than 5 years	50	Fine and others 1986

Table 12A-4. Case Management Interventions for Leprosy

Strategy	Level of Management			
	Household	Primary	Secondary	Tertiary
Secondary prevention or treatment	Diagnosis, medical	Diagnosis, medical	Diagnosis, medical	Diagnosis, medical
Treatment of complications[a]	Diagnosis, medical	Diagnosis, medical	Diagnosis, medical, surgical	Diagnosis, medical, surgical
Reconstructive surgery	n.a.	n.a.	n.a.	Diagnosis, medical, surgical
Psychotherapy and rehabilitation	n.a.	Diagnosis	Diagnosis, medical	Diagnosis, medical

n.a. Not applicable.
a. In many developing countries, the leprologists and plastic surgeons needed for treatment of serious complications are found only in tertiary facilities.
Source: Authors.

Appendix 12B. Cost-Effectiveness Analysis

A cost-effectiveness analysis will be used to evaluate the costs of a leprosy control program. Such an analysis differs from a cost-benefit analysis in that input (cost of the control program) is considered in monetary terms and output (benefits of the control program) is considered in nonmonetary terms, whereas in a cost-benefit analysis both input and output are considered in monetary terms. The results of a cost-effectiveness analysis might be expressed as cost per death averted or per year of healthy life gained rather than as a ratio of cost of the control program to savings resulting from preventing loss of productivity. This approach is useful when the goal is to compare the costs of alternative strategies to achieve certain health outcomes or to compare the expected effect of each dollar spent across different disease control programs, the latter being the goal here.

A Supercalc microcomputer spreadsheet model developed by Ralph R. Frerichs of the Department of Epidemiology, School of Public Health, University of California at Los Angeles, will be used to evaluate the cost-effectiveness of a leprosy control program. The model is based on earlier work done in Ghana by the Ghana Health Assessment Project Team (1981). The model output is direct cost per year of healthy life gained. No attempt is made in the model to quantify indirect costs (or savings from preventing indirect costs) in monetary terms. The cost per YHLG was calculated for two different components of a control program, that is, drug therapy and treatment of complications, first individually and then in combination. The parameters of the model are:

- Average age at onset (AO)
- Average life expectancy at onset (L)
- Average age at death for those who die of the disease (AD)
- Case-fatality proportion (CF)
- Proportion of disablement prior to death of those who die of the disease (DPD)
- Proportion of those who do not die of the disease but who are permanently disabled (CD)
- Average level of disablement of the permanently disabled (CDP)
- Temporary days of disability (T)
- Level of temporary disablement (TPD)
- Incidence (I)

These parameters are entered first for the situation in which no intervention is undertaken. Then the proportionate changes in these parameters after intervention are entered into the model. From these changes, the model calculates years of healthy life gained from the intervention. It is then a case of putting in the cost of the intervention and dividing it by the years of healthy life gained.

Parameters were estimated as follows, assuming no intervention. The estimates come from data for Myanmar or represent educated guesses arrived at by consensus of two of us (Htoon and Kosasih) who had experience treating leprosy patients in developing countries.

- *Average age at onset:* 29 years (taken from urban data in Yangon, Myanmar).
- *Average life expectancy (at age of onset):* 41.52 years (data for Myanmar males, WHO 1985a).
- *Average case fatality:* 0.001 (Walsh 1988).
- *Average age at death of those who die of the disease:* 39 years (educated guess).
- *Proportion of disablement prior to death:* 0.8 (educated guess); the proportion of disablement is proportionate reduction in functional ability.
- *Proportion permanently disabled:* 0.16 (Myint, Htoon, and Shwe 1990).
- *Proportion of disablement of permanently disabled:* 0.5.
- *Temporary disability days:* 30 days; temporary disability for leprosy represents days during which the patient has skin lesions and suffers the accompanying psychosocial consequences but has no physical disability (educated guess).
- *Proportion of disablement of temporarily disabled:* 0.05; it is assumed that during the period of temporary disability, the patient does not have full productivity because of the psychosocial consequences of the disease, but that his or her productivity is reduced only slightly, that is, by 5 percent, because there is no actual physical disability during this period (educated guess).
- *Incidence:* 3 per 1,000 per year in Myanmar (Burma, Ministry of Health 1985). For each case of the disease, the model calculates:

Days lost because of premature death (x1):

$$(1) \qquad x1 = CF \cdot [L - (AD - AO)] \cdot 365$$

Days lost because of disability before death (x2):

$$(2) \qquad x2 = CF \cdot (AD - AO) \cdot DPD \cdot 365$$

Days lost because of chronic disability among those who do not die of the disease (x3):

$$(3) \qquad x3 = CD \cdot L \cdot CDPD \cdot 365$$

Days lost because of temporary disability among those who do not die of the disease and are not permanently disabled (x4):

$$(4) \qquad x4 = (1 - CF - CD) \cdot T \cdot TPD$$

Total days of healthy life lost (DHLL) because of the disease is, then, the sum of these four parameters:

$$DHLL = x1 + x2 + x3 + x4$$

Total days of healthy life lost per 1,000 population is calculated by multiplying total days of healthy life lost by incidence per 1,000 population.

Then, considering an intervention, the days of healthy life gained (DHLG) per 1,000 population is calculated by the following formula:

$$DHLG/1{,}000 = DHLL/1{,}000 - [I \cdot PI \cdot (DHLL - DHLG)],$$

where PI is the proportionate change in incidence.

The model has been used to estimate the cost per YHLG for drug therapy and treatment of complications. Some specific limitations of the analysis presented below should be emphasized. The state of the leprosy literature precludes accurate estimation of the various parameters used as inputs in the model. Therefore, the numbers used represent "best estimates." No sensitivity analyses were done on these "before intervention" parameters. Sensitivity analyses were done, however, for the effects of the three components of the intervention. These analyses involve varying the value of uncertain parameters within an expected range to see how sensitive the output (in this case cost per YHLG) is to the changes in a parameter. Sensitivity analysis is useful in that it provides some information about the degree to which the estimate of cost per YHLG might be inaccurate as a result of our uncertainty about a parameter.

Appendix 12C. Cost-Effectiveness of Multidrug Therapy

The first analysis considers the costs and benefits of drug therapy alone. The drug regimens are those recommended by WHO for multibacillary and paucibacillary cases (see the section on case management). Prices are taken from UNICEF's *Essential Drugs Price List* for July through December 1991. As shown below, the cost of drugs to treat a paucibacillary case is $2.15. It is estimated that the cost of delivery of the drugs and supervision is an additional $5.85 (see below for calculation of delivery cost), bringing the total cost of treating a case to $8.00. The cost of drugs to treat a multibacillary case is $81.66. It is estimated that the cost of delivery and supervision is an additional $40.95, bringing the total cost of treatment to $122.61 per case. Considering that approximately 20 percent of cases are multibacillary and 80 percent are paucibacillary, the average cost per case is $30.92 (a weighted average).

This multibacillary-to-paucibacillary ratio of 20:80 is based on the 1988 *Annual Report of the Leprosy Control Program,* Ministry of Health, Burma. The ratio was estimated for a leprosy endemic area in which multidrug treatment is not in use. Because paucibacillary cases are to be discharged after six months of treatment, their number will be quickly reduced compared with the number of multibacillary cases, which require an average of three and one-half years of treatment. Only after some years of multidrug treatment will the multi-

bacillary-to-paucibacillary ratio reach 50:50. The ratio will be even higher if the new case-finding activity is poor that discharged cases are not being replaced by an equivalent number of new cases. The cost per year of healthy life gained from treatment is calculated to be $12.71 per YHLG.

Details of the Calculations

Cost per case was first calculated separately for treatment of multibacillary and paucibacillary cases. The WHO treatment regimens and the calculation of costs per case (with use of the *Essential Drugs Price List*) were as follows:

- *Paucibacillary cases:* 600 milligrams of rifampicin once a month for six months. Rifampicin comes in 300-milligram tablets, so twelve tablets of 300 milligrams are needed.

$$12 \cdot \$9.87/100 = \$1.18.$$

100 milligrams of dapsone daily for six months. Approximately 190 doses are needed.

$$190 \cdot \$5.10/1000 = \$0.97.$$

The cost per case of delivering the drugs is estimated in the following way (from Myanmar, Ministry of Health 1985: the cost of delivery, including salaries and traveling allowances, is estimated at 4,664,000 kyats for 1985. At the exchange rate of 7 kyats to the U.S. dollar, this is equal to 4,664,000 divided by 7, or $666,286. The total number of cases treated in 1985 in Myanmar was 221,125. Thus the cost of delivery per case is $666,286 divided by 221,125, or $3 per case per year. This figure includes the cost of supervision, but not of vehicles, because the latter are to be considered as part of the capital cost. As endemicity decreases, the delivery cost is likely to go up. This $3 per case per year is calculated under the assumption of high endemicity and represents the cost for an average of four visits by health care workers. Six visits are needed for paucibacillary cases, however, so the cost of delivery for a paucibacillary case will be $3 · 6/4 = $4.50. The additional cost for supervision of drug delivery is estimated to be 30 percent of the delivery cost, or $1.35.

Thus, the total cost of drug therapy for a paucibacillary case is equal to

$$\$1.18 + \$0.97 + \$4.50 + \$1.35 = \$8.00.$$

- *Multibacillary cases:* 600 milligrams of rifampicin once a month for three and one-half years (Dr. S. K. Noordeen, Chief Medical Officer, Leprosy, Division of Communicable Diseases, WHO, personal communication August 30, 1989). Rifampicin comes in 300-milligram tablets, so 84 tablets (2 · 42) are needed.

$$84 \cdot \$9.87/100 = \$8.29.$$

300 milligrams of clofazimine once a month for three and one-half years. Clofazimine comes in 100-milligram capsules, so 126 capsules (3 · 42) are needed.

$$126 · \$96.74/1000 = \$12.19.$$

100 milligrams of dapsone daily for three and one-half years, so 1,278 tablets (3.5 · 365) are needed.

$$1,278 · \$5.10/1,000 = \$6.52.$$

50 milligrams of clofazimine daily for three and one-half years (except the forty-two days on which a 300-milligram clofazimine dose is taken), so 1,130 capsules (3.5 · [365 - 42]) are needed. A price is listed only for 100-milligram capsules, so this price will be halved for the calculation.

$$1,130 · (\$96.74/2)/1000 = \$54.66.$$

The cost per case of delivering the drugs for a multibacillary case is estimated as above for paucibacillary cases. If it costs $3 per case for an average of four visits to deliver drugs in Myanmar, and if forty-two visits are necessary for a multibacillary case, the delivery cost for a multibacillary case will

be $31.50 ($3 · 42/4). Thirty percent of the drug delivery cost ($9.45) will be added to cover the cost of supervision of drug delivery.

So the total cost of drug therapy for a multibacillary case is:

$$\$8.29 + \$12.19 + \$6.52 + \$54.66 + \$31.50 + \$9.45 = \$122.61.$$

Note: This may be an overestimate of cost for some multibacillary cases because treatment may be needed for only two years.

• Given that approximately 80 percent of cases of leprosy are paucibacillary cases, and 20 percent are multibacillary cases, the average cost of treating a leprosy case can be estimated by taking a weighted average:

$$(0.80 · \$8.00) + (0.20 · \$122.61) = \$30.92.$$

In the first analysis, the following initial assumptions were made (based on best estimates):

• That treatment of multibacillary and paucibacillary patients would reduce by 33 percent the proportion of patients who do not die but are permanently disabled and would reduce by 60 percent the level of disablement of these cases.

Table 12C-1. Cost-Effectiveness of Treatment Programs for Leprosy

Parameter	Baseline	With interventions	
		Drug therapy	Complications
Average case fatality	0.001	No change	No change
Annual incidence (new cases per 1,,000 population)	3.00	No change	No change
Average age at disease onset (years)	29	No change	No change
Average life expectancy at disease onset (years)	41.52	No change	No change
Average age at death from leprosy (years)	39	No change	No change
Proportion disablement of fatalities	0.8	No change	No change
Proportion of survivors permanently disabled	0.16	0.67	No change
Proportion disablement of permantly disabled	0.5	0.4	0.8
Temporarily disabled			
Days of temporary disability	30	0.67	0.8
Proportion disablement during period of temporary disability	0.05	No change	0.8
DHLL/DHLG *per case*[b]			
From premature death	11.50	0.00	0.00
From disability before death	2.92	0.00	0.00
From permanent disability among survivors	1,212.38	887.47	242.48
From temporary disability among survivors	1.26	0.36	0.45
Total	1,228	888	243
Total per 1,000 population per year	3,684	2,663	729
Costs of intervention			
Per case (dollars)	n.a.	30.92	225.00
Per YHLG (dollars)	n.a.	12.71	338.06

n.a. Not applicable.
a. Expected proportionate increase or decrease as result of multiple drug therapy and treatment of complications.
b. For baseline, days of healthy life lost. For intervention, days of healthy life gained from reduction of listed parameter.
c. Represents 98.72 percent of total DHLL per case.
Source: Authors.

- That treatment would also reduce the number of days of temporary disability by 33 percent.
- That treatment would not affect any of the other parameters of the model. (Eventually treatment of patients would reduce the incidence by decreasing the numbers of patients who are acting as sources of infection. This idea will be explored in the sensitivity analysis.)

In table 12C-1 we summarize the cost-effectiveness of treatment according to the model.

Results

The average cost of treating a leprosy patient (regardless of type of leprosy) is $12.71 per YHLG. It must be mentioned that the cost of laboratory facilities needed for confirmation of diagnosis and for determination of bacteriologic status of patients at the end of the course of treatment is not included in this calculation. Neither is the benefit of reduced incidence, which would come in time if the treatment program is maintained (although this will be discussed below).

Sensitivity Analysis

A sensitivity analysis was done to determine how much the cost per YHLG would be affected by varying the effects of drug therapy on the proportion of patients who are permanently disabled, the proportion of disablement of the permanently disabled, the temporary disability days, and the incidence. The first three parameters were varied to allow for inaccuracy in "educated guesses" regarding the effect of multidrug therapy on these parameters. The sensitivity analysis shows whether it matters that the estimates might be inaccurate. Variation in incidence is also explored because incidence will be reduced if a drug therapy program is continued for several years, and the cost per YHLG will subsequently be decreased (depending on the discount rate).

The sensitivity analysis involved the changes shown in table 12C-2 (values were varied for one parameter at a time). The model proved to be relatively insensitive to these changes. As might be expected, when the minimum values are entered for all the parameters (except incidence) and the resulting cost

Table 12C-2. Effects of Drug Therapy on Cost per YHLG

Parameter	Reduction (percent)	Cost per YHLG (dollars)
Proportion permanently disabled	0.10–0.50	14.54–11.63
Disablement of permanently disabled	0.30–0.80	17.52–10.75
Temporary disability days	0.10–0.50	12.71–12.71
Incidence	0.30–0.70	12.71–12.71

Note: Values were varied for one parameter at a time.
Source: Authors.

per YHLG is compared with the cost per YHLG in the situation in which all the maximum values are entered, there is little difference between the two outputs ($25.15 per YHLG as opposed to $10.34 per YHLG). Finally, in recognition of the possibility that costs may have been underestimated in the model, the cost per case was varied to determine the effect on the cost per YHLG. When the cost per case was doubled, the cost per YHLG for chemotherapy was $25.42, still a reasonable figure. Even when the cost per case was tripled, the cost per YHLG for drug therapy was only $38.13.

Appendix 12D. Second Analysis: Treatment of Complications

In the second analysis we consider the costs and benefits of treating complications of leprosy, including treatment of reactions and ulcers, reconstructive surgery, and all forms of rehabilitation. Costs of treating the complications were estimated to be $225.00 per case by consensus of the two members of our group who had had experience treating leprosy patients in a developing country. It was further estimated that 10 percent of cases would have complications requiring treatment. The model calculates that it costs $338.06 per YHLG to treat the complications of leprosy. This makes the cost of the combination of drug therapy and treatment of complications $350.77 per YHLG ($12.71 per YHLG + $338.06 per YHLG), assuming there is no interaction between drug therapy and treatment of complications, which is a reasonable assumption. The cost of psychotherapy is not included in this analysis. Further details are provided below.

Details of the Calculations

- The cost of treating reactions with prednisolone was estimated to be $3 per case on average. The estimate is complicated by individual variation in clinical response. The duration of treatment may be as short as two to three months or longer than two years. Prednisolone is such an inexpensive drug, however, this wide variation in duration of treatment is not expected to be important.
- The cost of treating ulcers was estimated at $20 per case on average.
- The cost of reconstructive surgery was estimated at $200 per case, and the cost of rehabilitation was estimated at $2 per case.
- Therefore, the total cost per case of treating complications of leprosy was estimated to be:

$$\$3 + \$20 + \$200 + \$2 = \$225.$$

In the second analysis, the following assumptions were made (input and output of the model are shown in table 12C-1):

- That treatment of complications reduces the disablement of permanently disabled cases by 20 percent.

- That it reduces the days of temporary disability by 20 percent.
- That it reduces the disablement during temporary disability by 20 percent.
- That it does not affect any other parameters in the model.

Results

The cost per YHLG for treatment of complications was calculated to be $338.06. The cost per YHLG for drug therapy plus treatment of complications was thus $350.77 per YHLG ($12.71 per YHLG + $338.06 per YHLG), assuming no interaction between the two components of the control program.

Sensitivity Analysis

A sensitivity analysis was done to determine how much the cost per YHLG would be affected by varying the effects of treatment of complications on the proportion of disablement of patients who are permanently disabled, the temporary disability days, and the proportion of disablement of those who are temporarily disabled. These three parameters were varied to allow for inaccuracy of educated guesses of these values. Again, the sensitivity analysis shows whether it matters that the estimates might be inaccurate. The sensitivity analysis involved the changes shown in table 12D-1.

The model was sensitive to changes in proportion of disablement of patients permanently disabled, indicating that knowledge of the effect of treating complications is necessary to have confidence in the estimate of cost per YHLG given by the model. Changes in the temporary disability days and the disablement of the temporarily disabled have little effect on the output because initial values of these parameters are so low that even a 50 percent change in the values is a small amount. When the minimum values are entered for all the parameters, including incidence, and the resulting cost per YHLG compared with the cost per YHLG in the situation in which all the maximum values, including incidence, are entered, the same values are obtained ($676.05 per YHLG as opposed to $135.27 per YHLG).

Again, because costs cited in this analysis may have been underestimated, it may be useful to consider the output if the average costs of treating complications are doubled ($676.12 per YHLG) or even tripled ($1,014.18 per YHLG).

Table 12D-1. *Effects of Treatment of Complications on Cost per YHLG*

Parameter	Reduction (percentage)	Cost per YHLG (dollars)
Disablement of permanently disabled	0.10–0.50	674.86–135.38
Temporary disability days	0.10–0.50	338.20–337.64
Disablement of temporarily disabled	0.10–0.50	338.20–337.64

Source: Authors.

Appendix 12E. Cost Issues in Screening and Immunization

The cost per YHLG of a screening program was not considered in this analysis because the model used was not designed for this application. Additional parameters such as coverage of the population and sensitivity and specificity of diagnosis are needed if the model is to reflect the effect of a screening program. The cost aspect of the analysis is complicated by the fact that screening without treatment has no effect on disease control.

In lieu of a cost per YHLG measure of the cost-effectiveness of a screening program, some of the cost issues involved with screening will be discussed briefly. It was estimated (by the two members of our group who had experience treating leprosy patients) that the cost per person of screening by clinical exam would be approximately $0.10 (based on costs in Myanmar). The total cost of screening would then be calculated by multiplying the cost per person by the number of persons screened. Therefore, screening 1,000 people would cost $100. The number of cases that would be detected by screening (but that would have gone undetected without screening) would have to be considered. It was further estimated that a screening and treatment program would decrease age at onset by 10 percent, that it would decrease the proportion of cases who do not die but are permanently disabled by an additional 20 percent (over treatment alone), and that it would decrease the proportion of disablement of those who are permanently disabled by an additional 20 percent. The screening and treatment program would eventually decrease incidence because the cases would be caught and treated earlier, thereby shortening the period during which persons with the disease are transmitting it. Because some of the benefits of screening and treatment are future benefits, the cost should be discounted. The cost of screening programs is relatively high because many people who do not have symptoms of the disease must be screened so that the few who do have it are found. Thus, a screening program must be very effective to justify the cost.

The cost per YHLG of a vaccination program with BCG vaccine was not considered because the efficacy of BCG vaccine for leprosy prevention is so variable from area to area, and the appropriate vaccination schedule is still a matter of debate. Also, this cost would be shared by leprosy and tuberculosis control programs. The cost per dose of BCG vaccine is small (approximately $0.10 in developing countries, Walsh 1988), however, so prevention of even a small proportion of the expected number of leprosy cases might justify the use of the vaccine for leprosy control, especially when the efficiency of immunizing for both tuberculosis and leprosy is considered. Of course, delivery costs would have to be included in such an analysis.

Appendix 12F. Effect of Accuracy of Diagnosis

In the analysis of the cost-effectiveness of drug therapy (appendix 12C), perfect accuracy of diagnosis was assumed. In this analysis, another spreadsheet program will be used to calculate cost per identified true case of the disease at varying levels of sensitivity and specificity of diagnosis. Inputs for this spreadsheet include the following:

- True prevalence among those who see a health worker: 10 per 1,000 (WHO 1985a)
- Sensitivity and specificity of diagnosis: to be varied.
- Cost per YHLG of multidrug therapy: $30.92 as calculated in previous model

Outputs (table 12F-1) include the following:

- Prevalence of disease as diagnosed by health worker
- Predictive value of health worker diagnosis
- Cost per identified true case of disease

Results

The specificity drives the cost. Even at the relatively high levels of 90 percent sensitivity and specificity, cost per identified true case of disease increases steeply to $371.04, as compared with $30.92 for perfect accuracy of diagnosis. With

sensitivity and specificity equal to 50 percent, cost per identified true case of the disease increased 100-fold to $3,092.00.

Discussion

These results emphasize the need for training of health workers for accurate diagnosis. Unfortunately, current levels of sensitivity and specificity of diagnosis of leprosy are unknown. This knowledge is important for estimating costs more precisely.

Appendix 12G. General Comments about Cost-Effectiveness Modeling

It is important to note that cost per YHLG calculated by the model does not include the cost of education of the community about leprosy or of training health workers. As discussed earlier, education of the community is essential to the success of a control program. The costs of educating people about the disease are very difficult to estimate, however, and because they would probably be incorporated into other health education efforts, they would fall under the budget of multisectoral

Table 12F-1. *Effect of Sensitivity and Specificity of Diagnosis on Cost per Case of Treated Leprosy*

	Data entered by analyst			Data derived by computer		
True prevalence among persons visiting health worker (per 1,000)	Sensitivity of health worker's diagnosis	Specificity of health worker's diagnosis	Cost per case diagnosed by health worker (dollars)	Prevalence of disease diagnosed by health worker (per 1,000)	Predictive value of health worker's diagnosis	Cost per identified true case of disease (dollars)
10.00	0.99	0.99	30.92	9.91	0.500	61.84
10.00	0.90	0.90	30.92	99.01	0.083	371.04
10.00	0.90	0.80	30.92	198.01	0.043	711.16
10.00	0.90	0.70	30.92	297.01	0.029	1,051.28
10.00	0.90	0.60	30.92	396.01	0.022	1,391.40
10.00	0.90	0.50	30.92	495.01	0.018	1,731.52
10.00	0.80	0.90	30.92	99.01	0.075	413.56
10.00	0.80	0.80	30.92	198.01	0.039	796.19
10.00	0.80	0.70	30.92	297.01	0.026	1,178.83
10.00	0.80	0.60	30.92	396.01	0.020	1,561.46
10.00	0.80	0.50	30.92	495.01	0.016	1,944.10
10.00	0.70	0.90	30.92	99.01	0.066	468.22
10.00	0.70	0.80	30.92	198.01	0.034	905.51
10.00	0.70	0.70	30.92	297.01	0.023	1,342.81
10.00	0.70	0.60	30.92	396.01	0.017	1,780.11
10.00	0.70	0.50	30.92	495.01	0.014	2,217.41
10.00	0.60	0.90	30.92	99.01	0.057	541.10
10.00	0.60	0.80	30.92	198.01	0.029	1,051.28
10.00	0.60	0.70	30.92	297.01	0.020	1,561.46
10.00	0.60	0.60	30.92	396.01	0.015	2,071.64
10.00	0.60	0.50	30.92	495.01	0.012	2,581.02
10.00	0.50	0.90	30.92	99.01	0.048	643.14
10.00	0.50	0.80	30.92	198.01	0.025	1,255.35
10.00	0.50	0.70	30.92	297.01	0.017	1,867.57
10.00	0.50	0.60	30.92	396.01	0.012	2,479.78
10.00	0.50	0.50	30.92	495.01	0.010	3,092.00

Source: Authors.

health education programs rather than under that of a leprosy control program. As illustrated in appendix 12F, money spent training health care workers is money saved through reducing the number of false-positive cases diagnosed. We did not attempt to estimate the cost of this training.

It is also quite important to recognize that in the cost analysis presented in this chapter we have not considered the value of intangible benefits of a leprosy control program. Failure to consider such intangible benefits as prevention of psychological trauma when weighing the cost-effectiveness of a control program leads to serious underestimation of the benefits of such a program. This point was emphasized by Creese and Henderson (1980 p. 494): "Health programs characteristically have effects which, though important, are extremely difficult to measure and to value. Benefits such as reduced anxiety, pain, or discomfort are typical examples: these are desirable 'outputs' of the health system, but they are not readily comparable with other outputs such as increased productivity."

Appendix 12H.   Total Cost of a Leprosy Control Program

In the previous appendixes, the cost-effectiveness of various aspects of a leprosy control program was discussed. In those analyses, we were considering a one-year program to treat new cases (assuming existing cases were already under treatment). We did not include capital costs and the cost of case detection, primarily because the model we used was not designed to include such costs and redesigning the model would have been a complicated undertaking beyond the scope of this project. In the following analysis, we will discuss the capital costs and the cost of case detection in the context of a five-year leprosy control program. We will then add these costs to those calculated previously for chemotherapy and complications to give an estimated total cost for a leprosy control program.

Capital Costs

The calculation of annualized capital cost will be based on a hypothetical population of 100,000 in a hyperendemic area with leprosy prevalence of 10 per 1,000 population. The capital cost will include cost of vehicles, buildings, office equipment, and laboratory equipment. The total capital cost (C) was estimated to be $100,000. The lifetime of equipment and vehicles was estimated at 10 years. The social rate of discount (r) was taken as 3 percent. The annualized discounting factor was calculated as follows:

$$a(r,n) = \frac{[r(1+r)^n]}{[(1+r)^n - 1]}$$
$$= \frac{.03(1+.03)^{10}}{(1+.03)^{10} - 1}$$
$$= 0.1172.$$

The annualized cost, $a(r,n)$ C, is then:

$$a(r,n)\,\text{C} = 0.1172\,(\$100,000)$$
$$= \$11,720.00.$$

In a population of 100,000 in which the prevalence of leprosy is 10 per 1,000, one thousand patients would be under treatment. So the annualized capital cost per patient is:

$$\frac{\$11,720}{1,000} = \$11.72 \text{ per case.}$$

Cost of Case Detection

The cost of screening for case detection will be based on the same hypothetical population of 100,000 assumed above. Furthermore, it will be assumed that no screening has been done in the population in the previous five years. The screening team would consist of five workers, and sixty days per year for five years would be devoted to screening. It is estimated that such a team could screen 200 persons per day. Typical salaries for each such workers in a developing country would be $5 per day, with an allowance of $2 per day for travel (based on costs in Myanmar). New cases would be detected by the screening program workers at the rate of 3 cases per 1,000 screened. If the community was fairly isolated, after five years of the screening program, fewer cases would be detected because the screening and early treatment would lower incidence (the incubation period is five to seven years). We estimate that approximately half the cases would be discovered when they presented for treatment on their own initiative, rather than through the screening effort.

The total cost of the screening program per year would be as follows:

$$\text{Total cost} = (\text{salaries} + \text{travel allowance}) \times \text{no. workers} =$$
$$[(60 \cdot \$5.00) + (60 \cdot \$2.00)] \cdot 5 = \$2,100.00.$$

The total number of persons screened would be equal to 60 days x 200/day, or 12,000 persons. The estimated number of new cases detected would be equal to the screened population multiplied by the number of cases detected through screening, which we estimate to be 3 per 1,000, so 36 cases (12,000 · 3 per 1,000) would be detected by screening. Therefore, the screening cost per new case detected would be $2,100.00 per 36 new cases detected, or $58.34 per new case detected. An additional 36 cases would present on their own initiative for treatment. Before the screening program was started, there were 1,000 registered cases in the total population of 100,000 (prevalence, 10 per 1,000). Together, then, there are 1,000 registered cases plus 36 cases detected by screening plus 36 cases detected when they presented on their own initiative, or a total of 1,072 cases in the population of 100,000. The total cost of screening per case is, then, $2,100.00 per 1,072, or $1.96 per case.

Total Cost per Case of a Leprosy Control Program

To calculate the total cost per case of a leprosy control program, the costs of basic chemotherapy as well as treatment of complications must be added to the capital and screening costs.

COST OF BASIC CHEMOTHERAPY. As discussed in appendix 12C, the cost of treatment of uncomplicated leprosy is estimated at $30.92 per case, if it is assumed that 80 percent of cases are paucibacillary and 20 percent are multibacillary.

COST OF TREATMENT OF COMPLICATIONS. As discussed in appendix D, the cost of treatment of complications for each of those who need such treatment is estimated at $225.00. Only 10 percent of all patients are expected to need treatment for complications. Therefore, the cost of treating complications averaged over all cases, calculated by dividing the total cost for treating complications $(1,000 \cdot 0.1 \cdot \$225.00)$ by the total number of registered cases $(1,000)$, is $22.50 per case.

TOTAL COST PER CASE. The sum of the estimated costs of capital, screening, chemotherapy, and treatment of complications is used to estimate the total cost per case in the leprosy control program.

Annualized capital cost	$11.72 per case
Screening	1.96 per case
Chemotherapy	30.92 per case
Complications	22.50 per case
Total	$67.10 per case

Discussion

If the screening and treatment are successful, in five to seven years (roughly the length of the incubation period of leprosy), the number of cases detected will begin to decline as the rate of transmission is reduced. As this happens, the cost per case detected will increase.

Notes

The authors gratefully acknowledge Drs. S. K. Noordeen, Emmanuel Max, W. Felton Ross, Richard Morrow, and Paul E. M. Fine for their comments, which guided the development of this chapter.

References

Bagshawe, A., G. C. Scott, D. A. Russell, S. C. Wigley, A. Merianos, and G. Berry. 1989. "BCG Vaccination in Leprosy: Final Results of the Trial in Karimui, Papua New Guinea, 1963–79." *Bulletin of the World Health Organization* 67:389–99.

Bharadwaj, V. P., and K. Katoch. 1990. "An Overview of the Current Status of Serological Techniques in the Epidemiology of Leprosy." *Tropical Medicine and Parasitology* 41:359–60.

Bloom, B. R. 1990. "An Ordinary Mortal's Guide to the Molecular Biology of Mycobacteria." *International Journal of Leprosy and Other Mycobacterial Diseases* 58:365–75.

Bloom, B. R., and T. Godal. 1983. "Selective Primary Health Care: Strategies for Control of Disease in the Developing World. 5. Leprosy." *Reviews of Infectious Diseases* 5(4):765–80.

Boerrigter, G., J. M. Ponnighaus, and P. E. Fine. 1988. "Preliminary Appraisal of a WHO-Recommended Multiple Drug Regimen in Paucibacillary Leprosy Patients in Malawi." *International Journal of Leprosy and Other Mycobacterial Diseases* 56:408–17.

Browne, S. G. 1985. "The History of Leprosy." In R. C. Hastings, ed., *Leprosy*. Edinburgh: Churchill Livingstone.

Cellona, R. V., T. T. Fajardo, Jr., D. I. Kim, Y. M. Hah, T. Ramasoota, S. Sampattavanich, M. P. Carrillo, R. M. Abalos, E. C. dela Cruz, and T. Ito. 1990. "Joint Chemotherapy Trials in Lepromatous Leprosy Conducted in Thailand, the Philippines, and Korea." *International Journal of Leprosy and Other Mycobacterial Diseases* 58:1–11.

Convit, Jacinto, N. Aranzazu, M. Ulrich, M. E. Pinardi, O. Reyes, and J. Alvarado. 1982. "Immunotherapy with a Mixture of *Mycobacterium leprae* and BCG in Different Forms of Leprosy and in Mitsuda-Negative Contacts." *International Journal of Leprosy and Other Mycobacterial Diseases* 50:415–24.

Courtwright, P., and G. Johnson. 1988. *Blindness Prevention in Leprosy*. London: International Center for Eye Health.

Creese, A. L., and R. H. Henderson. 1980. "Cost-Benefit Analysis and Immunization Programs in Developing Countries." *Bulletin of the World Health Organization* 58:491–97.

Declercq E. and C. Gelin. 1991. "Global Evaluation of the Introduction of Multidrug Therapy." *Leprosy Epidemiological Bulletin* 6. WHO Collaborating Centre for the Epidemiology of Leprosy, Catholic University of Louvain, Brussels, Belgium.

Dharmendra. 1986. "Epidemiology of Leprosy in Relation to Control." *Indian Journal of Leprosy* 58(1):1–16.

Dominguez, V. M., P. G. Garbajosa, M. M. Gyi, C. T. Tamondong, T. Sundaresan, L. M. Bechelli, K. Lwin, H. Sansarricq, J. Walter, and F. M. Noussitou. 1980. "Epidemiological Information on Leprosy in the Singu Area of Upper Burma." *Bulletin of the World Health Organization* 58:81–89.

Ellard, G. A., P. T. Gammon, H. S. Helmy, and R. J. W. Rees. 1974. "Urine Tests to Monitor the Self-Administration of Dapsone by Leprosy Patients." *American Journal of Tropical Medicine and Hygiene* 23(3):464–70.

Fine, P. E., J. M. Ponninghaus, N. Maine, J. A. Clarkson, and L. Bliss. 1986. "Protective Efficacy of BCG against Leprosy in Northern Malawi." *Lancet* 1:499–502. (new series).

Ganapati, R., C. R. Revankar, and R. R. Pai. 1987. "Three-Year Assessment of Multi-drug Therapy in Multibacillary Leprosy Cases." *Indian Journal of Leprosy* 59(1):44–49.

Ghana Health Assessment Project Team. 1981. "A Quantitative Method of Assessing the Health Impact of Different Diseases in Less Developed Countries." *International Journal of Epidemiology* 10:73–80.

Gillis, T. P., and D. L. Williams. 1991. "Polymerase Chain Reaction and Leprosy." *International Journal of Leprosy and Other Mycobacterial Diseases* 59:311–16.

Hagan, K. J., and S. E. Smith. 1979. "The Reliability of Self-Administration of Dapsone by Leprosy Patients in Burma." *Leprosy Review* 50(3):201–11.

Irgens, L. M., and R. Skjaerven. 1985. "Secular Trends in Age at Onset, Sex Ratio, and Type Index in Leprosy Observed during Declining Incidence Rates." *American Journal of Epidemiology* 122:695–705.

Jacobson, R. R. 1985. "Treatment." In R. C. Hastings, ed., *Leprosy*. Edinburgh: Churchill Livingstone.

Jesudasan, K., M. Christian, and D. Bradley. 1984. "Relapse Rate among Non-lepromatous Patients Released from Control." *International Journal of Leprosy and Other Mycobacterial Diseases* 52:304–10.

Katoch, V. M., C. T. Shivannavar, K. Katoch, G. V. Kanaujia, and V. P. Bharadwaj. 1990. "Towards Clinical and Epidemiological Application of Advances in Molecular Biology of *Mycobacterium leprae*." *Tropical Medicine and Parasitology* 41:299–300.

Lechat, M. F. 1981. "The Torments and Blessings of the Leprosy Epidemiometric Model." *Leprosy Review* 52(supplement 1):187–96.

———. 1985. "Control Programs in Leprosy." In R. C. Hastings, ed., *Leprosy*. Edinburgh: Churchill Livingstone.

Lechat, M. F., C. Vellut, C. B. Misson, and J. Y. Misson. 1978. "Application of an Economic Model to the Study of Leprosy Control Costs." *International Journal of Leprosy and Other Mycobacterial Diseases* 46:14–24.

Lwin, Kyaw, T. Sundaresan, M. M. Gyi, L. M. Bechelli, C. Tamondong, P. G. Garbajosa, H. Sansarricq, and S. K. Noordeen. 1985. "BCG Vaccination of Children against Leprosy. Fourteen-year Findings of the Trial in Burma." *Bulletin of the World Health Organization* 63:1069–78.

Max, Emmanuel, and D. S. Shepherd. 1989. "Productivity Loss due to Deformity from Leprosy in India." *International Journal of Leprosy and Other Mycobacterial Diseases* 57:476–82.

Mittal, B. N. 1991. "The National Leprosy Control Programme in India." *World Health Statistics Quarterly* 44(1):23–29.

Muliyil, Jayaprakash, K. E. Nelson, and E. L. Diamond. 1991. "Effect of BCG on the Risk of Leprosy in an Endemic Area: A Case Control Study." *International Journal of Leprosy and Other Mycobacterial Diseases* 59:229–36.

Myanmar, Ministry of Health. 1985. *Annual Report of the Leprosy Control Program*. Yangon.

Myint, Tin, M. T. Htoon, and T. Shwe. 1992. "Estimation of Leprosy Prevalence in Bago and Kawa Townships Using Two-Stage Probability Proportionate to Size Sampling Technique." *International Journal of Epidemiology* 21:778–83.

Neik, S. S., N. D. Bhange, K. V. Sawant, and R. Ganapati. 1988. "A Bacteriological Assessment of Multibacillary Cases in Leprosy Colonies after 4-1/2 Years of Multidrug Therapy." *Indian Journal of Leprosy* 60(3): 393–99.

Noordeen. S. K. 1986. "BCG Vaccination in Leprosy." *Developments in Biological Standardization.* 58(A):287–92.

———. 1985. "The Epidemiology of Leprosy." In R. C. Hastings, ed., *Leprosy*. Edinburgh: Churchill Livingstone.

———. 1992. *Weekly Epidemiological Record* 67:153–60.

Noordeen, S. K., L. L. Bravo, and D. Daumerie. 1991. "Global Review of Multidrug Therapy (MDT) in Leprosy." *World Health Statistics Quarterly* 44(1):2–15.

Pearson, J. M., G. S. Haile, and R. J. Rees. 1977. "Primary Dapsone Resistant Leprosy." *Leprosy Review* 48(2):129–32.

Ramanan, R., P. R. Manghani, A. Ghorpode, and S. K. Bhagolinal. 1987. "Follow-up Study of Paucibacillary Leprosy on Multidrug Regimen." *Indian Journal of Leprosy* 59(1):50–53.

Ridley, D. S. 1974. "Histological Classification and the Immunological Spectrum of Leprosy." *Bulletin of the World Health Organization* 51:451–65.

———. 1977. *Skin Biopsy in Leprosy*. Basel: Ciba Geigy.

Stanley, S. J., C. Howland, M. M. Stone, and I. Sutherland. 1981. "BCG Vaccination of Children against Leprosy in Uganda: Final Results." *Journal of Hygiene* 87:233–48.

Talwar, G. P., S. A. Zaheer, R. Mukherjee, R. Walia, R. S. Misra, A. K. Sharma, H. K. Kar, A. Mukherjee, S. K. Parida, and N. R. Suresh. 1990. "Immunotherapeutic Effects of a Vaccine Based on a Saprophytic Cultivable Mycobacterium, *Mycobacterium w* in Multibacillary Leprosy Patients." *Vaccine* 8:121–29.

UNICEF (United Nations Children's Fund). 1991. *Essential Drugs Price List.* July–December, 1991. Copenhagen: Procurement and Assembly Centre.

Walsh, G. P., E. E. Storrs, W. Meyers, and C. H. Binford.1977. "Naturally Acquired Leprosy Like Disease in the Nine-Banded Armadillo." *Journal of the Reticuloendothelial Society* 22:363–67.

Walsh, J. A. 1988. *Establishing Health Care Priorities in the Developing World*. Boston: Adams Publishing Group.

Wardekar, R. V. 1968. "Sulphone Treatment and Deformity in Leprosy." *Leprosy in India* 40:161–71.

Watson, J. M. 1988. *Preventing Disability in Leprosy Patients*. London: Leprosy Mission International.

WHO (World Health Organization). 1977. *Fifth Report of the World Health Organization Expert Committee on Leprosy. Technical Report 607. Geneva.*

———. 1980. *A Guide to Leprosy Control*. Geneva.

———. 1982. *Chemotherapy of Leprosy Control Programmes*. Technical Report 675. Geneva.

———. 1985a. *WHO Demographic Yearbook*. Geneva.

———. 1985b. *Epidemiology of Leprosy in Relation to Control*. Technical Report 716. Geneva.

———. 1988a. *Sixth Report of the World Health Organization Expert Committee on Leprosy*. Technical Report 768. Geneva.

WHO (World Health Organization), Regional Office of the Western Pacific. 1988b. "Final Report of the Regional Working Group on Drug Policy and Operational Research in Leprosy Programs." ICP/BUM/005. Manila. Typescript.

13

Malaria

José A. Nájera, Bernhard H. Liese, and Jeffrey Hammer

Malaria is a collective name for different diseases that may result from infection by any parasites of the genus *Plasmodium*. Four species of malaria parasites naturally infect humans: *Plasmodium falciparum*, *P. vivax*, *P. malariae*, and *P. ovale*. The characteristics of the disease vary with the intensity of the infection, the host's level of immunity, the adequacy of and opportunity for treatment, and the parasite's susceptibility to it.

Transmission between humans occurs through the bites of certain species of mosquitoes of the genus *Anopheles*. In this cycle, the parasite matures and reproduces sexually in the anopheline mosquito (the vector), which is therefore, strictly speaking, the parasite's definitive host, and human beings are its intermediate host.

A Natural History: Parasite and Vector

The life cycle of the parasite follows a general pattern. The infecting parasite, an actively motile form called a sporozoite, is inoculated into the blood with the saliva of the biting mosquito. After about half an hour, the sporozoites invade liver tissue cells, where they develop and multiply. Small parasite forms called merozoites, capable of invading the red blood cells, burst into the blood—as many as 20,000 per successful sporozoite. The time needed to multiply in the liver, the pre-erythrocytic stage, varies with the parasite species: six to seven days for *P. falciparum*, fourteen to sixteen days for *P. malariae*, and seven to eight days for *P. vivax*, although some *P. vivax* parasites remain dormant in the liver for months, even a few years, in a form called hypnozoite. Once the parasites invade the red blood cells they initiate the cycle of development and multiplication that causes clinical manifestations of the disease. Disease symptoms are caused only by parasites in the blood. The late development of hypnozoites, therefore, gives the disease a long incubation period, or a pattern of cure alternating with repeated relapses, because common antimalarial drugs that may clear the blood of parasites are not effective against parasites in the liver. Merozoites invade red blood cells, where they grow and multiply to produce eight to twenty-four merozoites (depending on the parasite species), which rapidly invade new red blood cells. This development is accomplished in forty-eight hours for the so-called tertian

malarias (benign, if from *P. vivax* and *P. ovale*; malignant, if from *P. falciparum*) and seventy-two hours for the quartan (from *P. malariae*). This development takes place in the peripheral blood for *P. vivax*, *P. malariae*, and *P. ovale*. But with *P. falciparum*, only red blood cells infected with very young parasites (called ring forms) are found in the peripheral blood; those infected with developing or dividing parasites are sequestered in the capillaries of such internal organs as the brain and cause the severe manifestations typical of *P. falciparum*.

Some parasites do not follow the cycle of asexual reproduction just described. Instead, they differentiate into male and female gametocytes, which are eventually taken up by an *Anopheles* mosquito. In the mosquito they can mature, achieve fertilization, and multiply in the stomach wall, producing about 1,000 sporozoites, which burst into the mosquito's body cavity and finally invade the salivary glands. This sexual cycle takes between nine and thirty days or more, depending on the temperature and the parasite species.

Not all species of anophelines are vectors of malaria, and those that are vary greatly in their ability to transmit the disease. General or specific refractoriness may be due to many causes, for example, because the plasmodia is unable to develop or to invade the salivary glands, or because the mosquito cannot live long enough to complete the parasite's extrinsic cycle, or because the mosquito has so little contact with humans (for example, is so unlikely to bite humans) that it is unlikely to bite a human after becoming infected. Of the roughly 400 species of *Anopheles*, only about 60 are vectors of malaria under natural conditions; some 30 of these are of prime importance.

As for all mosquitoes, the habitat of the immature *Anopheles* is water. Eggs are all laid on or on the edge of water and hatch in two to three days to produce larvae (wrigglers). Larvae develop through five aquatic stages—four larval and one pupal—to produce adult flying mosquitoes. Only the female mosquito bites; it does so because it needs blood for its eggs to mature. The male feeds on vegetable juices. Mating occurs only once, soon after the adult female emerges. The female stores the spermatozoa in a deposit called a spermatheca. The aquatic stages commonly last seven to twenty days, depending on the temperature. The adult female may live from a few days to well over a month, going through several cycles of blood feeds and egg laying (some 100 to 200 per batch), every two to four days. Survival and egg development depend mainly on temperature and relative humidity. In extreme climates mosquitoes may go into hibernation, which allows some of them to survive the winter in temperate climates.

Depending on the species, larval habitats vary enormously, reflecting mosquitoes' evolutionary adaptability. The habitats range from permanent to transient bodies of water; from fresh to brackish water; from standing water to flowing canals and open streams; from water in open sun to that in deep shade; from shallow pools to deep wells; from clean drinking water to water highly polluted with organic matter; from large open marshes to the tiny pools of water that collect between the leaves of bromeliads in plant axils, trees, rocks, crab holes, cattle footprints, or discarded artificial containers. But the characteristics of breeding places are rather narrowly defined for each species, so larval habitats can be modified for control of mosquito species.

The seasonal availability of breeding places and the great influence of weather conditions on mosquito activity and survival are largely responsible for the marked seasonality in mosquito population densities and malaria transmission in most areas outside of permanently humid tropical areas.

Specific behavioral characteristics of mosquitoes may also affect their vectorial ability. Mosquitoes' preferences for feeding on humans or animals and their frequency of feeding are important determinants of the probability of their transmitting malaria. Human dwellings and domestic animal shelters—particularly those with thatched roofs, dark corners, and many cracks in the walls—are good resting places in which mosquitoes can digest the blood they have consumed while their eggs mature. Such buildings favor mosquito survival but are also vulnerable to insecticidal spraying.

Malaria as a Disease

The chief symptom of malaria is fever, periodic bouts of which tend to alternate with days of less or no fever. The classical paroxysm of fever lasts eight to twelve hours, typically in three stages: cold shivering rigor, burning dry skin, and drenching sweat that lowers the temperature. This pattern is more typical of *P. vivax* (tertian periodicity) and *P. malariae* (quartan) than of *P. falciparum*, which typically involves prostrating fever, with brief and incomplete remissions, more often irregular than clearly periodic. Untreated, the acute attack is shorter than that of *P. vivax*; in fatal cases, death often occurs in two to three weeks and sometimes as soon as two to three days after the onset of symptoms. Repeated infections give rise to an immune response in the host which eventually controls the infection and the disease. Untreated or incompletely treated infections will produce several recrudescences, after long symptomless periods, from parasites surviving in the blood. By this mechanism alone, *P. falciparum* may persist for one or two years, whereas *P. malariae* has been reported to recrudesce up to fifty-two years after last exposure to infection. With *P. vivax*,

true relapses may occur, because latent hypnozoites will mature in the liver and invade the blood after other parasites have been completely eliminated from it. Without reinfection, *P. vivax* may persist for three to four years.

In the absence of other complicating factors, acute severity and mortality occur almost exclusively in *P. falciparum* infections. This parasite causes the surface of infected red blood cells to become adhesive and to be sequestered in the capillaries of internal organs, leading to the pathological changes responsible for cerebral malaria and the serious renal, hepatic, and gastrointestinal dysfunctions. Other severe complications such as shock, pulmonary edema, severe anemia and hemoglobinuria (or blackwater fever), are the results of more complex mechanisms.

P. falciparum malaria can lead rapidly to death, so it is important to recognize signs of severity early and refer the patient immediately for medical care. These signs include shock, anemia, convulsions, jaundice, hyperpyrexia, renal failure, impaired consciousness, spontaneous bleeding, macroscopic hemoglobinuria, and pulmonary edema or respiratory distress. Health services that suspect severe malaria should treat it as a medical emergency, providing immediate treatment and, whenever possible, laboratory monitoring of such signs of severity as hypoglycemia, parasite density, and an imbalance of fluids and electrolytes.

The risk of severe malaria is almost exclusively limited to those who are not immune. In highly endemic areas this risk affects children older than three to six months, who have lost the immunity transferred from their mother, up to the age of about five years, when surviving children have developed their own immunity. African health authorities report that in the last few years cerebral malaria is being seen increasingly often in older children and young adults. It has been suggested that this may be the result of urbanization and personal protection, which reduce the risk of infection and delay the development of immunity. Severity in adults is seen in areas of low endemicity, where people may reach adulthood without immunity. Equally at risk are immigrants and travelers from nonendemic areas—particularly laborers, who are often concentrated in camps, where nonimmunes and the infected live side by side in overcrowded conditions where the risk of transmission is high. Also at risk are pregnant women, possibly because natural immunity is depressed during pregnancy.

Most deaths from malaria occur in young children living in highly endemic areas of tropical Africa and the western Pacific islands. The most common causes of death are cerebral malaria and severe anemia. Malaria may also contribute seriously to the severity of other childhood diseases.

In pregnancy, *P. falciparum* malaria in the nonimmune may lead to death, abortion, premature delivery, or low birth weight. In the semi-immune inhabitants of highly endemic areas, malaria represents a serious risk in a first and second pregnancy. Pregnant women are more easily infected (and are susceptible to anemia, hypoglycemia, and other complications) because the placenta is a preferential site for parasite development. Malaria is an important cause of low birth weight and high neonatal mortality in first- and second-born children in endemic areas. It has been suggested that the build up of a total uterine immune response may account for the disappearance of these effects on subsequent pregnancies (McGregor 1982).

The Public Health Significance of Malaria

Roughly 110 million clinical cases of malaria develop annually. Some 270 million people are infected, carrying malaria parasites, although not necessarily developing symptoms. Indigenous malaria still exists in some 100 countries or areas. Accurate estimates are impossible because the accuracy of reporting varies considerably. Reporting from tropical Africa—where more than 80 percent of the clinical cases and 90 percent of the parasite carriers may be found—is especially irregular and fragmentary. Reported cases are believed to represent about 2 to 20 percent of the actual cases.

Geographical Distribution

Every year, in the *World Health Statistics Quarterly*, the World Health Organization (WHO) publishes an overview of the world malaria situation (map 13-1). The overview for 1990 (WHO 1992) indicates that the world population (about 5,300 million people) can be classified according to people's experience with malaria and their place of residence as follows:

- Areas in which malaria never existed or disappeared without specific antimalarial interventions: 1,431 million people, or 27 percent of the world's population.

- Areas in which endemic malaria disappeared after a specific campaign to control it was implemented and the area has remained malaria-free: 1,696 million people, or 32 percent of the world's population.

- Areas in which endemic malaria was reduced or even eliminated after control measures were implemented, but the disease was reinstated and the situation is unstable or deteriorating: 1,700 million people, or 32 percent of the world's population. This category includes zones (which include about 1 percent of the world's population) in which the most severe resurgence of malaria has recently developed as a result of significant ecological or social changes, such as sociopolitical unrest and agricultural or other exploitation of jungle areas.

- Areas in which endemic malaria remains basically unchanged and no national antimalaria program was ever implemented, because of the enormous difficulties of

Map 13-1. *Malaria Incidence*

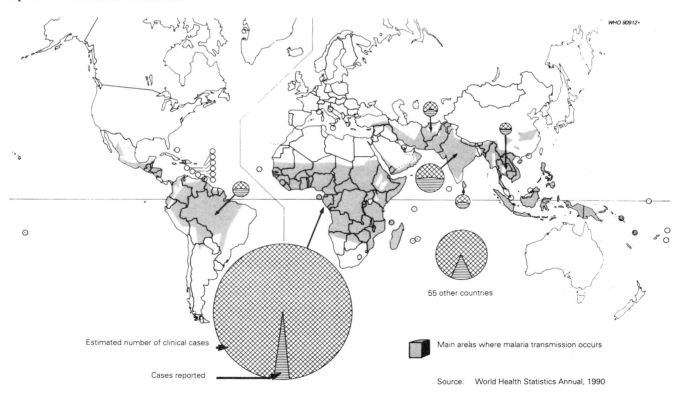

Estimated number of clinical cases

Cases reported

55 other countries

Main areas where malaria transmission occurs

Source: World Health Statistics Annual, 1990

Note: The designations employed and the presentation of material on this map do not imply the expression of any opinion whatsoever on the part of the World Health Organization concerning the legal status of any country, territory, city, or area or of its authorities, or concerning the delimitation of its frontiers or boundaries.
Source: Reproduced by permission of the World Health Organization, Geneva from *Weekly Epidemiological Record* 67 (22–23): 162–167/169–174 (1992).

achieving control: 500 million people, or 9 percent of the world's population. Malaria is most endemic in these areas, which contain 85 percent or more of the malaria cases in the world. These areas are mainly in tropical Africa; in some of them—including forested and medium-altitude areas—pilot projects were reportedly successful in interrupting malaria transmission, but in low savanna areas, particularly in the Sahel, no pilot projects ever reported full success.

Trends

The evolution of the malaria problem is traditionally described by the number of registered cases reported to WHO by member states. Figure 13-1, which excludes information on Africa because of inadequate, irregular reporting from that continent, shows the effect of the massive resurgence of malaria transmission in India in 1976 and its subsequent control. Changes in China are shown separately, because the Chinese started officially reporting to WHO only in 1977. China did not implement

a national malaria control program until it had developed a health infrastructure that has been considered a precursor of primary health care; the pattern of malaria incidence is similar to the pattern in countries that eradicated malaria (map 13-1). If India and China are not taken into account, the incidence of malaria in the world did not show a clear trend until the late 1970s, when it started a slow but steady deterioration. Data from India indicate that, after recovery from the 1976 epidemic, improvement slowed down and the situation seems to be stagnating.

The general pattern described here masks great local differences, not only in the intensity of the problem, but also in the pattern of its evolution over time. The geographical distribution of malaria is far from uniform; it can be seen that malaria clearly thrives in certain areas, and it may be said that it occupies definable socioecological niches. The limits of malaria foci are much more diffused than those for contagious diseases such as smallpox, however, so it is more difficult to target their control.

Figure 13-1. Number of Malaria Cases Reported, 1964–89

Number of Malaria cases reported
(millions)

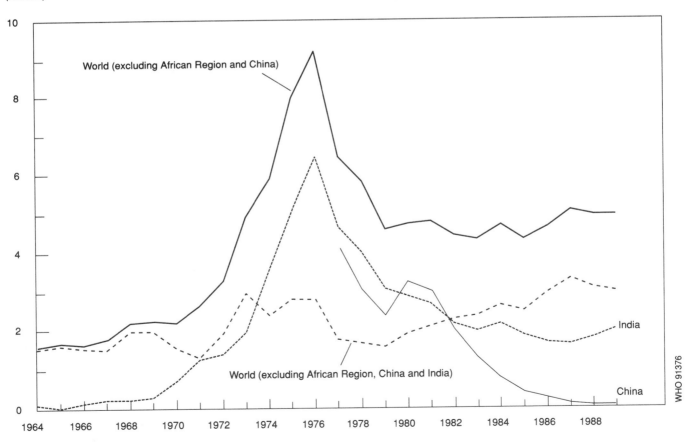

Morbidity in Tropical Africa

In the last decade African countries south of the Sahara have reported between 2 and 20 million cases a year to WHO; but extrapolating from fever and parasite surveys, it is estimated that 100 million clinical malaria cases may occur every year, and 275 million persons may carry the malaria parasite. The levels of endemic malaria are among the highest in the world. Extensive forest or savanna areas up to about 1,000 meters high, with rainfall of more than 2,000 millimeters a year, are classified as holoendemic. Areas between 1,000 and 1,500 meters high or lowland areas with 1,000 to 2,000 millimeters per year of rainfall are characterized as hyperendemic. As altitude increases above 1,500 meters or rainfall decreases below 1,000 millimeters per year, malaria becomes less endemic, concentrating in progressively smaller valleys or where favorable microclimatic conditions and mosquito-breeding places exist or are created by such human activities as irrigation, dam construction, and the establishment of fish ponds. Of course, altitude and rainfall are only rough indicators of malaria's endemicity; other factors, such as temperature, humidity, the distribution of rains, and the slope and permeability of the soil, also play important roles.

As endemicity decreases, the potential for epidemic outbreaks increases because fewer people have a chance to develop immunity. Equally, in areas of marked seasonality, as in the dry savanna of the Sahel, the transmission season, even if it occurs every year, takes on the characteristics of seasonal epidemics, at least as it affects younger age groups. Severe, large-scale epidemics occur in areas that have been free from transmission for several years in a row, and they exhibit a secular periodicity determined by the semicyclic occurrence of prolonged heavy rains or other climatological determinants. Such epidemics have been historically reported in high-altitude areas following abnormally warm and rainy summers. Such was the dramatic epidemic in the highlands of Ethiopia in 1958, which caused more than 3 million cases and claimed an estimated 150,000 deaths. They also occur in dry areas after abnormally heavy and prolonged rains, as in the epidemic of 1975 in Gezira and Central Sudan and the 1988 epidemic in Khartoum and Northern and Eastern Sudan. In 1988–90 a number of epidemics, or serious exacerbations of endemicity, occurred in several highland areas of Africa, particularly in Botswana, Madagascar, Rwanda, Swaziland, and Zambia.

In the high plateau of central Madagascar increasingly extensive and severe epidemics occurred between 1986 and 1988, reaching dramatic proportions in the first four months of 1988, when tens of thousands of people died. One of the main causes of this series of epidemics was that the DDT spraying campaign of the 1960s and early 1970s seems to have eliminated the main vectors of malaria A. *funestus* and A. *gambiae sensu stricto* so that malaria transmission was interrupted for about twenty years. But after spraying was discontinued and because of other opportunistic circumstances, both species progressively spread in the high plateau.

Smaller and more localized malaria epidemics have occurred when colonization efforts or agricultural or other economic development projects in endemic areas have attracted nonimmune populations from nonmalarious areas. This happened in the late 1950s, for example, when the lowlands of Kigezi (Uganda) began to be colonized by people from the overpopulated highlands, resulting in a tragic malaria epidemic with extremely high mortality. This led to the establishment in 1959 of one of the few successful malaria eradication pilot projects in Africa (de Zulueta and others 1961). In the last few years malaria endemicity has reportedly spread in the highlands of Amani in Tanzania. This increased transmission has been attributed to the active colonization of those areas and the subsequent intensification of agriculture and the attendant terracing and leveling of the land in and around human settlements, which increased potential anopheline breeding places (Matola, White, and Magayuka 1987).

Another possible factor in the apparent increase in epidemic potential in the last few years in the highland areas in Africa is the so-called greenhouse effect, by which the accumulation of carbon dioxide and other gases in the atmosphere may retain heat. In Madagascar the average temperature in the coastal areas was 0.5 degree centigrade warmer than in the previous thirty years; in the high plateau the difference was about 1 degree centigrade. These figures may not be fully comparable because data for the high plateau may be influenced by local ecological changes, such as the growth of Antananarivo. Still, an increase of even 0.5 degree centigrade could increase the potential transmission period in marginal areas, which might change a normally nonmalarious area into one subject to seasonal epidemics (de Zulueta 1988).

Morbidity in Other Malarious Areas

Outside tropical Africa, most malarious countries have similar reporting systems that permit some degree of comparison. As for the intensity of the problem, about 80 percent of the 5.01 million cases reported to WHO in 1990 (not including tropical Africa) are concentrated in eleven countries. They are, in decreasing order of total number of reported cases, India, Brazil, Afghanistan, Sri Lanka, Thailand, Indonesia, Viet Nam, Cambodia, China, Solomon Islands, and Papua New Guinea. These countries represent 65 percent of the population living in the world's malarious areas, excluding tropical Africa. India and Brazil, with only 26 percent of the population, report 46 percent of the cases. With only 34 percent of the population, the first seven countries report 70 percent of the cases. And within these countries, malaria is focused in certain areas. In India, for example, six states (Orissa, Uttar Pradesh, Punjab, Madhya Pradesh, Gujarat, and Assam) have 66 percent of the cases. In Brazil, 97 percent of the cases are in Amazonia, which has only 15 percent of the country's population; two states (Rondônia and Pará) report 70 percent of the cases, and four municipalities in Rondônia and four in Pará report more than 60 percent of the cases in those states.

These countries and areas show great variability not only in the intensity of the problem but also in its evolution in time. Cases reported annually to WHO since the mid-1960s show distinct patterns:

- Malaria declined and the situation has remained favorable in Algeria, China, Costa Rica, Cuba, Egypt, Korea, peninsular Malaysia, Morocco, Panama, Paraguay, and Tunisia.
- Malaria increased markedly in certain areas in Afghanistan, Bangladesh, Belize, Bhutan, Bolivia, Brazil, Cambodia, Colombia, French Guiana, Guatemala, Guyana, Madagascar, Mexico, Myanmar, Nepal, Papua New Guinea, Peru, the Philippines, Saudi Arabia, Solomon Islands, Thailand, Vanuatu, and Viet Nam.
- The incidence of malaria has oscillated—at relatively short cycles and with a quasihorizontal general trend, at least since the early 1960s—in Argentina, El Salvador, Honduras, Indonesia (the outer islands, reporting since 1970), Iran, Malaysia (Sabah), Nicaragua, Surinam, and the Republic of Yemen.
- In the last twenty years, one or two relatively short but significant resurgences, followed by renewed control, have occurred in the Dominican Republic, Ecuador, Haiti, India, Indonesia (Java and Bali), Iraq, Libya, Malaysia (Sarawak), Mauritius, Oman, Pakistan, Somalia, Sri Lanka, Syria, Turkey, Venezuela, and Yemen.

The only purpose of this preliminary classification is to stimulate analysis of the patterns of change. Groupings are based on total numbers of reported cases, and the fact that two countries appear in the same group does not indicate similarities in other epidemiological characteristics.

Except for India and China (which are significant producers of cases because of their great size) and Sri Lanka (which may be changing from a pattern of periodic resurgence because of sociopolitical unrest), most large producers of cases are in the second group. These countries are characterized by recent efforts to increase the exploitation of natural resources (through agricultural colonization of forest or jungle areas) or by civil war or sociopolitical conflict (including illegal drug trade) and large movements of refugees or other mass migrations. Eight of the eleven main producers of cases have been on that list since at least 1986.

All the countries in the first group, where malaria has declined, have shared a degree of social stability and socioeconomic development, including health services accessible to the public. The countries in the third group have suffered periodic bouts of malaria, followed by remobilized control efforts, after which the situation improved but could not be maintained, so malaria recurred. This pattern of "fire fighting" may progressively improve matters in the more developed areas as people become less tolerant of epidemics and health services become more responsive. In marginal areas, the response is nearly always late and possibly ineffective, because it often comes when the epidemic is naturally declining.

Drug Resistance and Proportion of P. falciparum

The proportion of *P. falciparum* in endemic areas outside tropical Africa, where *P. falciparum* remains the predominant species, was 38 percent in 1990 (compared with 15 percent in the early 1970s). In the last few years there has been an increased selection and progressive dispersal of *P. falciparum* parasites resistant to antimalarial drugs, because these drugs are used increasingly as prophylactics and for self-medication, usually in insufficient doses (see map 13-2). The problem of drug resistance has been particularly alarming in Africa; in recent years it has spread across the continent and is now developing rapidly in West African countries. Its continual intensification hampers efforts to provide adequate treatment in rural areas. It is difficult to assess how much to attribute this phenomenon to the migration of resistant parasites and how much to local selection, because both mobility and drug consumption have increased considerably. For some time the widespread use of chloroquine was advocated as the most effective way to reduce deaths from malaria in Africa; chloroquine, it was said, should be treated as a commodity and not as a drug. In many places in Africa people use chloroquine more often than aspirin for minor fevers and aches. Chloroquine has, no doubt, helped reduce deaths from malaria, but maintaining this gain will require targeting antimalarial drugs to those actually suffering from malaria, particularly in areas where resistant parasites require the use of more toxic and less affordable drugs.

Mortality

Most deaths from malaria occur in tropical Africa. As in all highly endemic areas, deaths occur most among the young. Maternal immunity transmitted to infants may reduce mortality in the first three to six months of life, but this effect may be masked in areas of marked seasonality. Past studies indicated mortality rates between ten and thirty per thousand in infants and between about seven and eleven per thousand in children one to four years old. In 1962 the WHO Regional Office for Africa estimated that every year between 200,000 and 500,000 African children die from malaria (Pampana 1969). In 1969, Bruce-Chwatt put that figure at about 1 million, a figure extensively quoted ever since. Molineaux (1985), reviewing the effect on infant mortality of some malaria control projects, especially in Kisumu (Kenya) and Garki (Nigeria), concluded that malaria was responsible for about 20 to 30 percent of infant deaths. Greenwood and others (1987), studying deaths from malaria in the Gambia, concluded that the mortality rate from malaria was 6.3 per 1,000 for infants and 10.7 per 1,000 for children one to four years old, representing 10 percent of the deaths of children less than a year old and 25 percent of deaths for children one to four.

There are signs that in some parts of Africa general infant and malaria-specific mortality may be declining, often independently of specific interventions, reflecting social develop-

Map 13-2. *Areas where Chloroquine-Resistant* Plasmodium Falciparum *has been Reported*

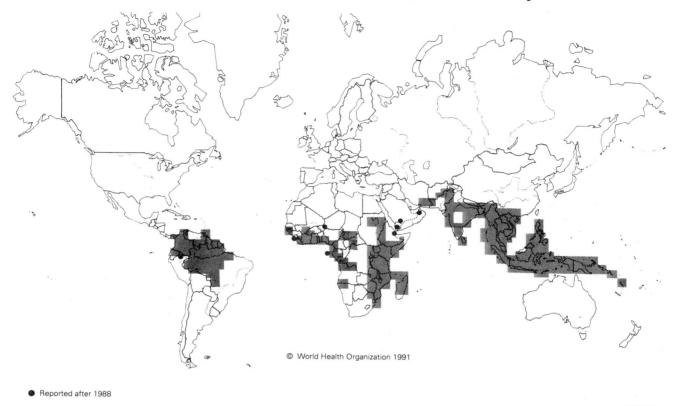

● Reported after 1988

© World Health Organization 1991

WHO 91363

Note: The designations employed and the presentation of material on this map do not imply the expression of any opinion whatsoever on the part of the World Health Organization concerning the legal status of any country, territory, city, or area or of its authorities, or concerning the delimitation of its frontiers or boundaries.

Source: Reproduced by permission of the World Health Organization, Geneva from *Weekly Epidemiological Record* 66 (22): 162 (1991).

ment and general education. Studies in the Congo and Burkina Faso in the late 1970s indicated that malaria-specific mortality might be lower than expected in areas where, some decades ago, malaria was a significant cause of infant mortality. The authors (Vaise and others 1981) attributed their findings to the widespread, albeit indiscriminate, use of antimalarial drugs. Often these drugs were used in doses inadequate to eliminate parasites but effective enough to produce a clinical cure and prevent death, even if collectively such use could be contributing to the selection of drug-resistant parasites. The wide availability of antimalarial and other active drugs has also been identified as possibly contributing to the general decline in infant mortality observed in the Kisumu area of Kenya. There, between 1972 and 1976, infant mortality reportedly declined from 157 per 1,000 to 93 per 1,000 during an effective malaria control program (spraying fenitrothion inside houses). Between 1981 and 1983, a decline in postneonatal mortality (from 73 to 67 per 1,000) and a marked drop in the mortality of children of one to four years (from 25 to 18 per 1,000) were recorded after implementation of a program of community-based antimalaria treatment. But most of that decline was attributed to a measles epidemic in 1981–82; malaria-specific

mortality, being relatively low, did not change significantly in the year of intervention. This study (Spencer and others 1987) confirmed in a small rural area the general observation that differences in child mortality can be explained largely by differences in maternal education, which no doubt influences the amount of drug use but, more important, improves hygiene and general living standards. Differences in infant mortality between districts in Kenya, as reported in the 1979 census, ranged from 38 to 153 per 1,000. When spraying in Kisumu ended, in 1976, the area did not return to the previous infant mortality rates. Infant mortality rates for the district in which this area is located declined from 220 in 1959 to 181 in 1969 and to 147 in 1979 (Spencer and others 1987).

Deaths from malaria outside tropical Africa occur mainly among nonimmunes who become infected by *P. falciparum* and get sick where appropriate diagnosis and treatment are unavailable. This happens especially to newcomers to endemic areas, such as agricultural workers, laborers, gold and gem miners, and prospectors in recently colonized or other frontier areas of economic development. Most affected are young adults, although whole families of settlers may be affected—for example, in the tropical jungles of South America (especially the basins of the Amazon and the Orinoco), in the outer islands of Indonesia, Sabah, Kalimantan, and, on a smaller scale, throughout the tropics. In the Brazilian Amazon, an estimated 6,000 to 10,000 people a year die from malaria (J. Fiusa Lima, personal communication, 1990).

Possible Patterns of Morbidity and Mortality: 2000, 2015

Malaria transmission is focal and depends on the dynamics between humans and the vector, parasite, and environment. More important, it depends on the effectiveness of control efforts, socioeconomic development, and political stability. It is thus quite risky to generalize about future patterns of morbidity and mortality. Given the increasing resistance of the parasite to antimalarial drugs, however, treatment of malaria in the future will be more difficult and less effective, thereby increasing the risk of both morbidity and mortality. Although new drugs are being investigated, and work is progressing on various potential malaria vaccines, alternative first- or second-line drugs or a vaccine are, even under optimistic circumstances, several years away.

Furthermore, population instability in areas in which there is the potential for malaria transmission is usually associated with an increasing burden of illness, including mortality due to malaria. This instability might result from political conflicts, economic development or relocation schemes, migration because of population pressure, or natural disasters. Examples from Brazil, Thailand, Indonesia, and Sri Lanka may illustrate different facets of this problem. To the extent that development projects ignore effects on health or that political conflicts create large refugee populations, malaria is likely to increase in each such local situation. Conversely, adequate socioeconomic development and political stability will facilitate effective and sustainable malaria control.

As to patterns of morbidity and mortality in the future, it is safe to predict that there will be more morbidity and possibly mortality as a result of malaria in several areas, but how much more and, more specifically, which regions will bear most of the burden, is less obvious. Well-documented case studies could serve as examples of potentially devastating effects, given similar scenarios in other areas of the world (that is, Brazil, Madagascar, Sudan, Indonesia, Afghanistan, Sri Lanka, and so on).

But most important in view of the presently deteriorating worldwide malaria situation referred to earlier, a forceful effort to rehabilitate, activate, or develop new malaria control activities in those countries most affected is crucial. Without such an effort malaria patterns in the year 2000 will be entirely different and substantively worse than the ones predicted.

Economic Costs of Malaria

The economic costs of malaria theoretically would include its effect on the economy and economic development, on the local community, on the household, and on the individual.

There have been few community-based methods used to evaluate the economic effect of malaria. The study by Conly (1975) highlights the problems encountered in attempting to quantify the effect on economic development resulting from the difficulty of collecting and processing data on a sufficiently large population and the complexity of the interactions of the parameters measured.

COSTS OF MORTALITY AND MORBIDITY. The costs that malaria imposes are borne through increased mortality and through high morbidity rates. The effect of mortality will vary with the age distribution of deaths, which in turn vary by ecological zones. In Africa, where most deaths are among infants and young children, the effect of and the perception of mortality will be different from other areas, where the deaths are among the main breadwinners or primary caretakers of families. Mortality and morbidity among adults are high in areas of low to moderate endemicity. See Over and others 1989 on the consequence of adult deaths.

MALARIA AND PRODUCTIVITY. Public health activities have been justified as improving productivity ever since debates about the "laziness disease" at the beginning of this century (Garcia 1981). Malaria is a classic example of a debilitating disease that impairs productivity. As the most prevalent disease in the poorest rural areas, malaria produces recurrent infections with attacks of fever in the warm and rainy seasons, when most workers are needed to collect crops. Often, affected people also suffer from malnutrition and other infections and lack of medical care. In areas subject to epidemics, these also tend to strike at times of peak demand for agricultural work.

The focus of much of the research has been on attempting to measure the effects of bouts of illness on lost output of workers. This research has been reviewed in Barlow and Grobar 1986. Research on the physical effect of the disease can be found in Conly 1975; Malik 1966; Russell and Menon 1942; and van Dine 1916. Days of disability per case of malaria estimated in these studies range from five to twenty. Other physical measures include effects on output or land cleared. Audibert (1984) sets values for the former varying from 0 to 1.5 for the elasticity of output of rice with respect to malaria prevalence, whereas Bhombore, Brooke Worth, and Nanjundiah (1952) found a reduction of 60 percent in cropped area in families with malaria. Conly (1975) traces a variety of adjustments in farm families in Paraguay, including increases in labor input per unit output as well as reallocations of land and hired labor. The reallocations of land entailed replacement of crops of high value whose crop season was malaria prone with crops of relatively low value whose crop season was not. De Castro (1985) finds that such reallocations may include an increase in the workload of healthy family members. Although this may be seen as an ameliorative factor which reduces the net effect of the disease, it may simply mean that some costs of the disease are borne by others besides those who are ill. In Southern Rhodesia it has been estimated that the loss of manpower to malaria was 5 to 10 percent of the labor force, with the heaviest incidence at the peak of agricultural production.

Estimates are much lower in highly endemic areas, where anyone who survives childhood can generally tolerate a malaria infection, showing only minor symptoms at most, although malaria is an important contributing factor in severe anemia. Brohult and others (1981), in a study in Liberia, found no detectable loss of physical ability in people with malaria parasites in their blood, but they did find a marked correlation between anemia and loss of physical ability.

It is a common convention in the literature to use the parameter of seven days of work lost to disability per bout of malaria in assessing a program when the parameter is not independently estimated (see Niazi 1969; Quo 1959; San Pedro 1967/68; and Sinton 1938); when independently estimated, the parameter varied between five and fifteen days. A further issue, raised by Wernsdorfer and Wernsdorfer (1988), is the undermining of the effectiveness of investment in education. In highly endemic areas, where adults normally have acquired sufficient immunity to make the symptoms less severe, schoolchildren are more severely affected. Judging the degree of impairment caused by illness would be hard to do and one can only wonder at the cost. Macdonald (1950) estimated that the learning of 35 to 60 percent of children may be impaired by malaria.

Other studies emphasize direct financial benefits from activities made possible by eradication or control. These are also surveyed in Wernsdorfer and Wernsdorfer (1988). Malaria has hurt economic development projects as well as armies at war and police forces or border patrols in endemic areas. Malaria had to be overcome for the successful construction of the Panama Canal and most roads and railways in tropical countries, for the agricultural development of the Roman campagna and the Venezuelan llanos, for the building of railways and roads in tropical areas, and for the protection of armies from World War I through Viet Nam. Agricultural development and mining in tropical jungle areas, which attract workers from densely populated, often nonmalarious, areas, form one of the particular problems associated with malaria. An example of research into the benefits of malaria control in this situation is given by Griffith, Ramana and Mashaal (1971), who estimate the increased profits derived from allowing workers to enter new areas for mining. Forgone profits are the measure of the cost of disease. Sinton (1938) documents many cases in India where malarious regions prevented an expansion into new territories, resulting in substantial losses in forgone earnings. Demographic changes since then, however, have probably made such opportunities for expansion much rarer in the subcontinent.

DISTRIBUTION OF COST. Litsios (1990) highlights the uneven distribution of malaria risk across a population. Data from Adana, Turkey (Yumer 1980), for example, show that anopheline bites per person were five times more frequent in the tents of migrant workers than in the houses of village residents. Malaria has been concentrated among migrant laborers in most areas where there is extensive cultivation of cotton and sugar cane and in some areas where coffee, bananas, and rice are cultivated. Litsios (1990, p. 8) concludes that "as malaria becomes a problem to be primarily found in marginal or fringe areas, it becomes a problem that is identified with marginal people." This can be seen by the tendency in some countries to associate malaria with "foreigners" or minority migrant groups, who are then accused of being responsible for carrying the parasites into areas that might otherwise be malaria-free. In endemic areas the burden of malaria is also borne disproportionately by the poor.

PROBLEMS IN MEASURING COST. The focus on days lost from work or output forgone is oddly narrow. With regard to welfare, two alternative measures would be preferable. The first is the compensating variation in income, or, the amount one would be willing to pay to avoid having the disease altogether. The second is the equivalent variation, the willingness to accept, or the amount one would need to be paid to accept having the disease. In many contexts, these two measures are similar, but in cases in which possible mortality is involved the latter could generate much larger measures of costs than the former. Willingness to pay is bounded by ability to pay or lifetime earnings. In practical application, it would be limited by borrowing constraints as well. Willingness to accept is under no such limitation. Either of these measures would capture the subjective, even psychological effect of the disease. In any case, using a measure which respects personal preferences would be more inclusive than simply including the instrumental effects of the disease on the productive capacity of the worker. There are a number of objections to using these alternative concepts. They require defining which set of preferences (before or after falling ill) is relevant for the comparison. The most important criticism, though, is that obtaining this number requires a significant research effort. Such calculations have been made in the literature on environmental effects but are not widely used. It is possible to infer a lower bound, though, by calculating the total costs required to obtain treatment. The total costs borne by families and individuals include payments for treatment, time and transport costs in seeking treatment, time costs for family members who look after the patient, and time and money costs of preventive action taken by households and the community. These costs vary greatly with variables such as access to primary health care, national drug distribution policies, the presence of chloroquine resistance, the level of malaria endemicity, the behavior and bionomics of the local vector(s), and whether or not malaria is perceived as a serious health problem by the local community. There are two main sources of underestimation. First, this calculation misses costs before treatment is sought. Second, there are those (inherently hard to measure) who have decided that the costs of seeking treatment are too high in relation to the costs of letting the disease run its course. For them, there is still a relevant cost and degree of necessary compensation. For people in remote areas, or those afflicted at peak agricultural seasons (when implicit wages are high, both for the person falling ill or, in the case of children especially, for those needing to accompany the person), or (more difficult to evaluate) those who are uninformed about treatment prospects, these costs can be high.

In their careful study of Thailand, Kaewsonthi and Harding (1986) attempted, among other things, to measure the costs borne by patients in seeking care. These were dubbed "external costs," that is, external to the malaria control organization. They amounted to $20 per positive case, or nine times the average wage. This estimate is for people presenting at the malaria clinic and therefore does not include those who have handled the disease in other ways. This study includes costs entailed in seeking local treatment before travel to the clinic. These amounted to 15 percent of the costs per positive case and are a component of the full cost to those who do not seek formal treatment. The degree of underestimation of the cost to sufferers is probably quite high. Time lost before and after seeking treatment can be considerable and varies with the quality (primarily speed) of service provided. This varies substantially within Thailand, let alone across countries.

Because the costs of malaria are borne disproportionately by the poor, there are further issues of aggregating individual costs into social costs. Whether disease averted should be weighted by the income of the sufferer, because of social welfare consideration or the possibility of successfully seeking treatment, is an ethical issue to be appraised by policymakers.

In summary, Andreano and Helminiak (1988, p. 35) state that "despite the many studies and the excellent work by Barlow and Conly, which represent methodological advances in the study of tropical diseases, we remain woefully ignorant of the social and economic effect of malaria in those countries of the world where it is prevalent." They also emphasize that findings in many of these studies cannot be easily generalized from one area to another.

Malaria Control

The idea of eradicating malaria, postulated as early as 1916, gained currency after World War II. Malaria epidemics had devastated parts of southern Europe, and DDT had been extremely effective in controlling not only those epidemics but also endemic malaria in both temperate and tropical areas, including Venezuela, British Guiana, and Taiwan. The Expert Committee on Malaria of the newly created World Health Organization, in its first five reports, adopted a cautious attitude, expressing concern about increasing reports of technical problems and of some disappointing results in the use of DDT, particularly in Africa. But the goal of eradicating malaria became irresistible, and the impending resistance to DDT was seen as a reason for racing to eradicate malaria before resistance developed. In 1954 the Pan-American Sanitary Conference adopted a continental plan to eradicate malaria from the Americas. In 1955 this plan was extended to the world by the World Health Assembly (WHA). In 1956, the Sixth Expert

Committee formulated a strategy for eradicating malaria (WHO 1957).

Soon after the WHA resolution and the report of the Expert Committee, most countries of the Americas, Europe, North Africa, Asia, and the Pacific officially declared that their antimalaria programs were eradication campaigns. In retrospect we can see that many of these programs were short on epidemiological knowledge and administrative capacity. These deficiencies were overlooked because of the programs' humanitarian appeal, the sense of urgency, and the feeling, shared by many, that peer pressure could shake the chronic apathy of the health services.

As anticipated, tropical Africa and some parts of Southeast Asia posed problems, because of their high endemicity, primitive state of development, and lack of human and economic resources. Successes elsewhere, although slower than expected, were still remarkable. But as more and more areas advanced into their program's consolidation phase, the expectation that a surveillance mechanism would maintain areas malaria-free, after spraying was interrupted, was not fulfilled. Resurgences occurred increasingly often in the consolidation and maintenance phase, particularly in Central America and Southeast Asia. And at the end of the decade a massive epidemic broke out in Sri Lanka, where malaria had been almost eradicated. Evidence began to accumulate that, although it was possible to reduce and even interrupt malaria transmission by spraying insecticide in large areas, it was difficult if not impossible to establish effective surveillance without a solid health infrastructure.

Finally, in 1969, after reexamining the global strategy of eradicating malaria, the World Health Assembly reaffirmed that eradication was the ultimate goal but stated that, in regions where eradication was not yet feasible, control of malaria with the means available should be encouraged and may be a necessary and valid step toward that goal (WHO 1969).

Unfortunately, after fifteen years of strictly regimented antimalaria action, health authorities—even malariologists—were reluctant to introduce the necessary changes in the programs while the concept of malaria control, and an acceptable global strategy for it, remained undefined. The Expert Committee provided only sketchy guidance on how to transform an ineffective malaria eradication program into a control program, emphasizing that "the objectives in these areas would be to consolidate the gains so far achieved, to extend the programme to areas where protection would give maximum socioeconomic benefit and to protect high risk groups" (WHO 1974, p. 30). Unfortunately, in most countries it was thought that the only way to consolidate gains achieved was to maintain as many routine activities as could be afforded, without making the necessary investment to evaluate their local effectiveness.

The formulation by WHO in 1978 of a strategy to develop a health care infrastructure included malaria control among its essential elements (WHO/UNICEF 1978). In line with these developments, the thirty-first World Health Assembly adopted a strategy of malaria control aimed at least at reducing mortality and the negative social and economic effects of the disease, preventing or controlling epidemics, and protecting malaria-free areas, with the ultimate objective of eradicating the disease whenever feasible (WHO 1978).

Malaria Control Measures

The most common antimalarial measures are (a) chemical control through residual intradomiciliary spraying with DDT or other insecticides and, in selected instances, aerial spraying or local fogging, (ultra low volume); and (b) the treatment of fever cases with antimalarials. These activities are sometimes supported by limited environmental management measures mostly in urban areas where such measures can be easier to implement than in rural ones. They involve drainage or filling of water bodies. Water-level fluctuations or intermittent irrigation are used in some large development schemes. For all practical purposes biological control measures are presently of little relevance. In addition to these active intervention measures, all control programs undertake active or passive malaria surveillance. Specific antimalarial measures can be classified according to their mode of action and the scope and scale of their use (table 13-1).

Two substantially different approaches may be pursued in malaria control.

* Improving general health services to ensure adequate diagnosis, access to health care, and treatment for individual malaria cases, as well as promoting personal and community protection. The aim of this approach is to eliminate deaths from malaria and to reduce the severity and duration of illness associated with it.
* Establishing the capability for long-term control of malaria transmission, control and prevention of epidemics, and progressive reduction of malaria endemicity (particularly in areas affected by *P. falciparum*).

The two approaches are in no way mutually exclusive, and ideally they should be complementary; however, they differ greatly in their requirements for specialized services. Whereas the former is a basic requirement in all malarious areas, the second would be developed progressively, according to the intensity of the problem and resources available.

New Perspectives for Control

In 1985 the thirty-eighth World Health Assembly expressed its continuing concern about resurgent malaria and, in particular, about the apparent inadequacies of existing malaria control strategies. Consequently, the WHO Expert Committee on Malaria (WHO 1986) reviewed the global malaria situation and attempted to develop further the epidemiological approach to malaria control, which had been proposed by the Expert Committee in 1979, giving particular emphasis to socioeconomic factors. Within the epidemiological approach is the recognition that variability among diverse malaria situations is the result of a multitude of factors, which will also affect the effectiveness of control measures. Mapping the distribution of these determining factors would constitute a "stratification" of the local malaria problem and would provide a useful framework for selecting and testing appropriate sets of control interventions.

Identification of Malaria Patterns

In practice, the identification of all relevant epidemiological factors has not come easily to control program managers. They are often not equipped to analyze and interpret the massive quantities of epidemiological, parasitological, and entomological information that need to be collected—and to use this information to define appropriate control actions. In particular, those in charge of control programs have generally lacked the ability to see specific malaria situations in their economic and social context; that is, to analyze the relationships between patterns of human occupation and exploitation of the environment and trends in malaria transmission.

Nevertheless, accumulated experience and some specific studies of problem areas showed that there are identifiable ecological and social situations in which malaria is not only more frequent and serious but also more difficult to control. In the Brazilian Amazon, for example, economic, social, environ-

Table 13-1. Malaria Control Measures

Action	Individual and family protection	Community protection
Reduction of man-mosquito contact	Bednets, repellents, protective clothing, screening of houses	Site selection, zooprophylaxis
Destruction of adult mosquitoes	Use of domestic space spraying	Residual indoor insecticides, space spraying, ultra-low volume sprays
Destruction of mosquito larvae	Peridomestic sanitation, intermittent drying of water containers	Larvicide for water surfaces, intermittent irrigation, sluicing, biological control
Source reduction	Peridomestic sanitation, small-scale drainage	Environmental sanitation, water management, drainage
Destruction of malaria parasites	Early diagnosis and treatment, chemoprophylaxis	Establishment of diagnosis and treatment facilities, chemoprophylaxis for pregnant women, mass treatment
Social participation	Motivation	Health education, community participation

Source: Adapted from Bruce-Chwatt 1985.

mental, and political factors have converged to produce three epidemiological patterns, collectively referred to as "frontier malaria" (Marques 1988; Sawyer and Sawyer 1987; Wilson and Alicbusan-Schwab 1991). These patterns are found in the now famous "garimpos" (gold-mining areas), in areas of new agricultural settlement, and in the rapidly expanding periurban areas of the region. Although found in less than one in ten municipalities, they account for more than 80 percent of all malaria cases reported. Similarly, most malaria situations throughout the world, when viewed in their social and economic context, fall into a few main types.

It has been suggested (Nájera 1981, 1989) that it is possible to recognize and describe a limited number of prototypes or typical patterns, synthesizing, from a global perspective, those observations in different countries, complemented with summaries of control experiences in such situations. These descriptions of epidemiological patterns (which have been referred to as "prototyes" or "malaria paradigms") could help health planners in the important task of designing and implementing appropriate sets of control measures, either to develop new programs or to adapt existing ones.

Malaria Patterns and Specific Ecological Conditions

The main determinants of malaria transmission (vector density and survival, human-vector contact and duration of parasite development in the vector) are dependent on availability of surface water and climate, which in turn have also influenced the distribution of rural populations and their agricultural activities. It is therefore possible to identify major differences in the epidemiology of malaria associated to the main types of ecological areas, which would provide a first characterization of the epidemiological pattern, unless man has sufficiently disturbed the environment and introduced some of the patterns referred to in the next heading.

THE AFRICAN SAVANNA. *Characteristics*: the African savanna represents the highest malaria endemicity in the world. The factors responsible for high levels of continuous transmission include propitious climatic conditions for vector breeding and the presence of such highly efficient vectors as A. *gambiae* and A. *funestus*. This pattern is characterized by high frequency of illness among young children and pregnant women, high childhood mortality, and high frequency of asymptomatic infections in older children and adults. Transmission may become seasonal in areas with less rainfall and at higher altitudes. Recently, the malaria problem has been aggravated by the rapid spread of drug resistance across the African continent.

Control: in the African savanna the most important goal of malaria control is to reduce the effect of the disease by providing effective treatment to all people suffering from malaria, which will require extension of services and health education to improve their use by the population. Pilot projects, aimed at the interruption of transmission in savanna areas, have been only partially successful, and institutional problems have constrained expansion of vector control programs (Bruce-Chwatt

1979 and Bruce-Chwatt and Archibald 1959 [Sokoto]; Foll and others 1965 and Nájera and others 1973 [Kankiya]; and Wilson 1960 [Pare Taveta]). There are some areas or population groups, however, in which vector control may be feasible; in particular it may be possible to introduce effectively insecticide-impregnated bed nets or curtains.

PLAINS AND VALLEYS OUTSIDE AFRICA. *Characteristics*: these areas correspond to the classic descriptions of malaria as a rural disease, being more intense in the poorest areas and in periods of economic depression. As in the African savanna, transmission may be from continuous to seasonal, depending on latitude, altitude, and aridity. The risk of transmission tends to increase with the introduction or extension of irrigation, but it considerably decreases with good water management and the improvement of farming techniques, houses, and animal shelters. In most of these areas malaria was brought under control by the early eradication campaigns, and vector control has continued over the last three decades. These areas show low endemicity and should continue to do so unless disturbed by civil unrest, insurgence, or war, which would not permit the functioning of health services.

Control: in most instances, it will be possible to maintain this favorable situation through the continuing development of their health and epidemiological services and by their ability to detect and control potential risk situations.

FOREST AND FOREST FRINGE AREAS. *Characteristics*: the extensive forest areas of Africa, South America, and Southeast Asia have increased in importance as the exploitation of forest resources has intensified. Malaria risks are associated with the type of human activity which modifies the microenvironment and the relation of humans and vectors to it. Nomadic and seminomadic tribal populations of forest areas, engaged in gathering and hunting, are generally too dispersed and mobile to sustain intense transmission. In the fringe of the forest or deforested areas, sedentary populations tend to be engaged mainly in agriculture, but they also use the forest to collect firewood and for hunting. In Africa the main malaria vectors, A. *gambiae* and A. *funestus*, follow man into the forest and, although they are more easily controlled than in the savanna, they are able to maintain the same levels of very high endemicity. In Asia and the Americas, settled population groups, engaged in regular agricultural activities in deforested areas, have a different malaria experience from that of those engaged in forest activities. The former suffer mostly from P. *vivax* infection and tend to have much lower malaria incidence, easily controllable with residual insecticides. In contrast, those engaging in activities at the edge of or inside the forest have a high risk of acquiring P. *falciparum* malaria.

Control: residual insecticides are practically ineffective against the highly exophylic (outdoor biters) forest vectors. Protection has been traditionally dependent on the use of drugs, often excessive and irregular, because of the absence of organized curative services. When international borders run across these areas, as is common in South America and Southeast Asia, there may be a concentration of illegal activities, which make areas even less accessible to programmed control. Chloroquine-resistant *P. falciparum* originated in areas of this type, both in the Colombian-Venezuelan and the Thai-Cambodian borders (Field 1967). Today more effective means of personal protection, such as pyrethroid-impregnated bed nets and repellents, offer a possibility of complementing the partial effect of currently available antimalarial drugs and eventually reducing the dependence on chemoprophylaxis.

HIGHLAND FRINGE AND DESERT FRINGE. *Characteristics*: altitude, drainage, and temperature are limiting factors in both mosquito breeding and in parasite development in the mosquito. Therefore, these factors have an important effect on the potential for malaria transmission along the fringes of highland areas. The highlands themselves, which tend to have less transmission of malaria, often are characterized by high population density and pendular migration between the highlands and neighboring valleys. These neighboring areas, which offer economic opportunities on plantations or in other development projects, often have more transmission. Unusually warm rainy seasons may cause serious epidemics in highland areas of low endemicity, resulting in high mortality (for example, East Africa and Madagascar in 1987–90). In Southeast Asia, vectors which breed in foothill streams (for example, A. *minimus* and A. *fluviatilis*) are more efficient vectors than those in the plains. Therefore, the foothills in such areas tend to be more malarious than the plains. In transitional zones adjoining deserts, the lengthy dry season also limits vector proliferation and malaria. Also, the populations of such areas tend to be dispersed and nomadic; epidemics may occur in years of exceptional rainfall or with the introduction of irrigation.

Control: as everywhere, effective disease treatment is fundamental in both highland and desert fringe areas. In addition, surveillance for the monitoring of epidemic risk indicators, and for the early detection of epidemics, is crucial. In different areas, different responses may be feasible. These responses may include a combination of preventive vector control, strengthening of treatment facilities, and mass fever treatment.

SEASHORE AND COASTAL MALARIA. *Characteristics*: the most typical situation is found where the mosquito vector breeds in brackish waters. Such mosquitoes are generally less efficient as vectors than those of neighboring inland areas, as is true of A. *melas* and A. *merus* in Africa and A. *aquasalis* in South America. Still, in Southeast Asia and the Pacific, A. *sundaicus* and A. *farauti* are responsible for serious malaria transmission. In some coastal areas, as in Central America and Mexico, freshwater-breeding mosquitoes may cause intense seasonal transmission by breeding profusely in estuaries closed during the dry season by a sand bar.

A frequent form of economic development in coastal areas is the establishment of tourist resorts, which often make important investments, not only in malaria control, but also in pest mosquito control, for the protection of the installations. The development of tourism often attracts more people than those that can make a living from the existence of the tourist resort, creating situations similar to those of periurban slums.

Control: disease control in tourist resorts is similar to that in urban areas. For rural coastal populations, whether they are engaged in agriculture or fishery, the basic measure should be case management and engineering methods, such as opening or flushing estuaries, land reclamation for agriculture or tree plantation, regulation of water courses, and so on.

URBAN MALARIA. *Characteristics*: except for some cities in southern Asia, where A. *stephensi* is fully adapted to the urban environment, malaria transmission does not occur in well-established, densely populated urban areas. Nevertheless, many tropical cities are surrounded by rapidly growing slums, which are basically a high concentration of shelters in what is still primarily a rural environment. Such situations increase the risk of malaria transmission. Eventually a high contamination of surface waters may prevent anopheline breeding before urbanization reaches the slum areas. Malaria transmission in urban areas varies considerably in space and time, but in certain situations it may be very high.

Control: malaria control in urban areas relies on environmental sanitation, in order to eliminate existing mosquito-breeding sites and prevent the creation of new ones. In addition, human-vector contact can be reduced through improved house construction and personal protection.

Malaria Patterns Associated with Specific Occupations or Social Conditions

There are a number of socioeconomic activities which create major disturbances of the environment, attract large numbers of temporary workers, or disrupt the social structure and therefore the health care system. All these activities transform the basic epidemiological parameters, as determined by the physical ecology of the area. The new malaria patterns so created may be not very extensive in area or may not persist very long in the same location, but where and when they occur, they may represent authentic epidemiological explosions and often leave marked sequelae of environmental degradation when they are abandoned.

AGRICULTURAL COLONIZATION OF JUNGLE AREAS. *Characteristics*: areas of new colonization attract displaced people either from cities or from densely populated areas that often have low malaria endemicity. Many people have, therefore, no or little acquired immunity and suffer severely from malaria when exposed to the high-transmission risk in the jungle environment. The effectiveness of vector control based on intradomiciliary spraying is limited in these areas because shelters are generally precarious and the vector does not always feed or rest indoors. Social services in these areas are weak or absent. In time, the situation tends to improve as these settlements become more developed. This pattern is found in Brazil, parts of India, and the outer islands of Indonesia (Binol 1983; Marques 1988). The agricultural settlement of large new areas is usually accompanied by the rapid growth of supporting urban centers as well. These centers attract large numbers of poor, often unemployed or underemployed migrants, who settle in precarious conditions on the urban periphery. This explosive periurban growth is also associated with high levels of malaria transmission (Sawyer 1986; Sawyer and Sawyer 1987).

Control: traditionally, protection has been dependent on the use of drugs, especially during the initial phases of settlement. The use of drugs, however, has often been excessive and irregular because of the absence of health services in these remote areas. Residual insecticides have proven less effective against highly exophilic forest vectors. In some areas traditional vector control activities may be possible. Furthermore, measures for personal protection, such as pyrethroid-impregnated bed nets and repellents, may be introduced in combination with appropriate information and health education.

GOLD AND GEM MINING. *Characteristics*: malaria is usually serious in remote forest areas among populations of miners who migrate frequently between existing mining areas, new mining areas, and urban and rural areas (for example, in Brazil and Venezuela). Occupation of these areas is often temporary, and investment in basic infrastructure and services is rare, especially in countries in which small-scale mining is illegal. *P. falciparum* drug resistance is frequent (for example, the Thai-Cambodian border, the Colombia-Venezuela border, and the Brazilian Amazon). Because they have tended to penetrate deeply into frontier areas, these gold and gem miners have often exposed highly vulnerable indigenous peoples to malaria and other diseases, with disastrous consequences.

Control: in these areas malaria control activities are exceedingly difficult. Case management is clearly a priority. Recently, attempts have been made to introduce insecticide-impregnated curtains and bed nets. In high-risk areas lacking any health facilities, it may sometimes be appropriate to establish specialized malaria clinics.

MIGRANT AGRICULTURAL LABOR. *Characteristics*: cotton, sugar, and large-scale rice cultivation often require large contingents of temporary labor for planting and harvesting. The workers generally live in crowded, unsanitary camps where mosquitoes abound and precarious shelters offer little protection against the malaria vector. Because of heavy pesticide use for agriculture, often sprayed by airplanes (especially in cotton farming), vector resistance to a broad spectrum of insecticides is common.

Control: disease control requires case management and the application of residual pesticides, where possible, and in some cases aerial pesticide application is very effective. In addition, personal protection measures, such as the use of insecticide-impregnated bed nets, can sometimes be applied. If irrigation practices allow, drainage, biological control, and other measures to reduce vector breeding may be indicated.

DISPLACED POPULATIONS. *Characteristics*: sociopolitical disturbances (such as wars, unrest, famines) often create situations in which the civilian population suffers a lack of basic supplies, destruction of houses, and considerable displacements, and even temporary or permanent housing in refugee camps. These situations, combined with the disruption of health services, may cause epidemic outbreaks even in areas previously well under control. These outbreaks particularly affect the civilian population; the military and police contingents are likely to benefit from organized control in their camps and chemoprophylaxis while in action.

Control: in these situations control depends on the size and organization of the refugee population and the intensity of the problem. It may be possible to consider mass fever treatment, temporary chemoprophylaxis, and even spraying of shelters. Sometimes relocation of camps and some sanitation measures are possible.

Patterns and Measures for Control

The matrix in table 13-2 relates the patterns identified above with control measures that have or have not proven effective in malaria control programs. This table is neither comprehensive nor prescriptive; its intent is to help operationalize the concept of epidemiological stratification.

It must be noted that the diagnosis and treatment of cases, including the management of drug resistance, applies equally to all patterns. Case management and drug treatment, which in most cases represents the care of fever, without specific diagnosis, are dependent on the structure of the general health care system. Diagnosis and treatment should be undertaken by the general health services; in areas in which such services are weak or nonexistent, such as in forest fringe areas and frontier areas, special fever-treatment posts or malaria clinics may be needed. Transmission control interventions should be used selectively wherever they are affordable and can achieve sustainable results.

Vector control operations have relied overwhelmingly on spraying of residual insecticides. The effectiveness of residual spraying varies substantially with the biting and resting behavior of the mosquito vector, the type of housing, and the habits of the people. A control measure which is receiving increasing attention is the use of insecticide-impregnated bed nets or curtains.

Other techniques of vector control play a more restricted role but, where indicated, may be highly effective. Space or aerial spraying is seldom used and is rarely justified. Larvicides are feasible only with easily identifiable breeding places. Techniques of source reduction, such as drainage and water management, can be the measures of choice in urban and periurban areas and economic development projects. They are normally too costly, however, for widespread use.

Residual Practices from Malaria Eradication Programs

Many malaria control programs continue to depend on practices held over from the eradication era that require adjustment. Indoor spraying of residual insecticides, the main

Table 13-2. Patterns Associated with Ecological and Social Conditions

Control intervention	Major ecological conditions							Specific occupations/ social conditions		
	African savannah	Plains and valleys outside frica	Forest and forest fringe	Highland and desert fringe	Seashore and coastal	Urban	Agricultural colonization of forest	Gold mining	Migrant agriculture labor	Displaced populations
Management of clinical malaria										
Diagnosis and treatment	+	+	+	+	+	+	+	+	+	+
Care of treatment failures	+	+	+	+	+	+	+	+	+	+
Protection of pregnant women										
Chemoprophylaxis	+	–	+	–	–	–	+	–	–	–
Bednets and personal protection	+	+	+	+	+	+	+	+	+	+
Vector control										
Residual spraying	–	Selective	Selective	Epidemic control	Selective	Limited	Selective	–	Limited	Epidemic control
Fogging ULV	–	–	–	–	+	Limited	–	–	Limited	+
Impregnated bednets or curtains	+	+	+	–	+	–	+	+	–	–
Environmental control										
Drainage and source reduction	–	–	–	–	+	+	–	–	+	–
Larviciding	–	–	–	–	+	+	–	–	+	–
Biological control	–	–	–	–	Limited	+	–	–	+	–
Surveillance										
Epidemiological surveillance	+	+	+	+	+	+	+	+	+	+
Monitoring epidemic risk	–	+	+	+	–	–	–	+	+	+
Health education	+	+	+	+	+	+	+	–	–	–

Source: Authors.

control activity of eradication programs, consumes a large part of present program budgets. In principle, coverage with residual insecticides should be complete and regular to achieve significant reduction or interruption of transmission. Today's spraying is seldom regular because most budgets do not provide enough insecticide to cover all cycles; they are rarely complete because people often refuse to allow continuous routine spraying. Therefore, more selective, targeted, and cost-effective use of pesticides is needed.

Many malaria control programs continue the practice of case detection as the main mechanism to diagnose and treat malaria. This procedure, devised for the confirmation of the disappearance of malaria during the consolidation phase of a malaria eradication program, aims at the collection of a blood slide from every fever case in the population by a system of periodic house visits and the collaboration of all outpatient clinics of the health services. All fever cases are also given a single dose (presumptive) treatment to be followed by a full (radical) treatment, if the blood slide is positive, when the result from the laboratory becomes available, normally weeks or months later.

The consequence of insisting on a thick blood film for every fever case is that malaria microscopists are overwhelmed with negative slides, the examination of which not only takes most of their time but could also distract them and cause them to miss positives. The diagnosis is, most often, late, so it cannot

help in the diagnosis of the cause of fever, and the radical treatment of positives, when offered, may no longer be needed. Reports to WHO indicate that 150 million slides are collected each year, with an average positive result of 3 to 5 percent. Great efforts are made in some malaria programs to maintain a network of laboratories staffed by reasonably trained microscopists, engaged most of the time in the diagnosis of ambulatory fevers. But those in charge of the programs do not feel responsible for making competent microscopy available in the medical care establishments for the diagnosis and monitoring of treatment of suspected severe malaria cases; case detection continues to serve mainly an epidemiological purpose and does not contribute to improve the quality of care delivered by the health services.

The epidemiological services of the malaria programs were designed to confirm that malaria had been eradicated, and were organized to achieve the direct confirmation that the parasite reservoir had been eliminated. Indirect indicators of risk were overlooked. As a result, malaria programs have a poor record for early detection, let alone the prediction, of malaria epidemics. Whereas poorly organized general health services, reporting abnormal increases of fever cases, detected a number of epidemics reported in the literature, the malaria program case-detection mechanisms operating in the area detected no abnormality until months later, when slides had been examined, the results reported, and the reported cases consolidated and analyzed at the center. Often these mechanisms are unable to detect abnormal situations before they become large enough to overcome the dilution effect of consolidated reporting, as practiced by centralized malaria programs. General health services and local authorities are more sensitive and more likely to demand action in response to peripheral complaints, if encouraged to do so.

Interventions: Patterns, Cost-Effectiveness, and Choice

The nature of the different scenarios has a strong effect on the choice of appropriate policies to combat malaria. Calculations of cost-effectiveness need to be made in each specific circumstance. The value of calculating cost-effectiveness of interventions is to help policymakers make decisions about competing uses of resources. The steps in any such analysis are the following: (a) identify the policy instrument which is actually under the control of the decisionmaker; (b) determine the relation between the policy instrument and the measure of outcome desired; (c) pursue the activity until the marginal effectiveness per unit of marginal cost falls to a level comparable to other uses of funds. Each of these components is problematic and each is sensitively related to the epidemiological pattern in which decisionmakers find themselves.

INTERVENTIONS. Often, the set of available policy options is clear. Still, there is sometimes confusion about what is actually controlled by the government. For example, chemoprophylaxis for pregnant women and insecticide-impregnated bed nets are included as control interventions. These are policies which promote the use of techniques of control, such as information, education, and communication activities (IEC) for prenatal care (in conjunction with a protocol for drug prescriptions); a subsidy on the sale of bed nets; active distribution of (free) materials; and an IEC campaign on appropriate use. Strictly speaking it is these latter policies which should be evaluated on the basis of costs and effectiveness.

Organizational, political, and social factors implicit in some of the patterns define or impose limits on the appropriate policies. For example, the policies involved with management of clinical malaria are specific to the structure of the general health care system. Costs associated with malaria are sensitive to the organization of the health system. Mills (1987) compares the costs of provision in vertical programs with those in integrated programs in Nepal and finds that the higher the volume of cases, the more similar the costs of the two organizational policies will be. In areas where caseloads are low, integrated programs can have substantial cost savings, because personnel can switch to other health needs as appropriate.

One decision concerning provision of treatment (for all complaints, not just malaria) would be the density of location of health centers, or, more realistically, the location of new centers. The difficulty in separating care for malaria from care for anyone who presents with fever is sharply defined in this case. Although probably the most important factor in the care of malaria in endemic areas, such decisions cannot possibly be made with regard to malaria alone. To the extent that malaria generates a large proportion of visits to health centers, however, this could argue for shorter distances to clinics in new areas of agricultural development (in relation to more stable communities) because of the greater severity of the disease in these areas, even though the set of appropriate interventions is the same for the two settings. Again, this is part of a much larger problem. In general, the interventions involved with case management are not specific to malaria and include protocols for the public health facilities; the regulation, taxation, or subsidization of drugs and private health care providers; and recommendations on care for these providers. Benefits accrue to the system from any of these interventions, but attributing them to malaria is misleading.

RETURNS TO SCALE. Costs per measure of outcome (deaths averted, discounted healthy life years gained) vary substantially with the level of activity of the intervention. Certain features of intervention programs are relatively fixed and therefore independent of scale of operation (facilities, staff salaries in the short run), others are variable and proportional to outputs, and still others rise more than proportionately with output. Assessing the (marginal) cost per unit of outcome achieved needs to be assessed in each context. At a global level, Molineaux (1988) speculates that there may be "decreasing returns," because many early programs of malaria reduction were recognized as having strong effects, whereas recent efforts have been more disappointing.

PORTFOLIO OF INTERVENTIONS. For a number of alternative policy options in malaria control, there is good reason to expect diminishing returns to most single activities and, therefore, to expect effective policies to entail a package of instruments. The cost of vector control activities will rise with expansion as a result of decreasing densities of vectors and of people. Costs of case management operations will rise also with decreasing frequency of cases and the eventual need for either public information or IEC campaigns, which are costly. Barlow and Grobar (1986) suggest that the great uncertainty surrounding cost estimates argues that a combination of policies need to be used in parasitic-disease control programs. This is an analogy to financial management in which a "portfolio" of instruments should be used to reduce the risk of the entire program's resulting in failure. Here, we argue that for malaria, at least, a combination of policies would be desirable even with accurate information, because of diminishing returns from any one instrument.

VECTOR CONTROL. The cost-effectiveness of residual spraying varies substantially with the endemicity of the disease in the locale and with the degree of intensity of use. In regions of low to medium endemicity, where either the elimination of the disease or a substantial reduction in prevalence in humans as a result of reductions in vector capacity is possible, the effectiveness of vector control may be high. It may also have thresholds or regions of "increasing returns" near levels at which eradication is possible. Generally, however, there are good reasons to expect rising marginal costs associated with increasing workers hired for spraying. With decreasing density of housing units and increased distance from facilities in urban or regional centers, costs per house protected will rise as more person-hours will be needed for more remote areas. Similarly, small regions with high densities of the vector will be cheap to reach, whereas expansion to wider areas will become costly. Within a region, the cost per house protected will rise as a result of decreasing chemical effectiveness on the vector pool. Refusal of populations to have their dwellings sprayed also make improvements on the margin more difficult.

Other techniques of vector control play a much more restricted role. Space or aerial spraying is seldom used, except for urban epidemics or to interrupt short transmission seasons, and is rarely justified on cost grounds. Larvicides are feasible only with easily identifiable breeding places and are thus of limited use. Other source reduction techniques such as drainage and land management techniques can have significant effects in mainly urban areas, planned human settlements, or economic development projects, but they cannot be a significant part of widespread control operations.

CLINICAL MANAGEMENT. The cost of chemotherapy depends on both the costs of treatment itself and the costs (both to the health care system and to the individual) of getting the patient to seek treatment. For self-diagnosis (for over-the-counter purchases of chloroquine) or for spontaneous presentation at a health care facility, these costs are generally quite modest, although they depend on the availability of drugs and distances to facilities. For a target population of malaria sufferers who do not seek help in either of these forms, expansion of chemotherapy requires the use of information campaigns designed to encourage people to seek timely care or active case-detection methods, which are usually very expensive.

As to the effectiveness of drug treatment, to date, the use of chloroquine has been a remarkably effective and cheap method of dealing with the disease. People have been able to obtain the drug easily, and much treatment has taken place outside the formal health care system. One consequence of this may well have been the speeding of the progress of chloroquine resistance, that is, that marginal costs of chloroquine had been higher and increasing all along. The spread of chloroquine-resistant malaria has changed the picture substantially. Not only do the drugs cost more, but they also require more professional supervision; and some of them run into more serious problems of compliance with drug regimens. At 1987 prices (for one adult course of drug treatment), with chloroquine, the costs are $0.23 per person; with sulfadiazine/pyrimethamine, $0.50; with mefloquine/sulfadoxim/pyrimethamine, $1.20; and with quinine and tetracycline, $3.00. Drug treatment is likely to continue to be the principal antimalaria weapon. The possibility of multiple resistance and the difficulty of extending suitable health care to more remote rural areas, however, are two reasons why the cost of malaria control will continue to increase, if it is based on the indiscriminate use of antimalarial drugs.

PERSONAL PROTECTION. To some degree, the government can rely on public information messages to increase people's use of protective measures or to influence their use of drugs. The protective measures include bed nets, perhaps impregnated with insecticides, and modification of evening activities and clothing. For bed nets, a subsidy on their sale is also a possibility. Although bed nets themselves have been shown to reduce disease, the prospects for increasing their use remain unknown. Some people (more educated or concerned) may be quite easy to reach, but increasing usage of these measures to any great extent is probably expensive. To the extent that behavior does change, however, it can increase the effectiveness of antivector campaigns.

More rational use of antimalarial drugs should help to slow the spread of resistance, which has been encouraged by excessive and inappropriate use. To the extent that behavior can be changed by public information campaigns, this effect can be ameliorated. What this might cost and how much it might be worth require research geared to helping operations.

COST ANALYSIS FOR DECISIONMAKING. Most countries with malarious regions have in place some institutions designed to address the problem. The activities which are undertaken by these institutions depend partly on the local needs but also on history, cultural acceptability, and political concerns. The most practical use of cost information is its ability to assist the managers of the local malaria public health facility to make better incremental decisions in environments where they are constrained. When specific activities are proposed for a specific area, costs can be gauged relatively easily, because changes in scale are not at issue. Incremental benefits can also be appraised with regard to the local epidemiology and institutional and administrative conditions. Costing exercises in these cases can greatly improve allocation divisions by managers. Good examples of this use is the work done by Kaewsonthi and Harding (1986) in Thailand and by Mills (1987) in Nepal. In these studies, comparisons between techniques of vector control and between vector control and therapy are made clearer by careful costing procedures at local levels, and practical recommendations for improvements are made. Mills, for example, was able to suggest a reduction in active case-detection methods and an increase in malaria clinics (or other treatment facilities), observing that either of these activities looked better than spraying.

Estimate of Cost-Effectiveness

From data in the papers by Barlow and Grobar (1986) and Mills (1987), we calculated the costs per year of life saved and cost-benefit ratios for a variety of countries (tables 13-3 and 13-4). The most striking feature of these numbers is their variability. Indeed, the differences between the studies are so marked that it would be hard to make any generalizations about them at all. The costs per case prevented ranged from $2.10 to $259 (in 1987 dollars), and the cost-benefit ratios, from 2.4 to 146. The higher cost-benefit figures make malaria control seem of utmost importance. The lower figures bring it into competition with many other government programs as well as with many estimates of the marginal deadweight loss from tax

Table 13-3. Cost-Effectiveness Ratios in Malaria Control

Source	Country	Method	Cost per case prevented (1987 dollars)	Cost per death averted (1987 dollars)	Cost per discounted DALY saved with various case-fatality rates			
					2%	1%	0.5%	Observed
Barlow 1968	Sri Lanka	Insecticide	—	78	—	—	—	2.8
Cohn 1973	India	Insecticide	2.10	—	3.6	7	14	—
Gandahusada and others 1984	Indonesia	Insecticide	83–102	—	142–174	284–349	564–693	—
Hedman and others 1979	Liberia	Vector control and chemotherapy	14	—	24	48	95	—
Kaewsonthi and Harding 1984	Thailand	Vector control and chemotherapy	27–74	—	46–127	92–253	183–502	—
Mills 1987	Nepal	Vector control and chemotherapy	1.30–172	—	—	—	—	2.8–255
Molineaux and Gramiccia 1980	Nigeria	Vector control and chemotherapy	259	—	443	886	1,759	—
Ortiz 1968	Paraguay	Insecticides	60	—	103	205	407	—
Walsh and Warren 1979	Developing countries	Vector control	—	990	—	—	—	34

— Data not available
Source: Barlow and Grobar 1989; Mills 1987; authors' calculations.

collection (the systematic undervaluation of costs of government sources). Part of the explanation of the wide range of variation is not very illuminating. Differences in data quality, the assumptions used in the analyses (for example, the estimation of mortality avoided), the definition of the relevant costs, the length of time studied, the discount rate applied, and the coverage and purpose of the original intervention account for much of this variation. As one example, in the Garki Project study (Molineaux and Gramiccia 1980), which generated the figure of $259 per case averted per year, the costs of the extensive research and monitoring exercise which accompanied the intervention are included in the program costs. Similarly, some of the studies included administrative costs, whereas others used only the cost of materials. Some costs were calculated on the basis of small pilot projects (Gandahusada and others 1984) and others on the basis of national efforts (Barlow 1968).

The last four columns of table 13-3 contain calculations of the cost per discounted disability-adjusted life-year (DALY) saved for differing assumptions concerning the case-fatality rate for those cases in which the study does not explicitly present that value. The numbers are sensitive to this assumption, much more so than to any other parameter in the DALY calculation. Any attempt to calculate the cost per discounted DALY saved by the program requires locally relevant estimates of case-fatality rates.[1]

There are more important, systematic reasons, however, to expect average costs per unit of output to vary substantially between studies: (a) differences in the ecological, epidemiological, and social characteristics between areas; (b) wide variations over time within areas of the incidence and severity of malaria; (c) variations in the organizational structure of control programs; and (d) differences in the intensity of application of the interventions being appraised.

Table 13-4. Cost-Benefit Ratios in Malaria Control

Source	Country	Method	Cost
Barlow 1968	Sri Lanka	Insecticide	146
Griffit, Rampana, and Mashaal 1971	Thailand	Chemoprophylaxis	6.5
Khan 1966	Pakistan	Eradication program	4.9
Livandas and Athanassatos 1963	Greece	Eradication program	17.3
Niazi 1969	Iraq	Eradication program	6.0
Ortiz 1968	Paraguay	Insecticides	3.6
San Pedro 1967	Philippines	Eradication program	2.4
Democratic Republic of Sudan 1975	Sudan	Control program	4.6

Source: Barlow and Grobar 1986.

Priorities

Our perception of malaria has been changing rapidly over the past decades. Malaria is not, as once was thought, evenly spread over the geographic areas in which it is prevalent. Instead, it is highly focal, primarily affecting the hardest areas to reach, and it is intimately linked to development efforts such as agricultural development, road building, fiscal incentives, and colonization projects. Furthermore, malaria, which once was easily treatable with chloroquine, has reemerged as a new disease called drug-resistant malaria. Drug-resistant malaria has been spreading, and serious problems in treatment are becoming more and more common. Finally, parasite distribution has not remained stable, but there is a general increase and a general shift from the more benign tertial malaria caused by *P. vivax* to the fatal tropical malaria caused by *P. falciparum*.

Taking into account the epidemiology of malaria at present, the prevalent trends in the past fifteen to twenty years, and the prevailing level of endemicity in Africa south of the Sahara, it is reasonable to believe that a considerable deterioration of the situation is to be expected before the end of this century, unless a more serious control effort is made. Even if vaccines, new drugs, or new insecticides are developed, in view of the time required for their final testing in the field, they are unlikely to have a significant effect on malaria in the 1990s. The most critical activities that could accelerate the progress in malaria control can be summarized as follows:

• In countries of Asia, the Americas, and North Africa, in which organized malaria control activities have been carried out for nearly three decades, the priority should be on reassessment of activities. Replanning of programs must be based on epidemiological analysis, and at the same time, necessary changes in the organization and administration of these programs must be implemented.

• In countries of Africa south of the Sahara, priority should be given to the extension of coverage of population by the health care system. At the same time, a nucleus of malaria specialists should be trained and selective control programs started. This should allow realistic planning and implementation of malaria control activities. The implementation of any control activity on a larger scale should be preceded by epidemiological field study that would contribute to the better understanding of the local epidemiology of malaria.

Human Resources Development

At the beginning of the malaria eradication program a significant effort was made to train the personnel needed for the program, but, as programs became staffed and because malaria was expected to disappear soon, technical people and, especially, professionals in medical and biological sciences became progressively scarce. It has been said that the global malaria eradication program did not eradicate malaria but did eradicate malariologists. Moreover, training for eradication was definitely oriented toward the execution of the highly standardized program tasks and operations. The training of malariologists did not give them the epidemiological background needed to adapt to changing situations, to solve problems, to manage uncertainty, or to adapt or change control methods and strategies.

To meet current needs and achieve sustainable control, it is essential to create the manpower needed and to reorient human resources, not only to apply standard solutions to recognized problems, but also to identify and find a solution to future problems. In that way we may be able to avoid repeating the cycle described in 1927, in the Second Report of the Malaria Commission of the League of Nations: "The history of special antimalarial campaigns is chiefly a record of exaggerated expectations followed sooner or later by disappointment and abandonment of work."

National training programs should be supported and coordinated to ensure, through technical collaboration between countries, that all countries are able to do the following:

• Maintain a corps of adequately trained professionals with the necessary epidemiological expertise to understand the malaria problem and to adapt control strategies and programs to new situations.

• Train and orient general health services staff in the clinical management of malaria, recognition and treatment of severe and complicated malaria, monitoring of drug resistance, and collection and management of epidemiological information.

• Develop appropriate training methods for nonprofessional workers and community health workers so they can better manage fever and promote personal protection and an improved environment.

• Promote the development of curricula in schools of medicine and schools of public health to include new strategies of malaria control and to increase their ability to stay abreast of the latest information on the diagnosis and treatment of malaria.

The development of new or improved methods or materials for malaria control—in particular, antimalarial drugs and potential vaccines—should continue to receive the highest priority. This view, which is widely supported and, to an important extent, has shaped the UNDP/World Bank/WHO Special Programme for Research and Training in Tropical Diseases' (TDR) research priorities, was recently reconfirmed by the National Academy of Sciences/Institute of Medicine report on malaria.

Research

The most damaging effect of the malaria eradication years was probably the neglect of malaria research and malariology's lack of appeal as a career to young scientists and epidemiologists. In the words of McGregor (1982 p. 126), "throughout the world support for further research into malaria, even that concerned with insecticides and chemotherapeutics, contracted swiftly. Worse still, the apparently imminent demise of a once important disease removed the necessity for training scientists in malariology. It took 10 more years and a war to halt this tragic trend." The reawakening of interest in malaria research showed a marked bias toward new technological developments through laboratory-based research, mostly in chemotherapy, immunology, genetics, and the genetic control of vectors and the possible use of mosquito pathogens.

In particular, since 1976 the UNDP/World Bank/WHO Special Programme for Research and Training in Tropical Diseases (TDR) has assumed a key role in coordinating and funding malaria research. It has made malaria its first priority and continues to provide technical drive toward development of new tools for control.

Actually, most available antimalaria interventions are far from ideal, not only in effectiveness but in their suitability for incorporation into long-term policies or the everyday practices of peoples and communities. Moreover, many of them have lost much of their original effectiveness because resistant strains of parasites or anophelines have developed. We must improve our understanding of the epidemiology of malaria and of problems such as parasite and vector resistance. We must improve the tools of epidemiological investigation so we can identify problems in the field, plan and evaluate potential solutions, and more effectively target interventions to problems. We must understand and monitor social and economic processes that may influence the epidemiology of malaria and facilitate or hamper the effectiveness of potential control measures. And we must come to understand how these processes may facilitate the incorporation of malaria control in developing a health infrastructure.

Funding for malaria control programs shrank when people began to recognize that malaria could not be eradicated, when the "basic health services" strategy in developing a health infrastructure did not succeed, and when no successful models developed for incorporating malaria control into the primary health care strategy. Malaria and general public health services exhibited a nearly universal reluctance to redefine their responsibilities toward the malaria problem.

Research may provide new and improved technologies needed to extend the feasibility of control, may provide epidemiological tools that improve efficiency of control, and may show better ways to combine interventions in more effective and efficient strategies. But it is also necessary that any new tool be validated in the field and field tested to determine its applicability in disease control. It is important that researchers try to find better ways to integrate new and old tools for control. It is important to use health systems research to find the best ways to incorporate new methods of control into the health infrastructure and deliver them to individuals and communities. And as part of the strategy of primary health care, we must test ways to control malaria through research and development.

Malaria control and malaria research have drifted apart over the years. While malaria control programs continued their fight using an established set of tools, research institutions moved off in search of new technological solutions, and both were under increasing financial constraints. Support for malaria research contracted during the eradication years (McGregor 1982), even for research on pesticides and drugs, but support has been revived. This renewed research effort, however, has shown a marked bias toward laboratory research and toward the development of new technologies in chemotherapy, immunology, genetics, the genetic control of vectors, and the potential use of mosquito pathogens.

In some parts of the world, control programs and research institutions have developed a curious rivalry: programs are almost defensively entrenched in the use of established methods, such as residual spraying, whereas researchers uncritically proclaim as alternatives what should be seen as complementary techniques. On the whole, researchers have undertaken projects that are of little relevance to ongoing control operations and the specific problems of control institutions. At the same time, control programs, which often collect massive amounts of valuable information, have lacked the capacity to select research priorities and carry out research projects.

Given the present status of malaria and malaria control programs, we recommend that priority be given to research in the following areas:

Epidemiology. Research is needed to improve our epidemiological tools and understanding and thereby improve our ability to identify problem areas and better target control interventions. In particular, we must understand and monitor social and economic processes that may influence the epidemiology of malaria and facilitate or hamper the effectiveness of potential control measures.

Technology. Research is needed to develop and field-test new control technologies and new combinations of old interventions in order to increase efficiency and cost-effectiveness of control programs.

Organization and management. Research is needed on the organization and management of control programs in order to develop more effective and efficient organizational structures and management processes.

Health infrastructure. Research is needed on health systems to examine the potential and means for effective participation of the general health services in malaria control, in particular in epidemiological surveillance, diagnosis and treatment, and community mobilization. Many countries have embarked on a process of decentralization of health services that could impart negatively on the effectiveness of vertical malaria control programs. These countries, in particular, will need to move cautiously and study carefully the alternatives for increasing the capacity of the general health services to assume new responsibilities in disease control.

Notes

1. For purposes of presentation, the other parameters in the DALY calculation were assumed to be twenty-nine discounted years gained per death averted, eight days of illness, and a 10 percent quality-of-life adjustment for nonfatal cases. Except at very low case-fatality rates, the calculations are quite insensitive to large ranges in the assumed values of these three parameters.

References

Andreano, Ralph, and Thomas Helminiak. 1988. "Economics, Health, and Tropical Disease: A Review." In A. M. Herrin and P. L. Rosenfield, eds., *Economics, Health, and Tropical Diseases*. Manila: University of the Philippines, School of Economics.

Audibert, M. A. 1984. *Agricultural Non-Wage Production and Health Status: A Case-Study in a Tropical Milieu*. Aix-en-Provence: Université d'Aix-en-Provence, Centre d'Economie de la Santé.

Barlow, Robin. 1968. *The Economic Effects of Malaria Eradication*. Ann Arbor: University of Michigan, Bureau of Public Health Economics.

Barlow, Robin, and L. M. Grobar. 1986. "Cost and Benefits of Controlling Parasitic Diseases." PHN Technical Note 85-17. Population, Health, and Nutrition Department, World Bank, Washington, D.C.

Bhombore, S. R., C. Brooke Worth, and K. S. Nanjundiah. 1952. "A Survey of the Economic Status of Villagers in a Malarious Irrigated Tract in Mysore State, India, before and after DDT Residual Insecticidal Spraying." *Indian Journal of Malariology* 6(4):355–66.

Binol, K. 1983. "Transmigration and Health in Connection with Tropical Disease in Indonesia." *Southeast Asian Journal of Tropical Medicine and Public Health* 14:58–63.

Brohult, J., L. Jorfeldt, L. Rombo, A. Björkman, P. O. Pehrson, V. Sirleaf, and E. Bengtsson. 1981. "The Working Capacity of Liberian Males: A Comparison between Urban and Rural Populations in Relation to Malaria." *Annals of Tropical Medicine and Parasitology* 75:487–94.

Bruce-Chwatt, L. J. 1969. "Malaria Eradication at the Crossroads." *Bulletin of the New York Academy of Medicine* 45(10):999–1012.

———. 1979. "Man against Malaria: Conquest or Defeat." *Transactions of the Royal Society of Tropical Medicine and Hygiene* 73:605–17.

———. 1985. *Essential Malariology*. 2d ed. London: Heinemann Medical Books.

Bruce-Chwatt, L. J., and H. M. Archibald. 1959. "Malaria Control Pilot Project in Western Sokoto, Northern Nigeria: A Report on Four Years' Results." In *Proceedings of the Sixth International Congress of Tropical Medicine and Hygiene, 1958*, Vol. 7. Lisbon: Instituto de Medicina.

de Castro, Bonita. 1985. "Development of Research-Training Project in Socio-economics of Malaria in Colombia." Report to TDR Programme, World Health Organization, Geneva. Typescript.

Cohn, E. J. 1973. "Assessing the Costs and Benefits of Anti-malaria Programmes: The Indian Experience." *American Journal of Public Health* 63:1086–96.

Conly, G. N. 1975. *The Impact of Malaria on Economic Development: A Case Study*. Scientific Publication 297. Washington, D.C.: Pan-American Health Organization.

van Dine, D. L. 1916. "The Relation of Malaria to Crop Production." *Scientific Monthly* (November): 431–39.

Field, J. W. 1967. "Resistance to the 4-aminoquinolines in the Malaria Infections of Brazil and South East Asia." WP/ScG/1. Working paper presented to the World Health Organization Scientific Group on Chemotherapy of Malaria, April 25–May 1, Geneva.

Foll, C. V., C. P. Pant, and P. E. Lietaert. 1965. "A Large Scale Field Trial with Dichlorvos as a Residual Fumigant Insecticide in Northern Nigeria." *Bulletin of the World Health Organization* 32:531–50.

Gandahusada, S., G. A. Fleming, Sukamto, T. Damar, Suwarto, N. Sustriayu, Y. H. Bang, S. Arwati, and H. Arif. 1984. "Malaria Control with Residual Fenitrothion in Central Java, Indonesia: An Operations-Scale Trial Using Both Full and Selective Coverage Treatments." *Bulletin of the World Health Organization* 62:783–94.

Garcia, J. C. 1981. "The Laziness Disease." *History and Philosophy of the Life Sciences* 3:3–59.

Greenwood, B. M., A. K. Bradley, A. M. Greenwood, P. Byass, K. Jammeh, K. Marsh, S. Tulloch, F. S. J. Oldfield, and R. Hayes. 1987. "Mortality and Morbidity from Malaria among Children in a Rural Area of The Gambia, West Africa." *Transactions of the Royal Society of Tropical Medicine and Hygiene* 81:478–86.

Griffith, D. H. S., D. V. Ramana, and H. Mashaal. 1971. "Contribution of Health to Development." *International Journal of Health Services* 1(3):253–70.

Hedman, P., J. Brohult, J. Forslund, V. Sirleaf, and E. Bengtsson. 1979. "A Pocket of Controlled Malaria in a Holoendemic Region of West Africa." *Annals of Tropical Medicine and Parasitology* 73:317–25.

Kaewsonthi, S., and A. G. Harding. 1986. "Cost and Performance of Malaria Surveillance: The Patients' Perspectives." *Southeast Asian Journal of Tropical Medicine and Public Health* 17:406–12.

League of Nations, Malaria Commission. 1927. *Principles and Methods of Antimalarial in Europe*. 2d General Report of the Malaria Commission. CH/MAL/73, III Health 1927, III 5. Geneva.

Litsios, Socrates. 1990. "Feasibility of Malaria Transmission Control: Economic Aspects." Paper presented to the 2d World Congress on Health Economics, September 11–14, Zurich.

Macdonald, G. 1950. "The Economic Importance of Malaria in Africa." WHO/MAL/60,AFR/MAL/CONF.16. World Health Organization, Geneva.

MacGregor, I. A. 1982. "Malaria: Introduction." *British Medical Bulletin* 38:115–16.

Malik, I. H. 1966. *Economic Advantages of Anti-Malaria Measures Amongst the Rural Population*. Publication 137. Lahore: Board of Economic Inquiry.

Marques, A. C. 1988. "Main Malaria Situations in the Brazilian Amazon." Superintendency for Public Health Campaigns, Ministry of Health, Brasilia. Typescript.

Matola, Y. G., G. B. White, and S. A. Magayuka. 1987. "The Changed Pattern of Malaria Endemicity and Transmission at Amani in the Eastern Usambara Mountains, North-eastern Tanzania." *Journal of Tropical Medicine and Hygiene* 90:127–34.

Mills, Anne. 1987. "Economic Study of Malaria in Nepal: The Cost Effectiveness of Malaria Control Strategies." Evaluation and Planning Center, London School of Hygiene and Tropical Medicine.

Molineaux, Louis. 1985. "La lutte contre les maladies parasitaires: Le problème du paludisme, notamment en Afrique." In J. Vallin and A. Lopez, eds., *La lutte contre la mort*. Travaux et Documents 108. Paris: Presses Universitaires de France.

———. 1988. "The Epidemiology of Human Malaria as an Explanation at Its Distribution, Including Some Implications for Its Control." In W. H. Wernsdorfer and I. A. McGregor, eds., *Malaria: Principles and Practices of Malariology*. New York: Churchill Livingstone.

Molineaux, Louis, and G. Gramiccia. 1980. *The Garki Project: Research on the Epidemiology and Control of Malaria in the Sudan Savanna of West Africa*. Geneva: World Health Organization.

Nájera, J. A. 1981. "La epidemiología y los problemas de la lucha antimalarica en las Américas." In *Pan-American Health Organization: Malaria en las Américas.*, OPS Scientific Publication 405. Washington, D.C.: Pan-American Health Organization.

———. 1989. "Global Malaria Situation." WPR/MAL(1)/89.14. World Health Organization, Geneva.

Nájera, J. A., G. R. Shidraw, J. Storey, and P. E. Lietaert. 1973. "Mass Drug Administration and DDT Indoor-Spraying as Antimalarial Measures in Northern Savanna of Nigeria." WHO/MAL/73.817. World Health Organization, Geneva.

Niazi, A. D. 1969. "Approximate Estimates of the Economic Loss Caused by Malaria with Some Estimates of the Benefits of the MEP in Iraq." *Bulletin of Endemic Diseases* 2:28–39.

Ortiz, J. R. 1968. "Estimate of the Cost of a Malaria Eradication Program." *Bulletin of the Pan-American Health Organization* 64:14–17.

Over and others. 1992. "The Consequences of Adult Ill-Health." In R. G. A. Feachem, Tord Kjellstrom, C. J. L. Murray, Mead Over, M. A. Phillips, eds., *The Health of Adults in the Developing World*. New York: Oxford University Press.

Pampana, E. 1969. *A Textbook of Malaria Eradication*. London: Oxford University Press.

Quo, W. K. 1959. In "Malaria Information." MAL/INFORM/46. World Health Organization, Geneva.

Russell, P. F., and M. K. Menon. 1942. "A Malario-economic Survey in Rural South India." *Indian Medical Gazette* 77:167–80.

San Pedro, C. 1967/68. "Economic Costs and Benefits of Malaria Eradication." *Philippine Journal of Public Health* 12:5–24.

Sawyer, D. 1986. "Malaria on the Amazon Frontier: Economic and Social Aspects of Transmission and Control." *Southeast Asian Journal of Tropical Medicine and Public Health* 17:342–45.

Sawyer, D., and Sawyer, D. 1987. "Malaria on the Amazon Frontier: Economic and Social Aspects of Transmission and Control." CEDEPLAR, Federal University of Minas Gerais, Belo Horizonte.

Sinton, J. A. 1935/36b. "What Malaria Costs India? Nationally, Socially, and Economically." *Records of the Malaria Survey of India* 5:413–89.

———. 1935/36c. "What Malaria Costs India? Nationally, Socially, and Economically." *Records of the Malaria Survey of India* 6:96–169.

———. 1938. *What Malaria Costs India*. Government of India Health Bulletin 26. New Delhi.

Spencer, H. C., D. C. O. Kaseje, W. H. Mosley, E. K. N. Sempebwa, A. Y. Huong, and J. M. Roberts. 1987. "Impact on Mortality and Fertility of a Community Based Malaria Control Programme in Saradidi, Kenya." *Annals of Tropical Medicine and Parasitology* 81(supplement 1):36–45.

Vaisse, D., R. Michel, P. Carnevale, M. F. Bosseno, J. F. Molez, P. Peelman, M. T. Loembe, S. Nzingoula, and A. Zoulani. 1981. "Le paludisme à *Plasmodium falciparum* et le gène de la drépanocytose en Républque Populaire du Congo. 2. Manifestations cliniques du paludisme selon la parasitémie et le genétype hémoglobinique." *Médecine Tropicale* 41(4):413–23.

Walsh, J. A., and K. S. Warren. 1979. "Selective Primary Health Care: An Interim Strategy for Disease Control in Developing Countries." *New England Journal of Medicine* 301:967–74.

Wernsdorfer, W. H., and I. A. McGregor (eds.). 1988. *Malaria: Principles and Practice of Malariology*. New York: Churchill Livingstone.

Wernsdorfer, G., and W. H. Wernsdorfer. 1988. "Social and Economic Aspects of Malaria and Its Control." In W. H. Wernsdorfer and I. A. McGregor, eds., *Malaria: Principles and Practice of Malariology*. New York: Churchill Livingstone.

WHO (World Health Organization).1957. *Expert Committee on Malaria: Report of the Sixth Session*. Technical Report 123, Geneva.

———. 1969. "Reexamination of the Global Strategy of Malaria Eradication." *Official Records of the World Health Organization* 176:106–26.

———. 1974. *Expert Committee on Malaria: Report of the Sixteenth Session*. Technical Report 549, Geneva.

———. 1978. "Malaria Control Strategy." Report by the Director-General. A31/19. Geneva.

———. 1986. *Expert Committee on Malaria: Report on the Eighteenth Session*. Technical Report 735, Geneva.

———. 1992. "World Malaria Situation in 1990." WHO *Weekly Epidemiological Records* 22:161–67; 23:169–74.

WHO (World Health Organization)/UNICEF (United Nations Children's Fund). 1978. "Primary Health Care." Report of the International Conference on Primary Health Care. Alma Ata, U.S.S.R., September 6–12, Geneva.

Wilson, D. B. 1960. "Report on the Pare Taveta Malaria Scheme 1954–59," Dar-es-Salaam.

Wilson, J. F. and A. Alicbusan-Schwab. 1991. "Development Policies and Health: Farmers, Goldminers, and Slums in the Brazilian Amazon." Working Paper 1991-18. World Bank Environment Division, Washington, D.C.

Yumer, R. 1980. "Influence du statut socio-économique sur la morbidité paludéenne: un essai de mesure." Ph.D. diss., Université des Sciences Sociales, Faculté des Sciences Economiques, Grenoble.

de Zulueta, J. 1988. "Report on a Mission to Madagascar." Travel report to World Health Organization, Geneva.

de Zulueta, J., G. W. Kafuko, J. R. Cullen, and C. K. Pedersen. 1961. "The Results of the First Year of a Malaria Eradication Pilot Project in Northern Kigezi (Uganda)." *East African Medical Journal* 38(1):1–26.

14

Dengue
(with Notes on Yellow Fever and Japanese Encephalitis)

Donald S. Shepard and Scott B. Halstead

Dengue, yellow fever, and the viral encephalitides (principally Japanese encephalitis) are acute, sometimes lethal infections which, with regard to morbidity and mortality, constitute the most significant arthropod-borne viral diseases of man. These viruses are all in the same taxon and share important biological similarities. Infections with wild or live-attenuated viruses result in lifelong immunity. Each virus is mosquito-transmitted and, therefore, typically causes diseases of place. Yellow fever and dengue share the same urban mosquito vector, *Aedes aegypti*; in some parts of Africa, related *Stegomyia* mosquitoes are more important for yellow fever transmission. Japanese encephalitis (JE) is transmitted by the rice-paddy breeding *Culex tritaeniorhynchus* and related species, which are distributed across the Asian land mass from Japan through India.

Arthropod-borne viral diseases are transmitted by injection of infected saliva during the bite of mosquitoes which, after ingesting blood containing virus, have survived sufficiently long for the virus to multiply in tissues, including the salivary gland. Following an incubation period in humans of a few days to a week or more, illness begins acutely, usually with fever, headache, myalgia, inappetence, and varying gastrointestinal symptoms. In its severe form, yellow fever evolves to an acute hepatitis, complicated by acute vascular permeability, hemorrhage, and renal failure; dengue evolves to dengue hemorrhagic fever/dengue shock syndrome (DHF/DSS), characterized by acute vascular permeability and bleeding. Japanese encephalitis involves acute central nervous system disease, commonly with altered cerebration, coma, and paralysis. In all three, the acute illness stage lasts for a week or more; severe findings and death or recovery occur promptly with yellow fever and DHF/DSS, but prolonged incapacitation is a frequent outcome of Japanese encephalitis.

Historically, case-fatality rates for yellow fever, dengue hemorrhagic fever, and Japanese encephalitis have been as high as 80 percent, 50 percent, and 60 percent, respectively. Today, in Africa, case-fatality rates for yellow fever are thought to be in the range of 0.5 to 6 percent; in tropical Asia, case-fatality rates for DHF/DSS are 1 to 5 percent; and in continental and South Asia, rates for Japanese encephalitis are 20 to 40 per-cent. Complication rates are extremely low for yellow fever and dengue, but for JE, long-term sequelae include personality disorders, reduced learning ability, gait abnormalities, and severe incapacitating paralysis. These occur in 25 to 40 percent of surviving patients.

In tropical Asia, DHF/DSS is almost exclusively confined to children under the age of fifteen years with a modal age of five to seven years. Male-to-female case and death ratios are approximately 1:1.2. Yellow fever epidemics in West Africa, Ethiopia, and Sudan have involved children and young adults with slightly more cases in males than females. Jungle yellow fever in Latin America involves principally young, adult males who work in or at the forest fringe. In China, under conditions of high enzootic transmission, Japanese encephalitis is a disease of children, principally five years of age and under; in Southeast Asia, an area of intermittent transmission, children up to fifteen years are vulnerable and, in South Asia, where virus is transmitted episodically, persons up to fifty years of age acquire encephalitis.

The primary risk factor for acquiring any of these diseases is living in areas where vector mosquitoes breed. Water storage in houses and promiscuous disposal of modern industrial trash permit *Aedes aegypti* breeding. *Culex tritaeniorhynchus* breeds in wet rice paddies. Children, females, Caucasians, and Orientals are the populations most at risk for DHF/DSS. There is no evidence to suggest that age, sex, or the innate susceptibility of blacks plays a part in the case-fatality rates of yellow fever. Japanese encephalitis is more severe and has higher case-fatality rates in children than adults and in Caucasians and blacks than Orientals.

In the remainder of this chapter we discuss all these conditions, describing their public health significance, economic effects, opportunities for better case management and prevention, and future priorities. We treat dengue in the greatest depth, presenting an empirical cost-effectiveness analysis. Dengue was selected for this more detailed analysis, and some original data were collected, because this condition poses the most difficult policy questions. Although there are current and prospective technologies with considerable potential to control the disease, their feasibility and cost in relation to the competing demands remains an open question.

Public Health Significance

Trends in the spread of epidemics and the levels of disability and death are the main public health concerns.

Morbidity and Mortality Levels and Trends, Circa 1985

Annually, jungle yellow fever is responsible for about 200 cases and 40 deaths in the tropics of the Western hemisphere, principally in adult males. Intermittent rural and urban epidemics occur in Sub-Saharan Africa (West, Central, and East). Much of African experience with yellow fever is unreported. During the 1987 Nigerian epidemic in Oyo State, 805 cases and 416 deaths were reported, but surveys of three involved villages suggested that as many as 120,000 cases and 24,000 deaths may have occurred (De Cock and others 1988). Another outbreak in the same year in Niger State in northern Nigeria may have been of similar dimensions (Nasidi and others 1989). Forty percent of cases were children under ten years; 30 percent were adults. The male-to-female ratio was 1.4:1. Yellow fever epidemics occur irregularly. The fifteen-year trend is toward increasing epidemic frequency, increasing involvement of urban areas in Nigeria, and extension to South Nigeria.

Attack rates of severe dengue illness have steadily increased. In 1987, more than 600,000 cases of dengue hemorrhagic fever with 24,000 deaths were reported from Southeast Asian countries. Ninety-nine percent of cases and deaths were in children under fifteen years. The male-to-female ratio is 1:1.2. In the Americas, dengue transmission has increased dramatically since 1963. There are four types of dengue, DEN 1, 2, 3, 4, and all four are now endemic in the Caribbean basin, and epidemic dengue has occurred in all South American countries except Argentina, Uruguay, and Chile. In 1981, DHF/DSS resulted in 116,000 hospitalizations in Cuba. Venezuela reported 50 deaths and 1,000 cases in a 1989–90 dengue outbreak, its first in many years (PAHO 1990). Brazil experienced thousands of cases in its first recent epidemic in 1986 (Schatzmayr and others 1986; Secretária de Estado de Saúde e Higiene 1986) and had a second resurgence in 1991. Attack rates in Southeast Asia have increased from 15 per 100,000 to 170 per 100,000 during the period 1970–87. In Thailand and Viet Nam, attack rates in 1987 were 3,700 and 6,400 per 100,000, respectively. Perhaps one-half of this increase is due to better case recognition and the fact that milder disease not reported earlier is now being reported (inflation of case identification). Nonetheless, cases reported are from medical facilities and signify use of diagnostic and curative services.

Cases of Japanese encephalitis have been reported in China, mainland Southeast Asia, and South Asia. Annual cases and deaths are estimated at 25,000 and 10,000, respectively, 70 percent in children below the age of fifteen years. The ratios of male-to-female cases and deaths are 1.1:1. There have been dramatic increases in epidemic occurrences of Japanese encephalitis in India, Nepal, Sri Lanka, and Thailand in the 1970s and 1980s. In this same period, JE has virtually disappeared from Japan, the Republic of Korea, and Taiwan (China) as a result of widespread use of effective vaccines. Annual cases in China have decreased from 100,000 to 25,000.

Morbidity and Mortality in 2000 and 2015

All three diseases are showing a tendency to increase absolutely with increasing population, but at a rate inversely proportionate to prosperity.

YELLOW FEVER. In Africa, there is increased risk of urban yellow fever transmitted by *Aedes aegypti*. For the past forty years, disease has predominantly affected rural areas, where it has been transmitted by other *Stegomyia* vectors. Attack rates and the area of involvement in Africa will increase with population and inversely with gross domestic product per capita.

DENGUE. Unless vaccine or nationwide vector control programs are implemented, the absolute number of cases of dengue will expand with population and growth of cities. Increases in gross domestic product per capita should reduce attack rates through improved standards for residential dwellings.

JAPANESE ENCEPHALITIS. Without incorporation of JE vaccine into the World Health Organization's (WHO's) Expanded Programme on Immunization (EPI) in South and Southeast Asia, attack rates will increase with population.

Economic Costs

Costs include those of treating the sufferers directly and the indirect social costs.

YELLOW FEVER. Yellow fever entails the same kinds of costs as those associated with dengue fever (see below): vector control, diagnosis and outpatient treatment of mild cases, and intensive care of the severely ill patients. Finally, there are costs associated with loss of work of adults ill themselves or attending children, and loss of life.

DENGUE. Costs include those associated with vector control, vaccination, diagnosis and outpatient treatment of mild cases (which are ten to fifty times more common than reported severe cases), and intensive care of the severely ill, including intravenous fluids, blood or plasma transfusion, and polypharmacy, with average hospital stays of five to ten days for severe cases. Adults lose work to attend to children's illness. Finally, there are costs associated with loss of life.

The literature contains no previous studies on the cost-effectiveness of dengue control. The literature on the economic consequences of dengue includes a study by Von

Allmen and others (1979) from Puerto Rico, in which the economic cost of the island's dengue fever epidemic of 1977 is calculated. Included are direct costs for medical care and vector control measures and indirect costs for lost production due to illness and absenteeism by patients and by parents caring for sick children. The population was 3 million. Direct costs ranged between $2.4 million and $4.7 million. Indirect costs ranged from $3.7 million to $10.9 million, with total costs of the epidemic ranging between $6.0 million and $15.6 million. Expenditure on patient care and vector control measures is considered to be in the range of 7.8 to 20.2 percent of the total expenses.

Gubler and others have also studied this epidemic and estimated costs to be an order of magnitude higher, ranging between $100 million and $150 million, in medical costs, control efforts, lost work, and lost tourism since 1977 (D. J. Gubler, personal communication 19 October 1992).

Kouri and others (1989) have estimated the cost of the 1981 DHF/DSS outbreak in Cuba (with a population of 10 million) at $103 million. In this outbreak more than 116,000 persons were hospitalized within a little over 3 months. It is remarkable that in such a short period more than 1 percent of the Cuban population required intensive care in a hospital setting. Included were direct costs for patient care and control of the vector of $41 million and $43 million, respectively, and indirect costs, including lost production of $14 million and disability payments of $5 million.

Much lower direct costs were estimated for the 1980 epidemic of DHF/DSS in Thailand, which included hospitalizations and deaths. Mosquito abatement costs and hospitalization costs, almost entirely for children, were $6.5 million (Matsurapas 1981; Halstead 1984).

Soper and others planned and executed with military-like precision environmental vector control in Brazil, and the efforts were replicated throughout the Americas (Soper and others 1943). Chan (1985) provides a thorough description, including a cost analysis, of the Singapore vector control program based on Soper's principles. The most important element of the program is source reduction—elimination of breeding sources for mosquitoes. Trained, uniformed public health officers are authorized to enter premises, inspect for, and destroy breeding sources. Destruction of breeding sources includes removing water-collecting refuse and sealing water storage containers. This environmental program is supplemented, in times of epidemics, by chemical control—fogging premises that have or are near places that have high *Aedes aegypti* indexes. Public health education, primarily through pamphlets, seeks to motivate and teach the population to eliminate breeding sites. During outbreaks, television, radio, and newspapers provide additional publicity. Moreover, Singapore enacted the Destruction of Disease-Bearing Insects Act (Act 26 of 1968) to require that persons comply with directives of the commissioner of health to eliminate breeding sources. Violations are punishable by fines. Chan reported that the environmental (*Aedes*) control program cost three to four

Singapore dollars per person per year in 1973 to 1974, or $1.36 to $1.82 (Chan 1985). In 1988 prices, based on a 5 percent annual inflation, the amount is $2.69 to $3.60. In the early 1980s, following a dengue epidemic, Cuba also embarked on a program of environmental vector control at a total (not annual) cost of $6.00 to $10.00 per capita.

JAPANESE ENCEPHALITIS: The average hospital stay for persons with JE is two weeks. Forty percent of survivors are physically or mentally crippled and require one to five years rehabilitation; 10 percent of these require chronic care.

Prevention

Some measures can be taken immediately, others await improved technology.

Lowering or Postponing Disease Incidence

Elements of a preventive strategy are as follows:

YELLOW FEVER. Risk factors principally are overpopulation, rural to urban migration, vector prevalence, and inadequate domestic water supply or sewage disposal. There are two preventive strategies: (a) production, purchase, distribution, and use of yellow fever vaccine; and (b) control or eradication of *Aedes aegypti* (in Africa, limited to urban vectors). The potential effectiveness of either of these two strategies is 100 percent. The current price of yellow fever vaccine (excluding costs of administering the vaccine) is $0.20 to $2.00 per dose.

DENGUE. The strategy is the same as for yellow fever except vaccine development is in progress and outcome is not known. Dengue transmission can be interrupted by eliminating the mosquito vector (*Aedes aegypti* or *Aedes albopictus*) which carries the virus. Two methods are possible: chemical control—killing adult mosquitoes by means of chemical insecticides—and environmental control—elimination of sites for breeding of the mosquito which transmits dengue fever (Chan 1985). As Chan points out, the high fecundity of the mosquitoes means that they can quickly replace their population. Chemical control must be repeated several times per year and, even then, may be of limited effectiveness.

Environmental control, though more difficult, appears to be far more effective (Chan 1985). Rubbish, such as old tires, must be removed from the area; water storage vessels must be covered and cleaned regularly; and the presence of the mosquito must be diligently monitored. These activities require initial capital costs to set up an infrastructure, educate the population about control measures, establish rewards and sanctions for implementing them, and train the necessary environmental control personnel. Recurrent costs are the costs of operating this infrastructure.

We collected original data on the costs of vector control in several countries. Thailand launched a large-scale effort, which, so far, has been unsuccessful. The cost-effectiveness of this strategy will depend on the extent to which control efforts can be reduced following an initial success. Although good data are not yet available, we will attempt in this chapter to produce useful estimates.

One of the most important contributions to the eradication of the mosquito is the implementation of cleanup campaigns. Organized primarily by the national or city agencies, vector control requires community support. For example, in Puerto Rico, cleanup campaigns are organized for an urban neighborhood with a population of about 50,000 people. Cleanup campaigns start with large public education campaigns to raise awareness. These campaigns require the cooperation of the leaders of each community, who work directly with state and city officials. Householders agree to take responsibility for cleaning each premise. Special teams are formed for public areas (parks, cemeteries) and difficult places (slums and junkyards). City cleanup workers provide trash bags, cleaning utensils, and pick-up trucks to collect garbage. A neighborhood campaign generally requires two to three weeks of preparation and two to three days of trash removal activities.

In response to a dengue outbreak that peaked in June 1978, Puerto Rico began the Anti-Dengue Program with funds from the Comprehensive Employment and Training Act. From August 1978 through September 1980, the number of workers increased from 300 to 900 under the Higienización Ambiente Físico Inmediato program. The workers were paid the current minimum wage of $600 per month. Thus, the annual cost of salaries for the clean-up campaign was about $4.3 million, or $1.30 per capita.

JAPANESE ENCEPHALITIS. Vaccine is the only preventive strategy for combating Japanese encephalitis. The current regimen is three doses of killed, purified vaccine. Currently, it is given to children in Korea, China, Japan, and Taiwan (China). In South and Southeast Asia, the wholesale cost is $2.30 per dose; in Southeast Asia, for children living in JE enzootic areas, two doses are recommended. As yet, there is limited distribution in South and Southeast Asia.

Possible Changes in Preventive Technology

Some improvements in technology may be available by the year 2000, some not until 2015.

YELLOW FEVER. For yellow fever, an improved vaccine is not anticipated by the year 2000. Improvements in vaccine production technology and increased production in developing countries could reduce the price and improve efficiency at delivery.

DENGUE. For dengue, a safe and effective genetically engineered vaccine is not likely by the year 2000, but it is likely by 2015. To date, research on development of a vaccine has been performed in Thailand, supported principally by the Southeast Asia Regional Office of the World Health Organization in New Delhi, India. The planned live-attenuated tetravalent dengue vaccine is likely to have a manufacturing cost of at least $10 to $20 per dose and require refrigeration during shipment and storage. It will have a very short shelf-life once rehydrated from the lyophilized product. In this respect, it will be similar to yellow fever and measles vaccines.

Costs of the vaccine strategy include capital costs for vaccine development and operating costs for vaccine manufacturing and delivery. A tetravalent live-attenuated dengue vaccine will be expensive to produce, but delivery costs should not be excessive because the vaccine will require only two doses and will be given primarily in cities. In all likelihood, the first dose of dengue vaccine will be administered with measles vaccine and added to the existing infrastructure of the Expanded Programme on Immunization for children.

JAPANESE ENCEPHALITIS. For Japanese encephalitis, one or more live-attenuated vaccines are likely to be available by 2000; genetically engineered vaccines are also likely to be available. The reduction in cost of a genetically engineered vaccine as compared with a live-attenuated vaccine will be marginal, although a one-dose live-attenuated vaccine will greatly decrease delivery costs.

Good Practice and Actual Practice

Good practice is not always within reach financially, and actual practice may not always be effective.

YELLOW FEVER. Vaccine-induced antibody barrier is quite effective in preventing urban yellow fever in Latin America. In the seven or eight African countries in which it has been used, vaccination effectively controls yellow fever. Vector control in Africa is almost completely ineffectual.

DENGUE AND JAPANESE ENCEPHALITIS. Except for those in Cuba and Singapore, modern *Aedes aegypti* control programs to combat dengue are in disarray. In contrast, excellent vaccine programs to combat JE operate in Japan, Korea, and Taiwan (China), and a good program has been activated in China. No widespread use of vaccines exists in Southeast and South Asia.

How Much Should Reasonably Be Done?

No countries have had the opportunity to examine health investments in relation to projected costs to the economy of yellow fever, dengue, or Japanese encephalitis. Yellow fever and JE, which involve adults or result in prolonged incapacitation, respectively, tend to make headlines and create hysteria. This has been the principal reason for government action in the past. Fear, political pressure, and the technical capacity of the society for vaccine production or vector control have dictated the actions adopted.

It is likely that domestic production of JE vaccine in Thailand and India would result in purchase and use of the product, whereas continued dependence on imported vaccine will result in temporization in adopting a national vaccination policy. Eradication of *Aedes aegypti* throughout the entire Western hemisphere currently offers the only preventive strategy for control of dengue and yellow fever.

Case Management

This section discusses opportunities there may be for improvements in case management.

Dengue

Palliation is the objective of medical intervention of DHF/DSS, which is characterized by loss of fluids internally through leaky capillaries and occasionally, severe hemorrhaging. Intensive hospital care is required and can successfully reduce the case-fatality rates of DHF/DSS. Management of the leaky capillary syndrome is complicated. In some cases treatment with fluid or fluid and plasma is useful, in other cases whole blood. Incorrect treatment can lead to heart failure and a substantial risk of mortality. To improve case management and reduce case-fatality rates, fundamentally soundly educated physicians and nurses are required, modern state-of-the-art and reliable laboratory facilities are essential, and adequately functioning pharmacies and a safe and resourceful blood supply system are required. Resources involved are capital resources for training of personnel and rehabilitating facilities and equipment and subsequently for increased operating costs of the maintenance of these facilities and equipment. In addition, good managers are needed to ensure that the facilities, equipment, and personnel remain available at optimum preparedness. Realistic levels of turnover must be included.

Theoretically, such improvements in case management can be costed and analyzed as if they were dedicated solely to the treatment of DHF/DSS. That is, we could calculate the cost of an education program solely for DHF/DSS, the costs of strengthening of laboratories, pharmacies, and wards solely for this condition. In practice, such a program might be undertaken to strengthen case management for other infectious diseases and would entail training, rehabilitation of facilities, and the like for several infectious diseases simultaneously. The cost and effectiveness would be greater than for treatment of dengue, and economies of scale may be realized.

Yellow Fever and Japanese Encephalitis

Intensive hospital care is also required for yellow fever. For Japanese encephalitis, palliation is necessary in addition to intensive hospital care, which may be followed by prolonged physical rehabilitation or even institutionalization.

Cost-Effectiveness of Dengue Control

We look at different combinations of factors that may affect overall costs of dengue control.

Structure of the Model

In this section we seek to quantify the cost-effectiveness of dengue control over the long run in those areas of the world at risk of the disease. As mentioned above, currently two strategies are available to control this disease—improved case management and vector control. In the future, a third strategy—vaccinations—may also become available. As preventive strategies, vector control and vaccinations (if and when available) would reduce the incidence of disease and thus reduce both morbidity and mortality. Case management primarily reduces mortality, with a small benefit in morbidity.

Combinations of strategies are also possible. Case management may be combined with either chemical or environmental vector control. In addition, case management, vector control, or both may be combined with vaccinations (if and when a vaccine is available). The costs of vector control or vaccination are not affected by other strategies. The cost of case management, however, is reduced by the presence of one or more of the preventive programs because the costs of case management depend on the number of cases. Vector control or vaccinations reduce the number of cases.

The effectiveness of combinations were calculated according to the principle that each control strategy eliminates a certain proportion of the deaths still remaining after other strategies have been applied. That is, the effectiveness of a combination of strategies is the product of the effectiveness fractions of each.

Dengue Epidemiological Scenarios

Studies of the cost-effectiveness of disease control must begin with prognoses of evolution of disease in the absence of any control measure. For dengue, these prognoses vary widely, according to conditions for dengue transmission and previous population exposure to one or more dengue viruses. Four different epidemiologic scenarios are possible. They are listed below, in order of increasing severity.

- Endemic dengue fever, in which disease is relatively silent except for dengue fever in young adults. Children are seen in doctors' offices with mild fevers. The situation in Brazil in 1987 through 1989 and in Puerto Rico during the past decade illustrated this scenario.

- An epidemic of dengue fever occurring in a largely susceptible population. This results in high morbidity in adults, absenteeism, loss of tourism, some hospitalization, a handful of hemorrhagic cases, and deaths. Brazil's outbreak in 1986 illustrated this situation.

- An epidemic of DHF/DSS occurring for the first time. Such an epidemic results in high morbidity and mortality in children and adults. This is a one-time-only occurrence and not a stable state. Examples are the Cuban epidemic of 1981, in which half of deaths and cases were in children, and the Venezuelan epidemic of 1989–90.

• Endemic DHF/DSS. In this scenario there is continuous high morbidity and mortality, limited to children. The situation in Thailand is an illustration.

In establishing a potential scenario for calculating the costs of dengue, it seems most appropriate to choose the endemic steady state of DHF/DSS (the last of the four epidemiologic scenarios). This situation results when there is unlimited abundance of *Aedes aegypti*. It is the most extreme scenario and the one which control is designed to avoid. Because present evidence suggests that only tropical Asia and tropical America are at risk of DHF/DSS, this cost-effectiveness study is targeted to hypothetical populations in these regions. Operationally, we have defined these regions as all of Central and South America and the Caribbean, and South and Southeast Asia. The core part of these regions contains 2.22 billion people (420 million in the Americas and 1.8 billion in Asia east of Pakistan [World Bank 1990]).

The calculational procedure of the model is concerned with the aggregate population of a country at risk. In the analysis of the vaccination strategy, the fact that a vaccine confers benefit only to the extent that it is used is taken into consideraion. Thus, following a model developed to aid in the analysis of vaccination programs (Shepard and others 1986), we multiply the efficacy of the vaccine and the coverage to arrive at the effectiveness of a vaccination program. For the purposes of the model, "coverage" means the correct administration of a vaccine. Thus, the word incorporates factors of diagnostic accuracy, provider compliance, and patient compliance, which are treated separately in some other studies.

As with other cost-effectiveness studies in the Health Sector Priorities Review, the model applies to a hypothetical population of one million persons of all ages in a country at risk of dengue. The model first estimates baseline results for costs and health effects if no control strategy is applied. It then estimates results assuming individual or combined strategies are applied.

All economic data for the model are expressed in constant 1988 U.S. dollars. The model uses fully allocated costs, rather than marginal costs, for all inputs. This method is appropriate because costs are being considered over the long run in many countries; results are being used to inform policies that are concerned with the creation or dismantling of whole programs, in which marginal considerations may not apply. The data also need to be comparable with companion cost-effectiveness studies.

The main measure of health benefits are disability-adjusted life-years (DALYs) in the standard population of one million. This measure combines a loss in life expectancy and in quality of life as a result of dengue. Future costs and health benefits are both discounted at a rate of 3 percent per year.

Feasible Applications in Each Setting

In any meaningful application of the model, only potentially feasible interventions should be included. The designation of which interventions are potentially feasible depends on the country and time frame in which the application is set.

The country is important because the levels of development of the health delivery system vary widely among nations. For one of the interventions in the model, case management, benefits depend critically on the level of sophistication of the health delivery system. In this analysis, we have categorized the health delivery system as either "developed" or "not developed" (or unevenly developed). Developed systems are ones which meet five criteria: (a) most of the population has access to quality primary health services; (b) the population is sufficiently sensitized to acute problems such as dengue that a severely ill child will receive medical care within twelve hours; (c) personnel in primary and first-level referral facilities are sufficiently trained that they can generally stabilize an acute illness and refer a case for definitive care when needed; (d) an acutely ill child can reach a secondary health facility within twelve hours; and (e) referral facilities have the technical development, personnel, and equipment to perform current treatments safely and effectively. Health systems without this capacity are termed "not developed." Because of the level of development of the health system required to implement effective case management for dengue, this strategy has proved feasible only in countries with strong health delivery systems.

For example, improved strategies of case management have been implemented in Thailand during the past thirty years. During this period the case-fatality rate from dengue hemorrhagic fever has fallen from 5.8 percent in 1958–65 to 0.5 percent in 1986–89. In general, children are promptly referred in emergencies. Physicians with the equivalent of United States specialty training who have adequate laboratory back up are on duty in a pediatric intensive care unit twenty-four hours per day. Nursing staff are skilled in managing pediatric emergencies and inserting intravenous lines to rehydrate children in emergency with minimal risk of infection.

In other countries in southeast Asia, such as Myanmar, Cambodia, Lao People's Democratic Republic, and Indonesia, the overall level of development of the health delivery system does not meet the criteria we have listed above. Although a few centers provide excellent care, success with improved case management has not been achieved on a national scale. Although this discussion of applications is based on countries, future extensions of it could consider regional policies based on variations within a country.

A country's mortality rate of children under five years of age serves as a good proxy for the level of development of its health system. We would expect that most countries which the United Nations Children's Fund (UNICEF) characterizes as having "middle" or "low" under-five mortality rates (70 or less per 1,000 live births) would have strong health systems, whereas most countries with "high" or "very high" rates (greater than 70) probably have variable health systems. Thailand and Indonesia had under-five mortality rates of 34 and 97, respectively, as of 1990 (Grant 1992), so their rates are consistent with this classification.

The time frame of an application is important because it determines the status of vaccine development. We have characterized vaccine status as either "available" or "not available." As of 1992, dengue vaccines appear ready for final testing and development by a vaccine manufacturer. Nevertheless, no vaccine is currently available for general use. It is assumed in the "vaccine available" case that current development efforts are successfully completed and that a vaccine for mass use is available. If current efforts continue successfully, this would be about 1997.

Up to four single interventions are considered in this cost-effectiveness model:

- Case management improved (C)
- Immunization against dengue virus (I)
- Vector (the *Aedes aegypti* mosquito) chemically controlled (V)
- Environmental vector control (E)

Because the two types of vector control would be duplicative, they are considered exclusive. Otherwise the single interventions can be combined up to three at a time.

The combinations of development of the health delivery system and availability of vaccine create four settings or cases: no vaccine in a developed and in an undeveloped health system and available vaccine in a developed and in an undeveloped system. In table 14-1 we show the various policies available in each setting. Even in the most constrained setting (no vaccine in a developed system), more than one policy is available. In the most inclusive setting (vaccine available in an undeveloped system), ten choices are possible.

In the analysis of the cost-effectiveness of potentially feasible alternatives, we consider two criteria: dominance and relative cost-effectiveness. The dominance criterion means that some interventions or combinations can be eliminated in some settings because they are inferior to another intervention (or mixture of interventions) on both costs and effectiveness. The relative cost-effectiveness criterion indicates the important policy tradeoffs between resources allocated to dengue control and results. These concepts will be clarified and displayed graphically in the context of specific numerical results below.

To evaluate the alternative policies, a cost-effectiveness model was applied with the best available data from the literature, case studies in Puerto Rico and Brazil, and subjective estimates. The cost-effectiveness model is specified in detail in the three appendixes to this chapter.

Results

Using the model described above, we projected the results of applying each policy to a population of one million people. The results are expressed in the cost and benefits per year of application in figures 14-1 through 14-5. The benefits are expressed either in deaths averted or disability-adjusted life-years (DALYs) saved. Baseline data are for the absence of any control policy and are considered to be those with no costs and no health benefits. In table 14-2 we show the results for all the dengue control strategies. Here all the policies (both single and combination) are listed alphabetically, regardless of their feasibility in a particular setting.

Examination of the data in table 14-2 shows that the interventions in the combined policies interact nonlinearly. For example, the combination VC averts fewer deaths than the sum of V and C. The cost is also somewhat less than the sum of the costs. This is so because any preventive strategy, such as V, reduces the number of cases requiring treatment. Thus, the benefit and added costs from better treatment are both less than when there were more cases.

The results of applying the model in each of the four settings are shown in graphic form in figures 14-1 through 14-5. The main part of the analysis, summarized in the first four figures, presents the results in cost per disability-adjusted life-year. In these figures, each feasible policy (a single intervention or combination of interventions) is denoted by a square or a dot. The letters above the square or dot are the label for the policy, as described in table 14-2. All the figures begin with the baseline (no control), which entails zero cost and zero health benefits.

Table 14-1. Interventions for Dengue Control in Developed and Undeveloped Health Systems

Vaccine availability	Developed health system	Undeveloped health system
No vaccine	Vector chemically controlled (V) Environmental vector control (E)	Case management improved (C) Vector chemically controlled (V) Environmental vector control (E) Environmental control and case management (EC) Vector chemically controlled and case management (VC)
Vaccine available	Immunization (I) Vector chemically controlled (V) Environmental vector control (E) Immunization and vector chemically controlled (IV) Immunization and environmental control (IE)	Case management improved (C) Immunization (I) Vector chemically controlled (V) Environmental vector control (E) Environmental control and case management (EC) Vector chemically controlled and case management (VC) Immunization and case management (IC) Immunization and vector chemically controlled (IV) Immunization and environmental control (IE) Immunization, case management, and environmental control (ICE)

Source: Authors.

Figure 14-1. DALYs *Saved without Vaccine Available in Undeveloped Health System*
(per 1 million population)

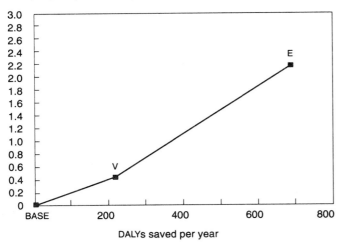

Note: BASE = Baseline; *Efficient policies* : V= Vector chemically controlled, E = Environmental vector control.
Source: Authors' cost-effectiveness model

In calculating DALYs, each death averted was 25.5 discounted years, which becomes 25.5 DALYs. No quality adjustment was required for deaths, because if a person survives an episode of DHF/DSS, he or she will not have any long-term impairment. By comparison, the regular (undiscounted) life expectancy at age 6, calibrated to areas at risk of dengue, is 63.8 years.

In figure 14-1, only three policies are shown: BASE, V, and E. These are the only feasible policies in countries without a developed health system and without a vaccine available. The position of policy E at the right of the graph shows that it is the most effective of the feasible policies in this setting. The fact that it is also the highest on the vertical axis indicates that it is also the most costly policy. The slope of the line segment from the baseline to the first policy (V) corresponds to the cost-effectiveness of that policy, in average cost per DALY saved. According to table 14-2, this cost-effectiveness ratio is $1,992. It is the ratio of the net cost of that intervention (approximately $435,000) divided by its effectiveness (219 DALYs saved), also shown in table 14-2.

Chemical vector control is technically a more cost-effective policy than the alternative of environmental control, which costs $3,129 per DALY, because its cost-effectiveness ratio is lower. That is, a given amount of money can buy more DALYs if spent on V rather than E.

An ideal policy would fall in the lower right corner of this graph—substantial health benefits and minimal costs. A poor policy would lie in the upper left corner—few benefits but high costs. The frontier of current efficient policies, shown by the solid line, is obtained by connecting those currently available policies for which no other policy is closer to the lower right corner. Thus, the baseline, V, and E form the frontiers of current efficient policies.

Figure 14-2 is an analogous graph for the situation in which no vaccine is available in a developed health system. Improvement in case management is a feasible intervention, both alone

Table 14-2. *Efficacy and Costs of Interventions for Dengue*
(per 1 million population)

| Intervention | Deaths averted | DALYs saved from | | | | Net cost ($000) | Average cost per DALY($) | Average cost per death ($) |
		Mortality	Morbidity	Total	Percent			
Baseline (BASE)	0.00	0	0	0	0	0	0	0
Case management improved (C)	21.74	554	3	557	92	327	587	15,042
Environmental vector control (E)	22.52	574	118	692	95	2,172	3,139	96,461
Environmental control and case management (EC)	23.61	602	118	720	100	2,189	3,040	92,712
Immunization (I)	16.44	419	86	505	69	727	1,440	44,251
Immunization and case management (IC)	23.10	589	87	676	97	828	1,224	35,827
Immunization, case management, and environmental control (ICE)	23.68	604	123	727	100	2,959	4,071	124,968
Immunization, case management, and vector chemically controlled (ICV)	23.28	594	98	692	98	1,250	1,806	53,691
Immunization and environmental vector control (IE)	23.34	595	122	717	98	2,954	4,117	126,537
Immunization and vector chemically controlled (IV)	18.62	475	97	572	79	1,180	2,062	63,372
Vector chemically controlled (V)	7.11	181	37	219	30	435	1,992	61,234
Vector chemically controlled and case management (VC)	22.33	569	39	609	94	664	1,091	29,754

Source: Authors' cost-effectiveness model.

Figure 14-2. *DALYs Saved without Vaccine Available in Developed Health System*
(per 1 million population)

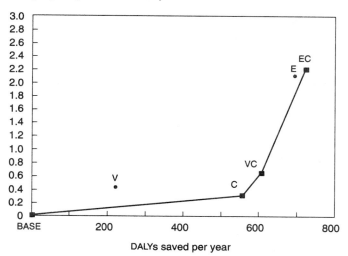

Note: BASE = Baseline; *Efficient policies*: C = Case management improved, VC = Vector chemically controlled and case management, EC = Environmental control and case management; *Inefficient policies:* V = Vector chemically controlled, E = Environmental vector control.
Source: Authors' cost-effectiveness model

and combined with other interventions. The efficient policies (C, VC, and EC) are shown by squares. These results show that case management is now the most cost-effective policy. It saves one DALY for $587, about a third of the cost of achieving this benefit with policies V or E, respectively. Case management is also a powerful policy, being able to save 92 percent of the morbidity imposed by dengue in the cohort. It must be emphasized, however, that this seemingly attractive policy is feasible because of and is dependent on a developed health system.

Policymakers often face the choice between the most cost-effective policy and the most effective policy. In the case of dengue control, an efficient policy that would yield still greater benefits is a combination of chemical vector control and case management (VC). As shown in table 14-2, policy VC saves 609 DALYs, compared with 557 saved by policy C. At a cost of $1,091 per DALY, policy VC is somewhat less cost-effective than policy C. The next step in effectiveness is to replace chemical by environmental vector control as an addition to case management (policy EC). The number of DALYs gained by this policy (720) is virtually the entire burden of dengue, but the cost for the cohort of one million persons ($2,172,000) would be substantial.

Although policy V is still feasible in the case of no vaccine in an undeveloped health system, economically it is no longer efficient. A partial application of the case management strategy to part of the population of one million persons could achieve the same benefit in DALYs at a lower cost than policy

V. In technical terms, a combination of BASE and C dominate policy V. This dominance is shown graphically by the fact that the line from BASE to C passes underneath the dot for policy V. In these figures, efficient strategies are shown by squares, whereas dominated policies are shown by dots. Strategy V is not economically efficient because this strategy was considered only 30 percent effective. Because the dengue-carrying mosquito breeds quickly, populations reduced by chemical spraying have been found to return quickly.

The technique of incremental cost-effectiveness analysis is useful to illustrate the tradeoff between cost-effective and effective policies. In table 14-3 we present this analysis in tabular form. The tradeoff is judged by the number of additional DALYs gained in relation to the additional cost incurred. The ratio of the additional cost to the additional gain in DALYs is the incremental cost-effectiveness ratio. For example, the comparison between policies VC and C show an incremental gain of fifty-one DALYs at an incremental cost of $337,000. The incremental cost-effectiveness ratio is $6,568, corresponding to approximately $337,000 per fifty-one DALYs. Graphically, this ratio corresponds to the slope of the line segment from C to VC. This line segment is substantially steeper than that from BASE to C, showing that the cost to save each of these few additional DALYs is quite high. In common parlance, it illustrates the decreasing marginal returns of larger investments in dengue control while holding the population fixed. Only efficient policies are listed in table 14-3, because they are the only ones to which incremental cost-effectiveness applies.

Figure 14-3. *DALYs Saved with Vaccine in Undeveloped Health System*
(per 1 million population)

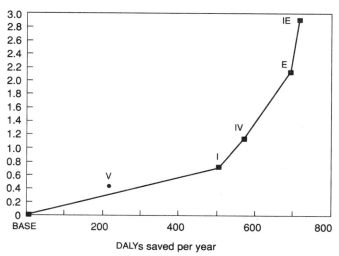

Note: BASE = Baseline; *Efficient policies*: I = Immunization, IVS = Immunization and vector chemically controlled, IE = Environmental vector control, E = Immunization and environmental control; *Inefficient policies*: V = Vector chemically controlled.
Source: Authors' cost-effectiveness model

Figure 14-4. DALYs *Saved with Vaccine in Developed Health System*

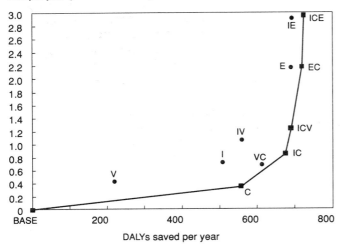

Note: BASE = Baseline; *Efficient policies*: C = Improved case management, IC = Vaccination and case management; ICV = Vaccination, case management, and vector chemically controlled, EC = Environmental vector control and case management, ICE = Vaccination, case management, and environmental vector control; *Inefficient policies*: V = Vector chemically controlled, I = Immunization, VC = Vector chemically controlled and case management, IV = Immunization and vector chemically controlled, E = Environmental vector control, IE = Immunization and environmental control.
Source: Authors' cost-effectiveness model

Figure 14-3 introduces the case in which a dengue vaccine is available, but the health system is still not developed. As explained in the appendix 14C, a dengue vaccine is expected to be 95 percent effective in protecting persons who receive it. In a population, however, its effectiveness is limited by a coverage of only 73 percent, the rate obtained for the third dose of DPT according to 1990 UNICEF data. As of 1992, a vaccine is expected to be available in three to five years, assuming the final development continues as planned. For this analysis, we have taken the longer estimate, giving a target date of 1997. Immunization is the most cost-effective strategy, followed by IV, E, and IE. Again, strategy V is not economically efficient. The incremental cost-effectiveness analysis comparing policies E and IE shows that adding immunization onto environmental control is not particularly cost-effective. The incremental cost per DALY gained is $30,927.

In figure 14-4, we present the analysis for the case in which the full range of alternatives is available. A vaccine is available and the health system is developed. Again, case management is the most cost-effective strategy. It is interesting that none of the preventive single interventions—immunization, chemical vector control, or environmental vector control—was economically efficient alone. Each was dominated by a combination of strategies that include case management. The immunization result is because of the relatively high cost of immunization of $40.87 per person; the cost is a result of the

assumed high cost of the vaccine itself ($17.50 per dose) and the need for two doses. The relatively high cost of vector control arises because vector control must be practiced for the entire population every year, whereas case management affects only sick patients.

A sensitivity analysis for vaccination showed immunization would become as cost-effective as case management if the cost of the series were to drop to $18.00. Allowing $3.07 (in future value) for the two vaccination contacts, as assumed in the base case, this would leave about $7.00 per dose for the vaccine itself. The dramatic drop in the price of hepatitis B vaccine illustrates that such a drop is possible. Initially introduced at a prohibitive price of $100.00 per dose, a plasma-derived hepatitis B vaccine is now available for only $1.00 per dose for bulk purchase by developing countries. A sensitivity analysis on case management showed that if the base cost of hospitalization episode (TREAT) rose from $200.00 to only $438.00, it would no longer be the most cost-effective strategy.

The analysis for the case in which vaccine is available in a developed health care system was also calculated in cost per death averted, as shown in figure 14-5. Although the numbers change, the demarcation between dominated and efficient policies, and the ordering among the efficient policies remains the same. The advantage of policy C over policy I in cost-effectiveness is seen more dramatically in deaths averted,

Figure 14-5. *Deaths Averted with Vaccine in Developed Health System*
(per 1 million population)

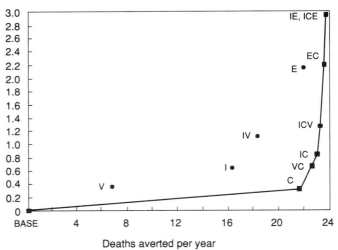

Note: BASE = Baseline; *Efficient policies*: C = Improved case management, VC = Vector chemically controlled and case management, IC = Vaccination and case management; ICV = Vaccination, case management, and vector chemically controlled, EC = Environmental vector control and case management, ICE = Vaccination, case management, and environmental vector control; *Inefficient policies*: V = Vector chemically controlled, I = Immunization, IV = Immunization and vector chemically controlled, E = Environmental vector control, IE = Immunization and environmental control.
Source: Authors' cost-effectiveness model

Table 14-3. Incremental Cost-Effectiveness of Interventions for Dengue Control

Intervention	DALYs saved	Net cost ($000)	Average cost per DALY ($)	Average cost per death ($)	Additional DALYs gained	Additional cost ($000)	Incremental cost per DALY ($)
No vaccine and health system not developed							
Baseline (BASE)	0	0	0	0	0	0	0
Vector chemically controlled (V)	219	435	1,992	61,234	219	435	1,992
Environmental vector control (E)	692	2,172	3,139	96,461	474	1,737	3,668
No vaccine but developed health system							
Baseline	0	0	0	0	0	0	0
Case management improved (C)	557	327	587	15,042	557	327	587
Vector chemically controlled and case management (VC)	609	664	1,091	29,754	51	337	6,568
Environmental control and case management (EC)	720	2,189	3,040	92,712	111	1,524	13,696
With vaccine but health system not developed							
Baseline (BASE)	0	0	0	0	0	0	0
Immunization (I)	505	727	1,440	44,251	505	727	1,440
Immunization and vector chemically controlled (IV)	572	1,180	2,062	63,372	67	452	6,754
Environmental vector control (E)	692	2,172	3,139	96,461	120	992	8,278
Immunization and environmental control (IE)	717	2,954	4,117	126,537	25	781	30,927
With vaccine and developed health system							
Baseline (BASE)	0	0	0	0	0	0	0
Case management improved (C)	557	327	587	15,042	557	327	587
Immunization and case management (IC)	676	828	1,224	35,827	119	501	4,217
Immunization, case management, and vector chemically controlled (ICV)	692	1,250	1,806	53,691	16	422	26,363
Environmental control and case management (EC)	720	2,189	3,040	92,712	28	939	33,643
Immunization, case management, and environmental control (ICE)	727	2,959	4,071	124,968	7	770	112,933

Note: Only policies that are feasible and economically efficient are listed.
Source: Authors' cost-effectiveness model.

because the number of deaths averted does not count the morbidity avoided by vaccinations.

Under both criteria, deaths averted and DALYs, case management remains the most cost-effective first strategy. The cost per DALY gained, $587, is comparable to the per capita income of an average low-income developing country. Thus, case management of dengue fever, although not as cost-effective as some of the other interventions examined in this collection, is still reasonable and cost-effective for all but the very poorest country. The cost per death averted, $15,042, is also an acceptable investment for a middle-income country. Among the preventive interventions, immunization, at $1,440 per DALY gained, is the most cost-effective policy.

Finally, the analysis adds future interventions to those under consideration. Case management remains the most cost-effective program, but the next intervention is to add immunization to case management (IC). That is, we first make sure treatment facilities can do a good job; then we add the preventive component. These results are opposite to the usual adage that prevention is cheaper than cure. With case management, we have a good argument for cure. Prevention is expensive and is directed to a condition that is relatively rare when both epidemic and nonepidemic years are averaged.

Priorities

On the basis of our analysis, we recommend policies in two areas. First, applying existing knowledge, we recommend measures for cost-effective control of dengue. Second, we examine how operational research could allow better disease control in the future.

Priorities for Resource Allocation

Policies differ among the three mosquito-borne diseases. For the two for which effective vaccines are available (yellow fever and Japanese encephalitis) the major questions concern overcoming the technical and financial constraints to vaccination.

DENGUE. Policies for dengue control vary with time and the level of development of a country's health system. In the case in which no vaccine is available and the health system is not developed, chemical vector control was most cost-effective ($1,992.00 per DALY), although not very effective in an absolute sense. Environmental vector control, through reduction of breeding sites, is the only other alternative. As practiced in Singapore, this policy proved highly effective but somewhat costly ($2.25 per person per year, even after excluding costs for controlling nuisance mosquitoes). It would be highly effective, and only slightly less favorable on cost-effectiveness than controlling mosquitoes through spraying.

In the case in which no vaccine is available but the health system is developed, the cost-effectiveness analysis suggests that case management is the most cost-effective policy ($587 per DALY). The analysis suggests that this method should be undertaken first. For additional control, chemical or environmental vector control should be added.

In the case in which a dengue vaccine is assumed to be available (beginning in 1997) but a country's health system is not developed, immunization would be the most cost-effective alternative at $1,440 per DALY. In the model, we estimated a relatively high cost for the assumed two-dose series for this vaccine of $40.87 per person vaccinated. If this price dropped with increasing volume, the cost-effectiveness of this option could improve substantially. For example, if the price per dose of vaccine dropped from its assumed value of $17.50 to $7.00, then immuniztion would become as cost-effective as case management.

In the case in which a dengue vaccine is available and the health system is developed, all policies would be technically feasible. Case management proved to be most cost-effective at a cost per DALY of $587, but immunization would be a valuable addition at an incremental cost of $4,217 per additional DALY gained. Case management and vaccination would be expensive for the countries with the lowest income. Many countries at risk of dengue in Asia and South America are middle- or upper-middle-income countries. For them, dengue control is a reasonable part of their health priorities.

An important caveat is that our analysis of vector control captures only direct patient benefits. Thus, certain secondary benefits of vector control are not captured or are incompletely measured. They include reduction in the nuisance and discomfort of mosquito bites, possible reduction in transmission from fewer infected people, and a possible reduction in the risk of other vector-borne diseases, such as yellow fever. The impact on yellow fever would be only a theoretical advantage in most regions of the world, however. The other, less tangible benefits, cannot be valued within the scope of this chapter.

Although a thorough sensitivity analysis has not been done, the cost-effectiveness of case management depends on the availability of moderately priced, high-quality referral hospital care. We assumed that the base cost of treating DHF/DSS was $200 per case (for an average hospital stay of five days) and that improved case management would raise this cost fivefold. If the base cost were about twice as high ($487 per case), the cost-effectiveness of case management would then be equal to that of vaccinations.

One factor in favor of each of these control programs is that they can be implemented on localized scales. Improvements in case management could be implemented at a single hospital. Vector control, whether chemical or environmental, could be implemented at the level of a single city, and in part, at a neighborhood level. The delivery of a vaccine, once it has been developed, can be directed to receptive populations. Thus, although the cost-effectiveness of dengue control policies may not place them in the highest priority for low-income countries, they certainly are feasible for middle-income countries and particularly for middle-class populations within middle-income countries.

Finally, the choice between preventive and curative policies involves ethical issues. Some public health officials feel that a society has an obligation to prevent disease if it can reasonably do so, even if curative policies appear somewhat more cost-effective in the short run. The public's willingness to undertake future preventive measures would be an additional benefit.

YELLOW FEVER. Partly because of its high case-fatality rate and partly because yellow fever has been controlled on a hemispheric basis both by vector control and by vaccination, modern societies regard epidemics of yellow fever as intolerable. In Africa, adequate supplies of potent yellow fever vaccine must be on hand for preventive immunization programs and to combat yellow fever epidemics. Nigeria, repeatedly affected by epidemics, still depends heavily on an antiquated manufacturing facility established by the Rockefeller Foundation in 1939. It is quite possible that batches of this vaccine have relatively poor thermostability compared with those produced by other manufacturers and that they still contain avian leukosis virus. Some lots may be contaminated with other organisms. Nigeria and other African countries also import vaccine from Brazil, Senegal, and France. Even potent yellow fever vaccine is extremely dependent upon an intact cold chain; on adequate supplies of jet injectors, needles, and syringes; and on trained vaccinators. All are at present inadequate. The authors recommend the following steps to address these problems:

- Funds should be made available to purchase and stockpile potent yellow fever vaccine.
- An effective delivery system is needed. Success in building a sustainable delivery system for EPI will also permit routine or emergency delivery of yellow fever vaccine.
- Yellow fever vaccine should be incorporated into the EPI program for those countries in Africa at risk of yellow fever.

JAPANESE ENCEPHALITIS. Public outcries and political pressures for action seem to be particularly powerful against this disease. Nonetheless, many affected nations have postponed the purchase of sufficient quantities of vaccines needed to immunize all at-risk children. This is largely because of the high cost in hard currency of Japanese-manufactured killed vaccines (at least $4.60 to $6.90 just for vaccine alone). India and Thailand, with Japanese assistance, are investing in domestic vaccine manufacturing facilities. These will require huge colonies of laboratory mice. There is reason to doubt, based on past performance, that output of vaccine will be sufficient for national needs. Estimates of current and projected costs and losses resulting from Japanese encephalitis might contribute to rational investment policies, whether for domestic manufacture or for vaccine importation.

Priorities for Operational Research

Priorities for operational research focus on ways to control the mosquito, development of vaccine (for dengue) improvement of vaccines (for yellow fever and Japanese encephalitis).

DENGUE. First, careers in vector control need to be entirely reconstituted. The leaders and experienced veterans of the Latin American *Aedes aegypti* campaigns have disappeared without replacements. Second, politically acceptable, cost-effective methods of *Aedes aegypti* control or eradication are needed. Third, research on cost-effective, efficacious, safe, and thermally stable vaccines requires adequate funding. Current programs are very poorly funded.

YELLOW FEVER. A second-generation genetically engineered vaccine might overcome the present requirement for lyophilization.

JAPANESE ENCEPHALITIS. First, a potent, safe, thermally stable live-attenuated vaccine is needed. A reasonable candidate has been developed in China. This requires internationally acceptable phase I, II, and III testing and introduction into the affected countries of Thailand, Myanmar, Nepal, Bangladesh, India, and Sri Lanka. Second, investments, both technical and financial, are needed in vaccine production capacities in most of these affected countries.

Appendix 14A. Definitions of Variables in the Cost-Effectiveness Model

The model involves the following parameters:

Morbidity and mortality
STAND.POP: The number of persons in the standard population (an arbitrary size) to which the model is applied. Here STAND.POP is one million persons of all ages.
CASES: Number of dengue infections without vaccination or vector control in the hypothetical birth cohort (all births within the standard population in one year).
SHOCK.R (Shock rate): Proportion of dengue infections that progress to dengue shock syndrome.
FATAL: Case-fatality rate of DSS 1960–65.
CLINICAL: Proportion of dengue infections which are clinically apparent.
DUR: Average duration of clinical illness, expressed in disability-adjusted life-years.

COHORT: Number of persons in one year's birth cohort in the standard population.

Effectiveness of interventions
YEAR.D: Discounted remaining life expectancy of a person at the average age of death of a fatal dengue case.
SALVAGE: Proportional reduction in case-fatality rate of DHF/DSS after improved case management.
SHORTEN: Proportional reduction in duration of illness among hospitalized cases after improved case management.
VACC.EF (vaccine efficacy): Proportional reduction in number of cases.
COVERAGE: Proportion of birth cohort vaccinated.
VCTRC.EF: (vector chemical efficacy): Proportional reduction in number of cases from chemical vector control.
VCTRE.EF: (vector environmental efficacy): Proportional reduction in number of cases from environmental vector control.

Costs of case management
TREAT: Current cost per case of treating hospitalized DHF/DSS.
IMPROVE: Cost as a multiple of TREAT per case of DHF/DSS of improved case management, converted to future value as of the average expected age at death from dengue.

Costs of vaccines
DEVELOP: Annualized expected development cost for cohort until successful development.
VACCINE: Vaccination cost per person vaccinated, converted to future value as of the average age at death from dengue.

Costs of vector control
VECTORC: Cost per person per year in target population of chemical vector control, including amortization of initial costs.
VECTORE: Cost per person per year in target population of environmental vector control, including amortization of initial costs.

The model also uses the following intermediate variables:

DEATHS: Number of dengue deaths in the standard population in one year with a specified control program.
D.AVERTED: The number of deaths averted in the standard population in one year.
D.BASELINE: The number of dengue deaths in the baseline situation of no dengue control program.
DALY.MORB: The number of disability-adjusted life-years saved through morbidity averted.
DALY.MORT: The number of disability-adjusted life-years saved through mortality averted.
YEAR.D: The discounted life expectancy at the average age at which one otherwise would have died of dengue.

Appendix 14B. Relationships in the Cost-Effectiveness Model

We look at these relationships in the context of deaths averted, disability-adjusted life-years saved, and aggregate costs.

Deaths Averted

The number of deaths is expressed as the product of the three factors: the number of infections times the proportion of those infections which progress to the potentially fatal condition of DHF/DSS times the proportion of DHF/DSS cases which are fatal. For consistency with the formulas in the computer spreadsheet in which this model was written, multiplication is shown by an asterisk. The equations below show how this principle applies to each of the control strategies.

Single interventions
At the baseline (policy BASE):

$$\text{D.BASELINE} = \text{CASES} \cdot \text{SHOCK.R} \cdot \text{FATAL.}$$

With case management improved (policy C):

$$\text{DEATHS} = \text{CASES} \cdot \text{SHOCK.R} \cdot \text{FATAL} \cdot (1 - \text{SALVAGE}).$$

With immunization or vaccination (policy I):

$$\text{DEATHS} = \text{CASES} \cdot (1 - \text{VACC.EF} \cdot \text{COVERAGE}) \cdot \text{SHOCK.R} \cdot \text{FATAL.}$$

With vector chemically controlled (policy V):

$$\text{DEATHS} = \text{CASES} \cdot (1 - \text{VCTRC.EF}) \cdot \text{SHOCK.R} \cdot \text{FATAL.}$$

With environmental vector control (policy E):

$$\text{DEATHS} = \text{CASES} \cdot (1 - \text{VCTRE.EF}) \cdot \text{SHOCK.R} \cdot \text{FATAL.}$$

Two-way combinations
With vaccination and case management (policy IC):

$$\text{DEATHS} = \text{CASES} \cdot (1 - \text{VACC.EF} \cdot \text{COVERAGE}) \cdot \text{SHOCK.R} \cdot (1 - \text{SALVAGE}) \cdot \text{FATAL.}$$

With vector chemically controlled and case management (policy VC):

$$\text{DEATHS} = \text{CASES} \cdot (1 - \text{VCTRC.EF}) \cdot \text{SHOCK.R} \cdot (1 - \text{SALVAGE}) \cdot \text{FATAL.}$$

With environmental vector control and case management (policy EC):

$$\text{DEATHS} = \text{CASES} \cdot (1 - \text{VCTRC.EF}) \cdot \text{SHOCK.R} \cdot (1 - \text{SALVAGE}) \cdot \text{FATAL.}$$

With immunization and vector chemically controlled (policy IV):

$$\text{DEATHS} = \text{CASES} \cdot (1 - \text{VACC.EF} \cdot \text{COVERAGE}) \cdot (1 - \text{VCTRC.EF}) \cdot \text{SHOCK.R} \cdot \text{FATAL.}$$

With immunization and environmental vector control (policy IE):

$$\text{DEATHS} = \text{CASES} \cdot (1 - \text{VACC.EF} \cdot \text{COVERAGE}) \cdot (1 - \text{VCTRC.EF}) \cdot \text{SHOCK.R} \cdot \text{FATAL.}$$

Three-way combinations
With immunization, case management improved, and vector chemically controlled (policy ICV):

$$\text{DEATHS} = \text{CASES} \cdot (1 - \text{VACC.EF} \cdot \text{COVERAGE}) \cdot (1 - \text{VCTRC.EF}) \cdot \text{SHOCK.R} \cdot (1 - \text{SALVAGE}) \cdot \text{FATAL.}$$

With immunization, case management improved, and environmental vector control (policy ICE):

$$\text{DEATHS} = \text{CASES} \cdot (1 - \text{VACC.EF} \cdot \text{COVERAGE}) \cdot (1 - \text{VCTRC.EF}) \cdot \text{SHOCK.R} \cdot (1 - \text{SALVAGE}) \cdot \text{FATAL.}$$

Number of deaths averted
For each strategy, the number of deaths averted is

$$\text{D.AVERTED} = \text{D.BASELINE} - \text{DEATHS.}$$

DALYs Saved

The number of disability-adjusted life-years saved with each policy is the sum of the number saved through deaths averted and through morbidity avoided or reduced. That is, for all interventions, the overall number of DALYs saved is

$$\text{DALY.MORT} + \text{DALY.MORB.}$$

The prevention strategies (vector control and vaccination) avoid morbidity, whereas case management shortens the morbidity of serious cases. The DALYs saved through deaths averted are

$$\text{DALY.MORT} = \text{D.AVERTED} \cdot \text{YEAR.D.}$$

On the basis of experiences in Thailand (Halstead 1980b), the number of cases hospitalized is assumed to be twice the number experiencing dengue hemorrhagic shock or dengue shock syndrome.

Single interventions
Because case management benefits only hospitalized cases, only these cases experience a reduction in morbidity. The number of DALYs saved through shortened morbidity in case management (policy C) is

$$\text{DALY.MORB} = \text{CASES} \cdot 2 \cdot \text{SHOCK.R} \cdot \text{SHORTEN} \cdot \text{DUR.}$$

Infections with dengue virus, like some other infections, are not always clinically apparent. The benefit of reduced morbidity applies, of course, only to clinically apparent cases. For chemical vector control (policy V), the morbidity avoided is

$$\text{DALY.MORB} = \text{CLINICAL} \cdot \text{CASES} \cdot \text{VCTRC.EF} \cdot \text{DUR.}$$

Similarly, for environmental vector control (policy E), the morbidity avoided is

$$\text{DALY.MORB} = \text{CLINICAL} \cdot \text{CASES} \cdot \text{VCTRC.EF} \cdot \text{DUR.}$$

Immunizations are assumed to lower the attack rate of dengue but not to affect the severity of a dengue infection. Thus, for immunizations (policy I) the morbidity avoided is

$$\text{DALY.MORB} = \text{CLINICAL} \cdot \text{CASES} \cdot \text{VACC.EF} \cdot \text{COVERAGE} \cdot \text{DUR.}$$

Two-way combinations
When chemical or environmental vector control and case

management are combined, the benefits from cases avoided are supplemented by shorter morbidity for the hospitalized cases among those that still occur. The morbidity avoided from chemical vector control combined with better case management (policy VC) is

$$\text{DALY.MORB} = \text{CLINICAL} \cdot \text{CASES} \cdot \text{VCTRC.EF} \cdot \text{DUR} + \text{CASES}$$
$$\cdot (1 - \text{VCTRC.EF}) \cdot 2 \cdot \text{SHOCK.R} \cdot \text{SHORTEN} \cdot \text{DUR}.$$

Similarly, the morbidity avoided from environmental vector control combined with better case management (policy EC) is

$$\text{DALY.MORB} = \text{CLINICAL} \cdot \text{CASES} \cdot \text{VCTRC.EF} \cdot \text{DUR} + \text{CASES}$$
$$\cdot (1 - \text{VCTRC.EF}) \cdot 2 \cdot \text{SHOCK.R} \cdot \text{SHORTEN} \cdot \text{DUR}.$$

With immunization and the vector chemically controlled (policy IV) the morbidity avoided is

$$\text{DALY.MORB} = \text{CLINICAL} \cdot \text{CASES} \cdot \text{VCTRC.EF} \cdot \text{DUR} + \text{CASES}$$
$$\cdot (1 - \text{VCTRC.EF}) \cdot \text{VACC.EF} \cdot \text{COVERAGE} \cdot \text{DUR}.$$

With immunization and environmental vector control (policy IE) the morbidity avoided is

$$\text{DALY.MORB} = \text{CLINICAL} \cdot \text{CASES} \cdot \text{VCTRC.EF} \cdot \text{DUR} + \text{CASES}$$
$$\cdot (1 - \text{VCTRC.EF}) \cdot \text{VACC.EF} \cdot \text{COVERAGE} \cdot \text{DUR}.$$

With both vaccination and case management (policy IC), the morbidity avoided would be

$$\text{DALY.MORB} = \text{CLINICAL} \cdot \text{CASES} \cdot \text{VACC.EF} \cdot \text{COVERAGE}$$
$$\cdot \text{DUR} + \text{CASES} \cdot (1 - \text{VACC.EF} \cdot \text{COVERAGE})$$
$$\cdot 2 \cdot \text{SHOCK.R} \cdot \text{SHORTEN} \cdot \text{DUR}.$$

Three-way combinations

With immunization, case management improved, and vector chemically controlled (policy ICV):

$$\text{DALY.MORB} = \text{CLINICAL} \cdot \text{CASES} \cdot (\text{VACC.EF} \cdot \text{COVERAGE}$$
$$+ \text{VCTRC.EF} - \text{VACC.EF} \cdot \text{COVERAGE} \cdot \text{VCTRC.EF})$$
$$\cdot \text{DUR} + \text{CASES} \cdot (1 - \text{VACC.EF} \cdot \text{COVERAGE})$$
$$\cdot 2 \cdot \text{SHOCK.R} \cdot \text{SHORTEN} \cdot \text{DUR}.$$

With immunization, case management improved, and environmental vector control (policy ICE):

$$\text{DALY.MORB} = \text{CLINICAL} \cdot \text{CASES} \cdot (\text{VACC.EF} \cdot \text{COVERAGE}$$
$$+ \text{VCTRC.EF} - \text{VACC.EF} \cdot \text{COVERAGE} \cdot \text{VCTRC.EF})$$
$$\cdot \text{DUR} + \text{CASES} \cdot (1 - \text{VACC.EF} \cdot \text{COVERAGE})$$
$$\cdot 2 \cdot \text{SHOCK.R} \cdot \text{SHORTEN} \cdot \text{DUR}.$$

Aggregate Costs

The aggregate costs are expressed as the number of people in the standard population receiving each service times the unit cost of that service.

Single interventions
Baseline (policy BASE):

$$\text{COSTS} = \text{CASES} \cdot \text{SHOCK.R} \cdot \text{TREAT}.$$

With improved case management (policy C):

$$\text{COSTS} = \text{CASES} \cdot \text{SHOCK.R} \cdot \text{TREAT} \cdot \text{IMPROVE}.$$

With vaccination (policy I):

$$\text{COSTS} = \text{CASES} \cdot (1 - \text{VACC.EF} \cdot \text{COVERAGE}) \cdot \text{SHOCK.R} \cdot \text{TREAT}$$
$$+ \text{DEVELOP} + \text{VACCINE} \cdot \text{COVERAGE} \cdot \text{COHORT}.$$

With vector chemically controlled (policy V):

$$\text{COSTS} = \text{CASES} \cdot (1 - \text{VCTRC.EF}) \cdot \text{SHOCK.R} \cdot \text{TREAT}$$
$$+ \text{STAND.POP} \cdot \text{VECTORC}.$$

With environmental vector control (policy E):

$$\text{COSTS} = \text{CASES} \cdot (1 - \text{VCTRC.EF}) \cdot \text{SHOCK.R} \cdot \text{TREAT}$$
$$+ \text{STAND.POP} \cdot \text{VECTORE}.$$

Two-way combinations
With vaccination and case management (policy IC):

$$\text{COSTS} = \text{CASES} \cdot (1 - \text{VACC.EF} \cdot \text{COVERAGE}) \cdot \text{SHOCK.R} \cdot \text{TREAT}$$
$$\cdot \text{IMPROVE} + \text{DEVELOP} + \text{VACCINE} \cdot \text{COVERAGE} \cdot \text{COHORT}.$$

With vector chemically controlled and case management (policy VC):

$$\text{COSTS} = \text{CASES} \cdot (1 - \text{VCTRC.EF}) \cdot \text{SHOCK.R} \cdot \text{TREAT}$$
$$\cdot \text{IMPROVE} + \text{VECTORC} \cdot \text{STAND.POP}.$$

With environmental vector control and case management (policy EC):

$$\text{COSTS} = \text{CASES} \cdot (1 - \text{VCTRC.EF}) \cdot \text{SHOCK.R} \cdot \text{TREAT} \cdot \text{IMPROVE}$$
$$+ \text{VECTORE} \cdot \text{STAND.POP}.$$

With vaccination and environmental vector control (policy IE):

$$\text{COSTS} = \text{CASES} \cdot (1 - \text{VACC.EF} \cdot \text{COVERAGE}) \cdot (\text{VCTRC.EF})$$
$$\cdot \text{SHOCK.R} \cdot \text{TREAT} + \text{DEVELOP} + \text{VACCINE} \cdot \text{COVERAGE}$$
$$\cdot \text{COHORT} + \text{STAND.POP} \cdot \text{VECTOR}.$$

With immunization and vector chemically controlled (policy IV):

$$\text{COSTS} = \text{CASES} \cdot (1 - \text{VACC.EF} \cdot \text{COVERAGE}) \cdot (\text{VCTRC.EF})$$
$$\cdot \text{SHOCK.R} \cdot \text{TREAT} + \text{DEVELOP} + \text{VACCINE} \cdot \text{COVERAGE}$$
$$\cdot \text{COHORT} + \text{STAND.POP} \cdot \text{VECTOR}.$$

Three-way combinations
With vaccination, case management, and vector chemically control (policy ICV):

$$\text{COSTS} = \text{CASES} \cdot (1 - \text{VACC.EF} \cdot \text{COVERAGE}) \cdot (1 - \text{VCTRC.EF})$$
$$\cdot \text{SHOCK.R} \cdot \text{TREAT} \cdot \text{IMPROVE} + \text{DEVELOP} + \text{VACCINE}$$
$$\cdot \text{COVERAGE} \cdot \text{COHORT} + \text{STAND.POP} \cdot \text{VECTORC}.$$

With vaccination, case management, and environmental vector control (policy ICE):

$$\text{COSTS} = \text{CASES} \cdot (1 - \text{VACC.EF} \cdot \text{COVERAGE}) \cdot (1 - \text{VCTRC.EF})$$
$$\cdot \text{SHOCK.R} \cdot \text{TREAT} \cdot \text{IMPROVE} + \text{DEVELOP} + \text{VACCINE}$$
$$\cdot \text{COVERAGE} \cdot \text{COHORT} + \text{STAND.POP} \cdot \text{VECTORE}.$$

Appendix 14C. Numerical Values of Input Parameters

Parameter values are listed alphabetically below. For each parameter, we give the best estimate and the basis of that estimate. If no units are shown, the parameter is a pure dimensionless number. Values are shown in the form in which they are entered into the model. Thus value of CLINICAL below (16 percent) is shown as the decimal share 0.16.

CASES: 52,400 dengue infections in standard population per year. We estimated two infections per person per lifetime. Thus, CASES equals two times COHORT. Although a dengue infection confers immunity to the type of dengue virus which caused the infection, the person is still at risk of the remaining three of the four types of dengue virus. This is a long-term average level. During the 1981 dengue outbreak, Cuba (with a population of 10 million persons) had 2.36 million infections (based on serological data), or an infection rate of 236,000 per million population (Guzman and others 1990). Epidemics result from a buildup of susceptible persons. The long-term rate for CASES is about one-fifth of the Cuban rate.

CLINICAL: 0.16. This share is based on clinical data for DHF/DSS in children from Thailand (Halstead 1980b).

COHORT: 26,200 persons born per year in the standard population. The birth cohort size is the weighted average of the crude birth rate in the countries at risk of dengue. This was calculated as a weighted average of the crude birth rate per 1,000 population in countries with at least 1 million persons, based on data (generally for 1988) in the *World Development Report* (World Bank 1990). The value of this parameter corresponds to a crude birth rate of 26.2 per 1,000 population per year.

COVERAGE: 0.73. This is the overall coverage of DPT-3 among one-year-old children in developing countries at risk of dengue in 1987–88 (Grant 1990). If and when a dengue vaccine is developed, it will probably be offered to children through the delivery mechanism of the Expanded Programme on Immunization.

DEVELOP: $2,488. According to a study by the Institute of Medicine, Vaccine Development (1986), the cost of research and development to try to produce a useful dengue vaccine was estimated at $25 million; the probability of success was 0.75; when estimates were compiled in approximately 1985, twelve years were then thought to be required to license and adopt the vaccine. That is, the projected target year was 1997. During the past decade, researchers in Thailand, who have received about $5 million in external support from the Rockefeller Foundation and the Italian government, and the equivalent of several million dollars of in-kind support from the Thai government, have now produced a tetravalent vaccine in the laboratory and tested it successfully on 200 volunteers. (Replication of this research in an industrial country today would have cost about $100 million.) Final development, full-scale testing in humans, and development of production methods and capacity re-

main. These steps are estimated to require a further investment of $25 million and require five more years from 1992. Thus, the target date remains 1997. Because the average age at death was six (as described below), there is an additional five-year delay from administration of the first dose at age one until a death is potentially averted. Thus deaths will not be averted until ten years in the future (five for development plus five after administration).

In full use in a stable (long-term) situation, the vaccine would be offered to the birth cohort in all countries at risk of dengue. The population of countries at risk of dengue is 1,210 million people, or 1,210 times the standard-size calculation of 1 million people used in this analysis. To make costs commensurate with the timing of benefits, the future value of the expenditure needs to be calculated, at the time the vaccine would be in full use. Furthermore, because the success of research is not certain, the expenditure needs to be adjusted for the expected chance of success, now estimated at 90 percent. Because research and development is a capital cost, the expenditure must also be annualized over its expected useful life and rescaled for the birth cohort. We assign a twenty-year useful life to the current research effort, on the grounds that an improved vaccine would be available after that time. Several other important vaccines, such as measles and polio vaccines, have benefited from substantial improvements over this period. Thus, the cost per cohort was calculated as:

$$\$25,000,000 \cdot (1.03)^{(5+5)} / (1,210 \cdot 0.90 \cdot \text{annualizing factor}) = 2,488$$

where the annualizing factor is the present value of 1 for twenty years at 3 percent interest.

DURATION: 0.0148 year. A clinical episode of DHF/DSS is estimated to last nine days. This time counts the patient's inability to pursue his or her usual activities before, during, and after treatment. This duration is slightly longer than Osani's (1983) estimate of six days for dengue fever and the policy of the Brazilian social security system, which allows a worker seven days of authorized disability for a case of dengue fever (Kiela, personal communication, Everardo Chagas Hospital, Rio de Janiero, July, 1989). As Brazil then had virtually no DHF, the mean duration should be lower than in areas in which this complication occurred widely. The ill person has a fever, severe aches, and is generally prevented from working or carrying out his or her usual activity. Except for the minority of cases that progress to DHF/DSS, the victim can remain at home and is conscious but feels extremely uncomfortable. In cases that progress to hemorrhagic fever, the patient may be in shock for part of the illness. We have assigned a quality level of 0.4 to this acute illness on a scale where 0 denotes death and 1 perfect health. Thus, the morbidity loss is converted to an annual equivalent as $9/365 \cdot (1 - 0.4)$.

FATAL: 0.058. This rate was the case-fatality rate of DSS cases in Thailand in 1958–65, before good treatment became available (Halstead 1980a). On the basis of 158 deaths in 116,000 hospitalized patients, Cuba's case-fatality rate in hospitalized cases was 0.0014 during its 1981 dengue epidemic (Kouri and others 1987). Cuba has a good health system, so its case-fatality rate should reflect the effect of SALVAGE. Undoubtedly, the hospitals included some cases that were not DHF/DSS.

IMPROVE: 5. This is the estimated ratio of costs in a referral specialty hospital to those in a typical secondary hospital.

SALVAGE: 0.917. This rate of salvage of hemorrhagic cases is based on experience in Thailand following improvement in hospital care. It is the reduction in the former case-fatality rate of 0.058 (see FATAL, above) to the rate in 1986–89 of 0.0048.

SHOCK.R: 0.0078. This is the average of the rates of DHF/DSS (corrected to include only cases meeting WHO criteria) in Thailand in 1962 and Cuba in the epidemic of 1981. Thailand's rate was 7.5 DHF/DSS per 1,000 persons, calculated from the experience at Children's Hospital (Halstead 1980b). Cuba's rate of 0.0080 is based on 20,000 DHF/DSS compared with 2,360,000 infections during the epidemic (Guzman and others 1990).

SHORTEN: 0.25. Good clinical management improves the DHF/DSS patient's rehydration, shortens the period of shock, reduces bleeding, and hastens return to normal function.

STAND.POP: 1,000,000 persons. The size of the standard population (total of all age groups). The population of one million was chosen for consistency in comparing dengue with other interventions. Any other convenient size could be chosen, but the value of COHORT would have to be modified accordingly.

TREAT: $200. The cost of treating one case of dengue hemorrhagic fever is based on $40 per hospital day (the average in Brazil) times five days (the average for Thailand) of hospital care per case of DHF/DSS.

VACCINE: $40.87. The vaccine is expected to require two doses; the first at age one and the second five years later. This schedule is expected to offer protection at least through the period of greatest risk, from infancy through youth, if not longer. Because the vaccine contains four antigens to protect against all four dengue types, it is relatively complex to produce. In the study on vaccine development for the developing world by the Institute of Medicine (1986), estimated possible dengue vaccine costs ranged from $12.00 to $48.00. We now estimate a cost per dose of $10.00 to $25.00 with a midpoint of $17.50 for the vaccine itself. In addition, administration of the first dose at age one was assumed to cost $0.50, because it could likely be given during the contact for another vaccine, such as measles. The second dose, at age six, was assumed to require a separate contact. Because this might be done on a mass basis in schools, however, the delivery cost could be modest. We estimate a cost for this contact of $2.50, which is consistent with the per contact costs found in cost studies of the Expanded Programme on Immunization if all doses are considered (Shepard and others 1986). The combined two-dose cost is:

$$(17.50 + 0.50) \cdot (1.03)^5 + (17.50 + 2.50) = 40.87.$$

VACC.EF: 0.95. The Bureau of Biologics standard for immunogenicity (and efficacy) of live-attenuated viral vaccines in the United States is 95 percent. Tetravalent dengue vaccine would not be released until it is at least that effective.

VCTRC.EF: 0.30. Areas with vigorous efforts at vector control appear to have avoided outbreaks of dengue fever, whereas such outbreaks appear to have occurred in areas that lacked such programs. For example, Venezuela suffered a DHF/DSS epidemic in 1989–90 after apparently lax control programs. The Brazilian state of São Paulo, which has had a well-organized dengue control program, including clean-up campaigns, has had minimal dengue cases. Puerto Rico's ongoing spraying programs have helped to prevent large epidemics, although dengue still continues on the island.

VCTRE.EF: 0.95. The efficacy is based on the success of the control program in Singapore, which combined environmental control (elimination of breeding sites), education, localized chemical fogging, a law prohibiting conditions for disease-bearing insects, and slum clearance. Prior to the establishment of a vector control unit, dengue epidemics occurred annually. In 1966, for example, 630 cases were reported and 24 persons died of DHF. In a small epidemic a decade later (1978), only 2 deaths were reported. If the cycle of five-year epidemics had continued, another epidemic would have occurred in 1983, but none happened (Chan 1985). Thus the control program reduced both the severity and frequency of dengue epidemics. Puerto Rico controlled dengue to low levels in 1973 when large numbers of workers were hired to clean up neighborhoods under the War on Poverty's Comprehensive Employment and Training Act.

VECTORC: $0.46. This per capita cost is the average of per capita costs of dengue control in 1988 in Brazil ($0.25) and Puerto Rico ($0.67) based on original field studies. Although environmental control was used occasionally in these two areas, both relied primarily on chemical control during this year, especially spraying of streets and placement of abate or temefos in places where water collects.

VECTORE: $2.25. In the Singapore program, described above (Chan 1985), the cost was approximately $3.00 per capita. Environmental vector control not only reduces the risk of dengue but also reduces the population of *Culex* mosquitoes, whose bite is itchy and annoying. Because the dengue-carrying *Aedes aegypti* mosquitoes are smaller, their bite is less noticeable. Thus, the cost of effective vector control needs to be allocated between dengue and control of nuisance mosquitoes. To perform this calculation, we obtained figures from New Orleans, Louisiana, a city known to spend public funds on control of nuisance mosquitoes.

The expenditure ($1 million) and denominator (500,000 persons) in New Orleans give a per capita expenditure of $2.00 We interpret this amount as a revealed preference of willingness to pay for control of nuisance mosquitoes. In trying to extrapolate this result to Singapore, we assumed that this expenditure would be slightly income elastic, as is health expenditure generally. Assuming an income elasticity of 0.3 and using the fact that Singapore's per capita income ($7,500) is half that of New Orleans, we estimate that the per capita willingness to pay for control of nuisance mosquitoes would be $0.75, or one-quarter of the total per capita spending on environmental vector control. Subtracting this amount leaves a per capita expenditure of $2.25 allocated to dengue control.

YEAR.D: 25.5 years. In Southeast Asia, where there are good data on the age distribution of dengue deaths (Halstead 1969), the average age at death was about six years, and we have used this age for all areas at risk of dengue. We calibrated a model life table to the areas at risk of dengue. The calibration was based on the model West life table, which best fit the weighted average life expectancy for areas at risk of dengue. The West table best describes an "average" mortality pattern, and it is recommended when "no reliable information on the age pattern of mortality is available" (Newell 1988, p. 138). The weighted average (based on countries with a population of one million or more at risk of dengue), was 66.3 years (World Bank 1990). This average was best fit by the Level 20 model table, which yields a life expectancy of 65.6 years. We estimated remaining discounted life expectancy at age 6 years, using a discount rate of 3 percent. This estimation used 5-year age intervals beyond age 10, with a maximum at age 102.5 years.

Notes

The authors are indebted to Dr. Francisco Ramos for leading the case studies of Brazil and Puerto Rico, to Dr. Duane Gubler and Dean Jamison for valuable comments and suggestions, to Dr. Antonio Carlos Rodopiano de Oliveira, former director of the Superintendencia de Campanhas de Saúde Pública (SUCAM) in Brazil for assistance in the Brazilian case study, to Dr. Carl Kendall for facilitating financial arrangements, and to Arayan Trangarn for data about Thailand. This work was supported in part by the Rockefeller Foundation through the Harvard Institute for International Development and Johns Hopkins University.

References

Chan, K. L. 1985. *Singapore's Dengue Haemorrhagic Fever Control Programme: A Case Study on the Successful Control of* Aedes aegypti *and* Aedes albopictus *Using Mainly Environmental Measures as a Part of Integrated Vector Control.* Tokyo: Southeast Asian Medical Information Center.

De Cock, K. M., T. P. Monath, A. Nisidi, P. M. Tukei, J. Enriquez, P. Lichfield, R. B. Craven, A. Fabujé, B. C. Okafor, C. Ravaonjanahary, A. Sorungbe. 1988. "Epidemic Yellow Fever in Eastern Nigeria, 1986." *Lancet* 2:630–33.

Grant, J. P. 1990. *The State of the World's Children, 1990.* New York: Oxford University Press.

————. 1992. *The State of the World's Children, 1992.* New York: Oxford University Press.

Guzman, M. G., G. P. Kouri, J. Bravo, M. Soler, S. Vazquez, and L. Mosier. 1990. "Dengue Hemorrhagic Fever in Cuba, 1981: A Retrospective Seroepidemiologic Study." *American Journal of Tropical Medicine and Hygiene* 42:179–84.

Halstead, S. B. 1980a. "Dengue Haemorrhagic Fever—A Public Health Problem and a Field for Research." *Bulletin of the World Health Organization* 58:1–21.

————. 1980b. "Immunological Parameters of Togavirus Disease Syndromes." In R. W. Schlesinger, ed., *The Togaviruses.* New York: Academic Press.

————. 1984. "Selective Primary Health Care: Strategies for Control of Disease in the Developing World. 11. Dengue." *Reviews of Infectious Diseases* 6:251–64.

————. 1987. "Arboviruses of the Pacific and Southeast Asia." In R. Feigin and J. Cherry, eds., *Textbook of Pediatric Infectious Diseases,* 2d ed. Philadelphia: W. B. Saunders.

Halstead, S. B., J. E. Scanlon, P. Umpaivit, and S. Udomsakdi. 1969. "Dengue and Chikungunya Virus Infection in Man in Thailand, 1962–1964. 4. Epidemiologic Studies in the Bangkok Metropolitan Area." *American Journal of Tropical Medicine and Hygiene* 18:997–1021.

Institute of Medicine. 1986. *New Vaccine Development.* Vol. II, *Establishing Priorities, Diseases of Importance in Developing Countries.* Washington, D.C.: National Academy Press.

Kouri, G. P., M. G. Guzman, and J. R. Bravo. 1987. "Why Dengue Haemorrhagic Fever in Cuba? An Integral Analysis." *Transactions of the Royal Society of Tropical Medicine and Hygiene* 81:821–23.

Kouri, G. P., M. G. Guzman, J. R. Bravo, and C. Triana. 1989. "Dengue Haemorrhagic Fever/Dengue Shock Syndrome: Lessons from the Cuban Epidemic, 1981." *Bulletin of the World Health Organization* 67:375–80.

Matsuraspas, W. 1981. "The Results of Evaluations of DHF Prevention and Control Programs, 1977–1980" (in Thai). *Journal of Communicable Diseases* 7:327–47.

Nasidi, A., T. P. Monath, K. M. De Cock, O. Tomori, R. Cordellier, O. D. Olaleye, T. O. Harry, J. A. Adeniyi, A. O. Sorungbe, A. O. Ajose-Clocker, G. Van Derlan, and A. B. O. Oyediran. 1989. "Urban Yellow Fever Epidemic in Western Nigeria, 1987." *Transactions of the Royal Society of Tropical Medicine and Hygiene* 83:401–6.

Newell, C. 1988. *Methods and Models in Demography.* New York: Guilford.

Osani, C. H., P. A. Travassos, A. T. Tang, R. S. do Amaral, A. D. Passus, P. L. Tanil. 1983. "Surto de Dengue em Boa Vista, Roraima Nota Previa." *Revista Instituto Medicine Tropical São Paulo* 25:53–54.

PAHO (Pan-American Health Organization). 1990. "Status of Dengue Outbreak in Venezuela." Caracas.

Schatzmayr, H. G., R. M. Rogueira, and A. P. Travassos da Rosa. 1986. "An Outbreak of Dengue Virus at Rio de Janeiro." *Memorias do Instituto Oswaldo Cruz* 81:245–46.

Secretária de Estado de Saúde e Higiene. 1986. "Informe Epidemiólogico sobre Dengue" 1:1–7. Unpublished report, Brazilian Ministry of Public Health.

Shepard, D. S., L. Sanoh, and E. Coffi. 1986. "Cost-Effectiveness of the Expanded Programme on Immunization in the Ivory Coast: A Preliminary Assessment." *Social Science and Medicine* 22:369–77.

Soper, F. L., D. B. Wilson, S. Lima, and W. Sa Antunes. 1943. *The Organization of Permanent Nation-Wide Anti-*Aedes aegypti *Measures in Brazil.* New York: Rockefeller Foundation.

Von Allmen, S. D., R. H. Lopez-Correa, J. P. Woodall, D. M. Morens, J. Chikiboga, and A. Casta-Velez. 1979. "Epidemic Dengue Fever in Puerto Rico, 1977: A Cost Analysis." *American Journal of Tropical Medicine and Hygiene* 28:1040–44.

World Bank. 1990. *World Development Report, 1990.* New York: Oxford University Press.

15

Hepatitis B

Mark Kane, John Clements, and Dale Hu

Hepatitis B, one of the main diseases of mankind, is now preventable with safe and effective vaccines—the first vaccines against cancer. More than 2 billion individuals alive today have been infected at some time in their lives with the hepatitis B virus (HBV), and approximately 350 million are chronically infected carriers of this virus. These carriers are at high risk of serious illness and death from cirrhosis of the liver and primary liver cancer, diseases that kill more than 1 million carriers per year (Maynard, Kane, and Hadler 1989). Primary liver cancer caused by HBV infection is one of the top three causes of cancer death in much of Africa, Asia, and the Pacific Basin (Parkin 1986). In addition, these carriers constitute a reservoir of infected individuals who perpetuate the infection from generation to generation.

Most people in Africa, eastern Asia, Southeast Asia, the Pacific Basin, the Amazon Basin, and parts of the Middle East become infected with this virus during childhood, either from an infected mother (perinatal transmission) or from another child. Infection during childhood is especially likely to lead to the chronic carrier state. In Europe, North America, much of Latin America, and Australia, hepatitis B infection is an important sexually transmitted disease and a significant cause of morbidity for health care personnel and certain other groups defined by lifestyle and occupation (CDC 1990).

Hepatitis B (HB) vaccines, if given prior to infection, can prevent disease and the carrier state from developing in almost all individuals. These vaccines have been used in more than 100 million persons and have proven to be among the safest, most immunogenic, and most effective vaccines yet developed. The vaccines are most effectively used as a routine part of the infant immunization schedule, although they can be used at any age.

Recent dramatic decreases in vaccine cost in developing countries (from $20 to $1–$2 per pediatric dose) have allowed public health officials to consider the mass use of these vaccines in infant immunization programs (Kane, Ghendon, and Lambert 1990), but it is still considerably more expensive than the other routine childhood vaccines. Although these vaccines have been widely used by health care workers in industrial countries and as a routine infant immunogen in countries with relatively more resources but in which the disease is endemic, international agencies and donors have not made the vaccines available to developing countries who are dependent on donors for the vaccines. An analysis of the reasons for this may shed light on the future of immunization as a viable public health strategy.

History and Epidemiology of HBV Infection

Hepatitis B virus infection leads to one of three outcomes in humans. An infected individual may die of fulminant hepatitis within days or weeks of clinical onset of disease, may recover after symptomatic or asymptomatic acute infection and develop lifelong immunity, or may become a chronic carrier, harboring a persistent infection which usually lasts for life. The age of infection is the primary factor in determining the outcome of HBV infection.

Approximately 25 percent of chronic carriers will die from cirrhosis or primary hepatocellular carcinoma (PHC), also called primary liver cancer (Beasley and Hwang 1984). Cirrhosis is usually preceded by chronic active hepatitis, which can cause years of morbidity and significant work loss. Death from cirrhosis and PHC usually occurs during the third to sixth decade of life, during the peak years of adult productivity.

Geographical Distribution

Hepatitis researchers have divided the world into areas of "high," "intermediate," and "low" HBV endemicity, basing this division on the prevalence of HBV markers and on the primary modes of HBV transmission. Areas of high endemicity include those in which most of the population becomes infected with the virus, usually during the perinatal period or during childhood. Various authors have used figures of 5 percent to 10 percent to define the lower limit of the prevalence of HBV carriers for this category. The upper limit of the prevalence of the carrier state is about 20 percent. Most countries included in this category have a carrier prevalence of 10 to 15 percent, and 50 to 95 percent of the population have serologic evidence of prior HBV infection. Africa, Asia east of the Indian Subcontinent, the Pacific Basin, the Amazon Basin, the Arctic Rim, the Asian Republics of the Commonwealth of Independent

States (CIS), and portions of the Middle East, Asia Minor, and the Caribbean are areas of high endemicity. Parts of eastern Europe such as Bulgaria, Romania, Albania, and Moldova have a carrier prevalence of between 5 and 10 percent in the general population.

Areas of intermediate endemicity generally have an HBV carrier prevalence of 2 to 5 percent, and 30 to 50 percent of the population have serological evidence of prior HBV infection. Some parts of southern and eastern Europe, the Middle East, western Asia through the Indian Subcontinent, and parts of Central and South America are included in this category. In these areas both child-to-child and adult-to-adult transmission occur. Acute viral hepatitis with jaundice is a primary cause of morbidity because a substantial proportion of infection occurs in older adolescents and adults, who are much more likely to present with acute clinical disease.

North America, western Europe, Australia, and parts of South America are considered to be areas of low endemicity. In these areas perinatal and child-to-child transmission is relatively uncommon, and most infections occur in adults through sexual activity, needle sharing during drug abuse, or during occupational exposure to blood. Acute hepatitis B is a significant cause of morbidity in many countries in this category.

Modes of Transmission and Outcome of HBV Infections

Understanding the outcome of HBV infection in children and adults is critical to designing effective control strategies. Young children rarely develop symptomatic HBV infection with jaundice, but about 25 percent of children infected before the age of seven will become carriers. The younger the child, the more likely it is that this will occur. Many carriers who acquire infection during childhood will live long enough to develop PHC after a latency period of thirty to sixty years. After the age of seven, children exhibit an adult pattern of disease outcome, with about 5 to 10 percent becoming carriers. Even if the duration of protection from HB vaccines were only seven years, children immunized early in life would be protected during the most critical period of HBV infection, and significant reductions in HBV transmission, cirrhosis, and PHC would occur.

Perinatal transmission is one of the most efficient and serious modes of HBV transmission (Stevens and others 1985). Perinatal transmission occurs from mothers who are positive for both the hepatitis B surface antigen (HBsAg) and the hepatitis B "e" antigen (HBeAg). More than 90 percent of these women are chronic HBV carriers, although women acutely infected with the virus during pregnancy may also transmit to their children. Mothers who are HBeAg-positive carriers have a 70 to 90 percent chance of infecting their newborns perinatally, and almost all these infected newborns become HBV carriers. Infected newborns rarely develop acute hepatitis, although there have been several reports of fatal fulminant hepatitis. These carriers form a pool of infectious individuals who will infect others in the community and eventually their own offspring. Infants of mothers who are HBeAg-negative carriers rarely become carriers through perinatal transmission.

Transmission from child to child, often called horizontal transmission, is responsible for the majority of HBV infections and carriers. Although the relative importance of the various modes of transmission from child to child have not been established, many hepatitis researchers believe that skin lesions such as impetigo, scabies, abrasions, and infected insect bites play an important role. These lesions provide a route for the virus to leave the body of infectious children and a route for it to enter the body of susceptible children with whom they have skin-to-skin contact, such as in wrestling or sharing the same bed. Other modes of transmission include reuse of unsterile needles and other medical and dental equipment, tattooing and other scarification procedures, sharing of household items such as toothbrushes, and sexual activity. Premastication of food and insect transmission have been postulated as modes of transmission but remain unproven.

The transmission of HBV to adults is the primary mode of transmission in regions of lower endemicity where large populations of susceptible adults are found. About one-third of infected adults develop clinical hepatitis B with jaundice, and 6 to 10 percent become chronic HBV carriers with a subsequent risk of chronic active hepatitis, cirrhosis, and PHC. Sexual transmission, both heterosexual and homosexual, accounts for the majority of adult transmission. In some Western countries, needle sharing by drug abusers is also important. Hepatitis B is the main infectious occupational hazard to health care workers in areas of low and intermediate endemicity. Transmission to patients by contaminated blood product and unsterilized reused medical and dental instruments also occurs. In addition, any of the modes of transmission discussed for child-to-child transmission may occur.

Hepatitis B Vaccines

Hepatitis B vaccines are alum adjuvented highly purified preparations of hepatitis B surface antigen, the glycoprotein that forms the outer coat of the hepatitis B virus. Hepatitis B surface antigen can either be purified from the plasma of HBV carriers (plasma-derived vaccines) or produced in yeast or mammalian cells by recombinant technology (recombinant vaccines). Hepatitis B vaccines are highly immunogenic, even in newborns, and can induce protective anti–hepatitis B surface antibody in 90 to 97 percent of healthy individuals, depending primarily on the age of the recipient.

Hepatitis B vaccines have been successfully used in field trials in many parts of the world where the immunogenicity of the vaccines in infants is usually measured at 95 to 99 percent. The protective efficacy of the vaccines against the development of disease or the carrier state is often 95 to 99 percent in cohorts of immunized infants.

Plasma-Derived Vaccines

In natural HBV infections, liver cells produce much more HBsAg than is needed to coat viral particles, and the excess HBsAg forms 22-nanometer spherical and long tubular particles. Plasma-derived HB vaccines are prepared by purifying HBsAg particles from the plasma of HBsAg-positive donors. These vaccines are inactivated to ensure that no infectious viral or other microorganisms are present, and then alum is added as an adjuvant. Plasma-derived vaccines, available since 1981, have an outstanding record of safety and efficacy and have been used in more than 70 million individuals.

Recombinant HB Vaccines

These vaccines are produced from HBsAg derived from yeast or mammalian cells in which replicating plasmids containing the viral HBsAg gene are inserted. The HBsAg forms spherical particles similar to the natural 22-nanometer spherical particle in both chemical composition and immunogenicity. Recombinant HBsAg for vaccines may be produced in almost unlimited amounts in brewery-like fermentation vats, so there need be no concern that lack of availability of antigen will compromise future vaccine supply. Manufacturers could produce tens of millions of doses in the next few years but will require firm commitments from vaccine purchasers before they make the capital investments to produce the more than 300 million doses necessary to provide this vaccine to the world's children.

HB Vaccines and Immunization

The single most important step in the global control of hepatitis B will be the integration of these vaccines into the Expanded Programme on Immunization (EPI). This integration was recommended by the Technical Advisory Group on Viral Hepatitis and the Global Advisory Group of EPI in 1987. In 1991 the Global Advisory Group set targets for the introduction of HB vaccine into national immunization programs (WHO/EPI 1992a, b, and c), and these targets were approved by the World Health Assembly in 1992. Targets call for all countries with a prevalence of carriers of 8 percent or greater to integrate HB vaccines into routine infant immunization programs by 1995: all other countries should have programs in place by 1997.

Integration of HB vaccines into routine infant immunization raises many practical questions which need to be addressed when the addition of a new antigen is considered. Hepatitis B vaccines have characteristics which make them ideal for the integration into EPI. They are flexible enough to integrate into immunization schedules without requiring additional patient visits, do not interfere with the immune response to currently used antigens, have an extremely low rate of unacceptable side effects, are immunogenic from birth with no interference from maternal antibody, and have shipping and storage characteristics similar to currently used antigens.

Compatibility with Other EPI Antigens

Coursaget and coworkers (1986, 1990) have shown that EPI antigens do not interfere with the immune response to HB vaccines, and conversely, that HB vaccines do not interfere with the response to BCG (bacille Calmette-Guérin), DPT (diphtheria-pertussis-tetanus), or inactivated polio, measles, and yellow fever antigens. Similar data are available from laboratory animal studies as well as from human trials in Italy, Senegal, Myanmar, and China.

Target Age

When HB vaccine is given to an infant of a carrier mother who is HBeAg positive, he or she has, in most cases, already been exposed to the virus, and the vaccine must provide postexposure prophylaxis. Plasma-derived HB vaccines alone have an efficacy of about 75 percent in preventing such infants from becoming carriers if the first dose is given soon after birth. This may be feasible if infants are delivered in hospitals or clinics, but it may be difficult to achieve at home deliveries unless they are attended by midwives specially trained to administer vaccine or unless there is very rapid reporting of births to vaccinators. A hepatitis B vaccine trial in Lombok, Indonesia, has successfully stimulated birth registration and achieved a high level of immunization of infants within one week from birth in an area where home delivery predominates. In another trial, in Long An County, China, midwives have been successfully trained to deliver the vaccine at the time of birth.

Infants of mothers who are not HBeAg-positive HBV carriers can receive the first dose of HB vaccine either near the time of birth with BCG, or with DPT-1, because many are protected by passive maternal antibody and because the risk of horizontal infection is low during the first few months of life.

Duration of Immunity

The duration of protection from HB vaccines is a crucial issue which will be understood only by carefully following long-term HB vaccine trials. Cohorts of immunized adults and older children followed for five to ten years show no evidence of clinical hepatitis B, antigenemia, the development of elevated liver enzymes, or the development of the carrier state, despite declining levels of serum antibodies. It is clear that protection against disease outlasts detectable serum antibody levels, although some individuals have developed antibodies to the hepatitis B "core" antigen (anti-HBc), indicating that subclinical infection has taken place.

It is unclear how long clinical protection against disease and the development of the carrier state will persist. Some experts believe that long-term, even lifelong protection against significant infection will occur following the immunologic "prime" provided by the initial vaccine series. Others think that loss of protection against significant disease will occur at some point and booster doses may be necessary. Further follow-up of immunized cohorts is indicated to answer to this question.

Number of Doses and Schedule

In early trials of HB vaccines and initial licensure of the product for adults, vaccine schedules were used that were not necessarily consistent with EPI schedules, and the vaccines were given at 0, 1, and 6 months or 0, 1, 2, and 12 months. For use in EPI, the vaccines should be given during existing visits to avoid the expense and trouble of additional patient contacts. Fortunately, the vaccines have proven themselves to be extremely flexible and capable of retaining their immunogenicity and efficacy in virtually any EPI schedule (Hadler and others 1989). The first dose should be given with BCG near birth, if possible, or with the first dose of DPT if there is no immunization contact at birth. The second dose should be given with the next dose of DPT, and the third dose with the third dose of DPT or at the time of the measles immunization.

Low-Dose and Intradermal Administration

Studies of healthy children and young adults in certain settings have shown good immunogenicity of doses of HB vaccines substantially lower than that for which the vaccines are licensed. Although there may be some savings in using one-half or even one-quarter the manufacturer's recommended dose, there is concern that many vaccine recipients may not get an immunologically sufficient dose under conditions which may be found in developing countries. These conditions include malnutrition, immunodeficiency, less than optimal administration, missed doses, and schedules which are not maximally immunogenic.

Some investigators have attempted intradermal administration of approximately one-tenth the recommended dose of HB vaccines in healthy adults and children; they have achieved relatively good rates of seroconversion but substantially lower geometric mean titers. Intradermal administration in infants was less successful, with lower efficacy in infants of carrier mothers and reports of difficulty in administration and pain in the recipients. Additional concerns include reliability of personnel in administering intradermal injections, and the use of extremely low doses of vaccines that may vary somewhat in potency. Intradermal administration of HB vaccines is presently not recommended by EPI and the Technical Advisory Group for Viral Hepatitis.

Immune Globulin

If hepatitis B immune globulin (HBIG) is given to newborns of HBeAg-positive mothers in addition to HB vaccines, the efficacy may be increased to 85 to 95 percent. Use of HBIG adds considerably to the cost of treatment because it is expensive ($25 to $50 per child) and because it requires serologic testing of mothers to determine their HBsAg status. Such testing is itself expensive and requires laboratories and prenatal testing programs that are generally unavailable in developing countries. For these reasons it is generally accepted that it is more cost-effective to devote resources to routine infant immunization and that most developing countries will elect to forgo the use of HBIG.

Stability and Temperature Requirements

Both plasma-derived and recombinant types of hepatitis B vaccines are adsorbed on aluminium salts. As with other such vaccine preparations, they should be protected from being frozen. At temperatures of 2 to 8 degrees centigrade, the vaccines appear to be stable for many years. Some plasma- and yeast-derived products appear to be relatively stable at higher temperatures. This raises the possibility that HB vaccines could be used in the field without a cold chain, something not previously contemplated for other EPI antigens. Such a proposal needs careful field testing before widespread implementation, but it opens up the possibility that the vaccines could be carried by those attending births in the home.

Currently, EPI recommends that the vaccines be handled in the same way as triple antigen (DPT), that is, kept between 2 and 8 degrees centigrade. A temperature-sensitive marker in the vaccine vial or on the exterior of the vial would be a helpful addition to the product. The marker would indicate if the vaccine had been frozen before use. Thus, with regard to the EPI cold chain, the vaccines are easy to integrate and need no new developments or conditions.

Storage Bulk

Vaccines that are delivered in vials which contain multiple doses are less expensive per dose and require less storage space than those which are packaged with few doses per vial. Wastage rates rise with increasing number of doses per vial, however, and this becomes an important issue while HB vaccines remain more expensive than other EPI antigens. There is concern that the cold-chain storage space in some locations will be exceeded if programs adopt HB immunization plans using vials containing few doses each. However, modeling done by EPI suggests that most cold chains could accommodate the addition of HB vaccines with little or no expenditure for additional equipment. Currently available HB vaccines vary enormously in packaging volume, and the World Health Organization (WHO) is working with manufacturers to develop efficient packaging standards. Careful calculations will need to be made to estimate space requirements before introduction of the vaccines.

Equipment

Hepatitis B vaccines are given by injection in the same manner as other EPI antigens: no special equipment is needed. The use of reusable equipment will require more episodes of sterilization and the replacement of equipment sooner. If disposable needles and syringes are used, three more per child will be needed. These items will have to be budgeted for and supplied appropriately.

Future Strategies to Increase the Efficiency of HB Immunization

Drop-out rates (parents not bringing their children for scheduled immunizations) between the second and third doses of DPT are significant, and a similar drop-out rate must be expected with HB vaccines. Any strategy that might reduce this drop-out rate would be advantageous. One possibility is the development of preparations which surround the antigen with a polymer which allows timed, slow release in pulses. This technology is, in theory, practical for HB vaccines and could mean that a single injection might be sufficient to immunize a child fully. Such research underlines the importance of developing a system which allows for the maximum number of antigens to be administered as early in life as possible.

Another way to increase the efficiency of immunization would be to use combined DPT and HB vaccines and DPT, IPV (inactivated polio vaccine), and HB vaccines; these are under development but will not be available for several years. Such vaccines would eliminate additional storage and delivery costs and would spare the recipient several additional injections. In Asia, an additional dose of univalent HB vaccine could be delivered at birth to prevent perinatal infection.

Strategies for Control

Recommended HB immunization strategies have differed in various regions of the world because of the different epidemiological patterns of HBV infection. When the vaccine became available in 1982, expert groups recommended universal infant immunization as the proper strategy for areas in which HBV infection was moderately or highly endemic, and immunization of "high-risk groups" as the recommended strategy for areas of lower endemicity.

Although high-risk individuals will undoubtedly benefit from immunization, there is now considerable doubt from both epidemiological and practical viewpoints that such high-risk-group strategies will ever lead to a significant reduction of HBV infection on a national or international scale. It is likely that universal infant immunization is the proper strategy for long-range control of HBV infection everywhere.

Hepatitis B Virus Control in Asia and the Pacific Basin

In the hyperendemic areas of Asia, about 7 to 10 percent of pregnant women are HBsAg-positive chronic carriers, and about 40 percent of these women are also HBeAg positive. Because the mothers of about 2.5 to 4 percent (40 percent of 7–10 percent) of Asians are HBeAg-positive carriers, and because about 10 to 15 percent of the population are carriers, it follows that 25 to 40 percent of carriers may have resulted from perinatal transmission. The majority of infection in the community and the development of the carrier state in the majority of carriers are the result of childhood infection which is not perinatal.

The need to treat infants of HBV-carrier mothers soon after birth poses a problem in areas in which there is no contact with immunization services until several weeks or months after birth. In such areas children born to carrier mothers who are HBeAg positive may not receive protection from the vaccines. Immunization programs in Asia will need to provide HB vaccines near birth to maximize the prevention of HBV-carrier children.

The problem of HBV infection and its relation to PHC is well understood by Asian health authorities, and HB control is high on their list of health priorities. Most countries in eastern Asia

and the Pacific Basin have begun infant immunization programs, which are presently at various stages. Countries with more health resources have embarked on national programs, whereas those with fewer resources have begun demonstration projects in selected areas with the intention of expanding them into national programs. Countries in this region which cannot afford vaccines are looking for donor support to allow them to begin immunization.

Hepatitis B Virus Control in Africa

In Sub-Saharan Africa, about 10 to 15 percent of the population are HBV carriers, and about 70 to 95 percent of the population show serological evidence of prior HBV infection. These prevalence figures are consistent in this region, and most experts do not feel that serological studies need to be done in each country before HB vaccine programs are begun. It may be necessary, however, to do such studies to convince health authorities that their country has an HBV problem of this magnitude.

The risk of a newborn infant acquiring HBV infection perinatally in Africa is much lower than that of his or her Asian counterpart (Mariner and others 1985). Although about 10 percent of women of childbearing age in Africa are HBsAg positive, only 10 to 15 percent of them are also HBeAg positive, so only about 1 to 1.5 percent of African children are born to HBeAg-positive mothers. For this reason perinatal transmission is much less common. In contrast, 70 to 90 percent of children become infected before the age of seventeen. In many countries in Sub-Saharan Africa, PHC is the first or second cause of cancer death in males.

Because perinatal transmission is uncommon, and because most African children are passively protected by maternal antibodies for about six months, the timing of the first HB vaccine injection is not critical. About 95 to 98 percent of fully immunized children would be protected whether the first dose were given at birth or at three months of age. Several studies are in progress in Africa which are designed to examine the question of optimal timing of doses.

Hepatitis B Virus Control of Intermediate Endemicity Areas

Less attention has been paid to HBV control in areas of intermediate endemicity than in areas of higher or lower prevalence. Public health officials in these areas often believe that immunization of health care workers and maternal screening with treatment of newborns of carrier mothers make up the proper strategy for control of hepatitis B. For reasons that will be discussed below, however, immunization of all newborns with HB vaccine is probably the only strategy that will provide long-term control.

Hepatitis B Virus Control in Areas of Low Endemicity

Since the availability of HB vaccines in 1981–82, strategies for HBV control have stressed the immunization of high-risk groups and the screening of pregnant women and treatment of the infants of HBV-carrier mothers. With few exceptions, the effect of this strategy has been the immunization of health care workers—about 85 percent of HB vaccines sold in the United States and Europe has been used in this group. Although it is certainly desirable to immunize these workers, cases of hepatitis B in health care workers represent fewer than 5 percent of reported cases in the United States, and it is unlikely that immunization of one small group will control HBV infection in the community (Alter and others 1990).

Intravenous drug abusers, those who acquire HBV infection through homosexual or heterosexual activity, and those who belong to ethnic minorities in which HBV infection has a higher-than-average prevalence are difficult to reach with health care services and are often infected before they go to any health setting where immunization could be offered (Kane and others 1989). For these reasons immunization of all infants and, in some areas, of adolescents for an interim period is now national policy in the United States (CDC 1991), Italy, and New Zealand and is being viewed by many experts worldwide as the only strategy that will provide long-term control of HBV infection even in areas of low endemicity.

Treatment of Chronic Sequelae of HBV Infection

There is no effective treatment for PHC, which is essentially 100 percent fatal even with tertiary care in industrial countries. Death occurs within one to four months of presentation in developing countries, so PHC itself does not carry with it prolonged morbidity (Beasley 1988). Most patients who die of PHC, however, have underlying cirrhosis, and many patients have had years of morbidity from their chronic liver disease. In industrial countries, PHC patients are often treated with chemotherapy, hepatic artery embolization, or surgery. Although these measures can prolong life for several months at great expense, the cure rate is extremely low.

Alpha-fetoprotein is a host protein produced early and in high quantities by PHC tumor cells. It is detectable with sensitive assays, and trials are in progress to assess its usefulness as a screening test for early detection of PHC at a stage when the tumor may be resectable. Trials in Alaska (McMahon and others 1990) and Shanghai have met with success in screening populations with this marker and resecting patients with early tumors. Japanese gastroenterologists use yearly ultrasound examinations of the liver in cirrhotic patients in a similar attempt to find curable early PHC tumors, which they treat with either surgery or ethanol injections. Alpha-fetoprotein and routine ultrasound screening are expensive, require knowledge of who in the population are carriers, and are not practical at this time in developing countries.

There is also no practical treatment for chronic hepatitis or the carrier state in developing countries. In industrial countries, liver transplantation is sometimes attempted to prolong the life of a cirrhotic patient or one with fulminant hepatitis, but this is not a reasonable option in developing countries. Interferon treatment is being tried to alter the natural history of carriers with chronic hepatitis. Treatment may cause an early seroconversion from HBeAg to anti-HBe, which may bring about histological and biochemical improvement in chronic liver disease, but only a few patients lose their HBsAg, which defines the carrier state. It is not known whether oncogenic progression to PHC will be affected by this treatment. The treatment requires six months of thrice weekly interferon injections, is expensive ($3,000 just for the drug), causes significant side effects in most patients, and is usually ineffective if the carrier state has been present since childhood, which is the usual situation in developing countries. If a country finds it difficult to prevent the development of a carrier with vaccine for $3 per child, it will probably not be able to treat hundreds of thousands or millions of carriers for thousands of dollars each.

Cost-Effectiveness Considerations

Although there are numerous publications on the cost-effectiveness of HB immunization of health care workers and of maternal screening for HBsAg in industrial countries, there are few published studies on the cost-effectiveness of universal infant HB immunization in industrial or developing countries, and the studies which exist do not use the outcome measure of disability-adjusted life-years (DALYs). Because immunization in industrial countries is not the issue of concern in this collection, it will be mentioned but not discussed in detail.

There are no effective treatment alternatives to immunization, although in industrial countries patients with severe chronic disease or PHC may receive expensive palliative treatment or treatment designed to slow or alter progression of disease. No one would argue, from a medical, ethical, or economic point of view that we should consider not preventing this disease in favor of treating infected individuals. The effect of treatment on economic analyses is greatly to increase the cost of not vaccinating in industrial countries.

In industrial countries, with a relatively low incidence of infection and high vaccine cost, immunization of health care workers (Mulley and others 1982; Lahaye and others 1987; Koplan 1986), immunization of other high-risk groups (Adler and others 1983), screening of pregnant women, and immunization of newborns of carrier mothers (Arevalo and Washington 1988; Kane and others 1988) have been shown to be cost effective and even cost saving. The author of one study in Greece (Hatziandreu and others 1991) and the investigators of several as yet unpublished studies in the United States have examined the cost-effectiveness and cost benefit of universal HB immunization in industrial countries of low and intermediate endemicity. (Personal communications [1992] from Dr. P. Coleman, Centers for Disease Control; Dr. B. Bloom, University of Pennsylvania; Dr. R. Anderson, University of London; and Dr. G. Ginsberg, Jerusalem Ministry of Health.) Taking into consideration the high cost of treatment and medical care in these countries, those researchers who attempted to do a cost-effectiveness analysis found that the strategy of universal immunization of infants was cost effective and cost saving if the cost of vaccine for public sector programs was less than that charged in the private sector.

In 1985 the Institute of Medicine published a comprehensive report on priorities for new vaccine development in developing countries (Institute of Medicine 1985). In its analysis, the burden of disease from HBV infection ranked second to *Streptococcus pneumoniae* among all infectious diseases considered. The researchers estimated that, in 1985, 572,650 deaths per year occurred from PHC, 246,239 deaths occurred from cirrhosis, and 3,347 deaths occurred from acute and fulminant HB infection. Unfortunately, they considered the probable cost of HB vaccine to be $30.00 per dose and did not perform a sensitivity analysis on vaccine cost. Because the cost of HB vaccine is now $0.65 to $2.00 per dose in developing countries, it would be useful to recalculate their outcome measures.

For developing countries, the authors of two cost-effectiveness studies (Maynard, Kane, and Hadler 1989; Hu 1990) have constructed decision trees to model the number of carriers and deaths from liver disease that will result from doing nothing and from integrating HB vaccines into EPI programs. These studies predict a cost per carrier prevented ranging from $65.00 to $100.00 and an undiscounted cost per death prevented ranging from $260.00 to $400.00 at a vaccine cost of $1.00 to $1.40 per dose. It is assumed in the studies that the delivery cost of the vaccine will add an additional one-sixth to the current EPI costs. In one analysis the undiscounted cost per death prevented drops to $75.00 if vaccine cost drops to $0.50 per dose, a level probably achievable now in very large purchases.

An important study of the cost-effectiveness of hepatitis B immunization in the Gambia, the only African country with routine infant HB immunization, has recently been prepared (Robertson and others 1992). The authors of this study used actual costs from the Gambian EPI program, and they used the HBV prevalence and incidence rates as measured by the Gambia Hepatitis Intervention Study. At an HB vaccine cost of $1.00 per dose, the marginal costs of adding the HB vaccine to the existing Gambian EPI averaged $4.23 per fully immunized child. The delivery costs, the cost of all inputs except vaccine, averaged only $0.28 per dose for a three-dose regimen.

The analysis revealed that at a vaccine cost of $1 per dose, the cost per carrier prevented was $30 to $40, and the undiscounted cost per death averted was approximately $150 to $200. Discounting raised the cost per death averted to approximately $1,000 to $1,400. Because the carrier state develops during early childhood in the Gambia, discounting is not a significant factor in the calculation of the cost per carrier averted. These results compare favorably with the cost-effectiveness of other vaccines in the Gambia. The authors of the study note that the cost per carrier averted is higher than the cost of preventing a case of measles or pertussis but much lower than the cost of preventing a case of neonatal tetanus, polio, or diphtheria (Robertson and others 1985). The cost-effectiveness of HB immunization in the Gambia also compared favorably with data on other EPI vaccines from other countries (WHO 1982; Barnum and others 1980).

We are aware of only one attempt at a cost-benefit analysis of HB immunization in a developing country (Zhy Yi Xu and Richard Mahoney, personal communication, August 1992). These researchers, who measured the cost benefit of routine HB immunization in China, found an extremely high benefit-to-cost ratio for vaccine use at a vaccine cost of approximately $1.00 per dose. They also calculated the cost per DALY gained for universal HB immunization in China, which they found to be $17.50 to $22.40, about one-half the cost calculated by Barnum and Greenberg (chapter 21, this collection).

There is an obvious need for additional cost-effectiveness and cost-benefit studies concerning the addition of HB vaccines to routine immunization programs in other areas of the world, and there is a need for researchers to convert their outcome measures to DALYs so that results are comparable with other interventions discussed in this collection. Nevertheless, the existing published and unpublished studies, whether based on modeling or actual country data, are quite consistent in finding that at present it costs only $20 to $60 to prevent, through a routine infant immunization program, the development of a chronic carrier of hepatitis B in countries of high endemicity. This finding, plus the cost per death prevented, discounted or undiscounted, places HB immunization among the most cost-effective health interventions available. It is equally important to realize that this intervention is possible within the existing framework of national immunization programs which are effectively delivering vaccines to 80 percent of the world's children.

Hepatitis B is a disease with a burden of morbidity and mortality comparable to measles, each having the potential to cause up to 3 percent of the mortality in a population. Hepatitis B vaccine, because it can be used at birth, is more effective than measles vaccine. Deaths from chronic hepatitis, however, usually occur during the third to sixth decade of life and are heavily discounted by the DALY method. Families in developing countries, however, might "discount" (in a noneconomic sense) the loss of a four-month-old child from measles and the death of a forty-five-year-old father in a much different way, because the loss of the father could have dire social and economic consequences for the entire family.

Hepatitis B Vaccine and Future Immunization Policy

Excellent HB vaccines have been available for ten years but are still not available to children in many developing countries. There is a serious problem in our ability to integrate a developed new vaccine into the international immunization system. The problem is not technical but relates to the willingness of donors to increase their contribution to add vaccines to national immunization programs that are dependent on donor support. A discussion of this issue must consider the economics and politics of vaccine development and delivery, and the goals and realities faced by private sector companies, international and nongovernmental organizations, donors, and industrial and developing countries.

The Expanded Programme on Immunization is a network of international, regional, national, and local immunization programs that deliver vaccine to approximately 80 percent of the world's children. Some of these vaccines are produced by laboratories in the public sector in various countries, and some vaccines are purchased from manufacturers by national governments, but approximately 50 percent of vaccines for children are purchased from private manufacturers by the United Nations Children's Fund (UNICEF), which must raise money from donors to purchase this vaccine. The cost fully to immunize a child varies from country to country, but it averages about $15. Most of this cost goes for salaries, equipment, training, and delivery of the vaccine: the cost of the vaccines themselves is less than $1 per fully immunized child.

Most vaccines are produced by private manufacturers in industrial countries, who are in business to make a profit. Yet prices obtained by UNICEF are only pennies per dose. How can such prices be obtained? Because manufacturers' books are not made public, the actual costs of production are proprietary information, but these prices can reflect little more than the marginal cost of production plus the cost of the vial and packaging. Some manufacturers claim that they can only provide low cost vaccine to UNICEF because they sell the same vaccine for much more in industrial countries. Indeed, in the United States and Europe, pediatric vaccines sell for between $5 and $20 per dose. A second reason for the relatively low cost is that these are older vaccines, whose costs for research, development, and capitalization have already been recovered.

Manufacturers of hepatitis B vaccine claim that this is a relatively new vaccine and that they are still recovering the very substantial costs of research, development, and marketing and the capital costs of the new production facilities. In addition, some manufacturers pay a substantial royalty per dose to other companies who developed the clones used to make the vaccine. They claim that they cannot sell this vaccine at prices comparable to the other EPI antigens. In industrial countries HB vaccine sells for between $5.00 and $20.00 per pediatric dose. In developing countries vaccine may be obtained for between $0.65 and $2.00 per dose. It is unclear how low this price would go if tenders for tens of million to hundreds of million doses were offered.

A vicious cycle exists between potential vaccine purchasers, such as UNICEF, and the manufacturers. Even at $1.00 per dose ($3.00 per child), UNICEF claims, the vaccine cost per fully immunized child would more than double and thus it cannot afford this vaccine. The manufacturers claim that without guaranteed substantial orders, they cannot make the investments to scale up production that would allow them to offer a lower price. Pooling of orders from a number of countries and competitive bidding with large orders should lead to significantly lower prices, which in turn would allow more countries to afford HB immunization. Pooled procurement would also ensure that participating countries received vaccine that met

WHO requirements and that uniform shipping and storage conditions were met.

Ministry of Health officials in countries that can afford the vaccine are often confused by contradictory information from manufacturers, local experts, international agencies, and nongovernmental organizations. They are variously advised to purchase plasma-derived vaccine, purchase recombinant vaccine, import and repackage bulk vaccine, produce their own plasma vaccine or recombinant vaccine, and enter into regional production or procurement schemes. National committees are often set up and given the task of sorting these options out, but the committees are often unable to come up with acceptable recommendations even after years of deliberation.

In many developing countries, children do not get vaccine unless it is provided by donors. The newer vaccines, with HB vaccine as the prototype, will cost more per antigen than the six vaccines currently supplied to EPI. Donors and international immunization authorities must increase the resources devoted to the purchase of new vaccines and fund new vaccine development if the world's children are to benefit from these technologic advances.

Transfer of Technology

A number of countries have expressed interest in local production of HB vaccines. In theory, local production of plasma-derived vaccines and the use of a readily available local material, HBsAg-positive plasma, which is identified during blood donation and is otherwise discarded, could make vaccines available at an estimated cost of $0.10 to $0.40 per dose (Mahoney 1990). The technology to produce plasma-derived HB vaccine has been successfully transferred to China, which has produced up to 20 million doses per year. Several countries, including China, are exploring the possibility of transfer of technology to produce recombinant HB vaccines.

Critics of transfer of technology point out that there are few instances of successful transfer of technology of biologicals in the public sector. They also point out that current producers in industrial countries could produce large volumes of additional vaccine at a marginal cost that is less than the cost of putting into place new transfer of technology schemes. There is concern that although a few well-trained scientists and engineers could produce a vaccine, the overall infrastructure to ensure that high-quality vaccine is consistently produced may not exist. There may not be consistent availability of good water, electricity, trained technicians, and reagent kits for quality control. National control authorities with independent, high-quality testing facilities and trained personnel may also not be present.

Proponents of the idea argue that although efficient production by a few large producers may be a good strategy in an ideal global economy, HB vaccines have been available for ten years, and most developing countries still cannot afford them. Hard currency considerations make it such that countries that cannot afford foreign vaccines may be willing to spend local currency to produce vaccine. Purchase from a few large producers also does nothing to reduce long-term dependence on foreign aid to supply vaccines. There has been much consolidation among large pharmaceutical firms, and vaccine production, not a very profitable enterprise compared with the production of other pharmaceuticals, could conceivably be dropped by many producers in the future.

Additional arguments in favor of transfer of technology include the economic benefits of developing a capability for production of biologicals and recombinant biotechnology. The production could be placed in the private sector, where there may be more motivation for efficient operation. Excess vaccine could be sold in the private sector or to neighboring countries to recoup part of the cost of production.

A significant obstacle to local vaccine production is the large initial cost of purchasing the technology, the equipment, and the plant. International funding agencies and donors should consider loans or grants to cover this period if an analysis of the economic aspects shows local production to be reasonable, and if competent national regulatory authorities exist to ensure that a high-quality product is consistently produced. In some countries, the level of technology and infrastructure seem adequate to produce an affordable, high-quality vaccine.

Conclusions

Hepatitis B vaccines have proved themselves to be stable, safe, immunogenic, and effective. There are no technical or scientific impediments to their immediate use. Indeed, the dimensions of the global problem of HBV infection make it clear that their use is a matter of urgency. As with all vaccines, research and development efforts must continue to improve the vaccine and its preparations, determine the most cost-effective strategies for delivering it, and lower the costs of production. The final task before us is to develop national programs and obtain financial resources to provide this important antigen to the world's children.

References

Adler, M. W., E. M. Belsey, J. A. McCutchan, and A. Mindel. 1983. "Should Homosexuals be Vaccinated against Hepatitis B Virus? Cost and Benefit Assessment." *British Medical Journal* 286:1621–24.

Alter, M. J., S. C. Hadler, H. S. Margolis, W. J. Alexander, P. Y. Hu, F. N. Judson, A. Mares, J. K. Miller, and A. Meyer. 1990. "The Changing Epidemiology of Hepatitis B in the United States: Need for Alternative Vaccine Strategies." *JAMA* 263:1218–22.

Arevalo, J. A., and E. Washington. 1988. "Cost Effectiveness of Prenatal Screening and Immunization for Hepatitis B Virus." *JAMA* 259:365–69.

Barnum, H. N., D. Tarantola and I. F. Setiady. 1980. "Cost Effectiveness of an Immunization in Indonesia." *Bulletin of the World Health Organization* 58:499–503.

Beasley, R. P. 1988. "Hepatitis B Virus: The Major Etiology of Hepatocellular Carcinoma." *Cancer* 61:1942–56.

Beasley R. P., and L.-Y. Hwang. 1984. "Epidemiology of Hepatocellular Carcinoma." In G. N. Vyas, J. L. Dienstag, and J. H. Hoofnagle, eds., *Viral Hepatitis and Liver Disease*. Orlando, Fla.: Grune and Stratton.

CDC (Centers for Disease Control). 1990. "Protection against Viral Hepatitis: Recommendations of the Immunization Practices Advisory Committee (ACIP)." *Morbidity and Mortality Weekly Report* 39(RR-2):1–26.

———. 1991. "Hepatitis B Virus: A Comprehensive Strategy for Eliminating Transmission in the United States through Universal Childhood Vaccination: Recommendations of the Immunization Practices Advisory Committee (ACIP)." *Morbidity and Mortality Weekly Report* 40(RR-13):1–25.

Coursaget, P., B. Yvonnet, E. H. Relyveld, J. L. Barrero, I. Diop-Mar, and J. P. Chiron. 1986. "Simultaneous Administration of Diphtheria-Tetanus-Pertussis-Polio and Hepatitis B Vaccines in a Simplified Immunization Program: Immune Response to Diphtheria Toxoid, Tetanus Toxoid, Pertussis, and Hepatitis B Surface Antigen." *Infection and Immunity* 51(3):784–87.

Coursaget, P., B. Yvonnet, E. Relyveld, A. Brizard, C. Bourdil, L. Bringer, E. Jeannée, S. Guindo, I. Diop-Mar, and J. P. Chiron. 1990. "Simultaneous Injection of Hepatitis B Vaccine with BCG, Diphtheria, and Tetanus Toxoids, Pertussis and Polio Vaccines." In P. Coursagel and M. J. Tong, eds., *Progress in Hepatitis B Immunization* London/Paris: Colloque INSERM/John Libbey Eurotext Ltd. 194:319–24.

Hadler, S. C., M. A. de Monzon, D. R. Lugo, and M. Perez. 1989. "Effect of Timing of Hepatitis B Vaccine Doses on Response to Vaccine in Yucpa Indians." *Vaccine* 7:106–10.

Hatziandreu, E. J., A. Hatzakis, S. Hatziyiannis, M. A. Kane, and M. C. Weinstein. 1991. "Cost-Effectiveness of Hepatitis B Vaccination in Greece: A Country of Intermediate HBV Endemicity." *International Journal of Technology Assessment in Health Care* 7(3):256–62.

Hu, D. 1990. "Integration of Hepatitis B Vaccine into the EPI." EPI/GAG/WP.14. Working paper for the Global Advisory Group of EPI. Cairo.

Institute of Medicine. 1986. *New Vaccine Development*. Vol II, *Establishing Priorities. Diseases of Importance in Developing Countries.* Washington, D.C.: National Academy Press.

Kane, M. A., M. J. Alter, S. C. Hadler, and H. S. Margolis. 1989. "Hepatitis B Infection in the United States: Recent Trends and Future Strategies for Control." *American Journal of Medicine* 87(supplement 3A):11s–13s.

Kane, M. A., Y. Ghendon, and P. H. Lambert. 1990. "1990—Where Are We: The WHO Programme for Control of Viral Hepatitis." In F. B. Hollinger, S. M. Lemon, and H. S. Margolis, eds., *Viral Hepatitis and Liver Disease: Proceedings of the 1990 International Symposium on Viral Hepatitis and Liver Disease*. Baltimore: Williams and Wilkins.

Kane, M. A., S. C. Hadler, H. S. Margolis, and J. E. Maynard. 1988. "Routine Perinatal Screening for Hepatitis B Surface Antigen." *JAMA* 259:408–9.

Koplan, J. P. 1986. "Assessment of New Vaccines in Immunization Programs." *Israel Journal of Medical Sciences* 22:272–76.

Lahaye, D., P. Strauss, C. Baleux, and W. Vav Ganse. 1987. "Cost-Benefit Analysis of Hepatitis B Vaccination." *Lancet* 2:365–69.

McMahon, B. J., S. R. Alberts, R. B. Wainwright, L. Bulkin, and A. P. Lanier. 1990. "Hepatitis B Related Sequelae: Prospective Study in 1400 Hepatitis B Surface Antigen Positive Alaska Native Carriers." *Archives of Internal Medicine* 150:1051–54.

Mahoney, R. T. 1990. "Cost of Plasma Derived Hepatitis B Vaccine Production." *Vaccine* 8:397–401.

Mariner, E., V. Barrois, B. Larouze, W. T. London, A. Cofer, L. Diakhate, and R. S. Blumberg. 1985. "Lack of Perinatal Transmission of Hepatitis B Virus Infection in Senegal, West Africa." *Journal of Pediatrics* 106(5):843–49.

Maynard, J. E., M. A. Kane, and S. C. Hadler. 1989. "Global Control of Hepatitis B through Vaccination: Role of Hepatitis B Vaccine in the Expanded Programme on Immunization." *Reviews of Infectious Diseases* 11(Supplement 3):S574–78.

Mulley, A. G., M. D. Silverstein, and J. L. Dienstag. 1982. "Indications for Use of Hepatitis B Vaccine, Based on Cost-Effectiveness Analysis." *New England Journal of Medicine* 307(11):644–52.

Parkin, D. M., ed. 1986. *Cancer Occurrence in Developing Countries*. International Agency for Research on Cancer (IARC) Scientific Publications 75. Lyons. Distributed for IARC by Oxford University Press.

Robertson, R. L., A. J. Hall, P. E. Crivelli, U. Lowe, H. M. Inskip, and S. K. Snow. 1992. "Cost Effectiveness Analyses of the Expanded Programme on Immunization (EPI) and of the Addition of Hepatitis B Virus Vaccination to the EPI of The Gambia." *Health Policy and Planning* (June).

Robertson, R. L., S. O. Foster, H. F. Hull, and P. J. Williams. 1985. "Cost Effectiveness of Immunization in The Gambia." *Journal of Tropical Medicine and Hygiene* 88:343–51.

Stevens, C. E., P. T. Toy, M. J. Tong, P. E. Taylor, G. N. Uyas, P. V. Nair, M. Gudavalli, and S. Krugman. 1985. "Perinatal Hepatitis B Transmission in the United States: Prevention by Passive-Active Immunization." *JAMA* 253:1740–45.

WHO (World Health Organization)/EPI (Expanded Programme on Immunization). 1982. "Expanded Programme on Immunization Cost Effectiveness." *Weekly Epidemiologic Record* 67(22):170–72.

———. 1992a. *Weekly Epidemiological Record* 67(3).

———. 1992b. *Weekly Epidemiological Record* 67(4).

———. 1992c. *Weekly Epidemiological Record* 67(5).

PART THREE

The Unfinished Agenda, II
Reproductive Health and Malnutrition

16

Excess Fertility

Susan Cochrane and Frederick Sai

The health priorities addressed in the other chapters of this collection have all been conditions that cause debility or death. Among these conditions are maternal and perinatal health problems. High fertility and close child spacing are a significant determinant of poor health of mothers and infants in the first week of life, as discussed in the chapter by Walsh and others and in the recent review of the National Research Council (NRC 1989). High fertility and close spacing also have consequences beyond the first week of life, at least up to age five, and have negative consequences beyond those immediate health consequences. They have negative consequences on the health and on the economic and social well-being of the family by diluting the resources available for each child and putting pressure on parents to work harder and save less. The balancing of the costs and benefits of fertility to the woman and, to a considerable degree, to the larger household is captured by her stated fertility preferences. High fertility may also have negative consequences for society as a whole. Fertility beyond which such negative consequences occur is deemed to be excess fertility. Such excess fertility is to be considered a health priority, not only because many of the negative effects are on health, but also because the delivery of family planning to prevent excess fertility is provided primarily through the health system and thus places claims on the system beyond those purely for health considerations.

The definition of excess fertility is, however, difficult, because some level of fertility is desirable from both the individual and the societal perspective. Excess fertility may be defined in several ways. From a health perspective, births to women who are too young or too old, who are of too high a parity, or who have pregnancies too closely spaced increase their own risks of mortality and poor health and those of their offspring. Births that fall into any of these categories could be considered excess. From a societal point of view, population growth rates above 2 percent are considered by many economists to be detrimental to development. Another way of defining excess fertility would be to consider what women themselves or their husbands report as excess fertility. The level of excess fertility differs substantially among these definitions. Very crude application of the first two definitions gives an estimated excess fertility of 14 to 25 percent of all births in the countries covered. The reports from individuals of their fertility prefer-ences indicate excess fertility of 30 percent. Not only do levels differ according to the definition, but the location of excess fertility differs even more dramatically. Because of these very substantial differences we shall pay considerable attention to the issue of definition in this chapter.

Two important conclusions can be drawn from the analysis in this chapter. First, improved spacing and the deferment of birth until reproductive maturity is achieved are more important for improving child survival than are other high-fertility behaviors. Second, the societal economic benefits of reducing fertility must be weighed against the costs of doing so, and these costs depend on the motivation of women to control their fertility. Thus, the individual and societal measures of excess fertility are linked.

In the first part of this chapter, we document the current levels and trends of fertility in the various regions of the world. We shall then use these levels to determine the levels of excess fertility by different definitions from the point of view of society as a whole. In the next part, we document the levels of excess fertility from the individual's perspective, and then we document the costs of excess fertility. Given the great discrepancy between the measures of excess fertility, it is necessary to provide a link between the measures that will provide useful policy guidance. This link will be made in the section on the costs of fertility regulation. Although we give considerable attention to the measurement of excess fertility, in the rest of the chapter we follow the outline laid out for the other chapters in the collection: the costs of excess fertility are examined, strategies and costs of preventing excess fertility are estimated and case management is discussed, and finally funding and research priorities are identified.

The Significance of Excess Fertility

The significance of excess fertility needs to be established to determine its priority as a health issue.

Levels and Trends in Fertility in the Developing World

The levels and trends in fertility in the developing world vary greatly between and within regions. In table 16-1, we report regional averages of total fertility rates (TFR), the crude birth rates (CBR), and rates of natural increase (RNIs) for the main regions of the world. In 1985, fertility in the developing world, whether measured by the crude birth rate or the total fertility rate, was lowest in Latin America and the Caribbean and in Asia, where rates were almost identical. Fertility was highest in Sub-Saharan Africa, where TFRs were almost twice as great as in Asia and Latin America. The Middle East and North Africa had rates closer to those in Africa than to the those in the areas of lower fertility.

The regional averages hide substantial variation. In table 16A-1 we provide levels and trends in fertility and the rate of natural increase for selected countries of the developing world.[1] These data show that in Sub-Saharan Africa, not only are growth rates quite high, often in excess of 3 percent, but in many cases they have increased substantially since the early 1960s. The reason for this is that although death rates have fallen from very high levels, crude birth rates have fallen little until very recently. Significant fertility declines have just recently been observed in Zimbabwe, Kenya, and Botswana. For Latin America and the Caribbean the pattern is different. The rate of natural increase has fallen in almost every case from 3 percent or higher to between 2 and 2.6 percent. This has been accomplished by decreases in birth rates that were so dramatic that they exceeded the great declines in death rates documented elsewhere in this collection.[2] Asia shows a different pattern with less uniformity. China, the Republic of Korea, and Thailand have had some of the most dramatic fertility declines ever recorded, the TFR falling almost 60 percent during the period, whereas Nepal has recorded no decline. Growth rates have remained constant in Bangladesh, have risen in Nepal, and have decreased substantially in China, Malaysia, the Philippines, Korea, and Sri Lanka. Although growth rates have not declined dramatically yet, TFRs have fallen substantially in Indonesia. The Middle East and North Africa display a mixed pattern as well, but on the whole fertility rates are higher than in Asia, there has been less decline, and growth rates are high. With the exception of Turkey, fertility and growth rates are lower in North Africa than in the Middle East for the countries in this sample.

Estimating Excess Fertility

This section discusses various ways of measuring excess fertility.

AGGREGATE MEASURES OF EXCESS FERTILITY. At the societal level, excessive population growth may have a number of negative effects, in particular on economic growth and on the environment. There is substantial debate on the effects of high rates of population growth on economic growth. (See the section "The Consequences of High Fertility," below, for more detail.) Sixty-five of 131 developing countries report that they perceive that their population is growing too fast (United Nations 1988).[3] Although each country has its own perception of what rate of growth is too high, a rule of thumb that was developed in The World Bank's *The World Development Report* (1984) was that a rate of natural increase in excess of 20 per 1,000, or 2 percent, was likely to be detrimental to economic development.

Even if it is agreed that a population growth rate above 2 percent is excessive, establishing a correspondence between the rate of population growth and the level of fertility is difficult because population growth reflects both fertility and mortality.[4] An alternative method of estimation is to identify excess fertility by the level of fertility that has negative health consequences. The accepted definition is that births too early (to women under eighteen), too late (to women over thirty-four), too frequently (closer than twenty-four months apart), and too many times (more than four children) are likely to be detrimental to maternal and child health.[5] The evidence on these consequences will be discussed in detail below. In the aggregate we could say that, using the rules of thumb, fertility is excessive if the rate of natural increase exceeds 2 percent, if the mother is younger than eighteen or older than thirty-four, if the births for one mother are closer than twenty-four months, and if the births for one mother exceed four.

Although it is easy to determine the extent to which the population growth exceeds 2 percent, it is quite difficult to determine how many births represent health risks. We do not know how many births are beyond the fourth parity, but if the average TFR is four, we know a substantial number of births are of fifth parity or higher.[6] We can also get very rough estimates of the percentage of births to women who are too old or too young from looking at age-specific birth rates. Although we will make rough estimates of the proportion of births that represent health risks, precise estimates are possible only from individual level data sets, because many women and births are in more than one risk category. There are, however, only three

Table 16-1. Projected Fertility and Rate of Natural Increase

Region	1985			2000			2015		
	TFR	CBR	RNI	TFR	CBR	RNI	TFR	CBR	RNI
World	3.4	27	17	2.9	23	14	2.6	20	1
Industrial countries	1.7	13	5	1.8	12	−3	2.0	12	1
Nonmarket economies	2.3	17	7	2.1	15	4	2.1	14	3
Latin America and the Caribbean	3.6	29	20[a]	2.5	21	14	2.2	18	7
Sub-Saharan Africa	6.4[a]	46	31[a]	5.4	40	29	4.0	32	23
Middle East and North Africa	5.6[a]	40	30[a]	4.3	32	24	3.1	26	19
Asia	3.3	27	18	2.6	21	13	2.2	17	9

a. Excess.
Source: World Bank data.

countries where individual level estimates have been made. In table 16-2, we summarize these estimates. None of the countries mentioned in the table has marriages involving very young women, but some other countries would have a much higher risk factor on this dimension. For these three countries, the risk factors differ substantially because of definitions. The proportion who are at risk because of high parity reflects the level of the TFR, being highest in Kenya and lowest in the Philippines.[7] The proportion of births beyond four can be calculated for selected countries for selected years from *The United Nations Demographic Yearbook* (United Nations 1986). These data are not generally available unless a system for registering vital statistics is in place or fertility surveys have been conducted. The available survey evidence is given in table 16-2. The United Nations (UN) data from registration of vital statistics show that the percentage of births beyond four ranges from about 2 percent in Korea to 30 percent in Egypt and Pakistan. The UN data for the Philippines shows a rate of 3 percent, whereas the survey data yields 19 percent. (See NRC 1989, p. 79, for a table showing how this proportion has declined dramatically in those countries which have had large fertility declines.) Using data from the World Fertility Surveys (WFSs), Hobcraft, writing in 1987, (cited in NRC 1989) has calculated the proportion of women with two or more births in which the preceding interval was less than two years. This proportion ranged from over 50 percent in Jordan, Costa Rica, and Colombia to about 20 percent in Senegal, Lesotho, and Korea. These last three countries show two patterns. The two African countries have long breastfeeding and postpartum abstinence to prevent close spacing of children, whereas Korea has very high levels of contraceptive use.

Therefore, we can identify excess fertility as the number of births needed to reduce the rate of natural increase to 2 percent, to reduce the TFR to four, or to eliminate births at high-risk ages.[8] Using the aggregate data in table 16-1 and data on age-specific fertility for the countries in table 16A-1, we find that there would be excess fertility of 14 percent, 16 percent, and 31 percent, respectively, by each definition.[9]

Looking at the individual countries one sees a pattern that is more mixed. In table 16A-1, the countries that have excess fertility by one definition or the other are noted. All countries of Africa are noted as having excess fertility on measures of both TFR and RNI. Excess fertility ranges from a 48 percent TFR and a 105 percent RNI in Kenya to a low of about 30 percent for both in Lesotho.[10] In Latin America and the Caribbean only four of the countries have TFRs above four, but all countries except Trinidad and Tobago have a RNI of 2 percent or greater. Brazil, Colombia, Guyana, Haiti, and Jamaica, however, have rates of 2 or 2.1 percent. Thus it is the other countries that have excess fertility of a substantial amount, ranging from over 30 percent in Paraguay to 20 to 25 percent in the Dominican Republic, Ecuador, and Venezuela. In Asia, excess fertility is greatest in Nepal and Bangladesh. India has marginal excess fertility. Malaysia and the Philippines have TFRs below four but have a RNI in excess of 2 percent. All the countries of the Middle East and North Africa in our sample except Turkey have excess fertility by both measures. The Middle East countries, however, have higher excess fertility than those in North Africa.

By using these measures for individual countries, it is possible to estimate the percentage of births in each region which fall into the excess category. These estimates are presented in table 16-3. The three measures give different estimates of the magnitude of high fertility. The TFR and the RNI indicate that about 14 to 16 percent of the births in the developing world outside China and India are excess. The data on births by age of mother indicate that about 30 percent of the births are in high-risk categories. By these measures the greatest excess fertility is in Sub-Saharan Africa, followed by the Middle East and North Africa. There is little excess in Asia and Latin America, where fertility rates have already fallen substantially, but a fifth to a quarter of births are to women under twenty or over thirty-four.

EXCESS FERTILITY AS REPORTED BY INDIVIDUALS. The usefulness of parents' stated fertility preferences has been questioned for many years and is still questioned by many. One argument is that parents tend to rationalize their actual fertility and thus are unlikely to report that they want fewer children than they already have. This may be true. Nonetheless, in survey after survey in recent years, many women have reported lower desired than actual fertility or that their last birth was unwanted.[11] Even more report that they want no more children. In addition, many who do want more children want to wait a significant period before the birth of their next child. Evidence of this kind can be used to get a first approximation of excess fertility. In table 16-4 we give the number of children desired by women according to surveys conducted in the late 1970s and early 1980s. We also report the actual TFR and the TFR that would have prevailed if preferences were realized or if all unwanted births had not occurred.[12]

Several observations emerge from the various data. Family size preferences and the proportion of families who want no

Table 16-2. Percentage of Women with Various High-Risk Factors for Another Birth
(percent)

Risk Factor	Kenya	Philippines	Zimbabwe
Too young[a]	1.4	3.6	4.4
Too old[b]	36.2	35.8	33.6
Too many births[c]	61.5	42.4	40.1
Births too soon[d]	48.3	32.3	29.6
Any risk factor	—	79.7	69.7

— Not available.

Note: World Bank estimates for TFR: Kenya, 7.7; Philippines, 3.9; Zimbabwe, 5.4.

a. Under eighteen in Kenya and Zimbabwe, under twenty in the Philippines.

b. Thirty-five and older.

c. Four or more births in Kenya and the Philippines, five or more in Zimbabwe.

d. Birth in the preceding twenty-four months in Kenya; open birth interval of less than fifteen months in the Philippines; less than fifteen months postpartum and not pregnant in Zimbabwe.

Source: Kenya and Zimbabwe, DHS reports. Philippines, Casterline 1990.

Table 16-3. Excess Fertility, Measured by National Demographic Data
(millions)

Region	Births in women under 20 and over 34		TFR > 4		RNI > 20	
	Percent	Number	Percent	Number	Percent	Number
Latin America	20	2,473,000	1	86	11	1,034,000
Sub-Saharan Africa	34	3,337,000	42	4,474,000	41	4,329,000
Middle East and North Africa	39	3,421,000	22	2,663,000	25	2,938,000
Asia[a]	26	3,686,000	9	1,409,000	7	1,138,000
Total[a]	31	12,917,000	14	8,632,000	16	9,439,000
Excess births[a] (millions)	12.9	12,900,000	8.6	8,600,000	9.4	9,400,000
Total births for countries covered (millions)	42	42,300,000	59.0	59,000,000	59.0	59,000,000

a. Excluding China and India. In 1985–90, there were 113 million births in the developing world on average annually and 65 million outside India and China.
Source: Authors' calculations from World Bank data.

more children vary greatly from place to place. In Sub-Saharan Africa fewer women say they want no more children, and the desired TFR (6.7 or 6.4) in table 16-4 is very close to the actual TFR (6.9). Even so, there are differences among countries, particularly among younger women. Ghana and Lesotho report substantially lower desired fertility among the youngest women. In Latin America, actual (4.7) and desired (3.7 or 3.8) family sizes are much lower than in Africa, but excess fertility is greater. In Asia, desired (3.7 or 3.3) and actual (4.7) TFRs are very close to those in Latin America and the Caribbean. The Middle East and North Africa have the most varied pattern among countries, actual and desired fertility being very low in Turkey and very high in the Republic of Yemen. On average the TFR is 6.2 for this region, and desired fertility ranges between 5.6 and 4.7. Therefore, using the conservative desired fertility measures cited above, we find that in a perfect contraceptive world, fertility could be lowered by at least one child per woman in Latin America and Asia, by between 0.2 and 0.5 children in Sub-Saharan Africa, and by between 0.6 and 1.5 in the Middle East and North Africa.

In table 16-5 we report the proportion of women who want no more children according to World Fertility Surveys (funded by UNEP and USAID) and more recent Demographic and Health Surveys (DHS funded by USAID). We also give the proportion who wish to postpone their next birth among those who do want more children. In every case in which there are data from two points in time, the proportion who want no more children has increased over the period. Kenya, where the proportion wanting no more children increased from sixteen to forty-nine, is the most dramatic example.

In table 16-6 we sum the individual measure of excess fertility by region. This estimate is obtained by taking the percentage difference between the actual TFR and the desired number of children and adding any births reported as unwanted and weighting it by the number of births in that country in a recent year. For the countries covered, 30 percent of the births are considered excess by the individual women themselves. This proportion exceeds 30 percent in every re-

gion except Sub-Saharan Africa. Overall, in the countries covered there were 11.6 million excess births in the average year in the late 1980s: 5 million in Asia outside China and India, 4 million in the Middle East and North Africa, and 2 million in Latin America. If these countries were representative of the entire developing world except China, which is a special case, there were 27 million excess births a year by the individual women's definition.[13]

The figures above, however, probably underestimate excess fertility for several reasons: first, as mentioned earlier, women are somewhat reluctant to report desired fertility below actual; second, fertility preferences are declining in many cases faster than actual fertility, as indicated by the fact that the proportion of women wanting no more children is increasing;[14] third, many women wish to space their births;[15] and fourth, to the extent that fertility preferences themselves reflect the cost of contraception these preferences would be reduced by increased access.

Another way of estimating excess fertility is to measure what fertility would be if contraception were perfect in all women who wish to stop childbearing or postpone their next birth. This is a much more difficult measure to obtain because of the rarer data on spacing and the need to run population projections with different usage levels.

A possible way of analyzing the extent of unwanted fertility is through model populations. In figure 16-1 we plot the relationship between the mortality level and the proportion of women who want no more children. Forty percent of the women in the countries with a crude death rate of ten or below want no more children, with the exception of Paraguay, where only a third want no more. The pattern is less uniform for the high-mortality countries. Twenty percent or less of the women in all the Sub-Saharan countries want no more children.[16] This also applies to Yemen, where 19 percent want no more. In most non-African high-mortality countries 30 to 40 percent of the women want no more children. Thus three model country types would be needed: high-mortality African countries and probably also high-mortality Middle Eastern countries, high-

Table 16-4. *Preferred Family Size and Total Fertility Rates in Relation to Desired Family Size*

Country	Preferred family size			Total fertility rate		
	Women 15–19	Women 45–49	All women	Usual TFR (no birth deleted)	Desired family size exceeded and birth deleted	Desired family size exceeded or last birth unwanted and birth deleted
Africa						
Benin	7.2	8.0	7.6	7.3	7.3	6.9
Cameroon	6.5	8.6	8.0	6.4	6.1	6.1
Côte d'Ivoire	7.5	9.6	8.4	7.2	7.2	7.0
Ghana	5.2	7.3	6.0	6.1	6.0	5.6
Kenya	6.6	8.7	7.2	7.9	7.6	6.9
Lesotho	5.6	7.3	6.0	6.0	5.6	5.3
Mauritania	8.3	9.4	8.8	7.5	7.1	6.8
Senegal	8.3	8.4	8.3	7.1	6.9	6.7
Sudan (North)	5.4	6.5	6.4	5.6	5.0	4.8
Latin America and the Caribbean						
Colombia	2.7	5.7	4.0	4.6	3.4	2.6
Costa Rica	3.5	6.1	4.7	3.5	3.0	2.6
Dominican Republic	3.4	6.0	4.7	5.2	3.8	3.0
Ecuador	3.1	5.6	4.1	5.2	4.1	3.1
Guyana	3.4	5.9	4.6	4.4	3.8	2.8
Haiti	2.8	4.3	3.6	5.6	4.3	2.8
Jamaica	3.3	4.8	4.1	4.4	3.4	2.3
Mexico	3.8	5.8	4.4	5.7	4.5	3.6
Panama	3.4	5.1	4.3	4.2	3.9	3.4
Paraguay	3.7	7.1	5.2	5.0	4.5	4.2
Peru	3.1	4.6	3.8	5.3	3.5	2.6
Trinidad and Tobago	3.2	4.8	3.8	3.2	2.5	2.4
Asia						
Bangladesh	3.7	5.0	4.1	5.4	4.6	3.1
Indonesia	3.3	5.4	4.2	4.3	4.0	3.6
Korea, Republic of	2.7	3.8	3.1	3.9	2.8	2.5
Malaysia	3.9	4.5	4.3	4.5	3.3	3.1
Nepal	3.6	4.3	3.9	6.1	5.4	4.5
Philippines	3.0	5.6	4.3	5.1	4.1	3.6
Sri Lanka	2.6	4.8	3.7	3.4	2.9	2.2
Thailand	2.9	4.4	3.6	4.3	3.2	2.6
Middle East and North Africa						
Egypt	4.2	4.7	4.1	5.0	3.6	3.1
Jordan	4.9	7.5	6.2	7.0	6.0	5.1
Morocco	4.3	6.6	4.9	5.5	4.4	3.7
Pakistan	4.0	4.5	4.2	6.0	4.3	3.9
Syria	5.0	7.1	6.1	7.4	6.3	5.6
Tunisia	3.7	4.4	4.1	5.5	4.1	3.6
Turkey	2.8	3.1	3.0	3.8	cc	2.4
Yemen, Rep. of	4.5	6.9	5.5	8.9	8.2	7.4

Note: Preferred Family size based on direct question; TFR based on synthetic cohort estimates of desired stopping points.
Source: Lightbourne 1987.

mortality Asian and Latin American countries, and low-mortality countries. Three artificial countries have been created to represent these types of countries; high-mortality Sub-Saharan countries, Libana; high-mortality Latin American or Asian countries, Banglapal; and low-mortality countries of Asia and Latin America, Colexico.

The excess fertility in these three model countries of a million population is given in table 16-7. The assumptions underlying these models are fairly straightforward. Three population types were developed of 1 million population each in 1990. They all had age structures, age-specific fertility and mortality rates, and patterns of marriage, breastfeeding, and contraceptive use specific to real countries of a general type. The number of births per year with current contraceptive use was projected for 1990 and 2000 as a base case. Then two alternative projections were made. In the first, all women who

Table 16-5. Currently Married Women Who Want No More Children or Who Wish to Postpone Children
(percent)

Country	Want no more		Wish to postpone[a]		DHS Year
	WFS	DHS	WFS/CPS	DHS	
Africa					
Benin	8	—	55	—	1982
Botswana	—	33	—	55	1988
Burundi	—	24	—	76	1987
Cameroon	8	—	—	—	1978
Côte d'Ivoire	4	—	38	—	1980
Ghana	12	23	—	70	1978/1988[b]
Kenya	16	49	—	68	1978/1989[b]
Lesotho	14	—	—	—	1977
Liberia	—	17	—	48	1986
Mali	—	17	—	50	1987
Mauritania	11	—	—	—	1981
Morocco	42	48	—	53	1987
Nigeria (Ondo State)	—	23	—	58	1986
Senegal	6	19	—	—	1986
Sudan	15	—	—	—	1978
Togo	—	25	—	71	1988
Tunisia	48	57	—	64	1978/1989[b]
Zimbabwe	—	33	—	61	1988
Latin America and the Caribbean					
Bolivia	—	72	—	48	1989
Brazil[c]	—	60	—	64	1986
Colombia	61	69	—	64	1976/1986[b]
Costa Rica	52	—	77	—	1976
Dominican Republic	52	63	—	51	1975/1986[b]
Ecuador	55	65	—	65	1979/1987[b]
El Salvador	—	63	—	68	1985
Guatemala	—	47	—	68	1987
Guyana	54	—	—	—	—
Haiti	42	—	—	—	—
Jamaica	48	—	—	—	—
Mexico	56	65	—	33[d]	1976/1987[b]
Panama	63	—	—	—	—
Paraguay	32	—	68	—	1979
Peru	61	70	—	60	
Trinidad and Tobago	46	55	—	55	1977/1987[b]
Venezuela	55	—	—	—	—
Asia					
Bangladesh	30	—	72	—	1976
Indonesia	40	51	—	73	1976/1987[b]
Korea, Republic of	74	—	36	—	1974
Malaysia	46	—	36	—	1974
Nepal	30	—	—	—	1976
Philippines	54	—	—	—	1978
Sri Lanka	62	65	—	60	1987
Thailand	61	66	—	61	1987
Middle East and North Africa					
Egypt	54	61	—	51	1988
Jordan	42	—	—	—	1976
Pakistan	43	—	—	—	1975
Syrian Arab Rep.	38	7.1	6.1	7.4	1978
Yemen, Rep. of	19	6.9	5.5	8.9	1979

— Not available.

a. Percentage of women who wish to postpone children for two or more years among those who want more children.

b. WFS/DHS.

c. Does not include currently pregnant women. Those who wish to postpone is defined as the percentage of women who prefer to wait one or more years among those who want more children.

d. Does not include currently pregnant women.

Source: WFS/DHS Surveys.

Table 16-6. Total Excess Fertility, Measured from Individual Responses

Region	Excess over desired fertility (number)	Excess of TFS (percent)
Latin America and the Caribbean	2,015,000	37
Sub-Saharan Africa	467,000	9
Middle East and North Africa	4,088,000	35
Asia[a]	5,062,000	31
Total excess births	11,632,000	30
Total excess births among births covered	38,971,000	n.a.

n.a. Not applicable.
a. Excluding India and China.
Source: Author.

claimed that they wanted no more children were assumed to be using perfect contraception.[17] The second alternative assumed that, in addition to those who wish to limit fertility, one-half of those women who wish to space their next birth are using perfect contraception.[18] It is surprising that by this measure high-mortality African countries have somewhat higher excess fertility than the high-mortality non-African countries. The reason for this is that current contraceptive use in Libana is much lower than in Banglapal. If spacing demand for contraception is included, Libana and Colexico have almost 40 percent excess fertility and Banglapal 26 percent. The relative importance of unmet need for contraception for spacing and for limiting, however, shows that

Figure 16-1. Relationship between Life Expectancy and Proportion of Women Wanting No More Children

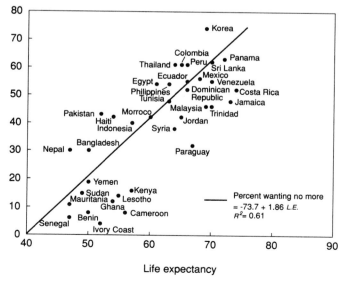

Percentage wanting no more children

Life expectancy

Percent wanting no more
= -73.7 + 1.86 *L.E.*
R^2 = 0.61

Source: Authors' calculations.

limiting is less important than spacing in the high-mortality countries.

ABORTION AS AN INDICATION OF EXCESS FERTILITY. The most extreme statement that a woman can make about excess fertility is to seek an abortion. It was because of the high incidence of complications from illegal abortion that the family planning movement began in the United States and many countries of Latin America. Because the data are of such poor quality, measures of the extent to which actual births exceed desired births cannot be derived from estimating the magnitude of abortion. The data are sufficient to give an indication of the extent to which current programs delivering contraception have been insufficient for controlling fertility to levels desired by women. (This issue is also treated under the section on case management.) The worldwide estimate of the number of abortions is between 40 million and 60 million (Henshaw 1987). It is estimated that at least 14 million occur in China and 11 million in the countries of the former U.S.S.R. Other industrial countries contributed about 4.5 million abortions. Estimates of abortion in developing countries are much less precise because abortions are more likely to be illegal there than in industrial countries. In developing countries, abortion appears to be highest in Latin America and Asia and lowest in Sub-Saharan Africa, where, as indicated above, desired family sizes are much greater. There is evidence that there are substantial differences in the incidence of abortion in the countries of Africa and that such incidence is increasing.

The Consequences of High Fertility

The consequences of high fertility are many, ranging from health consequences for mother and child to consequences for economic development.

HEALTH CONSEQUENCES OF HIGH FERTILITY. The health consequences of high fertility for mother and newborns are discussed in another chapter of this collection. In this chapter, we will discuss the health consequences beyond the first week of life. There is little debate in the literature that mortality of neonatal and postneonatal infants, and of children is positively correlated with women giving birth at too young an age, too old an age, too closely together or too many times. There is substantial debate about whether increased contraception will improve survival rates (Trussell and Pebley 1984; Bongaarts, Mauldin, and Phillips 1987, 1988; Potter 1988; Trussell 1988).[19] In this section, we will first examine the evidence of an association between high fertility and infant and child mortality. We will then discuss upper and lower limits on the costs of the deaths that may be averted by reduced fertility.

The hypothesized effects of high fertility on the survival of offspring arise from both biological and socioeconomic and behavioral factors. The biological factors arise most noticeably in the period immediately after birth and are assumed to explain why both very early and very late childbearing are detrimental to children as well as why close spacing may be problematic. High parity and close spacing are also believed to

Table 16-7. *Excess Fertility for Three Model Countries*

	1990		2000	
Scenario	Births	Excess (percent)	Births	Excess (percent)
Libana—High-mortality African or Middle Eastern country				
1. Current conception prevalence rate (CPR)	54,010	n.a.	74,810	n.a.
2. All who want no more children (using contraception)	46,470	n.a.	64,090	n.a.
3. Line 2 plus half of spacers	33,975	n.a.	46,655	n.a.
4. Excess: lines 1–2	7,540	14	10,720	14
5. Excess: lines 1–3	20,035	38	28,155	38
Banglapal—High-mortality Latin American or Asian country				
1. Current contraception prevalence rate (CPR)	46,540	n.a.	62,400	n.a.
2. All who want no more children (using contraception)	42,900	n.a.	57,450	n.a.
3. Line 2 plus half of spacers	34,635	n.a.	46,260	n.a.
4. Excess: lines 1–2	3,640	8	4,950	14
5. Excess: lines 1–3	11,905	26	16,140	26
Colexico—Low-mortality Asian or Latin American country				
1. Current contraception prevalence rate (CPR)	33,565	n.a.	43,031	n.a.
2. All who want no more children (using contraception)	26,397	n.a.	33,766	n.a.
3. Line 2 plus half of spacers	20,740	n.a.	26,434	n.a.
4. Excess: lines 1–2	7,168	21	9,265	22
5. Excess: lines 1–3	12,825	38	16,597	39

n.a. Not applicable.
Note: Calculated using target models with constant levels of proximate determinants of fertility, except contraceptive use. Current contraceptive prevalence was estimate to calculate number of births. The effectiveness was the level currently observed with the existing method mix. Assumes that all women who want no more children and half of those who wish to space children use perfectly effective contraceptives.
Source: Authors.

have the effect of diluting the household resources of maternal time and attention as well as family economic resources. Therefore, we should expect different patterns of effects depending on the age of the child as well as on the environment.

Data from the World Fertility Survey has been extensively analyzed by Hobcraft, McDonald, and Rutstein (1983, 1985) to show the relationships between childbearing patterns and the survival of offspring. In table 16-8 we show the average of thirty-five developing countries of the percentage increase in death rates from various reference groups for various categories of births. These estimated effects have been controlled for maternal age, spacing, parity, sex of the child, and the education of the household and thus cannot be attributed to different fertility patterns of women of different educational groups. (Detailed estimates for each country in the study are reported in tables 16A-2 through 16A-5.)

The effects of birth order generally come to mind when the effects of high fertility are mentioned. These effects are nonmonotonic and nonuniform across age groups. The first year of life has the highest risk for first births. The risk of dying for first births is 80 percent higher than for second and third births in the neonatal period and 60 percent higher in the postneonatal period. The fourth through sixth births do not show elevated mortality in the first year of life but do have 20 to 30 percent higher mortality in the second through fourth years. Births beyond six have 20 to 30 percent higher mortality at all ages. These patterns do vary substantially from country to country. Fourth through sixth births tend to be more disadvantaged in Latin America and the Caribbean than elsewhere. Births at parity seven or more are less disadvantaged in Asia and the Middle East than elsewhere, but even there, there are exceptions and the mortality of these high-parity births is more than 60 percent higher in Yemen and the Philippines than that for children of second or third parity.

Because of the much higher mortality of first births than any other group, the reduction of fertility through the reduction of higher-order births will not necessarily reduce infant mortality. This is so because a larger percentage of births will then be first births. We have found no conceptual resolution of this apparent paradox (Bongaarts 1988 and Trussell 1988).

The effects of maternal age are also nonmonotonic. The mortality of children of mothers under twenty is 30 to 60 percent higher than that of children whose mothers are twenty-five through thirty-four. Other evidence suggests that for children of women under eighteen these risks are even greater. The risks also differ between regions and are somewhat less elevated in Africa than elsewhere. Even there, there are countries, such as Tunisia, where the mortality risks of the neonates of these young mothers are greater than for the neonates of older mothers. These high risks persist until the child reaches two. The different patterns of risk for very young mothers reflect in part the selectivity of women who bear children at these young ages, which may not be completely captured by the control for education. Mortality risks are also higher for the children of women over thirty-four, but again this varies by region, being greatest in the Americas, less in Africa, and much less in Asia. Postponing the births of women until they reach the age of twenty and reducing the births after the age of thirty-four could possibly make important contributions to reducing mortality in a number of countries, all else being equal, but until more is known about who has children at these ages and the behaviors that affect their survival chances, it is difficult to judge the magnitude of effects.

It has been hypothesized that close spacing of children is detrimental to their health for two reasons. First, the biological effect on the mother of close spacing of children leads to depletion of her health and her ability to nurture and bring to term a baby of normal weight and her ability to breastfeed that baby adequately.[20] The second factor is the competition for household resources such as the mother's time and attention and the household's economic resources. From the analysis in table 16-8, it is clear that having a birth in the twenty-four months prior to the birth of the studied child raises substantially the child's risk of death. If that previous child survived, mortality of the subsequent child is increased by between 50 and 90 percent, depending on the age group under consideration. These relative risks show more consistency than those for parity and maternal age, especially for infants. There are, however, substantial differences between countries. The relative risks in North Africa and the Middle East seem to be particularly high because of close spacing. The elevation in mortality is much more dramatic if a previous child died, but this does not necessarily so much reflect the effect of the short birth interval as the high clustering of deaths within households. Close spacing of births after the birth of a child also show

an important correlation with higher mortality of toddlers and young children. One or more live births in the twelve months after a birth raises toddler mortality by about 130 percent and child mortality by 40 percent (tables 16A-1 through 16A-5).

Thus, the effects of spacing on child survival are both stronger and more consistent across countries than are the other effects of high fertility (Hobcraft, McDonald and Rutstein 1985; NRC 1989). For this reason, to get a rough estimate of the effect of family planning on child survival, we will concentrate on the effect of spacing on mortality. These estimates are tentative at best. We will estimate the effect of one year of contraceptive protection. Assuming an average of three months of natural protection from conception following a birth and nine-month gestation, it would take only twelve months of contraception protection to extend the birth interval to two years. In table 16-9 we summarize for a sample of countries the number of deaths averted in the first five years of a child's life from 1,000 years of contraceptive protection. The first estimates of deaths averted, method 1, are arrived at by comparing actual mortality of those children where there was no living birth in the preceding twenty-four months with the mortality of children when there was one surviving child.[21] The second estimate (method 2), which is generally smaller, is based on the Hobcraft and others (1985) estimates that control for age, parity, education, and spacing simultaneously. The low costs per death averted through the family planning of one year are estimated on the basis of 100 percent effective-

Table 16-8. Percentage by Which Mortality Rates of Births in Various Categories Exceed Those of Reference Group

Child	Births in previous 24 months[a]			Parity[b]			Mother's age[c]		
	One alive	One dead	Two or more	4–6	7 or more	1	20 or less	20–24	35 or more
Neonatal (0–1 month)									
Africa	69	278	289	1	27	114	18	0	18
Asia	82	259	362	–12	0	98	37	6	3
Latin America	53	319	209	15	44	40	37	12	27
Developing world	70	290	250	0	20	80	30	10	20
Postneonatal (1–12 months)									
Africa	65	261	233	7	27	49	38	15	0
Asia	100	215	384	2	31	70	32	6	–3
Latin America	99	256	203	3	43	62	65	27	7
Developing world	90	240	240	0	30	60	40	20	0
Toddler (1–2 years)									
Africa	19	97	62	17	14	–1	43	15	–4
Asia	83	145	81	25	31	5	44	–1	–7
Latin America	27	62	99	23	45	–8	98	46	11
Developing world	40	100	80	20	30	0	60	20	0
Child (2–5 years)									
Africa	48	67	38	18	18	–5	35	10	12
Asia	42	67	124	29	17	–12	52	16	22
Latin America	59	47	23	35	42	0	25	3	–15
Developing world	50	60	60	30	30	–6	40	10	10

a. Reference category is no birth.
b. Reference category is parity of two or three.
c. Reference category is age 25–34.
Source: Derived from Hobcraft, McDonald, and Rutstein, 1985.

ness and $7.70[22] costs per couple-year protection.[23] Because each year of couple protection does not result in a prevented birth, these figures are then adjusted for the average annual births per woman of childbearing age in the country under consideration. The high cost estimate assumes $18.00 per couple-year of protection.[24] These are then converted into disability-adjusted days of life gained.

There are substantial differences in the costs per death averted and the costs per disability-adjusted life-year gained. Not surprisingly, the lowest costs are in the highest mortality countries in the group, Pakistan and Bangladesh. More surprisingly, Egypt, which has a life expectancy at least five years above Pakistan, has similar costs, and Kenya, with life expectancy 3.5 years less than Egypt, has costs 50 percent higher. Diarrheal diseases may be an important factor in explaining these different patterns, because close child spacing may be linked to early weaning and higher mortality risks.

In summation, increased spacing of births probably represents the most important way to reduce mortality through family planning. Elimination of births at the youngest age groups is probably the second most important factor in reducing infant and child mortality. High parity and births to women over thirty-four have an effect that is less well established.

SOCIAL AND ECONOMIC COSTS OF EXCESS FERTILITY. Population growth affects economic development through its effects on savings and investment, technological change, changes in efficiency, and returns (increasing or diminishing) to scale.[25] In addition, population growth affects the resource base through resource depletion and pollution. The precise relationship between any one of these and population growth has yet to be firmly established and depends on current levels of population density, resource endowment, and the rate of population growth as well as on myriad policies from property rights in resources to agricultural subsidies (Kelley 1988; *The World Development Report* 1984; and NRC 1986 for comprehensive reviews).

The National Research Council concludes, "On balance, we reach the qualitative conclusion that slower population growth would be beneficial to economic development of de-

veloping countries" (NRC 1986, p. 90). The 1984 *World Development Report* concluded, "In short, policies to reduce population growth can make an important contribution to development (especially in the long run), but their beneficial effects will be greatly diminished if they are not supported by the right macroeconomic and sectoral policies. At the same time, failure to address the population problem will itself reduce the set of macroeconomic and sectoral policies that are possible, and permanently foreclose some long run development options" (WDR 1984, p. 105).

The costs of excess fertility, like its measurement, can be viewed by the family or society. The costs of children are primarily borne by the family. Therefore, the family's report of what is the desirable family size would incorporate the family's judgment of the desirable expenditure on children. The costs to the family of excess fertility would be measured by the costs of the marginal child to the family. Unfortunately, due to both methodological and data problems, the measurement of the costs of a child is rarely available for developing countries.[26] In addition to the costs of food, clothing, medical care, schooling, and housing, children in the family affect the amount of time a mother devotes to child care. These costs are borne by a number of adjustments in the household. Expenditure per child is reduced with increasing numbers, resulting in many cases of poor health in the children (the excess child and its siblings) and reduced school participation of all children. In addition to reduced expenditure per child, high fertility also results in efforts to increase family income.[27] The increase may come about through child labor or through added labor of the parents. An interesting body of evidence is accumulating on the higher labor participation of men in households with larger numbers of children. Finally, the adjustment to higher unwanted fertility can be made by reducing the savings of the household. (See King 1987 and Cochrane, Kozel, and Alderman 1990 for reviews of these issues.) The bottom line is that it is impossible to document the negative effects of high fertility on every dimension or every country. Thus there is not one cost of a child that can then be used to evaluate the savings from averting a birth for the individual household.[28] Therefore, it must be left to the household to establish its own evaluation

Table 16-9. Infant and Child Deaths Averted by 1,000 Couple-Years of Protection through Child Spacing and Associated Costs, Selected Countries

| | Deaths averted | | Cost per DALY saved (1988 dollars) | | | |
| | | | Actual[a] | | Adjusted[b] | |
Country	Actual[a]	Adjusted[b]	Low cost	High cost	Low cost	High cost
Pakistan	85	63	405/41	944/33	544/19	1,268/44
Mexico	40	34	1,532/53	3,570/123	1,794/62	4,189/144
Bangladesh	96	125	445/15	1,037/36	341/12	795/27
Philippines	40	38	1,667/58	3,907/135	1,764/61	4,110/142
Kenya	61	64	784/27	1,827/63	746/26	1,738/60
Egypt	111	131	483/17	1,125/39	413/14	962/33

a. Actual differences in mortality rates for births with and without a birth within previous twenty-four months. Other method uses adjusted rates.
b. Estimates controlled for the education, and parity of the mother.
Source: Author.

of the costs and benefits of children. These evaluations are reflected in their stated fertility preferences. The fact that at the family level the costs exceed the benefits in many cases is revealed by the evidence cited above that 30 percent of births are in excess of stated family size preferences.

The evidence above refers to the effect of an added child on the family. If that child is unwanted, the negative effects, particularly for the child, are probably much more severe even though they are less well documented. Some work has been done on this for the industrial world as part of the justification for publicly subsidized family planning programs. For example, women denied abortion in Prague were followed up for a period of twenty years. Forty-five percent of these mothers were dissatisfied with their child's development compared with 21 percent among controls. The children themselves perceived more problems in life and more disappointments in life, love,

and mental health (David 1986). Other data on how parents treat unwanted children have been documented by Shorter (1976), Ware (1976), and Scrimshaw (1978 and 1983). Evidence of infanticide, abandonment, neglect, and the selective provision of food and medical care to children has been drawn from historical and contemporary data from all geographic regions. Further evidence of the effect of unwanted children comes from a recent study in Ethiopia. It was reported that women whose births were described as unwanted were least likely to seek antenatal care (Kwast and others 1985).

The unwanted fertility of the unmarried woman is even more costly for both the mother and the potential child. Women lose out on educational and employment investments and are forced to choose between abortions (safe or unsafe), fostering out or adoption of children, and raising the child without economic support from the father. Little or no economic analysis has been done of the economic costs of fertility outside marriage in the developing world. The medical costs of unsafe abortion are discussed later in the chapter.

Society also bears some costs as a result of the birth of a child. The most obvious costs are those for education and health. If the state also takes on responsibility for food, shelter, safe water, and so on, through subsidies or public provision, the costs are commensurately higher. In the late 1950s and early 1960s efforts were made to calculate the savings from a birth averted. These most frequently took the form of estimating the consumption by children and adults and the earnings of an average adult and discounting the hypothesized streams of consumption and production. These efforts are reviewed by Ohlin (1967). Since any period of production is preceded by a period of consumption, these estimates were highly sensitive to the discount rate. Enke (1960) used rates of 10, 15, and 20 percent for a country like India and found the value of a birth averted was 3.8, 2.6, and 2.1 times the per capita annual income, respectively. Ohlin estimates that the value of a birth averted would be zero at a 4 percent discount rate, but twice per capita income at 6 percent. Alternative methodology was employed by Demeny (1965), who projected income using a macroeconomic model with different levels of fertility. He estimates that "gains from preventing a birth is of the order of magnitude of two per capita income" (Demeny 1965 cited in Ohlin 1967, p. 116).

More recent work has been less heroic and has focused only on public expenditure saved by preventing a birth.[29] Nortman and Lewis (1986) focused on the savings to the Mexican social security system from each peso spent on family planning. They documented that the cost per pregnancy per mother was 36,000 pesos and the cost of care for a child in the first year of life was 34,000 pesos.[30] In calculating a cost-benefit ratio, they also included the benefits of preventing incomplete abortions, which then had to be treated. The cost-benefit ratio was calculated to be nine pesos saved for pesos spent on family planning. For Indonesia, Chao and others (1985) analyzed the savings from expenditure averted for education and health by preventing a birth. A study by Kiranandana and others (1984) for Thailand estimated the savings in lower expenditure on

Table 16-10. Savings per Birth Averted in Three Types of Countries
(1987 U.S. dollars)

Expenditure	5 percent discount	10 percent discount
Libana—high-mortality African country		
Primary education	160[a]	84
Secondary education	147[b]	57
Health	129[c]	60
Total	436	201
Banglapal—high-mortality non-African country		
Primary education	160[d]	84
Secondary education	193[d]	74
Health	129[c]	60
Total	482	218
Colexico—low-mortality developing country		
Primary education	508[e]	354
Secondary education	492[f]	273
Health	564[g]	281
Total	1,564	908

a. Assumes universal six years of school. Capital costs at lowest 30 percentile for World Bank primary school projects. Buildings last thirty years. Recurrent cost 13 percent of average poor country per capita income.

b. Assumes 16 percent attend six years of secondary school. Capital costs at lowest 30 percentile of World Bank secondary school projects. Buildings last thirty years. Recurrent costs per year are twice those in primary education.

c. Assumes $6 per capita (as in China and Sri Lanka). Life expectancy is fifty-one years.

d. Assumptions as in note b., but 21 percent of children have six years of secondary education.

e. Universal six years of primary school. Capital costs at median for World Bank projects. Recurrent costs $100 p.a.

f. Assumes forty-five percent secondary enrollment. Capital costs at median for World Bank projects. School life thirty years. Recurrent costs twice those in primary education.

g. Assumes $28 per year for public expenditures per capita. Life expectancy is sixty-four years.

Source: World Bank estimates.

education, health care, housing and infrastructure, and social services. As long as programs are completely voluntary the benefits of a wanted child to the parents need not be included in the calculations for obvious reasons.

In table 16-10 we report the total savings and the savings per birth averted in education and health for the three model countries if all the unwanted births are averted.[31] The savings per birth averted are dramatically different between the high- and low-mortality countries but fairly similar for the two high-mortality countries. The rate of discount also makes a substantial difference in the savings. In a later section the savings per birth averted will be compared with the costs per birth averted.

Reducing Excess Fertility

The most direct strategy for reducing excess fertility is family planning, but delayed marriage, prolonged breastfeeding and abortion have significant effects as well.

Elements of Preventive Strategies

Strategies to prevent excess fertility have been very widely discussed in the literature. It is now accepted that general socioeconomic development leads to a lowering of fertility and therefore any programs aimed at fertility control will ensure the most rapid results if undertaken as a component of broader development efforts. A strategy for preventing excess fertility would have to be based on a careful analysis and appreciation of the proximate determinants of fertility in any given country or community and the relative value or relative contribution of each determinant within the system at any given point in time. Bongaarts (1978) has stated the following as the main determinants of fertility in any community:

- The patterns of marriage and consequently exposure to pregnancy
- Breastfeeding practices
- Abortions
- Contraception or direct fertility regulations activities

These proximate variables directly affect fertility. Socioeconomic factors, access to family planning, and economic opportunities, as well as legislation, affect fertility through these proximate determinants. Education is the most pervasive and best-documented factor affecting fertility through these multiple channels (Cochrane 1979; Cochrane and Zachariah 1983; United Nations 1988).

In many developing countries marriage patterns are varied and not easy to define. In traditional societies, women are generally expected to marry early and remain in marriage; their period of exposure to childbearing is thus very long. In many parts of Africa, for example, young women marry as early as age fifteen or younger—among some groups as early as onset of menarche—and remain married either to the same person or another person until they stop childbearing naturally.[32]

Widowhood is not a bar to remarriage, and polygamy ensures that women do not remain without partners for too long. Thus in most parts of Africa most fertile women are exposed to the possibility of childbearing throughout their reproductive life, except for periods of postpartum abstinence, which may be quite long in some traditional societies.

It is difficult to change behavior as basic as the initiation of sexual activity and marriage, but age of marriage does rise systematically with certain aspects of economic development. Developmental actions are taking place today which influence these types of marriage and which can be considered among possible strategies for decreasing fertility in many communities. Among these are general education and paid employment away from home. General education, particularly of girls, helps them to postpone getting married until they are in the later teens or early twenties. By postponing marriage they have less exposure to pregnancy and may have fewer children, if premarital fertility does not increase. Legislation may also have some effect on the age of marriage, but it must be accompanied by general reform of women's rights and enforcement mechanisms (Duza and Baldwin 1974).

Cultural taboos, such as a woman's leaving the husband's family after she has a baby and staying with her own family until the child can walk, or a woman's not having contact with her husband until the child has grown its milk teeth, are stipulations which ensured that children were spaced at intervals of three or more years. These taboos are breaking down with modernization and as husband and wife stay together in nuclear families in urban situations. In such situations, there is a clear need to replace the lost cultural taboos with technology to ensure child spacing.

Breastfeeding is considered the most important natural contraceptive. For breastfeeding to be a useful contraceptive on a community basis, it has to be prolonged and given on demand with the child being at the nipple whenever he or she wants, even at night. It is believed that the suckling at the nipple produces a nervous stimulus which then triggers the hypothalamus and pituitary axis to produce the necessary hormones which prevent ovulation. Therefore, efforts to promote breastfeeding must be considered an important contribution to efforts to help with the reduction of excess fertility. Recent guidelines indicate that breastfeeding is a highly reliable method of contraception until the child reaches six months of age, supplementary feeding is introduced, or menses returns. Under these circumstances breastfeeding is 98 percent effective. (See Consensus Statement on the Use of Breastfeeding as a Family Planning Method, *Lancet* 1988.) If any one of these events occurs, other forms of contraception should be introduced. Breastfeeding beyond any of these points will lower the probabilities of conception, but the degree of that reduction varies greatly from one woman to another. Thus, although prolonged breastfeeding, beyond six months, can suppress fertility for society as a whole, it is an unreliable individual contraceptive. During the course of development and with the increase in education, the practice of breastfeeding to maximize its antinatal effects tends to decrease. To counter this, it

Table 16-11. *Appropriateness of Contraceptive Method, by Stage in Reproductive Life Cycle*

Method	Before first birth (delay)	After first birth (spacing)	Completion of family
Oral contraceptive	Most appropriate	Appropriate	Inappropriate
Injectable hormone	Appropriate	Most appropriate	Least appropriate
Implant	Appropriate	Appropriate	Most appropriate
IUD	Inappropriate	Most appropriate	Appropriate
Condom	Most appropriate	Least appropriate	Inappropriate
Vaginal spermicide	Appropriate	Appropriate	Inappropriate
Diaphragm/cap	Appropriate	Appropriate	Inappropriate
Periodic abstinence	Appropriate	Appropriate	Inappropriate
Sterilization	Inappropriate	Inappropriate	Most appropriate

Note: Menstrual regulation and abortion are backups throughout reproductive life cycle.
Source: Hutchings and Sanders 1985.

is necessary to make family planning more available and to provide for the promotion of breastfeeding where possible (Huffman and Combest 1988; Green 1989; and Labbok and McDonald 1990 in the supplement to volume 31 [1990] of the *International Journal of Gynecology and Obstetrics*).[33]

The attitudes and practices of health personnel, particularly those attending delivery, can have an important effect on the establishment and continuation of breastfeeding and on appropriate weaning behavior. These practices are important as health interventions which have an externality of preventing pregnancy. It is impossible, however, to determine the cost-effectiveness of such interventions in reducing excess fertility.

Family planning programs depend on the availability and the acceptance of modern contraception. The programs themselves need to create demand as well as provide services. Demand creation can be divided into two types: indirect and direct. Indirect demand creation depends generally on social and economic development, issues within the domain of development planning generally and national social mobilization. Among specific efforts in this domain are activities that improve general education of the people and especially those which emphasize women's education, women's mobilization, and the improvement in the status of women through various activities, be these activities developed as direct projects for family planning programs or activities developed from other programs but relating to the improvement in the status of women or improvement of their economic opportunities. Such programs can indirectly lead women to seek and accept more readily assistance to control their fertility. Their effect can be strengthened when accompanied by special messages or information and communications activities aimed at highlighting awareness of the women about the importance of fertility regulation for their lives. In education generally, opportunities need to be taken to emphasize the relation between population and resources and population and the environment. Population dynamics need to be a part of every school program in developing countries at the present time. Girls and young women must also learn at an early age the consequences of high fertility for their own health and welfare and that of their children.

Direct demand creation is that incorporated in information, education, and communication (IEC) programs which provide information specific to family size preferences or family planning and contraception techniques and services. This can take many forms, from mass media campaigns to a series of smaller, more directed efforts. All available methods of communication may be used from a variety of ministries and agencies, ministries of health, youth, women's affairs, defense, industry, and agriculture, to name a few. All these need to go hand in hand with programs for the distribution of contraceptive supplies.

The delivery of services can take diverse forms. In many environments they have been most effective as part of maternal and child health programs. In other environments vertical or single function programs have proven most successful. The

Table 16-12. *First-Year Failure Rates of Birth Control Methods*

Method	Lowest observed failure rate[a]	Failure rate in typical users[b]
Chance (no method of birth control)	70	70
Tubal ligation	0.04	0.04
Vasectomy	0.15	0.15
Injectable progestin	0.25	0.25
Combined birth control pills	0.5	2
Progestin-only pill	1	2.5
IUD	1.5	4
Condom	2	10
Diaphragm (with spermicide)	2	13
Cervical cap	2	13
Foam, creams, jellies and vaginal suppositories	3–5	15
Coitus interruptus	16	23
Fertility awareness techniques (basal body temperature, mucus method, calendar, "rhythm," and douche)	2–20	20–30

a. Number pregnant by end of year among 100 women who start out the year using a given method and who use it correctly and consistently.
b. Number pregnant by end of year among 100 typical users who start out the year using a given method.
Source: CDC 1983.

Figure 16-2. *Estimated Annual Deaths Resulting from Pregnancy, Abortion, and Contraceptive Use, by Age of Woman*

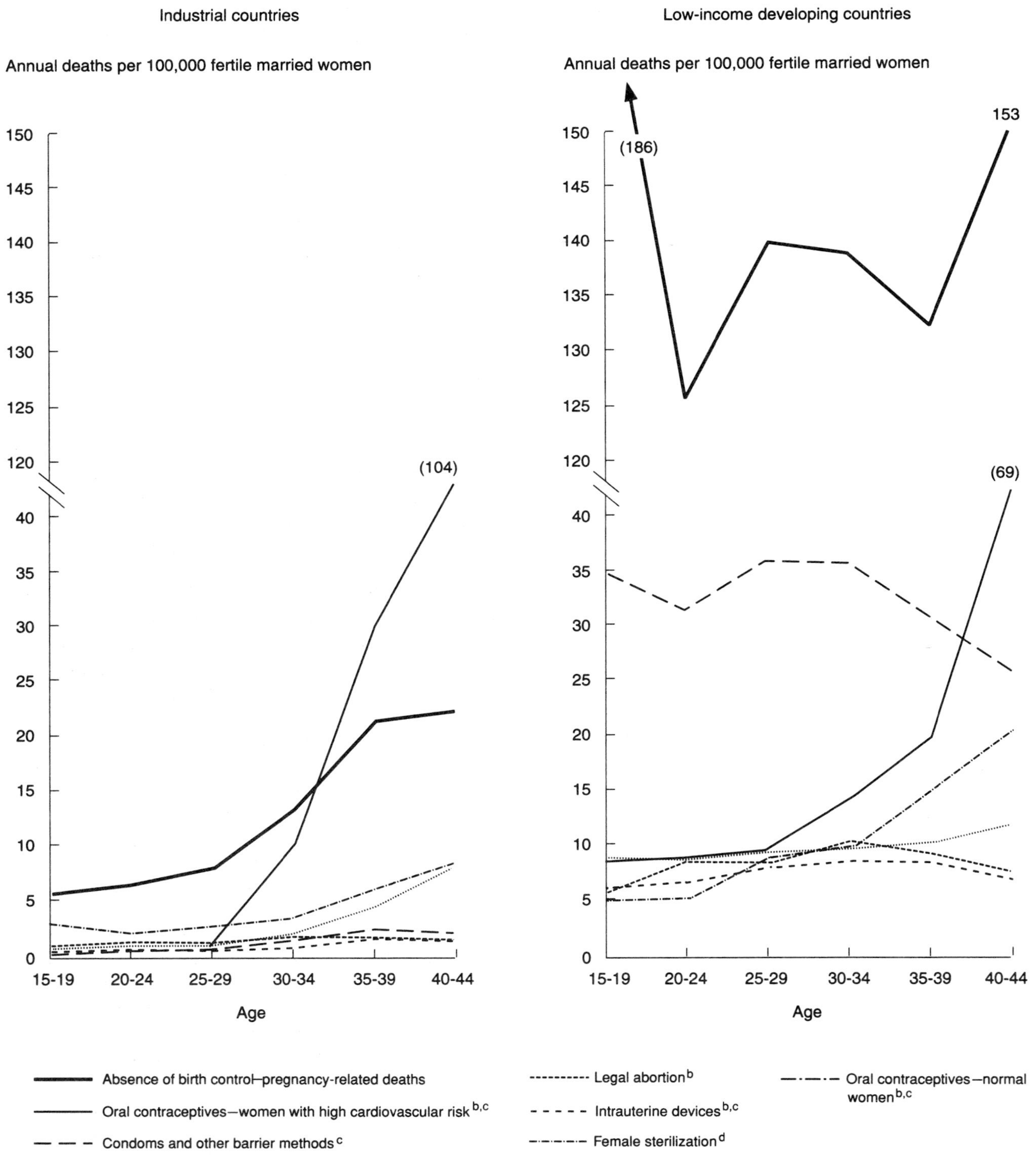

Industrial countries

Low-income developing countries

Annual deaths per 100,000 fertile married women

Annual deaths per 100,000 fertile married women

Legend:

— Absence of birth control–pregnancy-related deaths

— Oral contraceptives–women with high cardiovascular risk [b,c]

– – – Condoms and other barrier methods [c]

---------- Legal abortion [b]

- - - - Intrauterine devices [b,c]

–·–·–·– Female sterilization [d]

–·–··– Oral contraceptives–normal women [b,c]

Note: Maternal death estimates assume lower use-effectiveness rates in developing countries for all methods except the IUD.

a. Countries with per capita incomes less than $410 (U.S. dollars) and with average maternal mortality rates of about 350 deaths per 100,000 live births.

b. Method-related deaths.

c. Pregnancy-related deaths.

d. Procedure-related deaths, a one-time risk. Data that reflect deaths per 100,000 procedures rather than per 100,000 women overstate relative risks over time compared with other methods.

Source: Population Crisis Committee 1985, adapted from Potts, Speidel, and Kassel 1977.

Table 16-13. Relative Cost of Birth Control Methods

Method	Costs in initial year (U.S. dollars)	Subsequent product cost, per year (U.S. dollars)	Relative cost per CYP in initial year[c] (percent)	Relative cost per CYP amortized over average lifetime of method[a] (percent)
Oral contraceptive	2.17	2.17	100	100
Injectable hormone	3.51	3.51	162	162
Implant	16.23	n.a.	748	212
IUD	3.45	n.a.	159	42
Condom	3.88	3.88	179	179
Vaginal spermicide	5.76	5.76	265	265
Diaphragm/cap	4.75	0[b]	219	77
Female sterilization	8.91	n.a.	411	59
Male sterilization	6.68	n.a.	308	44
Menstrual regulation/abortion	4.45	n.a.	205	n.a.

n.a. Not applicable.

a. Percentages are based on estimated couple of years protection (CYP) initial year costs and are relative to cost of oral contraceptives.

b. In actual practice, spermicide use would add to the yearly cost.

c. Couple years of contraceptive protection.

Source: Hutchings and Sanders 1985.

one thing that has been learned is that there is no uniquely defined best delivery mode. Important though such clinic-based programs are, their outreach may be rather limited, especially in communities where the health services themselves are fairly restricted in their outreach. In such a situation there is a need to build outreach programs such as social marketing or community-based programs which ensure that the users themselves are closely involved with the family planning programs. Irrespective of the form of delivery system, there is a need to have a medical service with trained staff in what may be termed clinical contraception, such as the insertion of intrauterine devices (IUDs) or terminal methods such as vasectomy and tubectomy. Such a service provides for referral, backup, and training of the staff of other programs.

Primary prevention of excess fertility is thus based on a strategy of general social development with equity, in particular when such development targets women. Direct population education in communicating also helps, as does specific IEC for men and women of childbearing age. Family planning services providing information and contraceptive services at affordable prices help to ensure that the population is able to control its fertility. There are, however, other factors that inhibit that ability that need attention, from the empowerment of men and women to information on the real side effects of high fertility and contraceptive risks. The role of abortion in preventing excess fertility is more controversial and will be discussed later.

Costs and Efficacy of Family Planning

A wide variety of family planning methods is now available. They differ in their effectiveness and side effects as well as their costs (Holck and Bathija 1988; cited in WHO 1988). In table 16-11 we summarize appropriateness of various contraceptives to different phases of the reproductive life of a woman. In table 16-12 we summarize the failure rates for most modern methods

except the most recently developed implants.[34] In figure 16-2 we summarize the mortality risks from various methods. It is important to note how the relative risks between contraception and childbearing differ between developing and industrial countries. It is less easy to summarize the morbidity and other side effects of various methods. Most methods have some actual or perceived negative side effects. These effects and the importance attached to them differ greatly from one woman or couple to the next. It is also true that some methods have positive side effects, from reducing anemia (oral contraceptives) to prevention of sexually transmitted diseases to the reduction of the risk of some cancers (Lee, Peterson, and Chu 1990). Thus, programs that offer a wide mix of methods are able to attract a larger number of women than programs with a narrower range of methods. It is also clear that side effects of contraceptives, particularly oral contraceptives, differ according to a woman's age. This is another reason to have a program that has a wide method mix. Family planning methods vary substantially in commodity costs and personnel and infrastructure costs. The costs of various methods are too specific to be reviewed in detail here (see table 16-13 for the supply costs of various methods and those costs in relation to the cost of oral contraceptives). Of greater relevance are the program costs of serving a family planning user or preventing a birth. Reviews of program costs per user or per birth averted were compiled in preparation for the 1984 World Population Conference (Bulatao 1985 for a review and analysis of these costs). The costs include or should include the entire costs of promoting family planning use and of commodities, personnel, equipment, and facilities for the program. These cost estimates are in fact often simply derived by dividing expenditure in any given year by the number of users. Detailed cost analyses to give precise estimates are fairly rare. (Analyses by Barnum [1983] and Chernichovsky and others [1989] are exceptions. See Serageldin and others 1983 for a review of the issues in cost-benefit and cost-effectiveness analysis and Cochrane, Hammer, Janowitz, and Kenney 1990 for a review of newer cost estimates.)

For the purpose of this analysis the costs per user in the study by Bulatao (1985) and the costs per birth averted in the study by Cochrane and Zachariah (1983) will be used. Both of these are dependent on earlier work by Speidel (1983). The costs as collected refer to 1980, but they have been inflated to 1987 in table 16-14.[35] If economies of scale exist in the program, the average costs have probably dropped since 1980.[36] The costs per birth averted are related to the fertility preference of the women in the society. Regression analysis shows that the cost per birth averted drops by $66 for a one-child difference between the actual and desired TFR (table 16-4). As shown in figure 16-3, the cost per birth averted also decreases with an increase in the proportion who want no more children ($4.6 per 1 percent increase in the number wanting no more children).[37] Therefore, for the three hypothetical countries we can predict the costs of a birth averted by first determining the average life expectancy (fifty-one years for model countries Libana and Banglapal and sixty-four years for Colexico) and predicting the percentage wanting no more children (figure 16-1) and then projecting costs per birth averted from the equation in figure 16-3. One adjustment that must be made is that on average the countries with lower mortality have higher proportions of women who want no more children than do the primarily African countries. Best estimates indicated approximately 20, 30, and 45 percent of the women want no more children in the three models, respectively. The equation in figure 16-3 implies the costs per birth averted of $259, $213, and $144, respectively, in the three countries.[38] Comparing these costs with the savings of births averted in table 16-10, one finds that at the 5 percent discount rate, the costs of a birth averted is justified on the basis of economic savings to the government alone in all three models. At the 10 percent rate of discount, the costs of a birth averted would be fully justified in Colexico, marginally justified in Banglapal, and unjustified in Libana[39].

There are several caveats to be made with respect to the findings above: (a) the costs and savings are based on hypothetical country types, and actual estimates would have to be made in real circumstances; (b) the conclusions above apply only to the economic benefits of family planning, and the health benefits, which are substantial, as shown above, would be additional; and (c) the extent to which access to contraception would in fact alter family size preferences is yet to be established. To the extent that such an effect exists, the cost functions are incorrectly specified.

Technology and Future Changes

All existing contraceptives have some negative side effects or inconvenience; few methods allow male control or responsibility for the method, and some methods are unacceptable to certain religious groups. Thus technological development is needed for contraceptives. In addition there is continued uncertainty about the most effective and efficient delivery systems for family planning in different environments. We will briefly review changes that are currently on the horizon.

Many contraceptive technologies are currently being developed that may be useful eventually. The most promising for the 1990s is the implant. This provides highly effective contraception for up to five years with few side effects except irregular menstrual periods. It is, however, relatively expensive and requires skill in its implantation and even more skill in its removal.[40] Thus it is intensive in training and personnel at the beginning and end of use. Some research is under way on developing a biodegradable sheath which would eliminate the necessity of removal. A once-a-month injectable contraceptive, Cyclofem, is nearing commercial production and would eliminate the problem of irregular menstrual periods that occur with longer-term, hormonal methods. Other contraceptive methods being developed have less chance for immediate breakthrough because they are in earlier stages. The male pill is being developed in China under a cooperative program with the Rockefeller Foundation. Vaginal rings are also being developed, and the new RU486 provides some promise for future use. The Population Council, Family Health International, the Ford Foundation, the National Institutes of Health in the United States, the Rockefeller Foundation, and the Human Reproduction Programme (HRP) in WHO are the main actors in coordinating research on contraceptive technology. (See NRC 1990 for a review of the evaluation of contraceptive research and development.)

Despite the efforts of these organizations, the low level of funding for contraceptive development for low-income countries is a serious problem because private enterprise, which is a significant source of technological change, is not interested in developing contraceptives for that market. Three factors explain this lack of interest: (a) because many techniques that need to be developed for poor countries must, of necessity, be very low cost and low dosage, they will offer low profits; (b) because most contraceptive research is done in industrial countries and must be approved for use there to be profitable, the research is skewed toward contraceptives that reflect the relative risks of using contraceptives and the maternal risks in those countries (see figure 16-2); and (c) product liability laws are so stringent in many countries like the United States that new products face too many potential liability costs even if a product is developed and is sold. An example of how these risks distort research is the recent development of the contraceptive sponge in the industrial world. This method is too expensive, too inconvenient, and has too high a failure rate for poor countries, but it has very few possibilities of side effects for which a company could be sued (Population Crisis Committee 1985).

An important question to be addressed in the area of contraceptive technology in the next decade is the interaction of various methods and acquired immunodeficiency syndrome (AIDS). The condom serves both to prevent births and reduce the probability of contracting AIDS. For other methods the linkage between the spread of the disease and the use of the

Table 16-14. Costs of Averting a Birth through Family Planning
(1987 U.S. dollars)

Country	Cost per user	Cost per averted birth	
		Low	High
Bangladesh	29	102	109
Colombia	7	21	29
Costa Rica	22	71	160
Dominican Republic	17	50	69
Indonesia	12	49	64
Jordan	31	88	108
Kenya	100	350	386
Korea, Rep. of	12	53	77
Malaysia	21	69	92
Mexico	22	59	78
Nepal	80	330	364
Pakistan	15	77	81
Panama	36	136	231
Peru	10	34	38
Philippines	20	63	77
Sri Lanka	8	31	41

Source: Converted from 1980 figures in table 9 of Cochrane and Zachariah 1983, using standard indices of the Priorities Project.

methods is unclear and needs to be researched. All surgical methods require much close attention to cleaning of instruments and equipment when the AIDS virus is at all prevalent in society. This covers implants, sterilization, abortion, and IUD insertions. In addition, injections must be more carefully monitored to be sure that needles are not reused or are properly sterilized. The Human Reproduction Programme is sponsoring

Figure 16-3. Relationship between Costs per Birth Averted and Percent Wanting No More Children

Cost per birth averted

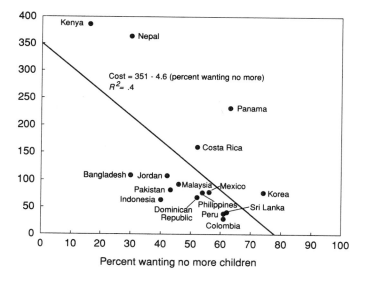

$$\text{Cost} = 351 - 4.6 \text{ (percent wanting no more)}$$
$$R^2 = .4$$

Source: Authors' calculations.

the development of a small, cheap vial-needle combination that is impossible to reuse for delivery of Cyclofem. Research is also needed on how various contraceptives affect the risk of contracting the human immunodeficiency virus or developing the disease by either changing sexual behavior, increasing the receptivity to the virus, or stimulating the development of the disease. Through HRP the World Health Organization is sponsoring some research in this area and has issued guidelines. These risks must be set against the risk of the more rapid onset of the disease that is stimulated by pregnancy and the transmission of the disease to the infant during pregnancy or delivery.

In the area of the management of the delivery system, attention is now being focused on two important aspects: improvement of service quality (Jain 1989; Bruce 1990), and developing delivery models in Sub-Saharan Africa, where demand for family planning is weaker and more oriented toward spacing births than stopping them and the health infrastructure is very weak. Other themes that are receiving considerable attention are the necessity of having an appropriate monitoring and evaluation system, the movement away from one-method programs (India), the appropriate role of the private sector (Indonesia), and the appropriate mix of family planning delivery and promotion (issues involving the ministries of health, ministries of information and education, and other important ministries and coordinating bodies in population and family planning). The commitment of the medical profession as well as national leaders to the delivery of family planning for health, equity, and economic considerations is also of crucial importance to the success of a delivery system. There exist serious shortcomings of actual practice over the best practice in family planning delivery, but it is also true that despite excellent synthesis work done by the National Academy of Science in its 1987 review by Lapham and Simmons and the Johns Hopkins University Population Reports there is still an enormous amount that needs to be done to clarify what the best practice is in different environments.

Reasonable Delivery Systems for Model Countries

In the two hypothetical high-mortality countries the lack of health infrastructure is a fundamental underlying constraint. In addition in Libana demand for contraception is less than in Banglapal. In both models it is necessary to develop the health delivery system. It is also essential to target efforts in family planning, but in the second model the targets can be broader. Providing condoms, pills, and other barrier methods through health centers and pharmacies and perhaps social marketing may be desirable and effective in urban areas. Sterilizations and IUD insertions should be done in district hospitals everywhere, but in Banglapal they may also be done in clinics if they have adequate staff and if staff members are available to handle side effects. Sterilization camps, particularly for vasectomies, may also be cost-effective, but politically sensitive. Injections can be done on a mobile team if a reliable system of delivery can be maintained to make regular trips. This latter function may be better carried out by a nongovernmental organization if the government logistics are weak. Such programs need to be backed up by information, education and communications programs that can advise on location of service and appropriate use and contraindications. This is particularly important where contraception use is low, because fear of side effects can seriously undermine the development of a program if there exists no referral agency to handle them.

In Colexico all the above can be used, but delivery of IUDs, sterilization, and injection can be done more routinely at lower levels of service because of higher demand and better health infrastructure. It is probably also essential to have either explicit policies on legal abortion or IEC on the dangers of abortion and medical facilities for treating incomplete abortions. This is likely to be more serious in Colexico because the much stronger demand to restrict fertility will lead to abortion in more cases of contraceptive failure.

Case Management: Unwanted Pregnancies

For pregnant women who want no more children or who wish to postpone the timing of a birth, the choice is between carrying the pregnancy to term or seeking an abortion. The type of costs of an unwanted pregnancy include: (a) the cost of abortion, (b) the cost of treating incomplete induced abortion, and (c) additional costs associated with unwanted pregnancies that are not associated with normal pregnancies. These latter costs are not well documented for industrial or developing countries.

There are enormous differences from country to country in laws covering abortion. Where it is legal, the method is relatively safe in the first trimester and the costs are mainly those associated with the abortion itself. Estimates from the UN indicate that about 40 percent of the women in developing countries have access to legal induced abortion. This ranges from 10 percent in Africa to 50 percent in Asia (40 percent in Latin America; United Nations 1988, table 38). The laws on abortion differ dramatically, however. In thirteen of ninety-six developing countries reviewed, it was illegal under all circumstances, and in only seven was it available on request. In the vast majority it is available for health reasons, but in most, only to save the life of the mother (forty-two of ninety-six). Thirty-five countries permit abortion for health reasons. Such laws permit wide latitude to doctors in preforming abortions and give access to safe abortion to most women who can pay doctors fees. The price of private legal abortion ranges from $16 in Bangladesh to $966 in Iraq. The normal range is between $100 and $200 in countries for which data are available (Ross and others 1988). Publicly provided abortions are free in a number of countries, but fees of under $100 are charged in several countries.

For women with no access to safe abortions, the cost of abortion complications must be added to the cost of the abortions themselves. It is impossible to get an estimate of the number of illegal abortions performed throughout the world or their cost. Evidence of abortion complications from hospital admissions is the best index. The "Population Reports" of July 1980 by Liskin compiled data on complications of abortions

up to that time. It estimated that, depending on the country, between 4 and 70 percent of maternal deaths in developing country hospitals were the result of complications of illegal abortion. A recent study on illegal abortion by Figa-Talamanca and others, assessed the medical costs of illegally induced abortion in urban hospitals in four developing countries. For Malaysia, 52 percent of the abortion cases admitted were estimated to be induced, whereas only 12 percent of those in Nigeria were. In Turkey, 41 percent were estimated to be induced. There are no estimates immediately available of the economic costs of those abortions, but the induced abortion cases experienced high costs in hospital days, units of blood administered, and cost of medication (table 16-15). The cost in disability and ill health from these illegal abortions has not been estimated.

Priorities

Priorities for resource allocation depend on the level of demand for family planning and the level of mortality.

Priorities for Resource Allocation

A considerable amount of evidence has been compiled in various sources on the unmet demand for family planning to limit births and to a lesser degree to space births (see table 16-5 for data; Westoff and Moreno 1989 for a deeper analysis for five Latin American countries). As discussed above, we estimate that about a third of the births in the developing world

Table 16-15. Cost-Related Indices of Induced and Spontaneous Abortions in Four Participating Centers[a]

Parameters, by center	Induced abortion	Spontaneous abortion
Mean length of hospitalization (days)		
Malaysia	4.8	4.5
Nigeria	10.5	7.5
Turkey	1.7	1.0
Venezuela		
Caracas	4.2	2.4
Valencia	5.3	2.5
Mean units of blood administered		
Malaysia	0.2	0.1
Nigeria	0.6	0.2
Turkey	—	—
Venezuela		
Caracas	0.5	0.2
Valencia	1.0	0.5
Relative cost of medication[b]		
Malaysia	1.9	1.0
Nigeria	—	—
Turkey	1.5	1.0
Venezuela	8.8	1.0

— Data not available.
a. Data refer to cases classified as shown in Table 16-6.
b. Computed by considering the spontaneous abortion cost equal to unity.
Source: Figa-Talamanca and others 1986.

outside China are unwanted, and excess fertility would be even higher if births that come too soon were to be included. This implies substantial unmet need for family planning.

It is difficult to estimate what would be necessary to meet all the need for family planning as expressed by individuals. The analysis above indicates that in areas where mortality is low or demand to limit family size is 30 percent or more the savings from public health and education expenses alone are sufficient to justify public expenditure on family planning to avert a birth.[41] Where the demand to limit the number of births is lower, as in much of Sub-Saharan Africa, the cost of averting a birth is much higher. Because of this the economic justification for supporting family planning is less compelling, but given much higher maternal, infant, and child mortality in these areas the health justifications are more important (see table 16-9 for the cost of averting an infant or child death through family planning for spacing). In addition, reducing mortality is an important factor in stimulating more demand for family planning.[42] Even in areas of low demand, however, at rates of discount of 5 percent it is justifiable that the public fully support the prevention of all births that are unwanted by the family.

The level of expenditure needed to eliminate all fertility that is unwanted by the family is difficult to calculate. The estimate in table 16-6 that 11.6 million births were unwanted in the countries for which we have data is, of course, an underestimate because those countries included only 39 million of the approximately 113 million births that occurred in the developing world in the average year in the late 1980s. The estimates in table 16-14 show an average estimate of about $125 per birth averted in 1987 prices. Preventing the 11.6 million births would cost $1.5 billion. If one can generalize from the WFS data, 30 percent of all births in the developing world are unwanted and preventing them would cost $4.2 billion per year. The United States Agency for International Development (USAID) estimates that $1.5 billion was spent on family planning in 1980 and that $3 billion would be needed in 1990 (Gillespie and others 1988). The USAID estimates imply that if the WFS figures are representative of the world as a whole, substantial increases in funding will still not be sufficient to cover current users plus all those women who want no more children and are not using contraception. Our estimate is that this figure would be $4.6 billion in 1987 prices. This could not cover the unmet need for contraception for spacing. Regardless of exact current resource needs in 1990, by the year 2010 the number of currently married women of reproductive age will have doubled according to USAID estimates. Therefore the expenditure on family planning in the developing world is substantially below what is needed to eliminate unwanted fertility by the estimates of individuals, and those resource requirements are increasing rapidly. The geographic distribution of expenditure is more controversial because of the large difference in geographic distributions of excess fertility by societal and individual estimates of excess fertility. Therefore we know that a substantial increase in expenditure in family planning is needed. There is, however, a large number of factors that are not known.

Priorities for Research

Research in contraceptive technology is needed primarily in the following areas: (a) reversible sterilization, (b) male contraceptive methods, and (c) understanding of the interaction between various contraceptives and AIDS. Reversible sterilization has high priority, not only to expand the range of choice of individuals, but also to meet the requirements of Islamic teachings on what is acceptable.[43] Male contraceptives are needed for a number of reasons. Evidence is accumulating that in many parts of the world husbands do not want significantly more children than their wives, and in some cases they want fewer (Mason and Taj 1987). Therefore it is important to provide them with more methods from which to choose. The interaction of contraception and AIDS is, as explained earlier, an important question in gaining access to the effectiveness and safety in contraceptives.

Although the lack of a perfect contraceptive for all users restricts use to some degree, there are important research questions that still need to be addressed in service delivery, not to mention motivation. As indicated earlier, a large number of women in the developing world who are motivated to limit their fertility or space their births are not using contraception, and many of them say that they do not intend to do so in the future. One important area of research is the ambivalence toward family planning. There has not been a large compendium of information from surveys on why women say they are not using or do not intend to use contraceptives, particularly among the women who want no more children or want to postpone their next birth.[44] Data that have been compiled indicate that there are wide differences in reasons for nonuse of contraception among those who do not want another child. In Nepal and Mexico the main reason was lack of knowledge of a source.[45] Fear of side effects was a prime reason in Asia and Latin America. In three countries of Latin America in the late 1970s, the cost of contraception was also a significant deterrent. Lack of access is not mentioned frequently in African surveys, although it is probably important. In addition, few of the surveys find the opposition of husbands a great problem. In the recent Demographic and Health Surveys, lack of knowledge of contraception was the main reason given in Ghana, conflict with religion and custom was given as an important reason for nonuse of contraception in Senegal, and health concerns about contraceptives were most important in Nigeria. Clearly more research is needed on why people who want to limit fertility do not use contraception. This work should focus on trying to design strategies for family planning delivery which are specific to the concerns of the country. Increasing attention is being given to the quality of service as a dimension of access that affects not only use but efficency of use and continuation.

A final area that needs attention is the determinants of family size preferences themselves. As indicated earlier, particularly in Sub-Saharan Africa, there is a discrepancy between what individuals may consider excess fertility and what might be excessive from the point of view of economic growth and development. It may well be that one reason for the large family size preferences is the lack of access to reliable family planning services. The effect of service access on family size preferences is not well studied in the literature. There is good theoretical reason to believe not only that the access to family planning affects the use of contraception among those who want to limit their fertility, but also that it directly affects whether they wish to limit it (Cochrane and Cochrane 1971 and 1974). The prior question of whether they perceive fertility as a choice is probably related to access as well, but this has not been well researched.

Finally, it is essential to gain a better understanding of contraception for spacing: its determinants and its demographic consequences. This knowledge is basic to the development of family planning services that are best suited to societies such as those in high-mortality countries of Africa, where there is low motivation to limit fertility but high motivation to space births. The role of breastfeeding in the fertility decisionmaking also needs to be more completely researched, especially with respect to spacing.

Appendix 16A. Tables

The tables in this appendix show the relationships between childbearing patterns and the survival of offspring, by country.

Table 16A-1. Total Fertility Rate, Crude Birth Rate, and Rate of Natural Increase, by Country

Country	1960–65			1970–75			1980–85			1985–90		
	TFR	CBR	RNI	TFR	CBR	RNI	TFR	CBR	RNI	TFR	CBR	RNI
Sub-Saharan Africa												
Benin	6.8	48	16	6.8	50	23	7.0	51	30	6.5[a]	49	33[a]
Cameroon	5.7	43	20	5.7	42	23	5.8	43	27	7.0[a]	48	35[a]
Côte d'Ivoire	6.6	43	18	6.7	45	24	6.7	46	30	7.0[a]	48	34[a]
Ghana	6.5	48	28	6.5	47	30	6.5	47	32	6.3[a]	45	32[a]
Kenya	8.1	57	35	8.2	57	39	8.1	55	41	7.7[a]	52	41[a]
Lesotho	5.8	43	20	5.7	43	33	5.8	42	25	5.8[a]	41	28[a]
Liberia	6.3	46	23	6.4	46	26	6.9	49	31	6.6[a]	46	33[a]
Mauritania	6.9	50	23	6.9	50	26	6.9	50	29	6.5[a]	48	30[a]
Nigeria	6.9	42	28	7.1	51	31	7.1	50	33	6.9[a]	50	34[a]
Senegal	6.7	47	21	6.7	47	25	6.5	46	37	6.5[a]	45	28[a]
Sudan	6.7	47	22	6.7	47	25	6.7	46	29	6.6[a]	45	29[a]
Latin America and the Caribbean												
Brazil	6.1	42	30	4.7	34	24	3.8	29	22	3.4	28	21[a]
Colombia	6.7	45	32	4.8	33	24	3.9	29	23	3.2	27	20[a]
Costa Rica	6.9	45	36	4.3	31	26	3.5	31	24	3.3	28	24[a]
Dominican Republic	7.3	48	32	6.3	42	31	4.2	33	25	3.8[a]	31	25[a]
Ecuador	6.9	46	31	6.0	41	30	5.0	35	31	4.3[a]	33	26[a]
Guyana	6.0	40	32	4.5	33	25	3.3	29	23	3.1	27	20[a]
Haiti	6.1	44	23	6.1	43	23	5.7	41	27	4.7[a]	35	22[a]
Jamaica	5.5	40	31	5.4	33	25	3.4	28	23	2.9	26	20[a]
Mexico	6.7	45	34	6.4	43	34	4.6	34	27	3.6	28	23[a]
Panama	5.9	41	31	4.9	36	28	3.5	28	23	3.1	26	23[a]
Paraguay	6.6	42	30	5.7	38	30	4.9	36	29	4.6[a]	35	21[a]
Peru	6.9	46	29	6.0	41	28	5.0	37	26	4.1[a]	32	29[a]
Trinidad and Tobago	5.0	38	31	3.5	27	20	2.9	25	18	2.8	26	23[a]
Venezuela	6.5	44	35	5.0	36	29	4.1	33	27	3.8	31	19[a]
Asia												
Bangladesh	6.7	47	25	7.0	49	28	6.1	45	27	5.5[a]	40	25[a]
China	5.9	38	21	4.7	31	22	2.4	19	12	2.4	21	14
India	5.8	42	23	5.4	38	22	4.3	32	19	4.3[a]	22	20[a]
Indonesia	5.4	43	21	5.5	41	24	4.1	32	19	3.6	29	18
Malaysia	6.1	43	30	5.1	35	24	3.9	31	24	3.5	28	22[a]
Nepal	5.9	46	21	6.5	47	25	6.3	42	23	5.9[a]	41	24[a]
Philippines	6.6	44	31	5.3	37	26	4.4	33	25	3.9	30	23[a]
Korea, Republic of	5.4	40	27	4.1	29	20	2.6	23	17	2.1	20	14
Sri Lanka	5.1	35	26	4.0	29	21	3.4	28	21	2.8	24	18
Thailand	6.4	44	30	5.0	35	26	3.5	28	20	2.8	25	17
Middle East and North Africa												
Egypt	7.1	45	25	5.5	38	22	4.8	37	25	4.5[a]	34	24[a]
Jordan	7.2	48	29	7.4	47	35	7.4	45	37	5.8[a]	38	32[a]
Morocco	7.2	50	30	6.9	46	30	5.1	36	25	4.3[a]	32	23[a]
Pakistan	7.2	48	26	6.5	44	26	5.8	43	28	6.7[a]	47	33[a]
Syrian Arab Rep.	7.5	47	31	7.5	45	33	7.2	47	38	6.8[a]	45	38[a]
Tunisia	7.2	47	29	6.1	37	24	4.8	33	23	4.3[a]	31	23[a]
Turkey	6.0	41	26	5.5	37	25	4.0	30	21	3.7[a]	29	21[a]
Yemen, Republic of	7.0	49	21	7.0	49	23	7.0	49	30	6.8[a]	49	29[a]

Table 16A-2. Estimate for Main Effects Parameters in Model of Neonatal Mortality

| Country | Base | Births in past 2 years | | | Births in the past 2–4 years | | | Mother's education | | Birth order | | | Mother's age at birth | | | Female child |
		One alive	One dead	Two or more	One alive	One dead	Two or more	Medium	High	Fourth to sixth	Seventh or more	First	Less than 20	20–34	35 or more	
Africa																
Senegal	−2.89	1.42	3.49	1.25	1.01	1.31	1.65	0.75	0.57	0.88	0.80	1.38	1.12	0.79	1.38	0.79
Benin	−2.89	1.02	2.72	2.34	0.79	1.55	1.07	0.81	0.42	1.21	1.75	1.07	1.23	1.13	0.76	0.81
Egypt	−3.71	2.46	4.10	4.22	1.21	1.86	1.88	0.74	0.53	1.28	1.28	3.06	1.19	1.30	1.57	0.75
Côte d'Ivoire	−2.90	1.07	2.36	1.39	1.06	2.01	1.60	0.69	0.29	0.91	1.07	2.27	1.26	1.06	1.20	0.69
Cameroon	−3.46	1.36	3.10	2.39	1.06	2.08	1.68	0.87	0.51	1.09	1.08	1.88	1.25	1.14	1.05	0.96
Mauritania	−3.60	1.75	3.67	5.75	1.03	2.53	1.62	1.63	1.14	0.79	1.21	2.05	1.06	0.77	1.21	0.61
Lesotho	−2.90	1.70	3.60	6.82	0.93	1.73	1.25	0.90	1.11	0.81	1.32	1.27	0.91	1.02	1.20	0.90
Kenya	−3.70	1.57	3.16	1.90	1.00	1.80	1.03	0.84	0.67	1.15	1.52	2.61	1.21	1.13	0.95	0.79
Morocco	−3.80	2.77	3.53	2.92	1.08	1.28	1.52	0.57	0.78	1.01	1.39	3.10	1.09	0.91	1.27	0.84
Sudan	−3.61	1.63	4.53	2.48	1.13	2.83	1.68	0.64	0.87	1.16	0.89	2.29	1.09	0.76	1.55	0.66
Ghana	−3.77	1.49	3.10	3.90	1.13	3.06	1.19	0.82	0.83	1.19	1.88	2.44	1.05	0.97	0.79	0.86
Tunisia	−5.50	2.03	8.08	11.36	1.65	3.97	3.46	0.96	0.01	0.64	1.07	2.25	1.65	0.97	1.26	1.06
Average	−3.56	1.69	3.79	3.89	1.09	2.17	1.63	0.85	0.64	1.01	1.27	2.14	1.18	1.00	1.18	0.81
Asia and the Pacific																
Yemen, Republic of	−3.22	1.25	2.72	2.77	0.91	1.02	0.96	0.63	0.83	1.02	1.62	1.49	1.73	1.39	0.61	0.72
Nepal	−2.88	1.58	2.32	1.42	1.02	2.10	1.67	0.80	0.63	0.95	1.15	1.60	1.49	1.17	1.02	0.91
Bangladesh	−3.01	1.99	3.94	3.71	1.14	1.54	1.65	0.89	0.76	0.71	0.90	2.59	1.09	0.85	0.57	0.94
Pakistan	−2.87	1.32	3.06	2.46	1.02	1.62	1.51	0.80	0.66	0.93	0.93	1.84	1.42	1.07	0.97	0.76
Indonesia	−3.50	1.99	2.36	3.19	1.13	1.90	1.77	0.76	0.73	1.05	1.22	1.49	1.72	1.17	1.02	0.82
Thailand	−3.92	2.20	3.97	5.87	1.48	2.61	2.59	0.88	0.39	0.98	1.03	2.80	1.43	1.25	1.22	0.87
Philippines	−3.91	1.62	2.32	2.53	0.68	1.88	1.07	0.90	0.68	1.57	1.65	1.54	1.25	1.05	1.25	0.72
Syrian Arab Republic	−4.81	2.48	7.77	9.39	0.90	2.29	1.08	0.86	0.64	0.90	0.79	3.63	0.89	0.79	1.08	0.84
Jordan	−3.76	1.92	4.26	4.95	0.87	2.05	1.35	0.89	0.73	0.70	0.88	1.90	1.06	0.72	1.00	0.99
Sri Lanka	−3.21	1.36	3.67	3.32	0.95	2.83	1.51	0.77	0.54	0.76	0.61	1.79	1.11	0.85	1.77	0.71
Korea, Republic of	−5.05	2.16	2.80	0.04	1.12	3.56	1.42	0.84	0.40	0.53	0.49	1.65	1.88	1.45	1.05	0.84
Malaysia	−4.49	1.92	3.94	3.78	1.13	3.56	2.48	0.78	0.34	0.47	0.76	1.46	1.38	1.00	0.79	0.73
Average	−3.72	1.82	3.59	3.62	1.03	2.25	1.59	0.82	0.61	0.88	1.00	1.98	1.37	1.06	1.03	0.82
Latin America and the Caribbean																
Haiti	−3.00	1.43	3.74	1.03	1.02	1.67	1.21	0.90	0.41	1.58	1.12	1.40	1.43	1.17	0.87	0.90
Peru	−3.46	1.97	3.29	2.83	1.19	1.88	1.67	0.55	0.42	1.13	1.05	1.67	1.36	0.84	1.06	0.70
Ecuador	−3.49	1.68	2.86	2.61	0.87	1.67	1.25	0.73	0.64	1.19	1.16	1.43	1.38	1.00	1.46	0.79
Colombia	−3.30	1.34	4.01	3.42	0.98	2.41	1.26	0.81	0.47	0.67	0.83	1.16	0.97	0.70	0.84	0.82
Mexico	−3.56	1.31	3.13	3.10	0.88	1.84	1.08	0.73	0.62	1.35	1.82	1.42	1.70	1.27	1.07	0.76
Costa Rica	−3.70	1.54	3.86	5.53	0.88	1.86	1.21	0.78	0.63	0.87	1.02	1.08	1.35	1.17	1.49	0.78
Guyana	−3.36	1.43	6.69	5.47	0.79	1.77	1.22	1.19	0.81	0.74	0.99	1.49	0.87	1.54	2.08	0.61
Panama	−3.60	1.72	5.75	3.56	0.81	1.42	0.54	0.49	0.55	1.49	1.01	1.80	1.11	0.95	2.53	0.79
Jamaica	−3.27	1.54	1.92	0.01	0.89	2.53	0.82	1.02	0.68	0.69	0.81	1.36	0.54	0.40	0.54	1.12
Trinidad and Tobago	−4.56	1.32	6.69	3.35	0.78	1.03	0.97	0.82	0.78	1.75	4.62	1.13	2.97	2.16	1.27	1.05
Average	−3.53	1.53	4.19	3.09	0.91	1.81	1.12	0.80	0.60	1.15	1.44	1.40	1.37	1.12	1.27	0.83
Europe																
Portugal	−4.30	1.21	9.49	5.58	0.75	2.51	2.23	0.86	0.84	1.30	0.72	2.59	1.12	0.94	1.67	0.61

Source: Hobcraft, McDonald, and Rutstein 1985.

Table 16A-3. Estimates for Main Effects Parameters in Model of Postneonatal Mortality

| Country | Base | Births in past 2 years | | | Births in the past 2–4 years | | | Mother's education | | Birth order | | | Mother's age at birth | | | Female child |
		One alive	One dead	Two or more	One alive	One dead	Two or more	Medium	High	Fourth to sixth	Seventh or more	First	Less than 20	20–34	35 or more	
Africa																
Senegal	-2.90	0.65	2.34	3.46	1.21	1.36	1.35	0.80	0.54	1.21	1.09	0.99	1.36	1.39	1.03	0.97
Benin	-3.05	0.91	3.03	2.14	1.40	2.05	1.36	0.66	0.99	1.20	1.30	1.40	1.36	0.97	1.07	0.92
Egypt	-3.26	2.08	2.83	3.16	1.17	1.67	1.84	0.99	0.70	0.96	0.93	1.75	1.36	1.06	1.14	1.17
Côte d'Ivoire	-2.88	1.21	2.16	1.46	1.04	1.63	1.70	0.86	0.67	1.17	1.13	1.45	1.32	1.09	0.84	0.89
Cameroon	-3.12	1.84	2.80	3.42	0.92	1.51	1.46	0.59	0.46	0.99	1.12	1.65	1.17	1.12	1.22	1.13
Mauritania	-3.47	0.90	2.92	2.10	0.66	1.40	0.81	1.04	1.52	0.88	1.86	1.00	1.20	0.94	1.04	1.17
Lesotho	-3.50	1.73	2.18	2.80	1.32	2.20	1.93	1.02	0.76	1.77	1.68	1.26	1.93	1.27	0.79	1.03
Kenya	-3.29	1.75	3.86	3.42	1.02	2.12	1.79	0.77	0.45	0.89	0.96	1.65	1.38	0.90	0.95	0.95
Morocco	-3.79	1.82	3.06	2.94	0.97	1.43	1.46	1.13	0.87	1.16	1.73	1.68	1.46	1.23	0.92	0.96
Sudan	-4.02	2.03	5.42	5.16	1.28	3.49	2.83	0.66	1.21	0.48	0.74	2.53	1.12	1.16	1.04	0.86
Ghana	-3.60	2.39	4.01	3.86	1.02	3.32	1.72	0.58	0.68	0.88	0.84	1.14	1.28	1.22	1.17	0.78
Tunisia	-4.91	2.51	8.67	6.05	0.80	1.58	1.58	0.81	0.01	1.23	1.88	1.42	1.57	1.42	0.73	1.01
Average	-3.48	1.65	3.61	3.33	1.07	1.98	1.65	0.83	0.74	1.07	1.27	1.49	1.38	1.15	1.00	0.99
Asia and the Pacific																
Yemen, Republic of	-3.07	2.44	4.22	4.01	1.12	1.49	1.36	0.79	0.39	0.94	1.19	2.14	1.51	1.09	1.20	0.90
Nepal	-2.88	1.27	1.97	3.82	1.19	1.84	1.67	0.88	0.76	1.07	1.23	1.39	1.54	1.30	0.84	0.99
Bangladesh	-3.03	1.79	2.12	2.03	0.99	1.75	1.23	1.08	0.99	0.73	0.97	1.65	1.14	1.05	0.94	0.78
Pakistan	-3.33	1.62	2.44	2.75	1.16	1.65	1.51	0.88	0.84	1.07	1.01	2.01	1.08	0.96	1.00	1.15
Indonesia	-3.00	2.01	2.44	1.77	0.98	1.92	1.51	0.57	0.28	0.93	0.79	1.54	1.11	0.90	1.13	0.82
Thailand	-3.70	1.95	3.39	2.64	1.11	2.12	1.99	0.82	0.33	0.82	1.19	1.62	1.04	0.89	0.76	1.06
Philippines	-3.39	2.01	2.39	5.05	1.11	1.39	1.35	0.74	0.42	0.84	0.99	0.86	1.07	1.01	1.21	0.75
Syrian Arab Republic	-3.87	2.53	4.39	4.57	1.16	1.97	1.54	0.73	0.37	0.97	1.21	2.59	1.36	1.27	1.16	1.04
Jordan	-4.29	3.94	3.97	8.17	0.99	1.26	1.84	0.65	0.73	0.93	1.05	2.48	1.34	0.92	0.59	1.16
Sri Lanka	-4.28	1.46	1.52	2.69	0.98	1.86	1.63	0.91	0.80	1.45	1.95	1.06	1.30	1.17	0.66	0.92
Korea, Republic of	-4.47	2.12	6.49	6.42	1.31	2.48	2.20	0.61	0.70	1.27	1.45	2.14	1.42	0.93	1.17	1.00
Malaysia	-3.42	0.90	2.46	2.20	0.80	1.80	0.79	0.85	0.39	1.21	2.64	0.89	1.92	1.27	0.96	0.64
Average	-3.56	2.00	3.15	3.84	1.07	1.79	1.55	0.79	0.58	1.02	1.31	1.70	1.32	1.06	0.97	0.94
Latin America and the Caribbean																
Haiti	-2.97	1.80	2.80	2.80	1.20	1.73	1.99	1.92	0.87	0.84	0.86	1.46	0.95	1.06	1.09	0.84
Peru	-3.21	2.14	3.03	3.03	1.08	1.82	1.72	0.58	0.32	1.03	1.07	1.49	1.46	1.12	0.98	0.90
Ecuador	-3.52	1.68	3.22	3.13	0.93	1.67	1.60	0.95	0.39	1.20	1.52	1.68	1.35	1.04	0.83	0.82
Colombia	-3.79	2.72	3.49	4.66	0.97	1.92	1.75	0.43	0.58	0.83	0.83	1.62	1.30	0.95	1.14	0.90
Mexico	-3.66	1.84	2.05	2.64	0.81	1.63	1.65	0.87	0.27	0.97	0.95	1.20	1.34	1.12	1.03	0.84
Costa Rica	-4.06	1.97	2.89	5.00	2.05	3.29	3.39	0.92	0.56	0.78	0.97	1.88	2.05	0.92	1.52	0.62
Guyana	-4.26	1.70	4.06	3.39	1.73	2.94	1.60	1.03	0.88	0.70	0.76	1.42	0.95	0.89	0.82	0.94
Panama	-4.88	1.16	0.77	0.73	1.21	2.27	0.68	0.74	0.39	1.23	2.80	1.13	2.61	2.86	0.82	1.13
Jamaica	-5.34	2.64	9.21	1.63	1.70	2.29	1.23	1.07	0.90	1.01	1.65	1.43	3.22	1.27	1.23	0.91
Trinidad and Tobago	-5.54	2.23	4.10	3.25	1.28	5.31	0.90	1.17	0.80	1.67	2.86	2.86	1.27	1.46	1.40	0.77
Average	-4.12	1.99	3.56	3.03	1.30	2.49	1.65	0.97	0.60	1.03	1.43	1.62	1.65	1.27	0.69	0.87
Europe																
Portugal	-3.85	2.01	0.42	4.35	1.06	0.99	2.05	0.59	0.30	0.85	0.87	0.70	2.48	1.72	1.38	0.90

Source: Hobcraft, McDonald, and Rutstein 1985.

Table 16A-4. *Estimates for Main Effects Parameters in Model of Toddler Mortality*

| Country | Base | Births in past 2 years | | | Births up to one year later | | Mother's education | | Birth order | | | Mother's age at birth | | | Female child |
		One alive	One dead	Two or more	Births	Pregnant	Medium	High	Fourth to sixth	Seventh or more	First	Less than 20	20–34	35 or more	
Africa															
Senegal	−2.44	0.54	1.11	0.75	0.01	0.95	0.75	0.44	1.21	1.36	1.05	1.28	1.00	0.87	1.02
Benin	−3.45	0.79	1.45	0.40	2.18	2.12	0.61	1.00	1.73	1.16	0.75	2.18	1.25	0.97	0.91
Egypt	−3.49	1.62	2.61	2.18	2.46	1.95	0.89	0.61	1.17	1.15	1.17	1.22	1.05	0.99	1.30
Côte d'Ivoire	−3.12	1.00	0.91	3.42	1.92	2.05	0.75	0.67	1.00	0.87	1.11	1.22	1.01	0.86	0.83
Cameroon	−3.30	1.46	2.39	0.61	3.35	1.42	0.77	0.59	0.90	0.78	0.84	1.42	0.97	0.73	0.90
Mauritania	−3.66	0.79	1.80	1.73	1.86	2.36	0.89	0.76	1.36	1.15	0.61	1.15	1.20	1.23	1.14
Lesotho	−3.23	1.04	1.58	2.48	3.39	2.86	0.87	0.56	0.78	0.83	1.12	1.36	1.51	0.87	0.62
Kenya	−3.36	1.43	1.86	1.60	2.01	1.36	0.52	0.53	0.96	0.97	1.09	1.23	0.88	0.92	0.82
Morocco	−3.95	1.82	2.77	1.60	2.01	1.48	0.38	0.00	1.19	1.26	0.84	1.49	1.45	0.98	1.04
Sudan	−3.73	1.04	3.06	1.12	1.92	1.84	0.90	1.42	0.90	0.94	0.87	1.35	0.89	1.46	0.70
Ghana	−3.67	1.26	1.65	0.00	4.95	1.79	0.73	0.55	1.22	1.28	1.21	1.43	1.04	0.84	0.82
Tunisia	−6.62	1.46	2.48	3.56	3.94	4.31	1.57	0.03	1.65	1.97	1.21	1.75	1.58	0.78	0.93
Average	−3.67	1.19	1.97	1.62	2.50	2.04	0.80	0.60	1.17	1.14	0.99	1.43	1.15	0.96	0.92
Asia and the Pacific															
Yemen, Republic of	−3.62	2.80	5.42	2.14	2.12	1.99	0.55	0.75	0.94	0.64	1.84	0.62	0.77	1.02	1.22
Nepal	−2.87	1.46	2.08	1.21	2.10	1.60	0.66	0.29	1.03	0.91	1.01	1.05	0.82	0.73	1.06
Bangladesh	−4.60	1.79	1.45	2.92	2.69	2.69	0.86	0.76	1.40	1.38	1.28	1.77	1.46	1.03	1.31
Pakistan	−3.91	1.48	1.73	0.99	2.14	1.86	0.79	0.21	1.32	1.40	0.83	1.60	1.31	0.89	1.40
Indonesia	−3.73	1.70	2.41	1.90	3.13	2.75	0.83	0.26	1.27	1.45	0.96	1.46	1.12	0.48	0.88
Thailand	−4.79	1.88	3.82	0.00	4.06	3.86	0.76	0.00	0.94	1.63	0.37	1.07	0.98	0.90	0.69
Philippines	−4.06	1.27	2.20	1.32	1.58	1.63	0.68	0.36	1.20	1.46	0.56	1.55	1.04	0.73	0.98
Syrian Arab Republic	−4.75	1.68	2.14	2.27	1.43	1.55	0.66	0.73	1.19	1.39	0.80	1.60	0.90	1.15	0.89
Jordan	−4.18	2.01	3.13	5.26	1.48	1.55	0.65	0.30	0.76	0.68	1.04	0.99	0.88	0.44	1.08
Sri Lanka	−5.67	1.52	1.34	2.34	4.14	0.78	1.06	0.68	2.61	2.61	1.57	2.66	1.77	0.81	1.13
Korea, Republic of	−6.49	2.97	2.56	0.07	4.66	5.47	0.71	0.23	1.58	1.16	2.32	1.88	0.70	1.86	2.72
Fiji	−5.13	2.18	0.01	3.10	1.17	0.33	1.79	1.49	0.86	0.43	0.82	0.97	0.12	0.33	0.66
Malaysia	−5.35	0.98	3.53	0.01	1.62	1.38	1.17	0.00	1.17	1.90	0.30	1.43	0.99	1.77	0.53
Average	−4.55	1.83	2.45	1.81	2.49	2.11	0.86	0.47	1.25	1.31	1.05	1.44	0.99	0.93	1.12
Latin America and the Caribbean															
Haiti	−3.34	1.06	2.20	6.17	1.02	1.22	0.00	0.89	1.13	0.63	1.13	1.03	0.84	1.09	0.76
Peru	−3.49	1.95	2.32	1.77	2.10	1.90	0.27	0.14	0.94	0.96	1.35	0.91	0.89	0.89	1.12
Dominican Republic	−3.78	1.45	1.34	3.29	3.42	1.39	0.58	0.23	1.14	0.87	0.43	1.52	1.22	1.09	1.27
Ecuador	−3.86	1.45	1.90	1.03	2.08	1.62	0.58	0.34	1.13	1.16	0.63	2.46	1.92	1.32	0.91
Colombia	−4.46	1.62	2.23	3.00	1.67	1.08	0.76	0.22	0.84	0.61	0.61	1.54	1.51	1.40	1.60
Mexico	−4.56	1.35	2.75	2.41	3.16	1.62	0.53	0.33	1.77	1.51	0.70	2.32	1.38	1.03	0.85
Paraguay	−4.54	1.19	0.57	0.01	1.72	1.75	0.76	0.54	1.07	1.28	0.55	1.17	1.77	1.08	0.69
Costa Rica	−4.76	0.96	2.12	2.92	2.34	1.17	0.44	0.28	1.30	2.14	0.85	2.61	1.62	0.92	0.98
Guyana	−6.36	1.19	2.16	2.48	1.67	2.29	1.60	1.38	2.48	3.32	0.78	4.66	1.22	2.03	0.76
Venezuela	−4.62	1.05	1.21	1.54	0.92	1.13	0.62	0.00	0.97	1.43	0.95	1.03	1.72	0.76	0.79
Panama	−4.39	1.15	1.27	1.28	2.23	0.80	0.57	0.30	1.21	1.48	0.83	1.34	1.14	1.06	0.98
Jamaica	−4.22	1.21	0.98	0.01	1.80	0.48	0.68	0.45	1.28	1.62	1.20	2.94	1.11	0.87	0.66
Trinidad and Tobago	−6.55	0.95	0.01	0.01	2.64	1.79	1.43	0.91	0.78	1.90	0.66	2.20	2.61	0.90	2.44
Average	−4.53	1.27	1.62	1.99	2.06	1.40	0.68	0.46	1.23	1.45	0.82	1.98	1.46	1.11	1.06
Europe															
Portugal	−6.50	4.10	6.82	0.01	5.64	1.21	0.35	0.32	1.75	1.08	0.98	5.64	1.54	2.08	1.09

Source: Hobcraft, McDonald, and Rutstein 1985.

Country	Base	Births in past 2 years			Births up to 1 year later			Mother's education		Birth order			Mother's age at birth			Female child
		One alive	One dead	Two or more	One or more alive	None alive	Pregnant	Medium	High	Fourth to sixth	Seventh or more	First	Less than 20	20–34	35 or more	
Africa																
Senegal	-2.34	0.70	0.83	0.00	0.89	0.67	0.00	0.73	0.22	0.83	1.17	0.91	1.12	1.15	0.72	1.05
Benin	-2.37	0.76	1.35	0.76	0.95	1.09	2.80	0.50	0.43	0.87	0.88	0.84	1.11	1.03	1.06	0.95
Egypt	-3.54	1.73	1.60	1.99	1.40	1.54	2.39	0.82	0.57	1.43	1.30	0.64	1.22	0.94	0.83	1.15
Côte d'Ivoire	-3.04	1.27	1.16	0.00	1.20	1.31	0.00	0.90	0.43	1.13	0.84	0.76	1.62	1.14	1.11	0.88
Cameroon	-2.90	1.28	1.86	1.16	0.95	1.58	1.57	0.63	1.97	1.27	1.46	1.51	0.79	0.87	0.95	1.03
Mauritania	-2.74	0.98	0.90	1.95	0.96	1.54	1.93	1.17	0.52	1.16	1.26	0.66	1.34	0.96	1.17	1.06
Lesotho	-3.47	2.97	0.75	0.01	0.92	0.64	0.01	0.63	0.49	1.43	0.45	1.12	1.73	1.68	1.14	0.68
Kenya	-3.57	1.21	1.70	1.75	0.99	1.09	0.83	0.59	0.74	1.05	1.49	0.78	1.40	0.96	1.16	0.95
Morocco	-4.06	1.84	1.63	2.69	1.01	1.79	2.69	0.27	0.00	1.39	1.55	1.17	1.52	1.07	1.11	0.84
Sudan	-3.68	1.19	1.36	1.73	1.19	3.03	1.93	0.52	2.29	1.21	1.23	0.71	1.26	0.86	1.54	1.27
Ghana	-3.61	1.54	1.15	0.00	1.35	2.97	1.09	0.30	0.38	1.03	0.85	0.99	2.10	1.27	1.55	0.96
Tunisia	-5.11	2.25	5.75	4.44	2.16	2.34	3.03	0.51	0.01	1.30	1.62	1.31	1.00	1.27	1.14	1.42
Average	-3.37	1.48	1.67	1.38	1.16	1.63	1.52	0.63	0.67	1.18	1.18	0.95	1.35	1.10	1.12	1.02
Asia and the Pacific																
Yemen, Republic of	-3.27	3.25	1.95	4.44	0.85	1.09	1.58	0.58	0.60	0.81	0.68	1.55	1.16	0.87	0.87	1.23
Nepal	-3.36	1.31	1.08	1.90	1.31	2.14	3.13	0.65	0.24	1.52	1.58	0.78	1.67	1.21	0.59	1.07
Bangladesh	-3.14	1.63	1.23	2.53	1.73	1.28	1.63	0.73	0.39	1.09	0.98	0.96	1.00	0.88	0.97	1.13
Pakistan	-3.42	1.52	1.28	1.46	1.05	1.49	1.08	0.68	2.61	1.11	0.97	0.76	1.43	1.17	1.20	1.31
Indonesia	-3.26	1.25	1.48	2.72	2.18	1.42	3.35	0.64	0.19	1.00	1.15	0.80	1.52	1.03	0.90	0.77
Thailand	-4.34	1.55	0.85	3.10	1.65	2.27	3.16	0.73	0.19	1.58	1.60	0.64	1.14	1.17	0.56	1.57
Philippines	-4.64	1.63	2.77	1.77	1.31	1.25	2.16	0.83	0.25	1.51	1.79	1.02	1.48	1.00	0.59	0.89
Syrian Arab Republic	-4.91	1.23	2.75	1.16	1.17	1.32	1.67	0.31	0.16	1.62	1.35	0.84	0.91	1.09	0.41	1.32
Jordan	-4.94	1.93	1.90	3.46	1.11	1.51	0.84	0.12	0.22	1.14	0.64	0.73	1.65	1.07	0.53	0.79
Sri Lanka	-4.10	1.08	0.79	0.50	1.72	2.32	0.46	0.68	0.35	1.21	1.73	0.56	1.14	0.85	0.55	0.96
Korea, Republic of	-6.08	0.59	3.35	0.03	1.70	0.02	0.03	0.61	0.44	0.76	0.21	2.05	1.51	2.97	4.95	0.88
Fiji	-5.38	0.67	1.04	301.87	0.81	0.00	0.00	1.12	1.73	1.14	0.77	0.28	0.54	0.97	1.04	1.05
Malaysia	-5.80	0.77	1.19	6.89	1.58	0.01	0.02	0.58	0.38	2.25	1.79	0.47	4.57	0.77	2.69	0.90
Average	-4.36	1.42	1.67	22.24	1.40	1.24	1.47	0.64	0.60	1.29	1.17	0.88	1.52	1.16	1.22	1.07
Americas and the Caribbean																
Haiti	-2.80	1.40	1.03	0.00	1.06	1.02	3.13	1.27	0.52	0.73	0.37	0.76	1.55	0.94	1.39	1.06
Peru	-3.93	1.35	1.21	1.48	0.98	1.42	4.35	0.30	0.15	1.46	1.65	0.73	2.27	1.39	0.95	1.20
Dominican Republic	-3.76	1.43	0.75	1.26	1.26	1.48	0.52	0.55	0.16	0.39	1.02	0.71	1.58	1.30	0.41	1.05
Ecuador	-4.01	1.07	1.54	1.90	1.55	2.77	2.41	0.54	0.34	0.98	1.12	0.68	0.89	1.31	0.84	1.09
Colombia	-3.90	1.31	1.52	0.85	1.28	1.93	4.62	0.62	0.18	1.08	0.88	0.92	1.04	0.83	1.55	1.02
Mexico	-3.98	0.88	0.91	0.74	1.05	0.78	4.22	0.32	0.05	1.27	1.03	0.80	1.46	0.64	1.05	1.19
Paraguay	-4.19	1.15	0.58	1.51	1.16	1.25	0.02	0.38	0.15	0.95	1.86	0.89	1.30	1.55	0.85	0.36
Costa Rica	-5.32	1.17	0.57	2.46	1.30	2.59	4.35	0.63	0.00	1.79	1.21	0.80	0.76	0.68	1.42	1.49
Guyana	-4.63	1.27	0.80	0.00	1.04	0.00	0.01	1.07	0.47	1.20	0.85	1.49	0.00	0.42	1.04	0.91
Venezuela	-5.56	2.14	0.01	5.75	1.09	3.25	4.85	0.38	0.12	1.88	1.36	2.41	1.30	1.63	0.01	1.23
Panama	-5.20	0.85	0.78	0.01	1.86	0.01	3.39	0.35	0.32	1.58	2.03	1.45	2.16	1.34	0.53	1.31
Jamaica	-7.51	6.11	8.76	0.04	2.59	0.01	0.01	0.19	0.21	3.74	2.61	24.53	0.78	0.56	1.04	1.51
Trinidad and Tobago	-7.81	0.48	0.70	0.02	2.86	20.49	31.19	0.00	1.55	0.49	2.46	1.19	1.14	0.79	0.00	2.66
Average	-4.82	1.59	1.47	1.23	1.54	2.85	4.85	0.51	0.33	1.35	1.42	1.00	1.25	1.03	0.85	1.24
Europe																
Portugal	-9.86	4.57	0.00	0.00	2.18	0.00	0.00	3.00	6.75	6.36	15.64	1.14	16.12	6.17	1.25	0.80

Source: Hobcraft, McDonald, and Rutstein 1985.

357

Notes

The authors would like to thank Dr. Julie Da Vanzo of Rand Corporation, Drs. Judith Fortney and Nancy Williamson of Family Health International and Ms. Jane Nassim and Mr. Rodolfo Bulatao of the World Bank for helpful comments. Several anonymous reviewers also provided useful insights. Any remaining deficiencies in the chapter are, of course, the responsibility of the authors.

1. The countries selected were, for the most part, countries in which survey data allow us to compare these aggregate measures of fertility and excess fertility with individual reports of excess fertility or the desire to cease childbearing. Unfortunately, China, India, and Brazil have no World Fertility Survey data sponsored by USAID and UNFPA available to draw on for comparisons, but Brazil has participated in the more recent Demographic and Health Survey, sponsored by USAID.

2. The dramatic nature of these declines in fertility can be observed by a decline by half in the TFR between the early 1960s and the late 1980s in Colombia, Costa Rica, and the Dominican Republic and by 40 percent or more in Brazil, Ecuador, Mexico, and Venezuela.

3. Half or more of the developing countries of all regions except central west Asia perceived their population growth as being excessive. None of the countries in the Economic and Social Commission for Africa (ESCWA) had that perception (United Nations 1989, p. 14).

4. Governments of 68 of 131 developing countries have reported to the United Nations that fertility is too high in their country (United Nations 1989, p. 14).

5. See the National Research Council's review for detailed discussion of the health consequences for women and children in developing countries of contraception and reproduction (NRC 1989).

6. This summation represents a simplification. In a period of transition, such as the baby boom in the United States after World War II, the TFR can be much higher than the average parity. Such a situation occurs if women have been postponing their first and second births and all women of different ages are having low-parity births at the same time.

7. It should be noted that in these microeconomic studies, the percentage at risk because of high parity is much larger than the percentage by which the TFR exceeds four. The reader should bear this in mind when interpreting the figures in table 16-3.

8. See footnotes to table 16-3 for descriptions of how the number of women in various categories are assigned to categories of excess births.

9. Asia's pattern is distorted by the very low fertility in China.

10. More recent data from Kenya would give lower excess fertility, 43 and 83 percent, respectively, by these measures but higher excess fertility by preference measures.

11. Although most surveys report data only for women, a number of surveys report men's family size preferences. Contrary to what is generally believed, men do not systematically report higher fertility preferences than women (Mason and Taj 1987). Perhaps the men do bear some costs of higher fertility by having to work harder to support larger families in those environments where marriages are stable.

12. Time constraints have not allowed the recalculation of these artificial TFRs for more recent years.

13. Bongaarts, Mauldin, and Phillips (1990) estimate unwanted fertility preferences for the developing world, including China, at 21 percent. In China and a number of countries in Africa, there is deficit fertility which has not been netted out of these estimates.

14. In every country the youngest women report lower fertility preferences than the oldest women. Part of this may result from reporting bias mentioned above and part from genuine declining preferences.

15. A birth postponed will reduce the rate of growth in the short term. In addition, many births that are postponed never take place.

16. More recent Demographic and Health Surveys show that more than 20 percent of the women wish to cease childbearing in Burundi, Ghana, and Ondo State in Nigeria.

17. The proportions of women who wish to limit their fertility in the three countries are 30 percent, 23 percent, and 64 percent, respectively. The proportions currently using contraceptives are 25 percent, 12 percent, and 53 percent, respectively.

18. Because many of those who wish to space a child will go on to have further births, there is no correct assumption that would allow the conversion of spacing into excess births. Therefore, one-half was chosen as an arbitrary figure. It is clearly incorrect to assume that all those who wish to space should be counted. Likewise it is incorrect to assume that the spacers account for no excess fertility. In these models, 26 percent, 38 percent, and 14 percent of the women wish to space their next birth.

19. The three main arguments why increased contraception will not improve survival rates are (a) that reducing high parity births will result in a larger proportion of births being first births and these births have even higher mortality than high-parity births; (b) that these correlations are not causative but are associated with other characteristics of the mother or family, such as low education and economic status; and (c) that changes in contraceptive use may be associated with other changes in behavior, such as the reduction of breastfeeding, which will cause increased health risks.

20. The biological mechanisms to explain these relationships have not been identified (Haaga 1989).

21. This is an underestimate to the extent that it ignores the intervals in which a child was born in the preceding twelve months and then died. In those cases, the causal issues are more complex. It also ignores the effect of the postponed birth on the mortality risk of previous children.

22. Here and throughout, 1987 U.S. dollars are used.

23. This estimate is based on the cost of Community-based distribution (CBD) programs as estimated from a number of countries by Cochrane, Hammer, Janowitz, and Kenney (1990).

24. This corresponds to a mid-range of costs for a couple-year of protection for clinic-based distribution of oral contraceptives and intrauterine contraceptive devices (Cochrane and others 1990).

25. The health costs of high fertility and close spacing of children are discussed in chapter 17, this collection. Family planning can reduce maternal mortality in two ways: (a) the fewer the births a woman has, the fewer her exposures to the risk of maternal mortality, and (b) by confining births to the healthiest age groups and spacing births to the best intervals, the risk of death associated with every birth that does take place is reduced. There exist various estimates of the effect of family planning on mortality. It has been estimated that 24 percent of maternal deaths could be averted by contraceptive use by fecund women not currently using contraception but desiring no more births (Sai and Nassim 1987).

There has been somewhat of a revision of position in the development community in the United States and the development agencies away from the dire predictions of the negative consequences of rapid population growth (NRC 1986) just at the time that some Latin American and French scholars and African politicians are becoming more concerned (Blanchet 1988; Paiva 1988).

26. See Birdsall, Cochrane, and Van der Gaag (1987) for a review of the methodological issues and estimates of child costs in industrial countries. See Lindert (1980) for a review of the estimates available for developing countries. In addition Deaton and Muelbauer (1986) have recently estimated the costs of a child in Sri Lanka and Indonesia.

27. One reason it is so hard to determine the consequences of high fertility is that the causation goes in two directions and income can affect fertility as well as the converse.

28. Neither is there a well-defined range of the cost of a child, since the effect of a child on his or her parents and other siblings varies substantially from one environment to another. Deaton and Muellbauer (1986) estimate that parents spend about 30 to 40 percent of what they spend on themselves on a child in Sri Lanka and Indonesia. Because they do not include the time or opportunity costs that the child imposes on others in the family, these expenditures are only part of the costs to a family of an additional child.

29. See King 1970 for an example for Jamaica.

30. The exchange rate between the peso and the U.S. dollar was 120 in 1983.

31. These estimates are too large to the extent that there are economies of scale, and thus marginal costs of a child are below average costs. The estimates are made assuming a government commitment to universal primary education

and a progression rate from primary to secondary education similar to current patterns in the country. Costs are obtained from two World Bank internal documents: "Comparative Education Indicators" for recurrent costs and "Unit Cost Estimates" for the capital costs. These costs have been inflated to 1987 as a base. Because no unit recurrent costs are available for secondary school we have assumed that the ratio of recurrent secondary recurrent costs to primary recurrent costs reflects the ratio of their respective capital costs per school place. There is no comparable measure of the health costs to be saved by a birth averted. *Financing Health Services in Developing Countries: An Agenda for Reform* (World Bank 1987) provided the per capita health expenditure for a range of countries that can be used as a first approximation. For the two poor, high-mortality countries the annual per capita public expenditure on health of Sri Lanka and China have been used, $6. For the low-mortality country an average of seven countries has been used, yielding $28 per capita. The education costs have not been adjusted to reflect the age structure of mortality. The education figures would be at least 17 percent lower if the probability of survival to age five were used to adjust the figures. The health expenditure for each country does reflect mortality to the extent that the number of years included depends on the life expectancy in the model country. A more sophisticated method would weigh health cost in each year by the survival cohort for that age. This would require information on expenditure by age, which is not available. The authors of chapter 17 in this collection are preparing estimates of costs that could be used in the calculations here as well if an age profile of expenditure were to be used.

32. In Northern Nigeria in 1981 the median age of first marriage was fifteen, which means that half the women are married by that age or earlier (*Nigeria Fertility Survey 1981/1982*, published in 1984 by the National Population Bureau).

33. The health benefits of breastfeeding are substantial but must be balanced against the time and nutritional costs to the mother. This is a topic that has been extensively discussed in the literature.

34. A more comprehensive list of failure rates by method and study is available in Trussell and Krost (1987). Their estimates include an estimate of failure rates for Norplant (a contraceptive implant) of 0.2 compared with 2 to 2.5 for oral contraceptives.

35. These estimates are taken from general data sets. For actual policy analysis in a country, detailed analysis of the family planning delivery system would be necessary.

36. There is some evidence that real costs per user have dropped since 1980 in Indonesia even when costs of the health delivery of the family planning program are included (World Bank 1990).

37. There are two main reasons why costs would drop the more women are motivated to cease childbearing. First, the more motivated the women, the more likely they are to be using contraception. If there are economies of scale, then costs would fall. Second, the more motivated women are, the less money needs to be spent on motivation and the less extensive the delivery system needs to be, because presumably the more motivated women will travel further to get services.

38. Using the lower estimate of costs per birth averted, one gets estimates of $238, $191, and $121, respectively.

39. The conclusions remain unchanged if the lower estimate of the costs per birth averted is used rather than the higher.

40. The cost of the materials alone is $17, which is high compared with approximately $2 a year for the oral contraceptive but almost identical to the five-year costs of injections. That cost has to be incurred up front, thus discouraging many programs.

41. These expenses cover universal primary education and public health expenditures per capita on the level of Sri Lanka and China.

42. Cochrane and Zachariah (1983) showed that reducing infant and child mortality was a more cost-effective way to reduce fertility than family planning in some very high mortality countries that had a low proportion of women wanting no more children. The data in that case applied to Kenya.

43. In Indonesia, for example, religious leaders have ruled that any irreversible change cannot be justified except on health grounds (World Bank 1990).

44. Johnson-Acsadi and Szykman (1980) and Ainsworth (1985) compiled data on the reason for nonuse of contraception for six and ten countries, respectively, from data from the late 1970s or early 1980s.

45. The data for Mexico were from 1978. It is interesting to note that once the government undertook support for family planning about that time, there was a rapid decline in fertility.

References

Ainsworth, Martha. 1985. *Family Planning Programs: The Client's Perspective.* World Bank Staff Working Paper 676, World Bank, Washington, D.C.

Barnum, Howard N. 1983. *Cost-Effectiveness of Family Planning Services in Nepal.* Technical Notes, RES 9. Population, Health, and Nutrition Division, World Bank, Washington, D.C.

Birdsall, Nancy, Susan H. Cochrane, and Jacques van der Gaag. 1987. "The Cost of Children." In George Psacharopoulos, ed., *Economics of Education: Research and Studies.* New York: Pergamon Press.

Blanchet, Didier. 1988. "Estimating the Relationship between Population Growth and Aggregate Economic Growth in LDCs: Methodological Problems." Paper presented at the meeting of the United Nations Expert Group on Consequences of Rapid Population Growth in Developing Countries. New York, N.Y., August.

Bongaarts, Jon. 1978. "A Framework for Analyzing the Proximate Determinants of Fertility." *Population and Development Review* 4:105–32.

———. 1987. "Does Family Planning Reduce Infant Mortality?" *Population and Development Review* 13:323–24.

———. 1988. "Does Family Planning Reduce Infant Mortality? Reply." *Population and Development Review* 14:188–90.

Bongaarts, Jon, W. Parker Mauldin, James F. Phillips. 1990. "The Demographic Impact of Family Planning Programs." Population Council Working Paper 17. New York.

Boulier, Bryan L. 1986. "Family Planning Programs and Contraceptive Availability: Their Effects on Contraceptive Use and Fertility." In Nancy Birdsall, ed., *The Effects of Family Planning Programs on Fertility in the Developing World.* World Bank Staff Working Paper 677, Population and Development 2. Washington, D.C.

Bruce, Judith. 1990. "Fundamental Elements of the Quality of Care: A Simple Framework." *Studies in Family Planning* 21(2):61–91.

Bulatao, Rudolfo A. 1985. *Expenditures on Population Programs in Developing Regions: Current Levels and Future Requirements.* World Bank Staff Working Paper 679, Population and Development 4. Washington, D.C.

Casterline, John B. 1990. "Integrating Health Risk Consideration and Fertility Preference in Assessing the Demand for Family Planning." World Bank consultant report. Washington, D.C.

CDC (Centers for Disease Control). 1983. "Family Planning Methods and Practices: Africa." Health Promotion and Education, Division of Reproductive Health, Atlanta, Ga.

Chao, Dennis N. W., John Ross, and David Piet. 1985. "Public Expenditure Impact: Education and Health, Indonesian Family Planning.": BKKBN/USAID, Jakarta.

Chernichovsky, Dov, Henry Pardako, David de Leeuw, Pudjo Raherje, and Charles Lerman. 1989. In "The Indonesian Family Planning Program: An Economic Perspective." Typescript. East Asia and Pacific Country Department 1 (Philippines).

Cochrane, Susan. 1983. "The Effects of Education and Urbanization." In R. A. Bulatao and Ronald D. Lee, eds., *Determinants of Fertility: A Summary of Knowledge.* Washington, D.C.: National Academy of Sciences.

Cochrane, Susan, and J. L. Cochrane. 1971. "Child Mortality and Birth: A Micro-Economic Approach." *American Statistical Association and Proceedings.*

———. 1974. "Child Mortality and Desired Number of Children and Births." *Australian Economic Papers,* 13.

Cochrane, Susan, Valerie Kozel, and Harold Alderman. 1990. *Household Consequences of High Fertility: The Case of Pakistan.* World Bank Discussion Paper 111. Washington, D.C.

Cochrane, Susan H., and K. L. Zachariah. 1983. *Infant and Child Mortality as a Determinant of Fertility: The Policy Implications.* World Bank Staff Working Paper 556. Washington, D.C.

Cochrane, Susan, Jeffery Hammer, Barbara Janowitz, and Genevieve Kenney. 1990. "The Economics of Family Planning." Typescript. Population, Health, and Nutrition Division; World Bank, Washington, D.C.

David, Henry P. 1986. "Unwanted Children: A Follow-Up from Prague." *Family Planning Perspectives* 18(3):143–44.

Deaton, Angus S., and John Muellbauer. 1986. "On Measuring Child Costs: With Applications to Poor Countries." *Journal of Political Economy* 94(4):720–44.

Demeny, Paul. 1965. "Investment Allocations and Population Growth." *Demography* 2:203–32.

DHS (Demographic and Health Surveys). Various years, Various countries. Columbia, Md.: Institute for Resource Development.

Duza, M. B., and C. S. Baldwin. 1974. *Nuptiality as an Area for Policy Intervention: A Comparative Perspective.* New York.: Population Council.

Enke, Stephen. 1960. "The Gains to India from Population Control: Some Money Measures and Incentive Schemes." *Review of Economics and Statistics* 17(2):175–81.

Figa-Talamanca, Irene, T. A. Sinnalhuvary, K. Yusaf, and Chee Kin Fong. 1986. "Illegal Abortion: An Attempt to Assess Its Cost to the Health Service and Its Incidence in the Community." *International Journal of Health Services: Health and Social Policy* 16(3):375–89.

Gillespie, Duff, H. E. Cross, J. G. Crowley, and S. R. Radloff. 1988. "Financing the Delivery of Contraceptives: The Challenge of the Next Twenty Years." *The Demographic and Programmatic Consequences of Contraceptive Innovations.* Committee on Population, National Academy of Sciences, Washington, D.C.

Green, Cynthia P. 1989. "Media Promotion of Breastfeeding: A Decade's Experience." Nutrition Communication Project, conducted by the Academy for Educational Development for U.S. Agency for International Development, Washington, D.C.

Haaga, John G. 1989. "Mechanisms for the Association of Maternal Age, Parity, and Birth Spacing with Infant Health." In National Research Council, *Contraceptive Use and Controlled Fertility.* Washington, D.C.: National Academy Press.

Henshaw, Stanley K. 1987. "Induced Abortion: A Worldwide Perspective." *International Family Planning Perspective* 13(1):12–15.

Hobcraft, John. 1983. "Child Spacing Effects on Infant and Early Child Mortality." *Population Index* 49(4):585–618.

———. 1987. "Does Family Planning Save Children's Lives." Paper prepared for the International Conference on Better Health for Women and Children through Family Planning. Nairobi, October 5–9.

Hobcraft, J. N., J. W. McDonald, and S. O. Rutstein. 1985. "Demographic Determinants of Infant and Early Child Mortality: A Comparative Analysis." *Population Studies* 39(3):363–86.

Holck, S., and H. Bathija. 1988. "Safety and Efficacy of Fertility Relating Methods." In E. Diczfalusy, P. D. Griffin, and J. Khanna, eds., *Research in Human Reproduction: Biennial Report (1986–1987).* Geneva: World Health Organization Special Programme on Research, Development, and Research Training in Human Reproduction.

Huffman, Sandra, and C. Combest. 1988. "Promotion of Breastfeeding: Yes, It Works!" Center to Prevent Childhood Malnutrition, Bethesda, Md.

Hutchings, Jane, and Lyle Sanders. 1985. "Assessing the Characteristics and Cost-Effectiveness of Contraceptive Methods." Paper 10. PIACT (Program for the Introduction and Adaption of Contraceptive Technology), Seattle, Wash.

Jain, Anrudh K. 1989. "Assessing the Fertility Impact of Quality of Family Planning Services." Population Council, New York.

Johnson-Ascadi, Gwendolyn, and Maurice Szykman. 1980. "Selected Characteristics of 'Exposed' Women Who Wanted No More Children but Were Not Using Contraception." In *Survey Analysis for the Guidance of Family Planning Programs.* Liège: Ordina.

Kelley, Alan. 1988. "Economic Consequences of Population Change in the Third World." *Journal of Economic Literature* 26:1685–1728.

King, Elizabeth M. 1987. "The Effect of Family Size on Family Welfare: What Do We Know?" In D. Gale Johnson and Ronald D. Lee, eds., *Population Growth and Economic Development: Issues and Evidence.* Madison: University of Wisconsin Press.

King, Timothy. 1970. *The Measurement of Economic Benefits from Family Planning Projects and Programs.* World Bank Working Paper 71. Washington, D.C.

Kiranandana, Thienchay, Suchada Kiranandana, Suwanee Surasieng Sunk, Rachanivran Uthaism in collaboration with others. 1984. "Planning for Family Planning Programs and Social Services in Thailand." Chulalongkorn University.

Kwast, Barbara, W. Kidav-Mariam, E. M. Saed, F. G. R. Fowkes. 1985. "Epidemiology of Maternal Mortality in Addis Ababa: A Community-Based Study." Paper presented at the World Health Organization International Meeting on Prevention of Maternal Mortality, November 11–15, 1985, Geneva.

Labbok, M. H., and M. McDonald, eds. 1990. "Proceedings of the Interagency Workshop on Health Care Practices Related to Breastfeeding." *International Journal of Gynecology and Obstetrics* 31(supplement 1).

Lancet. 1988. "Breastfeeding as a Family Planning Method." ii:1204–5.

Lapham, Robert and George Simmons. 1987. *Organizing for Effective Family Planning Programs.* Washington, D.C.: National Academy Press.

Lee, Nancy, Herbert Peterson, and Susan Chu. 1989. "Health Effects of Contraception." In National Research Council, *Contraceptive Use and Controlled Fertility.* Washington, D.C.: National Academy Press.

Lightbourne, Robert E. 1987. "Reproductive Preferences and Behavior." In John Cleland and Chris Scott, eds., *The World Fertility Survey: An Assessment.* London: International Statistics Institute.

Lindert, Peter H. 1980. "Child Costs and Economic Development." In Richard A. Easterlin, ed., *Population and Economic Change in Developing Countries.* Chicago: University of Chicago Press.

Liskin, L. S. 1980. "Complications of Abortions in Developing Countries," *Population Reports* Series F 7 (July).

Maine, Deborah. 1985. "Maternal Mortality in the Third World." *People* 12(2):6–8.

Mason, Karen Oppenheim, and Anju Malhotra Taj. 1987. "Gender Differences in Reproductive Goals in Developing Countries." Population Studies Center Research Report 87–105. University of Michigan, Ann Arbor.

National Population Bureau. 1984. *The Nigerian Fertility Survey Principal Report.* 2 Vols. London: International Statistical Institute.

Nortman, Dorothy. 1986. "Cost-Benefit Analysis of the Mexican Social Security Administration's Family Planning Program." *Studies in Family Planning* 17(1):1–6.

Nortman, Dorothy L., and Gary L. Lewis. 1986. "A Time Model to Measure Contraceptive Demand." In John A. Ross, ed., *Survey Analysis for the Guidance of Family Planning Programs.* Liège: Ordina.

NRC (National Research Council). 1986. Working Group on Population Growth and Economic Development, Committee on Population, Commission on Behavioral and Social Sciences and Education, eds., *Population Growth and Economic Development: Policy Questions.* Washington, D.C.: National Academy Press.

———. 1989. *Contraception and Reproduction: Health Consequences for Women and Children in the Developing World.* Washington, D.C.: National Academy Press.

———. 1990. *Developing New Contraceptives: Obstacles and Opportunities.* Washington, D.C.: National Academy Press.

Ohlin, Goran. 1967. "Population Control and Economic Development." Development Center for the Organization for Economic Cooperation and Development (OECD), Paris.

Paiva, P. D. 1988. "Rapid Population Growth and Economic Development in Latin America." Paper presented at the meeting of the United Nations

Expert Group on Consequences of Rapid Population Growth in Developing Countries, New York, August.

Population Crisis Committee. 1985. "Issues in Contraceptive Development." *Population.* Briefing paper 15 (May).

Population Information Program. 1980. "Complications of Abortion in Developing Countries." In *Population Reports: Pregnancy Terminations.* Series F 7. Baltimore: Johns Hopkins University.

Potter, Joseph E. 1988. "Does Family Planning Reduce Infant Mortality?" *Population and Development Review* 14:170–87.

Potts, Malcom, J. J. Speidel, and E. Kassel. 1977. "Relative Risks of Various Means of Fertility Control when Used in Less Developed Countries." In J. J. Sciarra, G. Zatuchni, and J. J. Speidel, eds., *Risks, Benefits, and Controversies in Fertility Control.* Arlington, Va. (1978. Hagerstown, Md.: Harper and Rowe.)

Ross, John A., Marjorie Rich, Janet Molzan, and Michael Pensak. 1988. "Family Planning and Child Survival: 100 Developing Countries." Center for Population and Family Health, Columbia University, New York.

Sai, Fred and Janet Nassim. 1987. "The Role of International Agencies, Governments, and the Private Sector in the Diffusion of Modern Contraception." *Technology in Society* 9:497–520.

Salkever, David, and Ismail Serageldin. 1983. "Cost-Benefit and Cost-Effectiveness Analysis in Population Programs: Its Role in Program Planning and Management." In Ismael Abdel-Hamid Serageldin, David S. Salkever, and Richard W. Osborn. eds., *Evaluating Population Programs: International Experience with Cost-Effectiveness Analysis and Cost-Benefit Analysis.* New York: St. Martin's Press; London: Croom Helm.

Scrimshaw, Susan. 1978. "Infant Mortality and Behavior in the Regulation of Family Size." *Population and Development Review* 4:383–404.

———. 1983. "Infanticide as Deliberate Fertility Regulation." In R. A. Bulatao and R. D. Lee, eds., *Determinant of Fertility in Developing Countries.* New York: Academic Press.

Serageldin, Ismail. 1983. *Evaluating Population Programs: International Experience with Cost-Effectiveness Analysis and Cost-Benefit Analysis.* New York: St. Martin's Press; London: Croom Helm.

Shorter, Edward. 1977. *The Making of the Modern Family.* New York: Basic Books.

Speidel, J. J. 1983. "Cost Implications of Population Stabilization." In Ismail Serageldin and others, eds., *Evaluating Population Programs: International Experience with Cost-Effectiveness Analysis and Cost-Benefit Analysis.* New York: St. Martin's Press; London: Croom Helm.

Trussell, James. 1988. "Does Family Planning Reduce Infant Mortality? An Exchange." *Population and Development Review* 14:171–78.

Trussell, James, and Kathryn Krost. 1987. "Contraceptive Failure in the United States: A Critical Review of the Literature." *Studies in Family Planning* 18(5):237–83.

Trussell, James, and A. R. Pebley. 1984. "The Potential Impact of Changes in Fertility on Infant, Child, and Maternal Mortality." *Studies in Family Planning* 15(6):267–80.

UN (United Nations). 1986. *Demographic Yearbook.* 38. New York: Department of International Economic and Social Affairs, Statistical Office.

———. 1988. *World Population Trends and Policies: 1987 Monitoring Report.* New York.

———. Population Division. 1987. *Fertility Behavior in the Context of Development: Evidence from the World Fertility Survey.* New York.

———. 1989. *Trends in Population Policy.* Population Studies 114. New York.

Ware, Helen. 1976. "Motivations for the Use of Birth Control: Evidence from West Africa." *Demography* 13(4):479–93.

Westoff, Charles F., and Lorenzo Moreno. 1989. "The Demand for Family Planning: Estimates for Developing Countries." Paper presented at the International Union for Scientific Investigation of Population (IUSSP) Seminar on The Role of Family Planning Programs as a Fertility Determinant, Tunis.

WFS (World Fertility Surveys). Various years. International Statistical Institute. The Hague.

World Bank. 1984. *Population Change and Economic Development.* (World Development Report, 1984). New York: Oxford University Press.

———. 1987. *Financing Health Services in Developing Countries: An Agenda for Reform.* Washington, D.C.

———. 1990. *Indonesia: Family Planning Perspectives in the 1990s.* World Bank Country Study. Washington, D.C.

WHO (World Health Organization). 1988. "Research in Human Reproduction, Biennial Report (1986–1987)." Special Programme on Research, Development, and Research Training in Human Reproduction.

17

Maternal and Perinatal Health

Julia A. Walsh, Chris M. Feifer, Anthony R. Measham, and Paul J. Gertler

More than 20 percent of the population in developing countries are women in their reproductive years (United Nations 1988). During a woman's life, one of the greatest risks to her health is childbearing. Pregnancy brings high risks of sickness, complications of delivery, disability, and death. Moreover, when pregnant women have complications, the infants these women bear are at increased risk of low birth weight, illness resulting from the complications of delivery, disability, and perinatal mortality. This chapter treats maternal and perinatal health problems together because they are inseparably linked: the main risk factors for disease and death among mothers and their newborns are the same. Not surprisingly, many of the interventions simultaneously improve both maternal and fetal health.

Maternal and perinatal mortality rates are indicators of the health of women of reproductive age and an indirect measure of the quality of the health care system. In many places health care during pregnancy is the only contact with modern medicine that a woman seeks. Obstetric services, therefore, represent a link to the general health care system and thus have an effect on present and future pregnancies and on the well-being of the entire family. High-quality supportive health services reinforce the family's use of preventive and promotive services in the future.

In table 17-1 we detail the risk factors for maternal and perinatal health problems. The main ones include illiteracy, poverty, poor nutrition, and low weight prior to pregnancy, minimal weight gain during pregnancy, first pregnancy or higher than fourth pregnancy (grand multipara), maternal age younger than twenty or older than thirty-four years, poor outcome of prior pregnancies, infections and illnesses during pregnancy, smoking, and inadequate health care during pregnancy and delivery. This complex web of social and medical factors suggests that health service solutions will be inadequate without concurrent attention to the other areas mentioned.

The health problems discussed in this chapter are more complex than many of the others covered in this collection. In the first place, they result from pregnancy, which is not a disease but is often a sought-after and highly desirable condition. Further, the lives of two people, mother and infant, are involved. Finally, events early in the life of the mother, years

before pregnancy was ever contemplated, will result in complications many years later. The factors that affect the mother and newborn can be divided into three: those that occur prior to conception, so that a woman enters into the pregnancy in a precarious state of health; those during pregnancy (prenatal care may eliminate these); and those during delivery. Good health care will decrease these hazards. To reiterate, illness in the mother puts the newborn at greater risk.

Unfortunately, prevention is relatively difficult: the lengthy list of causes of disease and social conditions associated with problems makes this evident. Obviously, no single, highly effective control measure, such as a vaccine, drug, or vector control method, exists. Attention to women's general health care needs and readily available prenatal and obstetric care, however, can prevent the preponderance of perinatal and maternal morbidity and mortality.

Public Health Significance

The size of the problem of maternal death and disability has been underestimated and poorly recognized. Data on deaths and complications of mothers have not been collected, nor have data on the consequences for family and child health.

Current Levels and Trends in the Developing World

Maternal deaths and illnesses, low birth weight, and perinatal deaths are underreported in most countries. The best figures for the developing world are merely estimates pieced together from multiple sources of varying degrees of reliability. Little information exists which would allow quantification of the severity and duration of disability.

MATERNAL MORTALITY AND MORBIDITY. The World Health Organization (WHO) estimates that 500,000 women annually die of complications of pregnancy and delivery. Ninety-nine percent of these deaths occur in the developing world. Maternal mortality is usually defined as death occurring while the woman is pregnant or within forty-two days of termination of pregnancy. The "maternal mortality ratio," the number of maternal deaths per 100,000 live births, ranges from 25 to

Table 17-1. Risk Factors for Maternal Morbidity and Mortality, Low Birth Weight, and Perinatal Mortality

Risk factor	Adverse Outcome			Preventive or treatment measures available
	Maternal morbidity and mortality	Low birth weight	Perinatal mortality	
Prepregnancy—Demographic risk factors				
Age (less than twenty; more than thirty-four)[a]	Yes	Yes	Yes	No
Race[b]	No	Yes	No	No
Low socioeconomic status[a,b]	Yes	Yes	Yes	No
Unmarried[b]	Yes	Yes	No	No
Low level of education[b]	No	No	Yes	No
Medical risk factors				
Number of children (none or more than four)[a]	Yes	Yes	Yes	Yes
Low maternal weight-for-height (poor nutritional status)[a]	Yes	Yes	Yes	Yes
Short paternal height	No	Yes	No	No
Diseases such as diabetes and chronic hypertension	Yes	No	Yes	Yes
Poor obstetric history[a,c]	Yes	Yes	Yes	No
Gynecologic abnormalities[d]	Yes	Yes	No	No
Maternal genetic and related factors[e]	No	Yes	No	No
Conception				
Male fetus[a]	No	Yes	Yes	No
Pregnancy—Medical risk factors				
Multiple pregnancy[a]	No	Yes	Yes	No
Poor weight gain (maternal and fetal)[a]	Yes	Yes	Yes	Yes
Anemia/abnormal hemoglobin	Yes	Yes	Yes	Yes
Malaria[a]	Yes	Yes	Yes	Yes
Streptococcus (group B) infection[a]	Yes	Yes	Yes	Yes
Sexually transmitted diseases[a]	Yes	Yes	Yes	Yes
Urinary tract infection	No	Yes	No	Yes
Rubella, cytomegalovirus	No	Yes	Yes	No
Respiratory and diarrheal disease	No	Yes	Yes	Yes
Short interpregnancy interval	Unknown	Yes	Yes	Yes
Induced abortion (especially illegal)[a]	Yes	No	No	Yes
Ectopic pregnancy[a]	Yes	No	No	Yes
Hypotension	No	Yes	No	No
Hypertension/pre-eclampsia/toxemia[a]	Yes	Yes	Yes	Yes
Low blood volume	No	Yes	No	No
First or second trimester bleeding	No	Yes	No	No
Placental abnormalities[a,f]	Yes	Yes	Yes	No
Hyperemesis	No	Yes	No	No
Oligohydramnios/polyhydramnios	No	Yes	Yes	No
Inadequate health care	Yes	Yes	Yes	Yes
Isoimmunization	No	Yes	Yes	No
Fetal anomalies	No	Yes	Yes	No
Incompetent cervix[a]	No	Yes	Yes	Yes
Spontaneous premature rupture of membranes[a]	No	Yes	Yes	Yes
Behavioral and environmental risk factors				
Unwanted pregnancy[a]	Yes	Yes	Yes	Yes
Smoking/tobacco use[a]	Unknown	Yes	Yes	Yes
Alcohol and other substance abuse[a]	No	Yes	Yes	Yes
Diethylstilbestrol (DES) and other toxic exposures[g]	No	Yes	Yes	No
High altitude	No	Yes	Yes	No
Absent or inadequate prenatal care[a,h]	Yes	Yes	Yes	Yes
Delivery				
Inadequate obstetrical care[a]	Yes	Yes	Yes	Yes
Iatrogenic prematurity[a]	No	Yes	Yes	Yes

Risk factor	Adverse Outcome			Preventive or treatment measures available
	Maternal morbidity and mortality	Low birth weight	Perinatal mortality	
Postpartum/neonatal period				
Inadequate care for mother[a]	Yes	No	No	Yes
Inadequate care for infant[a]	No	No	Yes	Yes

a. High relative risk and/or very common. Reflects the relative risk and the proportion of the population with the risk factor.
b. Closely associated factors with increased risk in different studies. The independent contribution of each factor is difficult to disaggregate.
c. Previous low-birth-weight-infant, maternal morbidity, perinatal morbidity, multiple spontaneous abortions, infertility treatment.
d. Small pelvis, female circumcision, uterine disease, tubal scarring secondary to sexually transmitted diseases and potentially leading to ectopic pregnancy, and similar problems.
e. For example, low maternal weight associated with own birth.
f. Such as placenta previa and abruptio placentae.
g. Including occupational hazards.
h. Prenatal care appears to decrease maternal and infant disease. However, it may have less effect than expected from comparisons of the outcome of pregnancy between women who attend prenatal care and those who do not. Those women who voluntarily choose prenatal care usually are healthier and have fewer risk factors.
Source: Authors.

1,660 in studies from developing countries, and averages 10 in industrial ones.[1] As reported in table 17-2, the highest overall ratio occurs in Africa (640); the ratios are lower in Asia (420) and in Latin America (270). Differences between countries, and between urban and rural areas, are blurred by the regional statistics, however. A recent study of the rural areas of the Gambia found a maternal mortality ratio of 2,200 (Greenwood and others 1987). The maternal mortality ratio measures the obstetric risk in a given pregnancy.

Table 17-2. Estimated Maternal Mortality, by Region

Region	Live births (millions)	Maternal deaths (thousands)	Maternal mortality rate (per 100,000 live births)
Africa	23.4	150	640
North	4.8	24	500
West	7.6	54	700
East	7.0	46	660
Middle	2.6	18	690
Southern	1.4	8	570
Asia	73.9	308	420
West	4.1	14	340
South	35.6	230	650
Southeast	12.4	52	420
East	21.8	12	55
Latin America	12.6	34	270
Middle	3.7	9	240
Caribbean	0.9	2	220
Tropical south	7.1	22	310
Temperate south	0.9	1	110
Oceania	0.2	2	100
Developing countries	110.1	494	450
Industrial countries	18.2	6	30
World	128.3	500	390

Note: Estimates for 1980–85 from UN demographic indicators of countries.
Source: WHO 1985.

The "maternal mortality rate" is the number of maternal deaths in one year per 100,000 women of reproductive age, usually age fifteen through forty-nine. This rate combines the fertility rate (births per thousand women of reproductive age) and the maternal mortality ratio defined above, so it is influenced both by the likelihood of becoming pregnant and by the risk of dying from that pregnancy. Improvements in both family planning and obstetric services affect the maternal mortality rate (Fortney 1987).

The lifetime risk of maternal mortality is many times greater than the ratio indicates because the ratio ignores the effect of repeated pregnancies. Each pregnancy adds to the total lifetime risk. In the developing world (excluding China) an average woman faces a lifetime risk of one chance in thirty-three that a pregnancy will result in her death. For those with serious risk factors or for those living in areas with inadequate health services and high fertility rates, the lifetime risk escalates greatly. The difference between industrial and developing nations is much larger for maternal mortality than it is for infant mortality: the risk of infant death is about 9 times greater in the least industrialized countries, but for maternal mortality the risk can be more than 100 times as great (WHO 1986).

Three-quarters of all maternal deaths can be attributed to one of three causes—hemorrhage, sepsis, or eclampsia (convulsions resulting from hypertensive disease during pregnancy)—though the route to these ends can vary. Most countries list five main causes of maternal mortality: hemorrhage, sepsis, eclampsia, abortion, and obstructed labor. Obstructed labor and abortion, however, usually lead to death from sepsis or hemorrhage. Moreover, differences in reporting can obscure underlying events. For example, Reich suggests that about one-quarter of all pregnancies worldwide end in induced abortions and result in up to 200,000 deaths (Reich 1987); however, these deaths may be coded as hemorrhage or sepsis. In table 17-3 we summarize the leading causes of death in several countries.

Death from hemorrhage can occur in less than an hour. Women far from health services are exposed to the greatest danger because they may not reach a hospital in time for

Table 17-3. Major Causes of Maternal Deaths, 1980–85
(percent)

Region	Hemorrhage	Sepsis	Eclampsia	Abortion	Obstructed labor/ruptured uterus	Other
United States	10	8	17	6	3	56
Cuba	6	19	12	15	..	48
Jamaica	23	9	30	10	3	25
Zambia (Lusaka)	17	15	20	17	..	31
Egypt (Menoufia)	29	11	5	4	..	51
Tanzania (four regions)	18	15	3	17	6	41
Ethiopia (Addis Ababa)	6	2	6	25	4	57
Bangladesh	22	3	19	31	9	16
Indonesia	46	10	5	7	..	32
India	18	14	16	14	3	35

.. Negligible.
Source: Calculated from Herz and Measham 1987.

transfusion or surgery. A study in China found, for example, that 60 percent of the maternal deaths in rural areas were from hemorrhage, in contrast to 25 percent in the urban areas (Zhang and Ding 1988).

Figure 17-1. Major Causes and Consequences of Prolonged or Obstructed Labor

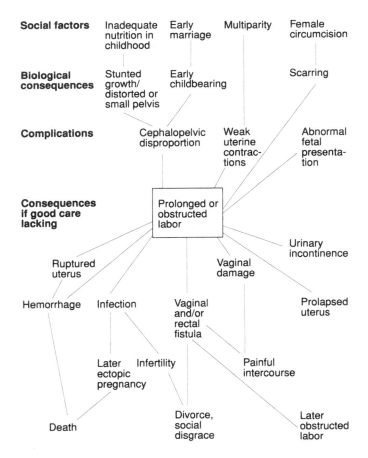

Source: Lettenmeier and others 1988.

The remaining one-quarter of maternal deaths include complications of illness that existed prior to pregnancy, such as hypertension, diabetes, and heart disease. Hepatitis, for example, causes hemorrhage or liver failure in pregnant women and is a significant cause of maternal death in many countries (China [Chen 1985]; Ethiopia [Kwast and Stevens 1987]; India [Rao 1985; Bhatia 1985]; Nigeria [Ojo and Savage 1974];) and in refugee camps in Somalia and Sudan (CDC 1987). Anemia impedes a woman's ability to resist infection or survive hemorrhage and may increase the likelihood of her dying in childbirth by a factor of four (Llewellyn-Jones 1965; Chi and others 1981). Additionally, latent infections, such as tuberculosis, malaria, and sexually transmitted and other genital infections, can become active during pregnancy and severely threaten the health of mother and baby.

The same complications which cause death can lead to chronic disability when they are less severe. The complications of obstructed or prolonged labor, postabortal or puerperal sepsis, and hemorrhage, for example, include fistulae (tears in the vaginal wall), stenosis (narrowing of the vagina), and uterine scarring or prolapse (Howard 1987). Fistulae (rectal, urethral, and vaginal) can cause foul-smelling discharge and social ostracism. Uterine scarring and prolapse can cause infertility. In figure 17-1 the antecedents and consequences of obstructed labor are presented, clearly illustrating the interconnectedness of reproductive complications. Other chronic disabilities include hypertension, chronic renal failure, and urinary incontinence. Some of these illnesses can cripple a woman, both physically and socially, for the rest of her life.

The incidence of pregnancy-related complications is poorly defined. The authors of the most-quoted study, that of a small village in India, found sixteen illnesses for every death (Datta and others 1973). If the incidence is similar elsewhere, then 3 to 12 percent of all pregnancies result in episodes of serious ill health in women. Other studies, from Zaria, Nigeria, and from China and Egypt, present widely differing results, ranging from 1 to 37 percent, depending on the population and survey methods (Li and others 1982; Mekhemar and others 1984; Harrison 1985).

Thus, complications of pregnancy and delivery cause an enormous burden of illness. Most of this burden can be averted, however, by perinatal and obstetric care. Maternal mortality has declined substantially with increasing use of hospitals for delivery. In Latin America and the Caribbean region, it has fallen by half since 1960 (Walker and others 1986). Despite these declines, deaths from illegal abortion represent a larger percentage here than in other regions (Royston and Lopez 1987). Trends in Asia and Sub-Saharan Africa are not known. About 25 percent of the deaths of women between the ages of twenty and thirty-four years result from maternity-related causes.

PERINATAL HEALTH PROBLEMS. At no other age is life so tenuous and the risk of death so great as in the perinatal period. Figure 17-2 illustrates the daily risk of death throughout infancy and childhood, from the perinatal period, which extends from delivery through the first week of life, until five years of age. Perinatal health reflects both the health of the woman and

Figure 17-2. Daily Mortality Rate for Infants and Children in Chaco Province, Argentina

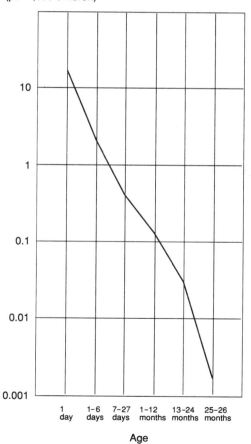

the quality of care during pregnancy, delivery, and the neonatal period. It is a key determinant of health and well-being for the rest of an individual's life. Compare the prospects of an infant of low weight born after a prolonged, difficult delivery (with substantial risk of hypoxic brain damage, or limb weakness from birth trauma, or pneumonia acquired from amniotic fluid infection) with those of a normal infant. In developing countries very little is known about the incidence of these perinatal disabilities and their consequences for the future well-being of both the child and family.

Seven million perinatal deaths occur annually—almost all in developing countries (Lopez 1990). These perinatal deaths include stillbirths (also called late fetal deaths) and deaths in the first week of life.[2] The perinatal mortality rate includes all births (stillbirths and live births) in its denominator. In most developing countries, it ranges between 40 and 60 per 1,000. High rates of 80 to 100 are found in the least industrialized and most disadvantaged countries. In industrial countries, rates range from 6 to 10 (Belsey and Royston 1987, quoting from WHO data banks). Perinatal deaths, particularly stillbirths delivered at home, are frequently underreported. As infant mortality declines, postneonatal deaths (up to twenty-eight days postpartum) decline more rapidly and perinatal deaths thus comprise a larger proportion of infant deaths. For example, the infant mortality rate in Mauritius declined from 70 in 1967 to 29 in 1982; the perinatal mortality rate declined from 67 to 34; however, perinatal deaths as a percentage of all late fetal deaths and infant deaths increased from 61 to 70 percent during the same period. In general, in developing countries, the perinatal mortality rate is almost the same as the infant mortality rate. Neonatal deaths, shared by both the perinatal and infant mortality statistics, approximate 50 to 60 percent of each of these statistics (Edouard 1985).

Perinatal mortality is largely determined by delivery care and the maturity of the fetus, as reflected by birth weight and gestational age. Studies of the relative effects of birth weight and gestational age on mortality suggest that birth weight is the predominant factor (McCormick 1985). Figure 17-3 demonstrates the dramatic rise in perinatal mortality among infants with a birth weight of less than 2,500 grams and more than 4,000 grams. These infants at the ends of the curve usually had gestational ages of less than twenty-eight weeks or more than forty-two weeks.

The main causes of perinatal mortality are infection of the amniotic fluid, congenital syphilis, abruptio placentae, fetal hypoxia of unknown cause, compression of the umbilical cord, premature rupture of membranes, obstructed labor, birth trauma, and congenital malformations. Up to 30 percent of deaths are due to "other" causes (Naeye 1980; Lucas and others 1983; Oyedeji and others 1983; McCormack and others 1987). Virtually all these deaths occur within the first year of life, primarily during the first few days of life.

Morbidity resulting from perinatal problems is difficult to quantify. The long-term consequences of low birth weight, one of the most severe perinatal health problems, are discussed below. Even less is known about the disabling effects of (a) lack of oxygen during labor and delivery that may cause cerebral

Figure 17-3. Neonatal and Postneonatal Deaths by Birth Weight

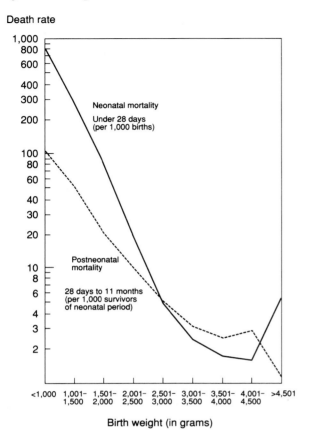

Death rate

Neonatal mortality
Under 28 days
(per 1,000 births)

Postneonatal mortality

28 days to 11 months
(per 1,000 survivors of neonatal period)

Birth weight (in grams)

Note: Deaths of single infants alive at birth, 1974–75, based on data from eight areas of the United States.
Source: Shapiro and others 1980.

palsy, mental retardation, or learning disabilities; (b) pulmonary dysfunction from scarring, respiratory infections, and prematurity; (c) congenital syphilis causing multiple organ and brain damage; (d) birth trauma injuring limbs, nerves, and internal organs; and (e) amniotic fluid infections which result in pulmonary, ocular, brain, and other organ damage. These acute and chronic disabilities have large social costs in health service use, family disruption, lost earnings, and long-term care.

Many infant deaths are potentially preventable by provision of prenatal and obstetric care to women. A clinico-pathological study of 702 perinatal deaths in Nairobi revealed that one-third were potentially preventable with better obstetric care (pregnant woman coming to the hospital earlier in the delivery process), because 38 percent of these were fresh stillbirths. More than 40 percent of deaths resulted from problems avoidable by early cesarean section or assisted delivery: birth trauma, ruptured uterus, cord prolapse, obstructed and prolonged labor, placenta previa, placental abruption, and eclampsia. In addition to these deaths, nearly 10 percent of the neonates died of infection acquired intrapartum, potentially avoidable with early treatment and prompt delivery following

rupture of membranes (Lucas and others 1983). Many of these same problems also cause maternal disease and death; improved obstetric care can prevent both maternal and perinatal morbidity and mortality.

Only a few researchers have examined the incidence of morbidity among neonates, but they have demonstrated its high frequency. In a Madras maternity hospital, with efficient obstetric and pediatric care, 20 percent of all babies suffered some illness and 4 percent died neonatally. The most common conditions were low birth weight (below 2,000 grams in 7.5 percent) and infections (in 8.3 percent). Obstetrical injuries and asphyxia affected only a few (2 percent) as a result of the quality of obstetric and pediatric care (Thirugnanasambandham and others 1986).

Reproductive tract infections from both sexually transmitted diseases and other genital infections are common and result in a substantial amount of perinatal as well as maternal disease (Kundsin and others 1988). In parts of Africa, more than 10 percent of pregnant women are seropositive for syphilis, but few are treated prior to delivery (Brunham and others 1984). In a study done in the 1940s prior to the availability of penicillin, syphilitic mothers experienced over 10 percent stillbirths and 20 percent infant deaths; more than 20 percent of the infants who survived had evidence of congenital syphilis, and only a third of the pregnancies resulted in a healthy child (Brunham and others 1984). Gonorrhea, chlamydia, and mycoplasma cause stillbirths, preterm delivery, and intrauterine growth retardation. Group B streptococci and bacterial vaginosis are associated with neonatal sepsis and low birth weight (Brunham, Holmes, and Eschenbach 1984; Berman and others 1981; Investigators of the Johns Hopkins Study of Cervicitis and Adverse Pregnancy Outcome 1989; Walsh and Hutchinson 1989; Wasserheit 1989). Most of these infections can easily be identified and treated before and during pregnancy to prevent these consequences.

As infant mortality has declined and prenatal and obstetric care have improved, the perinatal mortality rate also has declined but to a smaller extent. Among all infant deaths, however, the proportion from perinatal deaths has increased. As more women obtain skilled prenatal and delivery care, perinatal morbidity and mortality should continue to decline.

LOW BIRTH WEIGHT. The World Health Organization defines low birth weight as a birth weight less than 2,500 grams, because below this value birth weight-specific infant mortality begins to rise rapidly. Two main processes determine birth weight: duration of gestation and intrauterine growth rate, and both affect fetal, neonatal, postneonatal, and child mortality. When gestation lasts less than thirty-seven weeks, the infant is considered preterm. Intrauterine growth retardation (IUGR) is also called "small-for-gestational-age" or "small-for-dates" but has no standard definition. Commonly used definitions include: birth weight less than the tenth (or fifth) percentile for gestational age; birth weight less than 2,500 grams and gestational age greater than or equal to thirty-seven weeks; and birth weight less than two standard deviations below the mean value for gestational age.[3]

Unfortunately, most studies from developing countries do not distinguish IUGR from preterm infants (and even fewer disaggregate types of IUGR). Analysis of a small number of studies suggests that more than half of the cases of low birth weight in developing countries probably result from IUGR, whereas in industrial countries most of such cases result from preterm delivery. In 1982, of the 127 million infants born, 16 percent (20 million) weighed less than 2,500 grams and more than 90 percent of these infants were born in developing countries (see table 17-4 for reported mean birth weight and prevalence of low birth weight in selected countries). Western European countries have the lowest proportion (5 percent) of infants of low birth weight (Kramer 1987).

The lowest infant mortality rate occurs among infants weighing 3,000 to 3,500 grams (see figure 17-3) but rises dramatically among those below this weight and only slightly above this. In industrial countries the prevalence of neurodevelopmental handicaps among low-birth-weight infants is three times that for those of normal birth weight. The risk for infants of very low birth weight (1,500 grams or less) is ten times that for normal weight infants. Eight to 19 percent of infants of very low birth weight may be severely affected despite the availability of neonatal intensive care. Low birth weight strongly predicts school failure, but the household setting modifies the effect (which is less pronounced in advantaged households) (McCormick 1985). Comparable statistics are not available for developing countries.

Infants of low birth weight have twice the risk of congenital anomalies than those of normal weight, and infants of very low birth weight have three times the risk. Congenital anomalies and neurodevelopmental handicaps are not mutually exclusive. The proportion of infants affected with one or both ranges from 19 percent in infants of normal birth weight to 42 percent in those of very low birth weight; the proportion of infants severely affected is 2 to 14 percent (McCormick 1985). Low-birth-weight infants also suffer more pulmonary disease, use health services extensively (for neonatal care and subsequent physician visits), increase family health costs, and disrupt the normal functioning of the family.

Though the cause of the majority of low-weight births occurring in both developing and industrial countries remains unexplained, there are many important risk factors (see table 17-1). They are believed to include infant gender, race, ethnic origin, socioeconomic status, maternal height, prepregnancy weight, paternal weight and height, maternal birth weight, parity, history of prior low-birth-weight infants, gestational weight gain and caloric intake, general morbidity and episodic illness during pregnancy, reproductive tract infections (including sexually transmitted diseases), malaria, cigarette smoking (and tobacco chewing to a lesser extent), alcohol consumption, and in utero exposure to diethylstilbestrol.

From 1979 to 1982, the proportion of low-birth-weight infants appeared to decline globally from 16.8 to 16 percent. In developing countries it was reported to have declined from 18.4 to 17.6 percent, whereas in industrial nations it dropped from 7.4 to 6.9 percent. These are minimal declines and probably represent only improved data collection. Data from

Table 17-4. Mean Birth Weight and Prevalence of Low Birth Weight, Selected Countries

Country	Mean birth weight (g)	Low birth weight (percent)
Africa		
Egypt	3,200–3,240	7.0
Kenya	3,143	12.8
Nigeria	2,880–3,117	18.0
Tunisia	3,210–3,376	7.3
Tanzania	2,900–3,151	14.4
Zaire	3,163	15.9
Asia		
China	3,215–3,285	6.0
India	2,493–2,970	30.0
Indonesia	2,760–3,027	14.0
Iran, Islamic Rep. of	3,012–3,250	14.0
Iraq	3,540	6.1
Japan	3,200–3,208	5.2
Malaysia	3,027–3,065	10.6
Pakistan	2,770	27.0
Latin America		
Brazil	3,170–3,298	9.0
Chile	3,340	9.0
Colombia	3,912–3,115	10.0
Guatemala	3,050	17.9
Mexico	3,019–3,025	11.7
North America		
Canada	3,327	6.0
United States	3,299	6.9
Europe		
Czechoslovakia	3,327	6.2
France	3,240–3,335	5.6
Hungary	3,144–3,162	11.8
Norway	3,500	3.8
Sweden	3,490	4.0
United Kingdom	3,310	7.0

Source: Kramer 1987.

developing countries prior to 1979 are fragmentary; few neonates were weighed except in urban referral hospitals, and only a small proportion of births was under surveillance. National averages cannot be accurately estimated from these figures, and in any event, few of these statistics have been compiled.

Maternal and Perinatal Morbidity and Mortality in 2000

Future patterns of maternal and perinatal morbidity and mortality probably depend more on the number and proportion of women of childbearing age in the population and fertility rates than on specific factors such as hospital access. The World Health Organization made a series of projections assuming (a) no change in fertility and maternal mortality, (b) a reduction in fertility of 25 percent, and (c) halving of the maternal mortality ratios. In the first case, 600,000 maternal deaths would occur in the year 2000. If fertility were reduced by 25 percent, the number of deaths would drop to 450,000. By halving the mortality ratio, deaths would decrease to 300,000.

If fertility declined by 25 percent and the mortality ratio by half, then maternal deaths would shrink to 225,000 in the year 2000, fewer than half the deaths experienced in 1985.

The World Health Organization estimates continued declines in rates of low birth weight without citing the reasons for the expected decrease. Reduced fertility would result in fewer perinatal deaths and the decline in rate of low birth weight would reduce the perinatal mortality rate. By 2015 the perinatal mortality rate should decline from the 1985 level of 98 for males and 75 for females to 42 and 31 in developing countries (Lopez, chapter 2, this collection). This decline depends on an increase in skilled delivery services along with the decline in low birth weight.

Indirect Economic Costs

There is a dearth of information both on treatments used for maternal and infant morbidity occurring during pregnancy and delivery and on the effects this morbidity has on the women and infants, their families, the community, and health services. Though chronic morbidity may be more expensive than a quick death, mortality is complicated in that the death of the mother is usually accompanied by the death of the infant from that pregnancy. Ninety-five percent of the infants born to mothers who died in childbirth also died, according to a small study in Bangladesh (Chen and others 1974). A disabled mother confined to bed for severe anemia or renal failure might drain the family resources and compromise the health of family members, particularly the very young children, but there would also be long-range effects on the well-being of the entire family from the mother's death.

Although their efforts are often undervalued, women support families through their productive labor: cash crop labor, subsistence farming, and other remunerative work. Poorer women are more likely to be solely responsible for their families. Many regions experience high male outmigration for jobs, in effect leaving the women alone as the sole parent. The loss of the mother through death or disability then means the loss of the nurturer, provider, and de facto household head.

Treatment of low-birth-weight infants and neonatal illness can also drain the resources of the family and health service, particularly when neonatal intensive care is required. Indeed, when health resources are limited, health planners should weigh the cost of neonatal intensive care, which may benefit only a few infants, against the cost of improved preventive care for maternal and perinatal health, which would confer wider benefits. Even where neonatal intensive care units are absent, the increased health needs of sick and disabled infants are costly and time consuming.

Summary

Maternal and perinatal health (including low birth weight) are closely linked, and efforts to improve the health of either pregnant women or the newborn will have synergistic effects on the health of the other. Death and sickness among these population groups are common, and the effects of this ill health are pervasive and costly to society.

Risk Reduction prior to Conception

Reduction of risk prior to pregnancy is the most feasible way to improve maternal health.

Elements of Prevention Strategies

In order completely to eradicate reproductive risk, pregnancy would have to be eliminated. Because families and society obviously value and desire children, however, the goal should be to avoid unwanted pregnancies and to lower the risks when pregnancy occurs. Many steps can be taken to do this even before conception.

BETTER GENERAL HEALTH FOR WOMEN. In general, when women are healthier they are better equipped to handle pregnancy and their infants will be healthier. Good health for all women requires an integrated set of actions, including health services, community development, and education for female children.

Women need better services throughout their life. Nutrition is important at all ages so that a woman enters childbearing age with normal height, weight, pelvic size, and nutritional status. Nutrition programs can include a variety of components, for example, nutrition and health education, anemia screening and prevention (including iron and folate supplements), iodine supplementation, food supplementation, promotion of community and household gardens, and income supplements (Lettenmeier and others 1988). The choice of intervention depends on the most important nutritional deficiencies experienced in an area and the availability of resources.

It is also important to pay attention to those conditions affecting girls early in life that make pregnancy more risky. Rheumatic fever, for example, causes heart disease which can complicate childbirth. In Menoufia, Egypt, 16 percent of maternal deaths were due to cardiovascular disease; one-half of them involved a history of rheumatic fever (Fortney and others 1988). Infections of the reproductive tract and sexually transmitted diseases (STDs) also must be diagnosed and treated. These can cause scarring of the fallopian tubes that may result in infertility or ectopic pregnancy (an important cause of maternal death from hemorrhage) when conception occurs. These infections are also responsible for much morbidity as discussed earlier. Women are often uninformed about the symptoms, risks, and means to prevent STD infection.

The delay of reproduction until a woman is fully grown is very important and may be achieved by raising age at marriage, reducing the need for women to prove their fertility early, and giving more attention to male and female responsibilities in avoiding adolescent pregnancies. Economic and social development also makes it easier for people to obtain the resources required for good health and to maintain hygienic conditions to safeguard it. Careful attention to development policy choices can increase the probability that women will have lighter workloads and better food, both of which are extremely important in reducing the wear and tear on health, which is most felt during pregnancy and childbirth.

The status of women in society directly affects their health in many ways. For example, in some societies women are the last to get food in the family and the least likely to use health services. Education can be an important means to improve status. Most important, increasing the education of women indirectly increases the motivation and the means to attain improved health status and instills in each woman an awareness of her own health needs and the methods by which she may handle them. Educated women tend to marry later and are more likely to use family planning, prenatal, and obstetric services and to avoid dangerous traditional health practices (Harrison 1980; Kwast and others 1984; London and others 1985; and Monteith and others 1987). Maternal education substantially affects infant mortality rates (figure 17-4); one might expect similar results for maternal health, but this is not well documented.

FAMILY PLANNING. Family planning acts on maternal health through several mechanisms. First and most important, with fewer unwanted pregnancies, fewer women resort to illicit abortion. Second, a birth interval of more than two years has no proven effect on maternal morbidity and mortality, but it does improve the health of the infant. Still, longer birth intervals usually result in fewer total pregnancies for a woman and, therefore, fewer grand multiparas (more than five pregnancies). Third, targeted family planning can play a significant role by reducing the number of pregnancies in women most at risk of pregnancy complications, especially those under eighteen or over thirty-four years of age. Family planning includes education and access to a variety of contraceptive methods such as pills, condoms, intrauterine devices, and so on, plus availability of safe abortion. Because approximately 25 percent of maternal deaths result from unsafe abortion, the provision of safe abortion services to back up other contraceptive services is a highly effective and low-cost way to reduce maternal mortality (Blacker 1987).

The effect of family planning on maternal mortality depends on a country's stage in the demographic transition (Fortney 1987). If the number of unwanted pregnancies and the need for abortion are reduced, potential declines in maternal mortality range from 5 percent in Côte d'Ivoire to 62 percent in Bangladesh (Lettenmeier and others 1988). A general rule of thumb is that in countries in which fertility is already low, increased use of contraception will have relatively little effect on fertility and maternal mortality. These countries should focus maternal and perinatal health care strategies on obstetric improvements. It is also useful to look at both the maternal mortality ratio and rate; where the rate is high and the ratio is low, family planning is likely to have more effect on maternal deaths, especially if deaths due to abortion are high (Fortney 1987). Family planning is somewhat less effective and more costly, however, in societies in which women want large families.

As the total fertility rate declines, the proportion of grand multiparas declines, but the proportion of primiparas increases. These two trends have opposite effects on maternal mortality in industrial and developing countries. In industrial countries, a slight increase in maternal mortality results; however, in developing countries, the improvement in maternal health from the decline in grand multiparas outweighs the negative effect of the increase in primiparas.

Wider birth spacing has been recommended for improving maternal morbidity and mortality. Too many births too closely spaced seem to cause a general decline in the health and nutritional status of some women; this decline is called the maternal depletion syndrome. Whether this syndrome actually exists has been questioned (Winikoff and Castle 1987). Nonetheless, the freedom to plan the timing of offspring, and the education required to help a woman make this choice, are undeniably appropriate goals for any maternal health program.

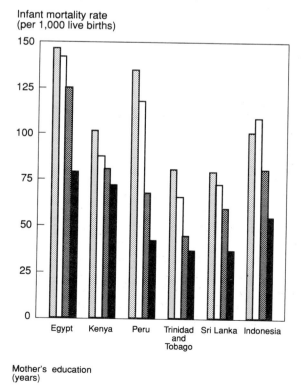

Figure 17-4. *Infant Mortality by Mother's Education, Selected Countries*

Infant mortality rate (per 1,000 live births)

Mother's education (years)

▦ 0   ▢ 1–3   ▨ 4–6   ■ 7+

Source: Starrs 1987.

Targeted family planning can help avoid pregnancies among women who are too young (less than eighteen), too old (over thirty-four), have already had many births (more than four), have an obstetric or medical history which places them at higher risk, or who do not want another pregnancy (Lettenmeier and others 1988). Locating such women and providing them with contraception will substantially reduce maternal mortality rates. Estimates for this reduction range from 25 to 50 percent of all maternal deaths (Maine 1981; Rinehart and others 1984; Blacker 1987; Maine and others 1987; Winikoff and Sullivan 1987).

Good Practice vs. Actual Practice—Where Are the Gaps?

Many developing countries have made remarkable progress in reducing maternal mortality. Their experiences provide clues to the most effective actions to take. Lettenmeier and others (1988) report that "Sri Lanka, through nearly universal education, raised the average age at marriage and increased the use of family planning, thereby reducing the number of risky pregnancies in adolescents and in older women with many children (Henry and Piotrow 1979). At the same time health care improved. The Sri Lankan maternal mortality ratio dropped from 555/100,000 in 1950 to 95 in 1980 (Royston and Lopez 1987)." Lettenmeier and others (1988) also report that "China lowered maternal mortality by substantially lowering birth rates, raising the age at marriage, and improving health care for pregnant women (Chen and Kols 1982). The maternal mortality ratio, at 25, now rivals that of industrial countries (WHO 1986)." These two success stories demonstrate the potential of multifaceted efforts to reduce maternal mortality and morbidity.

Despite recent gains in a few countries or among women of certain classes, most women in developing countries face social constraints in status and decisionmaking power which limit their ability to safeguard their own health (PCC 1988). Women in developing countries still lag behind men in educational attainment and literacy, as is evident in table 17-5, in which are also shown the regions of the world where women marry at young ages and have large families. Africa scores lowest for educating its women and age of marriage, and it has the highest fertility; maternal mortality is also highest in Africa. The Indian subcontinent (Middle South Asia) scores the next lowest and has maternal mortality rates nearly as high as Africa.

Poor nutrition is still a widespread problem among women despite recent efforts to provide food supplements and nutrition education. A survey of eighty developing countries in the early 1980s showed that between 20 and 45 percent of the women age fifteen through forty-four consumed insufficient calories daily (Hamilton and others 1984). Anemia incidence is even higher; up to 80 percent of the women of reproductive age in developing countries may be anemic (Royston 1982). Food supplementation programs have proved expensive and difficult to manage logistically. Furthermore, they have not generated data on their contribution to the reduction of maternal mortality or morbidity (Weston 1986). To compound matters, nutritional deficiencies are passed from generation to generation. The poorly nourished woman is more likely to give birth to an infant of low birth weight who in turn may never reach fully normal stature. When this infant becomes an adult, she may give birth to other low-birth-weight children or have obstructed labor from small pelvic size. Contrary to expectations, there has not yet been any evidence of change in the incidence of low birth weight in developing countries as a result of the large-scale food supplementation programs for girls and women prior to conception.

In table 17-6 we summarize possible actions of a maternal and child health program before conception occurs. The priorities for services include family planning, including contraception and safe abortion; integration of family planning into health services which can screen for and treat anemia, infections of the reproductive tract, sexually transmitted diseases, malaria, and other illnesses common in the particular locale; and health education through health centers and other avenues for the prevalent illnesses and for health risks such as poor nutrition and tobacco and alcohol use. Many of these screening, treatment, and education services obviously are needed during pregnancy as well. Wherever possible, all these priority services should be integrated into pregnancy care. Another alternative is to provide family planning and treatment for reproductive tract infections and STDs together and pregnancy care separately.

Pregnancy, Delivery, and the Neonatal Period

The strategy for maximizing good health during pregnancy requires access to health care.

Case Management of Pregnancy and Complications

The ability of the health system to decrease the effect of pregnancy complications depends upon the capacity to identify high-risk women, prevent complications or treat them, and refer for skilled obstetric care. When a complication presents itself in spite of prenatal care, back-up obstetrical referral facilities are required. It is difficult to identify all women who will have complications; for example, in a group of women with no risk factors receiving prenatal care in Canada, 10 percent of the women had obstetric complications and 19 percent of the neonates had complications (Moutquin and others 1987).

A maternity care program in rural Bangladesh which posted trained midwives at village health posts and referred complicated deliveries to a central maternity clinic reduced maternal mortality by 60 percent (Fauveau and others 1991). Even though the maternal mortality ratio remained high in the program area (1.4 per 1,000), the reduction suggests that midwives can improve maternal survival when given proper facilities, supervision, and referral facilities. The program was undertaken in an area with an already existing high-quality primary health care system, probably a key element in its effectiveness. The effect on perinatal mortality and costs must still be determined.

Table 17-5. Selected Sociologic Indicators, by Region

Region	Literate adults Male (percent)	Literate adults Female (percent)	Married women age 15–19 (percent)	Total fertility rate[a]
Africa	33	15	44	6.2
North	—	18	34	5.1
West	20	6	70	6.9
East	29	14	32	6.9
Central	35	9	49	6.2
Southern	55	56	2	4.7
Asia	56	34	42	3.5
Southwest	58	31	25	5.1
Middle south	44	17	54	4.7
Southeast	75	53	24	3.7
East	97	92	2	2.4
Latin America	76	70	16	3.6
Central	75	67	21	3.9
Caribbean	67	66	19	3.0
Tropical south	74	67	15	
Temperate south	93	91	10	3.5
Oceania	90	88	10	2.5
North America	99	99	11	1.8
Europe	96	93	7	1.7
Former U.S.S.R	100	100	10	2.4
World	67	54	30	3.5
Industrial countries	98	97	8	1.9
Developing countries	52	32	39	3.9

a. Number of children per woman.
Source: Starrs 1987; United Nations various years.

The generally accepted strategy for dealing with the complications of pregnancy and childbirth involves a regional network of community risk assessment through prenatal care and use of facilities at the first-referral level, usually a district hospital, for the management of high-risk cases and treatment of obstetrical emergencies. Due to the nature of transportation in the developing world, maternal health programs must address the need for emergency transfer. In some cases, maternity waiting homes for those with expected complications are proposed; in others, innovative methods for providing transportation are involved. Herz and Measham (1987) advocate stronger community-based prenatal, delivery, and family planning services (incorporating the preventive strategies described earlier), stronger referral facilities, and an alarm and transport system.

PRENATAL CARE. Prenatal care is cost-effective because it reduces the number of women requiring skilled obstetrical care by screening and treating women at risk of complications and referring them to other facilities if necessary. Prenatal care can also substantially reduce the proportion of low-birth-weight infants and the incidence of perinatal disease. These reductions depend, however, on identifying high-risk women early

in pregnancy and providing them with special care: for example, encouraging an appropriate diet, treating infections and other illnesses, and arranging skilled delivery for those requiring it. A study in Indonesia found that women who received no prenatal care were more than five times as likely to die than those who attended a prenatal clinic (Chi and others 1981). It is estimated that in the United States each dollar invested in equitable access to comprehensive prenatal care results in a savings of $3.38 in subsequent expenditure for the care of low-birth-weight infants (IOM 1985). Low birth weight and perinatal problems are less common among women who have prenatal care (Chi and others 1981; Donaldson and Billy, 1984; Brown 1985; Harrison 1985; IOM 1985; Trivedi and Mavalankar 1986; Winikoff 1988). Nevertheless, it has not been possible to identify the specific components of prenatal care which reduce these problems (IOM 1985; Winikoff 1988). Women who avail themselves of prenatal care tend to be better educated and in better general health beforehand, so any comparison of women who take advantage of prenatal care with those who do not will show that the former group is better off. Where general health care is not available to prevent or treat risk factors before conception, prenatal care becomes even more important.

Table 17-6. Preconception Services to Improve Maternal and Perinatal Health

Intervention	Effectiveness	Major drawbacks	Program feasibility
Nutrition Food supplementation	Benefit to mother has not been evaluated. Supplementation increases birth weight 30 to 200 g. Most effective in malnourished women.	Difficult to ensure that pregnant woman does not share the supplement with others or substitute it for usual diet.	High cost. Generally too expensive for large continuing programs. Works best with locally available, inexpensive foods and when combined with nutrition education. Having women eat supplement at local distribution site most effective.
Iron/folate supplementation before and during pregnancy	Highly effective if tablets taken regularly. Malaria and parasite treatment needed in endemic areas.	Gastrointestinal side effects and need to take tablets several times a day make compliance a problem. Hard to motivate asymptomatic women to take tablets.	Low cost. Easy to add to existing antenatal care or other health care that reaches women. No special storage facilities needed.
Iodized oil injections	One injection prevents iodine deficiency for three to five years, shrinks existing goiter.	To benefit infant, injections must be given before pregnancy.	Low cost. Easy to add to existing antenatal care.
Family Planning Change maternal age Allow for birth spacing Limit family size Avoid high-risk pregnancy Avoid unwanted pregnancies	All major methods highly effective if used regularly and correctly.	Long-term consistent use and continuity of supplies needed for some methods. Rumors and concerns about potential side effects may deter use. Specialized training needed to perform sterilizations and insert IUDs and implants. Cultural restrictions against use of family planning in some areas.	Moderate cost. Variety of methods allows delivery through many medical and nonmedical delivery systems. Users have choice of methods. Some methods can be distributed by briefly trained workers. Elaborate storage system not needed.
Health services Primary health care for STDs, reproductive tract infections, hypertension	Highly effective depending on content and use. Prevents tubal scarring, which can lead to infertility and ectopic pregnancy.	Services depend on local resources and endemic illnesses. Specialized training, diagnostic tests, and treatments required locally.	Moderate cost systems often in place due to Alma Ata conference and "Health for All" programs.
Health education Reproductive tract infections and STDs Poor health habits (tobacco, alcohol) Nutrition Signs of premature labor	Effect on maternal and perinatal health depends on content and use.	Community participation in education and adequate training of health educators.	Moderate cost systems often in place due to Alma Ata conference and "Health for All" programs.

Source: Lettenmeier and others 1988.

To some degree, the content of prenatal care must be adjusted according to local technologies, economics, and population needs. The prevailing health problems must be identified and care must be targeted to those at risk so that they are identified and treated. Prenatal programs in poor countries cannot hope to be as comprehensive as those recommended in industrial countries; managers of such programs must select carefully the components they will include for maximum efficiency and benefit. In table 17-7 we list the important components of prenatal care for developing countries and the lowest levels of the health care system at which this care can occur. At the community level, health workers can educate pregnant women about good nutrition, dangerous habits (tobacco and alcohol use), STDs, and about signs of premature labor and other complications so that women can get to the referral centers quickly (Iam 1989). At the primary level, health workers should be trained and resources available for health and nutrition education and for screening and monitoring for a variety of conditions. The choice of diseases to screen for depends upon the local disease burden. For example, in parts of Africa

Table 17-7. Prenatal Interventions for Preventing Maternal Morbidity and Mortality, Low Birth Weight, and Perinatal Mortality in Developing Countries

Level of care	Activity	Areas covered
Community	Educate	Nutrition; tobacco and alcohol use; signs of premature labor and other serious complications; self-referral for care
Primary	Monitor and treat or refer for skilled care	Uterine growth; weight gain; bleeding; presentation; hypertension; edema
Primary	Screen and treat or refer for skilled care	Reproductive tract infections; sexually transmitted diseases; diabetes; urinary tract infections; cardiac disease
Primary	Treat intercurrent illness	Diarrhea, respiratory infections, malaria, and other diseases
Primary	Provide preventive and nutritional care	Malaria prophylaxis in endemic areas; tetanus immunization; iron and folate supplements for anemia; nutritional supplements for malnourished women
Referral	Detect and treat	Premature labor; rupture of membranes
Referral	Skilled delivery	Small pelvic size; poor obstetric history; open cervix; other risk factors (such as age, parity)
Referral	Treat	Complications of spontaneous and induced abortions; ectopic pregnancies; hemorrhage

Source: Authors.

where STDs and malaria are prevalent, these problems must be addressed. Inexpensive diagnostic tests are available for many diseases: syphilis, gonorrhea, malaria, and anemia, among others. Unfortunately, for sexually transmitted diseases, even these diagnostic tests may be too expensive for widespread use. More operational research on diagnosis and treatment of STDs is urgently needed. All prenatal clinics should have the capacity to screen for high-risk pregnancy, perform pelvic examinations, immunize against tetanus, monitor uterine growth, provide iron and folate, and provide malaria prophylaxis. Depending on resources, other interventions, such as more comprehensive health education, should be provided. Trained birth attendants, not just family members or untrained traditional midwives, should assist all deliveries so that incipient complications can be treated or the woman rapidly transported to a referral center.

Most countries have an inadequate number of facilities and trained personnel for prenatal care, normal deliveries, transport to referral centers, and care of complications. The cost and effectiveness of investments in training and facilities expands when they can be used for other priority programs such as STD screening and treatment, family planning, and maternal and child health care.

REGIONALIZED CARE AND REFERRALS. Careful consideration of which health care personnel will deal with what level of complications is critical. Table 17-8 is an outline of a proposed system for regionalized care and referral for prevention of maternal mortality. A similar system can be used to prevent low birth weight and perinatal mortality by adding screening for a small number of other fetal risk factors (for example, tobacco and alcohol use, need for malaria prophylaxis, reproductive tract infections, and sexually transmitted diseases). Health care workers should be adequately trained to assess and handle any complication they may encounter. If referral is necessary, they must know how to stabilize and find transportation for the patient. Those in charge of programs may decide to allow traditional birth attendants (TBAs) to dispense drugs

(for example, oral ergometrine for hemorrhage), or have nurse midwives do surgical procedures (for example, cesareans) when emergency transportation is a practical impossibility or likely to be slow enough that local emergency treatment is a necessity.

The World Health Organization recommends that referral centers provide the following eight essential obstetrical services (Starrs 1987; Lettenmeier and others 1988):

• Surgical procedures: cesarean sections, draining abscesses, repairing high vaginal and cervical tears, removing ectopic pregnancies, emptying the uterus following incomplete abortion, symphysiotomies, and, in case of severe complications, rupturing the amniotic membrane to induce or quicken labor.

• Anesthesia: general, spinal, and local.

• Medical treatment: providing fluids and medications intravenously, treating shock, infection, preeclampsia and eclamptic seizures, and inducing labor.

• Blood replacement: transfusions of blood or other fluids for hemorrhage or surgery.

• Manual procedures for diagnosis and treatment: removing placentas manually, delivering by vacuum extraction or forceps, and using partographs to monitor labor.

• Family planning: tubal ligations, vasectomies, implanting and removing intrauterine devices and Norplant, other family planning methods.

• Special care for newborn babies: resuscitation, keeping warm, preventing low blood sugar, treating infections.

• Managing high-risk women: providing waiting homes close by. (This depends on prenatal screening for success.)

Better care during pregnancy, labor, and delivery potentially could reduce maternal mortality rates anywhere from 50 to 80 percent (Kwast and others 1984; Walker and others 1986; Lettenmeier and others 1988) and perinatal mortality rates by 30 to 40 percent (Lucas and others 1983; Kaumitz and others 1984). Most of the improvement would result from additional

Table 17-8. Selected Interventions at Primary and First-Referral Levels for Prevention of Maternal Morbidity and Mortality

Problem	Intervention	Health system level[a]
All causes of maternal mortality and morbidity	Family planning	Primary, first referral
	Prenatal care	Primary
	Supervised delivery	Primary
Hemorrhage	Risk screening, referral	Primary
	Other prenatal care, including treatment of anemia	Primary
	Oxytocics when placenta delivered[b]	Primary
	Intravenous fluids	Primary
	Transport to first-referral level	Primary
	Manual removal of placenta	Primary
	Blood typing of donors	First referral
	Blood transfusion	First referral
Infection	Risk screening, referral	Primary
	Tetanus immunization	Primary
	Clean delivery	Primary
	Antibiotics when membranes ruptured, if not delivered within twelve hours[b]	Primary
	Transport to first referral level	Primary
	Hysterectomy	First referral
Toxemia	Monitor symptoms, blood pressure, and urine for protein	Primary
	Bed rest, sedatives	Primary
	Transport to first-referral level	Primary
	Induction or cesarean section	First referral
Complications of abortion	Antibiotics[b]	Primary
	Transport	Primary
	Oxytocics	Primary
	Evacuation	First referral
	Hysterectomy	First referral
Obstructed labor and ruptured uterus	Risk screening, referral	Primary
	Partograph	Primary
	Transport to first-referral level	Primary
	Symphysiotomy	First referral
	Cesarean section	First referral

a. Primary level includes outreach programs and health dispensaries, posts, or centers. First-referral level usually is a district or cottage hospital with twenty or more beds and the capability of giving blood transfusions and performing cesarean sections.
b. Recommended experimental approach at the community level.
Source: Herz and Measham 1987.

training for those who attend most births and by organizing emergency systems for unexpected complications.

Recently, experts have suggested the use of three indicators for assessing the effectiveness of prenatal and delivery care: the ratio of fresh stillbirths to macerated stillbirths, the percentage of cesarean sections, and the ratio of scheduled deliveries (women identified as high risk during pregnancy and hospital delivery arranged) to emergency deliveries (Mark Belsey, personal communication, June 1991). The ratio of fresh stillbirths may indicate potentially avoidable deaths; a low rate of cesarean sections may suggest that additional maternal and perinatal disease and death may be preventable; and a low proportion of scheduled deliveries suggests that prenatal care and referral should be improved to identify better the women at risk and arrange for hospital deliveries prior to onset of complications. In European countries where the perinatal mortality ratio is

about 10 per 1,000 births, the ratio of fresh-to-macerated stillbirths is one to five. In contrast, in developing countries like Kenya, the ratio is one to three (Belsey and Royston 1987). Other countries, such as Mexico, suffer from excess cesarean sections with poor quality perinatal care and have high perinatal mortality (Bobodilla 1988).

The quality of postpartum and neonatal care is another concern. Women should be treated for infections and checked for hemorrhage, the health needs of the infant should be monitored, and counseling should begin to address future health needs to guarantee less risky deliveries the next time. Counseling should cover family planning, nutrition, need for rest, child care, and breastfeeding. This attention during postpartum visits of women to hospitals or health centers is especially important in those areas where women use clinic services only for maternal health needs. In table 17-9 the feasibility of the proposed services for a maternal and child health program is assessed. Neonatal intensive care is extremely expensive and therefore limited to highly specialized referral centers which can provide high-quality care. At the local level, birth attendants should know about clearing respiratory passages, early breastfeeding, sterile cutting and care of the umbilicus, and hydration of the infant when needed.

TRAINING OF TRADITIONAL BIRTH ATTENDANTS. About 70 percent of all babies in developing countries are delivered by traditional birth attendants (TBAs) or relatives (Lettenmeier and others 1988). Many women prefer TBAs even when modern health care facilities are available. Health workers need to work with TBAs to improve the quality of maternal care delivered and to increase the number of women obtaining prenatal care. With appropriate training and supportive supervision, TBAs can provide the basic care required by women who have normal deliveries. They must learn to use hygienic techniques, avoid harmful practices (for example, excessive force on the woman's belly or pulling the umbilical cord to withdraw the placenta), and make the woman comfortable while encouraging her to adopt practices such as breastfeeding immediately after delivery, keeping clean, and watching for signs of postpuerperal infection or hemorrhage.

Traditional birth attendants also need instruction in emergency care. The attendants must recognize warning signs, know how to stabilize the woman's condition, and be able to transfer her to the next level of care. The proportion of births, by region, attended by trained personnel is shown in figure 17-5. Africa uses trained personnel the least and has the highest maternal mortality rates.

Good Practice vs. Actual Practice—Where Are the Gaps?

Existing reproductive care for women falls far short of needs and lags far behind what we know is feasible (Ratnam and Prasad 1984). Access to high-quality family planning and abortion services remains limited. Few women in developing countries receive prenatal care. Worse still, the women who receive late or no prenatal care are most often young, primiparous, poor, of a racial or ethnic minority, and undernourished, and they are more likely to smoke or drink (Kramer 1987), all of which puts them at higher risk than average and more in need of care. Of the women who do receive prenatal care, most make only one visit to a health care center and that one relatively late in pregnancy (Williams and others 1985). Rural women are much less likely to receive prenatal care than urban women (table 17-10). In places where walking distance is short, more use has been made of clinics. The best results have been where women are within three kilometers of the clinic (Williams and others 1985).

In many places, clinics are available but women do not attend for various reasons. Because the regional referral networks rely on contact during pregnancy, low prenatal participation rates undermine the entire effort. Cultural barriers to services range from distrust of male clinicians to fears of turning

control over to insensitive clinic staff. Some women may consider hospitals or clinics places to die and so refuse to use them for preventive or routine health care; they resort to prenatal care only if they develop complications (Lettenmeier and others 1988; see also Bamisaiye, Ransome-Kuti, and Famurewa 1986; Leslie and Gupta 1989).

Systems to identify high-risk pregnant women in industrial countries have had poor sensitivity and specificity (IOM 1985). Even though most of the adverse pregnancy outcomes occur in women who have several of the risk factors mentioned in table 17-1, many maternal and fetal diseases occur in women with no easily identifiable risk factor. Because of this phenomenon, the sensitivity and specificity of systems based upon history and physical examination average about 60 percent (IOM 1985). These systems identify only about half of the women who eventually have low-birth-weight infants. A reasonably reliable system for classifying women who will have poor pregnancy outcome is needed to contain the cost of services so that those at high risk can receive special, and more expensive, care. An excess of women incorrectly identified as high risk means that scarce resources are used for the care of those who will not benefit from the service and may experience

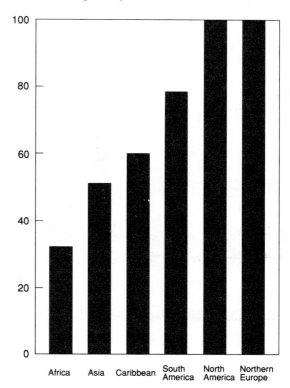

Figure 17-5. Births Attended by Trained Personnel, by Region

Births attended (percent)

Note: Reflects experience about 1982.
Source: Starrs 1987.

Table 17-9. *Maternal and Child Health Services for Management of Pregnancy*

Intervention	Effectiveness	Major drawbacks	Program feasibility
Antenatal[a]			
Antenatal care; screening and referral; monitoring of height, weight, blood pressure; checking for anemia, swelling, protein, presentation, and bleeding.	Women who receive antenatal care are three to five times less likely to die and also less likely to lose their child than women who do not get care. Low birth weight and perinatal complications also decline.	Appropriate screening criteria difficult to select. Village health care providers may have no formal training. Existing services underutilized.	High cost. Feasible if there are central referral hospitals. Special training may be needed. Community must be educated and involved so women will come for antenatal care.
Antenatal education: warning signs, nutrition, health habits	Difficult to assess. Studies of nutrition education found success in avoiding toxemia.	Scheduling education into busy clinic hours; getting women to attend.	Low cost. Can be done as home visits, through neighborhood organizations, TBAs.
Antenatal treatment of anemia, hypertension, infection, STDs, concurrent disease, complications of spontaneous abortion, ectopic pregnancies	Better to prevent these conditions or detect them early. Without this level of service, women will die.	Cost of diagnosis, medication, and training; getting services to appropriate levels.	Women already demand these services; they can be used as point of entry for general prenatal care. Some services can be done at primary level, others at referral level.
Antimalaria education and prophylaxis to endemic areas	Highly effective if taken regularly. Reduces low birth weight, anemia.	Weekly or monthly regimen for taking tablets throughout pregnancy makes compliance a problem. Only chloroquine is approved for pregnant women; best drug for areas with chloroquine-resistant malaria is controversial.	Low cost. Easy to add to existing antenatal care or other health care that reaches women. No special storage facilities needed. Women more likely to take medicine if assured it will not harm the baby or cause abortion.
Tetanus immunization	Eliminates most deaths from neonatal tetanus. Woman immunized as well.	Pregnant women need two injections at least four weeks apart, the second, at least two weeks before delivery. Toxoid must be kept cold. Some personnel may need special training to give immunizations.	Low cost. Coverage generally lags behind other childhood immunizations. Wider coverage possible if women could be immunized at all health centers.
Food supplementation	Benefit to mother has not been evaluated; benefits of supplementing women during pregnancy only have been evaluated. Increases birth weight 30 to 300 g. Most effective in malnourished women.	Difficult to ensure that pregnant woman does not share the supplement with others or substitute it for usual diet.	High cost. Generally too expensive for large, continuing programs. Works best when locally available, inexpensive foods used and when combined with nutrition education. Having women eat supplement at local distribution site most effective.
Iron/folate supplementation before and during pregnancy	Highly effective if tablets taken regularly.	Gastrointestinal side effects and need to take tablets several times a day make compliance a problem. Hard to motivate asymptomatic women to take tablets.	Low cost. Easy to add to existing antenatal care or other health care that reaches women. No special storage facilities needed.
Referral			
Mothers/ waiting homes	Reduced hospital maternal mortality rates in Nigeria and Cuba; other programs not evaluated.	Women may have to stay several weeks before delivery. Lack of transport to homes. Women more likely to come if they can bring their children. Need to maintain or possibly build homes.	Low cost. Done in at least ten countries. Requires good coordination between community programs and hospital. Food, bedding, and cooking utensils supplied by women's families.

Intervention	Effectiveness	Major drawbacks	Program feasibility
Transportation to hospital for obstetric emergencies	Many deaths from complications may be prevented by getting women to hospitals quickly.	Need to buy and maintain vehicles. Needs constant supply of parts, gasoline, drivers. Road building not planned to meet maternal health needs. Woman may need husband's permission to leave home.	High cost. In many places adequate roads will not be built fo years. Innovative communication and transport systems possible where roads are not available.
Delivery			
Regionalization; coordinate TBA, local health center, and specialized facilities[b]	Cost effective	Getting appropriate level of care, especially when unforeseen complications.	Cost depends on existing level of infrastructure. Can be added to any system.
Neonatal care	Detects and treats problems	None	High cost, depending on technology level.
Postpartum care	Most effective way to detect and treat postpartum infections and prevent secondary infertility.	Criteria for referral must be selected. Traditional practices may keep women at home for several weeks after birth. Existing services underutilized.	Low cost. Easy to add to existing antenatal care. Good opportunity to offer family planning. Best when home visits are a real possibility.
Training			
Training TBAs to provide antenatal care, screening, safe delivery	TBA performance improves or remains the same. Effect on maternal complication rates has not been evaluated.	Trainers need special skills and preparation. Supervision and refresher courses needed for TBAs. Delivery kits underutilized.	Moderate cost. Done in many countries. Most effective if community and formally trained health care providers are involved.
Training doctors, nurses, and others	Maternal health outcomes have not been evaluated.	Supervision and refresher courses needed. Degree of training needed that prepares personnel for rural posts. In-service training needs to be offered widely.	Moderate cost. In some countries nurses and nurse-midwives have been trained to perform obstetric surgery.

a. There is insufficient evidence to rate individual components of antenatal care.
b. Herz and Measham plan.
Source: Lettenmeier and others 1988.

complications from unnecessary diagnostic and therapeutic procedures. A misclassification as low risk, however, denies at-risk women access to beneficial services. Some of the systems evaluated classified more than half the women as high risk when the incidence of poor pregnancy outcome was less than 10 percent. These systems for classifying obstetrical risk were evaluated in populations where the average percentage of low-birth-weight infants is 6 percent.

The proportion of false positives and false negatives should decrease in developing countries where the incidence of the adverse outcome increases. For example, in developing countries where the incidence of low birth weight may be two to five times greater than in industrial countries, the predictive value of the screening systems should increase. Conversely, because maternal mortality occurs much less frequently than low birth weight and perinatal mortality, a risk assessment system set up solely to prevent maternal complications will misclassify (false positives and false negatives) a large proportion of women.[4] In order to have a successful maternal and perinatal health system, based on risk assessment and referral care, improved screening criteria are needed.

Delivery and postpartum care suffer from lack of use for reasons similar to those causing women to ignore prenatal care services. Delivery costs are a special barrier to formal services, which are also often competing against cultural norms favoring home delivery. Postnatal care is by far the least-used service; in 1982 only 5 percent of mothers in Costa Rica made one postpartum visit to a health care center, although nearly 97 percent delivered in hospitals (Lettenmeier and others 1988). In Jamaica only 37 percent of new mothers received postpartum care in 1981 despite the fact that the government there provides it free and locally through mobile clinics (WHO 1985). Various cultural factors cause the lack of demand for postpartum services, not the least of which is the widespread belief that new mothers must stay at home (Lettenmeier and others 1988).

There have also been many problems with programs for training TBAs. For example, the traditional compensation may be thought inadequate by the newly trained TBA, villagers may believe the attendant is paid through the health care system and not compensate her in the traditional way, and the training may be of limited use without an additional investment in supervision. For best results, the training must be part of a serious attempt to use available resources, not a potentially cheap solution for remote areas.

Emergency care suffers in many places from the lack of roads, reliable vehicles, restrictions on the use of gasoline, and lack of public transportation which would integrate a referral system. Some programs have developed innovative solutions to this problem: one community in rural Somalia has a flag on the road used to signal passersby when a woman needs a ride to the hospital (Lettenmeier and others 1988); Malawi developed bicycle-pulled stretchers; and Zambia gave women expecting complications free tickets for bus transportation (Favin and others 1984). The issue always is whether an emergency, if one arises, can be dealt with quickly enough.

Many prenatal care and delivery interventions have been recommended depending upon local problems and resources. The actual health effect of an intervention, however, depends on several factors: (a) rates of effectiveness, or the ability of an intervention to prevent or treat the problem; (b) accuracy of the diagnostic tests to identify those who would benefit from the intervention; (c) quality of care; (d) patient compliance; (e) coverage—in this case, the proportion of women using the service; and (f) frequency of the health problem. All these factors plus cost and feasibility should be considered by countries planning a system for improving maternal and perinatal health.

Strategies for Two Standardized Populations

In this section we use two hypothetical populations of one million persons to illustrate maternal and perinatal program strategies and priorities. The populations include a low-mortality country and a high-mortality country. Because of the close interrelationship of resource allocation for fertility control and the management of pregnancy, we present the prevention and case management illustrations in a unified separate section.

Low-Mortality Example

The first population, referred to here as Lomort (for low mortality), has already passed through much of the demographic transition. The fertility rate is 2.8, the infant mortality rate is 51 per 1,000 births, the perinatal mortality rate is 35.7 per 1,000 births (because about half of perinatal mortality occurs in the first week of life, about 35 percent of all infant deaths occur in the perinatal period), and life expectancy at birth is 64.4 years. We assume the maternal mortality ratio is about 200 deaths per 100,000 live births (inferred from WHO 1986) and that about 65 percent of women of reproductive age use contraceptives.

Table 17-10. *Women Reporting at Least One Prenatal Visit during Most Recent Pregnancy, Selected Countries*
(percent)

Country	Urban	Rural	Total
Sri Lanka	97	97	97
Dominican Republic	—	—	95
Liberia	91	77	83
Burundi	96	78	79
Thailand	94	74	77
Brazil	86	51	74
Ecuador	82	58	70
Colombia	83	59	69
Senegal	95	46	63
Guatemala[a]	56	26	34
Morocco	48	13	25

— Data not available.
Note: Based on demographic and health surveys in 1986 and 1987. Covers only pregnancies within five years preceding the survey. Interviewers asked women: "When you were last pregnant, did you see anyone for a check on that pregnancy?" Only those respondents checked by trained health care providers are indicated.
a. Only women checked by a doctor or nurse.
Source: Lettenmeier and others 1988.

Lomort has a reasonably well developed health system, a large proportion of women receive prenatal and delivery care from trained birth attendants, and the average standard of living is moderate. The effect of increasing contraceptive prevalence on maternal mortality in Lomort would be low. Increasing the use of contraception beyond the current level would be prohibitively expensive and the gains are unclear. Therefore, we consider other avenues in Lomort.

In order to bring the maternal mortality ratio down, perhaps to 25 per 100,000 live births, as in urban China, more investment is needed in obstetrical care and perhaps some important social reforms are required as well. China has achieved large reductions in adverse maternal events through its radical one-child policy for population control, higher age at marriage, and better health care for pregnant women. The China example underlines the importance of political will for health achievements at this level of development. China has widely available family planning services and a strong political commitment to maternal health, and it offers continuing education and motivational campaigns using different forms of persuasion (Chen and Kols 1982). Lomort could make substantial gains in maternal health with relative cost efficiency by improving the quality of existing services, focusing on use of the services, and coordinating with other sectors to implement social reforms which promote women's health.

Social reforms in particular can have a large effect on maternal health. Such reforms include legalizing abortion, raising the age of marriage, requiring universal education, and providing welfare to the worst-off, highest-risk groups. Latin American countries have maternal mortality ratios similar to Lomort's, and their revision of abortion policies could potentially save both lives and costs. In the early 1970s in Chile, 3,250 hospital-induced abortions cost $30,000 during a brief period when abortions were legalized. Researchers calculated a savings of more than $200,000 above earlier costs for emergency treatment of illegal abortion complications (Weston 1986). Cultural changes are equally important: researchers find that low use of maternal health services is often due to cultural perceptions of women's roles, which block the woman's ability to get care for herself (Leslie and Gupta 1989). There may also be traditional practices which are dangerous, female circumcision, for example, and women's health advocates are calling for national educational campaigns to discourage them.

Lomort's health sector might implement a ten-year, limited effort, safe motherhood program that emphasized health and nutrition education, hiring additional staff to extend community outreach and screening and to improve existing services and increase their use. The program would offer additional training for personnel; provide health and nutrition education campaigns; and examine facilities, emergency systems, and referral networks and renovate them as necessary. The cost estimates for this kind of effort are listed in table 17-11.

On the basis of experience in countries which have implemented similar efforts, we estimate that the program's effect on adverse events could be as much as a 65 percent reduction in maternal mortality and morbidity, a 20 to 25 percent reduction in the number of low-birth-weight babies, and a 35 percent reduction in perinatal mortality over the ten-year period. Table 17-12 contains before-and-after scenarios that use more conservative estimates of the progress which can be achieved. The table provides two sets of calculations for the achievements of a limited effort, in part because current gaps in knowledge keep us from knowing just what can be accomplished. For the lower estimate, we assume that the maternal mortality rate will be reduced by 25 percent, low birth weight will drop in incidence from 8 to 7.5 percent, and the perinatal mortality rate will be reduced by 12.5 percent; for the more optimistic scenario, we assume that maternal mortality will be reduced by 50 percent, the incidence of low birth weight will drop to 7 percent, and the perinatal mortality rate will be reduced by 25 percent. The total cost of the program for a population of one million would be about $480,000 annually, or about $0.48 per capita. The estimated cost per death averted (maternal and infant) ranges from $3,967 to $1,975, and the estimated cost per adverse event averted ranges from $1,103 to $550. Adverse events include deaths, episodes of maternal morbidity, and low-birth-weight babies.

The fertility rate and number of births have been held constant in table 17-12 in order to isolate the effect of improvements in prenatal and obstetric care alone. In reality, one would expect a further decline in fertility if services and community outreach were extended. The number of infant deaths and low-birth-weight babies avoided is much greater than the number of adverse maternal events in spite of the greater percentage of reduction in rates for women. This high-

Table 17-11. *Additional Annual Operating and Capital Costs for Maternal Health and Family Planning in Lomort, a Standardized Population of One Million, in Safe Motherhood Initiative: Limited-Effort Model*
(U.S. dollars)

Expenditures	Cost
Annual operating costs	
Staff	50,000
Transport	100,000
In-service training and supervision	75,000
Equipment and supplies	75,000
Health education, cultural campaigns	100,000
Monitoring and evaluation	20,000
Contingencies	30,000
Total	450,000
Cost per capita	0.45
Capital costs	
Training	200,000
Construction and upgrading	240,000
Vehicles	160,000
Total	600,000
Capital costs attributable to maternal health[a]	300,000
Annualized capital cost[b]	30,000
Annualized cost per capita	0.03
Total costs[c]	
Gross	480,000
Per capita[a]	0.48

a. Assumes half of total capital costs attributable to maternal health.
b. Assumes ten-year depreciation.
c. Annual operating costs plus annualized capital costs.
Source: Herz and Measham 1987.

lights the fact that safe motherhood programs benefit both women and their infants.

High-Mortality Example

Our second standardized population, Himort (for high mortality), can benefit substantially from relatively small investments in women's health. The ideal maternal and child health program would provide family planning services (including safe abortions, prenatal care, and training of traditional birth attendants and health personnel) and regional referral and emergency transportation systems. As mentioned earlier, efforts to increase female enrollment in schools and improve female nutrition would also contribute to better maternal and perinatal health.

Himort is at an early stage of development. A large area is desert and people are scattered in villages and nomadic settlements. Agriculture is limited and transportation is sparse. Another area is forested and has high humidity and seasonal

Table 17-12. Current Indicators of Maternal and Child Health in Lomort, a Standardized Population of One Million, in a Limited-Effort Safe Motherhood Program

Indicator	Before program	With limited-effort program	
		Conservative estimate	Moderate estimate
Demographics			
Population	1,000,000	1,000,000	1,000,000
Contraceptive prevalence (percent)[a]	65	65	65
Fertility rate	2.8	2.8	2.8
Crude birth rate	24.5	24.5	24.5
Births (number)	24,500	24,500	24,500
Morbidity and mortality			
Maternal mortality ratio (deaths per live 100,000 births)[b]	200	150	100
Perinatal mortality rate (deaths per 1,000 births)	35.7	31.2	26.8
Maternal deaths (number)	49	37	25
Maternal morbidity (number)[c]	784	592	400
Perinatal infant deaths (number)[d]	875	766	656
Low-birth-weight babies (number)[e]	1,960	1,838	1,715
Program effectiveness			
Births averted (number)	n.a.	0	0
Maternal deaths averted (number)	n.a.	12	24
Maternal morbidity averted (number)	n.a.	192	384
Perinatal infant deaths averted (number)	n.a.	109	219
Low birth weight averted (number)	n.a.	122	245
Costs (in U.S. dollars)			
Program cost	n.a.	480,000	480,000
Cost per capita	n.a.	0.48	0.48
Cost per death averted	n.a.	3,967	1,975
Cost per event averted	n.a.	1,103	550

n.a. Not applicable.
a. Among females age fifteen to forty-four.
b. Assumes that improved obstetric services result in 25 percent and 50 percent reductions in conservative and moderate estimates, respectively.
c. Number of maternal deaths multiplied by 16. Estimated ratio from Datta and others 1973.
d. Assumes that improved obstetric services result in 12.5 percent and 25 percent reductions in conservative and moderate estimates, respectively.
e. Predicted from regression (see appendix 17A). Assumes a 0.5 percent and 1 percent drop in low-birth-weight incidence in conservative and moderate estimates, respectively, resulting in 6.2 percent and 12.5 percent reductions in the number of low-birth-weight babies.
Source: Herz and Measham 1987.

floods. People crowd together on meager farming plots; communities are often isolated from each other by washed-out roads and unnavigable waterways. Some areas are more favored: conditions there are less harsh, people live in larger communities, health facilities are better developed, and roads are adequate.

Health services are scarce in Himort, with a few exceptions, constrained by inadequate staffing, supervision, and supplies. Family planning is virtually unknown, so there are very few modern contraceptive users except in the capital. Unsafe abortions are relatively common. Most women, about 90 percent, deliver at home; about 70 percent of births are attended by untrained traditional midwives or family members. The few better-off places are served by health centers and a district hospital, but maternal health is not given priority.

Life expectancy at birth is fifty-one years, the infant mortality rate is 129 deaths per 1,000 births and perinatal mortality is 51.6 deaths per 1,000 births (note that the ratio of perinatal mortality to all infant mortality is 0.4, lower than in Lomort because of the higher prevalence of infectious disease and

consequent infant deaths during the first year. This is an extremely conservative estimate of perinatal mortality [Edouard 1985]). Maternal mortality is believed to range from 800 to 1,400 per 100,000 live births in the various regions; health officials estimate a national average of 1,000 deaths. The total fertility rate is 6.9 and the crude birth rate is 49.5 (see table 17-13 for a summary of statistics). Use of modern contraception is low.

The problem facing Himort is how to improve maternal and perinatal health with severe limitations on resources, inadequate facilities, and inadequate transportation. Discussing a hypothetical situation similar to Himort, Herz and Measham (1987) proposed that the choice between "providing a little to many" and "providing more to a few" inadequately represents the dilemma. Little progress can be made in a situation like this without additional investment in community-level care, referral facilities, and transportation. Each region must individually assess its restrictions and needs and may need to plan an appropriate program which differs from those of other regions.

Table 17-13. Current Indicators of Maternal and Child Health in Himort, a Standardized Population of One Million

Indicator	Value
Demographics	
Population	1,000,000
Contraceptive prevalence (percent)[a]	0
Fertility rate	6.9
Crude birth rate	49.5
Births (number)	49,500
Morbidity and Mortality	
Maternal mortality ratio (deaths per 1,000 live births)	1,000
Perinatal mortality rate (deaths per 1,000 births)	51.6
Maternal deaths (number)	495
Maternal morbidity (number)[b]	7,920
Perinatal infant deaths (number)	2,554
Low-birth-weight babies (number)[c]	7,425

a. Among females age fifteen to forty-four.
b. Number of maternal deaths multiplied by 16. Estimated ratio from Datta and others 1973.
c. Predicted from regression (see appendix 17A). Represents 15 percent.
Source: Authors.

Among the options available to Himort are preventive activities as described earlier. In contrast to Lomort, family planning is the most cost-effective preventive activity that could be provided. Addition of some other cost-effective strategies discussed in earlier sections would improve cost-effectiveness, for example, STD screening and treatment. A second option would strengthen prenatal care and train birth attendants for pregnancy management. We begin by illustrating the likely costs and benefits of family planning alone and then discuss the implications of a broader maternal health program.

FAMILY PLANNING ALONE. If Himort did nothing to strengthen prenatal and delivery care but did offer family planning services, substantial improvements in maternal and infant health outcomes could result. There are a number of methods of providing family planning services, though social marketing, community-based distribution, postpartum projects, and voluntary sterilization services appear to be among the most cost-effective. Studies show costs in 1980 ranging from $1 per couple-year of protection for social marketing in Colombia to $90 for some clinic programs (Sherris and others 1985). A community-based delivery system, using traditional birth attendants and local health personnel, might be a good method for Himort. Such a program in rural Cheju Province in the Republic of Korea between 1976 and 1979, which also included free sterilization, resulted in a 20 percent increase in women who accepted contraceptives and a decline in the total fertility rate of more than 1.5 births in a period of five years, from 1975 to 1980. This program cost $0.47 annually per capita and $9.35 per couple-year of protection (Chen and Worth 1982; Park and others 1982).

In table 17-14 we present demographic data and health statistics for three scenarios: increases in the prevalence rate for contraception to 20 percent, 40 percent, and 60 percent, respectively. Through the increase in contraceptive users, fertility rates decline and the number of births is reduced, thereby reducing exposure to pregnancy risk. The maternal mortality ratio is held constant throughout table 17-14, however, emphasizing that unlike the maternal mortality rate, it is unaffected by overall changes in fertility. In spite of the constant maternal mortality ratio, maternal deaths and morbidity drop remarkably. Using the new fertility rates, calculated on the basis of the contraceptive prevalence rates, we have also derived revised rates of low birth weight. Perinatal infant death rates are assumed to drop 5 percent for every 20 percent increase in contraceptive prevalence. The number of low-birth-weight infants and infant deaths declines with reductions in fertility for the following reasons. First, with fewer births there is a smaller risk pool; second, in order to provide family planning services, health personnel increase their contacts with the community, which improves health outcomes; third, part of the demand for family planning results from social improvements, which also improve health.

The success of family planning efforts depends on program quality and acceptability, a strong demand-generation effort, method effectiveness, and consistent availability of supplies. Demand is increased by such changes as increasing the age at marriage, increasing female education, and employment patterns which decrease the value or necessity of children. The demographic changes presented in table 17-14 may occur over several decades. The fertility rate in Thailand fell by almost 40 percent in twenty-five years—one of the most rapid reductions recorded. The crude birth rate was about 44 in the early 1960s (Sherris and others 1985) and fell to 24.5 in 1985 (WHO 1986). The drop in birth rate predicted in the model, from 49.5 to 28.4, is consistent with experience in Thailand but could take many more years, depending on the setting. The assumption for the costs discussed in table 17-14 is that expenses increase exponentially as population coverage goals increase, but ignored in these estimates are adjustment costs, which could occur over long periods and which may be necessary for significant increases in contraceptive use to take place. The data in table 17-14 do show that the cost efficiency of family planning for improving maternal and perinatal health decreases as contraceptive prevalence increases. The cost per death averted ranges from $806 to $1,338 to $2,962 as contraceptive prevalence reaches 20 percent, 40 percent, and 60 percent of couples at risk.[5] Costs per adverse event averted range from $139 to $229 to $505. Adverse events include deaths, episodes of maternal morbidity, and low-birth-weight babies.

COMPREHENSIVE MATERNAL HEALTH PROGRAM. In this section two plans are proposed for Himort which go beyond family planning by including various maternal care and structural improvements to the health system. They assume that Himort has adopted the goal of a family planning prevalence rate of 20 percent and that it also undertakes additional reforms in the

Table 17-14. Effects on Maternal and Child Health of Three Scenarios Based on Contraceptive Prevalence Rates

Indicator	20 percent prevalence rate	40 percent prevalence rate	60 percent prevalence rate
Demographics			
Fertility rate[a]	5.3	4.3	2.6
Births (number)	41,170	34,183	28,381
Morbidity and mortality			
Maternal mortality ratio (deaths per 100,000 live births)	1,000	1,000	1,000
Perinatal mortality rate (deaths per 1,000 births)[b]	49	46.4	43.9
Maternal deaths (number)	412	342	284
Maternal morbidity (number)[c]	6,592	5,472	4,544
Perinatal infant deaths (number)	2,017	1,586	1,246
Low-birth-weight babies (number)[a,d]	5,764	4,444	3,406
Program effectiveness			
Births averted (number)	8,330	15,317	21,119
Maternal deaths averted (number)	83	153	211
Maternal morbidity averted (number)	1,328	2,448	3,376
Perinatal infant deaths averted (number)	537	968	1,308
Low birth weight averted (number)	1,661	2,981	4,019
Costs (in U.S. dollars)			
Program[e]	500,000	1,500,000	4,500,000
Cost per capita	0.50	1.50	4.50
Cost per death averted	806	1,338	2,962
Cost per event averted	139	229	505

Note: Prevalence rate is percent of women fifteen to forty-four using contraceptives.

a. Predicted from regression (see appendix 17A).

b. Assumes decreases in perinatal mortality rate from the original high of 51.6 through contraceptive prevalence rates of 20 percent, 40 percent, and 60 percent, are 5 percent, 10 percent, and 15 percent, respectively.

c. Maternal deaths times 16. Estimated ratio from Datta and others 1973.

d. Assumes incidence of low birth weight decreases for each 20 percent increase in contraceptive prevalence. With decreases in numbers of births, the result is total decreases in number of low-birth-weight babies of 22 percent, 40 percent, and 54 percent, respectively, for the 20 percent, 40 percent, and 60 percent contraceptive prevalence rates.

e. Longer time periods are needed to achieve higher rates of contraceptive prevalence and are likely to involve costs not included here.

Source: Authors.

area of maternal health care. The limited goal of a 20 percent prevalence rate for contraception was chosen because it is a reasonable accomplishment for a ten-year plan; higher goals would demand a longer time horizon and more resources and would involve much greater uncertainty.

The goals for a comprehensive maternal health program in Himort would differ according to the existing infrastructure, socioeconomy, and ecology of particular subareas. The first effort, a limited one, is most appropriate for the very poor, isolated desert and rain forest areas that make up the bulk of the country. The plan includes resources necessary for a limited prenatal care and birth attendant training program; this effort would be carried out in addition to the family planning effort, aiming for 20 percent prevalence. The second, moderate effort would best be applied in areas that are not as poor, are densely populated, have existing health facilities, including a hospital, and where women use health services more. The moderate plan includes the resources necessary for a moderate prenatal care and birth attendant training program; this is again in addition to the previously mentioned family planning effort. The goals of each effort are described below. We have adapted the program design and cost estimates, developed by Herz and

Measham (1987), who provide a more detailed discussion of these items.

The goals of the limited effort are to reduce the maternal mortality ratio by 20 percent through prenatal and delivery care and trained birth attendants. In addition, we expect the plan to reduce the incidence of low-birth-weight babies to 13 percent (dropping from 14 percent with family planning alone) and perinatal infant mortality by an additional 12.5 percent. These decreases would be the result of reducing the number of high-risk pregnancies and of providing better care to those who become pregnant. The limited plan would include the following elements:

- Upgrading of existing facilities to ensure the availability of maternal health care and the establishment of four more centers (two with cesarean section and surgical family planning capacity)

- Investment in an emergency transportation system, one four-wheel drive vehicle for each new center, so that more women can reach the existing service areas

- Introduction of risk screening and development of plans for at-risk women to deliver in health facilities;

three mobile units equipped with radios and staffed by three health care workers; and maternity villages where those referred to facilities for delivery can await the start of labor

- Strengthening of all community-based services by training all traditional birth attendants and providing them with basic medications, compensation for family planning activities, and radios, so that prenatal and uncomplicated delivery care is readily available

- Coordination of outreach so that facilities and trained personnel are efficiently used

- Conduct of research activities to identify the most effective strategies

- Depending on the community or region, other potential components include training nurse-midwives to enlarge the pool of health workers able to provide blood transfusions, surgical family planning, and cesarean sections; strengthening health services management and giving higher priority to maternal health; and encouraging community groups to become involved in women's health and safe motherhood.

The total cost of the program for a population of one million, including family planning program costs, would be about $980,000 annually, or about $0.98 per capita (see table 17-15 for breakdown of costs for the maternal health component alone). The cost per death averted (maternal and infant) is about $1,303, and the cost per adverse event averted is about $179.[6] Adverse events include deaths, maternal morbidity, and low-birth-weight babies.

The goals of the moderate effort are to reduce the maternal mortality ratio by 40 percent through prenatal and delivery care, facility development, and training of birth attendants. In addition, we expect the plan to reduce the incidence of low-birth-weight babies to 12 percent (dropping from 14 percent from family planning alone) and perinatal infant mortality by an additional 25 percent. These reductions are more conservative than most cited in the literature. The plan would include the following elements:

- Establishment of a community outreach system for prenatal care, which would provide nutrition advice and pregnancy risk screening, make appropriate referrals, and encourage use of health facilities

- An increase in the number of health posts to one for every 10,000 population, built with community assistance, and the training of all TBAs in outreach and routine care activities

- An increase in the number of health centers by the construction of five new ones in five years, to be used as referral centers for pregnancy complications

- Addition of ten maternity beds to the district hospital and an operating room with the capacity to handle high-risk deliveries, cesarean sections, and surgical contraception

- Training of additional health personnel at each level so that a regional network of services exists with increasingly

Table 17-15. Additional Annual Operating and Capital Costs for Maternal Health in Himort Safe Motherhood Initiative: Limited-Effort Model
(U.S. dollars)

Expenditure	Cost
Annual operating costs	
Staff	150,000
Transport	100,000
In-service training and supervision	50,000
Equipment and supplies	75,000
Health education	25,000
Monitoring and evaluation	20,000
Contingencies	30,000
Total	450,000
Cost per capita[a]	0.45
Capital costs	
Training	100,000
Construction and upgrading	340,000
Vehicles	160,000
Total	600,000
Capital costs attributable to maternal health[b]	300,000
Annualized capital cost[c]	30,000
Annualized cost per capita[a]	0.03
Total costs[d]	
Gross	480,000
Per capita[a]	0.48

Note:
a. Assumes population of 1 million.
b. Assumes half of total capital costs attributable to maternal health.
c. Assumes ten-year depreciation.
d. Annual operating costs plus annualized capital costs.
Source: Herz and Measham 1987.

complex services offered at health posts, health centers, and the hospital, respectively

- Development of an emergency transport system and training of all personnel for appropriate referrals.

The total cost of the program for a population of one million, including the cost of the family planning program, would be about $2 million annually, or about $2 per capita (see table 17-16 for breakdown of costs of maternal health components alone). The cost per death averted (maternal and infant) is about $1,554, and the cost per adverse event averted is about $258.[7] In table 17-17 we summarize the effect of and cost information for the family planning effort alone and the family planning effort plus limited and moderate obstetrics programs.

For the limited and moderate obstetrics programs, we assume some community contributions, and both programs are based on assumed correlations between improved prenatal care and birth outcomes. The call for emergency transport systems and care is in recognition of the fallibility of current risk-screening methods and the likelihood that some women will continue to use health services only when there is a problem.

Table 17-16. Additional Annual Operating and Capital Costs for Maternal Health in Himort Safe Motherhood Initiative: Moderate-Effort Model
(U.S. dollars)

Expenditure	Cost
Annual operating costs	
Staff	575,000
Transport	125,000
In-service training and supervision	150,000
Equipment and supplies	300,000
Health education	50,000
Monitoring and evaluation	50,000
Total	1,250,000
Cost per capita[a]	1.25
Capital costs	
Training	800,000
Construction and upgrading	3,600,000
Vehicles	600,000
Total	5,000,000
Capital costs attributable to maternal health[b]	500,000
Annualized capital cost[c]	25,000
Annualized cost per capita[a]	0.25
Total costs[d]	
Gross	1,500,000
Per capita[a]	1.50

a. Assumes population of 1 million.
b. Assumes half of capital costs attributable to maternal health.
c. Assumes ten-year depreciation.
d. Annual operating costs plus annualized capital costs.
Source: Herz and Measham 1987.

Summary of Hypothetical Examples

As the examples illustrate, efforts to improve maternal and perinatal health should involve appropriate combinations of family planning, prenatal care, and obstetric improvements. Health services should also give priority to screening and referral networks and emergency transportation systems. Screening for potential complications is used to direct high-risk women away from home delivery and into adequately staffed and equipped delivery facilities. Emergency transportation systems are also needed for cases in which screening was absent or produced a false negative.

In countries with high fertility, significant reductions in maternal and infant deaths result both from reductions in the number of pregnancies through family planning and from improved maternal care. Where fertility is already low, reductions result almost entirely from improved maternal and perinatal care. Altogether, the investments required for safer motherhood and healthier starts to life are relatively low, and the potential gains are great. Still, the health system must have the capacity to make services available to people in all parts of the country. Extending service coverage is especially critical for those countries whose current budget is allocated largely to the urban centers.

Finally, a word of caution is in order. The calculations presented here depend on heroic assumptions, because reliable data are lacking. We have found virtually no data on the effect of maternal health programs on maternal health, infant mortality, or low birth weight, nor were we able to separate perinatal from neonatal or general infant mortality. There is no clear scientific evidence that a particular component contributes to a specified decline in adverse events. We proposed goals for the hypothetical populations and presented program components without clear evidence of the magnitude of the effect of these measures. In sum, the declines in adverse outcomes that we have suggested are no more than best estimates of the likely effect of the measures proposed based on the limited evidence available from the literature.

Priorities

Finally, we recommend priorities for resource allocation, and for research.

Priorities for Resource Allocation

Maternal mortality, perinatal mortality, high fertility, and low birth weight are all high-priority problems. Technically feasible and affordable methods exist which can significantly reduce the incidence of perinatal and maternal disease and death and increase the prevalence of contraceptive use. Furthermore, investments in family planning and maternal and perinatal health compare favorably with other health investments, such as curative care, that are more costly but have a more limited effect on the population. Indeed, because maternal and perinatal health problems have long been neglected, they should be at the top of the priority list in most countries—especially those in which maternal mortality, neonatal mortality, and low birth weight are high (that is, South Asia and Sub-Saharan Africa).

As the examples set forth in the last section illustrate, the priorities for particular programs that target maternal and perinatal health depend on the demographic situation, particularly the fertility rate and level of contraceptive use, and on ecological and economic factors. When countries are deciding on the balance between maternal health and other health programs, they will find it worth considering that maternal health affects the health of infants, children, and the dependent elderly. The loss of a mother threatens family survival. The choice need not be between maternal health services and other programs; creative health administrators are able to incorporate the needs of women into primary or other health care programs.

The focus in this chapter has been on mortality and morbidity; the other side of the equation, the magnitude and quality of health, has largely been ignored. When safe motherhood programs are implemented, the priority should be to promote good health, not merely to avoid death. Countries should look at the quality of life for newborn children and the quality of life for women both during and after the reproductive period. These priorities will require intersectoral collaboration, strong

Table 17-17. Estimated Effect of Comprehensive Maternal Health Plan Alone and for Family Planning with Limited and Moderate Obstetrics Program in Himort

Indicator	Before program	Family planning only	Family planning and limited obstetrics program	Family planning and moderate obstetrics program
Demographics				
Population	1,000,000	1,000,000	1,000,000	1,000,000
Contraceptive prevalence (percent)[a]	0	20	20	20
Fertility rate	6.9	5.3	5.3	5.3
Crude birth rate	49.5	41.17	41.17	41.17
Births (number)	49,500	41,170	41,170	41,170
Morbidity and Mortality				
Maternal mortality ratio (deaths per 100,000 live births)	1,000	1,000	800[b]	600[b]
Perinatal mortality rate (deaths per 1,000 births)	51.6	49	47.8[c]	36.8[c]
Maternal deaths (number)	495	412	329	247
Maternal morbidity (number)	7,920	6,592	5,264	3,952
Perinatal infant deaths (number)	5,643	2,017	1,968	1,515
Low-birth-weight babies (number)	7,425	5,764	5,352	4,940
Program effectiveness				
Births averted (number)	n.a.	8,330	8,330	8,330
Maternal deaths averted (number)	n.a.	83	166	248
Maternal morbidity averted (number)	n.a.	1,328	2,656	3,968
Perinatal infant deaths averted (number)	n.a.	537	586	1,039
Low birth weight averted (number)	n.a.	1,661	2,073	2,485
Costs (in U.S. dollars)				
Program cost	n.a.	500,000	980,000	2,000,000
Cost per capita	n.a.	0.50	0.98	2.00
Cost per death averted	n.a.	806	1,303	1,554
Cost per event averted	n.a.	139	179	258

n.a. Not applicable.

a. Among females age fifteen to forty-four.

b. Assumes additional decreases of 20 percent and 40 percent for limited and moderate efforts, respectively, over the decreases achieved by family planning alone.

c. Assumes additional decreases of 12.5 percent for limited and moderate efforts, respectively, over the decreases achieved by family planning alone.

Source: Authors' calculations.

political will, and a willingness to recognize the importance and value of women.

Family planning and access to safe abortion as a backup are clearly a priority. Successful family planning programs require a demand for spacing children and limiting family size. Health improvements must be accompanied, therefore, by concomitant efforts to improve female education and women's economic opportunities. Declines in fertility will then make reproductive health care services more affordable.

Access to prenatal and competent obstetric care also merit high priority. The content of these services, their quality, and their use certainly influence their effectiveness. Indeed, merely improving the quality of existing care and increasing the use of existing services could have a substantial effect in many countries. A study in Jamaica concluded that 68 percent of maternal mortality could be prevented through improvements in the quality of care (Walker and others 1986).

Some suggested priorities for prenatal and delivery care follow: screening for high-risk women; tetanus toxoid immunization; iron and folate supplements; malaria prophylaxis in endemic areas; nutrition education and supplements for the most malnourished mothers; testing and treatment for repro-

ductive tract infection and STDs in high-incidence areas; referral of women developing complications during pregnancy to facilities able to provide higher-level care; and encouraging higher-risk women to deliver in hospital. Somewhat lower priorities for prenatal care are education aimed at decreasing alcohol and tobacco abuse; monitoring weight and blood pressure of women during pregnancy; educating for signs of premature labor; screening all women for sexually transmitted diseases and treating identified cases; and performing pelvic examinations to check gynecological anatomy in all women. High priorities for delivery care are providing hygienic delivery kits to birth attendants; training TBAs for delivery emergencies (includes use of oxytocics) and neonatal resuscitation; arranging regional referral systems for skilled obstetrical care and neonatal intensive care. In all countries, health personnel should locate favorable traditional practices and build on these for health promotion.

Priorities for Operational Research

Maternal and perinatal health are areas that have been severely neglected by researchers. The focus of programs which have affected the health of women (such as nutrition supplementation) has more often been on infant mortality. We have little evidence of the factors causing mortality rate declines, no measures of the economic effect of death or disability, nor any firm idea of the prevalence or duration of maternal and perinatal illness. There is insufficient information to relate different service components directly with effectiveness and cost. It goes without saying that more field research is needed in this area, and more programs should include an evaluation component.

Appendix 17A. Regression Equations Used in the Construction of Tables 17-11 through 17-17

Data from *World Development Indicators* (1988) were used to estimate the regressions used for tables 17-11 through 17-17. All equations include gross national product (GNP) to control for societal effects like education, nutrition, and general health status. The fertility rates, rather than crude birth rates, were used as independent variables because they are a better indicator of risks for adverse maternal events. By multiplying the fertility rate and the maternal mortality ratio, one can also derive a maternal mortality rate.

$$\ln(\text{birthrate}) = 4.92 - 0.009\,(\%\ \text{contraceptive prevalence}) - 0.17\ln(\text{GNP})$$
$$(22.84)\ (4.97)\ (4.37)$$

$$\ln(\text{fertility rate}) = 3.63 - 0.0035\,(\%\ \text{contraceptive prevalence}) - 0.32\ln(\text{GNP})$$
$$(21.65)\ (3.45)\ (13.24)$$

$$\ln(\%\ \text{low birth wt}) = 3.24 + 0.26\ln(\text{fertility rate}) - 0.19\ln(\text{GNP})$$
$$(4.75)\ (1.53)\ (2.71)$$

Notes

1. The World Health Organization uses the ratio but calls it a rate.

2. The number of fetal deaths included depends upon the lower limit set for fetal viability. Recently, the World Health Organization has recommended that perinatal statistics for international comparisons be restricted to fetuses and newborn infants with a birth weight of at least 1,000 grams (or, when the birth weight is not available, the gestational age of twenty-eight weeks or crown-to-heel body length of 35 centimeters) for both numerator and denominator for the perinatal mortality rate (Edouard 1985; *Lancet* 1991).

3. Intrauterine growth retardation can be subdivided into "disproportional" or "wasted" IUGR infants, whose length and head circumference are relatively normal for their gestational age but who are thin, with low weight-for-length and skinfold measurements; and "proportional" or "stunted" IUGR infants with proportional reductions in weight, length, and head circumference. The distinction seems to relate to an earlier and more persistent impairment in growth in the stunted group. "Wasted" infants seem to grow faster postnatally, catch up to normal size more rapidly, and have fewer severe cognitive deficits than the "stunted" ones. Unfortunately, large studies comparing the relative incidence of these two forms of IUGR have not been published.

4. The highest maternal mortality ratios are about 8 per 1,000, the highest perinatal mortality is about 100 per 1,000, and the maximum incidence of low birth weight is up to 500 per 1,000.

5. This calculation is very sensitive to the estimated perinatal mortality. If a higher initial estimate for perinatal mortality is used, then the costs per death averted would decrease almost 50 percent.

6. See note 6.

7. See note 6.

References

Bamisaiye, A., Olikoye Ransome-Kuti, and A. A. Famurewa. 1986. "Waiting Time and Its Impact on Service Acceptability and Coverage at an MCH Clinic at Lagos, Nigeria." *Journal of Tropical Pediatrics* 32:158–61.

Belsey, M. A., and Erica Royston. 1987. "Overview of the Health of Women and Children." Paper presented at the International Conference on Better Health for Women and Children through Family Planning, Nairobi, Kenya, October 5–9, 1987.

Berman, S. N., R. Harrison, W. T. Boyce, W. W. J. Haffner, M. Lewis, and J. B. Arthur. 1981. "Low Birthweight, Prematurity, and Postpartum Endometriosis." *Journal of the American Medical Association* 257:1189–94.

Bhatia, J. C. 1985. "Maternal Mortality in Anantapur District, India: Preliminary Findings of a Study." Family Health Division, World Health Organization, Geneva.

Blacker, J. G. C. 1987. "Health Impacts of Family Planning." *Health Policy and Planning* 2:193–203.

Bobodilla, Fernandez J. L. 1988. *Quality of Perinatal Medical Care in Mexico City*. Instituto Nacional de Salud Pública, Mexico City.

Brown, S. 1985. "Can Low Birthweight be Prevented?" *Family Planning Perspectives* 17:112–18.

Brunham, R. C., K. K. Holmes, and D. Eschenbach. 1984. "Sexually Transmitted Diseases in Pregnancy." In K. K. Holmes, P.-A. Mardh, F. Sparling, and P. J. Wiesner, eds., *Sexually Transmitted Diseases*. New York: McGraw-Hill.

CDC (Centers for Disease Control). 1987. "Enterically Transmitted Non-A, Non-B Hepatitis—East Africa." *Morbidity and Mortality Weekly Report* 36:241–44.

Chen, K., and George Worth. 1982. "Cost-Effectiveness of a Community-Based Family Planning Program in Cheju, Korea." Paper presented at the International Health Conference, June 14–16, 1982, Washington, D.C.

Chen, L. C., M. C. Gesche, S. Ahmed, A. I. Chowdhury, and W. H. Mosley. 1974. "Maternal Mortality in Rural Bangladesh." *Studies in Family Planning* 5:334–41.

Chen, R. J. 1985. "Maternal Mortality in Shanghai, China." Family Health Division, World Health Organization, Geneva.

Chen, P. C., and A. Kols. 1982. "Population and Birth Planning in the People's Republic of China." *Population Reports*, J, 25. Johns Hopkins University, Population Information Program, Baltimore.

Chi, I. C., T. Agoestina, and J. Harbin. 1981. "Maternal Mortality at 12 Teaching Hospitals in Indonesia: An Epidemiological Analysis." *International Journal of Gynecology and Obstetrics* 24:259–66.

Datta, S. P., D. K. Srinivas, R. V. Kale, and R. Rangaswamy. 1973. "Evaluation of Maternal and Infant Care in a Rural Area." *Indian Journal of Medical Sciences* 27:120–28.

Donaldson, P. J., and J. O. G. Billy. 1984. "The Impact of Prenatal Care on Birthweight." *Medical Care* 22:177–88.

Edouard, L. "The Epidemiology of Perinatal Mortality." *World Health Statistics Quarterly* 38(3):289.

Fauveau, Vincent, K. Stewart, S. A. Khan, and J. Chakraborty. 1991. "Effect on Mortality of Community-Based Maternity Care Programme in Rural Bangladesh." *Lancet* 338:1183–86.

Favin, M., B. Bradford, and D. Cebula. 1984. "Improving Maternal Health in Developing Countries." World Federation of Public Health Associations, Geneva.

Fortney, J. A. 1987. "The Importance of Family Planning in Reducing Maternal Mortality." *Studies in Family Planning* 18:109–15.

Fortney, J. A., I. Susanti, S. Gadalla, S. Saleh, P. J. Feldblum, and M. Potts. 1988. "Maternal Mortality in Indonesia and Egypt." *International Journal of Gynecology and Obstetrics* 26:21–32.

Greenwood, A. M., B. M. Greenwood, A. K. Bradley, K. Williams, F. C. Shenton, S. Tulloch, P. Bypass, and F. S. J. Oldfield. 1987. "A Prospective Survey of the Outcome of Pregnancy in a Rural Area of the Gambia." *Bulletin of the World Health Organization* 65:635–43.

Hamilton, S., Barry Popkin, and D. Spicer. 1984. *Women and Nutrition in Third World Countries.* New York: Praeger.

Harrison, K. A. 1980. "Approaches to Reducing Maternal and Perinatal Mortality in Africa." In R. H. Philpott, ed., *Maternity Services in the Developing World—What the Community Needs.* London: Royal College of Obstetrics and Gynecology.

————. 1985. "Childbearing, Health, and Social Priorities: A Survey of 22,774 Consecutive Hospital Births in Zaria, Northern Nigeria." *British Journal of Obstetrics and Gynecology* Supplement 5:1–119.

Henry, A., and P. T. Piotrow. 1979. "Age at Marriage and Fertility." *Population Reports,* M, 4. Johns Hopkins University, Population Information Program, Baltimore.

Herz, Barbara, and Anthony R. Measham. 1987. "The Safe Motherhood Initiative: Proposals for Action." World Bank Discussion Paper 9. Washington D.C.

Howard, Deborah. 1987. "Aspects of Maternal Morbidity: The Experience of Less Developed Countries." In *Advances in International Maternal and Child Health.* Vol. 7. London: Oxford University Press.

Iam, J. D. 1989. "Current Status of Prematurity Prevention." *JAMA* 262:265–66.

Investigators of the Johns Hopkins Study of Cervicitis and Adverse Pregnancy Outcome. 1989. "Association of *Chlamydia trachomatis* and *Mycoplasma hominis* with Intrauterine Growth Retardation and Preterm Delivery." *American Journal of Epidemiology* 129:1247–57.

IOM (Institute of Medicine). 1985. *Preventing Low Birthweight.* Washington D.C.: National Academy Press.

Kaunitz, A. M., C. Spence, T. S. Davidson, R. W. Rochat, and D. A. Grimes. 1984. "Perinatal and Maternal Mortality in a Religious Group Avoiding Obstetrics Care." *American Journal of Obstetrics and Gynecology* 150:826–31.

Kramer, M. S. 1987. "Determinants of Low Birthweight: Methodological Assessment and Meta-analysis." *Bulletin of the World Health Organization* 65:663–737.

Kundsin, R. B., and S. S. Hipp. 1988. *Impact on the Fetus of Parental Sexually Transmitted Disease.* New York Academy of Sciences, New York.

Kwast, B. E., W. Kidane-Mariam, E. M. Saed, and F. G. R. Fowkes. 1984. "Report on Maternal Health in Addis Ababa, Sept. 1981–Sept. 1983: A Community Based Survey on the Incidence and Etiology of Maternal Mortality and the Use of Maternal Services, and Confidential Inquiries into Maternal Deaths in Addis Ababa, Ethiopia." Save the Children Federation, Addis Ababa, Ethiopia.

Kwast, B. E., and J. A. Stevens. 1987. "Viral Hepatitis as a Major Cause of Maternal Mortality in Addis Ababa, Ethiopia." *International Journal of Gynecology and Obstetrics* 25:99–106.

Lancet. 1991. "Perinatal Mortality Rates—Time for Change?" 337:331.

Leslie, J., and G. Gupta. 1989. "Utilization of Formal Services for Maternal Nutrition and Health Care." International Center for Research on Women, Washington, D.C.

Lettenmeier, C., Laurie Liskin, C. A. Church, and J. A. Harris. 1988. "Mothers' Lives Matter: Maternal Health in the Community." *Population Reports,* L, 7. Johns Hopkins University, Population Information Program, Baltimore.

Li, B. Y., A. M. Dong, and J. R. Zhuo. 1982. "Outcomes of Pregnancy in Hong-qiao and Qi-Yi Communes." *American Journal of Public Health* 72 Supplement 9:30–32.

Llewellyn-Jones, D. 1965. "Severe Anemia in Pregnancy." *Australian and New Zealand Journal of Obstetrics and Gynecology* 5:191–97.

London, K., J. Cushing, John Cleland, J. E. Anderson, L. Morris, S. H. Moore, and S. O. Rutstein. 1985. "Fertility and Family Planning Surveys: An Update." *Population Reports,* M, 8. Johns Hopkins University, Population Information Program, Baltimore.

Lopez, A. D. 1990. "Causes of Death: An Assessment of Global Patterns of Mortality around 1985." *World Health Statistics Quarterly* 43:91–104.

Lucas S. B., J. K. G. Mati, V. P. Aggarwal, and H. Sanghvi. 1983. "The Pathology of Perinatal Mortality in Nairobi, Kenya." *Bulletin of the Society of Pathologists* 76:579–83.

McCormack, W. M., B. Rosner, Y.-H. Lee, A. Munoz, D. Charles, and E. H. Kass. 1987. "Effect on Birthweight of Erythromycin Treatment of Pregnant Women." *Obstetrics and Gynecology* 69:202–7.

McCormick, Marie. 1985. "The Contribution of Low Birthweight to Infant Mortality and Childhood Morbidity." *New England Journal of Medicine* 312:82–90.

Maine, Deborah. 1981. "Family Planning: Its Impact on the Health of Women and Children." Columbia University, Center for Population and Family Health, New York.

Maine, Deborah, Allan Rosenfield, M. Wallace, A. M. Kimball, B. E. Kwast, Emil Papiernik, and S. White. 1987. "Prevention of Maternal Deaths in Developing Countries: Program Options and Practical Considerations." Paper presented at the International Safe Motherhood Conference, Feb. 10–13, Nairobi.

Mekhemar, S., A. el Sharbibi, I. Mourad, and H. Riad. 1984. "High Risk Pregnancy among Women under 20 Years of Age in a Rural Community." In M. M. Fayad and M. I. Abdalla, eds., *Medical Education in the Field of Primary Maternal and Child Health Care.* Cairo: Egyptian Ministry of Health.

Monteith, Richard S., Charles W. Warren, Egberto Stanziola, Ricardo Lopez Urzua, and Mark W. Oberle. 1987. "Use of Maternal and Child Health Services and Immunization Coverage in Panama and Guatemala." *Bulletin of the Pan-American Health Organization* 21:1–15.

Moutquin, J. M., R. Gagnon, C. Rainville, L. Giroux, G. Amyot, R. Bilodeau, and P. Raynauld. 1987. "Maternal and Neonatal Outcomes in Pregnancies with No Risk Factors." *Canadian Medical Association Journal* 137:728–32.

Naeye, R. L. 1980. "The Role of the Pathologist in the Developing World." In R. H. Philpott, ed., *Maternity Services in the Developing World—What the Community Needs.* London: Royal College of Obstetricians and Gynecologists.

Ojo, O. A., and V. Y. Savage. 1974. "A Ten Year Review of Maternal Mortality Rates in the University College Hospital, Ibadan, Nigeria." *American Journal of Obstetrics and Gynecology* 118:517–22.

Oyedehi G. A., S. K. Olamijulo, and K. T. Joiner. 1983. "Experience at Wesley: 1,391 Consecutive Admissions into the Neonatal Unit (Hurfod Ward)." *Journal of Tropical Pediatrics* 29:206–12.

Park, C. B., J. A. Palmore, and L. J. Cho. 1982. "The Korean Experience." Paper presented at the 52nd Annual Meeting of the Population Association of America, April 28–May 1, 1982, San Diego, Ca.

PCC (Population Crisis Committee). 1988. "Country Rankings of the Status of Women: Poor, Powerless, and Pregnant." Briefing Paper 20. Washington D.C.

Puffer, R. R., and C. V. Serrano. 1973. "Patterns of Mortality in Childhood." Pan-American Health Organization, Washington, D.C.

Rao, A. B. 1985. "Maternal Mortality in India: A Review." Family Health Division, World Health Organization, Geneva.

Ratnam, S. S., and R. N. V. Prasad. 1984. "Inadequacies of Present Health Services and Strategies to Improve Maternal and Child Health in Developing Countries." *International Journal of Gynecology and Obstetrics* 22:463–66.

Reich, J. 1987. "The International Conference on Better Health for Women and Children through Family Planning." *International Family Planning Perspectives* 13:86–89.

Rinehart, W., A. Kols, and S. H. Moore. 1984. "Healthier Mothers and Children Through Family Planning." *Population Reports*, J, 27. Johns Hopkins University, Population Information Program, Baltimore.

Royston, Erica. 1982. "The Prevalence of Nutritional Anemia in Women in Developing Countries: A Critical Review of Available Information." *World Health Statistics Quarterly* 35:52–91.

Royston, Erica, and Alan D. Lopez. 1987. "On the Assessment of Maternal Mortality." *World Health Statistics Quarterly* 40:214–24.

Shapiro, S., M. C. McCormick, B. H. Starfield, J. P. Krischer, and D. Bross. 1980. "Relevance of Correlates of Infant Deaths for Significant Morbidity at 1 Year of Age." *American Journal of Obstetrics and Gynecology* 136:363–73.

Sherris, J. D., K. A. London, S. H. Moore, J. M. Pile, and W. B. Watson. 1985. "The Impact of Family Planning Programs on Fertility." *Population Reports*, J, 29. Johns Hopkins University, Population Information Program, Baltimore.

Starrs, Ann. 1987. *Preventing the Tragedy of Maternal Deaths*. A report on the International Safe Motherhood Conference, Nairobi, Kenya, February 1987. New York: World Bank, WHO, UNFPA.

Thirugnanasambandham, C., S. Gopaul, and T. Sivakumar. 1986. "Pattern of Early Neonatal Morbidity: Observations in a Referral Maternity Hospital." *Journal of Tropical Pediatrics* 32:203–5.

Trivedi, C., and D. Mavalankar. 1986. "Epidemiology of Low Birthweight in Ahmedabad." *Indian Journal of Pediatrics* 53:795–800.

United Nations. Various years. *Demographic Yearbook*. New York.

Walker, G. J. A., D. E. C. Ashley, A. M. McCaw, and G. W. Bernard. 1986. "Maternal Mortality in Jamaica." *Lancet* 1:486–88.

Walsh, J. A., and S. Hutchinson. 1989. "The Importance of Group B Streptococcal Disease in the Developing World." *Pediatric Infectious Diseases* 9:271–77.

Wasserheit, J. N. 1989. "The Significance and Scope of Reproductive Tract Infections for Third World Women." *International Journal of Gynecology and Obstetrics* Supplement 3:145–68.

Weston, Lynn. 1986. "Reducing Maternal Deaths in Developing Countries." Population, Health, and Nutrition Technical Note 86-19. World Bank, Washington, D.C.

WHO (World Health Organization). 1985. "Coverage of Maternal Care: a Tabulation of Available Information." Geneva.

———. 1986. "Maternal Mortality Rates: A Tabulation of Available Information." Family Health Division, Geneva.

Williams, C. D., Naomi Baumslag, and D. B. Jelliffe. 1985. *Mother and Child Health: Delivering the Services*. London: Oxford University Press.

Winikoff, Beverly. 1988. "Women's Health: An Alternative Perspective for Choosing Interventions." *Studies in Family Planning* 19:197–214.

Winikoff, Beverly, and M. A. Castle. 1987. "The Maternal Depletion Syndrome: Clinical Diagnosis or Eco-demographic Condition?" Population Council, New York.

Winikoff, Beverly, and Maureen Sullivan. 1987. "Assessing the Role of Family Planning in Reducing Maternal Mortality." *Studies Family Planning* 18:128–43.

World Development Indicators. 1988. Washington, D.C.: World Bank.

Zhang, L., and H. Ding. 1988. "Analysis of the Causes of Death in China." *Bulletin of the World Health Organization* 1988, 66:387–90.

18

Protein-Energy Malnutrition

Per Pinstrup-Andersen, Susan Burger, Jean-Pierre Habicht, and Karen Peterson

More than 500 million people are unable to meet their energy and protein requirements for an active and healthy life. They are almost all poor and most of them live in developing countries, particularly in South Asia and Africa. They cope with the deficiency by reducing energy and protein expenditure in growth, work, and leisure. As a result of growth faltering, the weight of about 170 million preschool children, or about one-third of all preschool children, is currently below two standard deviations of normal healthy weight for children at their age; they suffer from protein-energy malnutrition (PEM) and related diseases. About 24 million infants are born underweight (weighing less than 2.5 kilograms) each year, in large measure because of PEM in women during pregnancy and before.

About 5 million infants are unable to cope with growth faltering and low birth weight resulting from PEM and associated diseases; they die before they reach the age of five. This amounts to about one-third of all deaths of preschool children in developing countries. In addition, PEM during childhood and adulthood increases the cost of health and education and reduces school performance, labor productivity, and general economic growth. The estimated economic losses worldwide resulting from reduced labor productivity alone are $8.7 billion annually. Thus, although the contribution to child mortality is very serious indeed, it is only part of the damage that PEM is doing to individuals, households, and nations.

Protein-energy malnutrition is a result of either infectious diseases or insufficient intake of energy and protein or—most commonly—a combination of the two. Each of these two immediate causes of PEM is influenced by a number of factors, including sanitary conditions, the quantity and quality of water available, access to primary health care, household behavior, and access to resources. Although child care, breastfeeding, and weaning practices are of particular importance in avoiding PEM among children, poverty and lack of access to appropriate primary health care are the overriding constraints to good nutrition at the household level.

Some single interventions, including food supplementation for preschool children and pregnant women, have been successful in alleviating PEM in a cost-effective manner. Thus, the cost of perfectly targeted food supplementation for preschool children and pregnant women per child life saved was estimated at $1,942.00 and $733.00, respectively. These estimates correspond to $40.00 and $23.65 per disability-adjusted life-year; costs that compare favorably with the costs associated with interventions in the health area and reported in other chapters of this book. Food supplementation is also justified on grounds of economic efficiency. The benefit-to-cost ratio of food supplementation of preschool children was estimated to be 17.4, implying a return of $17.40 for each dollar invested in such programs after discounting for differences in the timing of investment and returns. Other successful single interventions include nutrition education based on the concept of social marketing in Indonesia and the Dominican Republic, and promotion of breastfeeding in several countries.

Still, because PEM is frequently a result of many interacting factors, the effect of single interventions may be limited. Integrated programs that are designed to deal with the adverse factors identified for a particular population and for which the necessary national and local capacity and infrastructure for program implementation exist or can be developed are likely to be more successful than single interventions. Several such integrated programs, including the Tamil Nadu Integrated Nutrition Program in India and the Iringa Program in Tanzania, have dramatically reduced PEM in preschool children in the program areas.

To be successful, efforts to alleviate PEM must be based on a solid understanding of the environment within which the nutrition problem exists, the factors causing the problem, and feasible solutions. Such understanding is best obtained by direct participation of intended beneficiaries in program design and implementation. Furthermore, a strategy to alleviate PEM should consider direct and indirect interventions as well as broader government policies, which, although not directed at nutrition, may have a significant nutritional effect.

The Public Health Significance of PEM

Three indicators are commonly used to estimate the prevalence of protein-energy malnutrition: (a) protein and energy intake in relation to requirements; (b) growth, weight, and height in relation to established standards; and (c) birth weight. Because PEM results from either insufficient intake of energy and protein or infectious diseases, or most commonly a combination of the two, the first indicator measures a critical determinant of the nutritional status rather than nutritional status itself. An intake of energy and protein adequate to meet requirements is necessary but not sufficient to alleviate PEM.

The combined effect of energy and protein intake and the prevalence of infectious diseases is reflected in the rate of growth of children and in the weight in relation to height in adults. Birth weight may be used as an indicator of the nutritional status of women during pregnancy and before. The three sets of indicators mentioned above are widely used for estimating the prevalence of PEM in populations, and they are the only ones for which information is available at country and international levels.

The interpretation of the figures for energy and protein intake for the purpose of estimating the prevalence of PEM is further complicated by variations in energy requirements among individuals and over time and by unobserved adjustments in energy expenditure, whether in response to intake or not. Individuals are considered undernourished when their energy intake is less than the minimum required to maintain good health and desired activity. The Food and Agriculture Organization (FAO) suggests that the minimum energy requirement for adults is 1.2 to 1.4 times the basal metabolic rate (FAO 1987).[1]

Although the rate of growth is a better indicator of the current nutritional status of children than attained weight or height in relation to the genetic potential for a particular age (usually reported as weight-for-height, height-for-age, and weight-for-age), the former is not usually available for populations. Children whose weight-for-height is below two standard deviations of growth standards for a well-nourished population are considered "wasted," implying malnutrition resulting from recent or current deficiencies in nutrient intakes or infectious diseases or both. Children whose height-for-age is below two standard deviations of growth standards are considered "stunted," implying malnutrition resulting from past or longer-term deficiencies or infections or both. Low weight-for-age, frequently the only available measure of malnutrition, may be evidence of wasting or stunting or both (WHO 1986).

PROTEIN AND ENERGY DEFICIENCIES. Using the cutoff point of 1.2 times the basal metabolic rate, which, as already mentioned, is likely to fall considerably below desirable energy intake levels, the FAO (1987) estimated that about 335 million people were undernourished during the period 1979–81, up from 325 million ten years before. In relation to the total population of the developing countries, however, the percentage of those undernourished decreased from 19 percent to 15 percent during the ten-year period (table 18-1). Using the same cutoff point, the Subcommittee on Nutrition of the Administrative Committee on Coordination (ACC/SCN) of the United Nations estimates that the number of undernourished people had increased to 360 million by 1983–85 (United Nations 1987). Updating these estimates with the 1989 population figures and adding a rough estimate of food poverty in China, Chen (1990) estimates that in 1989, 465 million people lived in households too poor to obtain the energy necessary for minimal activity among adults and for the healthy growth of children. A more recent ACC/SSN publication (United Nations 1992) estimates that 786 million people were consuming less than 1.54 BMR by the end of the 1980s, down from 976 million in the mid-1970s.

As shown in table 18-1, the majority of undernourished individuals are found in Asia—notably South Asia—although when the number of undernourished people are measured in relation to total population, the problem appears to be slightly more severe in Africa. During the 1970s, the prevalence of undernourished people increased considerably in Africa, decreased in the Near East, and remained almost constant in Asia and Latin America. No reliable data are available by region for the period since 1981.

ANTHROPOMETRY-BASED ESTIMATES. The authors of a recent study for the United Nations Children's Fund (UNICEF) estimate that 150 million children below the age of five years in developing countries, excluding China, or 36 percent of all such children, are underweight, that is, below two standard deviations of standard weight-for-age (Carlson and Wardlaw 1990). Chen (1990) estimates that the prevalence in China is 18 million, which, added to the number in the developing countries, yields a total of 168 million for the world as a whole. In 1992 the United Nations ACC/SCN estimated that this num-

Table 18-1. Undernourished Population of Developing Countries, by Region, 1969–71 and 1979–81

Region	Total population (millions)		Undernourished population[a] (millions)		Proportion of population undernourished (percent)	
	1970	1980	1969–71	1979–81	1969–71	1979–81
Africa	282	376	57	70	20	19
Far East	986	1,232	208	210	21	17
Latin America	278	357	36	38	13	11
Near East	159	210	23	16	15	8
Total[b]	1,708	2,179	325	335	19	15

a. 1.2 times BMR for adults and adolescents.
b. Ninety-eight developing market economies.
Source: FAO 1987.

Table 18-2. Prevalence of Malnutrition in Children under Five in Developing Countries

Region	Underweight[a]		Stunting[b]		Wasting[c]	
	Millions	*Percent*	*Millions*	*Percent*	*Millions*	*Percent*
Africa	29	26.6	39	35.3	11	10.2
South Asia[d]	73	45.2	66	41.3	16	9.8
Rest of Asia[e]	40	43.4	43	46.2	7	8.3
Americas	8	13.8	15	27.7	1	1.3
Total[e]	150	35.7	163	39.0	35	8.4

a. Children more than two standard deviations below the reference median for weight-for-age.
b. Children more than two standard deviations below the reference median for height-for-age.
c. Children more than two standard deviations below the reference median for weight-for-height.
d. Afghanistan, Bangladesh, Bhutan, India, Maldives, Nepal, Pakistan, and Sri Lanka.
e. Excluding China.
Source: Carlson and Wardlaw 1990.

ber was valid for the mid-1970s and that it had increased to 184 million (34 percent) by the end of the 1980s. According to Carlson and Wardlaw, stunting is more prevalent than underweight, whereas wasting is estimated to affect about 35 million children, or about 8 percent of all children under the age of five years in developing countries, excluding China (table 18-2). As shown in table 18-3, more than 15 percent of the underweight children are severely underweight. Severe stunting affects more than 40 percent of all stunted children.

Underweight and stunting are more prevalent in Asia than in the other regions both in absolute numbers of affected individuals and in relation to all children who are malnourished. When measured in relation to the total population of children, wasting is most prevalent in Africa. This is undoubtedly a reflection of the deterioration of the African food situation during the late 1970s and the 1980s. Comparisons between the above figures and estimates reported by the FAO (1987) in the Fifth World Food Survey support the notion of deterioration in the nutritional situation in Africa. More recent developments including widespread famine indicate further deteriorations. Thus, based on a direct comparison of

continents, it appears that the prevalence of wasting among African children below the age of five has increased from 4 million to 11 million children, or from 7 to 10 percent of all such children in the region, whereas the absolute prevalence stayed constant for Asia and decreased in Latin America. In view of the differences between the two sets of estimates with regard to data sources and methods, the results of such direct comparisons are prone to large errors and should be interpreted as only rough indications of change in the prevalence by region.

The prevalence of malnutrition among preschool children is generally higher in rural than urban areas. Thus, in an examination of data from ten countries, Kates and others (1988) found that the prevalence of underweight in rural children was 1.4 to 2 times the prevalence in their urban counterparts. This finding was confirmed by Carlson and Wardlaw (1990), who found that the prevalence of underweight in preschool children was higher in rural than in urban areas of all thirty-one countries studied. On the average, the rural prevalence was 1.6 times the urban prevalence.

The average rural prevalence of stunting was 1.5 times the urban prevalence, and all but one country shows a lower prevalence in urban than in rural areas. Wasting showed a different pattern, with almost one-third of the thirty-one countries having a higher prevalence in urban areas. On the average, the rural prevalence exceeded the urban prevalence but only by a factor of 1.2. Although a firm interpretation of this finding must await further research, it may be hypothesized that the smaller difference between urban and rural areas with respect to wasting, which indicates more recent nutrition insults, than with respect to stunting is an indication of a shift of the nutrition problem from rural to urban areas. The shift is due to rural-to-urban migration and deterioration in urban living standards, including reduced real wages, higher food prices, reduced government expenditure on primary health care, and increased unemployment, resulting from the economic crises and associated macroeconomic policy reforms currently undertaken in most developing countries.

Children are generally exposed to the highest risk of PEM and associated mortality during and immediately following the

Table 18-3. Prevalence of Severe and Moderate Malnutrition
(percent)

Indicator of malnutrition[a]	Severe[b]	Moderate[c]	Total	Severe malnutrition as percentage of severe and moderate
Underweight	5.6	30.7	36.3	15.4
Stunting	14.5	20.9	35.4	41.0
Wasting	0.8	5.4	6.2	13.4

a. Underweight refers to low weight-for-age. Stunting refers to low height-for-age. Wasting refers to low weight-for-height.
b. More than three standard deviations below the median for the reference population.
c. Two to three standard deviations below the median for the reference population.
Source: Carlson and Wardlaw 1990.

weaning period, that is, between six months and twenty-four months of age. It is during this period that the prevalence of underweight and wasting is the highest. Beyond the age of two years, the prevalence of wasting usually drops off sharply and the prevalence of stunting is maintained, reflecting a lack of catch-up growth and a reduced risk of acute malnutrition beyond the age of two years. These relationships are illustrated in table 18-4.

The prevalence of low birth weight is an indicator of malnutrition among women during pregnancy and before. Chen (1990) estimates that about 24 million infants are born underweight (defined as weighing less than 2.5 kilograms) every year. This figure corresponds to 16 percent of all births globally. The problem is most prevalent in Asia, where an estimated 29 percent of all infants are born underweight as compared with 16 percent in Sub-Saharan Africa, 11 percent in Latin America and the Caribbean, and 7 percent in the United States (McGuire 1988).

Functional Consequences

The large magnitude of malnutrition in developing countries has serious functional consequences for the affected individuals and their families as well as economic consequences for individuals, households, and nations. Although the ultimate consequence of malnutrition is death, increased mortality is only one of many reasons why malnutrition is undesirable and costly. Protein-energy malnutrition in children inhibits their growth, increases their risk of morbidity, affects their cognitive development, and reduces their subsequent school performance and labor productivity. In women during pregnancy and before, PEM contributes to morbidity and mortality and to low birth weight of their infants, which in turn increases the risk of malnutrition and mortality in infants. Such increased risk is also associated with PEM in women during lactation. Work capacity and labor productivity in adults are negatively affected by PEM during childhood and adulthood, and the economic consequences of PEM are the sum of these productivity losses, additional costs of health and other social programs necessitated by malnutrition, lower school performance, higher educational costs, and lost productivity of care givers because of child malnutrition.

Table 18-4. Prevalence of Malnutrition by Age
(percent)

Age (years)	Underweight	Stunting	Wasting
Less than one	14.7	18.0	4.8
One	30.4	35.3	9.4
Two	26.6	33.5	5.1
Three	24.1	34.5	3.4
Four	23.2	35.3	3.6

Note: For thirty-nine countries. Underweight refers to low weight-for-age; stunting refers to low height-for-age; wasting refers to low weight-for-height.
Source: Carlson and Wardlaw 1990.

MORTALITY AND MORBIDITY. According to estimates made by UNICEF (1988), PEM is a contributing cause of the deaths of about one-third of the 15 million children that die annually. In view of the complex interactions between PEM and diseases that play a role in child mortality, the effect of PEM is difficult to isolate. The relation between low birth weight and child mortality is well documented (Ashworth and Feachem 1985; Herrera 1985; Rasmussen and others 1985; Kramer 1987). The pattern of risk is associated with the length of gestation and size at birth. Mortality in the first year of life appears to be greater for premature infants than for those who are full-term but suffer intrauterine growth retardation (IUGR). The mortality risk for children age one to four years, however, is greater for infants with IUGR (Ashworth and Feachem 1985). In developing countries, as much as 80 percent of low birth weights are due to chronic IUGR, rather than premature birth (Villar and Belizan 1982; Villar and others 1986; WHO 1986; Puffer and Serrano 1987). The growth potential of infants with chronic IUGR is restricted because of the severity and length of in utero deficits (Villar and others 1984, 1986). Among low-birth-weight infants who are premature or suffered acute IUGR, catch-up growth is rapid in the first six to eight months of life (Davies and others 1979; Villar and others 1984; Peterson and Frank 1987) but only if nutritional supplies are adequate.

The attainable birth weight of infants of women who are stunted as a result of childhood malnutrition is constrained, and thus the lifelong cycle of chronic growth deficits is perpetuated (Herrera 1985). In developing countries, maternal height makes a significant independent contribution to birth weight, an effect mediated through IUGR, not prematurity (Kramer 1987). The coefficient for maternal height independent of weight on birth weight is approximately 7.8 to 10 grams per centimeter of mother's height (Thompson, Billewicz, and Hytten 1968; Tanner and Thompson 1970; Kramer 1987). In longitudinal studies of children in developing countries, maternal height predicted both height-for-age and weight-for-age in the second and third years of life, independent of other biological and social risk factors (Mata 1978; Balderston and others 1981; Kielmann and others 1983).

In epidemiological studies of the short-term mortality risk among hospitalized children, the proportion of deaths was significantly greater among severely malnourished children than among those who were moderately malnourished (Gomez and others 1956; McLaren and others 1969). Prospective community-based studies (Kielmann and McCord 1978; Chen and others 1980; Kasongo Project Team 1983; Bairagi and others 1985; Lindskog and others 1988; Yambi 1988) have generally demonstrated an increase in risk of death at weights-for-age less than 70 to 80 percent of the reference median (Kielmann and McCord 1978) and a sharp increase in mortality risk at weights-for-age less than 60 percent of the median, weights-for-height less than 70 percent of the median, and heights-for-age less than 85 percent of the median (Kielmann and McCord 1978; Chen and others 1980; Lindskog and others 1988; Yambi 1988). Children who were both severely wasted and stunted were at the greatest risk of death (Chen and others 1980).

Growth faltering (Bairagi and others 1985) and arm circumferences less than 75 percent of median (Sommer and Lowenstein 1975) also predicted increased mortality risk. Mortality rates and the predictive ability of nutrition indicators varied by age (Kielmann and McCord 1978; Kasongo Project Team 1983) and were greater among children of lower socioeconomic status and born to shorter and lighter mothers (Chen and others 1980; Chowdhury 1988). A recent synthesis of studies of the relation between child anthropometry and mortality indicates that the relationship holds even for mild to moderate malnutrition (Pelletier 1991a).

Numerous studies have shown an association between malnutrition and infectious disease, especially diarrhea, among children in developing countries. Only a limited number of the researchers, however, used longitudinal analyses to examine nutritional status as a predictor of diarrhea and infections; even fewer controlled for other factors associated with PEM that may have contributed to infections.

Among studies in which measurements of diarrhea incidence and duration over intervals of two to three months were included, malnutrition predicted either increased duration (Tompkins 1981; Black, Brown, and Becker 1984) or incidence (El Samani and others 1988; Sepúlveda, Willett, and Muñoz 1988) of diarrhea. This relationship remained constant when previous diarrhea and sociodemographic variables were controlled in the analysis (Ghai and Jaiswal 1970; Sepúlveda, Willett, and Muñoz 1988). Anthropometric deficits did not predict incidence of diarrhea among preschool children in two studies in which incidence over intervals of nine months or longer were measured (Chen, Huq, and Huffman 1981; Peterson and others 1988b). Thus, the evidence suggests that malnutrition in preschool children in developing countries predicts short-term risk of increased incidence and duration of diarrhea, but prediction of long-term risk has not yet been demonstrated. In addition, the evidence for a causal role of child malnutrition in other infectious diseases, including measles, malaria, and acute respiratory infections merits longitudinal analysis.

COGNITIVE DEVELOPMENT. Growth retardation affects the development of motor and mental functions. Severe PEM affects brain growth, attention span, and short-term memory as well as activity level, which in turn affects interaction with the care giver and the environment (McGuire and Austin 1987). Because of the interaction between sensory environment and PEM-induced growth failure, Pollitt (1987) suggests that cognitive development is best understood as the outcome of the social environment and health history and the interaction of these variables with the nutritional status of children. It appears that psychosocial stimulation often can override or minimize the effects on the cognitive potential resulting from PEM.

In developing countries, early malnutrition has been associated with later developmental delays among children (Pollitt 1987); but most of the variability in intelligence quotients (IQs) was explained by differences in socioeconomic status (Richardson 1980). Among severely malnourished Korean preschool children who were adopted into American homes, the mean IQ score at school age exceeded the average score for American children and was forty points higher than that reported for children from similar populations who were returned to their home environment (Winick and others 1975). Several studies have shown that children in industrial countries who suffered early malnutrition secondary to organic illness, independent of socioeconomic deprivation, did not exhibit low developmental or intelligence test scores at later ages (Pollitt 1987). Interventions that provided food alone to children at risk of PEM resulted in mild to insignificant improvements on cognitive development. In contrast, those interventions that combined health care and educational or psychosocial stimulation with nutritional supplementation appeared to have a significant effect on cognitive development (McKay and Sinisterra 1974; Cremer and others 1977; McKay and others 1978; Grantham-McGregor and others 1979; Grantham-McGregor, Stewart, and Schofield 1980; Grantham-McGregor, Schofield, and Harris 1983).

SCHOOL PERFORMANCE. Sensory deprivation because of PEM in preschool children results in impaired learning abilities, adverse behavior, poor school attendance, and grade repetition. On the basis of a review of more than fifteen studies undertaken in various developing countries and the United States, McGuire and Austin (1987) conclude that "better growth is associated with better preschool and school-age I.Q. It is also associated with learning-relevant behavior, early enrollment in school and better school achievement, all of which enhance the educational efficiency of and economic return on primary schools." Similarly, the ACC/SCN concludes that "Malnutrition and infection during the preschool period, interacting with environmental factors related to poverty, are critical determinants of later school performance" (United Nations 1990).

LABOR PRODUCTIVITY. Evidence from small controlled experiments show a clear causal relation between body size, aerobic capacity, and physical work capacity (Spurr, and others 1977; Spurr 1983, 1984). Because the strenuous work undertaken by a large share of the labor force in developing countries requires a great deal of physical energy, it seems reasonable to assume that the link between body size and work capacity would be reflected in a strong link between body size and labor productivity. Similarly, a strong link between energy intake of adults and their labor productivity would be expected. Evidence of both links have been found in a number of studies as reviewed by Martorell and Arroyave (1984), Latham (1985), Strauss (1985), Agarwal and others (1987), McGuire and Austin (1987), and Berg (1987). Methodological flaws in the results of many of the studies reviewed, however, make the interpretation of the findings difficult (Strauss 1985).

Four recent studies appear not to suffer from serious methodological flaws. Strauss (1986), in a study of a sample of farmers in Sierre Leone, and Sahn and Alderman (1988), in a study of Sri Lankan households, found a significant relation between household-level energy consumption and labor productivity. Neither of the two studies had data available on the height and weight-for-height of the workers and their individual energy consumption. Thus, the effects of nutritional status in childhood, past energy consumption during adulthood, and current energy consumption cannot be separated. Such separation was done by Deolalikar (1988) in a study of South Indian households. He found that labor productivity as measured by attained wages and farm output was highly responsive to weight-for-height of the worker. No such response was found with respect to height and contemporary energy intake. Thus, although more research is needed, it may be hypothesized that weight changes provide a buffer between changes in energy intake and labor productivity. The immediate effect of reduced energy intake is weight loss, which if continued will subsequently influence labor productivity.

Haddad and Bouis (1990) found a strong effect of childhood nutritional status—as represented by height—on the labor productivity of Philippine agricultural workers. The elasticity of height on productivity—as measured by wage—was estimated to be 1.38, implying that a difference of 1 percent in the height of adult workers is associated with a 1.38 percent difference in their wages.

The findings from the four studies are powerful because they permit an estimation of the economic losses associated with malnutrition. Taken with estimates of cost-effectiveness of various programs, they make it possible to estimate the net economic gains associated with efforts to alleviate malnutrition. A preliminary estimate of this nature is made in the next section. Still, more research is needed to verify these findings and to develop empirical evidence for various settings to strengthen the validity of such estimates.

ECONOMIC COSTS. On the basis of the Haddad and Bouis estimates discussed earlier, a rough preliminary estimate can be made of the economic losses resulting from forgone labor productivity due to PEM. According to tables 18-2 and 18-3, stunting affects 163 million preschool children, of which 41 percent are severely stunted. After the age of about twenty-two months, severely stunted children are 10 centimeters shorter than the median, whereas moderately stunted children are 7 centimeters shorter (WHO 1979). Stunting during childhood appears to translate to equal height deficiencies in adulthood (Martorell, in press). Assuming an average daily wage of $2.50 and 300 working days per year for the workers exposed to stunting in childhood and an average height of 160 centimeters (the average height of the Philippine sample on the basis of which Haddad and Bouis estimated the above-mentioned relation between height and productivity), we find that the total economic loss due to stunting is $8.7 billion annually, or about one-fourth of the total health expenditure of developing countries (see appendix 18A for the methodology used in the calculation).

In addition to the economic costs associated with nutrition-related mortality and productivity losses, household incomes and national economic growth are negatively influenced by

PEM through higher costs of or lower benefits from education, higher health costs, higher costs of social programs, and income losses as a result of care giving in households with malnourished members. No quantitative estimates are available for these costs.

Causes of PEM

Protein-energy malnutrition is caused by infectious diseases and insufficient intake of energy and protein to meet requirements (figure 18-1). The effect of each of the two is a function of the state of the other, and most individuals who suffer from PEM do so because of exposure to both. The prevalence and severity of infectious diseases are influenced by sanitary conditions, quality and quantity of water available, access to primary health care, behavior of households and individuals, energy and protein intake, and, in the case of children, by child care, breastfeeding, and weaning practices. Energy and protein intake is influenced by household access to food, food acquisition and allocation behavior, infectious diseases, and the three child-related factors mentioned above. Access to food, sanita-

Figure 18-1. *Principal Factors Affecting* PEM

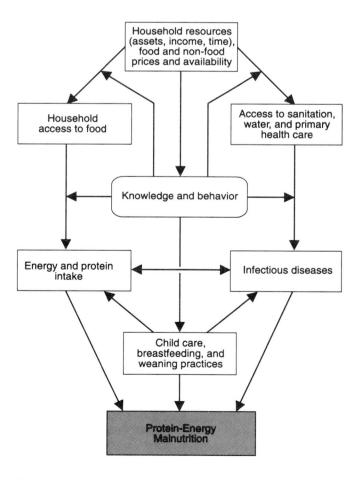

Source: Authors.

tion, water, primary health care, and knowledge is in turn influenced by household resources, that is, assets, income, and time, as well as the prices and availability of food and nonfood goods and services, including health care services at the community level.

Infectious Diseases

The effect of infection, especially diarrhea, on the nutritional status of poor children in developing countries has been well documented (Beisel 1977). Mechanisms by which diarrhea and other infections cause malnutrition include decreased food intake resulting from anorexia or food withholding, decreased nutrient absorption, increased metabolic requirements, and direct nutrient loss (Chen 1983; Keusch and Scrimshaw 1986). Epidemiological studies have demonstrated a negative relationship between infections—above all, measles, diarrhea, and malaria—and concurrent child growth in Latin America (Mata and others 1972, 1977; Martorell and others 1975; Mata 1978), Africa (Rowland and others 1977, 1988; Whitehead 1977) and Asia (Koster and others 1981; Kielmann and others 1983).

Evidence for the effect of respiratory infections on nutritional status is equivocal. No association has been reported by several authors (Rowland and others 1977; Whitehead 1977; Martorell and others 1975, 1983), although respiratory illness had as strong an effect as diarrhea on weight loss in Brazilian children (Leslie 1982). A recent longitudinal study (Rowland and others 1988) showed that lower respiratory tract infections were significantly associated with rate of weight gain in Gambian infants. After adjusting for the prevalence of disease, such infections accounted for one-quarter and diarrhea for one-half of the shortfall in attained weight compared with reference standards.

Intervention trials reviewed by Stephenson (1987) have pointed to the contribution by a number of parasitic infections to childhood growth retardation. With chemotherapy, children with parasitic infections showed small improvements in rate of weight gain, weight-for-height, and subcutaneous fat stores (Stephenson 1987). Other infections have not been shown to affect growth significantly, including infectious fevers (pertussis, chicken pox), skin and eye infections, and deep infections requiring antibiotic treatment (Martorell and others 1975; Rowland and others 1977; Whitehead 1977). Sample sizes for some of these studies were too small to pick up an effect, however, except for skin and eye infections.

The relative effect of infections and inadequate energy and protein intake on the growth of children in developing countries varies with the prevalence of infection (Martorell and Yarbrough 1983; Keusch and Scrimshaw 1986). In prospective studies, diarrhea incidence predicted height-for-age during periods of peak incidence, in the second and third years of life (Mata 1978; Balderston and others 1981; Kielmann and others 1983; Lutter and others 1989), but it did not explain variance in the weight or height of children studied before (Peterson and others 1988a) or after (Leslie 1982) the period of peak

incidence. Caloric intake (Balderston and others 1981) and weaning practices (Balderston and others 1981; Mata 1978) were as important as or more important than diarrhea incidence in multivariate models that explained variance in weights and heights of children from twelve months to thirty-six months of age. New findings from data collected in the 1970s in Guatemala and Bogotá indicate that the pernicious effect of diarrhea on growth is not seen if children are better fed during periods of diarrhea (Martorell, Rivera, and Lutter 1988; Lutter and others 1989; Rivera, Martorell, and Lutter 1989).

Energy and Protein Intake

Insufficient energy and protein consumption to meet desired expenditure results in reduced rate of growth, weight loss, reduced level of activity, or a combination of these. In children, the rate of growth is sensitive to both deficiency in intake and infection. Because of the synergistic relationship between food intake and infectious diseases, the expected growth response to improvements in one of the two may not be observed. Recent multivariate analyses have separated the effects of the two and shown strong growth responses to one or the other or both, depending on the context (Kennedy 1989; Von Braun, Puetz, and Webb 1989).

Child Care, Breastfeeding, and Weaning Practices

On the basis of a review of available literature, Huffman and Steel (in press) conclude that "few interventions have been shown to be as effective in preventing diarrhea among infants as breastfeeding." In view of the strong relation between diarrhea and PEM, this conclusion has obvious nutritional implications. Community- and hospital-based studies in a number of countries, including Brazil (Victora and others 1987), Peru (Brown and others 1988), Indonesia (Lambert 1988), India (Anand 1981), Costa Rica (Mata 1983), and the Philippines (Clavano 1982), all show that breastfeeding reduces the occurrence of diarrhea.

As discussed earlier, children are exposed to the highest risk of malnutrition and growth faltering during the weaning period from the age of six months to twenty-four months. Weaning foods commonly used are inadequate supplements to nutrients in breast milk and a source of contamination, contributing to an increased incidence of infectious disease (Scrimshaw and others 1968; Wyon and Gordon 1971; Barrell and Rowland 1979; Black and others 1982). Thus, where fecal contamination of the environment is widespread, prolonged full and partial breastfeeding is particularly important (Habicht and others 1988). In Brazil, delaying the introduction of solids promoted better growth in the first five months among the urban poor who had limited access to flush toilets, piped water, and refrigeration, presumably through reduced incidence of infectious disease. A recent study of infant feeding practices in a region of the Republic of Yemen that had a high prevalence of both acute and chronic PEM showed that breastfeeding had the strongest beneficial effect on weight-for-length and weight-for-age of infants age three months to six months (Jumaan and others 1989). The introduction of other foods was positively associated with weight-for-length only among children twelve to twenty-three months of age.

Child care is also of paramount importance during this period and beyond. Maternal child-rearing behaviors and attitudes, mother-child interaction, family social relationships, and stress have been associated with poor nutritional status in both industrial and developing countries in theoretical models (Williams 1962; Klein and others 1972; Caldwell 1974; Mata 1978; Herrera and others 1980; Rathbun and Peterson 1987). Maternal interaction with both family- and community-based networks has been associated with child growth outcomes in cross-sectional and longitudinal (Peterson and others 1988a) studies, suggesting that social support for the mother may be an important aspect of caretaking capacity and resourcefulness. These and related issues are further analyzed by Engle (in press).

Knowledge and Behavior

There is a strong association between maternal education and child nutrition and mortality, although the specific mechanisms through which the association operates is not fully understood (Leslie, in press). On the basis of a comprehensive review of available evidence, McGuire and Popkin (1990) conclude that the nutrition effects of maternal education are mediated through better management of household resources, greater use of available health care services, health behavior that compensates for a lack of such services, lower fertility, and more child-centered care-giving behavior.

Maternal Health and Reproductive History

Inadequate food availability to meet energy demands may adversely affect the health and nutritional status of mothers as well as that of their offspring. Maternal stunting due to early malnutrition and concurrent energy deficits can limit maternal work productivity and birth length and weight of the infant (Kramer 1987). Evidence suggests that the repeated demands of many pregnancies and close child spacing may deplete maternal nutritional status (Hamilton and others 1984; Merchant and others 1988), although further studies are needed on this topic. A large number of young children in the home may also adversely affect the nutritional status of the individual child (Kielmann and others 1983), independently of family socioeconomic status and maternal health and reproductivity history (Peterson and others 1988a), presumably because maternal time for child care and feeding must be shared by many.

Access to Sanitation and Water

Improved water and sanitation may affect PEM through a reduction in the transmission of pathogens, which in turn reduces diarrheal diseases. In addition, improved access to water may

affect PEM by reducing the time needed to acquire the water—usually a task performed by women and children—and by making more water available for household production of food (Burger and Esrey, in press).

Recent reviews (Esrey, Feachem, and Hughes 1985; Esrey and Habicht 1985, 1986; Esrey and others 1990; and Burger and Esrey, in press) found that improved water and sanitation are associated with decreased diarrheal diseases, improved nutritional status, and lower childhood mortality. The effect of improved water and sanitation on child morbidity and growth depends on the existing environmental conditions and the presence or absence of other related factors and programs that influence exposure to pathogens (Burger and Esrey, in press). For example, in Malaysia the introduction of flush toilets and piped water was found to have a greater effect on the mortality of nonbreastfed than breastfed infants, because breastfeeding reduced the exposure to pathogens (Habicht and others 1988). Similar interactions were found between improved water and sanitation and income and educational levels in several countries (Burger and Esrey, in press). On the basis of a review of past interventions, Esrey and Habicht (1986) conclude that water quantity has a greater effect on child morbidity than water quality in contaminated environments and that improved water quality may have little effect unless most other important routes of contamination are eliminated.

Evidence from several countries indicates that improved access to water increases the amount of time women spend on food production, processing, and preparation (Burger and Esrey, in press). Time saved in water collection may also be used in improved child care, income-generating activities, and other nutrition-related activities.

Household Access to Food

Household access to food is closely related to food consumption by individual household members, but intrahousehold food allocation does not necessarily parallel relative needs. Patterns of intrahousehold food distribution have been reviewed by several authors (Den Hartog 1972; Van Esterik 1984; Haaga and Mason 1987). Findings of preferential distribution of family food by age are equivocal and difficult to interpret because of differences in the outcome measures and the recommended dietary allowance schedule used (Haaga and Mason 1987).

The authors of some studies have shown that the adequacy of energy intake was greater in adults than for preschool children (Aligaen and Florencio 1980; Nutrition Economics Group 1982; Pinstrup-Andersen and Garcia 1990), whereas others demonstrated that children received a greater proportion of their recommended dietary allowance than adults (Nutrition Economics Group 1982; Van Esterik 1984), especially if total intake from both meals and snacks was computed (Harbert and Scandizzo 1982). The adequacy of the energy intake of children in relation to that of adults is influenced by family income and seasonal effects, including food shortages, lack of maternal time for child care and feeding, and the need for food for agricultural workers (Van Esterik 1984). Other feeding practices that may influence PEM in children include withholding solids from them during diarrhea (Taylor and Taylor 1976) and feeding them staples that have low energy density.

A sex bias in food distribution that favors males has been documented in the Middle East and South Asia (Van Esterik 1984; FAO 1987; Haaga and Mason 1987), whereas no such bias was found in Africa (Svedberg 1989; Von Braun, Puetz, and Webb 1989). The sex bias in South Asia is particularly important and deserves serious attention because of the high rates of malnutrition in that region. Differences in weaning and access to food (Van Esterik 1984) may be reflected as well in patterns of malnutrition and mortality (DeSweemer 1974; Chen and others 1980; Chen, Huq, and D'Souza 1981). A sex bias in food distribution is usually related to other factors, including age, lactation and pregnancy, birth order and sex of child in relation to siblings, maternal education, and family income (Abdullah 1983; Van Esterik 1984; Haaga and Mason 1987). Patterns of sex bias in food distribution and in nutritional and health status and survival may also be related to regional ecology, which determines the agricultural economy and the demand and perceived value of male as opposed to female labor (MacCormack 1988). Societies with an ideology of matrilineal descent (and greater investments in health and nutrition of women) seem to be found in high rainfall areas, which require labor-intensive hoe cultivation, whereas patrilineal descent is traditionally seen in dry-land plow regions of continents (MacCormack 1988).

Household Resources and Prices

Poverty is the most important determinant of PEM because it constrains household access to food, knowledge, sanitary living conditions, safe water, and appropriate health care (figure 18-1). Increasing household income among the poor results in expanded energy and protein consumption, stronger demand for education and health care, and improved living conditions (Pinstrup-Andersen 1985; Garcia 1988), although the effect of increases of income on energy consumption may be less than previously expected (Behrman 1988). Similarly, households respond to food price changes by adjusting household food consumption (Pinstrup-Andersen 1985).

As discussed above, changes in household food consumption influence that of high-risk household members, which in turn influences their nutritional status. Thus, evidence of causal effects for each of these steps implies a causal effect between income and nutritional status. Several researchers, including Garcia (1988) in the Philippines, Alderman (1990) in Ghana, and Sahn (1990) in Côte d'Ivoire, found a strong association between income changes and the nutritional status of preschool children. In addition to the importance of the absolute level of incomes and prices, fluctuations in incomes and prices, including seasonality, are important determinants of PEM in many rural areas (Payne 1985; Sahn 1989) and may

influence intrahousehold allocation of food (Van Esterik 1984).

The effect of higher incomes on nutrition may be insignificant in the short run in areas in which poor sanitation and lack of knowledge and primary health care are the most limiting constraints to good nutrition. In the longer run, however, higher incomes are likely to alleviate these constraints.

Interventions for Control of PEM

The factors that influence the two basic causes of PEM (inadequate intake of energy and protein and infectious diseases) may be manipulated by various interventions. In table 18-5 we list the most important factors, interventions, and related activities. Only the interventions related to intake will be discussed in this chapter.

Single Interventions to Improve Dietary Intake

Single interventions reviewed here include food supplementation of children and women as well as food price subsidies, income transfers, food fortification, and other broad programs and policies.

FOOD SUPPLEMENTATION. Food supplementation schemes are usually not designed in such a way as to permit credible evaluation of effect. Therefore, results from evaluation attempts such as those reported by Beaton and Ghassemi (1982) are difficult to interpret and do not permit inference regarding the biological effects per unit of food supplement. The synthesis undertaken here is limited to food-supplementation schemes designed in such a way as to permit a reliable estimation of effect. Four food-supplementation schemes for pregnant women in Colombia, the Gambia, Guatemala, and Taiwan (China) permitted such estimation (Lechtig and others 1975; Mora, Clement, Christiansen, Suescun, Wagner, and Herrera 1978; Mora, de Navarro, Clement, Wagner, de Paredes, and Herrera 1978; Lechtig and Klein 1979; Mora and others 1979; Herrera and others 1980; McDonald and others 1981; Delgado, Martorell, Brineman, and Klein 1982; Delgado, Valverde, Martorell, and Klein 1982; Overholt and others 1982; Mora 1983; Adair, Pollitt, and Mueller 1983, 1984; Prentice and others 1983; Adair and Pollitt 1985; Prentice and others 1987). The effect on dietary intake of supplementary food during pregnancy (detailed in table 18-6) was studied in relation to maternal weight gain, maternal activity, maternal body mass, and birth weight.[2]

Recent studies (Merchant, Martorell, and Haas 1990a, 1990b) of the nutritional stress of simultaneous pregnancy and lactation in poorly fed mothers show that mothers appear to absorb much of the deficit in energy by mobilizing their fat stores, and birth weight is little affected. Thus one might expect mothers more than their fetuses to benefit from the food supplementation. This was not the case. These studies showed little effect of supplemental food on maternal weight gain but did show a substantial improvement in mean birth weight,

Table 18-5. Causes and Interventions for Malnutrition

Causes	Contributing factors	Interventions	Activities
Inadequate intake of calories, protein, amino acids	Food (quantity and quality)	Resource transfer: supplementary foods	Food delivery to target individual or to family Feeding programs Nutrition rehabilitation
		Subsidies, transfer programs	Price subsidies Food stamps
		New foods	Weaning food preparation: processed and home preparation
		Fortification	Processing, marketing, and distribution Incentives (pricing)
		Agricultural production	Prices, incentives
	Income	Income generation	Income generation projects
	Knowledge	Nutrition education: information transfer, behavior change	Face-to-face (individuals and groups) Mass media
	Infant feeding	Promotion of breast-feeding	Training of health care personnel and mothers Restrictive legislation
	Time	Provision of child care	Support groups Day care centers
		Accessible cooking and water facilities	Better stoves Access to fuel Water projects
Nutrient losses, metabolic increases, and anorexia	Knowledge	Hygiene education	Face-to-face Mass media
	Water	Improved quality Improved quantity	Water projects, wells, pumps
	Feces	Latrines	Feces disposal
	Drugs	Drug administration	Distribution Prices
		Drug education	Training of health care personnel, individuals
	Vaccines	Immunization	Injections Distribution of vaccines
	Dehydration	Rehydration therapy: package or home remedy	Intravenous, nasogastric, oral (ORT)
	Medical care	Medical care	Medical care

Source: Authors.

which was greater the more malnourished the pregnant woman (table 18-7). Neither weight gain (Adair, Pollitt, and Mueller 1983; Adair and Pollitt 1985; Prentice and others 1987) nor measured activity patterns during pregnancy (Roberts 1982; Lawrence 1988) changed markedly in response to supplementation. Standardizing for the increase in total net caloric intake attributable to the supplement over the course of pregnancy (derived from values in table 18-6), we find that the improvements in birth weight per unit of increase in energy

intake ranged from a high of 34 grams per 10,000 kilocalories in Colombia to a low of 14 grams and 8 grams per 10,000 kilocalories, for males and females, respectively, in Taiwan (China).

Because of the relation between infant mortality and birth weight, improving the caloric intake of malnourished pregnant women through food supplementation can result in a lower infant mortality rate. The difference in incidence of low birth weight attributable to the increase in energy intake reported

Table 18-6. Supplementation during Pregnancy

Location	Period of supplementation	Treatment group	Maternal anthropometry Weight (kg)	Maternal anthropometry Height (cm)	Maternal intake Energy (kcal/day)	Maternal intake Protein (g/day)	Supplement distributed Energy (kcal/day)	Supplement distributed Protein (g/day)	Net intake Energy (kcal/day)	Net intake Protein (g/day)
Bogotá, Colombia	Third trimester	Supplement	—	150 ± 5	$1,646 \pm 630$[a]	37 ± 23[a]	856	38	133[b]	20[b]
		No supplement	—	150 ± 5	$1,606 \pm 665$[a]	37 ± 20[a]	0	0	33[b]	2[b]
	Low maternal weight-for-height[a]	Supplement	—	—	$1,589 \pm 632$[a,d]	35 ± 21[a,d]	856	38	334[b,e]	25[b,f]
		No supplement	—	—	$1,589 \pm 632$[a,d]	35 ± 21[a,d]	0	0	29[b,e]	1[b,f]
	Full-term	Supplement	—	—	$1,623 \pm 635$[a]	36 ± 19[a]	856	38	150[b]	9[b]
		No supplement	—	—	$1,621 \pm 655$[a]	37 ± 23[a]	0	0	48[b]	1
Taiwan (China)	Previous lactation and pregnancy	Supplement A	50 ± 5	155 ± 5	1,121[g]	37[g]	800	40	1,650[h]	64[h]
		Supplement B	49 ± 5	154 ± 5	1,197[g]	37[g]	80	6	1,206[h]	37[h]
Guatemala	Entire pregnancy	Atolé	48[d]	149 ± 5	$1,473 \pm 467$[g]	42 ± 13[g]	163[i]	11.5[i]	1,580	48
		Fresco	48[d]	149 ± 5	$1,411 \pm 467$[g]	42 ± 13[g]	59[i]	0[i]	1,492	42
Keneba, The Gambia	From sixteenth week	Postsupplement	50[d]	158[d]	—	—	1,300[j]	49[j]	1,898	—
		Presupplement	50[d]	158[d]	1,467	—	0	0	1,467	—
	Wet season	Postsupplement	50[d]	158[d]	—	—	1,500[j]	56[j]	1,838	—
		Presupplement	50[d]	158[d]	1,418	—	0	0	1,418	—

— Data not available.
a. In sixth month of pregnancy.
b. Difference between post- and presupplementation periods.
c. Less than 0.36 kg/cm.
d. For combined groups.
e. Significant difference between groups; $P < 0.005$.
f. Significant difference between groups; $P < 0.001$.
g. Home dietary intake; no initial dietary intake values reported.
h. Significant difference between groups; $P < 0.01$.
i. Content per 180 ml; offered ad libitum.
j. Maximum.

Source: Lechtig and others 1975; Mora, Clement, Christiansen, Suescun, Wagner, and Herrera 1978; Mora, de Navarro, Clement, Wagner, de Paredes, and Herrera 1978; Lechtig and Klein 1979; Mora and others 1979; Herrera and others 1980; McDonald and others 1981; Delgado, Martorell, Brineman, and Klein 1982; Delgado, Valverde, Martorell, Brineman, and Klein 1982; Overholt and others 1982; Mora 1983; Adair, Pollitt, and Mueller 1983, 1984; Prentice and others 1983; Adair and Pollitt 1985; Prentice and others 1987.

Table 18-7. *Supplementation during Pregnancy: Outcome*

Location	Treatment group	Incidence of LBW [a] (percent)	Maternal weight gain (kg)	Mean birth weight	Mean birth weight per intake (g/10⁴ kcal)[b]
Bogotá, Colombia	Supplement	8.7	—	$2,978 \pm 377$	34.1
	No supplement	11.0	—	$2,927 \pm 392$	n.a.
	Low maternal weight-for-height				
	Supplement	—	—	$3,014 \pm 379$[c]	55.4
	No supplement	—	—	$2,833 \pm 412$[c]	n.a.
	Full-term				
	Supplement	—	4.2 ± 1.8[d,e]	$3,003 \pm 354$[f]	35.4
	No supplement	—	3.5 ± 1.7[d,e]	$2,940 \pm 318$[f]	n.a.
Taiwan (China)	Males				
	Supplement A	—	7.5 ± 2.8[g]	$3,216 \pm 348$	13.8
	Supplement B	—	7.8 ± 2.5[g]	$3,161 \pm 364$	n.a.
	Females				
	Supplement A	—	7.5 ± 2.8[g]	$3,013 \pm 411$	8.0
	Supplement B	—	7.8 ± 2.5[g]	$2,981 \pm 321$	n.a.
Guatemala	Atolé[h]	—	—	$3,077 \pm 334$	21.0
	Fresco[i]	—	—	$3,027 \pm 461$	n.a.
Keneba, The Gambia	Postsupplement	8.0[e]	—	$2,891 \pm 27$[j,k]	16.0
	Presupplement	18.4[e]	—	$2,882 \pm 37$[j,k]	n.a.
	Wet season				
	Postsupplement	7.5[l]	—	$3,031 \pm 32$[e,j]	28.8
	Presupplement	23.7[l]	—	$2,842 \pm 48$[e,j]	n.a.

— Data not available.

n.a. Not applicable.

a. Birth weight less than 2,500 g.

b. Calculated from the net intake per day times an estimate of the total number of days supplemented during pregnancy. In Guatemala, women did not start receiving supplement until they recognized that they were pregnant, so birth weight per input is likely to be a slight underestimate.

c. Significant difference between groups; $P < 0.01$.

d. Third trimester.

e. Significant difference between groups; $P < 0.005$.

f. Significant difference between groups; $P < 0.001$.

g. Total group.

h. Atolé is a food supplement high in energy and protein.

i. Fresco, which has a low content of energy and no protein, was used as a control.

j. Adjusted for sex, parity, and gestational age.

k. Significant difference between groups; $P < 0.05$.

l. Significant difference between groups; $P < 0.002$.

Source: Mora and others 1979; Herrera and others 1980; McDonald and others 1981; Delgado, Martorell, Brineman, and Klein 1982; Mora 1983; Adair, Pollitt, and Mueller 1984; Prentice and others 1983; Adair and Pollitt 1985; Prentice and others 1987.

in table 18-6 varied from 2.3 percentage points in Colombia, where the incidence of low birth weight in the unsupplemented group was 8.7 percent, to 10 percentage points in the Gambia, where the presupplementation incidence (averaged over all seasons) had been 18 percent.

The selection of subgroups for targeted interventions on the basis of characteristics of those who are known to respond rather than the selection of subgroups on the basis of characteristics associated with malnutrition is likely to be much more effective. The response in birth weight to maternal food supplementation is greater among chronically and acutely malnourished women, as well as those who smoke. In Colombia, the mean birth weight of infants of women whose weight-for-height was low and whose diet was supplemented was 181 grams more than their counterparts whose mothers received no supplements (Mora 1983); in the total group, the difference in birth weight between the infants of those whose diets were supplemented and those whose diets were unsupplemented was only 51 grams. In Taiwan (China), "tall and thin" women who were below the median weight and above the median height had larger birth weight in response to supplementation than "short and thin" subjects (Adair and Pollitt 1985). The better response in tall, thin women to supplementation emphasizes an irreversible detrimental effect of stunting in women and points to an additional advantage of preventing stunting during childhood. Women may also be more responsive to food supplementation during periods of seasonal food shortage, as illustrated by results from the Gambia, where the gain in birth weight per unit of supplementation was higher during the wet season, when food availability is low (table 18-7).

In the studies conducted in relatively well nourished populations, supplementation of the diets of smokers had a greater effect on birth weight than the supplementation of those of nonsmokers (Rush, Stein, and Susser 1980a, 1980b; Kennedy and Kotelchuck 1984). This effect may be of importance in developing countries as smoking among women increases. If the effect of smoking on birth weight is a result of carbon monoxide and not nicotine or cyanide compounds (Kramer 1987), it may also be relevant among women who are exposed to smoke from wood stoves in poorly ventilated houses.

Studies of food supplementation in lactating women have shown mixed results. A well-implemented trial showing no effect (Prentice and others 1980; Prentice, Roberts, and Prentice 1983) may still be confounded by secular trends. The only randomized double blind trial conducted to date (Gonzalez and others 1991) of food supplementation in lactating women who had no supplementation during pregnancy showed a clear-cut increase in breast milk in a group of chronically malnourished women. The increase was larger among the initially most malnourished. This study also showed that women whose diet was supplemented prolonged full breastfeeding. These findings have implications not only for maternal and infant nutrition but also for birth spacing, because full breastfeeding postpones the return of fecundability much more than does maternal malnutrition (Kurz and others 1990).

Results of a recent observational study in Brazil point to a "weanling dilemma" for infants of poorly nourished mothers in contaminated environments (Martines and others 1988). Growth faltered at about three to four months of age among solely breastfed infants of poorly nourished mothers, whereas solely breastfed infants of well-nourished mothers maintained normal growth at this age (Martines and others 1988). The provision of solid food to the infants of poorly nourished mothers did not appear to be a solution, because diarrhea and other infections resulting from contamination of the foods had an even worse effect on growth than the inadequacy of maternal milk production (Martines and others 1988). Thus, where environmental sanitation is poor, postponing the introduction of weaning foods beyond the optimal period for infants in sanitary environments is less detrimental to infant growth than is the introduction of contaminated foods at that time. The "weanling dilemma" might be solved by improving the nutrition of the malnourished mothers so that growth of their infants does not falter, or by providing uncontaminated foods to infants. Empirical studies, however, have as yet not shown that either of these strategies improve infant growth.

Several studies that were sufficiently well designed to make estimations of the effect of food supplements on the growth of children (Gopalan and others 1973; Martorell, Klein, and Delgado 1980; Mora and others 1981; Martorell, Habicht, and Klein 1982) are reviewed here. Improved dietary intake among children as a result of the provision of supplementary food (detailed in table 18-8) has the potential to be partitioned into different biological responses, such as growth, activity, and compensation for energy lost during illness, although most studies reported only anthropometric indicators of growth. Behavioral changes resulting from provision of energy (Chavez and Martinez 1975; Chavez, Martinez, and Yaschine 1975) may also improve cognitive development, but that will be discussed in the section on integrated interventions, because well-designed studies which have measured this effect have also provided behavior-modifying interventions to the child.

Supplementation of children's diets improved both their weight and height (table 18-9). The response in growth depended on the age of the child, which determined both the magnitude and kind of deficiency, whether in protein or calories. Provision of supplemental food remedied these deficiencies to a marked but still imperfect degree. Taking into account the duration of supplementation (derived from table 18-8), we estimate the height difference to vary from a high of 5.0 centimeters per 100,000 kilocalories ingested by Guatemalan females age thirty-six months to a low of 0.8 centimeters per 100,000 kilocalories ingested by Indian children age forty-eight months to sixty months. The weight difference per supplement ingested ranged from a high of 800 grams extra per 100,000 kilocalories, attained by male Guatemalan children at thirty-six months of age, to a low of 40 grams extra per 100,000 kilocalories, ingested by Colombian children during the interval between eighteen months and thirty-six months of age.[3]

The variability in response to food supplementation in these studies, particularly in weight, may be because of the differences in age groups supplemented, infant and child feeding practices, incidence of infectious diseases, and the duration of supplementation. The studies in Bogotá and Guatemala included the most complete data for examining the effects of supplementation on incremental growth at different ages. The differences in the resulting relative rates of growth in length and in weight between the supplemented and unsupplemented children were greatest between nine months and twelve months, during peak incidence and duration of diarrhea, followed by the weaning period from three to six months (Lutter and others 1990). Food supplementation also modified the negative effect of diarrhea on growth. Diarrhea was negatively related to growth in length in the unsupplemented group, but had no effect on length in the supplemented group (Lutter and others 1989). The effect of supplementation depended on the level of diarrheal disease, having a greater effect on length in those with the most diarrhea and no effect on children with low levels of diarrhea (Lutter and others 1989). Similarly, in Guatemala, in the villages provided with a protein and energy-enriched supplement, the effect of diarrhea on growth was attenuated (Martorell, Rivera, and Lutter 1988; Rivera, Martorell, and Lutter 1989).

Finally, children also responded differently to supplementation at different ages according to their body composition. In

Table 18-8. Supplementation to the Child

Location	Duration of supplementation	Treatment group	Age of child (months)	Home dietary intake[a] Energy (kcal/day)	Home dietary intake[a] Protein (g/day)	Total supplement distributed Energy (kcal/day)	Total supplement distributed Protein (g/day)	Net intake Energy (kcal/day)	Net intake Protein (g/day)
India	Fourteen months	Supplement	12–23[b]	700[b]	18[b]	310	3	310	3
		No supplement	12–23[b]	700[b]	18[b]	0	0	0	0
Bogotá, Colombia	From mother's last trimester to three years of age	Supplement	18	1,020 ± 706	24 ± 38	623	30.0	1,478 ± 711	58 ± 40
		No supplement	18	1,310 ± 445	36 ± 18	0	0	1,310 ± 445	36 ± 18
		Supplement	36	1,017 ± 373	24 ± 16	623	30.0	1,380 ± 453	48 ± 24
		No supplement	36	1,167 ± 476	27 ± 16	0	0	1,167 ± 476	27 ± 16
Guatemala	From mother's pregnancy to three years of age	Male							
		Atolé	15–36	785 ± 213	20 ± 6	163[c]	11.5[c]	941 ± 226	31 ± 8
		Fresco	15–36	814 ± 213	19 ± 6	59[c]	0[c]	840 ± 226	22 ± 8
		Female							
		Atolé	15–36	718 ± 213	20 ± 6	163	11.5	868 ± 226	21 ± 8
		Fresco	15–36	756 ± 213	19 ± 6	59	0	779 ± 226	8 ± 8

a. Home dietary intake values are likely to be an underestimate of the intake the population would normally consume, since some of the home diet is probably displaced by the supplement.
b. For entire population.
c. Per 180 ml, fed ad libitum.
Source: Gopalan and others 1973; Martorell, Klein, and Delgado 1980; Mora and others 1981; Martorell, Habicht, and Klein 1982.

Table 18-9. *Supplementation to the Child: Outcome*

Location	Treatment group	Age of child (months)	Initial measurements Stature[a] (cm)	Weight (kg)	Final measurements Stature[a] (cm)	Weight (kg)	Increment Stature[a] (cm)	Weight (kg)	Outcome + Input[b] Stature[a] (cm/10^5 kcal)	Weight (kg/10^5 kcal)
India										
	Supplement	12–24	—	—	—	—	9.3[c]	2.35[c]	2.1	0.49
	No supplement	12–24	—	—	—	—	6.5[c]	1.71[c]	n.a.	n.a.
	Supplement	24–36	—	—	—	—	9.5[c]	2.34[c]	1.3	0.48
	No supplement	24–36	—	—	—	—	7.8[c]	1.71[c]	n.a.	n.a.
	Supplement	36–48	—	—	—	—	9.1[d]	2.04[d]	1.3	0.35
	No supplement	36–48	—	—	—	—	7.4[d]	1.58[d]	n.a.	n.a.
	Supplement	48–60	—	—	—	—	8.4[e]	1.86[a]	0.8	0.37
	No supplement	48–60	—	—	—	—	7.3[e]	1.38	n.a.	n.a.
Bogotá, Colombia	Supplement	18–36	75.1 ± 2.7	9.48 ± 1.09	87.5 ± 3.4[f]	12.35 ± 1.40[e]	12.4	2.87	1.5	0.05
	No supplement	18–36	73.5 ± 3.1	9.06 ± 1.04	85.3 ± 4.4[f]	11.88 ± 1.19[e]	11.8	2.82	n.a.	n.a.
Guatemala										
	Male									
	Atolé	36	84.3 ± 4[g]	11.6 ± 1.3[g]	86.9 ± 3.9[c]	12.4 ± 1.3[c]	—	—	2.8	0.79
	Fresco	36	84.3 ± 4[g]	11.6 ± 1.3[g]	85.1 ± 3.9[c]	11.9 ± 1.3	—	—	n.a.	n.a.
	Female									
	Atolé	36	84.3 ± 4[g]	11.6 ± 1.3[g]	85.9 ± 3.9[c]	11.9 ± 1.3[c]	—	—	5.0	0.70
	Fresco	36	84.3 ± 4[g]	11.6 ± 1.3[g]	83.1 ± 3.9[c]	10.8 ± 1.3	—	—	n.a.	n.a.

— Data not available.

n.a. Not applicable.

a. Some studies reported recumbent length, and others reported standing height. The use of length or height makes no difference to the net outcome, because it is determined by the difference between measurements.

b. Input is calculated as the kilocalories of supplement ingested per day dimes the duration of supplementation. In Colombia, the intake was the average of the intakes at eighteen and thirty-six months. In Guatemala, where infants also receive breast milk, the amount of supplement is likely to be less; the duration of supplementation therefore was considered to be the period between twelve and thirty-six months.

c. Significant difference between groups; $P < 0.001$.

d. Significant difference between groups; $P < 0.01$.

e. Significant difference between groups; $P < 0.05$.

f. Significant difference between groups; $P < 0.005$.

g. Total population.

Sources: Gopalan and others 1973; Martorell, Klein, and Delgado 1980; Mora and others 1981.

Guatemala, children of high weight-for-length at six months (Rothe, Rasmussen, and Habicht 1988) had higher weight gain, and at eighteen months of age (Marks 1989) had better linear growth in response to supplementation than children of low weight-for-length. At thirty months of age, this response was reversed; children of low weight-for-length responded with better linear growth (Marks 1989). The better linear growth of fatter children at younger ages in response to supplementation could be explained by two potential mechanisms: (a) protein is more limiting in younger children, or (b) younger children need to build up fat reserves before they can respond with better linear growth. Further research is needed to test either of these hypotheses.

FOOD SUBSIDIES AND TRANSFERS. Food price policy, food subsidies, and food-related transfer programs influence the ability of households to acquire food (Pinstrup-Andersen 1985). Evidence from studies in more than a dozen countries shows that food price subsidies and food stamp programs have increased incomes and improved food consumption among the poor, particularly but not exclusively in urban areas (Pinstrup-Andersen 1988). In many of the countries studied, the transfers from such programs contributed 15 to 25 percent of total income of the poorest 10 to 20 percent of the population reached. In general, each 1 percent increase in the income of the poor results in a 0.2 to 0.4 percent increase in household energy consumption and a somewhat higher percentage increase in the consumption of protein. Thus, although the effect varies among countries and population groups, food subsidy programs that add 20 percent to the purchasing power of the poor can be expected to increase their energy consumption by 4 to 8 percent. The effect will be higher among the poorest and most destitute.

The extent to which increases in household food consumption lead to improved nutritional status depends on the degree to which malnourished household members share in the increase and on the relative importance of food deficiency and infectious diseases. If food deficiency is not the only limiting constraint to improved nutrition, increased food consumption may have little or no effect. In Egypt, for example, existing food subsidies contributed to high levels of food consumption even among the poor. Malnutrition was still significant, however, because the effect of poor sanitation and diarrhea on growth were not effectively addressed (Alderman and Von Braun 1984; Alderman, Von Braun, and Sakr 1982).

Empirical evidence on the effect of food subsidies and price policies on the nutritional status of preschool children is limited. Kumar (1979) found that the weight-for-age of children in Kerala, India, would fall by 8 percent if the existing subsidized food ration scheme was discontinued. Similarly, food subsidies contributed significantly to increases in energy and protein intake and weight-for-age of preschool children in the Philippines (Garcia and Pinstrup-Andersen 1987).

WEANING FOODS. The risk of PEM and PEM-related mortality is particularly high during the weaning period. Programs to im-

prove weaning practices frequently involve the promotion of improved weaning food, whether made from local foods or commercially premixed (Gibbons and Griffiths 1984). Researchers who studied projects promoting weaning foods in Haiti (Berggren 1981) and Burkina Faso (Zeitlin and Formación 1981) found strong positive effects on the nutritional status of children. The affordability of weaning foods is an important consideration, and emphasis should be placed on locally available foods. Successes from recent integrated interventions may reflect a positive effect of improved weaning foods. Attempts to isolate the nutrition effect of each of a number of interventions, such as weaning foods, that form part of an integrated program may not be warranted because the effect of one is heavily influenced by the presence of others.

FORTIFICATION. Although fortification may be effective in alleviating deficiencies in micronutrients, fortification to alleviate PEM has not generally been successful. Amino-acid fortification has been tried in a number of populations. In many cases, however, little or no effect was detected, partly because the programs were not designed in such a way that they could be evaluated and partly because the staple foods on which fortification was tested—for example, wheat in Tunisia and rice in Thailand (NAS 1988)—were less likely to lead to a critical imbalance in amino acids than other staples, such as corn, cassava, or sweet potatoes. Thus, the additional protein provided was most likely converted to energy.

AGRICULTURAL PRODUCTION. Agricultural programs and policies may have important nutrition implications through their effect on incomes of the rural poor, food prices to be paid by poor consumers, time allocation by members of poor households, energy and protein expenditure, infectious diseases, and food consumption by high-risk individuals (Mebrahtu, Pelletier, and Pinstrup-Andersen, in press). Positive nutrition effects may be increased and negative ones alleviated by including in the design of such programs and policies consideration of how each of these six factors will be affected.

Agricultural research and technology have contributed to large increases in food production in many developing countries during the last twenty-five years, most notably in Asia and Latin America (Pinstrup-Andersen 1982). These increases have resulted in higher incomes for farmers and landless workers as well as lower food prices for consumers. Low-income farm families with members at risk of PEM have participated in these income gains, and the lower food prices have been particularly important for poor consumers, because they spend a large share of their income on food (Pinstrup-Andersen and Hazell 1985). Although evidence from other sources shows that incomes and food prices are closely associated with the nutritional status of household members, implying a positive nutrition effect of agricultural research and technology, no studies have been done to establish the link directly.

The authors of recent studies of projects to increase the commercial agricultural production by small farmers in the Gambia, Guatemala, India, Kenya, the Philippines, and

Rwanda (Alderman 1987; Kennedy and Cogill 1987; Von Braun, Hotchkiss, and Immink 1989; Von Braun, Puetz, and Webb 1989; Bouis and Haddad 1990; and Von Braun, de Haen, and Blanken, 1991) found strong positive effects on farm incomes and family food consumption. The effect on the nutritional status of preschool children was also positive but small, in some cases statistically insignificant. The results of these studies demonstrate that agricultural projects may be powerful in alleviating the household resource constraints to good nutrition but may have little effect on nutrition unless other constraints, such as infectious diseases and adverse household behavior, are removed at the same time.

INCOME GENERATION. Protein-energy malnutrition is closely associated with poverty, and increased household incomes are important for improved nutrition. Still, as illustrated above, additional income is not always sufficient for its elimination. There are several reasons for this. In the short run, additional income is likely to increase access to food but may have little effect on general sanitary conditions, knowledge, and access to and use of health care. In the absence of good sanitation and health care, additional food may have little nutritional effect. In the longer run, increased income is likely to improve living conditions, reduce health risks, and improve nutrition, particularly if accompanied by better information and behavioral changes. In the meantime, increased access to food may have a significant effect on nutrition only if primary health care and programs to modify household behavior and improve sanitary conditions and access to more and cleaner water are introduced as well.

Another reason why income increases may not be as effective as expected is that households may be unaware that a nutrition problem exists, they may lack knowledge and information about how best to use additional income for nutritional improvements, or they may be faced with extreme scarcity of other basic necessities which compete with nutrition for household resources. In such cases, growth monitoring or nutrition education may be needed along with efforts to assist households in meeting other basic needs.

The nutrition effect of income increases may also be less than expected because women allocate more time to income generation and less to child care, cooking, and other nutrition-related activities. In such cases, programs to increase the productivity of women's time within or outside the household are needed. Finally, intrahousehold income control may be in the hands of household members who place low priority on nutrition improvement.

NUTRITION EDUCATION. Several researchers have completed reviews of the effect of nutrition education programs during the last few years, including Whitehead (1973), Zeitlin and Formación (1981), Hornik (1985), Johnson and Johnson (1985), and Cerqueira and Olson (in press). The general conclusion from these reviews is that well-designed and well-implemented nutrition education programs can bring about behavioral changes that contribute to improved nutrition at

relatively low cost. In low-income households, such programs are most likely to be successful when the behavioral changes can be accomplished without additional resources (Hornik 1985). The interaction between resource availability at the household level and the opportunity for nutritional improvement through behavioral changes is an important consideration in the design of nutrition intervention programs. In very poor households, constraints on resources may prohibit behavioral changes and thereby limit the effectiveness of nutritional education.

Cerqueira and Olson (in press) argue that lack of success in many past nutrition education programs is due in large part to the influence of the traditional medical model, that is, curative rather than preventive. Recent participatory models with or without the use of mass media have contributed to significant nutrition improvements in several countries, including Indonesia (Zeitlin and others 1984), the Dominican Republic (USAID 1988), Tanzania (UNICEF 1988), and India (Shekar 1991). In most of these cases growth monitoring played an important role as a source of information for the education effort, and in some but not all of these programs nutrition education was closely integrated with other interventions (Cerqueira and Olson, in press). Thus, nutrition education offers great promise for nutritional improvements through behavioral changes when (a) the design and implementation is based on a thorough understanding of the environment within which the intended beneficiaries live and of the constraints they face, including those that limit behavioral changes; (b) the target community is intimately involved in the design and implementation of the complete set of interventions; and (c) household resource constraints are alleviated.

PROMOTION OF BREASTFEEDING. Breastfeeding contributes significantly to reduced infections and malnutrition in infants and children. Promotion of breastfeeding has been successful in increasing the rate of breastfeeding (Feachem and Koblinsky 1984). Maternal behavioral response to breastfeeding promotion varies according to socioeconomic characteristics (Hardy and others 1982). Training and education of health professionals in the advantages of breastfeeding and in techniques to help mothers breastfeed have been successful in a number of countries (Huffman and Steel, in press), including Indonesia, Thailand, Panama, and the United States. Appropriate hospital delivery practices, community support groups, and arrangements permitting mother and infant to stay together while in the hospital have proved effective in increasing breastfeeding rates and the ways breastfeeding is practiced in several countries (Huffman and Steel, in press).

Integrated Interventions to Improve Dietary Intake

Synergism among interventions may result in integrated strategies' having effects different from the sum of the effect of each of the individual interventions. Substitution and complementarity between and among interventions often play an important role in determining the total effect of a set of interventions. On the basis of a review of nutrition education programs in developing countries, Hornik (1985) concludes that nutrition education generally has been most successful when combined with increased household resources. Complementarity between nutrition education and food supplementation has been demonstrated by Gilmore and others (1980) in Morocco, and Garcia and Pinstrup-Andersen (1987) found complementarity between nutrition education and food price subsidies in the Philippines. Developmental education to influence maternal knowledge, behavior, and time spent with the child appears to increase the effect of food on growth and cognitive development. Home visits by fieldworkers to stimulate learning and development and positive caretaker-child interaction among families participating in the Bogotá Nutrition and Child Development Project (Herrera and others 1980) resulted in a growth in height of 1.3 centimeters more in children in the supplemented group who had received stimulation than in those who had not (Lutter 1987). This effect on height-for-age persisted at six years of age (Super and others 1989).

The main effect of stimulation was stronger than the main effect of supplementation in the Bogotá study for almost all the indexes of cognitive development tested (Cremer and others 1977). The highly significant interaction of supplementation and stimulation (Cremer and others 1977), points to the synergism of food and behavioral stimulation interventions. Similarly, behavioral stimulation had a much larger effect on cognitive development than dietary supplementation in children in Cali, Colombia (McKay and Sinisterra 1974, McKay and others 1978), although these results may be biased because participants were explicitly told the nature and the expected outcome of the study. Stimulation of severely malnourished children in a hospital also had similar effects (Grantham-McGregor and others 1979; Grantham-McGregor, Stewart, and Schofield 1980; Grantham-McGregor, Schofield, and Harris 1983).

Integration of efforts to improve nutrition and health in small-scale projects has positively affected nutrition and mortality (Gwatkin, Wilcox, and Wray 1980; Lamptey and Sai 1985). Two recent integrated projects—the Tamil Nadu Integrated Nutrition Program in India and the Iringa Project in Tanzania—have been particularly successful in reducing child malnutrition. Thus, TINP is estimated to have reduced the prevalence of severe malnutrition among children six months to thirty-six months old by one-third to one-half the prevalence that existed at the beginning of the project. The continued effect of TINP and another nutrition project in the region is estimated to be a 50 percent reduction of the prevalence of malnutrition among children less than five years old (World Bank 1990). An equally impressive result was obtained by the Iringa Project, which is estimated to have reduced severe and moderate malnutrition in the project area by 70 and 32 percent, respectively (UNICEF 1989; Yambi and others 1989).

Case Management of Severe Malnutrition

Most of the interventions previously described can be considered preventive because a diagnosis of severe malnutrition need not be among the criteria for receiving treatment. Nutritional status may be used to target interventions such as food supplementation, but the goal of the selection procedures is to prevent severe PEM and its consequences rather than to provide rehabilitation once it occurs. Severely malnourished children are commonly treated in two types of facilities: hospitals and nutrition rehabilitation (or mothercraft) centers.

In hospitals generally, the case-fatality rate of severe malnutrition has been reported to be approximately 25 percent (McLaren and others 1969; Cook 1971). Most studies of hospital-based case management of severe PEM on which these rates are based were conducted more than twenty years ago. In the interim, new methods of treatment and feeding schedules with better potential to reduce this high case-fatality rate have been developed (Waterlow and others 1978; WHO 1981). The effectiveness of these innovations will depend on adequate training and sufficient time and personnel to administer the frequent feedings required for rehabilitation. Follow-up upon release from the hospital is necessary to avoid relapse. Reported case-fatality rates ranged from 15 to 37 percent, but they dropped to nearly zero in the twelve-month period if "conscientious efforts were made for follow-up" (Cutting 1983, p. 121).[4]

Nutrition rehabilitation centers vary from those incorporated into a highly technical medical infrastructure to those completely separate from medical facilities (Beaudry-Darisme and Latham 1973). The case-fatality rates in a four-month period ranged from 0 to 6 percent (Beghin and Viteri 1973).

The effect of length of attendance at rehabilitation centers on nutritional status was retrospectively examined in two different countries, with equivocal findings (Beaudry-Darisme and Latham 1973). In Haiti, improvement in the median weight-for-age by the time of discharge and ability to maintain it one year after discharge were significantly greater in those who attended the centers for two months than for those who attended for one month. The mean percentage of Guatemalan children who attained and maintained the median weight-for-age was the same regardless of length of attendance.

Still, the above outcomes are all the result of poor planning or management rather than intrinsic biological constraints on recovery. In a well-managed trial in Guatemala, all malnourished children recovered when they received 10 percent or more of their recommended energy intake from food supplementation (Rivera, Habicht, and Robson, in press).

Questions yet to be resolved are what referral criteria would be most appropriate and under what conditions are the two types of facilities most useful to rehabilitate severely malnourished children when preventive efforts fail. A comparison of the relative effectiveness of hospitals and nutritional rehabilitation centers indicated that nutrition rehabilitation centers were more effective in curing malnutrition, although the outcome measure was not specified (Cook 1971). The criteria for hospital admission and prognosis may have been different for the two types of facilities, however, because hospitals usually deal with severe malnutrition, whereas rehabilitation centers handle less severe cases. This type of comparison is not useful in determining clinical criteria for referral of children from nutritional rehabilitation centers to hospitals. Perhaps because the costs are so high, the further study of criteria for referral has been grossly neglected.

Cost, Cost-Effectiveness, and Benefit-Cost

While direct costs of nutrition intervention are frequently reported, total costs and benefits are difficult to estimate. This section provides rough estimates only.

FOOD SUPPLEMENTATION. As shown in table 18-10, the cost of food supplementation varies among programs. Such variation provides little indication of cost-effectiveness, however, because the programs vary in nature and presumably in nutrition effect. As expected, the cost is lowest for food subsidy schemes that depend on the market for food distribution and include no other program components, such as those in the Philippines, Sri Lanka, and Egypt, and highest for integrated programs implemented by the public sector, such as the Tamil Nadu and the Colombian programs.

These cost estimates provide an input into assessments of cost-effectiveness. On the basis of the estimates presented in table 18-10, it seems reasonable to assume a cost of $0.20 per 1,000 calories transferred in programs that provide no other services. This rough overall estimate is used in an assessment of cost-effectiveness and a benefit-cost analysis presented below.

Two cost-effectiveness analyses are reported here. Both assess the cost of averting a child death by means of food supplementation. The first, which relates to food supplementation for preschool children, is based on the relation between food supplementation and child growth, shown in table 18-9, and the relation between the weight-for-age of preschool chil-

dren and their rate of mortality estimated for five countries and synthesized by Pelletier (1991). The result from the assessment, which should be interpreted as rough magnitudes rather than exact figures because of the assumptions made, is that the cost of averting a death is $1,942, which converts to a cost of $62.65 per disability-adjusted life-year (DALY). The second refers to food supplementation of pregnant women and is based on the relation between food supplementation and birth weight shown in table 18-7 and the relation between birth weight and infant mortality shown by Walsh and others (in press). If we assume a gain of 300 grams in the birth weight per 100,000 calories transferred to pregnant women (table 18-7) and a decrease of 9 per 1,000 in the child mortality rate for each 100-gram increase in the birth weight (approximated from Walsh and others, in press), the cost per child death averted is estimated at $733.00, or $23.65 per DALY. The assumptions made and the methodology used in this assessment are explained in appendix 18A.

The benefit-cost analysis is based on the elasticity of labor productivity of 1.38 with respect to height of the worker, reported by Haddad and Bouis (1990) and discussed in an earlier section of this chapter, and the estimated relation between food supplementation and height of preschool children (table 18-9). Estimates of the latter vary from 0.8 to 5.0 centimeters per 100,000 calories transferred. For this analysis, an estimate of 2.0 is used. This corresponds to the finding for Indian children age one to two years (table 18-9). The sensitivity of the result to the choice of estimate is tested by using estimates of 1.0 and 3.0 centimeters per 100,000 calories transferred. As above, a cost of $0.20 per 1,000 calories transferred is assumed. The cost associated with an increase in height of 1.0 centimeter is then the cost of 50,000 calories, or $10.00. Under the assumptions of a daily current wage of $2.50

Table 18-10. Cost of Food Transfers in Various Types of Programs

Program type	Country	Year	Cost per 1,000 calories delivered (U.S. dollars)	Source
Food subsidy	Brazil	1980	0.30	Berg 1987
Food subsidy	Colombia	1981	0.79	Berg 1987
Food subsidy	Egypt	1982	0.18	Alderman and Von Braun 1984; Kennedy and Alderman 1987
Food subsidy	Mexico	1982	0.42	Kennedy, Overholt, and Haddral 1984
Food subsidy	Philippines	1984	0.09	Garcia 1988
Food subsidy	Sri Lanka	1982	0.10	Edirisinghe 1987
MCH and feeding	Bolivia	1988	0.12	World Bank 1989
MCH and feeding	Brazil	1980	0.53	Berg 1987
MCH and feeding	Colombia	1982	0.38	Anderson and others 1981; Kennedy and Alderman 1987
MCH and feeding	Costa Rica	1982	0.60	Anderson and others 1981; Kennedy and Alderman 1987
MCH and feeding	Dominican Republic	1982	0.20	Anderson and others 1981; Kennedy and Alderman 1987
MCH and feeding	Ecuador	1988	0.21	World Bank 1989
MCH and feeding	Guatemala	1988	0.33	World Bank 1989
MCH and feeding	Honduras	1988	0.36	World Bank 1989
MCH and feeding	India (Tamil Nadu)	1985	0.69	Berg 1987
MCH and feeding	India	1982	0.20	Anderson and others 1981; Kennedy and Alderman 1987
MCH and feeding	Pakistan	1982	0.38	Anderson and others 1981; Kennedy and Alderman 1987
MCH and feeding	Paraguay	1988	0.90	World Bank 1989
MCH and feeding	Peru	1988	0.32	World Bank 1989
MCH and feeding	Uruguay	1988	0.24	World Bank 1989

Source: See last column.

and 300 working days per year, the annual current benefit is estimated at $6.45. Still, these benefits will begin only after the child enters the labor market, for example, at the age of eighteen years. Assuming a 2 percent annual rate of increase in the real wage, we find that the wage rate will have increased to $3.43 per day, or $1,030 per year, for the year the person enters the labor market. Thus, an investment of $10.00 in a child age six months to eighteen months will generate an income stream beginning sixteen years later and continuing for the duration of the productive life of the worker, say, until age fifty-five. This annual income stream will begin with $8.84 at age eighteen and end with $18.06 at age fifty-five. At a real discount rate of 3 percent, the present value of such an income stream is estimated to be $174.00, which, compared with the initial investment of $10.00 yields a benefit-cost ratio of 17.4. This is above most other investments made by the public sector. Reducing the effect of food supplementation from 2.0 centimeters to 1.0 centimeter per 100,000 calories resulted in a benefit-cost ratio of 8.7, whereas an increase to 3.0 was associated with a benefit-cost ratio of 26. Thus, even at the lower estimate of the effect of food supplementation on height, the return on investment in the growth of preschool children through food supplementation is high. The methodology used is presented in appendix 18A.

Estimates by Selowsky and Taylor (1973) for Chile and by Selowsky (1981) for Colombia also suggest high economic returns to government programs to improve child nutrition. In another study in Chile, Torche (1981) estimated that the economic return from a food supplementation program exceeded the discount rate of 17 percent usually applied to determine the economic viability of investment projects in the government sector. Additional studies of this nature are urgently needed to provide evidence of the economic return from nutritional improvements compared with the economic return from alternative investment and to increase the understanding of how to design nutrition interventions with high economic payoff.

NUTRITION EDUCATION. There is little reliable quantitative evidence on the cost-effectiveness of nutrition education. It may be difficult or impossible to isolate the effect of nutrition education when such education is an integral part of an intervention program. In such cases it may make more sense to evaluate the complete program, as discussed in the next section.

Two recent nutrition education programs provide information on costs and cost-effectiveness. Both are based on the social marketing strategy and both have been effective in improving nutrition. In Indonesia, the cost was $3.90 for each participant and $9.80 for each child whose nutrition was improved. In the Dominican Republic, the Applied Nutrition Education Program included about 9,000 children and cost about $23.00 per child annually. The prevalence of malnutrition, defined as weight-for-age below 75 percent of standard, decreased from 12.2 to 6.9 percent in a two-year period (1984–86). The cost per child removed from malnutrition was estimated at about $500.00 (USAID 1988). One reason for this

relatively high cost estimate is that, although severely malnourished children were most closely monitored, program resources were provided to all children, of which only 12 percent were classified as malnourished at the start of the program. If the program could be targeted to the malnourished only, the cost would be reduced considerably without a reduction in the effect as measured. Alternatively, the cost-effectiveness is likely to be higher in populations with a higher prevalence of malnutrition. Furthermore, only benefits associated with the movement of children from below to above the cutoff of 75 percent of standard were considered, and nutritional improvements occurring within each of the two groups were ignored.

INTEGRATED PROGRAMS. Several recent integrated health and nutrition programs, including the Tamil Nadu Integrated Nutrition Program and the joint WHO/UNICEF Nutrition Support Program in Iringa, Tanzania, have been successful in significantly reducing PEM. The cost of removing a child from moderate and severe malnutrition was estimated to be $33 in Tamil Nadu (Ho 1985) and $46 in Iringa (estimated on the basis of data in UNICEF 1988). Using the methodology reported in the appendix, we estimated the cost per averted child death in Iringa to be $2,560, corresponding to a cost per DALY of $82.

COSTS OF CASE MANAGEMENT.The costs of case management of moderate to severe protein-energy malnutrition are considerably higher than the costs of prevention. Beaudry-Darisme and Latham (1973) compared the costs of rehabilitation centers in two different countries using standardized food and salary costs. The mean cost per child with a positive change in weight-for-age above the control was $605 in Haiti and $2,672 in Guatemala and was even higher for the decreased incidence of severe PEM above the control group at $3,627 in Haiti and $5,344 in Guatemala. In a comparative review of rehabilitation centers and hospitals, costs for the period of recuperation varied from $46 to $54 in Guatemala to $120 in Costa Rica in rehabilitation centers (Beghin and Viteri 1973). In urban Uganda the cost of recuperation was $78 in the recuperation center and $120.00 in the hospital (Beghin and Viteri 1973). In a study of six Latin American countries, the cost per bed-day at a hospital ranged from 4.5 to 18 times the cost per child per day at a rehabilitation center (Beghin 1970). Still, the severity of the PEM, the criteria employed for referral, and the duration of recovery, among other factors, could account for some of the difference in cost. Costs varied from $117.60 for inpatient hospital treatment for kwashiorkor for two weeks to $77.00 for a six-week inpatient stay that included educating the mother.

Strategies and Priorities

An effective strategy must identify and combine programs and policies that are likely to have the greatest sustained effect on the nutritional status of a particular population group or groups per unit of resources spent. The design of such a strategy is difficult because of strong synergisms, such as those between food intake and infectious diseases and between purchasing power and nutrition knowledge. These synergisms imply that the effect of changes in one factor may be slight unless other factors are changed simultaneously. Furthermore, because the nature, causes, and relative rewards of particular interventions vary among population groups, across countries, and over time, the strategy must be tailored to a particular set of circumstances. No one strategy is likely to be optimal for all population groups.

A national strategy to alleviate PEM should consider direct nutrition interventions, such as food supplementation and nutrition education; indirect interventions, such as programs to improve primary health care, sanitation, and water availability; and broader policies and programs, such as those involving price, income, credit, interest rate, and employment policies and those influencing asset ownership and user rights. Such broader policies are likely to exercise powerful influences on the nutritional status of the poor, even though they may not be explicitly addressed to nutritional concerns. Their nutrition effects—positive or negative—should not be ignored. This is particularly important because poverty, with its associated unsanitary living conditions and lack of access to sufficient food, health care, and information, is clearly the overwhelming determinant of PEM. As mentioned earlier, however, policies and programs with the sole goal of increasing incomes have not been as effective in alleviating malnutrition in the short run as expected.

The choice, design, and implementation of nutrition intervention programs should be made within the context of existing policies and expected changes in them, because specific policies benefit some groups of the poor and hurt others, thereby changing the needs and the appropriate target groups for nutrition programs. The most appropriate program choice, design, and implementation strategy will depend on existing economic policies as well as opportunities for policy change.

The specific strategy and related programs and policies must be tailored to each location and time period. Ideally, the most appropriate government support will be identified through effective participation by communities and target households in problem diagnosis, program implementation, and monitoring. With or without such participation, however, the choice, design, and implementation of nutrition intervention programs should be preceded by (a) identification of the target groups, assessment of the constraints to good nutrition with which they are faced, an assessment of their food acquisition and allocation and health-seeking behavior, and identification of opportunities for nutrition improvement; (b) assessment of institutional and administrative capabilities for program implementation; and (c) identification of sources of financing. Two vehicles for the generation of the relevant information— growth monitoring and nutritional surveillance—have shown great promise, not only for information generation, but also as mechanisms with which to identify, coordinate, and integrate interventions and policies into an effective strategy.

Growth monitoring by itself is not an intervention; rather it is a tool to coordinate appropriate interventions to promote growth in an individual child. Most of the successful integrated programs mentioned earlier include growth monitoring as a tool to integrate intervention activities. From the success of these programs it appears that growth monitoring and promotion can be an important instrument in an integrated strategy. Furthermore, the cost of adding growth monitoring to nutrition intervention programs is small (Griffiths 1985).

In their review of the early attempts at growth monitoring, Gopalan and Chatterjee (1984) came to the conclusion that much of the failure to achieve the promised potential of growth monitoring was due to the difficulty of interpreting the growth curve and the consequent lack of appropriate follow-up action. The Applied Nutrition Education Program in the Dominican Republic among others has demonstrated that training workers to implement specific activities to address specific patterns on the growth chart can be successful (USAID 1988). This is, however, but one of the constraints to be overcome to make growth monitoring successful (Ruel, in press).

Just as growth monitoring can be used to integrate health and nutritional interventions at the level of the individual, so nutritional surveillance can be used to plan and implement interventions in populations and coordinate and integrate these interventions to make them more effective and less costly (Mason and others 1984; Tucker and others 1989). Like growth monitoring, nutritional surveillance does not by itself prevent or cure malnutrition. Instead it provides the relevant information for the choice, design, and correct timing, synchronization, and concatenation of effective interventions. Because the relation between information and interventions effective for the population level is much less clear than it is between information and growth monitoring at the individual level, it is not surprising that no useful evaluations of effect have been done on nutritional surveillance. In the absence of such evaluations no firm conclusions can be drawn regarding the nutrition effects of nutritional surveillance. The relatively narrow form in which nutritional surveillance efforts have been operationalized in the past, however, suggests that any positive effects which have taken place are far short of the potential (Pelletier, in press). As illustrated by the willingness of the private sector to pay for market information, decisionmakers value relevant information. Information plays an important role in guiding government decisions related to food and nutrition (Alderman, in press). Thus, nutrition surveillance activities that make relevant and timely information available to decisionmakers is likely to result in better interventions. Because the cost of nutritional surveillance is such a small fraction of the cost of the interventions, the potential cost of wrong decisions, and the cost of maintaining the capability of intervening in crises that the generation of the type of information provided by effective nutrition surveillance should be encouraged.

The interaction between interventions and the socioeconomic and cultural environment within which they are introduced as well as the interaction among types of interventions and the synergism among factors influencing nutrition are of paramount importance in designing the strategy. This implies that integrated or concurrent interventions are more likely to be successful than single ones. Still, integrated interventions require institutional and administrative capabilities and infrastructure that are frequently in short supply.

In countries in which the necessary capabilities and infrastructure are available or can be developed as part of the program, integrated health and nutrition programs combined with favorable government policies offer great promise. Each program should be tailored to the particular circumstances but a combination of growth monitoring; nutrition education that emphasizes breastfeeding, child spacing, and weaning practices; financial and technical assistance for the production and distribution of weaning food; distribution of food stamps to participating households; and overall primary health care may form the core of most programs or part of the menu of options for consideration. Active community and target group participation in various aspects of program design and implementation is important for long-term sustainability, and separate but related efforts to assist the target groups in strengthening their income-generating capacity are needed to reduce the need for future outside financial support.

In countries in which the institutional and administrative capabilities and infrastructure are weak, less complex programs should be pursued. For example, in areas that have health posts, if insufficient food intake is a constraint to good nutrition, the distribution of food stamps to low-income mothers who bring their preschool children to the posts should be considered. Such a strategy was successful in urban and rural areas of Colombia and in both remote and less remote rural areas of the Philippines (Garcia and Pinstrup-Andersen 1987). Using food stamps instead of the more traditional food supplementation relieves the health system of physically distributing the food, a job for which it is not well equipped, without removing the food-related incentive for coming to the health post.

Rather than repeating the many other examples of appropriate interventions already discussed, we will only suggest that the introduction of any such intervention in a particular community should be preceded by a sound assessment of the situation and that the intended beneficiaries should participate in that assessment.

It should be stressed that attempts to set up large-scale nutrition programs that exceed the institutional and administrative capabilities have failed in the past and will fail if tried again. Instead, emphasis should be on strengthening these capabilities, including training at all levels and the building of nationwide primary health care systems, which may become the conduits for integrated nutrition and health programs. Such linkage will be successful only if nutrition is given a more prominent role in primary health care. At the same time, nutritional improvements should be pursued through policies and programs that require less administrative and institutional capabilities and infrastructure, such as price, income, and employment policies; credit and technical assistance to low-income people; basic training and education; and small-scale intervention programs. Such programs may be very cost-effective if designed by and for the community target groups with outside support.

In view of the above, high priority should be placed on strengthening the capacity of households, communities, and government agencies to assess the nutrition situation, to diagnose the problem, to identify the critical constraints to good nutrition, and to design, implement, and monitor strategies most appropriate for a particular situation. Priority should also be placed on making available to program designers and implementors information and technologies needed to ensure success in such strategies.

International assistance to reduce PEM should focus on the strengthening of this capacity through a combination of training, technical assistance, research, technology transfer, and financial support to cover program costs. The nature of each of these activities and the correct combination needs to be defined for each country and community. The overriding priority of international aid agencies and national governments should be to ensure that each community and each country is capable of defining, implementing, and obtaining financing for the most appropriate strategy and associated policies and programs. That—and not a specific technology or intervention—is the magic bullet to be applied across countries and communities.

In support of these priorities for action there is a need for operationally relevant research on a number of topics. First, a better understanding is urgently needed of how to make more effective the generation of useful information to support decisions by mothers, communities, and government agencies. For this purpose, research is needed to determine (a) how best to generate such information, for example, various formulations of growth monitoring or alternative sources of information for mothers and cost-effectiveness of various methods of nutrition surveillance for communities and government agencies; (b) how best to integrate information generation with the design and implementation of interventions and broader policies and programs; and (c) how best to analyze, interpret, and make available information, including the most appropriate institutional arrangements.

Second, there is an urgent need for sound evaluations of the nutritional effect of various formulations of integrated nutrition programs; of how such effect is influenced by the socioeconomic and cultural environments, including existing nutrition-related policies; and of how information from such evaluation can be generalized for use in the guidance of programs elsewhere.

As shown earlier, virtually all scientifically sound information about the effect of nutrition interventions refers to single interventions. Yet, the complex set of interacting determinants and strong synergism between and among various factors influencing the nutritional status lead to the conclusion that single interventions may not provide the most cost-effective strategy. Evidence from various integrated programs support this conclusion. Much more solid evidence is needed, however, to guide the design and implementation of the most appropriate integrated programs for the future.

Third, current attempts to deal effectively with the nutrition problem are hampered by a lack of a clear understanding about the most appropriate role of each group of key actors within a given socioeconomic and political environment. In some cases, agencies of national governments try to do what would be done more cost-effectively by the mother or the community, whereas in others, unreasonable expectations are placed on mothers to solve problems that can only be solved by agencies of a national government.

Attempts to provide predetermined solutions or magic bullets to solve problems that are poorly diagnosed frequently fail. Conversely, universal magic bullets are useful to remove certain constraints. The issue is to identify the constraints most effectively alleviated by generalized solutions and those requiring more specific solutions and to allocate available resources accordingly.

To do this, sound knowledge about household behavior related to food acquisition and intrahousehold allocation as well as health and nutrition-seeking activities is essential. Erroneous assumptions about the response of households to external influences frequently result in policies and programs that are poorly designed, poorly implemented, and cost-ineffective. Insufficient knowledge about the constraints to good nutrition at the household level adds to the problem. Finally, a better understanding of household coping strategies will greatly increase the ability to design appropriate strategies.

Research is also needed on the appropriate role of community action in alleviating health and nutrition problems. What type of action is likely to be most useful in various socioeconomic and political environments, and how can such action be most appropriately supported from outside the community? A great deal of lip service has been paid to community participation in primary health care and nutrition programs. In fact, much of such participation has been limited to the implementation of externally designed and controlled interventions. Community participation in problem diagnosis and the choice, design, and implementation of health and nutrition-related action that is sustainable without external material support has not been widespread, and research is needed to improve the understanding of how community action may be most effective.

With regard to research on the role of each of the key actors, there is an urgent need to improve existing knowledge about institutional and political economy factors and how these factors, including the behavior of various public and private sector agencies and groups, affect nutrition and nutrition interventions. The poor and malnourished usually possess very little political power and, although altruism may play a role, government action to alleviate poor nutrition effectively is likely to come about only if the nation as a whole or politically powerful groups within are perceived to gain. Therefore, the poor and malnourished must establish coalitions with more powerful groups. Furthermore, efforts to alleviate malnutrition must be institutionalized if they are to receive the necessary political support. Finally, information must be available to show the potential benefits to the various groups and to society as a whole, including additional analysis of the economic cost of malnutrition and cost-benefit and cost-effectiveness analyses of nutrition interventions.

Fourth, operational research is needed on a number of interventions to make available better information about what types of programs are likely to be most cost-effective under what conditions and for which population groups.

Fifth, certain biological and behavioral research is needed on the magnitudes and determinants of PEM among adult women, including but not limited to maternal depletion and how modifications in household behavior and access to resources may influence the nutritional status of women. This area has been almost totally ignored in the past. Finally, there is an urgent need for research on how best to deal with the increase of PEM as a result of economic crises and reforms and socioeconomic transitions, such as urbanization and associated changes in dietary patterns.

The above list of priorities for resource allocation and operational research should not be interpreted as being all-inclusive. Because PEM is influenced by such a complex set of factors, many more priorities could be listed. We have tried to list those that we feel are most important. We have not listed priorities associated with diseases discussed in other chapters in this collection, although many of them (for example, diarrhea and measles), are of great importance in PEM.

Appendix 18A. Estimating Nutritional Benefits

This appendix summarizes various ways to estimate nutritional benefits.

Estimating Economic Losses from Stunting

Carlson and Wardlaw (1990) report that 163 million preschool children are stunted. Of these, 41 percent, or 66.8 million, are severely stunted, whereas the rest, 96.2 million, are moderately stunted. Assuming a normal distribution and the standard deviation reported by WHO (1979), the height of severely and moderately stunted children at the age of two years is 10.0 and 7.0 centimeters below standard height, respectively. Martorell (in press) found that the absolute stunting in childhood measured in centimeters translates to an equal reduction in the height of adults. On the basis of a study of a sample of rural workers in the Philippines, Haddad and Bouis (1990) estimated the elasticity of labor productivity with respect to height of the workers to be 1.38; that is, a 1 percent difference in height is positively associated with a difference of 1.38 percent in labor productivity as measured by the actual wage received. The average height of the sample workers was 160.0 centimeters. Thus, 10.0 and 7.0 centimeters correspond to 6.25 and 4.38 percent of the height, respectively. Multiplying the elasticity and the height reduction due to childhood stunting yields estimated losses in labor productivity of 8.63 percent for severely stunted and 6.04 for moderately stunted individuals. Assuming a daily current wage of $2.50 and 300 working days annually, we arrive at an annual current wage income of $750.00 per person. The total economic loss as a result of stunting is then estimated as the total number of children stunted times the economic gain per individual, or a loss of $4.32 billion as a result of severe stunting and a loss of $4.36 billion as a result of moderate stunting. These figures yield a total annual economic loss of $8.68 billion.

Estimating Benefit-Cost Ratio of Preschoolers' Food Supplement

On the basis of results reported in table 18-9 it is assumed that a food transfer of 100,000 calories to malnourished preschool children results in an addition of 2.0 centimeters to the height of the child and that this height addition is maintained in adulthood. With reference to table 18-10, it is further assumed that the cost of the food supplementation program is $0.20 per 1,000 calories transferred. Thus, the cost per centimeter is $10.00. Using the above-mentioned estimates from the study by Haddad and Bouis (1990), one centimeter is equal to 0.625 percent of the height of the workers studied, and the corresponding increase in wages would be 0.625 x 1.38, or 0.86 percent. Under the above assumptions regarding daily wage and number of working days per year, this amounts to $6.45 per worker annually. Assuming that this wage gain begins at the age of eighteen, that is, seventeen years after the food supplement was received, and continues to age fifty-five, and using a discount rate of 3 percent and an annual increase in real wages of 2 percent, we arrive at $174.00 as the present value of the gain per worker, or a benefit-cost ratio of 17.4. For the purpose of sensitivity analysis, we estimated the benefit-cost ratios associated with height gains of 1.0 and 3.0 centimeters per 100,000 calories. The corresponding benefit-cost ratios are 8.7 and 26, respectively.

Estimating Cost per Child Death Averted by Supplement

Assuming a normal distribution and the standard deviation reported by WHO (1979), we estimated the prevalence of severe and moderate malnutrition from the average weight of the preschool children participating in food supplementation (table 18-9) prior to the supplementation (7.6 kilograms) and after a hypothetical average weight gain of 0.5 kilograms, which according to table 18-9 is brought about by a transfer of 100,000 calories. Based on the different mortality rates reported by Pelletier (1991) for severe and moderate underweight and using the prevalence of underweight reported in table 18-3, we estimated the effect of a weight gain of 0.5 kilograms on the overall mortality rate to be 1.03 percentage points. Considering this estimate as the reduction in the probability of dying, we estimated that the average cost of averting a child death would be $1,942, the cost of transferring 100,000 calories times 100 divided by 1.03.

Notes

1. These levels are not likely to be sufficient to cover energy expenditure associated with work and other activities desired by most people. Thus, they should be considered suboptimal in most cases.

2. Measurable responses may be less than expected by a purely factorial addition because physiological adaptations during pregnancy, such as changes in the resting metabolic rate and thermogenesis, may be altered by protein-energy malnutrition. Some of the improvement in dietary intake might be channeled into meeting the energy costs of these physiologic changes.

3. Weight at ages other than eighteen months and thirty-six months is not reported for Colombia in table 18-8 because the corresponding dietary intake was not reported for other ages.

4. The "conscientious efforts" were not specifically described.

References

Abdullah, M. 1983. "Dimensions of Intra-household Food and Nutrient Allocation: A Study of a Bangladesh Village." Ph.D. diss., University of London.

Adair, Linda S., and Ernesto Pollitt. 1985. "Outcome of Maternal Nutritional Supplementation: A Comprehensive Review of the Bacon Chow Study." *American Journal of Clinical Nutrition* 41:948–78.

Adair, Linda S., Ernesto Pollitt, and W. H. Mueller. 1983. "Maternal Anthropometric Changes During Pregnancy and Lactation in a Rural Taiwanese Population." *Human Biology* 55(4):771–87.

———. 1984. "The Bacon Chow Study: Maternal Nutritional Supplementation and Birth Weight of Offspring." *American Journal of Clinical Nutrition* 34:2133–44.

Agarwal, D. K., and others. 1987. "Nutritional Status, Physical Work Capacity, and Mental Function in School Children." Scientific Report 6. Nutrition Foundation of India, New Delhi.

Alderman, Harold. 1987. *Cooperative Dairy Development in Karnataka, India: An Assessment.* Research Report 64. International Food Policy Research Institute, Washington, D.C.

———. 1990. "Nutritional Status in Ghana and Its Determinants." Working Paper on Social Dimensions of Adjustment in Sub-Saharan Africa 3. World Bank, Washington, D.C.

———. In press. "Information as an Input into Food Policy Formation." In Per Pinstrup-Andersen, David Pelletier, and Harold Alderman, eds., *Beyond Child Survival: Enhancing Child Growth and Nutrition in Developing Countries.*

Alderman, Harold, and Joachim Von Braun. 1984. *The Effects of the Egyptian Food Ration and Subsidy System on Income Distribution and Consumption.* Research Report 45. International Food Policy Research Institute, Washington, D.C.

Alderman, Harold, Joachim Von Braun, and Sakr Ahmed Sakr. 1982. *Egypt's Food Subsidy and Rationing System: A Description.* Research Report 34. International Food Policy Research Institute, Washington, D.C.

Aligaen, M., and C. Florencio. 1980. "Intra-household Nutrient Distribution and Adequacy of Food and Nutrient Intake of Filipino Urban Households." *Philippine Journal of Nutrition* 33:11–19.

Anand, R. K. 1981. "The Management of Breastfeeding in a Bombay Hospital." *Assignment Children* 55/56:167–80.

Anderson, Mary Ann, James Austin, Joe D. Wray, Marian F. Zeitlin. 1981. *Nutrition Intervention in Developing Countries, Study 1: Supplementary Feeding.* Cambridge: Oelgeschlager, Gunn, and Hain.

Ashworth, A., and R. G. Feachem. 1985. "Interventions for the Control of Diarrhoeal Disease Among Young Children: Prevention of Low Birth Weight." *Bulletin of the World Health Organization* 63:165–84.

Bairagi, Radheshyam, Mridul K. Choudhury, Young J. Kim, and George T. Curlin. 1985. "Alternative Anthropometric Indicators of Mortality." *American Journal of Clinical Nutrition* 42(2):296–306.

Balderston, J. B., A. B. Wilson, M. E. Friere, and M. S. Simonen. 1981. *Malnourished Children of the Rural Poor.* Boston: Auburn House.

Barrell, R. A. F., and M. G. M. Rowland. 1979. "Infant Foods as a Potential Source of Diarrheal Illness in Rural West Africa." *Transactions of the Royal Society of Tropical Medicine and Hygiene* 73:85–90.

Beaton, George H., and Hossein Ghassemi. 1982. "Supplementary Feeding Programs for Young Children in Developing Countries." *American Journal of Clinical Nutrition* 35:864–916.

Beaudry-Darisme, M., and M. C. Latham. 1973. "Nutrition Rehabilitation Centers: An Evaluation of Their Performance." *Journal of Tropical Pediatrics and Environmental Child Health* 19:299–332.

Beghin, I. D. 1970. "Nutritional Rehabilitation Centers in Latin America: Critical Assessment." *American Journal of Clinical Nutrition* 23:1412–17.

Beghin, I. D., and R. E. Viteri. 1973. "Nutritional Rehabilitation Centres: An Evaluation of Their Performance." *Journal of Tropical Pediatrics and Environmental Child Health.* 19:404–16.

Behrman, Jere. 1988. "Nutrition and Incomes: Tightly Wedded or Loosely Meshed?" Pew/Cornell Lecture Series on Food and Nutrition Policy. Ithaca, N.Y.: Cornell Food and Nutrition Policy Program.

Beisel, W. R. 1977. "Resume of the Discussion Concerning the Nutritional Consequences of Infection." *American Journal of Clinical Nutrition* 30(8):1294–1300, August.

Berg, Alan. 1987. *Malnutrition: What Can Be Done?* Baltimore: Johns Hopkins University.

Berggren, Gretchen. 1981. "Home-Prepared Food Supplements, Mothercraft Centers, and Nutrition in Haiti." *Food and Nutrition Bulletin* 3(4):29–33.

Black, R. E., Kenneth H. Brown, and Stan Becker. 1984. "Malnutrition is a Determining Factor in Diarrheal Duration, But Not Incidence, in a Longitudinal Study in Rural Bangladesh." *American Journal of Clinical Nutrition* 39(1):87–94.

Black, Robert E., Kenneth H. Brown, Stan Becker, A. R. M. Abdul Alim, and Michael H. Merson. 1982. "Contamination of Weaning Foods and Transmission of Enterotoxigenic *Escherichia coli* Diarrhoea in Children in Rural Bangladesh." *Transactions of the Royal Society of Tropical Medicine and Hygiene* 76:259–64.

Bouis, Howarth E., and Lawrence J. Haddad. 1990. *Effects of Agricultural Commercialization on Land Tenure, Household Resource Allocation, and Nutrition in the Philippines.* Research Report 79. International Food Policy Research Institute, Washington, D.C.

Brown, Kenneth H., Robert E. Black, Guillermo Lopez de Romaña, and Hilary Creed de Kanashiro. 1988. "Infant Feeding Practices and Their Relationship with Diarrheal and Other Diseases in Huascar (Lima), Peru." *Pediatrics* 83:31–40.

Burger, Susan, and S. A. Esrey. In press. "Water and Sanitation: Health Benefits to Children." In Per Pinstrup-Andersen, David Pelletier, and Harold Alderman, eds., *Beyond Child Survival: Enhancing Child Growth and Nutrition in Developing Countries.*

Caldwell, B. M. 1974. "The Malnourishing Environment." In J. Cravioto, L. Hambraeus, and B. Vahlquist, eds., *Early Malnutrition and Mental Development.* Uppsala: Swedish Nutrition Foundation.

Carlson, Beverley A., and Tessa M. Wardlaw. 1990. "A Global, Regional, and Country Assessment of Child Malnutrition." UNICEF Programme Division. Staff Working Papers 7. New York.

Cerqueira, Maria Teresa, and Christine M. Olson. "Nutrition Education in Developing Countries." In press. In Per Pinstrup-Andersen, David Pelletier, and Harold Alderman, eds., *Beyond Child Survival: Enhancing Child Growth and Nutrition in Developing Countries.*

Chávez, Adolfo, and Celia Martinez. 1975. "Nutrition and Development of Children from Poor Rural Areas v. Nutrition and Behavioral Development." *Nutrition Reports International* 2(6):477–89.

Chávez, A., C. Martinez, and R. Yaschine. 1975. "Nutritional Behavioral Development and Mother-Child Interaction in Young Rural Children." Federation of American Societies for Experimental Biology. *Federation Proceedings* 34(7):1574–82.

Chen, Lincoln C. 1983. "Interactions of Diarrhea and Malnutrition." In Lincoln C. Chen and Nevin S. Scrimshaw, eds., *Diarrhea and Malnutrition: Interactions, Mechanisms, and Interventions.* New York: Plenum Press.

Chen, Lincoln C., A. K. M. A. Chowdhury, and S. L. Huffman. 1980. "Anthropometric Assessment of Energy-Protein Malnutrition and Subsequent Risk of Mortality Among Preschool-Aged Children." *American Journal of Clinical Nutrition* 33:1836–45.

Chen, Lincoln C., Emdadul Huq, and Stan D'Souza. 1981. "Sex Bias in the Family Allocation of Food and Healthcare in Bangladesh." *Population and Development Review* 7(1):55–70.

Chen, Lincoln C., Emdadul Huq, and Sandra L. Huffman. 1981. "A Prospective Study of the Risk of Diarrheal Diseases According to the Nutritional Status of Children." *American Journal of Epidemiology* 114:284–92.

Chen, Robert S., ed. 1990. "The Hunger Report: 1990." Brown University, Alan Shawn Feinstein World Hunger Program, Providence, R.I.

Chowdhury, A. K. M. A. 1988. "Child Mortality in Bangladesh: Food Versus Health Care." *Food and Nutrition Bulletin* 10(2):3–8.

Clavano, N. R. 1982. "Mode of Feeding and Its Effect on Infant Mortality and Morbidity." *Journal of Tropical Pediatrics* 28:287–93.

Cook, R. 1971. "Is Hospital the Place for Treatment of Malnourished Children?" *Journal of Tropical Pediatrics and Environmental Child Health* 17(1):15–25.

Cremer, H. D., A. Flórez, L. de Navarro, L. Vuori, and M. Wagner. 1977. "The Influence of Food Supplementation and/or Psychological Stimulation on Mental Development." *Nutrition and Metabolism* 21:358–71.

Cutting, W. A. M. 1983. "Nutritional Rehabilitation." In D. S. McLaren, ed., *Nutrition in the Community.* New York: John Wiley and Sons.

Davies, D. P., P. Platts, J. M. Pritchard, and P. W. Wilkinson. 1979. "Nutritional Status of Light-for-Date Infants at Birth and its Influence on Early Postnatal Growth." *Archives of Disease in Childhood* 54:703–6.

Delgado, H. L., Reynaldo Martorell, E. Brineman, and R. E. Klein. 1982. "Nutrition and Length of Gestation." *Nutrition Research* 2:117–26.

Delgado, H. L., V. E. Valverde, Reynaldo Martorell, and R. E. Klein. 1982. "Relationship of Maternal and Infant Nutrition to Infant Growth." *Early Human Development* 6:273–86.

Den Hartog, A. P. 1972. "Unequal Distribution of Food Within the Household." *Nutrition Newsletter* 10:8–17.

Deolalikar, A. B. 1988. "Nutrition and Labor Productivity in Agriculture: Estimates for Rural South India." *Review of Economics and Statistics* 70(3):406–13.

De Sweemer, Cecile. 1974. "Growth and Morbidity." Ph.D. diss., Johns Hopkins University.

Edirisinghe, Neville. 1987. *The Food Stamp Scheme in Sri Lanka: Costs, Benefits, and Options for Modification.* Research Report 58. International Food Policy Research Institute, Washington, D.C.

El Samani, F. Z., W. C. Willett, and J. H. Ware. 1988. "Association of Malnutrition and Diarrhea in Children Aged Under Five Years." *American Journal of Epidemiology* 128:93–105.

Engle, Patrice. In press. "Child Care and Preschool Nutrition." In Per Pinstrup-Andersen, David Pelletier, and Harold Alderman, eds., *Beyond Child Survival: Enhancing Child Growth and Nutrition in Developing Countries.*

Esrey, S. A., R. G. Feachem, and J. M. Hughes. 1985. "Interventions for the Control of Diarrhoeal Disease Among Young Children: Improving Water Supplies and Excreta Disposal Facilities." *Bulletin of the World Health Organization* 63:757–72.

Esrey, S. A., and Jean-Pierre Habicht. 1985. "The Impact of Improved Water Supplies and Excreta Disposal Facilities on Diarrheal Morbidity, Growth, and Mortality Among Children." In S. A. Esrey, Jean-Pierre Habicht, and

W. P. Butz, eds., *A Methodology to Review Public Health Interventions: Results from Nutrition Supplementation and Water and Sanitation Projects.* Cornell International Nutrition Monograph Series 15. Ithaca, N.Y.: Cornell Food and Nutrition Policy Program.

———. 1986. "Epidemiologic Evidence for Health Benefits from Improved Water and Sanitation in Developing Countries." *Epidemiology Reviews* 8:117–28.

Esrey, Steven A., J. B. Potash, L. Roberts, and C. Shiff. 1990. *Health Benefits from Improvements in Water Supply and Sanitation: Survey and Analysis of the Literature on Selected Diseases.* Technical Report 66. Water and Sanitation for Health Project, Arlington, Va.

FAO (Food and Agriculture Organization). 1987. *Fifth Annual World Food Survey.* Rome.

Feachem, R. G., and M. A. Koblinsky. 1984. "Interventions for the Control of Diarrhoeal Diseases Among Young Children: Promotion of Breastfeeding." *Bulletin of the World Health Organization* 62:271–91.

Garcia, Marito. 1988. "Food Subsidies in the Philippines: Preliminary Results." In Per Pinstrup-Andersen, ed., *Food Subsidies in Developing Countries: Costs, Benefits, and Policy Options.* Baltimore: Johns Hopkins University Press.

Garcia, Marito, and Per Pinstrup-Andersen. 1987. *The Pilot Food Price Subsidy Scheme in the Philippines: Its Impact on Income, Food Consumption, and Nutritional Status.* Research Report 61. International Food Policy Research Institute, Washington, D.C.

Ghai, O. P., and V. N. Jaiswal. 1970. "Relationship of Undernutrition to Diarrhea in Infants and Children." *Indian Journal of Medical Research* 58:789.

Gibbons, Gayle, and Marcia Griffiths. 1984. "Program Activities for Improving Weaning Practices." Information for Action Issue Paper Prepared for UNICEF. World Federation of Public Health Associations, Geneva.

Gilmore, J. W., C. C. Adelman, A. J. Meyer, and M. C. Thorne. 1980. "Morocco: Food Aid and Nutrition Education." Project Impact Evaluation 8. United States Agency for International Development, Washington, D.C.

Gomez, F., R. Galvan, S. Frenk, J. C. Muñoz, R. Chavez, and J. Vazquez. 1956. "Mortality in Second and Third Degree Malnutrition." *Journal of Tropical Pediatrics* 2:77.

Gonzalez-Cossio, T., Jean-Pierre Habicht, H. Delgado, and K. M. Rasmussen. 1991. "Food Supplementation during Lactation Increases Infant Milk Intake and the Proportion of Exclusive Breast Feeding." Federation of American Societies for Experimental Biology. FASEB *Journal.*

Gopalan, C., and Meera Chatterjee. 1984. *Use of Growth Charts for Promoting Child Nutrition: A Review of Global Experience.* Special Publication 2. Nutrition Foundation of India, New Delhi.

Gopalan, C., M. C. Swaminathan, V. K. Krishna Kumari, D. Hanumantha Rao, and K. Vijayaraghavan. 1973. "Effect of Calorie Supplementation on Growth of Undernourished Children." *American Journal of Clinical Nutrition* 26:563–66.

Grantham-McGregor, Sally, William Schofield, and Linda Harris. 1983. "Effect of Psychosocial Stimulation on Mental Development of Severely Malnourished Children: An Interim Report." *Pediatrics* 7(22):239–43.

Grantham-McGregor, Sally, Marie E. Stewart, Christine Powell, and W. N. Schofield. 1979. "Effect of Stimulation on Mental Development of Malnourished Child." *Lancet* 2:200–1.

Grantham-McGregor, Sally, Marie E. Stewart, and W. N. Schofield. 1980. "Effect of Long-Term Psychosocial Stimulation on Mental Development of Severely Malnourished Children." *Lancet* 2:785–89.

Graves, P. L. 1976. "Nutrition, Infant Behavior, and Maternal Characteristics: A Pilot Study in West Bengal, India." *American Journal of Clinical Nutrition* 29:305–19.

Griffiths, Marcia. 1985. "Growth Monitoring of Preschool Children: Practical Considerations for Primary Health Care Projects." Information for Action Issue Paper prepared for UNICEF. World Federation of Public Health Associations, Geneva.

Gwatkin, Davidson, Janet R. Wilcox, and Joe D. Wray. 1980. *Can Health and Nutrition Intervention Make a Difference?* Overseas Development Council, Washington, D.C.

Haaga, J. G., and J. B. Mason. 1987. "Food Distribution Within the Family: Evidence and Implications for Research and Programmes." *Food Policy* 12(May):146–60.

Habicht, Jean-Pierre, Julie DaVanzo, and William P. Butz. 1988. "Mother's Milk and Sewage: Their Interactive Effects on Infant Mortality." *Pediatrics* 81:456–61.

Haddad, Lawrence J., and Howarth E. Bouis. 1990. "The Impact of Nutritional Status on Agricultural Productivity: Wage Evidence From the Philippines." *Oxford Bulletin of Economic Statistics* 53(1):45–68.

Hamilton, Sahni, Barry Popkin, and Deborah Spicer. 1984. *Women and Nutrition in Third World Countries.* New York: Praeger Press.

Harbert, Lloyd, and Pasquale Scandizzo. 1982. "Food Distribution and Nutrition Intervention: The Case of Chile." Working Paper 512. World Bank, Washington, D.C.

Hardy, Ellen E., Ana M. Vichi, Regina C. Sarmento, Lucila E. Moreira, and Celia M. Bosqueiro. 1982. "Breastfeeding Promotion: Effect of an Educational Program in Brazil." *Studies in Family Planning* 13(3):79–86.

Herrera, M. G. 1985. "Maternal Nutrition and Child Survival." Paper presented to UNICEF Conference on Child Health and Survival, Harvard School of Public Health, May 30–31, Boston.

Herrera, M. G., J. O. Mora, B. de Paredes, and M. Wagner. 1980. "The Effects of Nutritional Supplementation and Early Education on Physical and Cognitive Development." In Ralph R. Turner and Hayne. W. Reese, eds., *Life-Span Developmental Psychology: Intervention.* New York: Academic Press.

Ho, Teresa J. 1985. *Economic Issues in Assessing Nutrition Projects: Costs, Affordability and Cost Effectiveness.* Population, Health, and Nutrition Technical Note 85-14. World Bank, Washington, D.C.

Hornik, R. C. 1985. *Nutrition Education—A State of the Art Review.* State of the Art Series. Nutrition Policy Discussion Paper 1. Administrative Committee on Coordination, Subcommittee on Nutrition, United Nations, New York.

Huffman, Sandra, and Adwoa Steel. In press. "The Impact of Child Survival Interventions on Child Growth." In Per Pinstrup-Andersen, David Pelletier, and Harold Alderman, eds., *Beyond Child Survival: Enhancing Child Growth and Nutrition in Developing Countries.*

Johnson, David W., and Roger T. Johnson. 1985. "Nutrition Education: A Model for Effectiveness, A Synthesis of Research." *Journal of Nutrition Education* 17(supplement 2)1–44.

Jumaan, A. O., M. K. Serdula, D. F. Williamson, M. J. Dibley, N. J. Binkin, and J. J. Boring. 1989. "Feeding Practices and Growth in Yemeni Children." *Journal of Tropical Pediatrics and Environmental Child Health* 35:82–86.

Kasongo Project Team. 1983. "Anthropometric Assessment of Young Children's Nutritional Status as an Indicator of Subsequent Risk of Dying." *Journal of Tropical Pediatrics and Environmental Child Health* 29:69–75.

Kates, R. W., Robert S. Chen, T. E. Downing, Jeanne X. Kasperson, Ellen Messer, and Sarah R. Millman. 1988. *The Hunger Report: 1988.* Brown University, Alan Shawn Feinstein World Hunger Program, Providence, R.I.

Kennedy, Eileen T. 1989. *The Effects of Sugarcane Production on Food Security, Health, and Nutrition in Kenya: A Longitudinal Analysis.* Research Report 78. International Food Policy Research Institute, Washington, D.C.

Kennedy, Eileen T., and Harold Alderman. 1987. *Comparative Analysis of Nutritional Effectiveness of Food Subsidies and Other Food-Related Interventions.* International Food Policy Research Institute, Washington, D. C.

Kennedy, Eileen T., and Bruce Cogill. 1987. *Income and Nutrition Effects of Sugarcane Production in Southwestern Kenya.* Research Report 63. International Food Policy Research Institute, Washington, D.C.

Kennedy, Eileen T., and Milton Kotelchuck. 1984. "The Effect of WIC Supplemental Feeding on Birth Weight: A Case-Control Analysis." *American Journal of Clinical Nutrition* 40(3):579–85.

Kennedy, Eileen T., C. Overholt, and C. Haddral. 1984. *Effect of a Milk Subsidy on the Distribution of Benefits within the Household.* International Food Policy Research Institute, Washington, D.C.

Keusch, G. T., and N. S. Scrimshaw. 1986. "Control of Infection to Reduce Malnutrition." In J. A. Walsh and K. S. Warren, eds., *Strategies for Primary Health Care*. Chicago: University of Chicago Press.

Kielmann, A. A., C. E. Taylor, R. L. Parker, W. A. Reinke, D. N. Kakar, and R. S. S. Sarma. 1983. "Child and Maternal Health Services in Rural India: The Narangwal Experiment." In *Integrated Nutrition and Health Care*. 1. Baltimore: Johns Hopkins University Press.

Kielmann, A. A., and C. McCord. 1978. "Weight-For-Age as an Index of Risk of Death in Children." *Lancet* 2:1247–50.

Klein, R. E., H. E. Freeman, J. Kagan, Charles Yarbrough, and Jean-Pierre Habicht. 1972. "Is Big Smart? The Relation of Growth to Cognition." *Journal of Health and Social Behavior* 13:219.

Koster, F. T., G. C. Curlin, K. M. A. Aziz, and H. Azizul. 1981. "Synergistic Impact of Measles and Diarrhea on Nutrition and Mortality in Bangladesh." *Bulletin of the World Health Organization* 59:901.

Kramer, M. S. 1987. "Determinants of Low Birth Weight: Methodological Assessment and Meta-Analysis." *Bulletin of the World Health Organization* 65:663–737.

Kumar, S. K. 1979. *Impact of Subsidized Rice on Food Consumption and Nutrition in Kerala*. Research Report 5. International Food Policy Research Institute, Washington, D.C.

Kurz, K. M., K. M. Rasmussen, and Jean-Pierre Habicht. 1990. "Maternal Nutritional Status Has a Small Influence on Length of Postpartum Amenorrhea among Guatemalan Women." Federation of American Societies for Experimental Biology. *FASEB Journal* 4(4):A1160.

Lambert, J. 1988. "Pakistan: Update on Breastfeeding." *Mothers and Children* 7(2):5–6.

Lamptey, Peter, and Fred Sai. 1985. "Integrated Health/Nutrition/Population Programmes." In Margaret Biswas and Per Pinstrup-Andersen, eds., *Nutrition and Development*. London: Oxford University Press.

Latham, M. 1985. "The Relationship of Nutrition to Productivity and Wellbeing of Workers." Paper presented to the Workshop on Political Economy of Nutrition Improvement, June 10–13, 1985, Coolfront, W.V.

Lawrence, M. and R. G. Whitehead. 1988. "Physical Activity and Total Energy Expenditure of Child-Bearing Gambian Village Women." *European Journal of Clinical Nutrition* 42:145–60.

Lechtig, Aaron, Jean-Pierre Habicht, Hernán Delgado, Robert E. Klein, Charles Yarbrough, and Reynaldo Martorell. 1975. "Effect of Food Supplementation During Pregnancy on Birth Weight." *Pediatrics* 56:508–20.

Lechtig, A., and R. E. Klein. 1979. "Maternal Food Supplementation and Infant Health: Results of a Study in Rural Areas of Guatemala." In Hugo Aebi and Roger G. Whitehead, eds., *Maternal Nutrition During Pregnancy and Lactation*. Bern: Hans Huber.

Leslie, Joanne. 1982. "Child Malnutrition and Diarrhea: A Longitudinal Study from Northeast Brazil." Ph.D. diss., Johns Hopkins University School of Hygiene and Public Health.

Leslie, Joanne. In press. "Improving the Nutrition of Women in the Third World." In Per Pinstrup-Andersen, David Pelletier, and Harold Alderman, eds., *Beyond Child Survival: Enhancing Child Growth and Nutrition in Developing Countries*.

Lindskog, U., P. Lindskog, J. Carstensen, Y. Larsson, and M. Gebre-Medhin. 1988. "Childhood Mortality in Relation to Nutritional Status and Water Supply: A Prospective Study from Rural Malawi." *Acta Pediatrica Scandinavica* 77:260–68.

Lutter, C. K. 1987. "Nutritional Supplementation: When is It Most Effective in Promoting Growth Among Malnourished Infants and Children." Ph.D. diss., Cornell University.

Lutter, C. K., J. O. Mora, Jean-Pierre Habicht, K. M. Rasmussen, D. S. Robson, and M. G. Herrera. 1990. "Age-Specific Responsiveness of Weight and Length to Nutritional Supplementation." *American Journal of Clinical Nutrition* 51:359–64.

Lutter, C. K., J. O. Mora, Jean-Pierre Habicht, K. M. Rasmussen, D. S. Robson, S. G. Sellars, C. M. Super, and M. G. Herrera. 1989. "Nutritional Supple-

mentation: Effects on Child Stunting Because of Diarrhea." *American Journal of Clinical Nutrition* 50:1–8.

MacCormack, C. P. 1988. "Health and the Social Power of Women." *British Journal of Science and Medicine* 26:677–83.

McDonald, E. C., E. Pollitt, W. Mueller, A. M. Hsueh, and R. Sherwin. 1981. "The Bacon Chow Study: Effect of Nutritional Supplementation on Maternal Weight and Skinfold Thicknesses During Pregnancy and Lactation." *British Journal of Nutrition* 51:357–69.

McGuire, Judith S. 1988. *Malnutrition: Opportunities and Challenges for A.I.D.* United States Agency for International Development, Washington, D.C.

McGuire, Judith S., and J. E. Austin. 1987. "Beyond Survival: Children's Growth for National Development." In *Assignment Children*. 2:1–51.

McGuire, Judith S., and Barry M. Popkin. 1990. *Helping Women Improve Nutrition in the Developing World: Beating the Zero Sum Game*. Technical Paper 114. World Bank, Washington, D.C.

McKay, H., and L. Sinisterra. 1974. "Intellectual Development of Malnourished Preschool Children in Programs of Stimulation and Nutritional Supplementation." In Joaquin Cravioto, Leif Hambraeus, and Bo Bahlquist, eds., *Early Malnutrition and Mental Development: Symposia of the Swedish Nutrition Foundation 12*. Swedish Nutrition Foundation Stockholm: Almquist and Wiksell.

McKay, Harrison, Leonardo Sinisterra, Arlene McKay, Hernando Gomez, and Pascuala Lloreda. 1978. "Improving Cognitive Ability in Chronically Deprived Children." *Science* 200:270–78.

McLaren, Donald Stewart, Emmanuel Shirajian, Herminé Loshkajin, and Sossy Shadarevian. 1969. "Short-Term Prognosis in Protein-Calorie Malnutrition." *American Journal of Clinical Nutrition* 22:863–70.

Marks, G. C. 1989. "The Relationships of Body Weight and Composition in Preschool Children." Ph.D. diss., Cornell University.

Martines, J. C., Jean-Pierre Habicht, A. Ashworth, and B. R. Kirkwood. 1988. "Exclusive Breast-Feeding and Growth: When Should Supplements be Introduced." Typescript.

Martorell, Reynaldo. In press. "Promoting Healthy Growth: Rationale and Benefits." In Per Pinstrup-Andersen, David Pelletier, and Harold Alderman, eds., *Beyond Child Survival: Enhancing Child Growth and Nutrition in Developing Countries*.

Martorell, Reynaldo, and G. Arroyave. 1984. "Malnutrition, Work Output, and Energy Needs." Paper presented at the International Union of Biological Sciences Symposium, Ciba Foundation, London.

Martorell, Reynaldo, Jean-Pierre Habicht, and R. E. Klein. 1982. "Anthropometric Indicators of Change in Nutritional Status in Malnourished Populations." In Barbara Underwood, ed., *Proceedings Methodologies for Human Population Studies in Nutrition Related to Health*. National Institutes of Health Publication 82-2462. Washington, D.C.: U.S. Government Printing Office.

Martorell, Reynaldo, Jean-Pierre Habicht, Charles Yarbrough, A. Lechtig, R. E. Klein, and K. A. Western. 1975. "Acute Morbidity and Physical Growth in Rural Guatemalan Children." *American Journal of Diseases of Children* 129(11):1296–1301.

Martorell, Reynaldo, R. E. Klein, and H. Delgado. 1980. "Improved Nutrition and Its Effects on Anthropometric Indicators of Nutritional Status." *Nutrition Reports International* 21(2):219–30.

Martorell, Reynaldo, J. Rivera, and C. K. Lutter. 1988. "Interaction of Diet and Disease in Child Growth." Paper presented at the 4th International Human Lactation Meeting, Nov. 16–19, 1988, San José, Costa Rica.

Martorell, Reynaldo, and Charles Yarbrough. 1983. "The Energy Cost of Diarrheal Diseases and Other Common Illnesses in Children." In Lincoln C. Chen and Nevin S. Scrimshaw, eds., *Diarrhea and Malnutrition: Interactions, Mechanisms, and Interventions*. New York: Plenum Press.

Mason, John B., Jean-Pierre Habicht, H. Tabatabai, and V. Valverde. 1984. *Nutritional Surveillance*. Geneva: World Health Organization.

Mata, L. J. 1978. *The Children of Santa Maria Cauque: A Prospective Field Study of Health and Growth*. Cambridge, Mass.: MIT Press.

————. 1983. "Promotion of Breastfeeding, Health, and Growth Among Hospital-Born Neonates, and Among Infants of a Rural Area of Costa Rica." In Lincoln C. Chen and Nevin S. Scrimshaw, eds., *Diarrhea and Malnutrition: Interactions, Mechanisms, and Interventions*. New York: Plenum Press.

Mata, L. J., R. A. Kromall, J. J. Urrutia, and B. Garcia. 1977. "Effect of Infection on Food Intake and the Nutritional State: Perspectives as Viewed from the Village." *American Journal of Clinical Nutrition* 30:1215–27.

Mata, Leonardo J., Juan José Urrutia, Constantino Albertazzi, Olegario Pellecer, and Eduardo Arellano. 1972. "Influence of Recurrent Infections on Nutrition and Growth of Children in Guatemala." *American Journal of Clinical Nutrition* 25:1267–75.

Mebrahtu, Saba, David Pelletier, and Per Pinstrup-Andersen. In press. "Agriculture and Nutrition." In Per Pinstrup-Andersen, David Pelletier, and Harold Alderman, eds., *Beyond Child Survival: Enhancing Child Growth and Nutrition in Developing Countries*.

Merchant, Kathleen, Reynaldo Martorell, and Jere Haas. 1990a. "Consequences for Maternal Nutrition of Reproductive Stress Across Consecutive Pregnancies." *American Journal of Clinical Nutrition* 52:616–20.

————. 1990b. "Maternal and Fetal Responses to the Stresses of Lactation Concurrent with Pregnancy and of Short Recuperative Intervals." *American Journal of Clinical Nutrition* 52:280–88.

Merchant, Kathleen, and others. 1988. "Frequent Reproductive Cycling." *Progress in Food and Nutrition* 12(4).

Mora, José. 1983. "Supplementary Feeding During Pregnancy: Impact on Mother and Child in Bogotá, Colombia." In B. A. Underwood, ed., *Nutrition Intervention Strategies in National Development*. New York: Nutrition Foundation, Academic Press.

————. In press. "Integrated Programs for Primary Health Care and Improved Nutrition." In Per Pinstrup-Andersen, David Pelletier, and Harold Alderman, eds., *Beyond Child Survival: Enhancing Child Growth and Nutrition in Developing Countries*.

Mora, J. O., J. Clement, N. Christiansen, J. Suescun, M. Wagner, and M. G. Herrera. 1978. "Nutritional Supplementation and the Outcome of Pregnancy. 3. Perinatal and Neonatal Mortality." *Nutrition Reports International* 18(2):167–75.

Mora, J. O., L. de Navarro, J. Clement, M. Wagner, B. de Paredes, and M. G. Herrera. 1978. "The Effect of Nutritional Supplementation on Calorie and Protein Intake of Pregnant Women." *Nutrition Reports International* 17(2):217–28.

Mora, J. O., B. de Paredes, M. Wagner, L. de Navarro, J. Suescun, N. Christiansen, and M. G. Herrera. 1979. "Nutrition Supplementation and the Outcome of Pregnancy. 1. Birth Weight." *American Journal of Clinical Nutrition* 32:455–62.

Mora, J. O., M. G. Herrera, J. Suescun, L. de Navarro, and M. Wagner. 1981. "The Effects of Nutritional Supplementation on Physical Growth of Children at Risk of Malnutrition." *American Journal of Clinical Nutrition* 34:1885–92.

National Academy of Sciences. 1988. *Amino Acid Fortification of Cereals: Results and Interpretation of Trials in Three Countries: A Report of the Task Force on Amino Acid Fortification of Cereals*. Cornell International Nutrition Monograph Series 20. Committee on International Nutrition Programs, Food and Nutrition Board, Commission on Life Sciences, National Research Council. Ithaca, N.Y.

Naylor, A. J., and R. A. Wester. 1985. "Lactation Specialist Training for Health Professionals From Developing Nations." Summary Report of Sessions 1–4, August 1983–January 1985. San Diego Lactation Program.

Nutrition Economics Group. 1982. *Intra-Family Food Distribution: Review of the Literature and Policy Implications*. United States Department of Agriculture, Office of International Cooperation and Development, Technical Assistance Division, Washington, D.C.

Overholt, Catherine, Stephen G. Sellers, José O. Mora, Belen de Paredes, and M. Guillermo Herrera. 1982. "The Effects of Nutritional Supplementation on the Diets of Low-Income Families at Risk of Malnutrition." *American Journal of Clinical Nutrition* 36:1153–61.

Payne, Philip R. 1985. "The Nature of Malnutrition." In Margaret Biswas and Per Pinstrup-Andersen, eds., *Nutrition and Development*. Oxford: Oxford University Press.

Pelletier, David. 1991. *The Relationship Between Child Anthropometry and Mortality in Developing Countries: Implications for Policy, Programs, and Future Research*. Cornell Food and Nutrition Policy Program Monograph Series 12. Ithaca, N.Y.

————. In press. "The Role of Information in Community-Based Nutrition Programs." In Per Pinstrup-Andersen, David Pelletier, and Harold Alderman, eds., *Beyond Child Survival: Enhancing Child Growth and Nutrition in Developing Countries*.

Peterson, K. E., and D. A. Frank. 1987. "Feeding and Growth of Premature and Small-For Gestational-Age Infants." In William Taeusch and Michael Yogman, eds., *Follow-Up Management of the High-Risk Infant*. Boston: Little, Brown.

Peterson, K. E., M. G. Herrera, and C. M. Super. 1988. "Sequelae of Growth Delay in Colombian Children Aged 0–36 Months." Paper presented to the Annual Meeting of the American Public Health Association, Boston.

Peterson K. E., C. M. Super, and M. G. Herrera. 1988. "Biological and Social Predictors of Nutritional Status at 6 Months of Age in Colombian Children at High Risk of Malnutrition." Proceedings of the Fifth International Congress of Auxology, Exeter, England.

Pinstrup-Andersen, Per. 1982. *Agricultural Research and Technology in Economic Development*. New York: Longman.

————. 1985. "Food Prices and the Poor in Developing Countries." *European Review of Agricultural Economics* 12(78):69–81.

————, ed. 1988. *Food Subsidies in Developing Countries: Costs, Benefits, and Policy Options*. Baltimore: Johns Hopkins University Press.

Pinstrup-Andersen, Per, and Marito Garcia. 1990. "Data on Food Consumption by High-Risk Family Members: Its Utility for Identifying Target Households for Food and Nutrition Programmes." In Beatrice Lorge Rogers and Nina P. Schlossman, eds., *Intra-Household Resource Allocation: Issues and Methods for Development Policy and Planning*. Tokyo: United Nations University Press.

Pinstrup-Andersen, Per, and Peter B. R. Hazell. 1985. "The Impact of the Green Revolution and Prospects for the Future." *Food Reviews International* 1(1):1–25.

Pollitt, E. 1987. "A Critical View of Three Decades of Research on the Effects of Chronic Energy Malnutrition on Behavioral Development." In Blat Schurch and Nevin S. Scrimshaw, eds., *Chronic Energy Deficiency: Consequences and Related Issues*. Lausanne, Switzerland: International Dietary Energy Consultancy Group (IDECG).

Prentice, A. M., T. J. Cole, F. A. Foord, W. H. Lamb, and R. G. Whitehead. 1987. "Increased Birth Weight After Prenatal Dietary Supplementation of Rural African Women." *American Journal of Clinical Nutrition* 46:912–25.

Prentice, A. M., S. B. Roberts, and A. Prentice. 1983. "Dietary Supplementation of Lactating Gambian Women. 1. Effect on Breast-Milk Volume and Quality." *Human Nutrition: Clinical Nutrition* 37:53–64.

Prentice, A. M., Susan B. Roberts, M. Watkinson, R. G. Whitehead, Alison A. Paul, Ann Prentice, and Anne A. Watkinson. 1980. "Dietary Supplementation of Gambian Nursing Mothers and Lactational Performance." *Lancet* 2(October–December 1980):886–88.

Prentice, A. M., R. G. Whitehead, M. Watkinson, W. H. Lamb, and T. J. Cole. 1983. "Prenatal Dietary Supplementation of African Women and Birth-Weight." *Lancet* 1:489–92.

Puffer, R. R., and C. V. Serrano. 1987. *Patterns of Birth Weight*. Scientific Publication 504. Pan American Health Organization, Washington, D.C.

Rasmussen, K. M., N. B. Mock, and Jean-Pierre Habicht. 1985. "The Biological Meaning of Low Birth Weight and the Use of Data on Low Birth Weight for Nutritional Surveillance." Working Paper Series 27. Ithaca, N.Y.: Cornell Nutritional Surveillance Program.

Rathbun, J. M., and K. E. Peterson. 1987. "Nutrition in Failure-to-Thrive." In R. F. Grand, J. L. Sutphen, and W. H. Dietz, eds., *Pediatric Nutrition*. Boston: Butterworths.

Richardson, S. A. 1980. "The Long Range Consequences of Malnutrition in Infancy: A Study of Children in Jamaica, West Indies." In B. Wharton, ed., *Topics in Pediatrics 2*. Nutrition in Childhood. Tunbridge Wells, Eng.: Pitman Medical.

Rivera, Juan, Jean-Pierre Habicht, and Douglas Robson. 1991. "Effect of Supplementary Feeding Upon Recovery from Mild-to-Moderate Wasting in Preschool Children." *American Journal of Clinical Nutrition* 54(1):62–68.

Rivera, J., Reynaldo Martorell, and C. K. Lutter. 1989. *Interacción de la Ingesta Dietetica y la Enfermedad Diarreica en el Crecimiento de los Niños*. Institute of Nutrition of Central America and Panama, Guatemala City, Guatemala.

Roberts, S. B. 1982. "Seasonal Changes in Activity, Birth Weight, and Lactational Performance in Rural Gambian Women." *Transactions of the Royal Society of Tropical Medicine and Hygiene* 76:668–78.

Rothe, G. E., K. M. Rasmussen, and Jean-Pierre Habicht. 1988. "The Predictors of Growth Response to Supplementation in Malnourished Children." Typescript.

Rowland, M. G. M., S. G. J. G. Rowland, and T. J. Cole. 1988. "Impact of Infection on the Growth of Children From 0 to 2 Years in an Urban West African Community." *American Journal of Clinical Nutrition* 47:134–38.

Rowland, M. G. M., T. J. Cole, and R. G. Whitehead. 1977. "A Quantitative Study into the Role of Infection in Determining Nutritional Status in Gambian Village Children." *British Journal of Nutrition* 37:441–50.

Ruel, Marie. In press. "Growth Monitoring as an Educational Tool, an Integrating Strategy, and a Source of Information: A Review of Experience." In Per Pinstrup-Andersen, David Pelletier, and Harold Alderman, eds., *Beyond Child Survival: Enhancing Child Growth and Nutrition in Developing Countries*.

Rush, D., Z. Stein, and M. Susser. 1980a. "Diet in Pregnancy: A Randomized Controlled Trial of Nutritional Supplements." (Original Article Series) *Birth Defects* 16:(3). New York: Alan Liss. Inc.

———. 1980b. "A Randomized Controlled Trial of Prenatal Nutritional Supplementation in New York City." *Pediatrics* 65:683–97.

Sahn, David E., ed. 1989. *Seasonal Variability in Third World Agriculture*. Baltimore: Johns Hopkins University Press.

———. 1990. *Malnutrition in Côte d'Ivoire: Prevalence and Determinants*. Working paper on Social Dimensions of Adjustment in Sub-Saharan Africa 4. World Bank, Washington, D.C.

Sahn, David E., and Harold Alderman. 1988. "The Effects of Human Capital on Wages and the Determinants of Labor Supply in a Developing Country." *Journal of Development Economics* 29(2):157–84.

Scrimshaw, N. S., C. E. Taylor, and J. E. Gordon. 1968. *Interactions of Nutrition and Infection*. Monograph 57. World Health Organization, Geneva.

Selowsky, Marcelo. 1981. "Nutrition, Health, and Education: The Economic Significance of Complementarities at an Early Age." *Journal of Development Economics* 9:331–46.

Selowsky, Marcelo, and Lance Taylor. 1973. "The Economics of Malnourished Children: An Example of Disinvestment in Human Capital." *Economic Development and Cultural Change* 22(2):17–30.

Sepúlveda, Jaime, Walter Willett, and Alvaro Muñoz. 1988. "Malnutrition and Diarrhea." *American Journal of Epidemiology* 127:365–76.

Shekar, Meera. 1991. *The Tamil Nadu Integrated Nutrition Project: A Review of the Project with Special Emphasis on the Monitoring and Information System*. Working Paper 14. Cornell Food and Nutrition Policy Program, Ithaca, N.Y.

Sommer, Alfred, and Matthew S. Loewenstein. 1975. "Nutritional Status and Mortality: A Prospective Validation of the QUAC Stick." *American Journal of Clinical Nutrition* 28:287–92.

Spurr, G. B. 1983. "Nutritional Status and Physical Work Capacity." *Yearbook of Physical Anthropology* 26:5–35.

———. 1984. "Physical Activity, Nutritional Status, and Physical Work Capacity in Relation to Agricultural Productivity." In Ernesto Pollitt and Peggy Amante, eds., *Energy Intake and Activity*. New York: Alan R. Liss.

Spurr, G. B., M. Barac-Nieto, and M. G. Maksud. 1977. "Productivity and Maximal Oxygen Consumption in Sugar Cane Cutters." *American Journal of Clinical Nutrition* 30:316–21.

Stephenson, L. S. 1987. *The Impact of Helminth Infections on Human Nutrition: Schistosomes and Soil-Transmitted Helminths*. London: Taylor and Francis.

Strauss, John. 1985. "The Impact of Improved Nutrition on Labor Productivity and Human Resource Development: An Economic Perspective." Paper presented to the Workshop on the Political Economy of Nutrition Improvement, June 10–13, 1985, Coolfront, W.V.

———. 1986. "Does Better Nutrition Raise Farm Productivity?" *Journal of Political Economy* 94:297–320.

Super, C. M., S. G. Sellers, J. O. Mora, B. de Paredes, and M. G. Herrera. 1989. "Weaning, Diarrhea, and the Transition to a Family Diet Among Colombian Infants at Risk of Malnutrition." Typescript.

Svedberg, Peter. 1989. "Undernutrition in Sub-Saharan Africa: Is There a Sex Bias?" Helsinki: Wider.

Tanner, J. M., and A. M. Thompson. 1970. "Standards for Birth Weight at Gestation Periods From 32 to 42 Weeks, Allowing for Maternal Height and Weight." *Archives of Disease in Childhood* 45:566.

Taylor, C. E., and E. M. Taylor. 1976. "Multifactorial Causation of Malnutrition." In D. S. McLaren, ed., *Nutrition in the Community*. London: John Wiley and Sons.

Thompson, A. M., W. Z. Billewicz, and F. E. Hytten. 1968. "The Assessment of Fetal Growth." *British Journal of Obstetrics and Gynecology* 75:903–16.

Tomkins, Andrew. 1981. "Nutritional Status and Severity of Diarrhoea among Preschool Children in Rural Nigeria." *Lancet* 1:860–62.

Torche, A. 1981. *Evaluación Económica del Programa Nacional de Alimentacio Complimentaria* (PNAC). Institute of Economics, Catholic University of Chile, Santiago.

Tucker, Katherine, David Pelletier, Kathleen Rasmussen, Jean-Pierre Habicht, Per Pinstrup-Andersen, and Frederick Roche. 1989. *Advances in Nutritional Surveillance: The Cornell Nutritional Surveillance Program 1981–1987*. Monograph 2. Ithaca, N.Y.: The Cornell Food and Nutrition Policy Program.

UNICEF (United Nations Children's Fund). 1988. *1983–1988 Evaluation Report of the Joint WHO/UNICEF Nutrition Support Programme in Iringa, Tanzania*. Government of the United Republic of Tanzania, World Health Organization, and United Nations Children's Fund, Dar es Salaam.

———. 1989. *The State of the World's Children*. New York: Oxford University Press.

United Nations. 1987. "First Report on the World Nutrition Situation." Administrative Committee on Coordination, Subcommittee on Nutrition, New York.

———. 1990. "Summary Report of the Sixteenth Session of the ACC/Subcommittee on Nutrition, February 19–23, 1990, Paris." UNESCO, Administrative Committee on Coordination, Subcommittee on Nutrition, United Nations, New York.

———. 1992. "Second Report on the World Nutrition Situation." ACC/SCN, New York.

USAID (United States Agency for International Development). 1988. *Growth Monitoring and Nutrition Education: Impact Evaluation of an Effective Applied Nutrition Program in the Dominican Republic*. Bureau for Science and Technology, Office of Nutrition, Washington, D.C.

Van Esterik, P. 1984. *Intra-Family Food Distribution: Its Relevance for Maternal and Child Nutrition*. Working Paper 18. The Cornell Nutritional Surveillance Program, Ithaca, N.Y.

Victora, C. G., J. Patrick Vaughan, C. Lombardi, S. M. C. Fuchs, L. P. Gigante, P. G. Smith, L. C. Nobre, A. M. B. Teixeira, L. M. Moreira, and F. C. Barros. 1987. "Evidence for Protection by Breastfeeding Against Infant Deaths from Infectious Diseases in Brazil." *Lancet* 2(August):319–21.

Villar, J., L. Altobelli, E. Kestler, and J. Belizan. 1986. "A Health Priority for Developing Countries: The Prevention of Chronic Fetal Malnutrition." *Bulletin of the World Health Organization* 64:847–51.

Villar, J., and J. Belizan. 1982. "The Relative Contribution of Prematurity and Fetal Growth Retardation to Low Birth Weight in Developing and Developed Societies." *American Journal of Obstetrics and Gynecology* 37:142–44.

Villar, J., V. Smeriglio, Reynaldo Martorell, C. H. Brown, and R. E. Klein. 1984. "Heterogeneous Growth and Mental Development of Intrauterine Growth-Retarded Infants During the First 3 Years of Life." *Pediatrics* 74:783.

Von Braun, Joachim, Hartwig de Haen, and Jurgen Blanken. 1991. *Commercialization of Agriculture under Conditions of Population Pressures: Production, Consumption, and Nutritional Effects in Rwanda*. Research Report 85. International Food Policy Research Institute, Washington, D.C.

Von Braun, Joachim, David Hotchkiss, and Maarten Immink. 1989. *Nontraditional Export Crops in Guatemala: Effects on Production, Income, and Nutrition*. Research Report 73. International Food Policy Research Institute, Washington, D.C.

Von Braun, Joachim, Detlev Puetz, and Patrick Webb. 1989. *Irrigation Technology and Commercialization of Rice in The Gambia: Effects on Income and Nutrition*. Research Report 75. International Food Policy Research Institute, Washington, D.C.

Waterlow, J. C., M. H. N. Golden, and J. Patrick. 1978. "Protein-Energy Malnutrition: Treatment." In John W. T. Dickerson and H. A. Lee, eds., *The Clinical Management of Disease*. London: Edward Arnold.

Whitehead, R. G. 1973. "Nutrition Education Research." *World Review of Nutrition and Dietetics* 17:91–149.

———. 1977. "Infection and Development of Kwashiorkor and Marasmus in Africa." *American Journal of Clinical Nutrition* 30:1281–85.

Williams, Cicely D. 1962. "Malnutrition." *Lancet* 2:342–44.

Winick, Myron, Knarig K. Meyer, and Ruth C. Harris. 1975. "Malnutrition and Environmental Enrichment by Early Adoption." *Science* 190:1173–75.

World Bank. 1989. *Feeding Latin America's Children*. Human Resources Division, Technical Department, Latin America and the Caribbean Region, Washington, D.C.

———. 1990. "INDIA—Tamil Nadu Integrated Nutrition Project Completion Report." World Bank, Washington, D.C.

WHO (World Health Organization). 1979. *Measurement of Nutritional Impact*. Report 79.1. Geneva.

———. 1981. "The Treatment and Management of Severe Protein-Energy Malnutrition." Geneva.

———. 1986. "Use and Interpretation of Anthropometric Indicators of Nutritional Status." *Bulletin of the World Health Organization* 64:929–41.

Wyon, J. B., and J. E. Gordon. 1971. *The Khanna Study*. Cambridge, Mass.: Harvard University Press.

Yambi, Olivia. 1988. "Nutritional Status and the Risk of Death: A Prospective Study of Children Six to Thirty Months Old in Iringa Region, Tanzania." Ph.D. diss., Cornell University.

Yambi, Olivia, Urban Jonsson, and Bjorn Ljungqvist. 1989. *The Role of Government in Promoting Community-Based Nutrition Programs: Experience From Tanzania and Lessons for Africa*. Pew/Cornell Lecture Series on Food and Nutrition Policy. Ithaca, N.Y.: Cornell Food and Nutrition Policy Program.

Zeitlin, Marian, and Candelaria S. Formación. 1981. "Nutrition Education." In *Nutrition Interventions in Developing Countries*. Cambridge, Mass.: Oelgeschlager, Gunn, and Hain.

Zeitlin, Marian, M. Griffiths, R. K. Manoff, and T. M. Cooke. 1984. "Household Evaluation, Nutrition Communication, and Behavior Change Component." Indonesian Nutrition Development Program. New York: Manoff International.

19

Micronutrient Deficiency Disorders

Henry M. Levin, Ernesto Pollitt, Rae Galloway, and Judith McGuire

Throughout the developing world high incidence of disease is associated with inadequate intake or absorption of micronutrients. Relatively minute quantities of each of the micronutrients are required for normal health status and well-being. If these nutrients are deficient, there are serious consequences for health, mental and physical. Because of known prevalence rates of deficiencies and ways of addressing them, we will focus in this chapter on three micronutrients: iron, iodine, and vitamin A. Deficiencies in other micronutrients are biologically significant—such as the effect of zinc on growth in certain disease states (Nishi and others 1980; Daeschner and others 1981), and the effect of vitamin B-6 on cellular immunity (Talbot, Miller and Kerkulirt 1987; Tomkins and Watson 1989)—but we know little about the extent of these deficiencies or how to attack them. Our purpose in this chapter, therefore, is to focus on iron, iodine, and vitamin A deficiencies and to assess global significance, public health importance, methods of prevention, and priorities within an economic framework in which costs, cost-effectiveness, and cost-benefit analyses are used. Much of what we learn about iron, iodine, and vitamin A will be useful in addressing other essential deficiencies in the future.

We will begin by discussing the global and public health significance of deficiencies in these micronutrients, including the magnitude and distribution of the deficiencies, their causes, and the implications for human health and development. We will then describe what is currently known about short- and long-term strategies and the proportion of potential beneficiaries actually covered by these programs. In the final section we will discuss issues for governments and other agencies in setting priorities for operations, institutions, allocation of resources, and research.

Public Health Significance

Micronutrient deficiencies are manifested by an array of disorders that have serious social, private, and economic costs to society.

Iron Deficiency

Iron is a mineral present in the body as a constituent of hemoglobin and in some enzyme and electron carriers. Because it cannot be made in the body, iron, like all essential nutrients, must be obtained from food.

MAGNITUDE AND DISTRIBUTION. It is generally thought that iron deficiency anemia is the most common nutritional deficiency in many developing countries, second only to protein-energy malnutrition (PEM) (Florentino and Guirriec 1984). Age and physiological status determine the degree of vulnerability of the individual: rapidly growing infants, children, and pregnant and lactating women are at high risk for deficiency. The Subcommittee on Nutrition of the Administrative Committee on Coordination (ACC/SCN) of the United Nations estimates that 1.3 billion people suffer from iron deficiency anemia (United Nations 1990). In table 19-1 this figure is disaggregated by region. Table 19A-1 contains available information on the prevalence of iron deficiency anemia by country, and table 19A-2 includes definitions for iron deficiency by age and sex.

CAUSES. Severe iron deficiency results in anemia (low hemoglobin level), which impairs the transport of oxygen and basic cell functions. People with mild iron deficiency may not have low hemoglobin (Hb) levels but yet have reduced body iron stores (ferritin) (Shils and Young 1988). "Iron deficiency" refers to any depletion of ferritin. An individual may be iron deficient without manifesting iron deficiency anemia, but all those with iron deficiency anemia are iron deficient. Anemia can also result from other nutrient deficiencies (for example, folate or vitamin B-12) or genetic abnormalities (for example, thalassemia). Folate deficiency is very commonly associated with iron deficiency anemia, so therapy usually includes a combined iron-folate tablet.

In populations in which the prevalence of iron deficiency anemia is high, the deficiency usually is the result of the

Table 19-1. Estimated Prevalence of Anemia by Geographic Region, Age, and Sex, 1980

Country	Children 0–4 years Percent	Number (millions)	Children 5–12 years Percent	Number (millions)	Men 15–59 years Percent	Number (millions)	Pregnant women 15–49 years Percent	Number (millions)	All women 15–49 years Percent	Number (millions)
Africa	56	48.0	49	47.3	20	23.4	63	11.3	44	46.8
Latin America	26	13.7	26	18.1	13	12.8	30	3.0	17	14.7
East Asia[a]	20	3.2	22	5.6	11	6.1	20	0.5	18	8.4
South Asia	56	118.7	50	139.2	32	123.6	65	27.1	58	191.0
Developing regions[a]	51	183.2	46	208.3	26	162.2	59	41.9	47	255.7

Note: Anemia is defined as a hemoglobin concentration below WHO reference values for age, sex, and pregnancy status.
a. Excluding China.
Source: DeMaeyer and Adiels-Tegman 1985.

interaction between dietary factors, chronic iron loss due to parasitic infections (for example, hookworm or schistosomiasis [Stephenson 1987]), or elevated needs (for example, during pregnancy and periods of rapid growth).

It is currently believed that diet is the most important factor determining iron status. Dietary factors include insufficient iron in the diet and poor bioavailability of dietary iron. There are two types of iron in foods: heme iron (present in animal flesh), of which about 20 to 30 percent is absorbed, and nonheme iron (present in plant sources), of which less than 5 percent is absorbed. Iron in breast milk is highly bioavailable, and up to 50 percent is absorbed (INACG 1979). People in developing countries derive most of their iron from nonheme sources, whereas those in industrial countries consume greater amounts of heme iron. The key dietary difference in iron status is its bioavailability rather than the absolute amount of iron in foods (INACG 1989). Absorption of nonheme iron can be improved up to 18 percent (DeMaeyer 1989) by the addition to the diet of ascorbic acid or foods containing ascorbic acid (Hunt and others 1990) or other acids, the addition to the diet of foods containing heme iron , or the removal from the diet of substances that inhibit iron absorption (DeMaeyer 1989). Some types of food processing, such as the fermentation of soy products, also seem to improve iron bioavailability (Macfarlane and others 1990). The recommended intake of iron for people by age and sex is given in table 19A-3. The upper value is needed by people who consume mainly nonheme iron.

Although parasitic infections also contribute to iron deficiency, the treatment of such infectious parasites alone is not the most cost-effective means of addressing iron deficiency anemia, because unless the parasites are removed, reinfection will take place. Hygiene education, footwear, and improved water supply and sanitation are needed (DeMaeyer 1989).

IMPLICATIONS FOR HUMAN HEALTH AND DEVELOPMENT. It had been assumed that iron deficiency in pregnant women did not put the fetus at risk because the fetus would have priority access to maternal iron stores (Bothwell and Charlton 1981). In a study in Benin, however, Hercberg and others (1987) found that when multiple indicators of iron status were used to assess maternal anemia there was a positive correlation between

maternal and infant iron deficiency. Increased prenatal and perinatal risk (low birth weight, prematurity, and mortality) has been associated with low levels of hemoglobin and hematocrit in the mother (Murphy and others 1986; Lieberman and others 1987, 1988; Brabin 1988).

In infants (6–24 months) and preadolescent children (9–11 years), iron deficiency anemia is associated with mild growth retardation (Lozoff 1982; Aukett and others 1986; Chwang, Soemantri and Pollitt 1988). Treatment of iron-deficient anemic infants (age 17–19 months [Aukett and others 1986]) and preadolescent children (age 8.2–13.5 years [Chwang, Soemantri, and Pollitt 1988]) has resulted in increased growth during the period of intervention. The causes of this growth retardation may be related to the general role of iron as an essential metabolic cofactor, its relation to immunocompetence (Higashi and others 1967; Klebanoff 1970; Chandra 1973; Mata 1977; Chandra and Puri, 1985; Dallman 1987), or its role in appetite, which decreases during iron deficiency (Basta and others 1979).

Iron deficiency anemia poses a developmental risk for cognitive dysfunction (for example, attention and concentration) in preschool and school-age children, and that risk factor is sufficiently severe to jeopardize educational attainment. The strongest and most consistent evidence of the effects of iron deficiency on cognition is found in clinical trials of preschool and school children who have been assessed for specific mental processes (for example, attention and concept formation) and school achievement. One example is a study by Soewondo, Husaini, and Pollitt (1989), which showed that anemic children three to six years old learned faster and formed appropriate concepts more efficiently after they were supplemented with iron than their placebo-fed anemic controls. In another set of studies, researchers in India (Seshardri and Gopaldas 1989) showed that when anemic children age five to fifteen were supplemented with iron, they performed better on tests for intelligence quotient (IQ), memory, visual perceptual organization, and clerical tasks improved than did anemic children who received a placebo.

Similar effects have been observed in the mental development scale scores of iron-deficient anemic infants (Lozoff and Brittenham 1985; Pollitt 1987). Iron-deficient anemic infants perform more poorly than iron-replete infants on the Bayley Scale of Mental and Motor Development (Lozoff 1989; Walter 1989), but the behavioral response to iron therapy is not consistent across different studies (Lozoff and Brittenham 1985; Lozoff and others 1982; Oski and others 1983; Aukett and others 1986; Lozoff 1989). No changes in mental test performance have been found among infants and children whose iron stores and circulating iron are depleted but whose Hb levels have remained constant. Conceivably, these changes are too subtle to be detected in small samples.

Higher morbidity has been noted in anemic pregnant women (Fleming 1989). Reasons for this may be that iron deficiency influences the risk of infection in distinct ways. It is associated with abnormalities in cell-mediated and nonspecific immunity (Higashi and others 1967; Klebanoff 1970; Chandra, 1973; Prasad 1979; Chandra and Puri 1985; Dallman 1987). The production of T cells is specifically compromised (Srikantia and others 1976; Bagchi, Mohanram, and Reddy 1980), and the capacity of neutrophils to kill bacteria is significantly diminished during iron deficiency (Walter and others 1986). Excess free iron in the serum has been associated with predisposition to infection, but this state results largely from injected iron rather than ingested iron (DeMaeyer 1989).

Because iron deficiency anemia compromises immunocompetence, it is likely to increase mortality among high-risk groups. This increase may not be attributable to immunodeficiency alone but also to circulatory failure (INACG 1989). The exact role that iron deficiency plays in mortality needs further definition.

There is a good deal of evidence that relates maternal mortality to severe anemia. In Maharashtra, India, 90 percent of all maternal deaths occurred in women with Hb levels of less than 7 grams per hundred milliliters of blood (Masani 1969, cited in Fleming 1989). In Nigeria, Harrison (1975) found that 4 percent of mothers with severe anemia (Hb levels of less than 5 grams per hundred milliliters of blood) died in childbirth. Some evidence suggests that 20 percent of all maternal deaths in West Africa and India (when blood transfusion was not available) were directly attributable to anemia and that additional mortality resulting from hemorrhage was indirectly caused by maternal anemia (Fleming 1989).

Iron deficiency impairs work performance through its effects on Hb and, possibly, myoglobin, which is involved in the transport of oxygen in muscle. There is a high negative correlation between Hb levels (grams of Hb per 100 milliliters of blood) and the percentage of increase in heart rate of a person on a treadmill (Gardner and others 1977). A strong positive relationship exists between Hb levels and potential maximum workload as measured in the Harvard Step Test. Performance improves after iron supplementation increases Hb to the expected normal level (Scrimshaw 1984).

Iron deficiency anemia adversely affected the work productivity of Indonesian rubber tappers until they received iron supplementation (Basta and others 1979). In a recent study in Indonesia, Suhardjo (1986) found that, following iron treatment, iron-deficient anemic women increased their productiv-

ity in picking tea leaves. In Kenya, Stephenson and others (1985) found an association between the intensity of the infection with Schistosoma haematobium, a direct cause of iron deficiency anemia, and physical fitness among school-age children.

Iodine Deficiency

Iodine, a mineral, is a component of two thyroid gland hormones which are necessary for normal metabolism.

MAGNITUDE AND DISTRIBUTION. The number of people estimated to be at risk of disorders from severe iodine deficiency is 680 million in Asia, 227 million in Africa, and 60 million in Latin America (see table 19-2). Prevalence is high in mountainous and flood-prone areas where iodine-deficient soils prevail. Although no age group or sex is immune to iodine deficiency, the fetus, women, and children seem to be most vulnerable to serious and irreversible consequences of deficiency (Hetzel 1988). A detailed disaggregation of the prevalence of iodine deficiency by country is given in table 19A-4.

CAUSES. The term "iodine deficiency disorders" (IDDs) covers the breadth of sequelae and is not limited to severe deficiency (Hetzel 1983). Iodine deficiency disorders result from inadequate intake of iodine either because the soils and water are iodine deficient or because certain naturally existing "goitrogens" in foods interfere with the individual's use of iodine. Iodine is essential for the formation of thyroid hormones [thyroxine (T_4) and 3,5,3'-triiodothyronine (T_3)], which are necessary for normal growth and development and for proper metabolic function. Recommended daily intake of iodine is about 150–300 micrograms (see table 19A-5). When the thyroid gland does not obtain enough iodine to make these hormones, it increases in size to compensate for the deficiency. The enlarged thyroid gland is called goiter.

IMPLICATIONS FOR HUMAN HEALTH AND DEVELOPMENT. Iodine deficiency affects reproduction. Some types of anovulation can be reversed by desiccated thyroid, which confirms the relation-

Table 19-2. Estimated Prevalence of Iodine Deficiency Disorders and Population at Risk, by Region
(millions)

Region	At risk	Goiter	Overt cretinism
Southeast Asia	280	100	4.0
Rest of Asia	400	30	0.9
Africa	227	39	0.5
Latin America	60	30	0.3
Eastern Mediterranean	33	12	—
Total	1,000	211	5.7

— Negligible.
Source: WHO 1990.

ship, known even in ancient times, between the thyroid gland and fertility (McMichael, Potter, and Hetzel 1980). In animals there is evidence of a significant increase in spontaneous abortions and stillbirths and a marked reduction in brain growth in the fetus when the mother is iodine deficient (Hetzel and Potter 1983). Conclusive evidence of these effects on human reproduction is weak; however, reduction in stillbirths and perinatal mortality and increased birth weight in Zaire (McMichael, Potter, and Hetzel 1980; Thilly 1981, as cited in Hetzel 1987), Papua New Guinea, Ecuador, and Peru (Clugston and others 1987) have been observed after implementation of iodine deficiency control programs. In Zaire the infant mortality rate for mothers given iodine supplementation during pregnancy was significantly less than for those who were not given iodine (Thilly and others 1980).

Severe iodine deficiency in utero can result in postnatal dwarfism, and people with goiter can be retarded in their physical development (Hetzel 1988). In addition to hindering growth, iodine deficiency also increases morbidity rates in children, especially from respiratory infection (Tomkins and Watson 1989). Phagocyte dysfunction (Chandra and Au 1981) and delayed immune response (Marani, Venturi, and Nasala 1985) have been reported.

It is known that the thyroid of the fetus does not become activated until the tenth week (Delong 1987); before that, development depends on the thyroid hormone of the mother (Hetzel and Potter 1983). Deleterious effects of maternal iodine deficiency on the fetus during this time include reductions in brain DNA and RNA (Hetzel and Potter 1983). Extreme deficiency results in severe mental retardation, known as cretinism, which can take several forms. The seriousness of cretinism is obvious, but from an economic development perspective the greatest concern in endemic areas is the possibility that even noncretinous children may be mentally and neurologically handicapped. This milder impairment might remain unnoticed within the community, but it can limit the social and economic growth of these communities (Stanbury 1987).

In endemic areas the performance of noncretinous children in cognitive and motor tests correlates positively with the mother's thyroid levels during the pregnancy of the respective offspring. For example, in the Western highlands of Papua New Guinea, serum thyroxine (T_4) during pregnancy was related to the offspring's performance at twelve years of age on tests of visual perceptual organization and visual motor coordination (Pharoah and others 1984).

Given the serious effects of iodine deficiency on the proper functioning of the brain, it is not surprising to learn that even mild deficiency may have irreversible effects. A study in the highlands of Bolivia of goitrous children age five and a half to twelve years failed to show a clear effect of iodized oil supplementation given twenty-two months earlier on IQ, visual motor coordination, and school performance (Bautista and others 1982). In contrast, the authors of a study in the Guizhou province of China (Yan-You and Shu-Hua 1985) of the effects of iodized salt on the hearing of otherwise normal seven- to eleven-year-old children one, two, and three years after pro-

phylaxis found significant positive effects of the intervention. The difference in these outcomes is probably related to the nature of the particular function of the central nervous system that was assessed and to the mechanism and timing of the deficiency. Some hearing loss associated with acquired hypothyroidism is correctable by increased iodine intake. Still, mild mental retardation resulting from impaired structural development of the brain during fetal life is probably irreversible. Thus, addressing iodine deficiency in reproductive-age women is of highest priority.

Because of the relation between IDD and intellectual capacity, productivity is adversely affected by iodine deficiency. After a salt iodization program in one Chinese village, the average income increased from 43 yuan per person in 1981 to 223 in 1982 to 414 in 1984, which was higher than the average for the district (Levin 1987). In addition, because mental and physical fitness improved, cereals were exported for the first time and men were fit enough to join the army after salt iodization. In Ecuador, Greene (1977) found that people with moderate iodine deficiency were consistently paid less for agricultural work than normal individuals. In summary, iodine deficiency has been associated with impaired reproduction, severe and mild mental retardation, growth inhibition, and reduced productivity.

Vitamin A Deficiency

Like all essential vitamins, vitamin A is an organic substance which the body cannot produce. Vitamin A is essential for normal vision, growth, and immune function and to maintain epithelial cells.

MAGNITUDE AND DISTRIBUTION. An estimated 42 million children under the age of six have mild or moderate xerophthalmia (West and Sommer 1987). About 250,000 to 500,000 children go blind annually and approximately 50 to 80 percent of those that go blind die within one year (Sommer 1982; IVACG 1989). In tables 19-3 and 19A-6 the prevalence of vitamin A deficiency is given by region and country. The age groups at highest risk for vitamin A deficiency are young children beyond weaning age (six months to six years), although older children and pregnant and lactating women are also affected. Prevalence peaks among two- to-four-year-old children (Eastman 1987). In some parts of the world it appears that boys are at higher risk than girls (Sommer 1982; Tielsch and Sommer 1984; DeMaeyer 1986), which may be a reflection of different cultural practices in rearing children or physiological differences (Sommer 1982). Prevalence is also greatest in low-income groups and during those seasons when food sources of the vitamin are scarce (Mamdani and Ross 1988). In table 19A-2, definitions for vitamin A deficiency are listed. Note that the population percentages in this table refer to those with severe vitamin A deficiency. There are currently no values for mild vitamin A deficiency.

CAUSES. Xerophthalmia and its cure through the diet were recognized in ancient times. It is only in the early part of this

Table 19-3. Estimated Prevalence of Vitamin A Deficiency, 1984–85

Region	Countries with deficiency[a]	Children aged 1–4 years (millions)	Children with mild to moderate deficiency[b] (millions)
Africa	16	53	7.9
Americas	5	38	5.6
Southeast Asia[c]	5	51	7.7
India	1	111	16.7
Mediterranean	3	7	1.0
Western Pacific	4	20	3.0
Total	34	280	41.9

a. Countries in WHO category A (significant problem with control programs in place 1984–85): Bangladesh, El Salvador, Haiti, India, Indonesia, Nepal, Philippines, Sri Lanka. Category B (significant problem but no control program 1984–85): Benin, Brazil (northeast states), Burkina Faso, Ethiopia, Malawi, Mali, Mauritania, Mexico, Oman, Sudan, Tanzania, Viet Nam, Zambia. Category C (probable problem but no assessment or program 1985–85): Afghanistan, Angola, Bolivia, Burma, Chad (north), Ghana (north), Kampuchea, Kenya, Lao P.D.R., Mozambique, Niger, Nigeria (north), Uganda.

b. Assumes 15 percent prevalence.

c. Excluding India.

Source: West and Sommer 1987.

century, when vitamin A was discovered, that the deficiency was first described in connection with physical growth and, later, with vision. In the more recent past greater attention has been placed on the association between the deficiency and infant and child morbidity and mortality. Traditionally, vitamin A deficiency has been defined as a severe reduction in vitamin A reserves along with clinical signs of the deficiency. Milder depletion may also be defined as deficiency, even though it does not result in changes in the eyes, because it may still have an important relationship to morbidity and mortality (West and Sommer 1987). Biochemically, even mild signs of deficiency in children are detected by a decrease in vitamin A reserves, with liver and serum levels less than 20 micrograms per deciliter (see table 19A-2).

Dietary sources of vitamin A include preformed vitamin A (retinol) from animal sources and beta-carotene and other carotenoids found in plant sources, which can be converted to vitamin A in the body. Retinol is the most active form of vitamin A, followed by beta-carotene and then the other carotenoids (see table 19A-5 on how these three compare). Vitamin A deficiency is caused by dietary inadequacy (see table 19A-5 for recommended intakes), by increased physiological requirements, and by cultural factors which determine individual availability and consumption. In countries in which the staple food is rice, a cereal without vitamin A, low-income groups are at high risk of vitamin A deficiency. Even in countries in which sources of the carotenoids exist, there may be high incidence of deficiency. In parts of Indonesia, for example, dark green, leafy vegetables (a rich source of beta-carotene) are commonly available, yet vitamin A deficiency is highly prevalent. This coincidence is partly explained by the low social value attributed to green vegetables (WHO 1982, as

cited in Mamdami and Ross 1988); partly by an inadequate source of fat, which facilitates the absorption of the carotenoids (United Nations 1985); and partly by protein inadequacy, which hinders vitamin A absorption, release, and transport (Mamdami and Ross 1988). Vitamin A transport is affected only when protein deficiency is severe (Sommer 1982). Intestinal abnormalities caused by bacterial infection or parasites can also interfere with the absorption of vitamin A. Respiratory infection and other diseases can increase the requirement for the vitamin and interfere with its intake through decreased appetite (United Nations 1985). In Africa, measles is often a precipitating factor in blindness due to vitamin A deficiency (Eastman 1987).

In addition, there are social and economic factors related to the deficiency (Mamdami and Ross 1988). For example, in urban Bangladesh a clear negative association has been noted between per capita income and vitamin A deficiency (Stanton and others 1986). Within low-income groups, however, such a correlation is often less obvious. Intrafamily food distribution patterns and, as noted, the low social value attributed to foods rich in vitamin A may determine risk in vulnerable groups.

Seasonal availability of vegetables and fruits often acts synergistically with other factors to precipitate deficiency. In countries such as the Philippines and Indonesia, dark green, leafy vegetables are generally unavailable when infections peak.

IMPLICATIONS FOR HUMAN HEALTH AND DEVELOPMENT. When pregnant women are deficient in vitamin A, severe xerophthalmia may develop in utero (Sommer 1982), which increases vulnerability to infection and death. Vitamin A deficiency also decreases fertility (Eastman 1987). Congenital malformations have also been related to experimentally induced vitamin A deficiency in animals. Less is known about the effects of vitamin A deficiency on congenital malformations in human beings, although some suggestive clinical observations exist (Wallingford and Underwood 1986), such as congenital xerophthalmia, anophthalmia, microphthalmia, and other ocular defects (IVACG 1986). Vitamin A overdose during early pregnancy may cause fetal absorption (Eastman 1987). For this reason it is generally recommended to give pregnant women no more than 1,000 micrograms of vitamin A at a time or to treat existing deficiencies with dietary sources of vitamin A (IVACG 1986).

The ocular signs of vitamin A deficiency fall under two categories: (a) night blindness due to the interruption of the dark adaptation process in the visual cycle; and (b) structural changes in the surface of the eye (Bitot's spots, drying, keratomalacia, ulceration, and so on) due to loss of secretory function in the mucosal epithelium in the conjunctiva of the eye and changes in the differentiation or maturation of specific epithelial cell types (Mamdami and Ross 1988). Night blindness, conjunctival dryness, and Bitot's spots are generally reversible, but more advanced stages are not and can result in lesions which cover the entire cornea, causing partial or total blindness. Once the disease has reached this extreme level of severity, the life of the child is endangered.

Both mild and severe forms of vitamin A deficiency are associated with increased morbidity, especially from respiratory and diarrheal disease (Sommer, Katz, and Tarwotjo 1984). The effects of vitamin A deficiency on cell-mediated immunity, antibodies, and secretory antibodies have been documented using both animal models and clinical data (Nauss 1986; Olson 1986; Chandra 1988). Conclusive information on its adverse effects on phagocytosis is not available.

It is known that measles and vitamin A deficiency have a complex reciprocal interaction. Vitamin A status is a determinant of the outcome of measles, especially in Africa, and measles, in turn, is a forceful precipitating factor in blindness (Eastman 1987). For example, measles was related to bilateral corneal ulceration in 78.9 percent of these cases (Ksanga, Pepping, and Kavishe 1985, as reported by Eastman 1987). In fact, the peak for vitamin A deficiency coincides with the peak for measles in children (Eastman 1987). An association between vitamin A deficiency and measles has also been found in Asia. In studies in Bangladesh (Cohen and others1985) and Indonesia (Sommer 1982), 10 percent and 37 percent, respectively, of children with keratomalacia had had measles within the previous four weeks. The intensity of the infection, and not a specific characteristic of measles, seems to be the determining factor in the high mortality observed among vitamin A deficient children (WHO/UNICEF 1987; WHO/EPI 1988b). The release of vitamin A from storage in the liver is apparently hindered by infection (DeMaeyer 1986). The effect on the immune system explains, in part, a well-documented association between vitamin A deficiency and growth retardation in animals (McLaren 1966, cited in West and Sommer 1987; Eastman 1987). In experimental animals vitamin A causes a cessation of bone growth along with loss of appetite (Eastman 1987).

Although conclusive information on mortality risks among children with all levels of vitamin A deficiency is not yet available (Wittpenn and Sommer 1986), it has been estimated that of the children with keratomalacia who remain untreated, 60 percent will die (West and Sommer 1987). Some studies show that even children with mild vitamin A deficiency have higher mortality rates than matched controls (Sommer and others 1983; Sommer and others 1986; Rahamathullah and others 1990). The cause of this is probably related to vitamin A's role in maintaining healthy mucosal tissue throughout the body and in the immune function. To confirm these findings similar studies are under way in other countries, and results should provide conclusive evidence on whether vitamin A deficiency increases the mortality risk in children (National Academy of Sciences 1987).

There are no known effects of vitamin A deficiency on the growth and development of the brain and intelligence. Blindness or partial blindness would obviously affect learning, especially in the classroom setting. To the extent that it increases morbidity, even mild vitamin A deficiency may affect school performance and productivity. At issue here is how many preschool- or school-age children with a history of xerophthalmia are left out of formal schools because of blindness due to vitamin A deficiency (Pollitt 1990). This question is particularly troublesome in Africa, where corneal scarring associated with measles is frequent (WHO/EPI 1988b). In Malawi and Tanzania, for example, half of the children attending schools for the blind reported a history of measles preceding total blindness (WHO/EPI 1988b).

To summarize, vitamin A deficiency has been linked with interference with ocular function, impaired growth and reproduction, and increased morbidity and mortality. Deficiencies in the three micronutrients are manifested by overlapping conditions. In table 19-4 we review the deficiency conditions for all three and show the similarities in the conditions for the micronutrients.

Micronutrient Interactions

The interaction of micronutrients can be viewed in two different ways. Deficiencies of the three micronutrients under discussion interact according to their geographic setting and according to how the micronutrients are metabolized.

Iron, iodine, and vitamin A deficiencies often occur in countries in which poverty limits dietary sources and in which geography limits the composition of food that normally would contain these micronutrients. Generally, these three micronutrient deficiencies occur simultaneously in certain areas of Africa, the Andes of South America, and in many parts of Asia (see tables 19A-1, 19A-4, and 19A-6).

Metabolism of the micronutrients may also be affected by dietary components. Protein-energy malnutrition interferes with iodine metabolism (Ingenbleek and De Visscher 1979; Gaitan, Mayoral, and Gaitan 1983). Other nutrients may also increase or inhibit the absorption or use of these micronutrients. Vitamin A and zinc deficiencies might interact synergistically (Baly and others 1984). Vitamin A deficiency also affects anemia (Bloem and others 1990). For example, in Guatemala, fortification of sugar with vitamin A resulted in improvement of hemoglobin levels (Mejia and Arroyave 1982). Because vitamin A seems to affect hemoglobin levels but not body stores, it might be involved in the synthesis of hemoglobin and red blood cells (Mejia and Chew 1988). Other components in foods may inhibit the use of dietary micronutrients, such as phytates in some plants, which inhibit iron absorption.

Prevention

Adequate consumption of the micronutrients through food is the best way of preventing micronutrient deficiencies. Recommended daily intake by age and sex is presented in table 19A-3 (iron) and table 19A-5 (iodine and vitamin A).

When the intake of these foods is limited, specific interventions are needed to prevent and address micronutrient deficiencies. Most micronutrient interventions represent both preventive and curative therapies. High-dose supplements, in particular, can be used to treat severe deficiency and to prevent deficiency in vulnerable age groups.

Table 19-4. Functional Effects of Essential Micronutrient Deficiencies

Effect	Deficiency		
	Iron	Iodine	Vitamin A
Morbidity			
Immune function	Yes	Unknown	Yes
Prevalence	Yes	Yes	No
Incidence	No	Unknown	Yes
Duration	No	Unknown	Yes
Severity	No	No	Yes
Mortality			
Infant	Yes	Yes	Yes
Child	Unknown	Yes	Yes
Maternal	Yes	Unknown	No
Other (fetal, early adult)	No	Yes	No
Mental development and learning disorders			
Brain development	Unknown	Yes	No
Aptitude	Yes	Yes	No
Intelligence quotient	Yes	No	No
Exploratory behavior	Yes	No	No
Attention span	Yes	Yes	No
Memory	Unknown	Yes	No
School achievement	Yes	Yes	Unknown
Learning disability (blindness, deafness)	No	Yes	Yes
Sensory impairment	Yes	Yes	No
Productivity			
Spontaneous activity	Yes	Yes	No
Endurance	Yes	No	No
Maximum aerobic capacity	Yes	No	No
Occupational productivity	Yes	Yes	No
Disability[a]	No	Yes	Yes
Growth	Yes	Yes	Yes
Reproduction			
Fertility	No	Yes	Yes
Miscarriage and stillbirth	Yes	Yes	Yes
Intra-uterine growth retardation	Yes	Yes	No
Prematurity	Yes	No	No
Congenital deformities (birth defects)	No	Yes	Yes

a. Such as blindness, mental retardation, or lack of motor coordination.
Source: Iron—DeMaeyer 1989; Iodine—Hetzel, Dunn, and Stanburg 1987; Vitamin A—West and Sommer 1987, Eastman 1987.

There are two main types of interventions to reduce micronutrient deficits: supplementation (the administration of pills, capsules or injections containing one or more of the micronutrients) and fortification (the addition of micronutrients to foods in processing). Other interventions, such as nutrition education and agricultural programs, can be used over the long term to promote the intake of these micronutrients by vulnerable groups.

Supplementation

Delivery of micronutrients through supplementation can be done in a variety of ways. The supplements can be taken orally or by injection. Typical iron supplementation programs are shown in table 19A-7. Some supplements must be taken daily (such as oral iron), whereas others can be taken at intervals of

three to five years, as is the case for iodized oil. The frequency depends mainly on the ability of the body to store the micronutrient (substantial in the case of iodine and vitamin A).

Although iron deficiency is usually treated with supplements from one of several iron compounds, ascorbic acid increases the absorption of nonheme iron from existing sources like maize, rice, wheat, or sorghum, in which the iron content is adequate but is in an unabsorbable form. Vitamin C supplementation and fortification can therefore be considered to be an iron intervention. When taken with such foods, ascorbic acid can increase the absorption of available iron by about 30 percent (Hallberg 1981; Berg and Brems 1986), or from about 5 percent to about 6.5 percent.

A significant challenge for prophylaxis or treatment through supplementation is compliance (taking the proper dosage at appropriate intervals). This is a problem particularly in iron supplementation, which requires the daily ingestion of iron tablets, sometimes with mild side effects (headache, nausea, and so on) in the initial weeks of supplementation. Side effects were thought to be an important detractor to compliance, but in recent iron studies in Thailand and Burma, only 10 to 15 percent of women taking iron complained of side effects (Charoenlarp and others 1988), and only a small proportion of those women failed to take supplements because of side effects. In another study, Griffiths (1980) found that when women were warned of possible side effects they were more likely to continue taking their iron supplements when side effects occurred. Ensuring compliance with iron therapy has been most successful in situations in which supplements are provided and ingestion is supervised, such as in the workplace and schools. But for persons who do not participate regularly in such institutions or who live in outlying areas, compliance and tablet availability are serious obstacles to success. A recent study of iron ingested in slow-release capsules (gastric delivery system [GDS]) showed that side effects did not differ between placebo, ferrous sulfate, and GDS. In addition, compliance did not seem to differ between ferrous sulfate or GDS even though the dosage for GDS was one pill per day and that for ferrous sulfate was two (Simmons 1990). The GDS iron was better absorbed, however.

When available, long-lasting, megadose supplements are superior to low-dose supplementation with respect to both cost and compliance. This is particularly true for injections of iodized oil, which provide protection for as long as four to five years, and oral doses of iodized oil, which are good for two years (Underwood 1983; Berg and Brems 1986). Large doses of iodine can cause adverse reactions (thyrotoxicosis, with such symptoms as increased heart rate, trembling, sweating, and weight loss [Hetzel 1988]), although this is not generally a significant problem because in most cases spontaneous remission will occur (Medeiros-Neto and others 1987). The highest risk of thyrotoxicosis is in people over forty, so giving supplements only to younger adults avoids most of this toxicity (Berg and Brems 1986). High doses of vitamin A are both toxic and teratogenic. Great care must be taken not to give vitamin A capsules at higher dosages than recommended or to women who might be pregnant (generally 1,000 micrograms or less). Vitamin A can be toxic even in children, so an alternative delivery scheme based on low, frequent doses is being investigated (Underwood 1989). As with any essential drug, micronutrient supplements need to be handled properly to ensure their stability, potency, availability, and proper use.

Fortification

Where essential micronutrient deficiencies are prevalent, dietary fortification is generally considered preferable to supplementation as a long-term strategy in controlling micronutrient deficiencies. The advantages of dietary fortification are that compliance is ensured if the appropriate carrier is selected. The cost of delivery of the micronutrients through food staples is far less than through the health system and can be partially or fully borne by the consumer. A crucial step in fortification is choosing the right food to fortify. Several criteria are used in selecting a particular food vehicle for fortification (Beaton and Bengoa 1976; Baker and DeMaeyer 1979):

- It must be a food that is consumed by the vast majority of the target population and in adequate amounts.
- It must be able to be fortified on a large scale and at relatively few centers, so the fortification can be adequately supervised.
- It must be stable under the extreme conditions likely to be encountered in storage and distribution.
- It must not interfere with the use of the nutrient, and the nutrient must not interfere with the food (that is, it must not be detrimental to flavor, shelf life, color, texture, or cooking properties).

Table 19-5 shows typical fortification programs for the three micronutrients under discussion. The usual food vehicles are salt or sugar because they tend to meet the four criteria. The food chosen for fortification is site specific; thus successful fortification programs have included wheat flour, skimmed milk, monosodium glutamate (MSG), infant foods, beverages, salt, and condiments (Clydesdale and Wiemer 1985). Foods commonly eaten only by specific subpopulations may prove to be satisfactory vehicles for targeting high-risk groups, such as small children. For example, in many industrial countries weaning foods are fortified with iron.

The fortification of salt with iodine has been practiced extensively in industrial countries. Many Latin American countries have passed legislation requiring iodization of all salt. Unfortunately, maintaining supplies of iodized salt has remained a problem in these countries. Political commitment at all levels of government and the community is needed for such legislation to be effective. A successful national program in Bolivia organized small salt producers into cooperatives, which made them more able to compete with larger

Table 19-5. Typical Fortification Program

Nutrient	Compound	Vehicle	Concentration	Source
Iron	Ferric orthophosphate	Salt	3.5 g/kg	Working group on fortification of salt with iron 1982
	NaFe EDTA	Sugar	13 mg/100 g	Viteri and others 1981
Iodine	Potassium iodate	Salt	15–40 ppm	Mannar 1987
Vitamin A	Retinol palmitate	Sugar	10 mg/g	Arroyave and others 1979

Source: See last column.

producers. This action increased their productivity, which in turn increased the availability of iodized salt, improving consumption of iodized salt and reducing the prevalence of goiter (Pardo 1990).

Fortification may not always be feasible, however, because of the lack of an appropriate carrier food available to at-risk groups, weak enforcement of fortification regulations, (Berg and Brems 1986), or excessive cost of the fortified food. The most appropriate carrier may also be a food that has unrelated health effects, such as hypertension and tooth decay, which are linked with the overingestion of salt and the consumption of sugar, respectively. In these cases other strategies may be required. Fortification is the best method available for solving micronutrient deficiency problems in the long term because of low cost, good coverage, and technical feasibility. The success of fortification in the long term hinges crucially on the regularity and enforcement capacity in the governmental departments responsible for food safety and quality. Without effective public and private oversight of the fortification system, the quality of a fortification program can deteriorate rapidly. Sufficient incentives and penalties for private industry and public regulators need to be set up to ensure longevity.

Double fortification of foods may be a way to address two micronutrient deficiencies in a cost-effective way. India has experimented with double fortification, using iron and iodine. Although the technology has not been completely worked out, double fortification offers hope in dealing with multiple micronutrient deficiencies in areas where several coexist.

Other Interventions

While supplementation and fortification are two of the main interventions used to address micronutrient deficiencies, there are a number of other interventions—nutrition education, breastfeeding promotions, agriculture, food processing, public health measures—that should be used either alone or along with supplementation and fortification efforts.

NUTRITION EDUCATION. Education of the consumer about nutrition is an important component of any micronutrient intervention. It is needed along with every fortification, supplementation, and food production program to guarantee that the intended beneficiary actually consumes the nutrients. Failure to educate the public and politicians to support fortification programs over the long term has been implicated as a significant reason for the failure of programs in Central and South America (Schaefer 1974, as cited in Thilly and Hetzel 1980). In both Guatemala and India, mass media and communication campaigns were required to create demand for fortified salt (Thilly and Hetzel 1980; United Nations 1987).

More general nutrition education is also important to increase intake of the micronutrients from the existing food supplies. Lack of maternal knowledge of the need for children to consume leafy green and yellow vegetables is associated with increased risk of nutritional blindness (Stanton and others 1986).

Breastfeeding promotion is important for micronutrient nutriture (as well as other nutrition and health benefits) because, if the mother is in good health, it is a good source of iron, iodine, and vitamin A. In addition, a protein in breast milk, lactoferrin, reduces free iron in the intestinal lumen and hence protects the infant against infection while simultaneously rendering the iron more absorbable (Tomkins and Watson 1989). Breastfeeding promotion is also important because vitamin A deficiency has been associated with the early cessation of breastfeeding (Stanton and others 1986). In Bangladesh the risk of a child's developing one or more signs of vitamin A deficiency is six times higher for a child younger than two years of age who is not breastfed (Mamdami and Ross 1988), and length of lactation was found to influence the risk of vitamin A deficiency in children in Ethiopia (de Sole, Belay, and Zegeye 1987, as cited in Mamdami and Ross 1988) and Indonesia (Sommer 1982).

Promoting the increased production and use of nutrient-rich local foods through agricultural programs and policies (improved marketing, greater dietary diversity, increased rural incomes) may prove invaluable to any program aimed at reducing the incidence of these deficiencies. Not surprisingly, in urban Bangladesh, risk of vitamin A deficiency in children was associated with poor intake of foods rich in vitamin A (Stanton and others 1986). In Bangladesh, families without gardens are more likely to have children with xerophthalmia than are those with gardens (Cohen and others 1985).

Research and development of new technologies to increase the micronutrient content of raw and processed foods and new high-nutrient varieties are also needed. For example, in processed foods the absorption of iron could be greatly increased by the addition of ascorbic acid or by the decrease of substances that compete with iron for absorption. Public health measures to alleviate environmental factors which exacerbate dietary deficiencies (Stanton and others 1986) may be recommended also.

Program Coverage

In tables 19A-1, 19A-4, and 19A-6 we give approximations for program coverage for iron, iodine, and vitamin A, respectively. As can be seen in table 19A-4, there is much activity in planning and implementing national programs to combat iodine deficiency disorders. Control programs usually involve either fortification or supplementation. Legislation to make iodization of food mandatory is more infrequent except in some Latin American countries in which legislation was passed several decades ago. It should be noted, however, that even with the passage of legislation, goiter has persisted in these countries, which indicates the difficulty in controlling and regulating industry to comply with the law. Knowledge of coverage for these iodization programs is scant, and even in a country such as Bhutan, where 100 percent of the salt is iodized, there are questions of whether or not this salt is reaching remote endemic areas and of whether the stability of iodine in the salt can be maintained at effective levels.

Vitamin A program activity has increased dramatically over the last several years, but gaps still exist in the knowledge of actual coverage in countries. Only a few countries have undertaken vitamin A fortification programs, making supplementation the most frequent option at present. Pilot studies in the Philippines for fortifying MSG with vitamin A have proved promising (Muhilal and others 1988; Muhilal, Muherdiyantiningsih, and Karyadi 1988). As for program coverage for iodine, program coverage for vitamin A is still underreported. Until such information is available, it will be difficult to gauge progress in combating the deficiency.

Control programs for iron deficiency are not well documented, even though iron supplementation presumably is part of standard practice in prenatal care. Considering the magnitude of the deficiency problem and the effects of iron deficiency, the lack of attention given to addressing the problem is surprising. Countries with active programs, such as India, have found difficulties in population compliance with a consequence of low coverage. More than 80 percent of those dropping out of iron supplementation programs cited discontinued supplies of tablets as the reason for noncompliance (United Nations 1990). Much more needs to be done to document exact prevalence and geographic location of iron deficiency so that control programs can be effectively targeted to those most at risk. Better program design is also needed to meet present problems.

Case Management

Prevention is the best type of case management, but where severe deficiencies of iron, iodine, and vitamin A exist, case management is best handled by trained health personnel and may require hospitalization. Immediate attention should be given to correcting deficiencies upon diagnosis. The exception to this is cretinism, which is irreversible. Immediate attention should be given to the mothers of cretinous children to improve the outcomes of future pregnancies. With mild and moderate deficiency, case management can be supervised by community health workers. In table 19A-2 we show how severe deficiencies in iron, iodine, and vitamin A can be detected, and in table 19A-7 we give typical supplementation programs for all these micronutrients.

For anemic patients with circulatory failure or respiratory distress, blood transfusion is required. Because blood loss of a severely deficient person can precipitate shock or heart failure, it is of vital importance to increase the hemoglobin level of anemic pregnant women before and during labor. If a child experiences severe vomiting or diarrhea after taking oral vitamin A capsules, water miscible retinol palmitate injections can be used. Oil-based injections should not be used because they are metabolized too slowly to be effective in acute, severe deficiency (West and Sommer 1987).

Assessment of the Effect of Interventions

In order to determine the best solution for addressing micronutrient deficiencies, the prevalence, socioeconomic and geo-graphic distribution, and causality need to be assessed in each country. Priorities for resource allocation must be based on the nature of the problem (prevalence, severity, geographic distribution, causality), the cost-effectiveness of alternative solutions, the institutional capacity to carry out the interventions, and the cultural acceptability of solutions.

Cost-Effectiveness Analysis

Different delivery systems are associated with different costs and effectiveness. In this context, the term "costs" refers to the value of all resources required to deliver the micronutrients to the target population. The term "effectiveness" refers to program and biological effectiveness. Program effectiveness is the efficacy of the delivery system in providing adequate dose and coverage to those with deficits. Biological effectiveness is the efficacy of the dose to eliminate the deficiency. Cost-effectiveness is the cost per unit of change in the outcome of interest (West and Sommer 1984). The choice of a delivery system should depend heavily upon its relative cost-effectiveness, the most desirable strategies being those with the highest effectiveness relative to cost. An additional economic criterion is that of the cost-benefit relation for each intervention. Micronutrient interventions have both costs—the value of resources required for delivery of micronutrients to the appropriate populations—and benefits—the improved functioning of those populations through the elimination of micronutrient deficiencies. For example, decreases in vitamin A deficiency will reduce blindness, allowing affected populations to care more fully for themselves, to reduce needless expenditures on health care, to benefit from education, and to be more productive in the workplace. Reduction of iron deficiencies improves educational outcomes and work output in both the household and the workplace. Reduction of iodine deficiencies decreases the likelihood of cretinism and other disorders that burden society.

One criterion for determining where to make investments in a resource-scarce situation is to allocate resources to those endeavors in which the ratio of benefits of the intervention to costs exceeds alternatives. Costs can provide a measure only of the cost of delivery and not of the program and biological effectiveness. Any measure of cost-effectiveness must take into account both the cost and the effectiveness of the intervention. The methodologies involved in determining costs and benefits are included in appendix 19B. In appendix 19C we describe the criteria of effectiveness. In appendix 19D general methodologies for cost-benefit analysis are presented.

Any comparative analysis of cost-effectiveness should take account of costs properly accounted for to meet micronutrient needs among at-risk persons for a given period of time. In table 19-6 the costs per person are given for different interventions in 1987 dollars (column 3). Column 4 presents the data from column 3 corrected for the duration of the dose. We stress in appendix B the need to use an ingredients or resource recovery method to estimate costs. Moreover, we indicate some of the reasons that the costs of a given intervention in a particular context cannot necessarily be generalized to other contexts.

With respect to micronutrient requirements, there is no assurance that different interventions have the same success for the reasons stated in appendix B. The prevalence and severity of micronutrient deficiencies differ from site to site and affect the success (and costs) of an intervention. Different interventions cover requirements for different lengths of time. A year of fortification, for example, meets one year's requirements; oral iodine covers needs for two years; injected iodine covers needs for three to five years, depending upon the dosage; and vitamin A capsules are associated with four to six months of protection, although lower-dose vitamin A supplements are available for monthly dosing. Clearly, the cost per year must be adjusted for the duration of protection provided by the intervention. Finally, the cost per year must be adjusted for the benefit leakage. In a large-scale fortification effort, not all of the recipients will be at risk, so the cost per person at risk will be higher than the cost per recipient. Targeting more finely may not be cost-effective even if leakages are high. If only one-third of the population is at risk of micronutrient deficiency, the cost per each at-risk person will be three times as high as the average cost per person.

One of these adjustments is made in the last numerical column in table 19-6, where the estimated cost per person in the previous column is calculated on the basis of one year of protection. The enormous differences in estimated cost between fortification with iodine and iodized oil injections is narrowed considerably when the five-year period of protection for oil is taken into account. Even so, the differences in cost for oil injections are substantial among studies, which may be the result of real differences, of some of the site-specific differences, or of poor data. With respect to vitamin A capsules, the two studies show considerable agreement on costs. Because two

capsules must be taken per year, the cost per year of protection is twice that for the administration of a single capsule—the cost basis in each of the studies. The difference in the costs between the two iron fortification programs using sugar as the vehicle is due to the addition of ascorbic acid to the second program. Ascorbic acid costs fifteen to twenty times as much as ferrous sulphate. The high estimated cost for delivery of ferrous sulphate tablets is because of the relatively high personnel requirement for providing daily tablets and the active supervision and motivation needed to obtain compliance. If such tablets could simply be delivered every six months to households, the cost would fall much closer to the cost of distributing vitamin A capsules.

Over time the cost-effectiveness may change. Tilden and Grosse (1988) found that dietary modification programs were more cost-effective over twenty years than either supplementation or fortification programs and that supplementation was more cost-effective over time than fortification. In their analysis they showed that over a twenty-year time period dietary modification is more effective than supplementation, which is more effective than fortification in preventing blindness and death from vitamin A deficiency. It should be kept in mind that fortified foods and water are consumed by large numbers of people who are not at risk. Thus, the cost per at-risk person for supplementation and fortification is much closer than the differences shown in table 19-6, and the cost-effectiveness of the two strategies may not be very different once these adjustments are taken into account. This is especially true for vitamin A deficiency; the numbers of those at risk are small (children under five) in relation to the entire population, and thus targeted supplementation would be more cost-effective.

Table 19-6. *Cost of Micronutrient Interventions*

Nutrient form	Country and year	Cost per person (U.S. dollars)	Estimated cost per person (1987 U.S. dollars)	Estimated cost per person per year of protection (U.S. dollars)	Source
Iodine					
Oil injection	Peru 1978	1.30	2.30	0.46	Hetzel and others 1980
Oil injection	Zaire 1977	0.35	0.67	0.14	Hetzel and others 1980
Oil injection	Indonesia 1986[a]	1.00	1.05	0.21	Irie and others 1986
Water fortification	Italy 1986	0.04	0.04	0.04	Squatrito and others 1986
Salt	India 1987	0.02–0.04	0.02–0.04	0.04	Mannar 1987
Vitamin A					
Sugar fortification	Guatemala 1976	0.07	0.14	0.14	Arroyave and others 1979
Capsule	Haiti 1978	0.13–0.19	0.23–0.34	0.46–0.68	Austin and others 1981
Capsule	Indonesia and Philippines 1975	0.10	0.21	0.42	West and Sommer 1984
Iron					
Salt fortification	India 1980	0.07	0.10	0.10	Cook and Reusser 1983
Sugar fortification	Guatemala 1980	0.07	0.10	0.10	Viteri and others 1981
Sugar fortification	Indonesia 1980	0.60	0.84	0.84	Levin 1985[b]
Tablets	Kenya and Mexico 1980	1.89–3.17	2.65–4.44	2.65–4.44	Levin 1985

a. Per injection.
b. From data provided in Derman and others 1977.
Source: See last column.

An additional way of measuring cost-effectiveness across a variety of health and nutrition interventions is to use a common outcome measure and estimate the costs per unit of that outcome. Throughout this collection, the disability-adjusted life-year gained is one measure of universal applicability. It is also possible to use cost per life saved or cost per unit of economic productivity gained.

The cost-effectiveness of achieving these outcomes with micronutrient interventions is shown in the tables in appendix 19E and summarized in table 19-7. Using the current prevalence of deficiencies commonly observed in developing countries and certain assumptions about demographics, death and disability, coverage and effectiveness (75 percent), the discount rate (3 percent), and life expectancy (seventy years), we calculated the discounted cost per disability-adjusted life-year gained based on available costs of micronutrient control programs.[1] For calculations of productivity, the annual wage rate was assumed to be $500, unemployment was assumed to be 25 percent, and disabilities were assumed to be the same as the health disabilities in table 19E-1. No adjustment was made for increased cost of feeding a more productive worker or for the employment replacement effect of increased productivity.

Cost-Benefit Analysis

Cost-benefit analysis for all micronutrients, although performed on a limited number of countries, suggests that both supplementation and fortification are good investments.

IRON. Levin (1985) estimated the benefits and costs of both medicinal supplementation and dietary fortification with iron-deficient populations on the basis of data from Indonesia, Kenya, and Mexico. Benefits accrued primarily from higher work output associated with normalization of hemoglobin levels in anemic populations. A remarkable degree of consistency was found in eight studies of work output related to hemoglobin levels. The elasticity of work output with respect to rises in Hb was between one and two: that is, an increase in Hb of 10 percent was associated with a rise in work output of 10 to 20 percent.

The pecuniary value of additional work output was estimated by first ascertaining the probable rise in Hb associated with particular interventions. This rise in Hb was converted into an increase in individual work output by applying the elasticities from the studies mentioned above. Because at least some of the rise in individual work output will simply replace the work output of others in a labor surplus economy, the social benefits will be less than the sum of the individual increases in productivity. That is, some workers will no longer be needed and will be unemployed as the output of other workers increases. Therefore, only half of the increase in work output was assumed to be a net increase in social productivity.

The net increase in social productivity was valued according to the wages that would be required to produce that additional output. The total value of productivity was adjusted to a per capita level by dividing by the entire population, including the portion of the population that was not economically active. Finally, the results were adjusted for the estimated effects of improved iron status on outputs other than work productivity. These include lower morbidity and mortality, greater physical stature, higher productivity outside of the workplace, improved quality of leisure time, greater learning and faster school advancement, and increased feelings of well-being. Especially important is the additional work output in the household and in peasant agriculture, which is not accounted for by the value of additional output in labor markets. This adjustment raised the value of total benefits by 50 percent above those of just the market-based work benefits.

Costs were estimated for fortification strategies in which both salt and sugar were used as examples of dietary vehicles. Supplementation was based on the assumption that iron supplements were one of four different dietary or health interventions delivered by a health system. Both the average cost per intervention was estimated as well as the marginal cost of the iron supplements alone. The cost of fortification was based on data from field trials. The cost of supplementation was based on the use of village health auxiliaries, various modes of transportation, facilities, and the cost of the supplements. An additional cost in both types of interventions resulted from the higher energy needs of workers who produce a larger work

Table 19-7. Return on Nutrition Investments

Intervention	Cost per life saved (U.S. dollars)	Discounted value of productivity gained per program dollar	Cost per disability-adjusted life-year gained (U.S. dollars)
Iron deficiency			
Supplementation of pregnant women only	800	24.70	12.80
Fortification	2,000	84.10	4.40
Iodine deficiency			
Supplementation of reproductive-age women only	1,250	13.80	18.90
Supplementation of all people under sixty years	4,650	6.00	37.00
Fortification	1,000	28.00	7.50
Vitamin A deficiency			
Supplementation of children under five years only	50	146.00	1.40
Fortification	154	47.50	4.20

Source: Based on table 19E-1.

output. This cost was estimated on the basis of the additional calorie input required for the additional work output, calculated from the cost of the additional rice or cornmeal required to produce those calories.

The benefits and costs were compared under a wide range of scenarios, including Hb increases, elasticities of work output with respect to Hb changes, costs of the interventions, and so on. Benefits in relation to costs were found to be highest in Mexico and lowest in Indonesia, with Kenya occupying the middle position. In all cases and under all reasonable conditions the benefits of both fortification and supplementation exceeded the costs by a wide margin. Under an intermediate set of conditions—neither the most optimistic nor the most conservative—the benefit-cost ratio for fortification varied from seven to one for Indonesia to forty-two and seventy to one for Kenya and Mexico, respectively. For supplementation, including the costs of both the ferrous sulphate and the prorated costs of the delivery system, the intermediate range of benefit-cost ratios was four, twenty-three, and thirty-eight to one for Indonesia, Kenya, and Mexico, respectively. Even under the most pessimistic assumptions, the benefits of the interventions exceeded their costs, often substantially.

IODINE. In table 19-8 we provide an overall map of the various documented effects on both human and animal populations of reductions in iodine deficiency disorders as well as the various benefit categories. In theory, it is only necessary to translate the effects into benefits and to place monetary values on them to compare them with the costs of an intervention. Unfortunately, the lack of field trials that incorporate data collection in the various benefit domains limits the application of cost-benefit analysis to this area. Nevertheless, two benefit-cost studies for iodine interventions provide illustrations of what appear to be substantial benefits in relation to costs. Correa (1980) did a benefit-cost analysis of reducing mild iodine deficiency in children. Benefits were assumed to be based on the higher earnings associated with reducing the mental effects of iodine deficiency, whereas costs were derived for the interventions necessary to reduce iodine deficiency. He first used data from a variety of sources to assess the relation between iodine deficiency and the IQ of children. He then used an independent source of data on the relation between IQ and earnings for a sample of adult men in Chile to project the earnings effects for the children with higher IQs due to iodine sufficiency. According to his calculations, the benefits, seen as improvements in lifetime earnings, of reducing mild iodine deficiency among children exceeded considerably the costs of the interventions; however, we should be cognizant that the estimates are based on diverse data sets and heroic assumptions that connect them.

More recently, the authors of two studies of screening and treatment of congenital hypothyroidism in the United States (Barden and Kessel 1985; ICCIDD/WHO 1989) showed benefits equal to three times the costs when benefits were the savings in institutional care, foster care, special education, productivity losses, and other requirements of caring for a retarded child. Both studies are limited with regard to a comprehensive

understanding of benefits and costs associated with IDD control in those areas of the world with substantial at-risk populations, but they do suggest a high payoff from iodine interventions.

VITAMIN A. A relatively comprehensive cost-benefit study of a vitamin A intervention for reducing xerophthalmia was undertaken by Popkin and others (1980). The study was based on Philippine data in which the social benefits of reducing xerophthalmia were viewed as increased income and the reduction in costs of outpatient care because fewer children would die, go blind, or become sick due to the disease. The assumption was that xerophthalmia affects both the future productivity and the development of children ages one through fifteen. Higher mortality and total blindness from xerophthalmia lower the productive time, and increased morbidity, mortality, and partial blindness reduce future productivity. Reductions in prevalence also reduce treatment costs. Three types of interventions were analyzed for their costs and effectiveness in reducing xerophthalmia: mass dose capsules of vitamin A every six months; fortification of MSG with vitamin A; and a program of health and nutrition education, disease prevention through sanitation and immunization, and limited curative work. The benefits were found to be substantially greater than costs for the mass dose capsule and MSG fortification interventions, but costs exceeded benefits for public health interventions. For the mass dose capsule, benefits were from 2.4 to 3.4 times the costs. For fortification, the benefits were 6 to 21 times the costs. As mentioned previously, Tilden and Grosse (1988) found that over time, long-term programs, such as dietary modification, will be more cost-effective than shorter-term interventions, such as supplementation and fortification.

Strengthening Institutional Capacity

Many different institutions can be used to control micronutrient deficiencies. The most obvious is the infrastructure of the

Table 19-8. *Effects of Iodine Interventions*

Population	Physiologic effects	Benefits to society
Humans	*Reductions in:* Mental deficiency Deaf-mutism Spastic diplegia Squint Dwarfism Motor deficiency Goiter	Higher work output Reduced costs of medical and custodial care Reduced educational costs because less absenteeism and grade repetition and higher achievement
Livestock	*Increases in:* Live births Weight Strength Health[a] Wool coat in sheep	Higher output of meat and other animal products Higher work output of animals

a. Less deformity.
Source: Hetzel and Maberley 1986; Levin 1987.

primary health care system, which is particularly important for supplementation programs. Expanded programs in immunization have been suggested as a vehicle for delivering supplements of vitamin A (WHO/EPI 1988a). Because vitamin A deficiency peaks in children two to four years of age, use of the existing Expanded Programme on Immunization (EPI) infrastructure may in fact make a lot of sense. Conversely, it may be preferable to put the supplementation in the hands of a village health worker. In that case the low-dose pump bottle may be the preferred delivery vehicle for vitamin A because the risk of overdosing is much lower. In some countries, health systems have low coverage, making it necessary to attack the problem differently. Nongovernmental organizations may also integrate micronutrient interventions into their programs, making an important contribution to the reduction of deficiencies in the groups in which they work. An alternative may be the school system, which can deliver micronutrients to the general community as well as children. Delivery to children is particularly relevant in view of the evidence that deficiencies in iodine, iron, and vitamin A affect the ability to learn. School feeding programs may increase attendance in schools and thus may increase the coverage of micronutrient interventions run through schools.

Markets can be used to distribute micronutrients either through fortification of food staples or increased agricultural production of micronutrient-rich food sources. The supply of micronutrients can be increased and, through consumer and nutrition education, demand and use can be expanded. Governments need to establish food regulatory institutions to ensure that fortification laws are being enforced.

Priorities for Resource Allocation

The most efficient way to allocate resources may be to give priority to vulnerable populations based on age, sex, and geographic region. Iron interventions should be targeted first to pregnant women and preschool children; vitamin A interventions should be targeted primarily to preschool children, but also to school-age children and pregnant and lactating women; and iodine interventions should be targeted to women of reproductive age and children.

The selection of a particular micronutrient intervention should be based on severity of deficiency, budgetary resources, and institutional capacity. Short-term solutions to frank deficiencies usually involve supplementation, which is easily targeted and quickly administered, but more comprehensive programs are needed (fortification, nutrition education, and food production). Food fortification, if it is feasible, will normally be the most cost-effective, long-term option in populations in which a high proportion is at risk because it entails only the marginal cost of adding the nutrient to a food staple, modifying the packaging, if necessary, to protect potency, and enforcing regulations. These marginal costs of fortification could be borne by producer, consumer, government, or some combination of these.

In some countries, fortification is not feasible because a suitable carrier cannot be identified. In others, regions that are populated by at-risk populations are so remote that transportation routes are not adequate to provide regular and continuing supplies of the fortified food. In both cases, mass dose supplements, fortification of the water supply, and the growth of nutrient-rich foods provide a basis for localized micronutrient programs.

The cost of supplementation is generally higher than that of fortification because of delivery, monitoring, and counseling. Supplements can be delivered by mobile health teams that visit villages periodically or by the primary health system and essential drug program.

Supplementation costs can be reduced by targeting programs only to those at risk and incorporating supplementation into existing programs, including EPI (WHO/EPI 1987). The compliance problem with iron supplements could be overcome by assigning a village health worker to provide health education to the villages with special emphasis on increasing the intake of the micronutrients.

Priorities for Operations Research

Although technology and operational experience are sufficient to implement micronutrient deficiency control programs now, more applied research is needed to improve the assessment and treatment of micronutrient deficiencies. Research is also needed on the oral supplements themselves. A slow-release iron supplement is needed which would obviate the need to take tablets every day. Development of a slow-release vitamin A supplement would minimize toxicity problems. Similarly, the technical system for fortifying salt with both iron and iodine is needed.

Another set of research issues relates to measuring the prevalence of micronutrient deficiencies. Surveys of micronutrient deficiencies are often outdated with respect to both the data themselves and the methodology used. The improved assessment of iodine status (thyroid stimulating hormone) from a drop of blood on filter paper can replace highly subjective goiter surveys and unreliable urinary excretion assessments. A new measure of iron status (transferrin receptors) exceeds the specificity of all other measures and can be done using a finger prick sample.

Further epidemiological research is needed on the incidence of multiple micronutrient deficiencies. Greater cost-effectiveness can be attained if ways are found to prevent more than one deficiency at a time. The potential of using a filter paper blood sample to analyze all three of the deficiencies under discussion would accelerate this research.

Much more information is needed about cost-effectiveness and institutional support. Although the data on iron are fairly strong, cost-effectiveness and cost-benefit data on vitamin A and iodine programs are weak. Effective enforcement of fortification programs needs further research, including the nature of legislation, the structure of regulatory bodies, and the mechanisms for inducing compliance. Finally, better data are needed on the functional effects of micronutrient deficiencies, especially those relating moderate deficiency to human resource development.

Summary and Conclusions

Iron, iodine, and vitamin A deficiencies are highly prevalent in developing countries. The existing data are sufficiently robust to conclude that these deficiencies result not only in increased mortality but also in increased morbidity, learning disabilities, reproductive wastage, and reduced work output. Yet cost-effective solutions exist and have been successful under a wide spectrum of conditions; supplementation and fortification are feasible but their appropriateness depends on local characteristics.

It is important to engage in long-term planning to control micronutrient deficiencies because the need will not diminish in the near future. Strategic planning requires an active assessment of institutional capacity and of the cost-efficiency of alternative methods. Sustainability is a central concern in designing any micronutrient deficiency control program. If supplementation or nutrition education are used, they need to be integrated into the health care system. Specific and targeted campaigns may work, but they are too costly in relation to integrating strategies into a more comprehensive health care approach. Micronutrients should not displace but rather complement protein-energy malnutrition as a key problem for health workers. Special attention should be given to organizational strengthening, including strong regulatory structures, if we are to win the battle against micronutrient deficiency disorders.

Appendix 19A. Prevalence, Programs, Recommended Intakes, and Indicators of Deficiencies

The tables in this appendix present detailed information on the iodine, iron, and vitamin A deficiencies discussed earlier in the chapter. Country-by-country statistics, which have been provided wherever possible, include data on current interventions.

Table 19A-1. *Prevalence of Iron Deficiency and Program Coverage by Country*

Country	Prevalence (percent)	Fortification Program status	Legislation	Program status[a]
Africa				
Benin	39.0[b]	None	None	None
Burundi	7.2[b]	None	None	None
Chad	25.0[b]	None	None	None
Ethiopia	6.0[b]	None	None	None
Kenya	6.0[b,c]	None	None	None
Mali	4.6	None	None	None
Sierra Leone	50.0	None	None	None
Tanzania	25.0[b,c]	None	None	None
Zambia	49.0[b]	None	None	None
Zimbabwe	45.0[b]	None	None	None
Asia				
Bangladesh	66.0[c]	None	None	None
Burma	82.0[b]	None	None	None
China	86.0[b,c]	None	None	None
India	69.0[b]	None	None	Under way[d]
Indochina	37.0[b]	None	None	None
Malaysia	83.0[b]	None	None	None
Nepal	24.1[b]	None	None	None
Philippines	37.5	None	None	Under way[e]
Sri Lanka	3.8[b]	None	None	None
Thailand	11.0[b]	None	None	None
Middle East				
Algeria	41.9[b]	None	None	None
Egypt	22.4	None	None	None
Lebanon	32.0[b]	None	None	None
Morocco	11.2[b]	None	None	None
Pakistan	20.0[b]	None	None	None
Syrian Arab Republic	47.0[b]	None	None	None
Tunisia	29.9	None	None	None
Latin America				
Argentina	16.0[b]	None	None	None
Bolivia	18.5[b]	None	None	None
Chile	20.0[b]	Under way	None	None
Costa Rica	7.0	None	None	Under way
Cuba	30.0[b]	None	None	None

(Table continues on the following page.)

Table 19A-1 (continued)

Country	Prevalence (percent)	Fortification Program status	Legislation	Program status[a]
Latin America (continued)				
Ecuador	46.0[b]	None	None	None
El Salvador	8.6[b]	None	None	None
Guatemala	National[f]	Under way	None	None
Guyana	40.0[b]	None	None	None
Jamaica	76.0[b]	None	None	None
Paraguay	76.0[b]	None	None	None

Note: The quality of data (sample size, age, region) necessitates caution when comparing countries.

a. Many countries distrubute iron tablets as part of MCH programs, but there are little data on coverage, compliance, effect, and so forth.

b. Regional or sporadic prevalence, or known regionally in some age groups and sexes.

c. Probable.

d. Twelve percent coverage.

e. Forty-five percent coverage.

f. Iron deficiency anemia prevalent nationally. Exact numbers not available.

Source: Chafkin 1984; Levin 1986; Hercberg and others 1987; Yepez and others 1987; Stekel 1987; Assami and others 1988; Prual and others 1988; Valyasevi 1988; Pollitt 1989; FAO undated; Florentino, undated; Seshadri and Gopaldas, undated.

Table 19A-2. Definition of Deficiencies

Group	Value	
Iron deficiency	*Hemoglobin (g / dL)*[a]	+
Children six months to six years		11.0
Children six to fourteen years		12.0
Adult males		13.0
Adult females, nonpregnant		12.0
Pregnant females		11.0
All ages	*Serum ferritin (mcg / L)*	
	< 10–12	

Iodine deficiency	Goiter prevalence (percent)	Median urinary iodine (mcg/g creatinine)
Mild		
Population	5–20	n.a.
Individual	n.a.	> 50
Moderate		
Population	21–29	n.a.
Individual	n.a.	25–50
Severe		
Population	> 29	n.a.
Individual	n.a.	< 25

Vitamin A deficiency
Population: children younger than six years (percent)

Night blindness (xN)[c]	1.0	
Bitot's spots (xIB)[c]	0.5	
Corneal scars, ulceration (x3A)[c] 0.01		
Xerophthalmia-related corneal scars	0.05	
Serum retinol < 10 mcg/dL	5.0	

Individual	Serum retinol (mcg/dL)	Liver retinol (mcg/g)
Mild deficiency		
Children	20	< 20
Adults	30	< 20
Severe deficiency		
Children	< 10	< 10
Adults	< 10	< 10

n.a. Not Applicable.

a. Hemoglobin values below which anemia is likely to be present in individuals living at sea level.

b. Prevalence of endemic cretinism is 1–10 percent.

c. Clinical abbreviation for stage of Xerothphalmia.

Source: West and Sommer 1987; DeMaeyer and Adiels-Tegman 1985; Hetzel 1988; DeMaeyer 1989.

Table 19A-3. Recommended Daily Intake of Iron, Based on Bioavailability in Diet

Age group	Absorbed iron requirement (mg/day)	Iron intake (mg/day) by quality of the diet[a]		
		Low bioavailability	Medium bioavailability	High bioavailability
4–12 months	0.96	32	16	9
13–24 months	0.61	20	10	5
2–5 years	0.70	23	12	6
6–11 years	1.17	39	19	11
Girls 12–16 years	2.02	67	34	18
Boys 12–16 years	1.82	61	30	16
Adult Males	1.14	38	19	10
Adult Females				
Pregnant	3.6	120	60	33
Lactating	1.31	44	22	12
Menstruating	2.38	79	40	22
Postmenopausal	0.96	32	16	9

a. As defined by Monsen and others 1978, a diet with low bioavailability contains no meat, fish, or poultry; none of the iron is heme iron, and 3 percent of total iron is absorbed. A diet with medium bioavailability contains 1 ounce of fish per day; four percent of the iron is heme iron, and 6 percent of total iron is absorbed. A diet with high bioavailability contains 3 ounces of beef per day; 21 percent of the iron is heme iron, and 11 percent of total iron is absorbed.
Source: DeMaeyer 1989.

Table 19A-4. Prevalence of Iodine Deficiency and Program Coverage, by Country

Country	Prevalence		Fortification			Supplementation program status
	Percent	Area[a]	Program status	Legislation (years)	Coverage (percent)	
Africa						
Angola	—	Regional	None	None	—	None
Benin	—	Regional	None	None	—	None
Botswana	63	Regional	None	None	—	Planned
Burkina Faso	7.7	National	None	None	—	Planned
Burundi	56	Regional[b]	Under way	None	—	Planned
Cameroon	59	Regional	None	None	—	Planned
Central African Republic	25	Regional	None	None	—	None
Chad	11	Regional	None	None	—	None
Comoros	40	Regional	None	None	—	None
Congo	—	Regional	Under way	1988	—	None
Côte d'Ivoire	18	Regional	None	None	—	Planned
Ethiopia	34	Regional	Under way	None	—	Under way
Gabon	1	National	None	None	—	None
The Gambia	—	Regional	None	None	—	None
Ghana	13	Regional	None	None	—	Planned
Guinea	15.4	National	None	None	—	None
Guinea Bissau	—	Regional	None	None	—	None
Kenya	15–72	National	Under way	1970	50	Planned
Lesotho	14.3	National	Planned	None	—	Planned
Liberia	—	Regional	None	None	—	Planned
Madagascar	18	Regional	None	None	—	Planned
Malawi	30–70	Regional	Planned	None	—	Under way
Mali	20	Regional	None	None	—	Planned
Namibia	—	Regional	None	None	—	None
Niger	13	National	None	None	—	Planned
Nigeria	40	Regional	None	None	—	Planned
Rwanda	19	Regional	Under way	None	—	Planned
Senegal	33	Regional	Under way	None	—	None
Sierra Leone	—	Regional	None	None	—	Planned
Somalia	—	Regional	None	None	—	None
Sudan	20	Regional	None	None	—	Planned
Swaziland	26	National	None	None	—	None
Tanzania	40	Regional	Under way	None	—	Under way
Togo	—	Regional	None	None	—	Planned
Uganda	—	Regional	None	None	—	None
Zaire	—	Regional	None	None	—	Under way
Zambia	27–81	Regional	Under way	1979	—	Planned
Zimbabwe	20	Regional	None	None	—	Planned

(Table continues on the following page.)

Table 19A-4 (continued)

Country	Prevalence		Fortification			Supplementation program status
	Percent	Area[a]	Program status	Legislation (years)	Coverage (percent)	
Asia						
Bangladesh	10.5	National	Under way	1989	55	Under way
Bhutan	64.5	National	Under way	None	100	Under way
Burma	14.3	National	None	None	—	Under way
Cambodia	30	National	None	None	—	Planned
China	—	Regional	Under way	None	87	None
India	7.3	National	Under way	1962	12	Planned
Indonesia	20	National	Under way	1976	51	Under way
Korea, Republic of	—	—	None	None	—	Planned
Lao PDR	—	—	None	None	—	Planned
Malaysia	—	Regional	Under way	None	0	None
Nepal	46.1	National	Under way	None	72	Under way
Papua New Guinea	40	Regional	Under way	1972	—	Planned
Philippines	14.9	National	Under way	None	—	Planned
Sri Lanka	19.3	National	Planned	None	0	Planned
Thailand	14.7	National	Under way	None	2	None
Viet Nam	34	National	Under way	None	5	None
Middle East						
Afghanistan	—	National	None	None	—	None
Algeria	—	Regional	Under way	None		Planned
Egypt	70	Regional	None	None	—	None
Iran	60	Regional	None	None	—	Planned
Iraq	80	Regional	None	None	—	Planned
Lebanon	50	Regional	None	None	—	Planned
Libya	20	Regional	None	None	—	Planned
Morocco	—	Regional	None	None	—	None
Pakistan	—	Regional	Under way	None	11–17	None
Tunisia	—	Regional	None	None	—	None
Latin America						
Argentina	15.6	National	Under way	1967	99	Under way
Bolivia	61	National	Under way	1967	20–80	Under way
Brazil	14.7	Regional	Under way	1977	—	None
Chile	18.8	Regional	Under way	1968	85	Under way
Colombia	1.8	Regional	Under way	1947	—	None
Costa Rica	3.5	National	Under way	1970	—	None
Cuba	30.3	Regional	None	None	—	Under way
Dominican Republic	80	Regional	None	None	—	None
Ecuador	36.5	Regional	Under way	1968	75–80	Under way
El Salvador	48	National	Under way	1961	17	Under way
Guatemala	10.6	National	Under way	1954	36	Under way
Honduras	17	National	Under way	1961	—	Under way
Mexico	—	Regional	Under way	1962	—	Under way
Nicaragua	20	National	Under way	1969	—	Under way
Panama	6	National	Under way	1966	47	Under way
Paraguay	18.1	National	Under way	1966	—	Under way
Peru	50–80	Regional	Planned	None	60	Under way
Uruguay	—	Regional	Under way	1961	—	Under way
Venezuela	21.3	National	Under way	1968	—	Under way

— Data not available.

Note: The quality of data (sample size, ages, region) necessitates caution when comparing countries.

a. Regional or sporadic goiter prevalence, or known regionally in some age groups; or national goiter prevalence or prevalent nationally in some age groups.

b. Probable.

Source: FAO no date; Hetzel 1987; United Nations 1987; PAHO/WHO/UNICEF 1988; Dunn (ed.) 1989a and 1989b; ICCIDD 1989; ICCIDD/WHO 1989; "Iodine Deficiency" 1989; Pollitt 1989; "Status of IDD" 1989; WHO 1989.

Table 19A-5. Recommended Daily Intake of Iodine and Vitamin A
(mcg/day)

Age group	Intake
Iodine	
All People	150–300
Vitamin A	
Infants younger than 1 year	300
1–3 years	250
4–6 years	300
7–9 years	400
10–12 years	575
13–15 years	725
16–19 years	750
Adult men and women[a]	750
Lactating women (first six months)	1,200

Note: Micrograms or retinol equivalents (RE) are currently used to measure retinol and the carotenoids. Previously, international units were used. To convert: 1 RE = 1 mcg retinol = 6 mcg all-trans beta-carotene = 12 mcg other provitamin A carotenoids = 10 IU provitamin A carotene = 3.33 IU of retinol.
a. Including pregnant women and lactating women after the first six months.
Source: FAO 1965; Hetzel 1988.

Table 19A-6. Prevalence of Vitamin A Deficiency and Program Coverage by Country

Country	Prevalence		Fortification		Supplementation program status
	Percent	Area[a]	Program status	Legislation	
Africa					
Angola	—	Probable	None	None	None
Benin	3.5	Regional	None	None	None
Botswana	—	Regional	None	None	None
Burkina Faso	—	National	None	None	None
Burundi	—	Probable	None	None	Under way
Chad	—	National	None	None	None
Côte d'Ivoire	—	Regional	None	None	Under way
Ethiopia	—	Regional	None	None	None
Ghana	—	National	None	None	Under way
Kenya	—	Probable	None	None	Under way
Madagascar	—	Regional	None	None	None
Malawi	3.9	Regional	None	None	Under way
Mali	—	National	None	None	Under way
Mauritania	2.3	Regional	None	None	Under way
Mozambique	—	National	None	None	Under way
Niger	—	National	None	None	Under way
Nigeria	—	Regional	None	None	Under way
Rwanda	—	Probable	None	None	None
Senegal	—	Regional	None	None	None
Somalia	11.0	Regional	None	None	Under way
Sudan	1.6	Regional	None	None	Under way
Tanzania	1.6	Regional	None	None	Under way
Uganda	—	Regional	None	None	Under way
Zaire	—	Regional	None	None	Under way
Zambia	—	Regional	None	None	Under way
Zimbabwe	—	Regional	None	None	None
Asia					
Bangladesh	4.9	National	None	None	Under way
Burma	—	Regional	None	None	Under way
Cambodia	—	Probable	None	None	None
China	—	National	None	None	None

(Table continues on the following page.)

Table 19A-6 (continued)

Country	Prevalence		Fortification		Supplementation program status
	Percent	Area[a]	Program status	Legislation	
Asia (continued)					
India	12–20	National	None	None	None
Indonesia	20.0	National	Under way	None	Under way
Lao PDR	—	Probable	None	None	None
Malaysia	—	Regional	None	None	None
Micronesia	10.0	n.a.	None	None	None
Nepal	1.0	National	None	None	Under way
Philippines	—	National	Planned	None	Under way
Sri Lanka	—	Regional	None	None	Under way
Thailand	—	Regional	None	None	None
Viet Nam	—	National	None	None	Under way
Middle East					
Afghanistan	—	Probable	None	None	None
Algeria	—	Regional	None	None	None
Egypt	—	Regional	None	None	None
Iran	—	Regional	None	None	None
Iraq	—	Regional	None	None	None
Jordan	—	Regional	Under way	1977	None
Morocco	—	Regional	None	None	None
Pakistan	—	Probable	None	None	Under way
Syrian Arab Republic	—	Regional	None	None	None
Yemen, Republic of	—	Regional	None	None	None
Yemen, Arab	0.57	Regional	None	None	None
Latin America					
Bolivia	—	Regional	None	None	None
Brazil	—	Regional	None	None	Under way
Costa Rica	—	Regional	Under way	Under way	None
Ecuador	—	Regional	None	None	None
El Salvador	—	Regional	None	None	Under way
Guatemala	—	Regional	Under way	Under way	Under way
Haiti	0.81	Regional	None	None	Under way
Honduras	—	Probable	Under way	Under way	None
Jamaica	—	Regional	None	None	None
Mexico	—	Regional	None	None	None
Nicaragua	—	Regional	Under way	None	None
Panama	—	Regional	Under way	Under way	None
Peru	—	Regional	None	None	None

— Data not available.

Note: The quality of data (sample size, ages, region) necessitates caution when comparing countries.

a. Either regional or sporadic prevalence or known regionally, or prevalent nationally, with clinical signs in children younger than six years.

Source: Arroyave 1982; Cohen and others 1985; FAO no date; IVACG 1989; Mathur and Kushwaha 1987; Pollitt 1989; Solon and others 1983; Underwood 1983; UNICEF 1988; United Nations 1985; WHO 1988a and 1988b.

Table 19A-7. Typical Supplementation Programs

Deficiency	Target group	Compound	Dose	Frequency
Iron				
Presumptive treatment	Pregnant women	Ferrous sulfate	200 mg	Twice daily
where prevalence of	Pregnant women	Folic acid	500 mcg	Daily
iron deficiency anemia	Children six months to five years[a]	Ferrous sulfate	10 mg/kg	Daily[b]
is moderate or high	School-age children	Ferrous sulfate	200 mg	Daily[b]
Presumptive treatment	Pregnant women	Ferrous sulfate	200 mg	Daily
where prevalence of	Pregnant women	Folic acid	250 mcg	Daily
iron deficiency anemia	Children six months to five years	Ferrous sulfate	3 mg/kg	Daily[b]
is mild	School-age children	Ferrous sulfate	100 mg	Daily[b]
Treatment of severe iron	Pregnant women	Ferrous sulfate	200 mg	Thrice daily for four weeks
deficiency anemia				
(hemoglobin less than	Pregnant women	Folic acid	250 mcg	Thrice daily for four weeks
7 g/dL)				

Deficiency	Target group	Compound	Dose	Frequency
	Children six months to five years	Ferrous sulfate	10 mg/kg	Daily
	Adults	Ferrous sulfate	200 mg	Twice daily
Treatment of moderate iron deficiency anemia (hemoglobin between 7 and 10 g/dL)	Pregnant women	Ferrous sulfate	200 mg	Twice daily
	Pregnant women	Folic acid	250 mcg	Daily
	Children six months to five years	Ferrous sulfate	3 mg/kg	Daily
	Adolescents	Ferrous sulfate	200 mg	Twice daily
	Adults	Ferrous sulfate	200 mg	Twice daily
Iodine	All	Iodinated oil-oral	2 ml	Two years
	All	Iodinated oil[c]	2 ml	Three to five years
	All	Iodinated oil-intratranscular	1 ml	Three years
Vitamin A	Children without xerophthalmia	Oil solution	20,000 mcg	Three to six months after age one year
	Children with xerophthalmia[d]	Oil solution	20,000 mcg	Diagnosis
			20,000 mcg	Next day
			20,000 mcg	Two to four weeks later, at clinical deterioration, or at discharge
	Pregnant women without dietary sources	Oil solution	1,000 mcg	Daily
	Lactating women	Oil solution	20,000 mcg	At parturition
			1,000 mcg	Daily

Note: All treatment is oral, unless otherwise specified.

a. Children younger than four months should be given only breast milk, which provides adequate iron. After four months, iron-containing weaning foods should be given. Low-birthweight infants require iron from two months age.

b. Short-course therapy.

c. Injected. A caveat for use of any injections is increased risk of AIDS transmission where needles are commonly reused and probability of sterilization is low.

d. Children younger than twelve months should receive half doses.

Source: IVACG 1986; Dunn 1987; West and Sommer 1987; DeMaeyer 1989; United Nations 1990.

Appendix 19B. Costs of Supplementation and Fortification

Before we review the costs of supplementation and fortification, it is important to review briefly the appropriate method for measuring costs. Although the notion of costs is often used quite casually in the health sector literature, it has a very specific meaning in the economics literature (Mishan 1976; Levin 1983; Mills 1985). It refers to the social value of all the resources, or ingredients, that are required to provide an intervention—even resources provided in kind. The proper method for ascertaining costs is first to specify the particular resources that are needed for a nutritional intervention, such as the facilities, personnel, materials, and micronutrients that are required. Second, the value or cost of each of the ingredients is derived from both market data, if these are available, and other determinants of economic value, such as shadow price (Mills 1985). These costs for all the ingredients are summed to determine the total cost of an intervention. The total cost can be divided by the overall population or another base to obtain the cost per participant of the intervention.

The determination of the cost of an intervention is independent of the issue of how it is financed. The cost is a measure of the value of resources that are used for the intervention, no matter who is paying for them. Although an analysis of who pays or should pay and how it should be financed is important, it is the subject of a separate analysis. It is important to get an accurate determination of the cost before addressing its financing.

Cost Estimation

Using the ingredients method of determining the cost of the delivery of medicinal supplements, such as iron, one must first select a delivery model. The usual model is that of a community- or village-based health care system in which there is a heavy use of local resources, such as health auxiliaries or community health workers. There is a considerable literature on village or community health workers (Djukanovic and Mach 1975; Hetzel 1978; WHO 1979; Bender and Yoder 1983). Such workers are people who have completed all or most of primary school and are literate in basic reading, writing, and computational skills. They typically come from the local community, so they relate well to the populations they serve. They can deliver nutritional supplements and provide information and advice on their use. They are able to offer inoculations and other specific health services for which they are qualified through short training programs, and they periodically have contact with more highly trained staff. Other ingredients for the supplementation model include facilities, equipment, transportation, and the micronutrient supplements themselves (Hetzel and others 1980; West and Sommer 1984; Levin 1985, 1986).

The costs of the fortification intervention are based on those of the micronutrient compounds as well as personnel, equipment, and special packaging required for the preparation and delivery of the fortified product (Arrojave and others 1979). The value of the food vehicle that is being fortified is not a cost of fortification but only the additional cost associated with the fortification process. To protect the micronutrient content associated with fortification, some products, such as fortified salt, must be packaged in more expensive bags than their unfortified counterparts.

Comparing Costs

The literature on micronutrient interventions contains cost estimates for both supplementation and fortification. Usually, these costs are expressed as the cost per person covered by the intervention. Thus, in theory, it would appear that one could readily compare the costs of injected supplements for iodine or vitamin A with the costs of orally administered supplements. Or one could compare the costs of fortification of different food vehicles with iodine, such as salt or water, or with iron, such as salt, sugar, wheat flour, or milk products. Then one could select those interventions that had the lowest cost per person for delivery.

For example, one of the most obvious features of table 19-6 is the large differences in the cost per person, even when standardized to 1987 dollars. Even for a single intervention, such as injections of iodinated oil, the cost per person varied from $0.67 to $2.30. The costs per person among different interventions for the same micronutrient differ even more.

Idiosyncratic Differences in Costs

In fact, comparisons of costs among studies cannot be used as a basis for determining the most efficient form of supplementation or fortification. The reason is that the costs in any particular study will—to some degree—be idiosyncratic because of the methodology used and the time and setting in which it was carried out (Mills 1985). It is important to summarize the sources of these idiosyncrasies to show why cost results from one study cannot necessarily be compared with another.

- *Methodological differences.* Different studies use different methodologies, from casual guesses at costs to rigorous cost accounting methods. Even among the latter there are differences in assumptions and methods based on different judgments. Unless a uniform method is used among studies, comparison is inappropriate.
- *Exchange rates.* The usual practice is to convert costs in local currencies to some standard monetary unit, such as U.S. dollars, that can be compared among studies. But exchange rates are distorted by speculation, government

intervention, dominance of particular commodity flows, and other factors that do not reflect the true value of resources in that standard monetary unit. The result is that some of the cost differences among interventions drawn from the experience of different nations may depend on fluctuating exchange rates that are not in competitive market equilibrium rather than on the "true" world value of those resources.

- *Time.* The usual cost comparisons among studies do not take account of the fact that often the studies were carried out at different times. Because prices change over time and follow different patterns among countries and because there are often no appropriate price deflators for standardizing them over time, the costs derived at different time periods are not strictly comparable even after adjusting for price-level changes.
- *Context.* A cost comparison between two different countries and situations will reflect the unique characteristics of those contexts. For example, it costs far less for health teams to go from village to village in a relatively flat region with good transportation than it does for them to travel in mountainous or jungle regions. Differences in population density affect costs profoundly because of the difficulties of reaching sparse and remote populations as compared with more compact ones. Tropical climates may pose additional costs for packaging and refrigeration of micronutrients than more temperate climates. The result is that some of the measured cost differences among interventions may derive from the differences in circumstances rather than intrinsic differences in costs.
- *Local price differences.* Some differences in costs among interventions in different countries and regions are due to differences in prices for the same commodities and labor. For example, the price of iodinated oil was found to be about 50 percent higher in Bolivia in 1985 than in France in 1983, a difference that cannot be explained by inflation (Dunn 1987). Among three countries in 1979, the cost of persons trained as vaccinators varied from $2.24 a day in Indonesia to $5.90 a day in Thailand, a considerable difference (Creese and others 1982). This is another reason that cost experiences in one country for a particular intervention might not reflect the costs of that intervention in another country.
- *Population base.* Some of the interventions are targeted to only the populations at high risk, such as is the case of iodinated oil in villages with a high incidence of goiter and low iodine in the soil. Others, such as the iodination of salt, are based on distributing a fortified product to the entire population, those in need of the intervention and those not in need. If only one-third of the population is in need of a particular intervention, the cost per person at risk is three times as high as the cost per capita in the population as a whole. Thus, the cost per person of interventions that reach only those who are at risk should not be compared with the much lower costs of those that reach the entire population, including those who are not at risk.

Appendix 19C. Criteria of Effectiveness

Some interventions will have a high success rate in obtaining repletion, such as injected or oral iodinated oil or oral capsules of vitamin A. Once ingested or injected, these interventions are almost invariably associated with iodine or vitamin A repletion. In contrast, medicinal supplementation with iron or dietary fortification does not always ensure repletion. Because the capacity of the body to store iron is limited, iron supplementation requires that the participant take iron daily. When administered in schools or workplaces, this compliance can be readily maintained. When it is necessary to depend on households continually to take iron supplements, it is not realistic to expect a high level of compliance. Thus, the cost of delivering the iron to households is not equivalent to the cost of obtaining iron repletion. Indeed, obtaining compliance may require continuing reinforcement through monitoring and persuasion by village health teams and other educational efforts.

The same is true with fortification. Not only is it necessary for all persons at risk to consume adequate amounts of the fortified food, but the food must have sufficient amounts of the micronutrient at the time of consumption. There may be a compliance problem when unfortified, local products compete with the nationally or regionally distributed fortified ones. In Ecuador it was necessary to mount a social marketing campaign to increase use of a fortified product such as iodinated salt because alternative salt sources were available at the local level (Manoff 1987). In tropical areas the hygroscopic nature of salt that is used for iodine fortification means that unless contained in watertight packaging until consumption, at least some of the iodine will be lost. Iodinated salt in jute bags showed a loss of three-quarters of its iodine in nine months (Mannar 1987). The type of packaging, the time it takes to get to consumers, and the use of open or closed containers by shops and consumers will determine potency. In very humid climates with highly undependable transportation and long periods before sale or consumption in open containers, the salt may lose virtually all its iodine.

Appendix 19D. Cost-Benefit Analysis

Cost-benefit analysis represents a technique for ascertaining whether micronutrient and other social interventions are worthwhile. Such interventions use scarce societal resources, which could be used to provide other types of social benefits. At a minimum, an intervention should not be undertaken unless its benefits exceed its costs. But because many investments have benefits that exceed costs, it is also important to consider whether the relation of benefits to costs exceed those—or are at least in the range of—alternative investments.

Although it would be desirable to have a standard cost-benefit methodology with precise rules for calculation for every situation, this is not the present case. The cost methodology is straightforward and is identical to the ingredients, or resource recovery, method that was outlined in appendix 19B for cost and cost-effectiveness studies. But although the conceptual methods for identifying and measuring benefits are well established (Creese and Henderson 1980; Mills 1985), the application of these methods depends crucially on a variety of judgments on both the measurement of benefits and their values. Some of the best work on cost-benefit analysis in the health sector is found in the area of immunization (Creese and Henderson 1980; Creese 1983), and many of the methods used there can be applied to micronutrients.

The basic method of estimating benefits is to identify the positive effects of micronutrient interventions on such areas as morbidity, work output, and educational benefits for children. The benefits of reduced morbidity are generally considered to be the savings in health care and the value of lost productivity; the benefits of work output can be measured with respect to additional days of productive work (in the labor market or household) and the additional productivity per day; and educational benefits include the value of additional student achievement and the reduction in the cost of special educational services or grade repetition. Some of these benefits also have implications for costs. For example, if iron-replete workers are able to put out more work effort to increase productivity, they will also need additional food to compensate for the higher expenditure of energy (Levin 1985, 1986).

As summarized in the earlier sections of this chapter, each of the micronutrient interventions has an effect on health, productivity, and other aspects of behavior. In theory, it is only necessary to translate the effects into benefits and to place monetary values on them to compare them with the costs of an intervention. Unfortunately, the lack of field trials that incorporate data collection in the various benefit domains limits the application of cost-benefit analysis to this area. Nevertheless, there exist studies for each of the three micronutrients that are both informative and suggest high returns. These are discussed in the main text of the chapter.

Appendix 19E. Costs and Benefits

The tables in this appendix show the costs and benefits of various interventions.

Table 19E-1. Assumptions in Calculating Costs per Disability-Adjusted Life-Year, Death Averted, and Income Enhancement

Parameter	Value
Program effectiveness (percent)	75[a]
Unemployment (percent)	25[b]
Life expectancy (years)	70
Discount rate (percent)	3
Annual wage rate (U.S. dollars)	500
Population (number)	100,000
Age distribution (number)	
0–1 year	3,900
1–2 years	3,250
2–3 years	2,340
3–4 years	1,950
4–5 years	1,560
5–9 years	12,000
10–14 years	9,000
15–59 years	57,000
60 years and older	7,000
Malnutrition rates (number and percent	
PEM	
Children younger than five	3,900 (30)
Adults stunted from childhood malnutrition	17,000 (30)
Iron	
Anemic children under age 15	18,000 (50)
Anemic adult men	7,250 (25)
Anemic pregnant women	2,520 (63)
Total population anemic	49,000
Iodine	
Population deficient	24,000 (24)
Cretinism	50 (0.4)[d]
Vitamin A	
Deficient children under six	1,950 (15)
Severely deficient children under six	40 (.27)
Severely deficient children under six dying	20 (.16)
Partially blind children under six	81 (0.060)
Totally blind children under six	41 (0.028)
Annual deaths from malnutrition (number)	
PEM-related causes in children under five	160
Severe anemia in women at childbirth	10
Stillbirths related to iodine deficiency	10
Neonatal deaths related to iodine deficiency	10
Children under five with vitamin A deficiency	40
Degree of disability (percent)[e]	
Undernutrition	10
Iron deficiency	20
Iodine deficiency	5
Cretinism	50
Partial blindness	25
Total blindness	50

a. Includes coverage as well as efficacy.
b. Adults age 15–59.
c. Includes 25,000 women of reproductive age, of whom 4,000 are pregnant.
d. One child is born with cretinism each year.
e. Health and productivity disability.
Source: Based on authors' assumptions.

Table 19E-2. Nutrition Program Costs for Population of 10,000

Intervention	Target group	Annual per capita cost (U.S. dollars)	Annual program cost (U. S. dollars)
Food supplements	Pregnant women Children 0–3 years	46	620,540
Nutrition education	Pregnant women	2	26,980
Food subsidy	Bottom quintile	30	600,000
Integrated nutrition PHC	Pregnant women	25	337,250
School feeding	Children 5–9 years	12	144,000
Iron			
Supplement[a]	Pregnant women	2	8,000
Fortification	Entire population	0.20	20,000
Iodine			
Supplement, selective	Women	0.50	12,500
Supplement, total	Entire	0.50	23,250
Fortification	Entire population	0.10	10,000
Vitamin A			
Supplement	Children 0–5 years	0.50	6,500
Fortification	Entire population	0.20	20,000

Note: Based on assumptions in table 19A-8.
a. Assumes six prenatal visits plus 200 iron tablets.
Source: Ho 1985; Levin 1985; Kennedy and Alderman 1987.

Table 19E-3. Costs and Effectiveness of Iron Intervention

Parameter	Iron supplementation of pregnant women	Iron fortification
Target group	Pregnant women	All people
Number	4,000	100,000
Average rate (percent)[a]	63	50
Per capita cost (U.S. dollars)[b]	2	0.20
Program effectiveness (percent)	75	75
Deaths averted	10	10
Immediate productivity gains (percent)	20	20
Program duration (days)	200	Year round
Program costs (U.S. dollars)	8,000	20,000
Discounted wage gains (U.S. dollars)	221,280[c]	1,682,720[d]
DALY gained	624	4,520
Wage gains divided by program cost	27.7	84.1
Cost per DALY (U.S. dollars)	12.80	4.40
Cost per death averted (U.S. dollars)	800	2,000

Note: Based on assumptions in table 19E-1.

a. Rate of anemia for iron supplementation of pregnant women; rate of iron deficiency for iron fortification.

b. Per pregnancy for iron supplementation; per participant for iron fortification.

c. Calculated as the product of the number of anemic participants times disability times wage times effectiveness times employment, plus the product of number of deaths times wage times employment times productive life expectancy; ([0.63 x 3990] x 0.2 x 500 x 0.75 x 0.75) + (10 x 500 x 0.75 x 21.3) = 141,400 + 79,880 = 221,280.

d. Calculated as the product of the number of adult participants times the rate of anemia times disability times effectiveness times employment times wage, plus the product of the number of deaths times wage times employment times productive life expectancy; (56,990 x 0.5 x 0.2 x 0.75 x 500) + (10 x 500 x 0.75 x 21.3) = 1,602,840 + 79,880 = 1,682,720.

e. Calculated as the product of the number of deaths times life expectancy, plus the product of disability times number of malnourished participants times effectiveness; (10 x 24.7) + (0.2 x 0.63 x 3990 x 0.75) = 247 + 377 = 624.

f. Calculated as the product of number of adult participants times the rate of anemia times disability times effectiveness, plus the product of the number of deaths times life expectancy; (56,990 x 0.5 x 0.2 x 0.75) + (10 x 24.7) = 4270 + 250 = 4520.

Source: Based on authors' assumptions.

Table 19E-4. Costs and Effectiveness of Iodine Intervention

Parameter	Iodine supplement: targeted coverage	Iodine supplement: mass coverage	Iodization of salt or water
Target group	Reproductive-age women	Everyone under age sixty	Everyone
Number	25,000	93,000	100,000
Average rate of iodine deficiency (percent)	24	24	24
Per capita cost (U.S. dollars)[a]	0.50	0.50	0.10
Program effectiveness (percent)	75[b]	75	75
Deaths averted	10[c]	10	10
Productivity loss (percent)			
Normal population	5	5	5
Cretins	50	50	50
Program duration	Year round	Year round	Year round
Program costs (U.S. dollars)	12,500	46,500	100,000
Discounted wage gains (U.S. dollars)	172,000[d]	280,000[e]	280,000[e]
DALY gained	660[f]	1,270[g]	1,335[h]
Wage gains divided by program cost (U.S. dollars)	13.8	6.0	28
Cost per DALY (U.S. dollars)	18.90	37	7.50
Cost per death averted (U.S. dollars)	1,250	4,650	1,000

Note: Based on assumptions in table 19E-1.

a. Per participant per year.   b. Prevents both neonatal death and cretinism.   c. Neonatal.

d. Calculated as the product of the number of participants times the rate of deficiency times disability times wage times effectiveness times employment rate, plus number who died times productive life expectancy times employment times wage for ten cretins, plus the product of frequency times productive life expectancy times employment times wage for ten deaths; (25,000 x 0.24 x 0.05 x 500 x 0.75 x 0.75) + (10 x 0.5 x 15.5765 x 0.75 x 500) + (10 x 15.5765 x 0.75 x 500) = 84,380 + 29,210 + 58,410 = 172,000.

e. Calculated as in note d; (57,000 x 0.24 x 0.05 x 0.75 x 0.75 x 500) + (10 x 0.5 x 15.5765 x 0.75 x 500) + (10 x 15.5765 x 0.75 x 500) = 192,380 + 29,210 + 58,410 = 280,000.

f. Calculated as the product of the number of participants times the rate of deficiency times disability times effectiveness, plus the product of disability times life expectancy for ten cretins, plus the life expectancy for ten deaths; (25,000 x 0.24 x 0.05 x 0.75) + (10 x 0.5 x 29) + 10 x 29 = 225 + 145 + 290 = 660.

g. Calculated as in note f; (93,000 x 0.24 x 0.05 x 0.75) + (10 x 0.5 x 29) + 10 x 29 = 837 + 145 + 290 = 1270.

h. Calculalated as in note f; (99,980 x 0.24 x 0.05 x 0.75) + (10 x 0.5 x 29) + 10 x 29 = 900 + 145 + 290 = 1335.

Source: Table 19E-1 using methodology described in d (above).

Table 19E-5. Cost and Effectiveness of Vitamin A Intervention

Parameter	Vitamin A supplementation[a]	Vitamin A fortification
Target group	Children under five	Entire population
Number	13,000	100,000
Average rate of vitamin A deficiency (percent)[b]	15	15
Per capita cost (U.S. dollars)[c]	0.50	0.20
Program effectiveness (percent)	75	75
Deaths averted (number)	20	20
Blindness averted (number)		
Total	4	4
Partial	8	8
Productivity loss (percent)		
Totally blind	50	50
Partially blind	25	25
Program duration	Year round	Year round
Program costs (U.S. dollars)	6,500	20,000[d]
Discounted wage gains (U.S. dollars)	140,188[d]	140,188[d]
DALY gained	696[e]	696[e]
Wage gain divided by program cost (U.S. dollars)	21.6	7.0
Cost per DALY (U.S. dollars)	9.3	29
Cost per death averted (U.S. dollars)	325	1,000

Note: Based on assumptions in table 19E-1.

a. Semiannual mass dose.   b. In children under five.   c. Per participant.

d. Does not include losses due to excess child morbidity. Calculated as the product of the number of deaths averted times the productive life expectancy times employment times wage, plus the product of the number of total blindness averted times productive life expectancy times disability times employment times wage, plus the product of the number of partial blindness averted times productive life expectancy times disability times employment times wage; (20 x 15.5765 x 0.75 x 500) + (4 x 15.5765 x 0.5 x 0.75 x 500) + (8 x 15.5765 x 0.25 x 0.75 x 500) = 116,824 + 11,682 + 11,682 = 140,188.

e. Calculated as deaths averted times discounted remaining life expectancy plus total blindness times disability times discounted remaining life expectancy plus partial blindness times disability times discounted remaining life expectancy; (20 x 29) + (4 x 0.5 x 29) + (8 x 0.25 x 29) = 696.

Source: Based on authors' assumptions.

Notes

1. In developing countries, 50 percent of children from birth to fourteen years, 25 percent of adult men and women, and 63 percent of pregnant women are iron deficient; 24 percent of the total population are iodine deficient, and 0.4 percent is cretinous because of iodine deficiency; 15 percent of children under five are deficient, 2.5 percent are severely deficient in vitamin A, 1.4 percent die of severe deficiency, 0.28 percent become totally blind, and 0.66 percent become partially blind.

Thirteen percent of the population of developing countries are under five years of age; 21 percent are five through fourteen; 57 percent are economically active adults, 44 percent of whom are women of reproductive age of whom 16 percent are pregnant; 7 percent are sixty years of age or over. Adults were assumed to be economically active between fifteen and fifty-nine years of age.

Excess mortality due to severe vitamin A deficiency was assumed to be 1 percent of the target age group, or about 41 percent of the severely deficient children; excess mortality due to iron deficiency was assumed to be 1 out of 400 pregnant women; excess mortality due to iodine deficiency was assumed to be 1 neonatal death out of 96 pregnancies of iodine-deficient women.

Partial blindness: 25 percent disability; total blindness: 50 percent disability; iron deficiency: 20 percent disability; iodine deficiency: 5 percent disability; cretinism: 50 percent disability.

Iron supplementation: $2.00 per pregnancy; iron fortification: $0.20 per capita per year; iodine supplementation: $0.50 per recipient per year; iodine fortification: $0.10 per capita per year; vitamin A supplementation: $0.50 per recipient per year; vitamin A fortification: $0.20 per capita per year.

References

Arroyave, G. 1982. "The Program of Fortification of Sugar with Vitamin A in Guatemala." In N. S. Scrimshaw and M. Wallerstein, eds., *Nutrition Policy and Implementation*. New York: Plenum Press.

Arroyave, G., J. R. Aguilar, M. Flores, and M. A. Guzman. 1979. "Evaluation of Sugar Fortification with Vitamin A at the National Level." Scientific Publication 384. Pan-American Health Organization, Institute of Nutrition of Central America and Panama, Washington, D.C.

Assami, M., S. Hercberg, S. Assami, P. Galan, A. Assami, and G. Potier de Courcy. 1988. "Iron and Folate Status in Algerian Pregnant Women." *Ecology of Food and Nutrition* 21:181–87.

Aukett, M. A., Y. A. Parks, P. H. Scott, and B. A. Wharton. 1986. "Treatment with Iron Increases Weight Gain and Psychomotor Development." *Archives of Disease in Childhood* 61:849–57.

Austin, J. E., T. K. Balding, D. Pyle, F. S. Solar, T. L. Fernandez, M. D. Latham, and B. M. Popkin. 1981. *Nutrition Intervention in Developing Countries: Fortification*. Study 3. Cambridge, Mass.: Gunn and Hain.

Bagchi, K., M. Mohanram, and V. Reddy. 1980. "Humoral Immune Response in Children with Iron-Deficiency Anemia." *British Medical Journal* 280:1249–51.

Baker, S. J., and E. M. DeMaeyer. 1979. "Nutritional Anemia: Its Understanding and Control with Special Reference to the Work of the World Health Organization." *American Journal of Clinical Nutrition* 32:368–417.

Baly, D. L., M. S. Golub, M. E. Gershwin, and L. S. Hurley. 1984. "Studies of Marginal Zinc Deprivation in Rhesus Monkeys. 3. Effects of Vitamin A Metabolism." *American Journal of Clinical Nutrition* 40:199–207.

Barden, H. S., and R. Kessel. 1985. "The Costs and Benefits of Screening for Congenital Hypothyroidism in Wisconsin." *Social Biology* 31:185–200.

Basta, S., D. Soekirman, D. Karyadi, and N. S. Scrimshaw. 1979. "Iron Deficiency Anemia and the Productivity of Adult Males in Indonesia." *American Journal of Clinical Nutrition* 32:916–25.

Bautista, A., P. A. Barker, J. T. Dunn, M. Sanchez, and D. L. Kaiser. 1982. "The Effects of Oral Iodized Oil on Intelligence, Thyroid Status, and Somatic Growth in School-Age Children from an Area of Endemic Goiter." *American Journal of Clinical Nutrition* 35:127–34.

Beaton, G. H., and J. M. Bengoa. 1976. *Nutrition in Preventative Medicine*. Geneva: WHO Nutrition Unit.

Bender, D., and D. Yoder. 1983. *The Village Health Worker in Review: An Annotated Bibliography*. Monticello, Ill.: Vance Bibliographies.

Berg, Alan, and Susan Brems. 1986. "Micronutrient Deficiencies: Present Knowledge on Effects and Control." Technical Notes 32. Population, Health and Nutrition Department, World Bank, Washington, D.C.

Bloem, M. W., M. Wedel, E. J. van Agtmaal, A. J. Speek, S. Saowakortha, and W. H. P. Schreurs. 1990. "Vitamin A Interventions: Short-Term Effects of a Single, Oral, Massive Dose on Iron Metabolism." *American Journal of Clinical Nutrition* 51:76–79.

Bothwell, T. H., and R. W. Charlton. 1991. *Iron Deficiency in Women*. International Nutritional Anemia Consultative Group, Washington, D.C.

Brabin, B. J. 1988. "Consequences of Maternal Anemia on Fetal and Early Infant Development in a Malaria Endemic Area: Perinatal Morbidity and Mortality." Paper presented at the International Nutritional Anemia Consultative Group meeting on Anemia and Pregnancy, November 14–16, 1988. Geneva.

Chafkin, S. 1984. "A Note on Iron Deficiency and World Bank Consideration Thereof." Unpublished report. Population Health and Nutrition Department, World Bank, Washington, D.C.

Chandra, R. K. 1973. "Reduced Bactericidal Capacity of Polymorphs in Iron Deficiency." *Archives of Disease in Childhood* 48:864–66.

———, ed. 1988. *Nutrition and Immunology*. New York: Alan B. Liss.

Chandra, R. K., and B. Au. 1981. "Single Nutrient Deficiency and Cell-Mediated Immune Responses. 3. Vitamin A." *Nutrition Research* 1:181–85.

Chandra, R. K., and S. Puri. 1985. "Trace Element Modulation of Immune Responses and Susceptibility to Infection." In R. J. Chandra, ed., *Trace Elements in Nutrition and Children*. Nestle Nutrition Workshop Series, no. 8. New York: Raven Press.

Charoenlarp, P., S. Dhanamitta, R. Kacwvichit, A. Silprasert, C. Suwanaradd, S. Na-Nakorn, P. Prawatmuang, S. Vatanavicharn, U. Nutcharas, P. Pootrakul, V. Tanphaichitr, U. Thanangkul, T. Vaniyapong, Thane Toe, A. Valyasevi, S. Baker, J. Cook, E. M. DeMaeyer, L. Garby, and L. Hallberg. 1988. "A WHO Collaborative Study on Iron Supplementation in Burma and Thailand." *American Journal of Clinical Nutrition* 47:280–97.

Chwang, L., A. G. Soemantri, and E. Pollitt. 1988. "Iron Supplementation and Physical Growth of Rural Indonesian Children." *American Journal of Clinical Nutrition* 47:496–501.

Clugston, G. A., E. M. Dulberg, C. S. Pandav, and R. L. Tilden. 1987. "Iodine Deficiency Disorders in South East Asia." In B. S. Hetzel, J. T. Dunn, and J. B. Stanbury, eds., *The Prevention and Control of Iodine Deficiency Disorders*. New York: Elsevier.

Clydesdale, F. M., and K. L. Wiemer, eds. 1985. *Iron Fortification of Foods*. Orlando, Fla.: Academic Press.

Cohen, N., H. Rahman, J. Sprague, M. A. Jahil, E. Leemhuis de Regt, and M. Mitra. 1985. "Prevalence and Determinants of Nutritional Blindness in Bangladeshi Children." *World Health Statistics Quarterly* 38:317–30.

Cook, J. D., and M. E. Reusser. 1983. "Iron Fortification: An Update." *American Journal of Clinical Nutrition* 38:648–59.

Correa, H. 1980. "A Cost-Benefit Study of Iodine Supplementation Programs for the Prevention of Endemic Goiter and Cretinism." In J. B. Stanbury and B. S. Hetzel, eds., *Endemic Goiter and Endemic Cretinism*. New York: Wiley.

Creese, A. L. 1983. "The Economic Evaluation of Immunization Programmes." In K. Lee and A. Mills, eds., *The Economics of Health in Developing Countries*. New York: Oxford University Press.

Creese, A. L., and R. H. Henderson. 1980. "Cost-Benefit Analysis and Immunization Programmes in Developing Countries." *Bulletin of the World Health Organization* 58:491–97.

Creese, A. L., N. Sriyabbaya, G. Casabal, and G. Wiseso. 1982. "Cost-Effectiveness Appraisal of Immunization Programmes." *Bulletin of the World Health Organization* 60:621–32.

Dallman, P. R. 1987. "Iron Deficiency and the Immune Response." *American Journal of Clinical Nutrition* 46:329–34.

Daeschner, C. W., III, M. C. Matustik, U. Carpentieri, and M. E. Hagggard. 1981. "Zinc and Growth in Patients with Sickle Cell Anemia Disease." *Journal of Pediatrics* 98:778–80.

Delong, R. 1987. "Neurological Involvement in Iodine Deficiency Disorders." In B. S. Hetzel, J. T. Dunn, and J. B. Stanbury, eds., *The Prevention and Control of Iodine Deficiency Disorders*. New York: Elsevier.

DeMaeyer, E. 1986. "Xerophthalmia and Blindness of Nutritional Origin in the Third World." Children in the Tropics 165. International National Children's Centre, Paris.

———. 1989. "Preventing and Controlling Iron Deficiency Anaemia through Primary Health Care." WHO Nutrition Unit, Geneva.

DeMaeyer, E., and M. Adiels-Tegman. 1985. "The Prevalence of Anemia in the World." *World Health Statistics Quarterly* 38:302–16.

Derman, D. P., M. H. Sayers, S. R. Lynch, R. W. Charlton, T. H. Bothwell, and F. G. H. Mayet. 1977. "Iron Absorption from Cereal-Based Meal Containing Cane Sugar Fortified with Ascorbic Acid." *British Journal of Nutrition* (2):261–69.

Djukanovic, V., and E. P. Mach, eds. 1975. *Alternative Approaches to Meeting Basic Health Needs in Developing Countries*. Joint United Nations Children's Fund/World Health Organization Study. Geneva.

Dunn, J. T. 1987. "Iodized Oil in the Treatment and Prophylaxis of IDD." In B. S. Hetzel, J. T. Dunn, and J. B. Stanbury, eds., *The Prevention and Control of Iodine Deficiency Disorders*. New York: Elsevier.

Dunn J., ed. 1989a. "Status of IDD." IDD (International Council for Control of Iodine Deficiency Disorders) *Newsletter* 5:1.

———. 1989b. "IDD in Southeast Asia." IDD (International Council for Control of Iodine Deficiency Disorders) *Newsletter* 5(2):1–24.

———. 1989c. "Staus of IDD Control in Ten East, Central and South African Countries." IDD (International Council for Control of Iodine Deficiency Disorders) *Newsletter* 5(1):1–8.

Eastman, S. J. 1987. "Vitamin A: Deficiency and Xerophthalmia: Recent Findings and Some Programme Implications." *Assignment Children* 1987-3 UNICEF, New York.

FAO (Food and Agriculture Organization). 1965. "Report of a Joint FAO/WHO Expert Group on Vitamin A." FAO Food Policy and Nutrition Division/WHO Nutrition Unit.

———. 1970. "Report of a Joint FAO/WHO Expert Group on Iron." FAO Food Policy and Nutrition Division/WHO Nutrition Unit.

———. 1989. "Nutrition Country Profiles, 1988–89." Food Policy and Nutrition Division.

Fleming, A. F. 1989. "Consequences of Anaemia in Pregnancy on the Mothers." Liverpool School of Tropical Medicine, Department of Tropical Medicine and Infectious Diseases, Liverpool, Eng.

Florentino, R. F. 1988. "Nutritional Anemia Control Program in the Philippines." Case Study presented at the International Nutritional Anemia Consultative Group (INACG), November 14.

Florentino, R. F., and R. M. Guirriec. 1984. "Prevalence of Nutritional Anemia in Infancy and Childhood with Emphasis on Developing Countries." In Abraham Stekel, ed., *Iron Nutrition in Infancy and Childhood*. Nestle Nutrition Workshop Series 4. New York: Raven Press.

Gaitan, J. E., L. G. Mayoral, and E. Gaitan. 1983. "Defective Thyroidal Iodine Concentration in Protein Calorie Malnutrition." *Journal of Clinical Endocrinology and Metabolism* 57:327–33.

Gardner, G. W., V. R. Edgerton, B. Senewiratne, R. J. Barnard, and Y. Ohira. 1977. "Physical Work Capacity and Metabolic Stress in Subjects with Iron Deficiency Anemia." *American Journal of Clinical Nutrition* 30:910–17.

Greene, L. S. 1977. "Hyperendemic Goiter, Cretinism, and Social Organization in Highland Ecuador." In L. S. Greene, ed., *Malnutrition, Behavior, and Social Organization*. New York: Academic Press.

Griffiths, M. 1980. Concept Testing Nutrition Communication and Behavior Change Components. Vol. 1. Unpublished report on the Indonesia Nutrition Development Program. Manoff International.

Hallberg, L. 1981. "Effect of Vitamin C on the Bioavailability of Iron from Food." In J. N. Counsell and D. H. Hornig, eds., *Vitamin C*. Englewood, N.J.: Applied Science Publishers.

Harrison, K. A. 1975. "Maternal Mortality in Anemia in Pregnancy." *West African Medical Journal*: 27–31.

Hercberg, S., P. Galan, M. Chauliac, A. M. Masse-Raimbault, M. Devanlay, S. Bileoma, E. Alihonou, I. Zohoun, J. P. Christides, and G. Potier de Courcy. 1987. "Nutritional Anaemia in Pregnant Beninese Women: Consequences on the Haematological Profile of the Newborn." *British Journal of Nutrition* 57:185–94.

Hetzel, B. S., ed. 1978. *Basic Health Care in Developing Countries: An Epidemiological Perspective*. Oxford: Oxford University Press.

———. 1983. "Iodine Deficiency Disorders and Their Eradication." *Lancet* 2(8359):1126–29.

———. 1987. "An Overview of the Prevention and Control of Iodine Deficiency." In B. S. Hetzel, J. T. Dunn, and J. B. Stanbury, eds., *The Prevention and Control of Iodine Deficiency Disorders*. New York: Elsevier.

———. 1988. "The Prevention and Control of IDD." State-of-the-Art Series, Nutrition Policy Discussion Paper 3. Administrative Committee on Coordination, Subcommittee on Nutrition, United Nations, New York.

Hetzel, B. S., and G. F. Maberley. 1986. "Iodine." *Trace Elements in Human and Animal Nutrition* 2:139–208.

Hetzel, B. S., and B. J. Potter. 1983. "Iodine Deficiency and the Role of Thyroid Hormones in Brain Development." In I. E. Dreosti and R. M. Smith, eds., *Neurobiology of the Trace Elements*. Vol. 1, *Trace Element Neurobiology and Deficiencies*. Clifton, N.J.: Humana Press.

Hetzel, B. S., C. H. Thilly, R. Fierro-Benitez, E. A. Pretell, I. H. Buttfield, and J. B. Stanbury. 1980. "Iodized Oil in the Prevention of Endemic Goiter and Cretinism." In J. B. Stanbury and B. S. Hetzel, eds., *Endemic Goiter and Endemic Cretinism*. New York: John Wiley and Sons.

Higashi, O., Y. Sato, M. Takamura, and M. Oyama. 1967. "Mean Cellular Peroxidase (MCP) of Leukocytes in Iron Deficiency Anemia." *Tohoku Journal of Experimental Medicine* 93:105–9.

Ho, T. J. 1985. "Economic Issues in Assessing Nutrition Projects: Costs, Affordability, and Cost Effectiveness." Technical Note 85-14. Population, Health, and Nutrition Department, World Bank, Washington, D.C.

Hunt, J. R., L. M. Mullen, G. I. Lykken, S. K. Gallagher, and F. H. Nielsen. 1990. "Ascorbic Acid: Effect on Ongoing Iron Absorption and Status in Iron-Depleted Young Women." *American Journal of Clinical Nutrition* 51:649–55.

ICCIDD/WHO (World Health Organization). 1989. "Report on the Developments in IDD Control in Africa Region." Paper presented at the ICCIDD 4th Annual Meeting, March 11–12, 1989, New Dehli.

INACG (International Nutritional Anemia Consultative Group). 1977. *Guidelines for the Eradication of Iron Deficiency Anemia*. Washington, D.C.

———. 1979. *Iron Deficiency in Infancy and Childhood*. Washington, D.C.

———. 1989. *Guidelines for the Control of Maternal Nutritional Anemia*. Washington, D.C.

Ingenbleek, Y., and M. De Visscher. 1979. "Hormonal and Nutritional Status: Critical Conditions for Endemic Goiter Epidemiology?" *Metabolism* 28(1):9–19.

Irie, M., Kuroda, K. Nakamura, K. Tsuboi, S. Takeda, K. Inoue, K. Enomoto, M. Arifs, P. Adji, and R. Djokomoeljanto. 1986. "Study of Endemic Goiter in Indonesia: Thyroid Function, Goiter Prevalence, and Control Programs." In G. Neto-Medeiros, R. M. B. Maciel, and A. Halpern, eds., *Iodine Deficiency Disorders and Congenital Hypothyroidism*. Ache, Indonesia.

IVACG (International Vitamin A Consultative Group). 1989. "Report on the National Symposium and 13th IVACG Meeting," Katmandu, Nepal, November 5–10.

Kennedy, E. T., and H. H. Alderman. 1987. "Comparative Analyses of Nutritional Effectiveness of Food Subsidies and Other Food-Related Interventions." Joint WHO/UNICEF Nutrition Support Program. International Food Policy Research Institute, Washington, D.C.

Klebanoff, S. J. 1970. "Myeloperoxidase: Contribution to the Microbicidal Activity of Intact Leukocytes." *Science* 169:1095–97.

Ksanga, Pauline, Free Pepping, and Festo Kavishe, comps. 1985. "Proceedings of a Workshop in the Control of Vitamin A Deficiency and Xerophthalmia in Tanzania." Tanzanian Food and Nutrition Center Report 980. Dar es Salaam, Tanzania.

Levin, H. M. 1983. *Cost-Effectiveness: A Primer*. Beverly Hills, Calif.: Sage Publications.

———. 1985. *A Benefit-Cost Analysis of Nutritional Interventions for Anemia Reduction*. Population, Health, and Nutrition Technical Note 12. Population, Health, and Nutrition Department, World Bank, Washington, D.C.

———. 1986. "A Benefit-Cost Analysis of Nutritional Programs for Anemia Reduction." *World Bank Research Observer* 1(2):219–46.

———. 1987. "Economic Dimensions of Iodine Deficiency Disorders." In B. S. Hetzel, J. T. Dunn, and J. B. Stanbury, eds., *The Prevention and Control of Iodine Deficiency Disorders*. New York: Elsevier.

Lieberman, A., K. J. Ryan, R. R. Monson, and S. C. Schoenbaum. 1987. "Risk Factors for Racial Differences in the Rate of Premature Births." *New England Journal of Medicine* 317:743–48.

———. 1988. "Association of Maternal Hematocrit with Premature Labor." *American Journal of Obstetrics and Gynecology* 159:107–114.

Lozoff, B. 1989. "Methodological Issues in Studying Behavioral Effects on Infant Iron-Deficiency Anemia." *American Journal of Clinical Nutrition* 50(supplement):641–54.

Lozoff, B., and G. M. Brittenham. 1985. "Behavioral Aspects of Iron Deficiency." *Progress in Hematology* 14:23–53.

Lozoff, B., G. M. Brittenham, F. E. Viteri, and J. J. Urrutia. 1982. "Behavioral Abnormalities in Infants with Iron Deficiency Anemia." In E. Pollitt and R. Leibel, eds., *Iron Deficiency: Brain Biochemistry and Behavior*. New York: Raven Press, 183–95.

Lozoff, B., G. M. Brittenham, F. E. Viteri, A. W. Wolff, and J. J. Urrutia. 1982. "The Effects of Short-Term Oral Iron Therapy on Developmental Deficits in Iron-Deficient Anemic Infants." *Journal of Pediatrics* 100:351–57.

Macfarlane, B. J., W. B. Vander Riet, T. H. Bothwell, R. D. Baynes, D. Sieganberg, U. Schmidt, A. Tal, J. R. N. Tayler, and F. Mayet. 1990. "Effects of Traditional Oriental Soy Products on Iron Absorption." *American Journal of Clinical Nutrition* 51:873–80.

McMichael, A. J., J. D. Potter, and B. S. Hetzel. 1980. "Iodine Deficiency, Thyroid Function, and Reproductive Failure." In J. B. Stanbury and B. S. Hetzel, eds., *Endemic Goiter and Endemic Cretinism*. New York: Wiley. 445–60.

McLaren, D. S. 1966. "Present Knowledge of the Role of Vitamin A in Health and Disease." *Transactions of the Royal Society of Tropical Medicine and Hygiene*. 60:436–62.

Mamdami, M., and D. A. Ross. 1988. "Vitamin A Supplementation and Child Survival: Magic Bullet or False Hope?" Evaluation and Planning Centre for Health Care, 19. London School of Hygiene and Tropical Medicine.

Mannar, M. G. Venkatesh. 1987. "Control of Iodine Deficiency Disorders by Iodination of Salt: Strategy for Developing Countries." In B. S. Hetzel, J. T. Dunn, and J. B. Stanbury, eds., *The Prevention and Control of Iodine Deficiency Disorders*. New York: Elsevier.

Manoff, R. K. 1987. "Social Marketing: New Tool to Combat Iodine Deficiency Disorders." In B. S. Hetzel, J. T. Dunn, and J. B. Stanbury, eds., *The Prevention and Control of Iodine Deficiency Disorders*. New York: Elsevier.

Marani, L., S. Venturi, and R. Nasala. 1985. "Role of Iodine in Delayed Immune Response." *Israel Journal of Medical Science*. 21:864.

Masani, K. M. 1969. *Proceedings of the International Seminar on Maternal Morbidity, Family Planning, Biology of Reproduction*. Purandare and C. L.

Jhaveri, eds. Bombay: Federation of Obstetric and Gynaecological Societies of India.

Mata, L. 1977. *The Children on Santa Maria Cauque*. Cambridge, Mass.: MIT Press.

Mathur, G. P., and K. P. Kushwaha. 1987. "Vitamin A Deficiency: Review Article." *Indian Pediatrics* 24:573–81.

Medeiros-Neto, G., R. Djokomoeljanto, M. Benmiloud, M. C. DeBlanco, M. Irie, T. Z. Lui, C. R. Ackardt. 1987. "The Monitoring and Evaluation of Iodine Deficiency Control Programs: Report of an ICCIDD Committee." In B. S. Hetzel, J. T. Dunn, and J. B. Stanbury, eds., *Prevention and Control of Iodine Deficiency Disorders*, New York: Elsevier.

Mejia, L. A., and G. Arroyave. 1982. "The Effect of Vitamin A Fortification of Sugar on Iron Metabolism in Preschool Children in Guatemala." *American Journal of Clinical Nutrition* 36:87–93.

Mejia, L. A., and F. Chew. 1988. "Hematological Effect of Supplementing Anemic Children with Vitamin A Alone and in Combination with Iron." *American Journal of Clinical Nutrition* 48:595–600.

Mills, A. 1985. "Economic Evaluation of Health Programmes: Application of the Principles in Developing Countries." *World Health Statistics Quarterly* 38:368–82.

Mishan, E. 1976. *Cost-Benefit Analysis*. New York: Praeger Publishers.

Monsen, E. R., L. Hallberg, M. Layrisse, D. M. Hegsted, J. D. Cook, W. Metz, and C. A. Finch. 1978. "Estimation of Available Dietary Iron." *American Journal of Clinical Nutrition* 31:134–41.

Muhilal, A. Mudeana, E. Azis, S. Saidin, A. B. Jahari, and D. Karyadi. 1988. "Vitamin A-Fortified MSG and Vitamin A Status: A Controlled Field Trial." *American Journal of Clinical Nutrition* 48:1265–70.

Muhilal, D. Permeisih, Y. R. Idjradinata, Muherdiyantiningsih, and D. Karyadi. 1988. "Vitamin A-Fortified MSG and Health, Growth, and Survival of Children: A Controlled Field Trial." *American Journal of Clinical Nutrition* 48:1271–76.

Murphy, J. F., J. O'Riordan, R. G. Newcombe, and E. C. Coles. 1986. "Relation of Haemoglobin Levels in First and Second Trimesters to Outcome of Pregnancy." *Lancet* 1:992–94.

National Academy of Sciences. 1987. "Prevention and Control." Food and Nutrition Board, Committee on International Nutrition Programs, Subcommittee on Vitamin A Deficiency, Washington, D.C.

Nauss, K. M. 1986. "Influence of Vitamin A Status on the Immune System." In J. C. Bauernfeind, ed., *Vitamin A Deficiency and Its Control*. London: Academic Press.

Nishi, Y., F. Lifshitz, M. A. Bayne, F. Daum, M. Silverberg, and H. Aiges. 1980. "Zinc Status and Its Relation to Growth Retardation in Children with Chronic Inflammatory Bowel Disease." *American Journal of Clinical Nutrition* 33:2613–21.

Olson, J. A. 1986. "Physiological and Metabolic Basis of Major Signs of Vitamin A Deficiency." In J. C. Bauernfeind, ed., *Vitamin A Deficiency and Its Control*. London: Academic Press.

Oski, F. A., A. S. Honig, B. Helu, and P. Howanitz. 1983. "Effect of Iron Therapy on Behavior Performance in Nonanemic, Iron Deficient Infants." *Pediatrics* 71:877–80.

PAHO (Pan-American Health Organization)/WHO (World Health Organization)/UNICEF (United Nations Children's Fund). 1988. "Expanded Program for the Control of Iodine Deficiency Disorders in Latin America." Washington, D.C.

Pardo, A. S. 1990. "The Pronalcobo: The National Program to Fight against Goiter in Bolivia." A Case Study prepared for the Population, Health, and Nutrition Division, World Bank, Washington, D.C.

Pharoah, P. O. D., K. J. Connolly, R. P. Ekins, and A. B. Harding. 1984. "Maternal Thyroid Hormone Levels in Pregnancy and the Subsequent Cognitive and Motor Performance of the Children." *Clinical Endocrinology* 21:265–70.

Pollitt, Ernesto. 1987. "Effects of Iron Deficiency on Mental Development: Methodological Considerations and Substantive Findings." In F. Johnston, ed., *Nutritional Anthropology*. New York: Alan R. Liss.

————. 1989. "Report of a Mission on a Nutrition Component for the World Bank's Basic Education Project in the Dominican Republic." Population and Human Resources Department, World Bank, Washington, D.C.

————. 1990. *Malnutrition and Infection in the Classroom*. Paris: UNESCO.

Pollitt, Ernesto, and R. Leibel, eds. 1982. *Iron Deficiency: Brain Biochemistry and Behavior*. New York: Raven Press.

Popkin, B. M., F. S. Solon, T. Fernandez, and M. C. Latham. 1980. "Benefit-Cost Analysis in the Nutrition Area: A Project in the Philippines." *Social Science and Medicine* 14:207–16.

Prasad, A. S. 1979. "Leucocyte Function in Iron-Deficiency Anemia." *American Journal of Clinical Nutrition* 32:550–52.

Prual, A., P. Galan, L. De Berris, and S. Hercberg. 1988. "Evaluation of Iron Status in Chadian Pregnant Women: Consequences of Maternal Iron Deficiency on the Haemotopoietic Status of Newborns." *Tropical Geographical Medicine* 40:1–6.

Rahmathullah, Laxmi, Barbara Underwood, Ravilla Thulasiraj, Roy Milton, Kala Ramaswamy, Raheem Rahmathulleh, and Ganeesh Babu. 1990. "Reduced Mortality among Children in Southern India Receiving a Small Weekly Dose of Vitamin A." *New England Journal of Medicine* 323(14):929–35.

Schaefer, A. E. 1974. "Status of Salt Iodination in PAHO Member Countries." In J. T. Dunn and G. A. Medeiros-Neto, eds., *Endemic Goiter and Cretinism: Continuing Threats to World Health*. Report on the 4th Meeting of the Pan-American Health Organization Technical Group in Endemic Goiter. Pan-American Health Organization, Pan-American Sanitary Bureau, Regional Office of the World Health Organization, Washington, D.C.

Scrimshaw, N. S. 1984. "Functional Consequences of Iron Deficiency in Human Populations." *Journal of Nutritional Sciences and Vitaminology* 30:47–63.

Seshadri, S., and T. Gopaldas. N.d. "Magnitude and Implication of the Problem of Nutritional Anemia." University of Baroda, India, Department of Food and Nutrition.

————. 1989. "Impact of Iron Supplementation on Cognitive Functions in Preschool and School-Aged Children: The Indian Experience." *American Journal of Clinical Nutrition* 50(supplement):675–86.

Shils, M. E., and V. R. Young. 1988. *Modern Nutrition in Health and Disease*. Philadelphia: Lea and Febiger.

Simmons, W. K. 1990. "Evaluation of a Novel Delayed-Release Formulation for Iron Supplementation in Pregnancy." Report 5. International Center for Research on Women. Washington, D.C.

Soewondo, M., M. Husaini, and E. Pollitt. 1989. "Effects of Iron Deficiency on Attention and Learning Processes in Preschool Children: Bandung, Indonesia." *American Journal of Clinical Nutrition* 50(supplement):667–74.

de Sole, B., Y. Belay, and B. Zegeye. 1987. "Vitamin A Deficiency in Southern Ethiopia." *American Journal of Clinical Nutrition*, 45:780–84.

Solon, F., R. Florentino, M. Latham, T. Fernandez, I. Panopio, and R. Guirriec. 1983. "Pilot MSG Fortification for the Control of Vitamin A Deficiency in the Philippines." In V. Tanphaichitr, W. Dahlan, V. Supharkarn, and A. Valyasevi, eds., *Human Nutrition: Better Nutrition, Better Life: Proceedings of the 4th Asian Congress of Nutrition, Bangkok*. Bangkok: Aksornsmai Press.

Sommer, A. 1982. *Nutritional Blindness: Xerophthalmia and Keratomalacia*. New York: Oxford University Press.

Sommer, A., E. Djunaedi, A. A. Loeden, I. Tarwotjo, K. P. West, R. Tilden, and L. Mele. 1986. "Impact of Vitamin A Supplementation on Childhood Mortality." *Lancet* 1:1169–73.

Sommer, A., J. Katz, and I. Tarwotjo. 1984. "Increased Risk of Respiratory Disease and Diarrhea in Children with Preexisting Mild Vitamin A Deficiency." *American Journal of Clinical Nutrition* 40:1090–95.

Sommer Alfred, Ignatius Tarwotjo, Gusti Hussaini, and Djoko Susanto. 1983. "Increased Mortality in Children with Mild Vitamin A Deficiency." *Lancet* (September 10):585–88.

Squatrito, S., R. Vigneri, F. Runello, A. M. Ermans, R. D. Polley, and S. H. Ingbar. 1986. "Prevention and Treatment of Endemic Iodine-Deficiency Goiter by Iodination of a Municipal Water Supply." *Journal of Clinical Endocrinology and Metabolism* 63:368–75.

Srikantia, S. G., C. Bhaskaram, J. S. Prasad, and K. A. V. R. Krishnamachari. 1976. "Anaemia and Immune Response." *Lancet* 2:307–9.

Stanbury, J. B. 1987. "The Iodine Deficiency Disorder: Introduction and General Aspects." In B. S. Hetzel, J. T. Dunn, and J. B. Stanbury, eds., *The Prevention and Control of Iodine Deficiency Disorders*. New York: Elsevier.

Stanton, B. F., J. D. Clemens, B. Wojtyniak, and T. Khair. 1986. "Risk Factors for Developing Mild Nutritional Blindness in Urban Bangladesh." *American Journal of Diseases of Childhood* 140:584–88.

Stekel, A. 1987. *Iron Nutrition in Infancy and Childhood*. Nestle Nutrition Workshop Series. New York: Raven Press.

Stephenson, L. S. 1987. *The Impact of Helminth Infections on Human Nutrition*. London: Taylor and Francis.

Stephenson, L. S., M. C. Latham, K. M. Kurz, D. Miller, S. N. Kinoti, and M. L. Oduori. 1985. "Urinary Iron Loss and Physical Fitness of Kenyan Children with Urinary Schistosomiasis." *American Journal of Tropical Medicine and Hygiene* 34:322–30.

Suhardjo. 1986. *The Effect of Iron Intervention on Work Productivity of Tea Pickers*. Bogor Agricultural University, Faculty of Agriculture, Bogor, Indonesia.

Talbot, M. C., L. T. Miller, and N. I. Kerkvlirt. 1987. "Pyridoxine Supplementation: Effect on Lymphocyte Responses in Elderly Persons." *American Journal of Clinical Nutrition* 46:659–64.

The Task Force for Child Survival. 1989. "Iodine Deficiency." *World Immunization News* 5(4):24–25.

Thilly, C. H. 1981. "Goitre et crétinisme endémiques: rôle étiologique de la consommation de manioc et stratégie d'éradication." *Bulletin de Académie Royale de Médecine Belgique* 136:389–412.

Thilly, C. H., and B. S. Hetzel. 1980. "An Assessment of Prophylactic Programs: Social, Political, Cultural, and Economic Issues." In J. B. Stanbury and B. S. Hetzel, eds., *Endemic Goiter and Endemic Cretinism*. New York: John Wiley and Sons.

Thilly, C. H., R. Lagasse, G. Roger, P. Bourdoux, and A. M. Ermans. 1980. "Impaired Fetal and Postnatal Development and High Perinatal Death-Rate in a Severe Iodine Deficient Area." In J. R. Stockigt and S. Nagataki, eds., *Thyroid Research 8. Proceedings of the Eighth International Thyroid Congress*. Canberra: Australian Academy of Science.

Tielsch, J. M., and A. Sommer. 1984. "The Epidemiology of Vitamin A Deficiency and Xerophthalmia." *Annual Review of Nutrition* 4:183–285.

Tilden, R. L., and R. N. Grosse. 1988. "Vitamin A Cost-Effectiveness Model." School of Public Health, University of Michigan, Ann Arbor. Typescript.

Tomkins, A., and F. Watson. 1989. *Malnutrition and Infection*. State-of-the-Art ser., Nutrition Policy Discussion Paper 5. Administrative Committee on Coordination, Subcommittee on Nutrition, United Nations, New York.

Underwood, B. A. 1983. *Nutrition Intervention Strategies in National Development*. New York: Academic Press.

————. 1986. "The Safe Use of Vitamin A by Women during Reproductive Years." Pamphlet from IVACG Secretariat, Washington, D.C.

————. 1989. Paper presented at International Vitamin A Consultative Group (IVACG) Annual Meeting, Kathmandu, Nepal.

UNICEF (United Nations Children's Fund). 1988. "Support to Vitamin A Deficiency Control Programs." New York.

United Nations. 1985. "Prevention and Control of Vitamin A Deficiency, Xerophthalmia, and Nutritional Blindness." Proposal for a ten-year program of support to countries. Administrative Committee on Coordination, Subcommittee on Nutrition, New York.

————. 1987. "A Global Strategy for the Prevention and Control of Iodine-Deficiency Disorders." Proposal for a ten-year program to support countries. Administrative Committee on Coordination, Subcommittee on Nutrition, New York.

————. 1990. "Controlling Iron Deficiency—Report of Joint ACC/SCN Workshop on Iron Deficiency Control, June 6–8, 1990. Dublin, Ireland." Administrative Committee on Coordination, Subcommittee on Nutrition, New York.

Valyasevi, Arec. 1988. "Delivery System for Iron Supplementation in Pregnant Women—Thailand Experience." Paper presented at the INACG (International Nutritional Anemia Consultative Group) Workshop November 14–16. Geneva.

Viteri, F. E., E. Alvarez, J. Bulux, H. Gonzalez, O. Pineda, L. Mejia, R. Batres, and B. Torun. 1981. "Iron Fortification in Developing Countries." *Progress in Clinical and Biological Research* 77:345–54.

Wallingford, J. C., and B. A. Underwood. 1986. "Vitamin A Deficiency in Pregnancy, Lactation, and the Nursing Child." In J. C. Bauernfeind, ed., *Vitamin A Deficiency and Its Control.* New York: Academic Press.

Walter, T. 1989. "Infancy: Mental and Motor Development." *American Journal of Clinical Nutrition* 50:655–61.

Walter, T., S. Arredondo, M. Arevalo, and A. Stekel. 1986. "Effect of Iron Therapy on Phagocytosis and Bactericidal Activity in Neutrophils of Iron-Deficient Infants." *American Journal of Clinical Nutrition* 44:877–82.

West, K. P., Jr., and A. Sommer. 1984. *Periodic, Large, Oral Doses of Vitamin A for the Prevention of Vitamin A Deficiency and Xerophthalmia: A Summary of Experiences.* Report of the International Vitamin A Consultative Group. The Nutrition Foundation, Washington, D.C.

————. 1987. *Delivery of Oral Doses of Vitamin A to Prevent Vitamin A Deficiency and Nutritional Blindness.* State-of-the-Art Series, Nutrition Policy Discussion Paper 2. Administrative Committee on Coordination, Subcommittee on Nutrition, United Nations, New York.

Wittpenn, J., and A. Sommer. 1986. "Clinical Aspects of Vitamin A Deficiency." In J. C. Bauernfeind, ed., *Vitamin A Deficiency and Its Control.* New York: Academic Press.

WHO (World Health Organization). 1979. *Training Utilization of Auxiliary Personnel for Rural Health Teams in Developing Countries.* Technical Report 633. Geneva.

————. 1982. "Control of Vitamin A Deficiency and Xerophthalmia." Technical Report 672. WHO Nutrition Unit, Geneva.

————. 1988. "Global Status for Vitamin A Deficiency." Geneva.

————. 1989. "Global Status of Iodine Deficiency Disorders." 1989. Report for World Health Assembly. WHO Nutrition Unit, Geneva. Typescript.

————. 1990. "Global Status of IDD." Report for World Health Assembly. WHO Nutrition Unit, Geneva. Typescript.

WHO (World Health Organization)/EPI (Expanded Programme on Immunization). 1987. *Potential Contribution of the Expanded Programme on Immunization to the Control of Vitamin A Deficiency and Iodine Deficiency Disorders.* Paper presented at the EPI Global Advisory Group Meeting, November 9–13, 1987, Washington, D.C.

————. 1988a. *Global Situation of Vitamin A Deficiency.* Geneva: WHO Nutrition Unit.

————. 1988b. *Programmes for the Control of Vitamin A Deficiency: The Role of the EPI in New Initiatives for the 1990s.* Geneva: WHO Nutrition Unit.

WHO (World Health Organization)/UNICEF (United Nations Children's Fund). 1987. "Joint Statement on Vitamin A for Measles." International Nursing Review 35(1):21.

Working Group on Fortification of Salt with Iron. 1982. "Use of Common Salt Fortified with Iron in the Control and Prevention of Anemia—A Collaborative Study." *American Journal of Clinical Nutrition* 35:1442–51.

Yan-You, W., and Y. Shu-Hua. 1985. "Improvement in Hearing among Otherwise Normal Schoolchildren in Iodine-Deficient Areas of Guizhou, China, Following Use of Iodised Salt." *Lancet* 2:518–19.

Yepez, R., A. Calle, P. Galan, E. Estevez, M. Davila, R. Estrella, A. Masse-Raimbault, and S. Hercberg. 1987. "Iron Status in Ecuadorian Pregnant Women Living at 2800 m. Altitude: Relationship with Infant Iron Status." *International Journal of Vitamin and Nutrition Research* 57:327–32.

PART FOUR

Emerging Problems

Sexually Transmitted Diseases
Cancers
Diabetes
Cardiovascular Disease
Injury
Cataract
Oral Health
Schizophrenia and Manic-Depressive Illness

20

HIV Infection and Sexually Transmitted Diseases

Mead Over and Peter Piot

The health programs of developing countries have not traditionally accorded a high priority to the prevention and control of diseases which are predominantly transmitted by sexual intercourse. With the realization that sex is the primary mode of transmission for the human immunodeficiency virus (HIV), however, international donors are helping national health ministries of developing countries allocate large human and financial resources to the fight against at least one sexually transmitted disease (STD). In many cases these programs for the prevention of acquired immunodeficiency syndrome (AIDS) are large enough to rival preexisting programs to prevent other diseases, like malaria and measles, which currently kill more people in most of these countries. By supporting this proposed expenditure pattern, the international donors and national health ministries have implicitly raised the priority attached to the prevention of STDs far above the position formerly occupied by this class of diseases. In addition, because of a growing awareness that at least one important cancer (cervical cancer) and a significant proportion of maternal morbidity and mortality result from STDs, there is a renewed interest in STD control in the public health community.

Our objective in this chapter is to examine the case for assigning a high priority to the prevention (primary and secondary) of the spread of STDs, including AIDS and its causative agent, HIV. Although it would be possible and in some ways more convenient to separate the discussion of AIDS from that of other STDs, a central theme of this chapter is the examination of the epidemiological, medical, and economic arguments for integrating AIDS prevention efforts with efforts to combat other STDs. Furthermore, the transmission dynamics of all STDs have strong similarities, which benefit from a common analytical examination. These considerations lead us to address AIDS and "classic STDs," or CSTDs, in the same chapter but often to separate the discussions into different sections.

The Epidemiology of STDs

Both CSTDs and HIV are mainly transmitted through sexual intercourse, although in many cases they may also be transmitted vertically from mother to child or by blood contact. More than fifty CSTDs have now been recognized, many of which were identified only during the last decades, partly as a result of improved laboratory techniques.

Distinctive Features of STD Epidemiology

A list of common sexually transmitted agents and the diseases they cause are presented in table 20-1. In this chapter, we focus on HIV infection and on selected CSTDs, including gonorrhea, genital chlamydial infections, syphilis, and chancroid. The contribution of the sexually transmitted human papilloma viruses to the causation of cervical cancer will not be discussed, although both in Africa and in Latin America the incidence of cervical cancer is among the highest in the world, and sexual activity is the main risk factor for this common neoplasm (Reeves, Brinton, and Brenes 1985; Rosenberg, Schultz, and Burton 1986; and Reeves, Rawls, and Brinton 1989).

An in-depth discussion of the biology and epidemiology of even the main STDs is beyond the scope of this chapter but can be found in several textbooks and monographs (Osoba 1987; Arya, Osoba, and Bennett 1988; Holmes and others 1989). Appendix 20A includes a summary of medical information on the individual diseases considered here.

The epidemiology of STDs is distinctive because of common behavioral and biological features. First, STDs typically have long latent or incubation periods before symptoms become apparent, during which transmission can occur. Second, the genetic structure of most STD agents varies so much that researchers have been unable to design a vaccine against them. Third, STDs are primarily spread by a class of behavior which is inherently resistant to change, because it is highly motivated, often clandestine, and varies so much both within and between social and ethnic groups.

A common biological feature of many of the microorganisms causing STDs is their unique and often exclusive adaptation to humans, the main mode of transmission being genital mucosal contact—for example, sex in most instances. Whether a microbial agent is mainly sexually transmitted in a given population, however, depends not only on its biology but also on behavioral and environmental conditions. Thus, in many developing societies some infections are mainly acquired in childhood because of low hygienic standards or poor living conditions,

Table 20-1. Important Sexually Transmitted Agents and Diseases

Agents	Disease or syndrome
Bacteria	
Neisseria gonorrhoeae	Urethritis, epididymitis, proctitis, bartholinitis, cervicitis, endometritis, salpingitis and related sequelae (infertility, ectopic pregnancy), perihepatitis; complications of pregnancy (e.g., chorioamnionitis, premature rupture of membranes, premature delivery, postpartum endometritis); conjunctivitis; disseminated gonococcal infection (DGI)
Chlamydia trachomatis	Same as *N. gonorrhoeae*, except for DGI; also trachoma, lymphogranuloma venereum, Reiter's syndrome, infant pneumonia
Treponema pallidium	Syphilis
Haemophilus ducreyi	Chancroid
Mycoplasma hominis	Postpartum fever, salpingitis
Ureaplasma urealyticum	Urethritis; low birth weight,,[a] chorioamnionitis[a]
Gardnerella vaginalis and others	Bacterial vaginosis
Calymmatobacterium granulomatis	Donovanosis
Group B β-hemolytic streptococcus[a]	Neonatal sepsis, neonatal meningitis
Viruses	
Herpes simplex virus	Primary and recurrent genital herpes; aseptic meningitis; neonatal herpes and associated mortality or neurological sequelae; spontaneous abortion, premature delivery
Hepatitis B virus	Acute, chronic, and fulminant hepatitis B, with associated immune complex phenomena and sequelae, including cirrhosis and hepatocellular carcinoma
Cytomegalovirus	Congenital infection; gross birth defects and infant mortality, cognitive impairment (e.g., mental retardation, sensorineural deafness); heterophile-negative infectious mononucleosis; protean manifestations in the immunosuppressed host
Human papilloma virus	Condyloma acuminata, laryngeal papilloma in infants; squamous epithelial neoplasias of the cervix, anus, vagina, vulva, and penis
Molluscum contagiosum virus	Genital molluscum contagiosum
Human immunodeficiency virus	AIDS and related conditions
HTLV-1 (Human T-lymphotropic virus)	T-cell leukemia, lymphoma; tropical spastic paraparesis
Protozoon: Trichomonas vaginalis	Vaginitis; urethritis,[a] balanitis[a]
Fungus: Candida albicans	Vulvovaginitis, balanitis, balanoposthitis
Ectoparasites	
Phthirius pubis	Pubic lice infestation
Sarcoptes scabiei	Scabies

a. Causative relationship uncertain.
Source: Based on compilation of the literature.

whereas in industrial countries the same infections are mainly sexually transmitted among adults (hepatitis B, cytomegalovirus infection). In general, infections become more often sexually transmitted with an increasing standard of living, because opportunities for person-to-person transmission are decreasing during childhood.

Risk factors for STDs are directly related to patterns of sexual behavior. They include a large number of sex partners, a history of STDs, urban residence, being single, and being young (Piot and Meheus 1983). Prostitutes are named by up to 80 percent of male patients as the source of infection in some, but not all, developing countries as compared with less than 20 percent in Europe and North America (Rajan 1978; D'Costa and others 1985) and are probably an important reservoir of STDs in many parts of the world. Still, significant differences in sexual behavior patterns exist within continents and even within countries.

The highest rates of STDs are found in urban men and women in their sexually most active years, that is, between the ages of fifteen and thirty-five. On the average, women become infected at a lower age than men. Increasing urbanization with

disruption of traditional social structures, increased mobility for economic or political reasons, poor medical facilities, a large proportion of the population composed of teenagers and young adults (who have the highest incidence of STD), and high unemployment rates are all contributing to the high incidence of STDs and their complications and sequelae (Piot and Holmes 1989).

STDs Are Communicable

Preventing or curing one case of an STD often prevents many other cases. This obvious consequence of the fact that STDs are communicable introduces a complication into the analysis of the priority to assign to their prevention. It is not sufficient to weigh against the cost of preventing a case only the benefits of preventing that single case; the so-called "dynamic benefits" that accrue to others than the immediately affected individual must also be included.[1]

A key epidemiological concept in this connection is that of the "reproduction rate."[2] Defined as the number of new (or secondary) cases infected by an average case, the reproduction rate can be used to multiply the number of prevented primary cases in order to obtain a crude measure of the total beneficial effect of the prevention effort.[3] Clearly the inclusion of these extra cases among the benefits of an STD prevention program will increase the measured cost-effectiveness of preventive efforts. It can be argued that the failure of decisionmakers to consider sufficiently the benefits of the prevention of secondary and subsequent cases has contributed to the undervaluation of the priority to assign to CSTD control in developing countries. In contrast, it is clear that the present attention allocated to AIDS prevention is almost entirely due to fear of a high reproduction rate.

In addition to its importance in estimating the benefits of preventing a communicable disease, the reproduction rate plays a key role in the analysis of the future course of an epidemic. To understand this, consider that a communicable disease characterized by a reproduction rate less than unity is headed for extinction as each individual case fails to replace itself entirely in the population. Contrarily, a disease whose reproduction rate is greater than unity can be predicted to explode geometrically. For any communicable disease in the early stages of an epidemic, the value of the reproductive rate (R) can be simply calculated as the product of three parameters: the probability of infection on each contact (Q), the number of contacts per time period between an infected person and a susceptible one (a), and the duration of infectivity of the infected person (D). Note that the first of these three values is primarily determined by characteristics of the disease, whereas the second is primarily behavioral. The third parameter, the duration of infectivity, is typically affected by both the biology of the particular disease and the effectiveness of public health strategies for either curing or isolating the infective individual. Later in this chapter we use estimated reproduction rates or their analogues both to characterize epidemic patterns and to estimate benefits of case prevention.

The Dynamics of Sexual Transmission

A turning point in the public health perspective toward STDs occurred with the realization in the late 1970s that a key distinction between STDs and other epidemics is the importance of the *heterogeneity* of sexual behavior in understanding the disease process. The simplest useful characterization of heterogeneous sexual behavior, introduced to the analysis of gonorrhea epidemics in 1978 by Yorke, Hethcote, and Nold (1978), is to posit two separate groups, a "core group" of highly sexually active individuals and a "noncore group," which is much less so. The characterization becomes more realistic as the number of groups is increased or as the behavior of individuals is allowed to vary within a group. However characterized, the heterogeneity of sexual behavior plays an extremely influential role in determining both the course of an STD epidemic and the choice of control strategy.

The definition of the reproduction rate and its importance as a simple indicator of the likely future course of an epidemic of any communicable disease were described earlier. The relationship $R = QaD$ can be applied directly to characterize the course of an STD epidemic, where a is interpreted as the rate of acquisition of new sexual partners and that rate is the same for all members of the population. If each individual in the population, however, has a different rate of sexual partner change, a_i, then it is not sufficient to use the average of these rates in order to estimate R. Instead, Anderson and May (1988) have shown that the heterogeneity in the sexual behavior, as measured by the variance of the a_i, adds substantially to the reproductive rate, and thus to the likely future rate of growth of the epidemic.[4] In addition, it is increasingly clear that there is considerable heterogeneity over time in the infectivity of individuals with HIV infection, adding to the complexity of the dynamics of viral spread in populations.

Current Levels and Trends in the Developing World

Reflecting the low level of priority assigned to CSTDs in most countries, data on the levels of CSTD infection in many populations in the developing world are poor and largely confined to selected groups (and samples of convenience). Therefore, the figures presented here should be considered as approximate and not necessarily representative for the general population. From a public health perspective, however, the overall prevalence or incidence rates in the general population may not be as critical as the size of the segment of the population that is at risk and the rate of infection in each risk group. For example, even if the nationwide prevalence of HIV infection in a country is low, there may still be a significant problem in the cities.[5]

CLASSIC SEXUALLY TRANSMITTED DISEASES. Two parameters important in estimating the burden of CSTDs are the prevalence of infection and the rate of complications and sequelae. The degree of health-seeking behavior and the quality of health services and STD control programs directly control the latter and, by reducing transmission, indirectly control the former.

In table 20-2, we present selected data on the prevalence of gonococcal and genital chlamydial infection and serologic evidence of present or past syphilis among samples of adult women in different parts of the world in the 1970s and 1980s. With the exception of the population-based surveys of women in Senegal and Uganda, the samples are drawn from the population of pregnant women. Although pregnant women imperfectly represent all adults, these data are as representative of the general population as one can get in the literature. Because infertile women are excluded from these series, there may be a bias to lower prevalence rates. Still, because the clinical manifestations of such CSTDs as gonococcal and chlamydial infection are less specific in women than in men, and their diagnoses therefore technically more complex, the prevalence rates of infection, but not necessarily the incidence rates, are usually higher in women than in men. Partly for this reason, morbidity and mortality rates from all CSTDs except syphilis are also much higher in women.

Table 20-2. Prevalence of Gonococcal and Genital Chlamydial Infection and Positive Serologic Test for Syphilis among Urban Pregnant Women

Country	Neisseria gonorrhoeae	Chlamydia trachomatis	VDRL/RPR TPHA/FTA-Abs[a]	Source
Africa				
Cameroon	15	n.a.	10	Nasah and others 1980; Kaptue and others 1990
Ethiopia	9	n.a.	n.a.	Perine and others 1980
Gabon	5.5	8.3	n.a.	Yvert and others 1984; Leclerc and others 1988
The Gambia	6.7	6.9	17.5, 7.2	Mabey and others 1984
Ghana	3.4	7.7	n.a.	Bentsi and others 1985
Kenya	7	8.9	3.8	Laga and others 1986b; Temmerman and others 1990
Mozambique	n.a.	n.a.	6.3	Liljestrand and others 1985
Nigeria	5.2	6.5	2.1	Okpere, Obaseiki-Ebor, and Oyaide 1987; Aladesanmi, Mumtaz and Mabey 1989; Fakeya, Onile, and Odugbemi 1986
Rwanda	5	16	4	Senyonyi 1987; Dabis and others 1989
Senegal	1.5	7	7.5	de Schampheleire and others 1990; Ndoye 1991[b]
Somalia	n.a.	n.a.	3	Jama and others 1987
South Africa	11.7	13	n.a.	Welgemoed and others 1986; Ballard, Fehler, and Piot 1986
Swaziland	3	n.a.	13.1	Meheus and others 1980; Guiness and others 1988
Tanzania	6[b,c]	n.a.	16.4	Cooper-Poole 1986
Uganda	18/2	n.a.	n.a.	Arya, Taber, and Nsanze 1980
Zaire	1.8	6.3	0.9	Luyeye and others 1990
Zambia	11.2	n.a.	14.3, 12.5	Ratnam and others 1982
Americas				
Chile	2	n.a.	n.a.	Donoso and others 1984
Jamaica	11	n.a.	n.a.	George 1974
United States	1/9[d]	n.a.	n.a.	Mtimavalye 1987
Asia				
India	10	n.a.	n.a.	Jha and others 1978
Malaysia	0.5	n.a.	n.a.	Mtimavalye 1987
Thailand	12	n.a.	n.a.	Mtimavalye 1987

n.a. Not applicable.

a. Test for *Treponema pallidum*, the etiologic agent for syphilis, was used for both diseases. Acronyms—VDRL: Venereal Disease Research Laboratoary/RPR: Rapid Plasma Reagin/TPHA: Teponema Pallidum Hemagglutination Assay/FTA: Fluorescrent Teponema Antibody.

b. Women in general population.

c. Low fertility district/high fertility district.

d. White/black.

Sources: See last column.

The morbidity of CSTDs occurs mostly between the ages of fifteen and forty-five years—not only the sexually most active period in life but also the most economically and demographically productive age. Geographic differences in prevalence are obvious from table 20-2, but extrapolations on the scale of a continent cannot be made. Prevalence data on genital ulcerations in the general population are not available from the developing world, but rates of 4 to 8 percent have been found in female prostitutes in Central and East Africa (D'Costa and others 1985; Laga and others 1989). Genital ulcers do not directly lead to mortality. Without treatment, the very painful chancroid lesions take two to three months to heal. The time between onset of disease and the individual's presentation at a medical facility is often two to four weeks in Sub-Saharan Africa (Plummer and others 1983).

In men, the incidence of both gonococcal and chlamydial infections may be very high (up to 20 percent annually between the ages of fifteen and forty-five years in high-risk groups). Because the associated morbidity (urethritis) is mostly limited in severity and duration (one to five weeks), delay before seeking treatment may be as long as two years (Population Information Program 1983). Mild to severe urethral stricture may occur after urethritis in up to 3 percent of men, with the time between onset of urethritis and acute urinary retention ranging between a few days and several years (Bewes 1973; Osegbe and Amaku 1981). Treatment is difficult and time consuming, and such cases constitute up to 80 percent of the practice of urologists in some parts of Africa (Bewes 1973). Acute and chronic epididymitis may occur in 1 to 10 percent of cases of urethritis and may be associated with long-term morbidity and infertility. The proportion of cases of infertility in the male due to CSTDs has not been well defined, but it is estimated at 20 to 40 percent in the developing world (Population Information Program 1983).

In women, uncomplicated cervical infection with *Neisseria gonorrhoeae* or *Chlamydia trachomatis* is usually associated with nonspecific genital signs and symptoms, which interfere only minimally with daily activities. Complicated disease and its sequelae are a significant cause of morbidity, however, and an important proportion of reproductive mortality, even in the United States (Grimes 1986).

Studies in Sweden have shown that 8 to 10 percent of women with gonococcal or chlamydial infection develop pelvic inflammatory disease (PID [Weström 1980]). The annual incidence of PID among urban women in Sub-Saharan Africa can be estimated at 1 to 3 percent between the ages of fifteen and forty-five, with incidence rates of 0.4 to 1.2 percent, and 0.4 to 1.5 percent for gonococcal and chlamydial PID, respectively (assuming that 20 to 40 percent of cases of PID are due to N. gonorrhoeae and 20 to 50 percent to C. trachomatis). Half of these cases occur during the puerperal period. The annual mortality directly attributable to PID in women of fifteen to forty-five years would then be 0.1 to 0.5 per 1,000 (assuming a 1 percent case-fatality rate). These figures are probably much lower in rural areas and in other parts of the developing world, but data are lacking.

The annual incidence of bilateral tubal occlusion (leading to infertility) is estimated at 0.3 percent to 1.5 percent in urban women in Sub-Saharan Africa, with gonococci and chlamydia each being responsible for 20 to 40 percent of cases (assuming a 15 to 40 percent risk of tubal occlusion after one episode of PID [Weström 1975; Weström and others 1979]). Whereas bilateral tubal occlusion is found in 50 percent of African women who are infertile, this is the case in only 14 to 20 percent of such women in Asia, Latin America, and the Middle East (Cates, Farley, and Rowe 1985).

The annual incidence of ectopic pregnancy in urban Africa resulting from PID is estimated at 0.01 to 0.04 percent, with an annual mortality rate of 0.001 to 0.005 percent for women between the ages of fifteen and forty-five (Urquhart 1979).

Finally, maternal mortality due to gonococcal and chlamydial infection (postpartum infectious complications) may be as high as 0.04 to 0.2 percent annually in Sub-Saharan Africa (with a maternal mortality rate of 0.5 to 1 percent and a 10 to 20 percent incidence of postpartum infections). Even in the United States, deaths due to STDs account for 20 percent of maternal mortality (Grimes 1986). In general, the overall mortality from STDs is not well defined. It is often a hidden mortality and morbidity because of a long latency period between the acute infection and the complication or sequela leading to death. In addition, the association between CSTDs and some of these complications is not well understood (Brunham, Holmes, and Embree 1989).

In neonates, conjunctivitis and respiratory disease are the main causes of morbidity due to N. gonorrhoeae and C. trachomatis infection in the mother. Their incidence depends on the prevalence of these infections in pregnant women. The occurrence of gonococcal ophthalmia neonatorum in neonates depends on whether effective eye prophylaxis is implemented at birth. Disablement from gonococcal neonatal infection is due to keratitis and blindness, and disablement from chlamydial infection results mainly from chronic respiratory disease.

Whereas prevalence rates of positive serologic tests for syphilis are available for numerous populations (see table 20-2), the morbidity and mortality due to the different stages of syphilis have not been documented for adults in the developing world. The consequences of syphilis for pregnancy have been better documented and are impressive. Approximately 10 to 12 percent of infants born to mothers with a positive syphilis serology will die during the neonatal period if untreated, yielding a mortality as high as 1 to 3 percent among under fours (in populations with a prevalence of a positive test for syphilis of more than 30 percent), in addition to a 20 to 25 percent stillbirth rate in the same group (Ratnam and others 1982; CDC 1986; Hira and Hira, 1987). Congenital syphilis is multiorganic and may result in severe physical and mental handicaps. Overall it occurs in 25 to 75 percent of exposed infants.

Trends for CSTDs and their complications between the early 1970s and the mid-1980s in the developing world are unknown. In Swaziland the prevalence rate of reactive syphilis serology among pregnant women remained at a level of approximately 30 percent between 1978 and 1987 (Ursi and others 1981; Guinness and others 1988), and in Rwanda the annual incidence of gonorrhea continuously increased among military recruits between 1981 and 1984 (Piot and Caraël 1988; see figure 20-1). Both sets of data suggest that the incidence of CSTDs in these countries remained at the same high levels during these periods. In contrast, the impressions gained from clinic-based data are that CSTD incidence has increased recently, particularly in urban populations.

HIV INFECTION. Because AIDS is a new disease, data on morbidity and mortality in the developing world are still fairly limited. Still, a growing set of data on the prevalence and incidence of HIV infection, as well as on the incidence of AIDS cases, is becoming available. The former data are probably the more important ones, because they indicate the number of

Figure 20-1. Gonorrhea Prevalence among Rwandan Military Recruits, by Months of Service

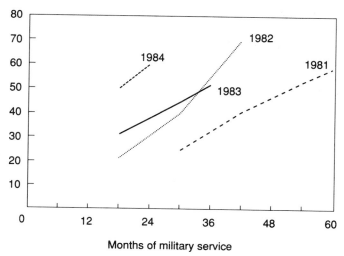

Cumulative percentage infected

Source: Piot and Caraël.

people who will develop AIDS in the next decades. For the sake of simplicity, we equate morbidity and mortality rates for AIDS, because no widespread effective treatment is available in the developing world.

There is considerable variation in the prevalence and incidence of HIV infection throughout the world, on a given continent and even within countries, making extrapolations speculative. For instance, the male-to-female ratio of AIDS cases is less than one in Zaire and Uganda, but two to four in both Côte d'Ivoire and Senegal (Piot and others 1990). These variations are often not well understood, and the elucidation of their causes may provide important clues for preventive programs. The interaction among demographic, behavioral, and political factors probably determine how and where HIV spreads.

The three modes of transmission of HIV include sexual intercourse, parenteral exposure to blood and blood products, and vertical transmission from mother to child. For Africa and the Caribbean, it is estimated that more than 80 percent of those who are infected with HIV acquired their infection heterosexually. In Latin America, homosexual men account for the majority of cases (15 to 80 percent) of HIV infection, but heterosexual transmission appears to be increasing in several countries in the region. Finally, in Asia, where the virus has been introduced more recently, HIV is spread mainly among people with multiple sexual contacts and among intravenous (IV) drug users. The latter group appears to be particularly vulnerable, as shown by the rapid spread of HIV infection among drugs users in Thailand and Burma (Phanuphak and others 1989). The features of these three epidemiologic patterns in the world are summarized in table 20-3.

The rate of transmission of HIV varies with the mode of acquisition and seems influenced by a number of parameters. Thus, it is thought that the basic risk of acquiring HIV infection through vaginal intercourse is 0.1 to 0.5 percent and through receptive anal intercourse is probably ten times higher (Piot and others 1987; Johnson and Laga 1988). In the presence of other STDs, however, particularly those associated with genital ulceration, both the susceptibility to HIV infection and the infectiousness of an HIV-infected individual are increased several fold (five to ten times [Piot and others 1988; Pepin and others 1989]). In addition, the infectivity of an HIV seropositive person seems to increase just before or when he or she develops clinical disease (Johnson and Laga 1988). This may at least partly explain why HIV has spread more quickly in the hetero-

Table 20-3. Three Epidemiologic Patterns of HIV Infection

Characteristic	Pattern I	Pattern II	Pattern III
Major group affected	Homosexual and bisexual men and IDU	Heterosexuals	Persons with multiple sex partners
Period when introduced or began to spread extensively	Mid-1970s or early 1980s	Early to late 1970s	Early to mid-1980s
Sexual transmission	Predominantly homosexual. Over 50 percent of homosexual men in some urban areas infected. Limited heterosexual transmission occurring, but expected to increase.	Predominantly heterosexual. Up to 25 percent of 20- to 40-year age group in some urban areas infected and up to 90 percent of female prostitutes. Homosexual transmission not a major factor.	Both homosexual and heterosexual transmission just now being documented. Very low prevalence of HIV infection even in persons with multiple partners, such as prostitutes (except in some areas of Southeast Asia and India).
Parenteral transmission	After homosexual transmision, intravenous drug abuse accounts for the next largest proportion of HIV infections, even in Europe. Transmission from contaminated blood or blood products not a continuing problem, but existing cohort of persons infected by this route before 1985.	Transfusion of HIV-infected blood is major public health problem. Nonsterile needles and syringes account for undetermined proportion of HIV infections.	Not a significant problem at present in most countries, but growing problem in IDU in Southeast Asia.
Perinatal transmission	Documented primarily among female IDU and women from HIV-1 endemic areas	Significant problem in those areas where 5 to 15 percent of women are HIV-1 antibody positive.	Currently not a problem.
Distribution	Western Europe, North America; some in South America, Australia, New Zealand.	Africa, Caribbean, some areas in South America.	Asia, the Pacific Region (except Australia and New Zealand), Middle East, Eastern Europe, some rural areas of South America.

IDU Injecting drug users.
Source: Piot and others 1988.

Table 20-4. Estimated HIV-1 Seroprevalence by Residence and High-Risk Category, Developing Countries, 1990
(percent)

Country	Residence Urban	Rural	High Risk[a]	Country	Residence Urban	Rural	High Risk[a]
Africa				*Africa (continued)*			
Angola	1.3[b]	—	14.2[b]	Sudan	0.0	—	16.0[d]
Benin	0.1	6.7	4.5[c]	Swaziland	0.0[c,d]	—	—
Botswana	0.8[c]	0.1[c]	1.2[c]	Tanzania	8.9	5.4	38.7
Burkina Faso	1.7[d]	3.1[b]	16.9[b]	Togo	—	—	—
Burundi	17.5	—	18.5[d]	Tunisia	0.0	—	1.9
Cameroon	1.1	0.4	8.6	Uganda	24.3	12.3	86.0[d]
Cape Verde	0.0	—	0.0	Zaire	6.0	3.6	37.8
Central African Republic	7.4	3.7	20.6	Zambia	24.5[d]	13.0[d]	54.0[d]
Chad	0.0	0.0	—	Zimbabwe	3.2[c]	1.4	—
Congo	3.9	1.0	34.3[d]				
Cote d'Ivoire	8.5[b]	3.3[b]	23.8[b]	*Latin America*			
Djibouti	0.3	0.0[d]	2.7	Antigua and Barbuda	—	—	1.7
Egypt	0.0	—	0.2	Argentina	0.3	0.1	5.8
Equatorial Guinea	0.3	0.3	—	Bahamas	0.5	—	—
Ethiopia	2.0	0.0	18.2	Barbados	0.1	—	—
Gabon	1.8	0.8	—	Bolivia	0.0	—	0.0
The Gambia	0.1	—	1.7[b]	Brazil	0.3	0.0	3.0
Ghana	2.2	—	25.2	Colombia	0.1	—	14.6
Guinea	0.6[b]	0.2	—	Costa Rica	0.0	—	0.0
Guinea Bissau	0.1	0.0	0.0[d]	Cuba	0.0	—	0.0
Kenya	7.8	1.0	59.2	Dominican Republic	1.6	—	2.6
Lesotho	0.1	—	—	Ecuador	0.0	—	0.0[d]
Liberia	0.0	0.0[c]	0.0[d]	Guadalupe	0.2	—	—
Libya	0.0	—	—	Guyana	—	—	0.0[d]
Madagascar	0.0	—	0.0	Haiti	4.9	3.0	41.9
Malawi	23.3	—	55.9	Jamaica	0.3	—	14.6[d]
Mali	0.4	—	23.0[b]	Martinique	0.5	—	38.9[d]
Mauritania	0.06	—	0.0	Mexico	0.7	—	2.2
Mauritius	0.0	—	—	Panama	0.0	—	0.0
Morocco	0.0	—	7.1[d]	Peru	0.1	—	0.3
Mozambique	1.1	0.8	2.6	Trinidad and Tobago	0.9	—	13.0
Namibia	2.5	—	—	Venezuela	0.0	0.0	—
Niger	—	—	5.8				
Nigeria	0.5	0.0	1.7	*Asia/Oceania*			
Rwanda	30.3	1.7	79.8[c,d]	Burma	—	—	1.9
Senegal	0.1[b]	0.0[d]	2.3[b]	India	0.1	—	18.1
Sierra Leone	3.6[b]	—	2.7[b]	Papua New Guinea	0.0	0.0[d]	0.7
Somalia	0.0	—	0.4	Philippines	0.0	—	0.1
South Africa	0.1	—	3.2	Thailand	0.0	—	0.2

— Data not available.
a. Prostitutes and clients, STD patients, or other persons with known risk factors.
b. Infection with only HIV-1 and dual infection (HIV-1 and HIV-2).
c. Data prior to 1986.
d. Data not necessarily reliable because small sample size (less than 100).
Source: U.S. Bureau of the Census 1991.

sexual population in Africa than in North America and Europe; genital ulcer disease seems to be more common in several African populations, and HIV has probably been present for a longer time among heterosexuals in Africa, resulting overall in a higher infectiousness of the HIV-infected population (Piot and others 1988).

Risk factors for HIV infection are generally those of other STDs, such as having a high number of sex partners, being single, having a history of STDs, and having sex with prostitutes or being a prostitute. Urban populations usually have much higher infection rates than rural populations (see table 20-4), though this may change when the epidemic spreads. Lack of circumcision has been claimed to be a risk factor for HIV infection in men, but this remains controversial (Van de Perre and others 1987; Simonsen and others 1988; Bongaarts and others 1989).

The efficiencies of transmission by a blood transfusion or by intravenous needle sharing are probably close to 100 percent. Because of a high rate of infection among young adults in several populations, and because of the incomplete availability of HIV antibody tests, HIV infection through blood transfusion makes up a larger proportion of cases of AIDS in pattern II countries than in Europe or North America. This is particularly the case in children, who are the main consumers of blood transfusions in large areas of the developing world, together with pregnant or parturient women. This is due to a high incidence of severe anemia caused by malaria or obstetrical problems (Greenberg and others 1988; Ryder and Mhalu 1988). In addition, indications for blood transfusion may not always be rational, and proper blood banks, involving voluntary, low-risk donors, are rarely functioning. Finally, there are now several reports of probable HIV transmission to blood donors through contaminated plasmapheresis equipment (Laga and Piot 1988).

Whereas it is often assumed that intravenous drug use is a prerogative of the rich West, the AIDS epidemic has dramatically shown that intravenous drug use is spreading rapidly in many developing countries. Thus, more than 40 percent of Thai IV drug users were infected by early 1989, as compared with 1 percent in 1987 (Phanuphak and others 1989). It is anticipated that similar outbreaks of HIV infection among IV drug users will occur in other developing countries. The role of contaminated medical injections in the spread of HIV infection is probably marginal (Piot and others 1988; Van de Perre and others 1987, Berkley 1991).

The rate of vertical transmission from mother to child is of the order of 25 to 50 percent in Africa, with women who are more advanced clinically being more infectious for their offspring (Lallemant and others 1989; Ryder and others 1989). Because of the mainly heterosexual spread of HIV in Africa, and increasingly in the Caribbean, a large and growing proportion of AIDS cases are infants and children. The incidence of AIDS is probably underestimated, however, because of technical problems in the diagnosis of AIDS and HIV infection in infants. In addition, there is growing evidence that an as yet unknown proportion of perinatally infected children do not become ill until the age of seven to ten years. This implies that it will take at least another decade before the full spectrum of morbidity and mortality of perinatally acquired HIV infection is known.

Although a limited number of anecdotal cases of HIV infection acquired through breastfeeding have been reported (Ziegler and others 1985; Colebunders and others 1988; Hira, Kamanga, and Bhat 1989), it appears that contaminated breast milk does not contribute significantly to the transmission of HIV infection from mother to child (Ryder and others 1990). Furthermore, Kennedy and others (1990) have convincingly argued that the health damage from bottle-feeding would probably exceed any gains from the averted transmission by breast milk.[6] Thus, there is currently no reason to modify current promotion of breastfeeding in HIV endemic areas in the developing world.

Finally, the effect of HIV infection on the natural history of childhood diseases, such as measles and malaria, is incompletely understood. Preliminary data suggest that HIV infection in children does not influence the response to childhood immunizations, though, again, it is not clear what the effect of HIV infection on protective immunity will be when the immune status of these children deteriorates (Mvula, Ryder, and Manzila 1989).

In pattern II countries, on which we focus (mainly Sub-Saharan Africa), the overall female-to-male ratio of people with HIV infection usually approaches one to one, though regional variations have been reported. A marked variation in sex ratio, however, has been found by age group in some countries (for example, Zaire), where HIV-seropositive women largely outnumbered men between fifteen and thirty years of age, whereas there were more infected men than women above that age (Ryder and Piot 1988). Several surveys in Africa have also found that the HIV seroprevalence rate is highest in individuals between twenty and forty years of age and that peak seroprevalence rates occur at a younger age in women than in men (Ryder and Piot 1988). This age pattern for both sexes combined is illustrated in figure 20-2; in the figure the HIV-1 seroprevalence rates are shown by age group as found in a national serum survey in Rwanda in 1986, in which a random cluster sampling method was used. The Rwandan data also indicate a higher infection rate for urban women than urban men (Rwandan Seroprevalence Study Group 1989).

In table 20-4 we summarize seroprevalence data in various groups of adults in different developing countries. The highest rates are consistently found in Central Africa, but epidemic foci start appearing in other parts of the continent as well, for

Figure 20-2. Seroprevalence of HIV-1 in Rwanda, by Age, Residence, and Gender, 1986

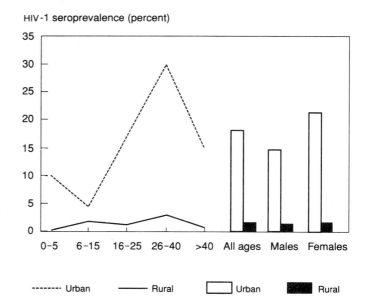

HIV-1 seroprevalence (percent)

Source: Bugingo and others 1988; Rwandan seroprevalence study group 1989.

instance, in Côte d'Ivoire. In addition, within each country, prostitutes are at a much higher risk of infection and constitute part of a "core" group of highly sexually active individuals whose special role in the epidemic is described below. In the Latin American cities homosexuals also show the higher prevalence rates associated with core groups.

Annual incidence rates of 0.5 to 1.8 percent for HIV infection among adults without particular risk factors have been documented in Central Africa (N'Galy and others 1988). Still, such rates were as high as 10 to 40 percent among highly exposed prostitutes in Kinshasa and Nairobi (Laga and others 1989; Plummer and others 1991).

In table 20-5 we present the cumulative number of cases of AIDS by continent reported to the World Health Organization (WHO) as of August 1989. The data from Africa in particular probably represent gross underestimations, and a figure of 250,000 AIDS cases by 1988 seems closer to reality. These morbidity data ultimately also indicate the number of deaths due to HIV infection.

Although HIV infection has been introduced recently in all populations (mid-1970s to mid-1980s), it has spread more rapidly in some than in others (figure 20-3). Possible patterns of morbidity and mortality during the next twenty-five years are difficult to predict because of inadequate knowledge of the natural history of the disease, of behavioral patterns in different populations, and of the potential changes in the relative contributions of different modes of spread of HIV. Based on current trends in some Latin American and Caribbean countries, however, it is anticipated that heterosexual transmission will become much more important in the Americas, and perhaps also in Asia, than it is at the present time. In the near future, it appears that proportionately more women and more poor people will be among those with HIV infection and AIDS.

Furthermore, dense urban populations with high rates of drug use or STDs, like those of Abidjan and Bangkok, may soon experience rapidly spreading HIV epidemics (De Cock, Pozter, and Odehouri 1989; Phanuphak and others 1989).

In 1989, WHO (1989c) estimated that by the year 2000 annual adult AIDS cases would rise from the present level of fewer than 100,000 per year to more than 800,000 per year. In the same survey it was estimated that adult HIV infections would rise to 13 million worldwide (Chin, Sato, and Mann 1989).

In addition to the morbidity directly caused by HIV infection, one should also consider the excess morbidity from other diseases as a result of HIV infection. This has already been documented for tuberculosis in the United States and several African countries, where the incidence of tuberculosis is rising as a result of the HIV epidemic (CDC 1989; Colebunders and others 1989; Standaert and others 1989).

Socioeconomic Correlates of HIV Infection

Information on the correlation, or lack of correlation, of STD incidence rates with socioeconomic indicators would be epidemiologically useful in several ways. First, such information could help in the effort to target interventions. Second, it could help us to understand the practices which spread the disease. And, finally, it could tell us more about the diseases' effects on society.

Unfortunately very little information has been available on STDs. Because individuals have incentives to hide an STD infection—and because the rich can hide these infections more successfully—any data on STD incidence or prevalence by social class were known to be suspect. With HIV infection, however, the situation has reversed itself. Because HIV/AIDS is

Table 20-5. Reported and Estimated Cases of AIDS, by Region and Stage of Development, 1990

Region	Reported cases		Estimated cases	
	Number	Per million population	Number	Per million population
Industrial countries				
United States and Canada	159,194	577.9	175,000	635.3
Europe	43,441	71.2	48,000	78.7
Australia	2,347	140.2	3,000	179.2
South Africa	650	17.8	1,000	27.4
Japan	294	2.4	300	2.4
New Zealand	207	61.7	200	59.6
Total	206,133	193.4	227,500	213.5
Developing countries				
Sub-Saharan Africa	81,833	173.0	648,000	1,369.7
Latin America and the Caribbean	31,943	71.7	275,000	617.3
Europe	2,462	13.9	52,000	293.7
North Africa and Mediterranean	686	1.5	1,000	2.2
Western Pacific	180	0.1	2,500	1.9
Southeast Asia	141	0.1	5,000	3.7
Total	117,245	27.7	983,500	232.8
Total	323,378	61.1	1,211,000	228.9

Source: Reported cases from World Health Organization 1991a; Chin, Global Programme on AIDS, WHO; Zachariah and Vu 1988.

Figure 20-3. Evolution of HIV Seroprevalence in Selected Populations of Developing Countries

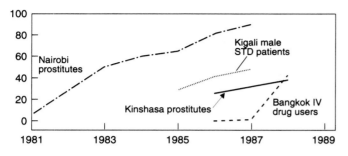

High-Risk Groups

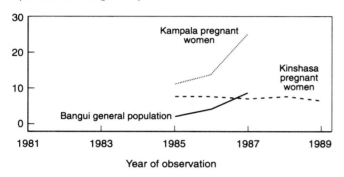

Low-Risk Groups

Year of observation

Source: Piot and others, 1990.

known to be fatal, wealthy people are alleged to have identified themselves in the hope of getting treatment. Thus, some have argued that estimated HIV infection rates by class are biased toward a higher infection rate for higher classes.

The data on this question are still scarce; we are aware of no data outside Africa. In table 20-6, however, we present information from three studies in three different African countries, all of which confirm the hypothesis of higher prevalence rates at higher income levels. These patterns might be explained by the relatively greater access of the rich to foreign travel or, alternatively, by greater rates of sexual partner change among higher-income adults. In either case, the pattern may dissolve as the epidemic spreads in a given population. Additional work is needed not only on prevalence rates but also, and especially, on incidence rates by social class so that public health officials can determine how best to target their control efforts.

It has been asserted, but not demonstrated, that the correlation between infection rates and higher social status is positive for men but negative for women.[7] Larson (1989) and Caldwell, Caldwell, and Quiggin (1989) advance an image of the sociosexual role of the African woman that predicts just such a possibility. In Larson's words:

Independence has not altered the ambivalence and outright hostility towards urban women generated during the colonial era. . . . Most East and Central African countries have taken actions to restrict urban women's activities. These range from the banning of miniskirts and other provocative clothing to more threatening actions such as attempts to bus unmarried women out of town or arresting unescorted women found on the streets or in bars hotels and cinemas at night (Larson 1989, p. 4).

As a result of these powerful negative incentives, there are many fewer young women than young men in the sexually most active age range in the urban centers of countries such as Côte d'Ivoire, Kenya, Rwanda, Burundi, and South Africa. It is natural to hypothesize that in these situations the demand by the young men for prostitution services is very high. In contrast, in cities which are relatively hospitable to young women, such as those of Zaire, Senegal, and Mali, the demand for sexual services can be expected to be smaller.

But the quantity of commercially supplied sexual services is determined by the supply as well as the demand. The supply will be high only if the potential suppliers have relatively few remunerative alternatives. We hypothesize that the number of women enrolled in secondary school per 100 men enrolled is a good indicator of the opportunity cost of the time of urban women.[8] In cities in which women are relatively well educated, we expect that, other things being equal, fewer women will become prostitutes and the HIV virus will spread more slowly.

More empirical evidence for the proposition that women's education and a high ratio of females to males might both contribute to reducing the prevalence of STDs is presented in figure 20-4. The upper-left panel of the figure displays a scatter plot of 1987 HIV prevalence rates against the urban ratio of females to males.[9] Note that the higher prevalence rates are associated with urban areas in which there are many fewer young adult women than men. The upper-right panel of figure 20-4 shows, for the same countries, the association between HIV prevalence and the ratio of female to male secondary education enrollment.[10] Here, the relationship is even more marked, with the highest seroprevalence rates observed in those countries with the poorest record on female education. For the smaller number of countries for which the infection rate of female prostitutes was known in 1987, the left lower panel of figure 20-4 demonstrates even more strongly the hypothesized effect of small female-to-male ratios—a high prevalence rate of HIV infection among prostitutes.

A multivariate regression of urban adult HIV seroprevalence rate on these two indicators of the status of women explains 48 percent of the variation in prevalence rates and is statistically significant at the 1 percent significance level. In this sample, each of the two variables, urban adult sex ratio and female education, contributes independently and significantly to explain variation in the seroprevalence level.[11]

Because this regression equation was estimated on a cross-section of cities, in some of which the HIV prevalence rates may still be rising, the relationship is likely to shift over time. Still,

Table 20-6. Relationship of Socioeconomic Status with Higher Rates of HIV Infection in Sub-Saharan Africa

Country	Date	Sample Population	Size	Socioeconomic indicator	HIV infection rate (percent)
Rwanda	1987	National sample of urban adults	1,255	Education	
				Primary or less	20.8
				More than primary	29.6
Zaire	1987	Employees of urban textile factory	5,951	Job	
				Worker	2.8
				Foreman	4.6
				Executive	5.3
Zambia	1985	Patients, blood donors, personnel of urban hospital	1,078	Years of education completed	
				0–4	8.0
				5–9	14.7
				10–14	24.1
				15 or more	33.3

Source: Melbye, Nselesani, and Bayley 1986; Bugingo and others 1988; Ndilu and others 1988.

the strong estimated effects of these two indicators of low female status on the prevalence of HIV infection are likely to persist. An implication is that one of the most promising ways to fight STDs over the longer run is to improve the education and increase the number of urban women.[12]

Public Health Significance of STDs

This section presents estimates of the burden of STDs and of the benefit of averting a case of CSTD and HIV infection.

Health Lost and Saved

Many other categories of diseases, as well as CSTDs and HIV, have substantial public health significance. In order to attach a priority ranking to STD interventions in a specific country, it is necessary to attempt to quantify the public health effect of STDs in comparison with other diseases in that country. Two broad methods are relevant. First, one can compute any of a variety of measures of the good health that is *lost* as a result of these diseases in comparison with others. Second, one can estimate the good health that would be *saved* by interventions on each category of disease.

The computation of the amount of good health lost due to each prevalent disease in a developing country was pioneered by the Ghana Health Assessment Project Team, hereafter referred to as GHAP (1981). The method the investigators used was to multiply a measure of the disability-adjusted life-years lost (DALYs) from a case of each disease by the annual incidence of that disease to obtain an estimate of the average annual burden of each disease on a typical member of the population.[13] Expressed as a formula, the equation for each disease is:

$$\text{DALYs} = \text{Cases/capita/year} \times \text{DALY/case}$$

By comparing estimates of DALYs per capita per year across diseases, one arrives at an estimate of the relative contribution of each disease to the total burden of ill health borne by a given population. Furthermore, these estimates indicate the total health benefit that would accrue from eradicating one of the diseases.

The example of smallpox notwithstanding, eradication is unfortunately not usually an option available to public health decisionmakers. Instead they are asked to make decisions at the margin, allocating 10 percent more of their resources to this prevention effort, perhaps by cutting resources on another effort. As GHAP recognized (1981), estimates of total burden are not useful for these marginal decisions. Instead decisionmakers need to know (a) how many disability-adjusted life-years could be saved for every case of the disease prevented or cured and (b) the relative costs of preventing or curing a case of each disease. In this section we present and interpret the burden measures, from both the static and the dynamic perspective. Then in the next two sections we turn to the second and perhaps more important issue, the estimate of the health effect of averting a case of an STD, again from both a static and a dynamic perspective.

The Static Burden of STDs

Analyses of the public health importance of sexually transmitted diseases have not typically accorded them great importance either in absolute terms or in relation to other infectious and parasitic diseases. For example, GHAP ranked "venereal disease" number 53 in order of the burden it imposed on the population of Ghana in the 1970s. Partly because of AIDS and partly because of a new understanding of how widespread the CSTDs are, especially in Africa, and how damaging their sequelae, opinion has begun to shift toward a more serious appreciation of the harm done by these diseases—and of the potential benefits of their alleviation. (See, for example, Curran 1980; Brown, Zacarias, and Aral 1985; Grimes 1986; Washington, Arno, and Brooks 1986; Washington, Johnson, and Sanders 1987; Wasserheit 1989).

Figure 20-4. Correlation of Urban HIV Infection with Gender and Schooling in African Countries, 1987

HIV seroprevalence in adults
(percent)

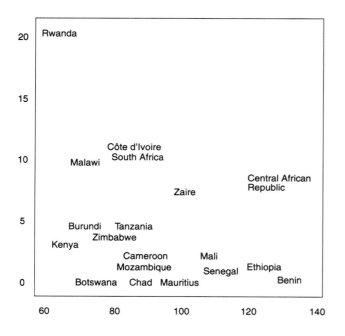

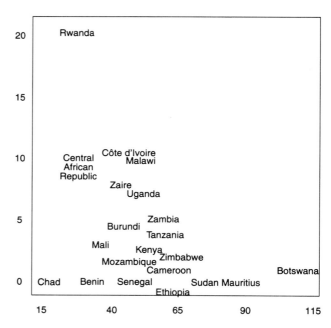

HIV seroprevalence in adults
(percent)

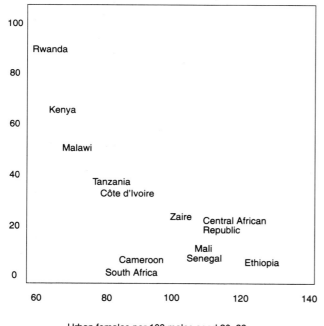

Urban females per 100 males aged 20 -39

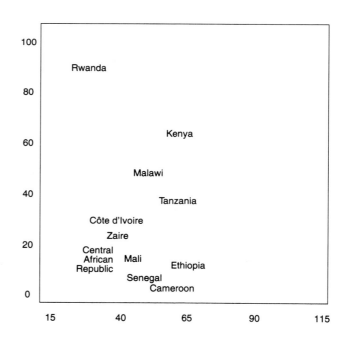

Secondary school enrollment of females per 100 males

Source: U.S. Bureau of the Census 1991.

In view of the heterogeneity of the epidemiological picture and the gaps in available information, it is difficult to discuss in detail the public health effect of STDs on any specific country. Instead we define a typology of countries according to the estimated prevalence rates of CSTD and HIV infection in the sexually active populations of their main urban centers. In table 20-7 we define nine patterns of STD prevalence and tentatively classify representative countries from Africa, Latin America, and Asia.

In order to compute estimates of the "burden" of each of the various diseases in model countries, we apply the method originally developed by GHAP (1981) and extended by Barnum (1987) and Over, Bertozzi, and Chin (1989), which is based on the above simple equation. In appendix 20A we present calculations of the number of disability-adjusted life-years lost per case for the STDs and other important diseases, which is one of the two pieces of the formula. The other necessary component is the estimated incidence rate for each disease. Because incidence rates of STDs are largely unknown, we "guesstimate" the age structure

of incidence for each STD in each of the two extreme urban settings described in table 20-7, a high-prevalence urban setting and a lowprevalence one. Our guesstimates appear in table 20-8, together with estimates for the other diseases which have been derived from the GHAP study of Ghana. The estimated STD incidence rates might apply anywhere in the world that an urban area can be characterized as in table 20-7. The estimated incidence rates for the other diseases, however, are specific to Ghana in the late 1970s and can only indicate the rough orders of magnitude of the burdens of these diseases in other times and places.

Multiplying the age-specific incidence rate of a disease (from table 20-8) by the disability-adjusted life-years lost per case from that disease at that age group (a calculation intermediate to obtaining the figures in table 20A-3), converting the result to days (by multiplying by 365), and, finally, computing the weighted average of these products across all age groups, with the age-group size as the weight, yields the estimated number of healthy life-days lost per capita per year from a given disease. In table 20-9 we present the results of this calculation, and in figures 20-5 and 20-6 we portray them.

The rather surprising feature in table 20-9 is that *the burden of STDs in a high-prevalence urban area is a substantial fraction of the entire disease burden of that population.* By itself, HIV ranks second on the discounted disability-adjusted life-days (DALD) criterion and moves up to first when lost days are weighted by their relative productivities. Furthermore, the sum of the burdens of HIV, syphilis, and chlamydia equals 85 DALDs and 63 productivity-weighted discounted disability-adjusted life-days (PDALDs) per capita, enough to place these STDs in aggregate at the top of the list in importance in an urban high-prevalence area. The eleventh ranking disease in table 20-9 and figures 20-5 and 20-6 is chlamydia, which attains its rank because of an extremely high incidence rate in ages fifteen to fifty and an assumption that 5 percent of cases are permanently disabled to the extent of 30 percent incapacity for women (crippling pelvic inflammatory disease) and 50 percent for men (severe urethral strictures). Only chancroid appears in these calculations to have an effect as small as that attributed by GHAP to all STDs together, but new information on the likely links between genital ulcers and the probability of transmission of HIV infection may promote chancroid far above its place here. (See the discussion below of the effect of genital ulcers on the transmission of STDs.) In contrast, in low-prevalence urban areas, syphilis is the most burdensome STD, and its burden is less than that of any of the top fifteen Ghanaian diseases.

The Short-Term Dynamic Burden of an STD Epidemic

In order to illustrate the essential features of dynamic STD epidemiology and to characterize the differences among epidemics of the different STDs, it is useful to experiment with two simple models of an STD epidemic. In this section of the chapter, these models extend our estimates of the burden of STDs by incorporating the fact that each case causes additional

Table 20-7. Urban Prevalence of HIV and CSTD, by Region

CSTD Prevalence[a]	Prevalence of HIV infection[b]		
	Low or unknown	Intermediate	High
Low or unknown	Cambodia	Angola	None
	Cape Verde	Botswana	
	China	Burkina Faso	
	Eastern Europe	Namibia	
	Middle East	Sierra Leone	
	Niger		
	Togo		
	Viet Nam		
Intermediate	India	Congo	None
	Senegal	Mali	
		Zaire	
		Zimbabwe	
High	Brazil	Cameroon	Burundi
	Colombia	Caribbean	Côte d'Ivoire
	Lesotho	Nations	Malawi
	Madagascar	Central African	Rwanda
	Mauritania	Republic	Uganda
	Mexico	Ethiopia	Zambia
	Nigeria	Gabon	
	Philippines	Ghana	
	Swaziland	Kenya	
		Mozambique	
		Tanzania	
		Thailand	

a. High: rates of gonorrhea among sexually active adults exceed 5 percent or prevalence of serological markers for syphilis exceed 10 percent in pregnant women. Intermediate: prevalence below these levels but at least 1 percent for both of these diseases. Other countries are categorized as "low or unknown."

b. Low or unknown: less than 1 percent. Intermediate: between 1 and 10 percent. High: more than 10 percent.

Source: Authors.

Table 20-8. Incidence of STDs and Other Important Diseases, by Age
(per 1,000 people)

Disease	Prevalence[a]	Sex	0–1	1–4	5–14	15–49	50–64	65+
					Age (years)			
Sexually transmitted disease								
Chancroid	High	Both	0	0	0	12.5	9	0
	Low	Both	0	0	0	1.25	0.9	0
Chlamydia	High	Male	50	0	0	50	5	0
	High	Female	50	0	0	37.5	0	0
	Low	Male	5	0	0	5	2.5	0
	Low	Female	5	0	0	3.75	0	0
Gonorrhea	High	Male	25	0	0	45	4.5	0
	High	Female	25	0	0	30	0	0
	Low	Male	2.5	0	0	5	0.45	0
	Low	Female	2.5	0	0	3	0	0
HIV	High	Both	20	0.5	2.5	15	2.5	0
	Low	Both	0.1	0	0	0.3	0	0
Syphilis	High	Male	25	0	0	20	2.5	0
	High	Female	25	0	0	20	2.5	0
	Low	Male	2.5	0	0.5	2	0.25	0
	Low	Female	2.5	0	0.5	2	0.25	0
Other diseases								
Birth injury	n.a.	Both	36	0	0	0	0	0
Cerebrovascular disease	n.a.	Both	0	0	0	3	9	12
Cirrhosis	n.a.	Both	0	0	0	1.2	1.2	1.2
Congenital malformations	n.a.	Both	21	0	0	0	0	0
Gastroenteritis	n.a.	Both	800	200	5	5	5	5
Injuries[b]	n.a.	Both	5	6	7.7	9	5	5
Malaria	n.a.	Both	600	100	0	0	0	0
Measles	n.a.	Both	375	150	0	0	0	0
Pneumonia, adult	n.a.	Both	0	0	0	12	13	15
Pneumonia, child	n.a.	Both	7	9	3	0	0	0
Prematurity	n.a.	Both	213	0	0	0	0	0
Severe malnutrition	n.a.	Both	8	6	0.5	0.1	0.1	0.1
Sickle cell	n.a.	Both	28	0	0	0	0	0
Tetanus (neonatal)	n.a.	Both	11.2	0	0	0	0	0
Tuberculosis	n.a.	Both	0.5	0.5	1	3	3	3

n.a. Not applicable.
a. For STD, urban areas of high or low prevalence in pattern II countries, defined by table 20-7.
b. Such as accidents.
Source: Authors; diseases not related to STDs, Ghana Health Assessment Project Team 1981.

future cases. In the next section these same models will be useful in estimating the effect of alternative interventions on the course of an epidemic of each STD.

The model presented first is a short-run model of the course of an STD epidemic within the confines of an enclosed stable population. Although this model reveals some features of an HIV epidemic, its focus is too short-term to represent fully the important effects of such a slow-acting disease. Thus, after exploring the implications of a short-term model, we turn to a presentation of a longer-term demographic model, which incorporates the interactions between an AIDS epidemic and the demographic features of a population.

The short-run model posits just two groups of individuals, a core and a noncore group, which have different sizes and different rates of sexual activity. To predict the pattern of an epidemic from the starting prevalence rates of infection in these two groups, it is sufficient to specify only two sets of

parameters, one set to describe the sexual behavior of the two groups and one to describe the medical characteristics of the disease to be modeled.

We characterize the sexual behavior of the two groups by making the following assumptions:

- The core group of highly sexually active people increases (both men and women) includes 1,000 individuals, only 2 percent of the 50,000 in the noncore group.

- Individuals in the core group are ten times as sexually active as those in the noncore group, with the former having a new sexual partner every five days and the latter every fifty days.[14]

- In choosing new sexual partners, individuals exercise no preference according to group but instead select randomly among all individuals who are choosing new partners during that time period.[15]

Table 20-9. Per Capita Annual Disease Burden of STDs and Other Diseases in Sub-Saharan Africa

Disease	Discounted disability-adjusted life-days lost		Discounted productive disability-adjusted life-days lost	
	Value	Rank	Value	Rank
Measles	68.9	1	45.1	2
HIVa	60.6	2	48.3	1
Malaria	55.1	3	35.2	3
Gastroenteritis	35.7	4	22.4	4
Syphilis[a]	15.9	5	9.3	5
Birth injury	12.4	6	7.7	6
Sickle cell	11.3	7	6.5	9
Prematurity	10.1	8	6.4	10
Pneumonia, child	9.7	9	7.1	7
Severe malnutrition	8.6	10	5.7	13
Chlamydia[a]	8.6	11	5.8	12
Cerebrovascular disease	7.9	12	6.6	8
Injuries (i.e., accidents)	7.5	13	6.0	11
Tuberculosis	5.2	14	4.1	14
Pneumonia, adult	4.8	15	4.0	15
Tetanus (neonatal)	4.2	16	2.6	17
Cirrhosis	3.7	17	3.0	16
Congenital malformation	3.6	18	2.2	18
Gonorrhea[a]	1.9	19	1.2	19
Syphilis[b]	1.3	20	0.7	21
HIV [b]	1.0	21	0.8	20
Chlamydia[b]	0.8	22	0.5	22
Gonorrhea[b]	0.6	23	0.4	23
Chancroid[a]	0.5	24	0.3	24
Chancroid[b]	0.05	25	0.03	25
Total non-STDs[c]	303		204	
Total STDs[a]	88		65	
Total STDs[b]	3.6		2.5	

Note: Burdens are summed over the entire population of both genders.

a. Sexually transmitted disease; high-prevalence urban area.

b. Sexually transmitted disease; low-prevalence urban area.

c. In addition to the listed non-STDs, this total includes forty-one other diseases, all with values of discounted DALDs and productivity-weighted discounted DALDs lost per capita less than 4.0.

Source: Ghana Health Assessment Prject Team 1981; authors.

These specific values were used by Hethcote and Yorke (1984, p. 38) in their gonorrhea model. For ease of reference, they are presented together with some other derivative parameters in table 20-10. It must be emphasized that these parameters are not considered to be representative of African populations. Although they were originally chosen by Hethcote and Yorke to characterize a North American gonorrhea epidemic, sexual behavior varies enormously in the United States just as it does in Africa, and these parameters are not known to be typical of a specific North American population either. The intention here is not to predict accurately every detail of an STD epidemic in Africa with a single model, a hopeless and senseless task. Rather, by presenting the results of simulations with this model, we intend to develop an analytical technique for approximating the public health effect of these diseases, *assuming the parameters of sexual behavior were known*. Because a great deal of effort is currently being expended to determine these quantities, before long it may be possible to substitute for the assumptions in table 20-10 some numbers based on empirical data.[16]

For the purpose of this modeling exercise, only two aspects of each disease are required, the probability of transmission per new sexual partner and the number of days that an infected person remains infective before recovering or dying.[17] In the first four rows of table 20-11 we summarize this information for six distinct STD epidemics to be modeled. In contrast to table 20-10, which is not intended to be particularly representative of a specific part of the world, the estimates in table 20-11 have been adjusted to approximate as closely as possible the medical characteristics of these diseases in Sub-Saharan Africa. Note that the probability of transmission of HIV infection on a single encounter is assumed to increase by a factor of three to five in the presence of genital ulcers. For this reason, we distinguish HIV in the absence of genital ulcers as a separately analyzed epidemic from HIV infection in their presence.

The parameters which represent the average duration of infectivity should be thought of as determined by the interplay of demand and supply for medical care. Factors which influence demand include the discomfort caused by the disease and socioeconomic characteristics of the infected individual. Dis-

Figure 20-5. *Static Burden of* STDs *in Relation to Other Diseases in a High-Prevalence African City*

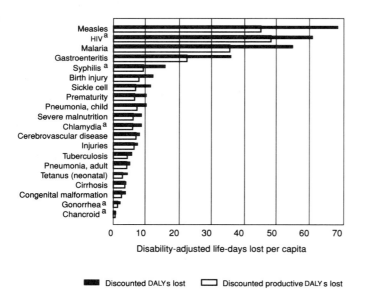

Disability-adjusted life-days lost per capita

■ Discounted DALYs lost   □ Discounted productive DALYs lost

a. Sexually transmitted disease.
Source: Authors' estimates; Ghana Health Assessment Project Team 1981.

comfort is known to vary by disease, by sex, and randomly across individuals. Socioeconomic factors which affect demand for medical care of an STD will include the income, education, geographical location, attitude toward STDs, and access to household resources of the infected individual. Sup-

ply considerations, such as the availability and quality of medical services, will also affect the duration of infectivity. Because we believe that the demand factors conspire with the supply factors in lengthening the duration of the average STD infection in many developing countries, we adopt assumed periods of infectivity which are roughly twice the durations typically found in industrial countries.

Because our model does not distinguish between the sexes, we must choose single values of the transmission probability and the duration of infectivity for each disease. Rows three and six of table 20-11 present these parameters, which are the averages of the parameters for the separate sexes.

A full statement of the model requires the specification of the equations of motion that determine the flows of individuals from the pool of susceptibles in a group (that is, the healthy, uninfected, nonimmune individuals) into the pool of infected in that group (that is, those individuals who suffer the consequences of the disease and are capable of transmitting it). In appendix 20B we present these equations and the derivations of the assertions made in the next few paragraphs.

Suppose the noncore group were isolated from the core. Under this assumption, row eight of table 20-11 shows the value of the reproduction rate in the noncore group for each simulated epidemic. Recall that a reproduction rate less than unity implies that the disease will fail to reproduce itself, dying out over time. Gonorrhea and chancroid would behave this way in the noncore group, because the reproduction rates in this group, in the absence of interaction with the core, would be 0.825 and 0.293, respectively. In contrast, note the particularly high value of 4.32 for the reproduction rate of HIV with ulcers in the noncore group. Also, note from row seven that

Figure 20-6. *Share of* STDs *in Total Disease Burden in a High-Prevalence African City, and Proportion of* STDs

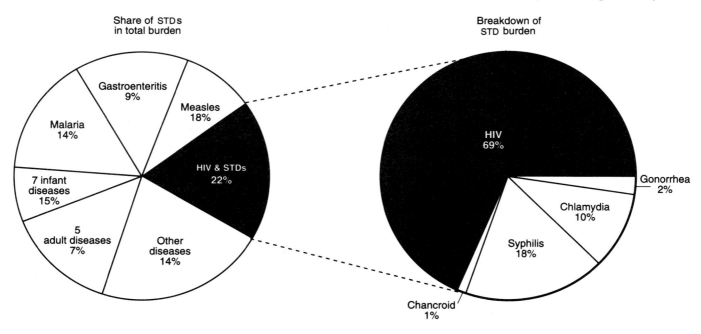

Source: Authors' estimates.

Table 20-10. Assumptions for Base Run of Core and Noncore Groups

| Parameter | Symbol[a] | Sexual activity risk groups | |
		Core	Noncore
Group size	N	1,000	50,000
New sexual partners per day	a	0.2	0.02
Total encounters per day per group	aN	200	1,000
Ratio of group encounters to total	b	0.167	0.833
Selectivity	G	0	0
Mixing coefficients	M_{1i}	0.167	0.833
	M_{2i}	0.167	0.833
Starting prevalence by group	I_0	0.2	0.01

a. See appendix 20B for the definitions of parameters not defined in the text. All these parameters are group specific except G, which is constant across groups.

Source: Authors' construction.

all the diseases can sustain themselves independently in the core.

Another important consequence derivable from the reproduction rate is the equilibrium level of prevalence of a disease in a single isolated group. Because infected individuals remain infected only D days, it is possible for an equilibrium to be established between the flows of individuals into and out of the infected pool. In appendix 20B we show that the equilibrium prevalence rate for an epidemic confined to a single group with reproduction rate R greater than one is simply expressed as $(R - 1)/R$. The fourteenth and fifteenth rows of table 20-11 present these rates, which would be approached asymptotically as the epidemic becomes endemic within a single group. Note the marked difference in equilibrium prevalence rates between the core and noncore groups for each disease, which is caused by the assumed tenfold difference in the rate of partner change of the two groups. The only exception to this pattern is the epidemic of HIV with ulcers, which, as distinct from HIV without ulcers, eventually becomes prevalent within more than 75 percent of the noncore as well as the core groups. This result derives from the extremely high value of the reproduction rate for this disease, which itself is due to the high probability of transmission combined with the long duration of infectivity for HIV—ten years.[18]

Table 20-11. Medical Parameters and Simulation Results for STDs

Parameter	Gonorrhea	Syphilis	Chlamydia	Chancroid	HIV without ulcers	HIV with ulcers
Transmission probabilities						
Male to female	0.6	0.250	0.4	0.350	0.03	0.1
Female to male	0.4	0.200	0.3	0.300	0.01	0.05
Q[a]	0.5	0.225	0.35	0.325	0.02	0.075
Duration of infectivity (days)						
Male	45	180	90	45	2,880	2,880
Female	120	270	240	45	2,880	2,880
D[b]	82.5	225	165	45	2,880	2,880
Reproductive rates[c]						
R (core)	8.25	10.1	11.55	2.93	11.5	43.2
R (noncore)	0.825	1.01	1.155	0.293	1.15	4.32
Contact number[d]	2.063	2.5	2.887	0.731	2.88	10.8
Parameters of equation of motion when selectivity, G, is set at 0[c]						
C_{11}	0.0167	0.0075	0.0117	0.0108	0.0007	0.0025
C_{12}	0.0833	0.0375	0.0583	0.0542	0.0033	0.0125
C_{22}	0.0083	0.0037	0.0058	0.0054	0.0003	0.0013
C_{21}	0.0017	0.0007	0.0012	0.0011	0.0001	0.0003
Equilibrium prevalence rates: isolated groups[e]						
Core	0.879	0.901	0.913	0.658	0.913	0.977
Noncore	0	0.012	0.134	0	0.132	0.769
Equilibrium prevalence rates: interacting groups[e]						
Core	0.684	0.778	0.822	0	0.822	0.972
Noncore	0.178	0.259	0.316	0	0.315	0.778

a. Average of male-to-female and female-to-male transmission probability per sexual partner.
b. Average of male and female durations of infectivity.
c. See appendix 20B for definitions.
d. Weighted average of R (core) and R (noncore).
e. Multiply by 1,000 for prevalence per 1,000.

Source: Rows 1, 2, 4, and 5 present results of a Delphi survey conducted by the authors. Other figures are authors' calculations; Hooper and others 1978.

As was pointed out earlier, the interesting feature of STD epidemiology is that the core and noncore groups do not remain isolated from each other but instead choose sex partners from the other group. Assuming that partners are selected from the two groups without prejudice in proportion to their availability (that is, the selectivity coefficient is 0 percent), Hethcote and Yorke (1984) show that the reproduction rate for the core-noncore model is simply the weighted average of the two individual rates.[19] This joint rate is called the "contact number" by Hethcote and Yorke and in table 20-11. If it is less than unity, as it is for chancroid, the disease will die out, not only in the noncore group, in which the reproduction rate is less than one, but also in the core group, in which it is greater than one. This occurs because the disease in the core is diluted by interaction between the core and noncore, making the disease unsustainable in either group. To produce the endemic levels of chancroid infection observed in African cities today, this simple model would require modified parameters, perhaps more active sexual behavior, a higher rate of transmission, or a longer duration of infectivity than we have assumed.

To explore the differences among the six different diseases, while holding constant the assumptions about sexual behavior, we simulate an epidemic of each disease from the same initial conditions. We start each epidemic at a prevalence rate of 1 percent among the 50,000 noncore and a prevalence rate of 20 percent among the 1,000 members of the core. The time paths of all six epidemics over a ten-year period are displayed in figure 20-7. In the graph in the left part of figure 20-7, only the core groups in the six epidemics are compared, whereas in the graph on the right side the results for the noncore groups are presented. In comparing the two graphs, keep in mind that 100 percent of the core is only 1,000 people, whereas 10 percent of the noncore, the upper limit of the vertical axis, represents 5,000 people. Because 2 percent of the noncore equals the entire population of the core, the data in figure 20-7 reveal that the size of any growing epidemic in the noncore quickly exceeds the total size of the core group.

When the model is simulated for ten years, five of the six epidemics closely approach their equilibrium levels in the core (chancroid at zero), whereas three do so in the noncore. Note that instead of disappearing entirely, as gonorrhea would have done in the absence of the core group, the prevalence of this disease rises to an equilibrium level of about 3 percent in the noncore. Similarly the prevalence of syphilis, which would have leveled off at the endemic level of 7.4 percent, instead reaches 28 percent at the end of the ten-year period. Although HIV spreads rapidly in the core even in the absence of ulcers, the large increase in its rate of spread in the noncore as a result of the ulcers is interesting indeed. Of course the simulated rate of spread assumes that the entire noncore (and core) populations suffer from genital ulcers. Because such ulcers are caused by syphilis, herpes simplex, and chancroid, a more realistic simulation for HIV might lie between the ulcers and no ulcers scenarios presented here. The dramatic difference between the

ulcer and the no ulcer scenarios lends credence to the hypothesis that a putative greater prevalence of genital ulcers in Africa than in Asia or Latin America accounts for the apparently more rapid heterosexual spread of AIDS in Africa.[20]

How "realistic" are the simulations presented here? The equilibrium prevalence rates of gonorrhea, syphilis, and chlamydia in the noncore are similar to prevalence rates estimated in some African capitals (see table 20-2). The estimated prevalence rate increase for HIV infection in the noncore group, from 1 percent to 10 percent in ten years, is remarkably similar to the epidemic's trend in some of the worst-hit African capitals (see figure 20-3).

How do the results of this modeling exercise change our understanding of the relative burden of STDs as presented above? One observation stands out. The total burden of an STD is likely to be unequally distributed between the core and the noncore groups, with the core group bearing a much larger per capita burden. The observation by Rothenberg (1983) regarding the relatively greater risk of STDs of inhabitants of urban as opposed to adjoining rural New York State communities is directly applicable to African countries. Table 20-4 and figure 20-2 both display the dramatic differences that have been found between the prevalence levels of HIV infection in urban and rural African communities. The World Health Organization's Global Programme on AIDS adopts the assumption that rural prevalence levels are about one-tenth those of urban areas (James Chin, in a 1988 article cited by Bongaarts and Way 1989).[21]

Although the model-generated values on the estimated trajectories of these epidemics cannot be used to predict actual prevalence rates, the behavior of the various epidemics depicted in figure 20-7 does capture some features of their real-world counterparts. In particular the modeled gonorrhea and syphilis epidemics demonstrate the lesson learned by STD modelers a decade ago, that the core group plays an important role in maintaining the prevalence rate of an epidemic in the noncore at levels substantially above those that would obtain without interaction with the core. In the next section of this chapter, we will use the simulations presented in figure 20-7 as a base against which to compare the effects of interventions. The results in this section suggest that policies which target interventions at the core group may be particularly promising candidates.

The Demographic Effect of AIDS Epidemic

Because the model used in the last section does not incorporate demographic changes, it is not suitable for modeling the long-run demographic burden of the HIV epidemic. Still, several models in the literature do incorporate an explicit model of heterosexually transmitted HIV infection into a demographic model of population growth. One of the first of these, by Bongaarts (1988, 1989), simulates the spread of the infection over twenty-five years in a population structured to resemble that of many African countries. Without the epidemic, the model country's population would continue to grow at 3 per-

Figure 20-7. Simulated STD Epidemics in Core and Noncore Groups

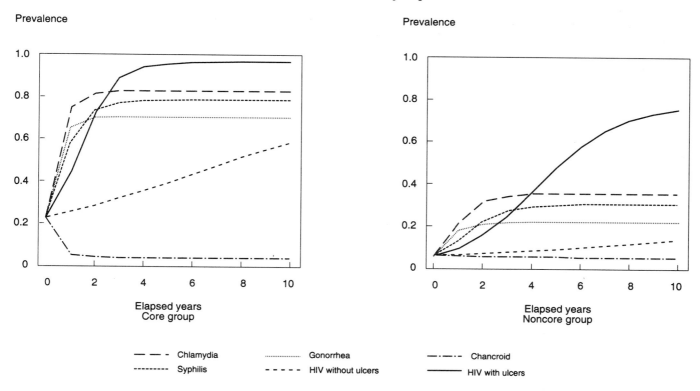

Source: Authors' estimates.

cent per year, birth and death rates would continue to fall, and life expectancy would continue to rise from its current level of forty-six by 0.3 years per annum.

Choosing hypothetical sexual behavior parameters and plausible epidemiological parameters, Bongaarts finds that, once introduced, the HIV epidemic reaches a stable dynamic equilibrium after about twenty-five years. By that time, the model predicts, the proportion of HIV-infected adults will stabilize at less than 30 percent, although approximately 55 percent of core-group females will be infected. Because Bongaarts's model assumes a latency period of 9.3 years, infected women have almost as many children as they would have had in the absence of AIDS. As a result the birth rate is unaffected by the epidemic and the increased perinatal and adult mortality offset one another, producing no change in the dependency ratio as a result of the epidemic.

What does change, of course, is the death rate. If the HIV prevalence rate in a given adult population is 10 percent and about 5 percent of those infected die each year, then the AIDS-related mortality in this population will be 5 per 1,000 more than it otherwise would have been. Each additional 10 percent in the infection rate similarly adds about 5 per 1,000 to the mortality rate. Because the baseline mortality rate for adults fifteen through forty-nine in Sub-Saharan Africa is 5 or 6 per 1,000, infection rates of 10 percent, 20 percent, and 30 percent will double, triple, and quadruple the adult mortality rates, respectively.

Bongaarts's model projects these increased mortality rates onto an entire national population in which the baseline mortality is currently about 19 per 1,000. Instead of declining from 19 to 13 per 1,000, as Bongaarts assumed would occur without AIDS, the death rate is predicted to rise to 26 per 1,000—twice what it would otherwise have been. With the birth rate's downward trend unchanged but the death rate increasing, Bongaarts's model projects the population growth rate to slow from 3 percent to 1.9 percent per year by the end of the twenty-five-year period.

This conclusion is remarkably robust to changes in two principal assumptions: the initial population growth rate and the severity of the epidemic. If the population growth rate were only 2.5 percent per year (lower than in any Sub-Saharan African country except Chad and the Central African Republic), the population growth rate would remain positive unless the seroprevalence rate attains the extremely high level of 45 percent among all adults (Bongaarts 1989, figure 7). With population growth rates at a more typical level of 3.0 percent or 3.5 percent, the epidemic severity required to shrink the population would be even higher—55 percent or 60 percent.

A second model combining epidemiologic and demographic features is by Anderson and others (1986). It predicts that population growth rates could eventually become negative if the initial incidence rate of HIV infection in the susceptible population exceeds the population growth rate. However, the incidence rates estimated from a few Central African cities exceed national population growth rates. For this reason, in this and later papers, Anderson and co-authors conclude that HIV infection could cause populations to stop growing within 30 to 100 years from the beginning of the epidemic. In their words, "[a] wide range of parameter values, all within the bounds suggested by current empirical studies, predicted asymptotically negative population growth rates" (Anderson and McLean 1988, p. 231).

These predictions of population shrinkage in African countries have received a great deal of attention. The incidence rates of HIV infection cited by the authors to support the plausibility of their assumptions, however, are all from studies of sexually active urban adults, some of whom were prostitutes. In fact, African populations are typically only 15 percent urban, and the unknown portion of women who are prostitutes is unlikely to exceed a few percentage points. Even an extraordinarily high incidence rate among all urban adults of 20 percent per year results in only a 3 percent incidence rate in the entire population if the rural 85 percent population remains uninfected, and this would be too low to result in negative population growth rates in most countries. If the incidence rate among urban adult susceptibles is instead under 2 percent per year, as it was estimated to be among the employees of the main hospital in Kinshasa, then negative population growth would require implausibly high rates of growth of infection in the rural population.

The Anderson-May-McLean models are parsimonious in portraying the interactions among demographic and epidemiologic variables. The models predict negative population growth, but only for implausible assumptions regarding the initial incidence rates of HIV infection in national populations.[22]

Recently the work of a team of modelers sponsored by the U.S. Department of State's Interagency Working Group on AIDS Models and Methods has come to fruition with the release of a model called the iwgAIDS model (Stanley and others 1989). Embodied in a user-friendly computer software package, the iwgAIDS model addresses such issues as transmission between prostitutes, their clients, and the wives of their clients and choice of sexual partners by age and location (that is, urban or rural), as well as transmission by blood transfusion, needle-sharing, and the vertical route from mother to infant. Although sufficiently flexible to project negative population growth, given sufficiently pessimistic, "worst case" assumptions, the intermediate scenario predicted by early runs of this model is a growth rate of 1.1 percent per year (Stanley and others 1989). More recently a careful attempt by the U.S. Bureau of the Census to characterize a "typical" African HIV epidemic over twenty-five years with this model predicts dramatic increases in adult mortality comparable to those predicted by the Bongaarts model and a fall in urban life-expectancy by nineteen years compared with the base case. At the end of twenty-five years, the national population growth rate is still growing at 2.2 percent per year, compared with 2.8 percent projected without the AIDS epidemic (Way and

Stanecki 1991). Future work with this model will characterize the likely epidemics in the harder-hit African countries and on Latin American and Asian countries, in which transmission patterns and the underlying population dynamics differ substantially from Africa.

For similar choices of parameters, all three models produce similar results regarding several key indicators of the long-term burden of the epidemic. First, both models agree that the dependency ratio, measured by

$$Dependency\ ratio = \frac{Number\ of\ people < 15\ or > 64}{Number\ of\ people\ 15\ through\ 64}$$

would not be greatly affected by the epidemic. This result at first seems surprising, in view of the anecdotal evidence from heavily affected areas of Tanzania and Uganda that AIDS is the "grandmother disease," because it kills adults, leaving orphaned children in the care of the grandparents. The explanation for this apparent contradiction lies in the distribution of the deaths. Because parental deaths precede child deaths in some households and follow them in others, the overall dependency ratio can remain relatively constant despite large increases in the number of orphans from the former households.

Still, the authors of all these models emphasize that any reductions in population growth rate caused by the HIV epidemic will be due to increased deaths primarily among young adults. Far from benefiting the population by reducing its growth rate, the consequent doubling or quadrupling of the mortality rate in individuals age fifteen through forty-four would have "disastrous effects on the health care system, the economy and the fabric of society" (Bongaarts 1988, p. 36). In the absence of a vaccine or effective treatment, these consequences can be prevented only by a concerted educational campaign designed to change sexual behavior. We will consider the possible design of such a campaign below.

The Gender-Specific Burdens of STDs

Do sexually transmitted diseases burden one sex more than another in developing countries? There are tentative answers to this question from both the static and the dynamic perspective.

Appendix 20A and table 20-8 include separate estimates for men and women of the STD mortality and morbidity rates in both high-incidence and low-incidence urban settings. Because the static burden calculations summarized in table 20-9 and figures 20-5 and 20-6 are intended to compare the effects of individual diseases, the effects on the two sexes are combined there. To the extent that appendix 20A and table 20-8 differentiate between the genders, we can return to them to estimate the ratio of the burden borne by women to that borne by men for each disease.

Because the statistics are based on pattern II urban areas, they ignore homosexual and IV drug transmission routes for HIV infection. In these pattern II countries, the ratio of male to female cases is close to unity for HIV transmission (see table 20-3). Therefore the data in appendix 20A and tables 20-8 and 20-9 are not able to discriminate between the effects of HIV transmission on men and on women. The effects of chancroid on the two sexes are also difficult to distinguish. For the remaining three diseases, however, the burden borne by each of the two sexes is presented in columns 4 and 5 of table 20-12, and a comparison of the per capita burden on women with that on men for each of the five STDs is shown in figure 20-8.

According to the data in table 20-12 and figure 20-8, women in a high-prevalence urban setting bear a total STD illness burden of 44.4 disability-adjusted life-days per capita per year, about 3 percent more than the burden borne by men. If human papilloma virus and its sequela, cervical cancer, had been included, and if our methodology permitted us to capture the earlier onset of HIV infection in women than in men (Ryder and Piot 1988), the excess burden on women over that on men would be greater.[23]

But these static calculations ignore the interactions between the presence of this disease and the socioeconomic positions of women in a population. Three types of such interactions are of concern. First, what are the effects of infertility caused by STDs on the future welfare of the affected individual—and how do such effects differ between men and women? Second, what have been the cultural adaptations to high prevalence of STDs and how have those adaptations affected the welfare of the two genders? Third, what has been the effect of these cultural adaptations, if any, on the spread of STDs and on consequent levels of infertility?

To do justice to any of these questions across all human cultures would require an extensive ethnographic survey, which space limitations do not permit. With respect to the first question, however, it is well established that a woman's value in a poor culture often hinges crucially on her presumed or demonstrated fertility. Although infertility clearly harms men as well, some cultures in which infertility is common have customs which protect an infertile man—but not an infertile woman—from its consequences. For example, in northwestern Tanzania, an infertile man may acquire an heir by being the

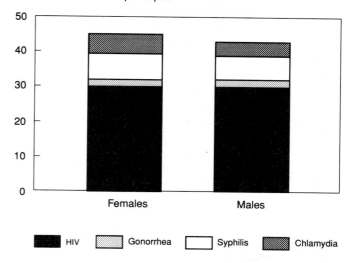

Figure 20-8. Annual Gender-Specific Burden of STDs

Discounted DALYs cost per capita

Source: Table 20-12.

first man to have intercourse with a woman after she gives birth. In this same culture, a husband may return an infertile wife to her parents and request the return of her bride-price (Reining 1972).

Whether a given cultural practice has developed in response to the high prevalence of STD-caused infertility would be extremely difficult to establish, even with an extensive ethnographic survey, because it would require longitudinal information specific to a given culture on both STD prevalence rates and the frequency of various cultural practices.[24] In the case of the practices just mentioned, however, it is hard to resist the interpretation that the practices have become more entrenched as a result of the high prevalence of STDs. Whatever their cause, it is clear that these cultural adaptations have resulted in an unequal sharing of the burden of infertility—imposing it more on the women than on the men.

The next link in the chain of causation is between such gender-biased adaptations to the prevalence of STDs and the

Table 20-12. Burden of STDs in High-Prevalence Urban Areas, by Gender

Disease	Average incidence (per thousand)		Discounted disability-adjusted life-days lost (per capita per year)			Discounted disability-adjusted life-years saved	
	Women	Men	Total	Women	Men	Women	Men
Chancroid	6.2	6.2	0.5	0.25	0.25	0.2	0.2
Chlamydia	9.5	12.4	8.6	4.8	3.8	1.3	0.8
Gonorrhea	7.3	10.8	1.9	0.9	0.9	1.0	0.7
HIV	8.5	8.5	60.6	30.3	30.3	19.5	19.5
Syphilis	5.8	5.8	15.9	8.2	7.7	3.9	3.7
Total	n.a.	n.a.	87.5	44.4	43.1	n.a.	n.a.
Average DALY saved per case selected	n.a.	n.a.	n.a.	n.a.	n.a.	5.6	4.7

n.a. Not applicable.
Source: Authors' calculations.

further spread of these diseases. In an exhaustive study of infertility in Sub-Saharan Africa, Odile Frank writes:

> Marital instability caused by infertility and the spread of venereal disease caused by marital instability and sexual mobility can form a vicious cycle. The movement of abandoned or rejected barren women to urban prostitution has been noted in Niger, Uganda, and the Central African Republic. Similarly, in many of these societies, marital and sexual mobility on the part of the women is interpreted as a desperate attempt to become pregnant, and tolerance on the part of society as a means to maximize their chances of doing so. . . . Once venereal disease was introduced into a community with some degree of sexual or marital mobility, its diffusion might have been assured by the existing customs. [Subsequently] the mobility itself [may have been] intensified to overcome the fertility effects (Frank 1983, pp. 22 and 26).

The existence of such a vicious cycle has recently been argued by Judith Wasserheit (1989), whose depiction of the causal links is reproduced as figure 20-9. To Wasserheit and Frank's argument, we add the intervening link of low status of women to their low education and their small numbers in urban areas, factors which the earlier discussion suggests cause, or create the preconditions for, urban prostitution. Furthermore, Wasserheit and Frank both argue that the resulting high level of infertility, far from damping the African population growth, exacerbates it by preventing individuals from confi-

dently postponing conception. In Frank's words, "[a]s long as infertility remains prominent in Africa, large numbers of individuals and some entire populations will remain thwarted in their ambitions to bear and raise children, and even larger numbers may resist both intrinsic and extrinsic pressures for fertility limitation in the face of the risk to which they see others exposed" (Frank 1983, p. 40).

Wasserheit draws an additional and more direct link between STDs and the success of family planning programs: "In the absence of accurate diagnosis and effective education and therapy [for STDs], it is far easier for a woman to blame her vaginal discharge on her contraceptive method than to entertain and address [other possibilities]. The net result is often that the woman drops her contraceptive method under the misimpression that the method caused an unrelated infection" (Wasserheit 1989, p. 10).

If the cost of a large population growth rate is borne disproportionately by women, then these arguments that STDs exacerbate the population growth rate reinforce the case that STDs affect women more than men. We leave as a challenge to others the quantification of these interaction effects.

Lowering or Postponing the Incidence of STDs

This section will discuss the principles and benefits involved in preventing STDs.

Figure 20-9. Interaction between Sociocultural and Physiological Factors in Reproductive Tract Infections in Developing Countries

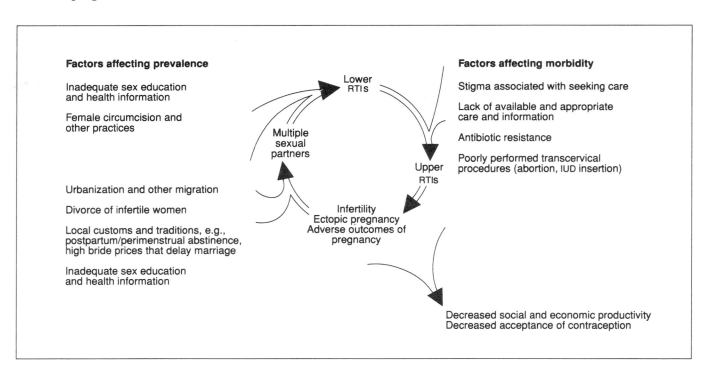

Source: Wasserheit 1989.

Principles of Primary Prevention of STDs

Principles of primary prevention follow, grouped by the form of transmission targeted.

TYPES OF PRIMARY PREVENTIVE STRATEGY. The four different modes of transmission of the HIV virus are sexual intercourse, mother-to-child (that is, "vertical"), transfusion of blood or blood products, and needles and other skin-piercing instruments. Each of these transmission modes applies to at least one CSTD as well as to HIV. Primary prevention strategies are designed to disrupt these modes of transmission, but a large number of different policies could contribute to this goal.

In table 20-13 we classify primary prevention strategies according to whether the indicated behavioral change is voluntary, mandatory, or only a passive response to environmental changes. This classification scheme, which has been borrowed from the field of injury prevention, directs our attention to the degree of coercion required to implement a policy and thus to the probable cost of the intervention.

Each of these three strategy categories corresponds to a distinctly different type of government policy. Voluntary be-havior modification can be encouraged only by information, education, and communication (IEC) campaigns and by individual counseling. Mandatory behavior modification requires the enactment and enforcement of government laws and regulations. Passive responses are the least intrusive of the three types of strategies, depending on government policies which change either the inherent likelihood of the risky behaviors or the risk attached to them.

In the rest of this subsection, available information on the effectiveness of interventions will be described for each transmission mode. By reference to table 20-13, each intervention can be associated with a voluntary, mandatory, or passive means of behavior modification.

PREVENTION OF SEXUAL TRANSMISSION: TARGETING. According to Hethcote and Yorke (1984, p. 32), "[i]n the early 1970s, the prevalent idea was . . . that everyone who was sexually active could get gonorrhea and, consequently, . . . that 'gonorrhea is everybody's problem.'" Then in the late 1970s public health opinion changed markedly in the United States, to the extent that the change was described by a WHO scientific working group in the following words: "This assumption is no longer in

Table 20-13. Interventions for Primary Prevention of STDs and HIV Infection, by Mode of Transmission and Form of Behavior Modification

Behavior modification	Mode of Transmission			
	Sexual intercourse	Mother-to-infant (vertical)	Transfusion of blood and blood products	Needles and other skin-piercing instruments
Voluntary (change demand by changing information or preferences)	*Encourage* Use of condoms or virucide Fewer sex partners Partner selection Partner notification by patient referral Sex education in schools Early treatment of STDs	*Offer* Voluntary screening of pregnant women Eye prophylaxis at birth, on request	*Encourage* Test of donated blood Recipient choice of donors Donor deferral Public information on low benefits and high risk of transfusion	*Encourage* Providers to sterilize reusable needles and to discard disposable ones Consumers to request sterile needles Providers to exercise caution with blood Needle exchange by IVDA
Mandatory (change external incentive structure by imposing quantity restrictions)	*Enforce* Regulation or prohibition of prostitution Quarantine of infected individuals Partner notification by provider referral	*Enforce* Screening of pregnant women Pregnancy counseling of infected women Contraceptive counseling	*Enforce* Provider compliance with transfusion criteria Blood screening and blood banking Eye prophylaxis	*Enforce* Destruction of disposable needles Regulation of handling of blood by HIV-positive patients Laws against IV drug abuse
Passive response to environmental changes (change external incentive structure through price restrictions)	*Increase* Subsidies for condoms and for STD treatment Tax or regulation of night clubs and alcohol Ratio of women to men in urban areas Jobs for single women Education for women	*Increase* Subsidies for condoms and for STD treatment Tax or regulation of night clubs and alcohol Ratio of women to men in urban areas Jobs for single women Education for women	*Prevent* Malaria, especially among children Anemia *Increase* Price of transfusions	*Provide* Needles that self-destruct after one use

Source: Authors' construction.

vogue in [the United States], and decisions for control are now based on the concept of the core of transmitters of disease which postulates that a relatively small proportion of the population is contributing to the maintenance of the epidemic and that it is precisely this group of transmitters that is particularly important [for disease control]" (WHO 1978, p. 116, as quoted in Hethcote and Yorke 1984)

Motivated to a remarkable degree by quasi-cost-effectiveness arguments derived from mathematical simulations, public health strategies against gonorrhea in the United States turned away from broad screening programs of the general population to focus on "targeted" control programs. Targeting strategies included partner notification in an attempt to identify and treat both the infector and the infectee(s) of the index case, rescreening of treated cases several months later to check for reinfection, and outreach activities to high-risk groups. Some examples of the arguments marshaled by mathematical models for such targeted activities include the following:

- Because diagnosed and treated cases are likely to be in the core group at high risk of reinfection, rescreening these cases several months after treatment is "approximately four times as effective per number of individuals tested as [would be the] screening [of randomly selected individuals from the general population] in reducing total incidence" (Hethcote and Yorke 1984, p. 32).

- Because the infectors of an identified case are more likely to have belonged to the core group than are infectees of that case, contact tracing, screening, and treatment lower disease prevalence more per discovered case if targeted at the former than the latter (Hethcote and Yorke 1984, p. 85).

- Under the hypothesis that a vaccination is developed which provides immunity to gonorrhea, but only for a short time, "post-treatment vaccination is about five times as effective per number of persons immunized as random vaccination in the population" (Hethcote and Yorke 1984, p. 33).

Empirical confirmation of the concept of the core group was presented by Rothenberg (1983):

The pattern of reported gonorrhea in upstate New York (exclusive of New York City) in the years 1975–80 is one of intense urban concentration, with concentric circles of diminishing incidence. The relative risk for gonorrhea in these central core areas, compared to background state rates, is 19.8 for men and 15.9 for women, but as high as 40 in selected census tracts. . . . Contact investigation data suggest that sexual contact tends to exhibit geographic clustering as well. These observations provide support for narrow focusing of epidemiologic resources as a major disease control strategy.

There are interesting parallels and contrasts between the history of public health thought regarding CSTDs and AIDS. It is natural to suppose that public health thinking about control strategies for HIV infection would build on the insights de-scribed above, taking maximum advantage of every available opportunity to target control activities. Instead the possibility of such targeting has been resisted with language which is reminiscent of the decades-old description of gonorrhea as "everybody's problem."[25]

The core is an epidemiological concept, rather than a precisely defined social group, and so identifying the core in a given population and reaching its members with education or treatment may be extremely difficult and costly. Because some prostitutes are relatively easy to identify, they are often the only part of the core that is reached. Countries like Ghana and Rwanda are conducting an AIDS-prevention program among their military personnel, demonstrating that targeting this part of the core group is sometimes politically feasible (Lamptey and Potts 1990). Clients of prostitutes are more difficult to reach, but some of them acquire a symptomatic STD and present themselves for treatment at a clinic. In general, men and women with an STD are by definition at risk, and they are a reasonably accessible group for HIV/STD prevention activities. Finally, sexually active adolescents can be reached through the school system and through formal and informal youth organizations and activities, such as sports clubs and popular concerts.

By selecting some groups for special attention, a targeting policy runs two risks: those targeted may be—or feel—stigmatized, and those not targeted may react with a false sense of security. Because, in contrast to CSTDs, HIV infection is incurable, policies to target prevention efforts at core groups or at infected individuals, for example, through contact tracing, can assume ominous political overtones. HIV-infected persons (HIPs) will lack confidence in the ability of a publicly operated contact-tracing program to maintain the confidentiality of its records. This fear is particularly well founded in developing countries, where the staff of the public health system is known by, and accessible to, most of the population, and traditions of bureaucratic anonymity and confidentiality are unknown. Once publicly identified, HIPs may lose substantial proportions of their civil rights, as either official or unofficial pressures attempt to isolate them from society. The problem is exacerbated in communities in which people continue to believe that AIDS might be transmitted by shaking hands, by eating out of a common bowl, or by other mundane, nonsexual social acts (Wilson and Mehryar 1991).

One strategy that has been effective in combating stigmatization has also appeared to contribute substantially to program success: peer counseling. Peers have been successful counselors in pilot projects with prostitutes in Kenya, Ghana, and Cameroon (Ngugi and others 1988; Lamptey and Potts 1990), with truck drivers in Tanzania, and with youth in Zaire.[26] Peers are not only better at communicating messages about safe sex; they are also better at finding other core group members in the first place. Thus their use can bring the otherwise prohibitive costs of finding core group members down to quite modest proportions. The section below elaborates on the cost of targeted and untargeted programs.

PREVENTION OF SEXUAL TRANSMISSION: INTERVENTIONS. Avoidance of sexual exposure to pathogenic microorganisms can be achieved in three ways: (a) avoidance of potentially infected sex partners (through sexual abstinence or mutual monogamy); (b) protection with a barrier method during sexual intercourse (condom use); (c) practicing only nonpenetrative sex ("safer sex"). All three methods depend entirely on individual behavior, which may be modified by various kinds of health education, targeted or not. Because of the strong effects of culture and religion on attitudes toward sex, the effects of health education on sexual behavior necessarily differ across societies or even across subgroups of a society. Methods as different as mass campaigns, school programs, and face-to-face counseling are being used in the primary prevention of STDs and HIV infection, implying widely varying personnel and recurrent cost requirements.

Although the incidence of HIV infection dropped spectacularly in selected groups of homosexual men in North America and Europe (Coutinho, van Griensven, and Moss 1989), how much of this decline can be attributed to health education programs is unclear. In the developing world, the effectiveness of health education on sexual behavior is even less understood. Targeted education programs in several African cities resulted in dramatically increased condom use among clients of female prostitutes, although this was not always associated with a decrease in the incidence of HIV (Lamptey and others 1988; Ngugi and others 1988; Laga and others 1989). The protection offered by a condom during intercourse with a person with an STD is unknown, but probably approaches 100 percent if properly used and if no breakage occurs.

Because spermicides and viricides can be controlled by the female partner, there has been substantial interest in the few studies to evaluate their in vitro activity against gonorrhea and chlamydial and HIV infection. There is some evidence that they protect against gonorrhea and chlamydia, especially when used in conjunction with a condom or diaphragm (Cole and others 1980; Austin, Louv, and Alexander 1984; Rosenberg, Schultz, and Burton 1986; Louv and others 1988). The authors of one study found no effect of contraceptive sponges on HIV acquisition in highly exposed prostitutes in Nairobi (Kreiss and others 1986). Therefore, it is premature to recommend them in the STD/HIV prevention program. Because of their potential importance in the primary prevention of STD and HIV, further research on this issue is a top priority.

Partner notification, also known as contact tracing, is an important element of CSTD programs. First vigorously promoted in the United States in the 1930s, tracing the sexual contacts of syphilis patients only began "in earnest [in] the 1940s when effective treatment for syphilis became available" (Bayer 1990, p. 125). Subsequently it became accepted in the United States as an essential component of the public health strategies against syphilis in the 1960s, gonorrhea in the 1970s, and chlamydia in the 1980s.

Partner notification acts to prevent the spread of a CSTD epidemic in two ways. First, the uninfected sexual contacts become aware of their risk and can protect themselves. Second, the infected contacts can be offered a cure. In addition, as argued earlier, sexual contacts of an index case are more likely than is the average CSTD patient to be members of the core group of transmitters.

The distinction between "mandatory" and voluntary partner notification is somewhat artificial because it is impossible to verify that an individual has named all sexual contacts. Partner notification programs can be more or less aggressive by varying the intensity of the interview and by offering the choice between (a) provider referral, in which the provider notifies the contact without revealing the identity of the index case; and (b) patient referral, in which the patient notifies the contact and advises the contact to seek counseling, testing, and, if necessary, treatment.

Policy prescriptions for HIV infection require a different perspective. Until recently, public health departments have not been able to offer any treatment or other incentive which might persuade exposed individuals to run the (real or perceived) risk of being identified and stigmatized as seropositive for HIV. Early experiments in Colorado showed that, in the United States, aggressive partner notification at a public health laboratory reduced the number of people asking to be tested. This finding supported worries that tying partner notification to testing would "drive the epidemic underground."

Now that zidovudine (AZT) has been found to retard the progression from HIV infection to AIDS, public health facilities able to offer AZT will for the first time be able to offer an incentive which will help to offset the fear of stigmatization. Furthermore, if distribution of AZT can be channeled through public health facilities with active partner notification programs, its availability will substantially improve the ability of these programs to trace contacts. In countries in which AZT can be afforded by the public health system, we expect the effectiveness of partner notification programs to rise dramatically. Even in the absence of a cure for HIV infection, the availability of AZT at public health facilities in a country may stimulate a movement of the AIDS control effort along the same path previously followed by CSTD control programs: that is, toward tightly targeted screening, rescreening, and partner notification programs and away from general public education (Clumeck and others 1989; Toomey and Cates, 1989).

Unfortunately for the application of such a strategy in developing countries, the price of AZT is extremely high. The current cost of $8,000 per patient-year may drop to $4,000 as a result of recent findings that a smaller dose gives the same effect as a larger one. That annual cost, however, exceeds the annual per capita gross national product (GNP) of almost all developing countries.

A remaining quandary is whether the individual who learns that he or she is seropositive for HIV will reduce high-risk sexual behavior. In American and European studies, knowledge of HIV infection has sometimes marginally decreased and sometimes actually increased high-risk behavior (Office of Technology Assessment 1988, p. 14; Van Griensven and others 1989). Until a medical treatment is available to reduce the infectivity of HIV-infected persons, the principal effect of partner notification programs on transmission may be to alert uninfected partners of their exposure and thereby motivate them to adopt safe sex practices. There is a pressing need for operational research on partner notification programs in diverse pattern II countries.

PREVENTION OF VERTICAL TRANSMISSION. For over a century, eye prophylaxis at birth has been the method of choice for the prevention of gonococcal conjunctivitis in the neonate. The method is simple and its effectiveness is 93 to 97 percent (Laga and others 1988; Laga and others 1989). It is officially recommended as a routine practice in most developing countries, although it is not always implemented (Laga and others 1986a and 1986b). Ocular prophylaxis at birth is not effective against chlamydial conjunctivitis, which is not a sight-threatening disease (Datta and others 1988; Hammerschlag and others 1989).

Detection and treatment of gonococcal and chlamydial infections in pregnant women may be the optimal strategy in controlling these diseases in mother and child, because it prevents transmission to the neonate as well as complications and sequelae in the mother. As discussed in appendix 20C, however, diagnosis of gonorrhea and chlamydial infection in women is technically demanding and as yet rarely available in the developing world. Such screening is more effective if targeted at women with higher prevalence rates for these infections, though this advantage may not outweigh the stigmatizing potential and lower social acceptability of selective screening. Moreover, attempts to delineate high-prevalence groups of pregnant women have met with variable success (Laga and others 1986a and 1986b; Braddick and others 1990). The prevention of neonatal chlamydial conjunctivitis and pneumonia is based on treatment of infected women, but, again, this is rarely practiced because of technical and fiscal reasons. Targeting screening activities for *C. trachomatis* infection (that is, to women below twenty years of age) has been recommended for the United States (Arnal and Holmes 1991).

Screening of pregnant women for evidence of syphilis is recommended in most countries of the world to prevent congenital syphilis. Although such screening is irregularly implemented, innovative programs involving primary health care workers using a simple and rapid assay for syphilis antibody (rapid plasma reagin test), have recently been initiated in Africa (Hira, Kamanga, and Bhat 1989).

Finally, screening pregnant women for HIV infection is increasingly used as a means of preventing perinatal HIV infection, although its application remains controversial in many countries and its effectiveness is unclear when the pregnancy is not interrupted (Braddick and Kreiss 1988).

PREVENTION OF TRANSFUSION-ACQUIRED HIV. Wherever possible, blood donations are being screened for syphilis and hepatitis B virus markers throughout the world—though the cost-effectiveness of screening blood donors for hepatitis B virus infection in hepatitis B endemic areas has been questioned (Ryder and others 1989). Storage of blood at 4 degrees centi-

grade for more than four days eliminates treponemes and could theoretically be used in countries in which no laboratory testing for syphilis is available. Areas without facilities for syphilis screening, however, do not usually have facilities for storing blood (Meheus and Deschryver 1989).

The prevention of transfusion-acquired HIV infection relies on four methods: (a) testing of all blood donations for HIV antibodies before transfusion and discarding donations that are HIV positive; (b) donor selection and recruitment (also known as donor "deferral") aiming at excluding donors presumably at high risk for HIV infection or at recruiting low-risk voluntary donors; (c) rational use of blood transfusion by the health service; (d) prevention of conditions which call for transfusion, especially severe anemia and childhood malaria. Improvement of prenatal care and the "safe motherhood" initiatives can reduce the need for peripartum transfusions, which are one of the main indications for blood transfusion in the developing world.

PREVENTION OF HIV TRANSMISSION BY SKIN-PIERCING TOOLS. Outbreaks of HIV infection in the Soviet Union suggest that intravenous injections may play an important role in the spread of HIV infection in some hospitalized populations (Pokrovski and others 1990). In general, the risk of infection from contaminated equipment is larger when prevalence among patients and staff is larger (Berkley 1991). Still, in contrast to other modes of transmission, the contribution of contaminated needles and syringes to the spread of HIV in pattern II countries is probably very small. Proper sterilization of reusable needles and syringes and use of disposable materials have been recommended to prevent the transmission of various microorganisms by injection.

Those who inject drugs are at increased risk for HIV infection through needle sharing and may be a source of infection for other population groups through sexual transmission. Prevention strategies for IV drug users are still largely experimental but mainly include prevention of IV drug use itself by health education, treatment of drug dependency, needle exchange programs, promotion of use of sterile or disinfected "works," and promotion of safer sex practices.

DEVELOPMENTS IN PRIMARY PREVENTION IN THE NEXT DECADE. A tremendous effort is being undertaken to develop a vaccine against HIV infection, though with little obvious success thus far. It is possible that such a vaccine will become available by the year 2000. Attempts to develop vaccines against gonorrhea and chlamydial infection have failed so far, and it is not expected that they will become available in the near future. A vaccine against syphilis seems even less likely.

Virucidal products for local genital prophylactic use will probably become available, but assessing their effectiveness will be difficult. Methods for barrier protection of women, such as the female condom, may become increasingly popular. As knowledge of people's sexual behavior and motivations increases, health education interventions may become more effective.

The Benefit of Averting a Case: Static Analysis

As explained earlier, unless a decisionmaker is considering the eradication of a disease, knowledge of the total burden of that disease is of less use to him or her than would be an estimate of the benefit of averting a single case. Coupled with information on the cost of averting a single case, this benefit measure would assist the decisionmaker to allocate resources. In the absence of interactions among different disease programs, the most cost-effective health resource allocation could be obtained by equating the health gained per dollar across all diseases.[27] The existence of these interactions prevents a straightforward application of this simple principle. Information on potential savings of disability-adjusted life-years from each averted case can still be a useful guide, which, together with ancillary information, can improve the effectiveness of health services in developing countries.

Earlier we defined the disability-adjusted life-years lost per capita per year from a given disease as a function of the discounted (productivity-weighted) number of disability-adjusted life-years lost per case of that disease; table 20A-3 provided these intermediate calculations which enabled the calculation of disease burdens for table 20-9. But the number of DALYs lost per case is also the estimated benefit of preventing, or of quickly curing, a single case of that disease. Thus, in order to estimate the health gain from averting a case of a disease, we need only turn back to table 20A-3 and reinterpret its content from this slightly different perspective. Figure 20-10 displays the results from table 20A-3 with diseases ranked in order of the disability-adjusted life-years (DALYs) saved per case averted.

Because the difference between the burden calculations done earlier and the benefit calculations in this section is to remove the effect of incidence rates, it is not surprising that conditions like sickle cell anemia, neonatal tetanus, and birth injury are favored by this change.[28] Each of these has a relatively low incidence compared with measles or malaria, for example, but each robs (an African) society of a great many life-years per case because its victims are so young. Discounting at 3 percent is not sufficient to offset this effect, so these diseases appear at the top of the list of benefits per case averted. Because of the high fourth-place ranking of HIV, however, STDs continue to hold a surprisingly high rank. Furthermore, note from figure 20-10 that adjustment for the relative productivity of the lost years raises HIV infection to first place among all the considered diseases.

Syphilis has been displaced by cirrhosis, cerebrovascular disease, tuberculosis, and several other diseases from its fifth-place ranking in figure 20-5. Although the other STDs rank much lower on the scale of benefits per case averted in this static analysis, the same caveat applies as was mentioned above: to the extent that chlamydia, gonorrhea, and chancroid predispose individuals to HIV infection, a portion of the benefit of averting a case of HIV should be attributed to the interventions which prevent the seemingly less important diseases.

Table 20-12 and figure 20-8 support the case that the static burden of STDs is slightly greater on women than on men in a typical high-prevalence urban setting. Another way to compare the genders is to ask how many disability-adjusted life-years would be saved on average by averting a case of STDs in each gender. According to the last columns of table 20-12, the static benefit is slightly higher when a case of chlamydia, gonorrhea, or syphilis is prevented or cured in a woman than if a similar case is prevented or cured in a man. Averaging these potential benefits with the equal benefits from preventing HIV or chancroid in a man or a woman yields an average static benefit of 5.6 disability-adjusted life-years for every case prevented in a woman, which is 19 percent more than the benefit of 4.7 DALYs of averting an STD in a man. Comparing either of these figures with the non-STDs in table 20A-3 or figure 20-10 shows that the benefit from curing an average STD ranks below tuberculosis and just above measles and malaria. When the unquantified interactions of STDs with a woman's socioeconomic status are added, STDs would rise even higher in importance.

The Benefit of Averting a Case: Dynamic Analysis

The above static analysis ignores the fact that each case of an STD prevented will, because of the contagiousness of the disease, prevent additional cases.[29] From the dynamic perspective, a health care intervention could achieve health benefits in two distinct ways. The simplest intervention is one that cures or prevents the infection of some people once. Such a "one-time" program might be implemented by a mobile clinic that visits a town once, never to return.[30] By changing the infection status of some people, a one-time program would

Figure 20-10. Static Benefit of Preventing a Case of STD and Other Diseases in Sub-Saharan Africa

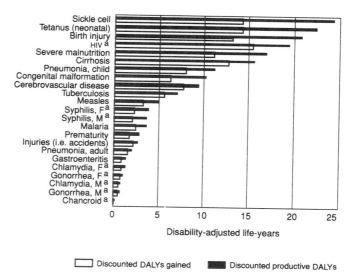

a. Sexually transmitted disease.
Source: Authors; Ghana Health Assessment Project Team 1981.

postpone ill health but would not prevent the epidemic from resuming its dynamic path toward equilibrium. The health benefits of a one-time program are due to the value of postponing an episode of ill health or a death. Because ultimately death can only be postponed, the benefits of such a one-time program should not be disparaged. Although temporary, they may nevertheless be considerable.

The second type of intervention is a sustained one that alters either the sexual behavior of the population or the disease-specific parameters. If maintained indefinitely, such changes will affect not only the epidemic's path toward equilibrium but the ultimate equilibrium prevalence rates themselves and therefore will have a permanent effect on the burden of the disease. Of course, a sustained intervention will typically require sustained budget support.

A CORE AS AGAINST A NONCORE STRATEGY. In order to examine the potential effect of a one-time intervention, we simulate an epidemic of each of the STDs in a population composed of two sexually active groups, the noncore and the core. We assume that the core comprises only 2 percent of the population but is five times more sexually active than the noncore and has a starting prevalence rate of 20 percent infection for each STD, compared with only 1 percent infection in the noncore.[31] Having simulated the course of each epidemic in the absence of intervention, we then simulate, for each STD, two different possible "one-time" interventions. In one of these we cure 100 individuals in the core and in the other we cure 100 individuals in the noncore. Then, by comparing each of these two alternative simulations with the base run, we compute which postpones more ill health and thereby best improves the health of the population.

Figures 20-11 and 20-12 portray the dynamic effect of preventing 100 cases of gonorrhea (figure 20-11) and of HIV (figure 20-12). Each figure contrasts the effect of preventing 100 cases in the core to preventing those cases in the noncore. For example, in figure 20-11 the top curve is calculated as the difference between the number of new cases of gonorrhea each month with no intervention and the smaller number if there is an intervention, which is applied only to the core group. In the sixth month after 100 core individuals are cured of gonorrhea, there are approximately 380 fewer new cases of gonorrhea, in the core and the noncore together, than if the intervention had not occurred. In contrast, if the 100 cures were effected in the noncore group, the number of cases averted during the sixth month in both groups would only be about 40. In table 20-14 we compare the simulated effects of the two types of prevention programs for all six epidemics.

The results of this dynamic simulation reveal several things about preventing cases of an STD that are hidden by the static analysis. First, note from figure 20-11 that the one-time cure of 100 gonorrhea cases, whether in the core or the noncore, has virtually no effect on the number of cases three years later. The beneficial effect of a one-time intervention is transitory, because of the speed with which this epidemic approaches its

equilibrium in the population. Similar patterns are displayed by the chlamydia, syphilis, and chancroid epidemics.

In contrast to the classic STDs, HIV has a much smaller probability of transmission per sexual contact (0.01 to 0.03 in contrast to 0.4 to 0.6 for gonorrhea) and a much longer duration of infectivity (eight years in contrast to up to one year for syphilis). These differences make an HIV epidemic much slower to reach equilibrium than any of the CSTD epidemics. As a result, as can be seen in figure 20-12, the beneficial effect on an HIV epidemic of an intervention is still apparent ten years after the intervention.

The pattern changes if the HIV epidemic occurs in a population that is saturated by genital ulcer disease (GUD). Assuming that GUD increases the transmission probability by a factor of four, the effect is greatly to speed the epidemic and therefore to speed the return of the epidemic's path to equilibrium after any one-time intervention. For this accelerated HIV epidemic, a one-time intervention results in fewer new cases each month for a period of about five years than would have occurred without the intervention. After about five years, however, the number of new cases each month would have begun to slow even without intervention, because so few uninfected people would have remained to be infected. As a result of the intervention, there are more uninfected people in the population after five years, so that the number of new cases can be slightly larger during the sixth and subsequent years than it would have been without intervention. Figure 20-13 shows that this pattern holds whether the intervention is in the core or the noncore group.[32]

THE ADVANTAGE OF TARGETING THE CORE. In order to measure the aggregate of all the ill health averted by the act of

Figure 20-11. *Dynamic Benefit of Curing or Preventing 100 Cases of Gonorrhea in the Core and the Noncore Groups*

New cases averted (per month)

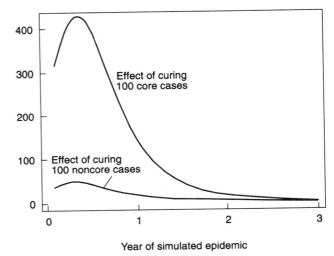

a. Cure in the initial intervention thereby preventing more infection.
Source: Authors.

Figure 20-12. Dynamic Benefit of Preventing 100 Cases of HIV in the Core and Noncore Groups when No Classic STDs Are Seen in the Population

New cases averted (per month)

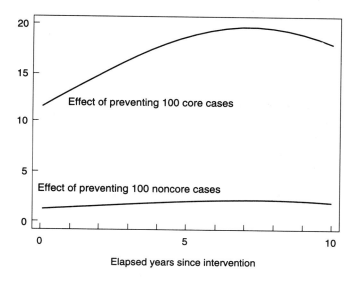

Elapsed years since intervention

Source: Authors.

preventing 100 cases today, we subtract in each month the number of new cases despite the intervention from the number predicted in the base run to have occurred in the absence of the intervention. Then we discount each of these averted future new cases back to the time of the intervention (at 3 percent per annum) and sum their discounted values to express the result as discounted new cases averted. Table 20-14 includes these figures for each disease and for each of the two interventions.

Consider again the disease gonorrhea. Despite the absence of any long-run effect on prevalence rate of either the core or the noncore one-time intervention, each of them does save a substantial number of case-years. Curing (or preventing) 100 initial cases in the noncore averts a total of 426 discounted future cases of gonorrhea (composed of 402 in the noncore and 24 in the core). Suppose, however, that the 100 cases prevented are instead extracted from the core group. In this case the total number of cases averted rises to 4,278, or ten times as many (of which only 231 are in the core). A policy of targeting the one-time intervention at the core averts ten times as many cases as would have been averted by a policy directed at the noncore. Furthermore, examination of the rest of table 20-14 shows that this result is robust across all the analyzed diseases.

The absolute number of discounted future cases averted by the one-time intervention is roughly similar for gonorrhea, chlamydia, and syphilis but is much smaller for chancroid (because it is less infective) and somewhat smaller for the slower epidemics of HIV with and without the exacerbation of genital ulcer disease. Note that preventing 100 cases of HIV has only slightly more effect when the HIV epidemic is exacerbated by GUD than when it is not. This is because the initially greater

effect in the presence of GUD is subsequently offset after year five as the epidemic accelerates back to its original path.

SENSITIVITY OF CORE STRATEGY TO ALTERNATIVE ASSUMPTIONS. The advantage of targeting the core highlighted in the above subsection is a significant result with potentially important policy ramifications. Because it is derived from a simulation based on specific parameter values, the question arises as to whether the result would hold under alternative assumptions. The exercise already varies the disease-specific assumptions across the six different simulated epidemics. We now examine the sensitivity of these results to changed assumptions about sexual behavior. We focus on two parameters from table 20-10, the selectivity coefficient (G) and the rate of sexual partner change (a).

As described above, the selectivity coefficient is the parameter which captures the degree of mixing between the core and noncore. The extreme values of 0 and 100 percent represent proportionate and zero mixing, respectively. The assumption of proportionate mixing (G = 0) used to this point in the chapter obviously does not represent the epidemiology of pattern I countries, in which homosexuals tend to be exclusively homosexual and IV drug users also represent a relatively (not entirely) isolated community. Proportionate mixing, however, may be a much more realistic representation of behavior patterns in pattern II countries.

Recall that the assumption of proportionate mixing implies that an individual chooses indiscriminately among core and noncore partners according to their availability for sexual contact. As table 20-10 shows, there are 1,000 noncore individuals available with whom to change partners each day and only 200 core individuals. Thus the assumption of proportion-

Figure 20-13. Dynamic Benefit of Preventing 100 Cases of HIV in the Core and Noncore when Transmission is Increased by Genital Ulcer Disease

New cases averted (per month)

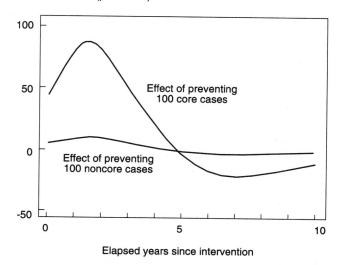

Elapsed years since intervention

Source: Authors.

Table 20-14. Dynamic Effects of Preventing 100 STD Cases in Core Rather than Noncore Group

Disease	Discounted new cases averted over ten years[a]		Ratio of core to noncore
	Targeting core group	Targeting noncore group	
Chancroid	810	83	9.8
Chlamydia	4,096	423	9.7
Gonorrhea	4,278	426	10.0
HIV without ulcers	1,744	180	9.7
HIV with ulcers	2,106	201	10.5
Syphilis	4,132	422	9.8

a. Sum of the savings in both the core and noncore group of an initial preventive or curative policy applied to only one group. The streams of saved cases are discounted at an annual rate of 3 percent.

Source: Authors' calculations.

ate mixing in this model implies that any individual in the core or the noncore has a five times greater chance of contacting a noncore than a core person. Among the sexually active groups in highly affected Sub-Saharan African cities described in Larson (1989) and Caldwell, Caldwell and Quiggin (1989), this scenario may indeed be quite realistic.

Still, what would happen if selectivity were greater than zero or if sexual behavior were less active? Repeated in the upper-left panel of table 20-15 are the effectiveness ratios from the right column of table 20-14. In the other three panels of table 20-15 are displayed the effects on these ratios of varying either the selectivity or the rate of partner change in the core. Note that none of the three alternative sets of sexual behavior parameters casts doubts on the greater effectiveness of a policy aimed at the core group. Indeed in no case does the ratio of the core to noncore effectiveness fall below 8.5, and in one case it rises to 55.5.[33]

COMBINING THE STATIC AND DYNAMIC BENEFITS. In the absence of an intervention, an epidemic causes a loss equal to the discounted sum of the losses from all future cases of the disease. If an intervention is effective, its benefit is to reduce the magnitude of this loss by reducing or postponing future cases. In the case of a one-time intervention like the one simulated here, prevalence rates of the STD epidemics ultimately reach the same levels as they would have reached without the intervention, only later. Thus the beneficial effect of the one-time intervention is to postpone these cases.[34]

In table 20-16 we combine the static estimates (from table 20A-3) of benefits from preventing or treating a case of each STD with the dynamic estimates (from table 20-14) of the discounted sum of averted future cases. Because the dynamic estimates are based on a ten-year simulation, they somewhat understate the estimated future effect of an intervention on an extremely slow epidemic, such as HIV in the absence of GUD. These estimates nevertheless show dramatically the substantial health benefits from the prevention or cure of the more serious STDs, such as syphilis and HIV infection, in contrast to the less serious, such as chlamydia and even gonorrhea. Recall,

however, that these estimates do not yet include the additional benefits of preventing or curing one of the CSTDs because of the consequent reduction of HIV transmission. The next subsection addresses this issue.

HEALTH BENEFITS WHEN STDs AFFECT HIV TRANSMISSION. The hypothesis that CSTDs affect the efficiency of HIV transmission is both biologically and epidemiologically appealing. When sexual contact occurs between an HIV-infected individual and a susceptible person, the presence of genital ulcer disease in either partner could plausibly increase the probability of HIV transmission by allowing the virus easier exit from the infected person or easier entry to the susceptible one. If STDs do increase the efficiency of HIV transmission, the higher STD prevalence rates in Sub-Saharan Africa would provide a partial epidemiological explanation for the faster increase in prevalence rates among heterosexuals in Africa than has been observed among heterosexuals in North America and Europe.

Whether STDs actually do increase the efficiency of HIV transmission is inherently difficult to demonstrate, because of the need to control properly for the frequency of sexual partner change. Without such control, an observed correlation between HIV infection and a past history of STDs could actually be due to the correlation of both variables with the degree of sexual activity. The researchers in several independent studies in both East and West Africa, however, have found large and statistically significant effects of STDs on the efficiency of HIV transmission, even after controlling for past sexual activity (Cameron and others 1989; Ryder and others 1990). Furthermore, investigators in a recent study in Zaire have found that even nonulcerative cases of gonorrhea and chlamydia increase the transmission probability (Laga and others 1990).

The simulations of an HIV epidemic both with and without ulcers in figures 20-12 and 20-13 demonstrate that, when an HIV epidemic is accelerated by STDs, the benefits of an inter-

Table 20-15. Sensitivity Analysis: Advantage of Preventing or Curing STD in the Core Group, Based on Selectivity and Rate of Partner Change

Rate of partner change	Disease	Selectivity (G)	
		0.0[a]	0.30
0.02[a]	Chancroid	9.8	20.5
	Chlamydia	9.7	9.0
	Gonorrhea	10.0	10.5
	HIV without ulcers	9.7	10.3
	HIV with ulcers	10.5	8.5
	Syphilis	9.8	9.5
0.04	Chancroid	20.1	22.6
	Chlamydia	17.1	11.2
	Gonorrhea	17.1	12.4
	HIV without ulcers	17.4	12.5
	HIV with ulcers	55.5	22.0
	Syphilis	17.0	11.5

a. Base value.

Source: Authors' calculations.

Table 20-16. *Discounted Disability-Adjusted Life-Years Saved per Case Prevented or Cured When Epidemics Independent: Core vs. Noncore*

Disease	Static benefit[a]	Dynamic benefit[b]		Total benefit[c]	
		Core	Noncore	Core	Noncore
Chancroid	0.2	1.6	0.2	1.8	0.4
Chlamydia	1.05	43.0	4.4	44.1	5.5
Gonorrhea	0.85	36.4	3.6	37.3	4.5
HIV without ulcers	19.5	340.1	35.1	359.6	54.6
HIV with ulcers	19.5	410.7	39.2	430.2	58.7
Syphilis	3.8	157.0	16.0	160.8	19.8

a. Benefit to only the cured or protected individual from curing or preventing a case of STD. Because the dynamic model does not distinguish the genders, the static benefits of averting a case in the two genders are averaged.

b. Benefit to people other than the cured or protected individual from curing or preventing a single case of STD. Computed by dividing the figures from table 20-14 by 100 and multiplying by the static benefit per case averted.

c. Benefit of a single cure or prevention to both the individual and to the people he or she would have infected. Computed by adding the static benefit to the dynamic benefit.

Source: Authors' calculations.

vention occur sooner and also decay more quickly. If the CSTDs could be somehow removed from a population in which they have been endemic, the rate of growth of HIV prevalence would slow dramatically, taking more than twice as long to reach its ceiling. But STDs cannot be magically removed; they must either be prevented or cured one at a time.

When STDs affect HIV transmission, the health benefits of curing or preventing a case of a CSTD should be larger than in the absence of such an interaction. To estimate the increased health benefit of curing or preventing a case of a CSTD in the presence of an HIV epidemic, we modify the simulation model used above to include an interaction between the STD being modeled and HIV. Because chancroid and syphilis cause genital ulcer disease, we assume that the probability of HIV infection when one partner has either of these diseases is five times larger than if neither is so infected. The nonulcerating diseases, gonorrhea and chlamydia, are assumed to increase infectivity by three and two times, respectively.[35]

Figure 20-14 illustrates the effects on the gonorrhea epidemic and also on a simultaneous HIV epidemic of an intervention which cures or prevents 100 cases of gonorrhea in the core group. In the top panel, the top curve charts the number of cases of gonorrhea averted each subsequent month as a result of this intervention, which totals 4,278, just as it does in table 20-14 as depicted in figure 20-11 above. The bottom curve in the top panel, although barely distinguishable from the horizontal axis, captures the indirect effect of curing gonorrhea cases on the HIV epidemic. The discounted sum of averted future cases of HIV infection is 425.1 over the ten-year span of the simulation.

The bottom panel of figure 20-14 graphs the same two epidemic paths as the top panel with one difference: each is multiplied by the static benefit per averted case to yield the flow of saved disability-adjusted life-years that result from curing 100 cases of gonorrhea. Because, according to figure 20-10 and table 20A-3, the static benefit per case of gonorrhea is only 0.85 disability-adjusted life-years (average of 0.7 for men and 1.0 for women) and is 19.5 disability-adjusted life-years per case of HIV infection, the flow of health resulting from

the intervention's indirect effect on the HIV epidemic outweighs that resulting from its effect on the gonorrhea epidemic. The transformation from cases averted to disability-adjusted life-years saved thus reverses the apparent importance of the two effects. The discounted sum of these health benefits are 3,646 disability-adjusted life-years from averted gonorrhea cases and 8,289 from averted HIV.[36] The total dynamic effect of averting 100 cases of gonorrhea in the core group is the sum

Figure 20-14. *Effect of Curing 100 Core Cases of Gonorrhea When Gonorrhea Increases HIV Transmission*

New cases averted (per month)

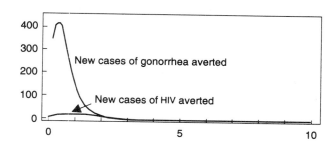

Disability-adjusted life-years saved (per month)

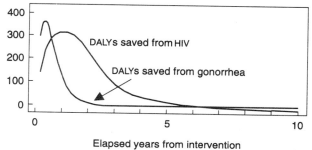

Elapsed years from intervention

Source: Authors.

Table 20-17. Dynamic Effects of an HIV Epidemic from Preventing 100 STD Cases in Core and Noncore Groups

Disease	Discounted new cases of HIV averted over ten years[a]		Ratio of core to noncore
	Targeting core group	Targeting noncore group	
Chancroid	275.9	17.4	15.9
Chlamydia	355.8	30.3	11.7
Gonorrhea	425.1	36.2	11.7
Syphilis	1,207.8	109.1	11.1

a. Sum of the averted cases of HIV infection in both the core and noncore groups from an initial prevention or cure of 100 cases of classic STD in only one of these groups. In addition to these health benefits, saving 100 cases of classic STD also reduces future cases of that STD.

Source: Authors' calculations.

of these two figures, or 11,935 disability-adjusted life-years. Adding this to the 85 disability-adjusted life-years gained for the lives of the individuals whose cases of gonorrhea were directly treated or prevented gives a total of 12,020 disability-adjusted life-years saved, or 120.2 disability-adjusted life-years saved per case of gonorrhea averted.

In table 20-17 we show the total cases of HIV averted when 100 cases of one of the CSTDs are cured or prevented in the core or the noncore group. These benefits are in addition to the benefits given in table 20-14. As might be expected, the indirect effects on averting cases of HIV, like the direct effects in table 20-14, are much greater when the intervention is targeted at the core group.

In table 20-18 we gather together the components to give the total health benefit, measured in disability-adjusted life-years saved, per case of each CSTD prevented or cured. The figures in table 20-18 are shown graphically in figure 20-15. Note the extraordinarily large health effect of preventing or curing a case of syphilis in the core group. By saving almost 400 disability-adjusted life-years per case cured or prevented, this intervention has an even greater effect on health than would the direct prevention of a case of HIV infection. The beneficial effects of interventions against all the other CSTDs are also

greatly increased in the presence of an HIV epidemic. These health benefits presented in table 20-18 and figure 20-15 are used later for the cost-effectiveness calculations.

BENEFITS OF A SUSTAINED INTERVENTION. Each STD is characterized in table 20-11 by a probability of transmission on a given sexual contact and by a duration of infectivity. Interventions which reduce either of these parameters for an STD in a given population will slow the epidemic and, if the intervention is permanent, will reduce the equilibrium incidence and prevalence rates in the population. Interventions which reduce the risk of transmission include circumcision (Bongaarts, Reining, and Conant, 1989; Moses and others 1989), the use of nonpenetrative sex, and, most important, the use of condoms.

Our method is analogous to that used above to model the effect of 100 cures. We use the same base runs for each epidemic to represent the situation without an intervention. Then we model two alternative interventions, one in the core and one in the noncore. The intervention consists of assuming that 100 people randomly drawn from the chosen (core or noncore) group are protected for one year from either becoming infected or from infecting others. In this way the probability that a susceptible person will acquire the transmission through contact with a person of a given group is reduced by the probability that at least one of the two partners is thus "protected."[37] The result is that, for a year, the rate of growth of the epidemics is slower than it would be in the absence of this intervention. At the end of the year the epidemic resumes its normal pace and the prevalence rate converges to the same equilibrium that it attains in the base scenario.

By protecting 100 people of the 1,000 in the core, we reduce the effective danger of sex with a core person by 10 percent. In contrast, protecting 100 people of the 50,000 in the noncore only reduces the danger of having sex with a noncore person by 0.2 percent. This difference is responsible for the dramatic difference in the effectiveness of the two interventions. Notice that a person-year of protection of a core individual in the presence of an HIV epidemic alone saves 56.6 DALYs, almost three times more than are saved by protecting a noncore person

Table 20-18. Discounted Disability-Adjusted Life-Years Saved per Case Prevented or Cured When STDs Affect HIV Transmission: Core vs. Noncore

Disease	Static and dynamic DALYs per case from classic STD only		Dynamic DALYs per case from averted HIV only[a]		Total DALYs saved per case of classic STD	
	Core	Noncore	Core	Noncore	Core	Noncore
Chancroid	1.8	0.4	53.8	3.4	55.6	3.8
Chlamydia	44.1	5.5	69.4	5.9	113.5	11.4
Gonorrhea	37.3	4.5	82.9	7.1	120.2	11.6
HIV without ulcers	359.6	54.6	n.a.	n.a.	359.6	54.6
HIV with ulcers	430.2	58.7	n.a.	n.a.	430.2	58.7
Syphilis	160.8	19.8	235.5	21.3	396.3	41.1

n.a. Not applicable.

a. Additional benefits of preventing or curing a case of a classic STD resulting from indirect prevention of HIV infection. Calculated by dividing the cases of HIV averted (table 20-16) by 100 and multiplying by 19.5, the static benefit of each case averted.

Source: Authors' calculations.

Figure 20-15. *Total Health Benefit of Averting a Case of Classic* STD *When* STD *Exacerbates* HIV *Transmission: Core vs. Noncore Strategy*

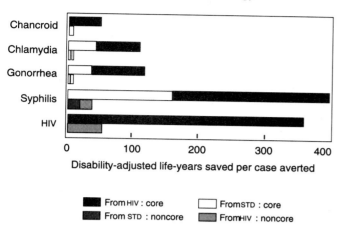

Disability-adjusted life-years saved per case averted

■ From HIV : core　　□ From STD : core
▨ From STD : noncore　▨ From HIV : noncore

Source: Table 20-18.

for a year. If the only STD epidemic is syphilis, which is much more infectious, protecting a core person for a year saves 141.7 DALYs, about twenty times more than would protecting a non-core person for a year. If the syphilis and HIV epidemics are both in the population simultaneously, however, protecting a core person saves a total of 384.6 DALYs, forty times more than would protecting a noncore person. Of the 384.6 DALYs saved, 141.7 are from syphilis, 56.6 are from HIV in the absence of any interaction with syphilis, and 186.3 are from HIV, because the slower syphilis epidemic has a smaller effect on HIV transmission.

The model estimates of a one-time intervention curing 100 people showed in table 20-18 that the intervention would have roughly ten times greater effect when targeted to the core than to the noncore. In table 20-19 it is shown that a sustained intervention which lowers transmission probabilities also has a larger effect when targeted at the core. But this time the advantage ranges from a multiple of forty for syphilis to a

multiple of seventy-four for chancroid. Unless the cost of targeting such a sustained intervention at the core is as much as forty times larger per person-year of protection than targeting it to the noncore, the data in table 20-19 lead us to predict that targeting to the core will be the more cost-effective strategy.

The modeling method used to generate the numbers in table 20-19 allows only one or two epidemics to be present simultaneously in the population. When there are more than two simultaneous epidemics, reducing transmission probabilities by protecting individuals, with condoms or otherwise, would have an even larger health benefit. Because the most important interaction is with HIV and because averted HIV infection provides most of the benefits of the sustained intervention, the effect of considering only two diseases at a time will be a minor understatement of the benefits of this intervention.

Costs of and Expenditure on Primary Prevention Programs

It would be useful to present cost and expenditure information on all forty-three of the interventions categorized in table 20-13 by the mode of transmission they are designed to interrupt. Unfortunately there is almost no information on either the cost of or the current expenditure on primary prevention of STDs in developing countries. In this section we present the fragmentary available information on the cost of a few of these interventions designed to interrupt three of the four modes of transmission: sexual intercourse, mother-to-infant, and blood transfusion. For lack of information on expenditure, we conclude the section by analyzing the budgeted expenditures in the Sub-Saharan countries' medium-term plans by 1988.

COST OF PREVENTING SEXUAL TRANSMISSION. Of the fourteen interventions listed in the first column of table 20-13, we focus our cost-effectiveness analysis on only one: the encouragement of condom use through social marketing. Both the costs and the effects of the other interventions are insufficiently well known to permit quantitative estimates.

Table 20-19. *Discounted Disability-Adjusted Life-Years Saved per Person-Year of Protection when* STDs *Affect* HIV *Transmission: Core vs. Noncore*

Disease	Static and dynamic DALYs per case from classic STD only		Dynamic DALYs per case from averted HIV only[a]		Total DALYs saved per case of classic STD	
	Core	Noncore	Core	Noncore	Core	Noncore
Chancroid	1.4	0.2	79.5	0.9	80.9	1.1
Chlamydia	52.3	2.3	144.4	1.9	196.6	4.2
Gonorrhea	64.9	2.4	210.3	2.8	275.2	5.2
HIV without ulcers	56.6	19.9	n.a.	n.a.	56.6	19.9
HIV with ulcers	156.0	21.5	n.a.	n.a.	156.0	21.5
Syphilis	141.7	6.5	242.9	3.3	384.6	9.7

n.a. Not applicable.

a. Obtained by multiplying the discounted sum of future cases averted over ten years as a result of the intervention, times the static benefit of each case averted, averaging the male and female values where they differ.

b. Additional benefits of a person-year of protection due to both the direct protection against HIV and the indirect prevention of HIV infection. The portion of this benefit due to the indirect effect through the reduced prevalence of the CSTD can be calculated by subtracting the numbers for HIV without ulcers in columns 1 and 2 from the numbers in columns 3 and 4.

Source: Authors' calculations.

Table 20-20. Two Condom Social Marketing Programs in Sub-Saharan Africa

Feature	Zaire	Tanzania
Location	Kinshasa	Six truck stops and two trucking companies
Start date	1989	1989
Baseline condom use	200,000 condoms sold privately per year at cost of $1 per condom.	Half of drivers had had more than fifty sexual partners in their lifetime. Condoms used consistently with casual partners by 42 percent of bar girls and commercial sex workers (CSW) and by 37 percent of drivers.
Accomplishments	13,000,000 condoms sold in two years at 6 cents per condom. Expect to sell 8,000,000 more in third year. Condoms now present in 7,000 of 9,000 targeted outlets.	Each truck stop is serviced by an average of 200 CSWs who use 20,000 condoms per month, or an average of 100 per CSW per month or four per night.
Total cost per year	About $2 million	$100,000 budget plus free condoms provided by National AIDS Control Program. Amortization of vehicles provided free by African Medical and Research Foundation (AMREF). Perhaps $750,000.
Total condom sales per year	About 8 million	2 million
Price per condom	6 cents in 1990, falling to 0.6 cents in 1991 as result of domestic inflation and devaluation.	No charge to customer
Cost per couple-year of protection		
Core[a]	$300	$456
Noncore[b]	$30	$45.60
Contractor	Population Services International	Family Health International/AIDSTECH

Note: All money in U.S. dollars.

a. Assumes four contacts per night, twenty-five nights per month. Cost per condom 25 cents in Zaire, 38 cents in Tanzania.

b. Assumes ten contacts per month. Cost per condom 25 cents in Zaire, 38 cents in Tanzania.

Source: Personal communications from Linda Cole, Family Health International, March 1991 (Tanzania) and from Richard Frenk, Population Services International, February, 1991.

The use of condoms by sexually active individuals with multiple sexual partners affects the STD epidemics by reducing the probability of sexual transmission on a given sexual contact. This probability, Q, is one of the four key behavioral parameters in the dynamic epidemiological model presented earlier.[38] The government-sponsored programs in several Sub-Saharan African countries have focused only on frequency of partner change, thereby failing to help and sometimes stigmatizing individuals who find it impossible to remain monogamous.

In many of these same countries, private organizations have informed prostitutes and others of means to reduce the danger of each sexual contact through the proper use of a condom. The cost of such programs is poorly understood. Sketchy information on programs funded by the United States Agency for International Development through AIDSTECH, Family Health International, is summarized in table 20-20. The subsidy costs of these condom social marketing programs for AIDS control range from $30 to $45 per year of protection for a noncore person in 1990 U.S. dollars, not including any money from cost-recovery efforts which remunerates the distribution network.

For comparison, the estimated cost of a couple-year of protection by condoms distributed by social marketing in family planning programs in Honduras and Bangladesh was recently estimated to be $14.77 and $6.55, respectively, in 1988 U.S. dollars, of which $4.59 and $5.90, respectively, were the net subsidy cost to the government (Bulatao 1985; Janowitz, Bratt, and Fried 1990). Because family planning programs presume that couples are monogamous, the cost of the condoms to protect a couple from conception for a year is roughly comparable to the cost of the condoms to protect one of these individuals from STDs for a year, assuming that person is in the noncore group. The difference of a factor of five to ten in average subsidy costs between the condom marketing programs aimed at STD prevention in Africa and the family planning programs in Latin America and Asia is partly due to the high overhead and substantial input of expatriate personnel during the start-up phase of the former. Perhaps as the STD prevention social marketing programs mature, the average annual subsidy per noncore person-year of protection will fall closer to the levels observed for the family planning programs. Still, the fact that AIDS prevention social marketing programs target high-risk groups may keep their average costs higher than the values attainable by family planning programs that target the noncore. We hypothesize that the budgetary (or subsidy) cost of a condom social marketing program targeted to the noncore will lie between the value of $5.00 per protected individual observed in the family planning programs and the value of $45.00 observed in the Tanzanian experiment in peer education. Whatever the cost per individual user in the noncore, we further hypothesize that the cost per protected individual will be ten times larger in the core group.

COST OF PREVENTING MOTHER-TO-INFANT TRANSMISSION. A major sequela of gonorrhea is gonococcal ophthalmia neonatorum, which can be inexpensively prevented by the application of an antibiotic to the eyes of the newborn immediately after birth. Because 3.5 percent of all live births in some African populations suffer from this potentially blinding disease, there is reason to consider a prophylactic application of antibiotic to the eyes of all neonates as part of a standard maternal and child health package. Laga, Meheus, and Piot (1989) have estimated the cost of applying an antibiotic (either silver nitrate or tetracycline) to the eyes of all newborn infants to be approximately $0.10 per newborn for silver nitrate and approximately $0.05 per newborn for tetracycline. On the basis of clinical trials of these alternatives in Nairobi, they estimate that silver nitrate prevents 40 of the 47 cases that would occur among 100 babies born of women with a gonococcal infection, whereas tetracycline would prevent 44 of the 47 cases. The calculation of the dollars per case of gonococcal ophthalmia neonatorum at different prevalence rates in the population is presented in table 20-21.

With respect to HIV infection, from 30 percent to 50 percent of the children born to HIV-infected women will be infected with HIV at birth. If those women could be counseled to prevent pregnancy or abort their fetus, one HIV-infected child would be prevented for every one to two uninfected children born. Unfortunately, anecdotal evidence suggests that many poor women, when informed that they are HIV-infected and of the probable consequences, prefer to continue bearing children. Our general position regarding mandatory programs—that they are unethical and counterproductive—seems particularly apt in the case of hypothetical programs to enforce or strongly encourage abortion of the fetuses of HIV-infected women. Thus we conclude that the only cost-effective way to prevent vertical transmission of HIV is to prevent the infection of the mother in the first place.

COST OF PREVENTING TRANSMISSION BY BLOOD TRANSFUSION. The average variable cost of an enzyme-linked immunosorbent assay (ELISA test) for the presence of HIV antibodies in the blood can be as low as $1 in a well-run laboratory in

a developing country which performs large numbers of such tests. Assuming another $1 per test for management overhead, the average total cost of such a test could be as low as $2. To obtain this low a cost in a developing country, however, requires good management, well-trained and well-managed technicians, and large volume. In rural areas of developing countries where none of these conditions obtain, an alternative test not requiring refrigeration is a rapid serologic test for HIV for which the average variable cost is as much as $4 per test, which becomes $5 with the addition of the same dollar for management overhead. Finally, a laboratory expert in Sub-Saharan Africa has informed the first author in confidence that the average total cost of blood screening in some Sub-Saharan African capitals can be as large as $10 per test.

Suppose that a perfect test to determine whether a unit of donated blood is infected with HIV costs $2 per blood sample tested. If 5 percent of donors are known to be infected, then it would require an average of twenty tests to find a single infected unit of blood. By eliminating this unit of blood and replacing it at no cost with an uninfected unit, a transfusion service has avoided transfusing a patient with HIV-infected blood at twenty times the cost of a blood test. In addition, suppose that three-quarters of the people to receive blood transfusions are HIV-negative before the medical emergency and subsequently survive the medical problem that caused them to need the blood. Then the cost of averting an HIV infection through blood screening is 4/3 of 20 times the cost of a single test, or $53 per HIV infection prevented. The general equation is:

$$\text{Cost per HIV infection averted} = \frac{\left(\dfrac{\text{Cost per test}}{\text{Prevalence rate}}\right)}{\text{Survival rate of transmission recipients}}$$

A more complete model of the cost-effectiveness of blood screening would relax many of the assumptions made in the above analysis. For example, the tests currently available are not perfect, especially under field conditions. They generate false positives and false negatives. Furthermore, infected units of blood cannot be replaced at no cost but cost as much as $5 each to replace. Elaboration of these more complete models with plausible values for the complicating parameters, however, raises the estimated cost per averted case of HIV infection by only a few percentage points. Therefore, for ease of exposition, we present here only the results of this extremely simple model.[39]

Shown in figure 20-16 on a logarithmic scale is the relation between the cost per averted case of HIV infection and the prevalence rate graphed for two different values of the cost per test, $2 and $10. At a prevalence rate of 5 percent and a test cost of $2, the cost of averting a case of HIV infection is $53 as in the above example. Note the dramatic effect of prevalence rate on cost. At one extreme, when the prevalence rate among donors is as high as 40 percent, as it might be for the donors that an urban prostitute would recruit from among her coworkers in a high-prevalence African city, screening can avert a

Table 20-21. Cost per Case Averted of Eye Infection from Gonorrhea, by Prevalence of Gonorrhea among Pregnant Women
(1989 U.S. dollars)

Therapy	Cost	Effectiveness	Prevalence of gonorrhea among pregnant women			
			0.001	0.01	0.10	0.25
Silver nitrate	0.10	0.85	111.11	11.76	1.18	0.47
Tetracycline	0.05	0.94	55.56	5.32	0.53	0.21

Source: Laga, Meheus, and Piot 1989.

case of HIV infection for only $7. At the other extreme, in areas of low prevalence, blood screening is a very expensive way to avert HIV infection, costing more than $6,000 per case averted. The left-most data point on the graph is at a seroprevalence rate of 4 per 10,000, or 0.04 percent.[40] All these costs are multiplied by five if the cost per test is $10 rather than $2. These higher costs are related to prevalence rates in the upper line in figure 20-16.

In any given country the possible sites for blood transfusion all have different prevalence rates among their donors and different laboratory conditions leading to different test costs. The lesson of figure 20-16 is that the cost-effectiveness of blood screening for averting cases of HIV infection will vary a great deal from one of these sites to another. Screening should begin at those sites where screening is most cost-effective and only be developed in the least cost-effective sites if the country is unable to avert cases of HIV or to save disability-adjusted life-years more cheaply in other ways.

BUDGET FOR PRIMARY PREVENTION OF HIV INFECTION. In table 20-22 we present the first-year budget of the sixteen Sub-Saharan African countries which were first to adopt such medium-term plans for AIDS prevention and control. With only partial minor exceptions, the first-year proposed expenditure has been fully funded, typically out of grants from bilateral donors, both directly and through the World Health Organization's Global Programme on AIDS (WHO/GPA).

In the third column of table 20-22 is the total (recurrent plus capital) central government health expenditure for those countries from which figures are available. The figures in the fifth column show that, in the average country, the medium-

Figure 20-16. Cost per HIV Infection Averted by Blood Screening, as a Function of Prevalence and Test Cost

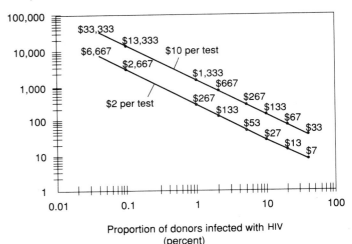

Cost per HIV infection averted (U.S. dollars)

Proportion of donors infected with HIV (percent)

Source: Authors.

term plan (MTP) will augment central government health expenditure by 6 percent. In Zaire and Rwanda the MTP represents a 20 percent increment to central government health expenditure, and in Uganda, Zambia, Tanzania, and Burundi the increment is about 10 percent.

One way to gauge the magnitude of these MTP budgets is to relate them to the estimated number of HIV-infected persons.

Table 20-22. Donor-Funded AIDS Prevention and Control Budgets in African Countries

Country	Year of MTP	First-year MTP budget[a]	Central government health expenditures	MTP as percent of government health expenditures	Estimated persons HIV positive	MTP budget per HIV-positive person
Uganda	1987	1,508	14,695	10.3	894.3	1.69
Zambia	1988	3,101	34,094	9.1	205.2	15
Zaire	1988	4,363	22,269	19.6	281.8	15
Central African Republic	1987–88	1,599	—	—	54.3	29
Rwanda	1987	2,922	13,680	21.4	81.5	36
Congo	1988	1,727	—	—	45.5	38
Tanzania	1987	3,945	51,250	7.7	96.6	41
Mozambique	1988	1,788	—	—	43.5	41
Cameroon	1988	1,841	86,593	2.1	33.2	55
Kenya	1987	2,940	120,335	2.4	44.5	66
Burundi	1988	1,719	14,925	11.5	15.0	115
Zimbabwe	1988–89	3,799	128,323	3.0	30.9	123
Botswana	1987	150	32,369	0.5	0.9	167
Senegal	1988	1,443	—	—	2.9	498
Mauritius	1988	242	26,045	0.9	0.1	2,420
Ethiopia	1988	3,137	45,480	6.9	0.1	31,370
Mean		2,264	36,879	6.0	114.4	20

Note: Budget and expenditures in thousands of 1987 U.S. dollars.
— Not available.
a. From first medium-term planning documents prepared by individual countries with WHO/GPA assistance.
Source: Bongaarts and Way 1989; World Bank 1989. See also note a, above.

The fifth column of the table contains the estimated number of HIPs in each country in 1987–88. From the data in the second and fifth columns, we arrive at that in the sixth column, the MTP budget per HIP, which ranges from less than $2 in Uganda to more than $31,000 in Ethiopia.

The appropriate budget allocation to a national AIDS control program depends on the cost of preventing a case of HIV infection in that country and on the alternative possible uses for the same budget resources. For an international agency such as WHO/GPA, the alternative expenditure for grant resources not spent in country X is expenditure on preventing HIV infection in country Y. Such an agency's goal might reasonably be to minimize the number of cases of HIV infection worldwide by maximizing the number of prevented cases each year. With a fixed global grant budget, this goal could be achieved only by equalizing the number of cases prevented per grant dollar across countries.

The cost per case of HIV prevented will vary across countries and within a country across interventions. As long as HIV prevalence rates are increasing, however, the number of people at risk of new infection will be roughly proportional to the number of people capable of infecting others in that country, that is, the number of HIPs. Thus a rational allocation of a global grant budget for AIDS control should approximately equate the MTP dollars per HIP across countries. Some variation in budget per HIP would remain because of the different institutional structures—and, therefore, the different costs of interventions—across countries. Still, the large variations in MTP budget per HIP revealed by the sixth column of table 20-22 demonstrate that the allocation of resources across these Sub-Saharan African countries is quite different from the prevention-maximizing allocation. Even ignoring the two extreme countries, Uganda and Ethiopia, the MTP budget per HIP is more than thirty times larger in Mauritius and Senegal than in Zambia and Zaire, a multiple too large to explain by differences in absorptive capacity. It is hard to escape the conclusion that the MTP budgeting process was driven by random political and other factors which bore little relation to a rational allocation of resources across countries.

There is a prior question, however—whether these large incremental expenditures can be effectively absorbed by the countries in question. Because the health expenditure of central governments rarely fluctuates by more than 2 or 3 percentage points in any given year, and then the fluctuation is usually spread over all the many preventive and curative programs in the ministry, it is not surprising that governments have had substantial difficulty launching such large incremental expenditure programs, amounting to as much as 10 to 20 percent of their health budgets, for a single disease. Although the key resource constraint over the short run has proved to be trained manpower, an additional limit to the absorptive capacity of national AIDS programs has been a lack of clear guidance on prioritizing interventions. The medium-term plan has typically enumerated a long list of desirable activities, including most of those listed in table 20-13, without ranking them by effectiveness or urgency. The result is that the small numbers of trained staff have been spread too thinly trying to do all these activities at once. We hope that analyses such as the present one will help guide the prioritization of activities and expenditure so that national AIDS programs can achieve greater health benefits (that is, save more disability-adjusted life-years) for their allotted budget.

Cost-Effective STD Prevention Strategies

Primary prevention of STDs requires the interruption of one or more of the modes of STD transmission displayed as column headings in table 20-13. Resources are not so plentiful, however, that countries can afford to press forward on all possible interventions simultaneously.[41] Instead, choices are required. In this section, we review the available primary prevention interventions and recommend some as likely to be more cost-effective than others. We retain from previous sections of this chapter the lesson that preventing a case of STD in the core will save many more subsequent cases than would preventing a case in the noncore.

In the first row of table 20-13, we present the voluntary behavioral changes, which can be stimulated by appropriately targeted information, education, and communication programs. These IEC programs typically affect the individual demand for a protective voluntary behavior, such as use of a condom or avoidance of a transfusion. They do so either by providing information or by changing preferences; sometimes they do both.

In contrast to voluntary behavior modification through IEC, mandatory and passive behavior modification typically occur through changes in the availability or price of a protective behavior or product, that is, on the supply side of a market. For example, either an enforced prohibition of prostitution or the provision of training and jobs for urban single women would reduce the supply, raise the price, and therefore reduce the frequency of commercial sex.

Although both mandatory and passive behavioral changes typically operate on the supply side, their mechanisms and effects are clearly distinct. Mandatory programs (such as the prohibition of prostitution) involve the enactment of laws and regulations which require the health-promoting behavior on penalty of fine or imprisonment. Examples outside the area of STD prevention include laws on speed limits and regulations concerning pollution control. To be effective, such laws and regulations must be enforced, which requires expenditure on government regulators. Furthermore, the regulators must be well paid and closely supervised to the point that their suborning is more costly to the would-be transgressor than is compliance with the laws. All these difficulties imply that mandatory behavior modification is best suited for short-term emergency control of easily observed, politically unpopular behavior.

Passive programs, in contrast, are typically slow to start but can be profound in their long-run influence on private decisions. If the government policies which support the passive program (such as improved job opportunities for women) are perceived to be permanent, they can induce individuals to choose different residential locations, careers, and family sizes and thus can profoundly affect the details of their lives.

The choice of a cost-effective package of primary prevention interventions must be conducted in two dimensions: choices are required both within modes of transmission (the columns of table 20-13) and between modes of transmission (the rows of the table). We begin with the sexual transmission mode, which is the sole mode of transmission for most CSTDs and accounts for more than 90 percent of all adult cases of HIV infection in pattern II countries.[42]

SEXUAL TRANSMISSION AND MANDATORY PROGRAMS. The privacy of sexual practices and the primacy of the sex drive make sexual behavior one of the least-suited activities for mandatory behavior modification. During World War II the United States conducted an excellent example of a failed mandatory policy when it attempted to enforce the prohibition against prostitution in order to halt the spread of STDs.

[After] thousands of women were institutionalized or detained [and] jails became overcrowded, Ness arranged for the creation of some 30 "civilian conservation camps" for young women as a means of relieving some of the pressure on existing facilities.[43] [But] despite the incarceration of thousands of prostitutes, it soon became clear that this could not in itself solve the venereal disease problem. Indeed, the effect of closing the red-light districts was sometimes disappointing to military officials. Increasingly, army physicians reported that prostitutes constituted only a minority of the soldiers' sexual contacts. In the Third Service Command, for example, only 19 percent of the infections could be attributed to prostitutes; in other communities even fewer infections could be so traced (Brandt 1987, p. 167).[44]

Thus, on practical grounds alone, we recommend against mandatory programs which rely on legal prohibitions. Furthermore, the consequences of such programs for civil liberties are likely to be unacceptable to democratic societies.[45]

SEXUAL TRANSMISSION AND CHANGED "PRICES." Setting aside mandatory programs as unlikely to be effective, we turn to policy choices categorized as either voluntary or passive. We believe that too little attention has been given to passive methods of modifying behavior in relation to that given to voluntary and mandatory ones. Among those listed in table 20-13, the potential effectiveness of subsidies to condom distribution through private channels has been demonstrated by a social marketing effort in Kinshasa, Zaire, which increased the sales of condoms in 110 pharmacies from 19,000 per month to 300,000 per month in only ten months (Lamptey and Goodridge 1991). Still, to our knowledge, the possibility of taxing alcohol served in public places in order to increase the cost of sexual partner change has not been studied.

More promising still are longer-run programs to improve the marriage, education, and job opportunities for women. It was demonstrated earlier that African cities with low female-to-male secondary enrollment ratios also had high rates of STD infection. To the extent that primary infertility caused by STDs prevents women from marrying or remaining married, programs to prevent or quickly cure STDs will help women avoid the stigmatization and rejection caused by infertility—and thus avoid recourse to prostitution. Education is a long-run strategy that will increase the woman's contribution to the development process, induce her to have fewer, healthier children, and improve her bargaining position in sexual relationships. Such a policy is an appropriate one to counter a slow, long-run epidemic like HIV infection that is exacerbated by low female education.

A somewhat shorter-run policy that has so far received little or no attention in national AIDS control programs is the creation of jobs for urban women. In a sampling of prostitutes in one Nigerian town, 67 of them reported that they would cease prostitution (an average of 4.4 paying clients per day) if they could find a job paying the equivalent of $15 a month (Williams, Hearst, and Udofia 1989). A possible example of an inadvertently beneficial effect on STD transmission of job creation for women is the "enterprise zones" of northern Mexico, where many of the young female employees are said to be grateful for these low-wage jobs as a welcome alternative to their former lives as prostitutes (personal communication from Sally Stansfield 1989).

Although the immediate effect of alternative female employment in urban areas of pattern II countries would be to reduce the supply and thereby raise the price of commercial sex for men, the longer-run effect would be to attract additional women to these urban centers. Still, on the basis of the statistical evidence presented earlier, we believe that this, too, would contribute to the control of STDs.

SEXUAL TRANSMISSION AND VOLUNTARY PARTNER NOTIFICATION. Although passive behavioral change seems to us the most promising long-run strategy by which to control sexual transmission, certain voluntary strategies, when tightly targeted at the core group, may also be cost-effective. As the first among these we designate voluntary partner notification, by both patient and provider referral. This method has proven increasingly effective in the control of CSTDs, especially after the availability first of salvarsan (in 1909) and then of penicillin (in 1943) made it possible to offer a cure to the sexual contacts of the index case. Some European countries, however, oppose partner notification programs for the CSTDs on the ground that, even when voluntary, they invade privacy.

Recently, some American states have been experimenting with partner notification in cases of HIV infection. Toomey and Cates' concise overview of U.S. practices points out that partner notification is far more effective than HIV screening of a population of STD patients in identifying new cases of HIV infection (1989). For example, compared with seroprevalence rates for HIV of 2.7 percent and 6.4 percent among STD patients in Virginia and Florida, seroprevalence rates among notified partners were 13.5 percent and 25.1 percent, respectively. The cost per index case in Virginia was $50 if the patient was asked to refer, and $64 if the public health staff conducted provider referral. In Colorado, researchers in a similar study using different methods found costs of $50 per index case without provider referral and $33 for each partner notified by the providers.[46] Because these figures, $33 to $65 per index case, consist largely of the cost of labor, they can be deflated to figures that would apply in poor pattern II countries by expressing them as 0.5 percent of GNP per capita.[47] If partner notification programs could be operated in pattern II countries at even 1 or 2 percent of local GNP per capita for each index case, the resources currently available for AIDS control could mount significant partner notification programs.

These American successes with partner notification were achieved before it was possible to offer any treatment for nonsymptomatic HIV infection. Now that AZT has been found to retard the development of the disease, these American programs will achieve even greater success. Although the high price of AZT will prevent its immediate wholesale provision to asymptomatic infected people of the pattern II countries, this technological advance nevertheless holds out hope for improved partner notification programs in either of two distinct scenarios.

First, suppose that the annual cost of a temporarily effective antiviral medication remains as high as it is now, several thousand dollars per year. In this case, a public health program in a poor developing country could afford to buy only a few such treatments next year. If the program could convince the public that these few treatments are to be allocated fairly to a few of those who are actively cooperating with prevention efforts, then the availability of even a small chance for a temporarily effective treatment could serve as a powerful inducement for behavioral change.[48]

But the price of antivirals is unlikely to remain constant. If it falls in price as fast as penicillin did after its discovery, antivirals will be 100 times cheaper by the mid-1990s (Brandt 1987, p. 170). At $40 per annual treatment, antivirals cannot be denied to the poor, severely affected pattern II countries. If they are tightly controlled by the government so that access to them is only through a public health clinic which aggressively pursues partner notification, then antivirals can substantially increase the effectiveness of partner notification efforts. The incidence of all STDs, including HIV, may be strikingly reduced.

Because partner notification may have significant ethical and practical problems and undesirable social and biological side effects, it may not be a feasible or recommendable approach to HIV control in many societies. Some issues which have to be resolved before initiating such a program include possible stigmatization of those notified, violation of privacy, potential for misuse by index cases, rejection of notified women by their partners (sometimes leading to prostitution), the need for a large corps of counselors and for medical facilities capable of monitoring the biological side effects of antiretroviral therapy, and an assurance of long-term sustainability and continuity. Preliminary results from counseling and partner notification efforts with HIV-infected pregnant women in

Africa are rather disappointing (Temmerman and others 1990). For all these reasons, we do not recommend partner notification as a primary strategy for HIV control at the moment, but we believe that pilot projects should be supported to address the issues discussed.

SEXUAL TRANSMISSION AND IEC PROGRAMS. The most cost-effective IEC program to inform the general public about STDs is targeted not at individuals at risk but at journalists. Using STDs as an excuse to sell newspapers by openly discussing sexual behavior, journalists and their editors have become willing collaborators with the public health authorities in STD control at least since President Franklin D. Roosevelt's surgeon general, Thomas Parran, broke taboos in the United States by publishing an explicit article on STDs in the Reader's Digest in 1936. More than 125 newspapers, many other magazines, and even the staid monthly the Ladies' Home Journal picked up the campaign, providing a wealth of free IEC (Brandt 1987, p. 141). In 1988 the British campaign against AIDS obtained 8 million pounds of free publicity in one month alone while spending only 3 million on its own campaign (United Kingdom, National Health Service 1988).

Any visitor to or resident of a developing country with an HIV epidemic is aware of how enthusiastically journalists there have picked up and reported any information about HIV infection, whether it is true or false. With respect to the media, the challenge for the national AIDS control programs in these countries is threefold: to prevent the publication of misinformation; to continue to provide new, interesting press releases expressed in lay language and accompanied by vivid graphics; and to broaden the discussion beyond HIV and AIDS to other STDs.

In our opinion, efforts to address publicly financed IEC campaigns to the entire population or even to all sexually active people are likely to be markedly less cost-effective in slowing STD epidemics than would the passive and voluntary programs described above. Evidence from a variety of national settings confirms that such IEC campaigns may improve knowledge and change attitudes but usually produce little if any behavioral change (Warner 1983; Hornik 1988). The IEC programs that are targeted at a specific subset of the core group may be a useful addition to the efforts described above.

For discussion of IEC campaigns, it is useful to cross-classify the population in two dimensions by "target group" and "access group." We define target groups as groups of individuals with homogeneous risk behavior, whose behavior change is the object of some STD intervention listed in table 20-13. Access groups are defined according to the means or channel by which we can gain access to them for the communication of IEC and training messages. In table 20-23 we present a classification of target groups as rows and access groups as columns.

The target group for behavioral change can be either the group at risk of infection or the group that controls the risk of infection. Information, education, and communication programs would be addressed to the former and training to the latter. In the rows of table 20-23, we identify three subgroups among those at risk: sexually active persons, health care consumers (at risk from transfusion or contaminated needles), and health care providers (at risk from accidental sticking by contaminated needles, and so on). In other rows of the table, we classify those controlling the risk of infection as health care providers or government officials. These latter groups administer and enforce mandatory or passive interventions. The target groups are, of course, of very different sizes. Although the relative sizes of the groups will vary from one urban setting to another, it is useful to note typical or "notional" relative sizes for the groups in table 20-23.[49]

In order to change the behavior of either the group at risk or the group controlling the risk, an IEC or training intervention must communicate, either through the mass media or face-to-face. The columns of table 20-23 identify subsets of the population reached by each of a selected set of access routes. Like the target groups, the access groups differ in size. Because the size of a specific access group can be varied, however (that is, by calling a meeting of unmarried workers in a given factory, or by targeting a media campaign to adolescents), it is not useful to associate even a national relative magnitude to each access group at this level of aggregation.

An IEC or training program aimed at a given access group will typically reach only some of the members of any target group but will also reach other individuals outside the target group. Define the "coverage" of a specific target group by an intervention as the proportion of the target group reached. Clearly, an intervention is to be preferred, other things being equal, if it reaches a large rather than a small proportion of the target group.[50] It is possible roughly to rank the coverage that messages aimed at each access group would achieve for each target group. For example, IEC efforts at bars or STD clinics may achieve relatively high coverage of female prostitutes, whereas IEC efforts at barracks, schools, and offices would do much less well on this measure.

Still, even if a message covers all of a target group, its effect on that group will be reduced if it also reaches large numbers outside the target. For example, a message on the desirability of using condoms with multiple sexual partners, when routed through the mass media, will lose credibility and plausibility to the prostitute, because she and her peers are a small percentage of those receiving the message. Define the "concentration" of a message on a target group as the percentage of all message recipients who are in the given target group.[51] Again, the concentration of a message routed through a given access group at a given target group can be roughly ranked. In the above example of a mass media campaign, we argue that the small concentration makes the campaign less effective, other things being equal. By focusing a message aimed at prostitutes via an access group defined by the clients of an STD clinic or by a red-light residential neighborhood, however, the message's concentration can be substantially increased. Thus concentration must be added to coverage as a desirable attribute of an IEC or training program.[52]

In the cells of table 20-23 we have tentatively classified the use of each access group to reach each target group as having a coverage and a concentration which are "high," "medium," or "low." As an example of how to read the table, consider an IEC program which attempts to change the behavior of prostitutes (the target group) by addressing all the clients of bars (the access group). Because such a program is likely to reach a high proportion of all prostitutes, it scores an "H" for "high" on coverage in the appropriate cell of table 20-23. A program addressed to the access group "saloon clients," however, will necessarily be diluted in its effect on prostitutes because of their small share in the population of such clients. Therefore this program scores an "L" for "low" on concentration in the same cell. If the goal of a program is to change the behavior of prostitutes, consideration should be given to reaching them through an STD clinic, especially one which might have a higher-than-average concentration of prostitutes, or in their residential neighborhood, in which we estimate both the coverage and the concentration to be "medium." If we assume that the goal of the IEC program is to slow the epidemics, preventing as many case-years of illness as possible per dollar of the IEC budget, the candidates for programs which hold the most promise are those which are targeted at part of the core group, have high coverage of and concentration on the targeted group, and provide a message which can be expected to interest and persuade many in the target group.

Consider, first, prostitutes who are part of the core. If we have guessed correctly on the entries in the first row of table 20-23, none of the access groups listed will provide both high coverage of and high concentration on this group. Furthermore, experience with female prostitutes in Nairobi, Kenya (Ngugi and others 1988); male bar workers in Bangkok, Thailand (Sittitrai 1990); and other groups has shown that even face-to-face contact fails to change the frequency of safe sex enough to slow the spread of the HIV virus. The most promising results from prostitutes came instead from peer training programs, in which trusted fellow prostitutes are the source of the persuasive message. A program like this in Cameroon increased the reported use of condoms (at least half the time) from 28 percent to 72 percent over a twelve-month period (Monny-Lobe and others 1989). Previous similar successes had been reported in Ghana (Lamptey and others 1988) and Mexico. The medium concentration that may be achieved in some red-light districts argues that these residential neighborhoods be the venue for these meetings.

The data in table 20-23 indicate that the clients of prostitutes are also likely to be hard to reach with high concentration, because they do not form a large percentage of any of these access groups. Because clients are a largely clandestine group in many countries, peer training programs are also likely to fail. Hence, we recommend against targeting them.

Like prostitutes, sexually active adolescents may respond relatively well to peer counseling and might otherwise be hard to reach. Because that portion of adolescents who are attending secondary school or a university are a particular critical national resource in pattern II countries, we recommend that they be targeted with particular vigor.

In contrast to the above groups, a message aimed at bar patrons is predicted to cover a large proportion of adults with

Table 20-23. Coverage and Concentration of IEC and Training Programs, by Target and Access Group

Target group		Access group					
Group	Size	Audience of mass media	Prisoners, soldiers, students, or workers in prisons, barracks, schools, or work sites	Sexually active adults at bars	Patients at general health care clinics	Clients and workers at family planning and STD clinics	Residents of a neighborhood
Groups at risk							
From sex							
Prostitutes	20	Low/low	Low/low	High/low	Medium/low	High/low	Medium/medium
Clients of prostitutes	100	Medium/low	High/low	High/low	Medium/low	High/low	Low/low
Sexually active adolescents	2,000	Low/low	Medium/low	Low/low	Medium/low	Medium/low	Low/low
Adults with multiple partners	2,000	High/medium	High/medium	High/high	Medium/low	Medium/high	High/low
From transfusions	10,000	Medium/high	Medium/high	Low/medium	High/high	Low/medium	High/high
From needles	5	High/low	Low/low	Medium/low	High/medium	High/high	Low/low
Group controlling risk							
Health care providers	5	High/low	Low/low	Medium/low	High/medium	High/high	Low/low
Government officials	5	High/low	High/medium	Medium/low	Low/low	Low/low	Medium/low

Note: Coverage is defined as the proportion of the target group reached by a message. Concentration is the proportion of those reached who are in the target group. "High" is defined as greater than two-thirds; "medium" is defined as one-third to two-thirds; "low" is defined as less than one-third. The estimated coverage precedes the estimated concentration; thus, the notation "high/low" means that using the indicated access group to target the indicated target group will have a high coverage but a low concentration.

Source: Authors' development of Hornik 1989a and 1989b.

multiple partners and to do so with high concentration. We recommend targeted IEC at this core group.

We explicitly assign a low priority to publicly financed IEC campaigns designed to change the sexual behavior of noncore groups, such as the health care consumers of table 20-23. Although some people in these other, lower-risk, populations may become infected with HIV through sexual intercourse, public programs are unlikely to deliver more effective messages than the privately financed media, and each public dollar spent here could be spent with greater effect on any of the programs discussed above.

It is extremely difficult to quantify all the above considerations. Still, the epidemiological model presented earlier can be used to arrive at a rough estimate of the relative cost-effectiveness of a particular kind of IEC program, one that is designed to increase the frequency of condom use. We assume that condoms are distributed with the assistance of a condom social marketing campaign which subsidizes IEC efforts that vary, depending on the campaign's target group.[53] For the noncore, the social marketing resources would be spent on the public media. To target the core, the campaign would employ peer counselors from among the high-risk population. In table 20-24 we present the estimated cost per disability-adjusted life-year saved by such an intervention depending on which STDs are present in the population, on the cost per person-year of the social marketing campaign, and on whether the program is targeted at the core or the noncore.

As predicted in the discussion of table 20-19, the immense increase in effectiveness attained by protecting core individuals rather than noncore is large enough to offset our assumption that the cost per person-year of protection will be ten times larger in the core. In table 20-24 we show costs per disability-adjusted life-year below \$1 for interventions targeted to the core group in the presence of certain epidemics. These costs compare favorably with those of other interventions.

PREVENTION OF TRANSMISSION FROM MOTHER TO INFANT. The World Health Organization estimates mother-to-infant transmission as the second most important transmission mode for HIV infection in pattern II countries, accounting for up to 11 percent of all cases. Obviously, prevention of HIV-infection in women also prevents these women from infecting their infants at no additional program cost. The question is whether additional resources should be reallocated to prevent infected women from conceiving or from giving birth.

As part of the program of notifying sexual partners, we recommend that HIV-infected women, especially if they are pregnant, receive extra, gender-specific, voluntary counseling which focuses on the risks of having seropositive babies and the costs of their care.[54] Recent experience from Kenya and Zaire suggests that the fertility rate of women who know they are infected with HIV is at least as great as that of uninfected women, despite counseling about their infection status and the risk of perinatal infection (Temmerman and others 1990). In addition, the illegality of abortion in many countries is a serious impediment to such a strategy.

Table 20-24. Cost per Discounted Disability-Adjusted Life-Year Saved for a Condom Subsidy Intervention: Sensitivity to Cost per Person Year of Protection and Core versus Noncore Strategy
(1990 U.S. dollars)

		Cost per year of protection	
Disease (group)	Disability-adjusted life-years saved per person-year of protection	\$50 in core group \$5 in noncore group	\$450 in core group \$45 in noncore group
Chancroid			
Core group	80.9	0.62	5.56
Noncore group	1.1	4.55	40.91
Chlamydia			
Core group	196.6	0.25	2.29
Noncore group	4.2	1.19	10.71
Gonorrhea			
Core group	275.2	0.18	1.64
Noncore group	5.2	0.96	8.65
HIV *without ulcers*			
Noncore group	56.6	0.88	7.95
Core group	19.9	2.51	22.61
HIV *with ulcers*			
Core group	156.0	0.32	2.88
Noncore group	21.5	0.23	2.09
Syphilis			
Core group	384.6	0.13	1.17
Noncore group	9.7	0.52	4.64

Source: First column from table 20-19; cost per person-year of protection from table 20-20; Janowitz, Bratt, and Fried 1990.

In table 20-21 we presented calculations of the cost per case of gonococcal ophthalmia neonatorum averted through the preventive application of silver nitrate or tetracycline. When the prevalence rate of gonorrhea among pregnant women is above 1 percent, a case of gonococcal ophthalmia neonatorum can be averted for less than \$6, if silver nitrate is chosen. Assuming that each averted case saves the affected child one disability-adjusted life-year, this preventive intervention buys disability-adjusted life-years for less than \$6 when prevalence rates are high.[55] Therefore, we recommend universal eye prophylaxis, without prior screening of the mother, in all areas in which gonorrhea prevalence rates are above 1 percent.

Finally, to prevent congenital syphilis, we recommend universal screening of pregnant women for serological markers of syphilis, followed by effective treatment of infected women.[56]

PREVENTION OF TRANSMISSION BY BLOOD AND BLOOD PRODUCTS. Because WHO estimates that only about 6 percent of all cases of HIV infection in pattern II countries are caused by transfused blood or blood products, the case for diverting resources from other prevention programs to this one must be based on sound cost-effectiveness analysis. We consider first mandatory then passive and voluntary policy interventions. Then we estimate the COST-effectiveness of blood screening under various circumstances.

The high incidence and severe consequences of malaria and anemia in many developing countries are discussed in other chapters of this collection. Blood transfusion has often been administered to these patients with little curative effect. Now, in pattern II countries, such patients incur the risk of HIV infection in addition to the other risks of these diseases.

In the area of blood transfusion, we depart from our aversion to mandatory policies to recommend one: a prohibition of the transfusion of unscreened blood except as a life-saving measure. According to Fleming (1988), such indications include the following:

- Profound anemia (hematocrit less than 4 grams per deciliter) with incipient cardiac failure
- Severe neonatal jaundice (serum bilirubin greater than 300 micromol/L
- Blood loss of more than 25 percent of total volume when the blood pressure and oxygen cannot be maintained by plasma expanders.

Each pattern II country should develop and enforce its own set of transfusion guidelines. Because the necessary enforcement effort is focused at secondary care institutions, it can be implemented in each such facility by a committee of senior physicians. The enforcement of this ban should be the top priority program for the prevention of infection by blood transfusion.

If additional public resources for transfusion remain after the above two programs have been implemented, the additional security which comes from a blood-screening program can be considered. When efficiently performed at a blood bank, blood tests now cost less than a dollar in Africa, which is less than 25 percent of the cost of a unit of blood in most African capitals. Furthermore, some laboratories are experimenting with the use of a single test to screen a vial of blood in which the samples of several individuals are pooled. With some of the available blood tests, a negative test result on the pool of five separate samples ensures that all individual samples are negative with a probability above .95. In areas of poor countries where blood bank facilities are unavailable or undependable and prospective donors must be screened on the spot, only the more expensive ($2.50–$4.00) rapid tests are useful for screening blood, and pooling is impractical (Laleman and others 1992). In this case, the screening will double the cost of blood. These considerations lead us to recommend that, once transfusion guidelines and donor recruitment programs are in place, a blood-screening program should be largely self-financing through patient fees, with appropriate sliding fee schedules to accommodate the indigent. Because user charges are already the de facto policy for blood screening in many African capitals, implementing such a policy will not be difficult. Both a centralized blood bank system and a decentralized strategy

using simple rapid tests should be considered (Laleman and others 1992). The choice between these institutional alternatives depends on the organization and capability of the local health system.

The second priority for the prevention of HIV infection from blood transfusion is to develop a corps of low-risk, voluntary donors who repeatedly donate blood in a given community. Such a policy will be more costly to administer than the laissez-faire ad hoc policies which required the patient's family to recruit a donor, but they will still be less costly and more cost-effective than would be the universal screening of all transfused blood.

Any effort to reduce the incidence of illnesses requiring blood transfusion will in a pattern II country also reduce the incidence of HIV infection. When this benefit is added to the intrinsic merits of these other programs, some of them will assume even higher priorities in national health promotion strategies than they would on their own merits. Such health problems include trauma (especially from road accidents), malaria, anemia, and adverse birth outcomes.

A quantitative analysis of the cost-effectiveness of blood screening should consider the cost per disability-adjusted life-year saved of donor deferral, donor recruitment, and training physicians to use more conservative criteria for transfusing. Unfortunately, costs of these varied strategies are not available. It is possible, however, to calculate the cost per DALY saved by blood screening under the simple assumptions used to construct figure 20-16. From table 20-16 we know that averting a case of HIV infection saves about 359.6 DALYs if the person is in the core group and only 54.6 DALYs if the person is in the noncore. Table 20-25 is constructed to combine these figures with the costs per case of HIV averted in figure 20-16, producing costs per DALY saved. Note that the argument for HIV screening in low-prevalence populations of poor countries is weak.

PREVENTION OF TRANSMISSION BY SKIN-PIERCING INSTRUMENTS. Fewer than 3 percent of all cases of HIV infection have been attributed to needles and skin-piercing instruments in pattern II countries. Furthermore, the costs of significant reform in this area seem high. We recommend that efforts here be restricted to a modest IEC campaign designed to stimulate health care consumers to insist on brand new or properly sterilized needles. In addition, health care providers should be educated about the importance of properly sterilized needles and, for their own protection, about safe methods of discarding them.

Case Management and Secondary Prevention

By treating CSTDs, further spread of the infection is prevented, and the risk of complications and sequelae in patients with an STD is reduced.

Goals of Case Management

Treatment of STDs benefits both the infected individual and, by reducing the reservoir of infected persons, the community

Table 20-25. Cost per Discounted Disability-Adjusted Life-Years Saved of Blood Screening

Sexual activity group of proposed blood recipient	Cost of blood test	Prevalence rate of HIV infection among blood donors			
		0.001	0.01	0.05	0.25
Core group	$2	7.42	0.74	0.15	0.03
	$10	37.08	3.71	0.74	0.15
Noncore group	$2	48.84	4.88	0.98	0.20
	$10	244.20	24.42	4.88	0.98

Note: See figure 16 and discussion. Costs include estimated overhead cost of managing blood screening service. From Table 20-26 we assume that each case of HIV averted in the core group saves 359.6 DALYs, while each case averted in the noncore saves 54.6 DALYs.
Source: Authors' calculations.

of uninfected people. Traditionally, early diagnosis and treatment (secondary prevention) have been the cornerstones of programs for the control of bacterial STDs, including syphilis, gonorrhea, and genital chlamydial infection. As effective antiviral chemotherapy becomes available against HIV infection and genital herpes, secondary prevention may become an increasingly important aspect of the control of viral STDs. In addition, it will be possible to increase greatly the life expectancy of patients with HIV infection. The overall goals of treatment of STDs are the following:

- To cure the actual disease
- To prevent complications and sequelae
- To prevent transmission of the treated disease
- To reduce the efficiency of HIV transmission

Principles of Case Management

The STDs caused by bacterial agents are all fully treatable by specific antibiotics. Still, case management of STDs is often of poor quality and ineffective in many, if not most, countries of the world. Furthermore, even the best treatment of viral STDs remains purely symptomatic or marginally effective and very expensive (for example, herpes). Problems in case management and secondary prevention of STDs are listed below.

- Health-seeking behavior (delay of diagnosis and treatment)
- Accessibility and quality of health care facilities
- Etiological diagnosis of syndromes (inadequate laboratories, lack of simple, inexpensive diagnostic tests)
- Antimicrobial resistance (gonorrhea, chancroid)
- Partner referral

Current case management guidelines are summarized in appendix 20C.

EARLY TREATMENT. Improving health-seeking behavior is a much neglected aspect of management strategies for STDs but

may be a critical element in the prevention of complications and sequelae through early diagnosis and treatment, as well as in the reduction of secondary cases of STD by the patient. Delays by men of several weeks and by women of several months before seeking treatment for an STD are not unusual. Health-seeking behavior is not only a function of attitudes toward disease and sex but also of the accessibility and quality of health care facilities dealing with STDs. These are often of poor quality, understaffed, and lacking even the most essential diagnostic tools and drugs. Whereas STDs can usually be managed at public primary health care facilities, patients often prefer to go to more expensive private physicians who for the most part are not offering a better standard of management. Training of health care workers in STD is also grossly inadequate in most medical schools.

DIAGNOSIS. A core problem in STD case management is the difficult etiological diagnosis of most syndromes, particularly in women. Thus, both gonococcal and chlamydial infection in the female are diagnosed by isolation of the bacterial agent, the simpler microscopic examinations not being adequate. Culture techniques are expensive and technically demanding and are beyond the competence or fiscal possibilities (reagents must be paid for in hard currency) of most laboratories in developing countries. Culture-independent techniques (enzyme immunoassay, immunofluorescent assays, DNA hybridization) for the diagnosis of bacterial and viral STDs have become available recently but are expensive and often still lack sensitivity and specificity. Clinical methods of diagnosing STDs by means of simple algorithms are being increasingly used (see appendix 20C). Thus far, however, these have failed effectively to diagnose gonococcal and chlamydial infections in women.

CASE FINDING AND SCREENING. Case finding and screening have traditionally been an important component of STD control programs. Their objective is to identify individuals who are infected, but are not symptomatic, in order to treat them before they develop complications and sequelae. As weapons for actively combating STDs, these two strategies must be compared with that of simply treating persons without diagnosis. In appendix 20C we analyze these two options for all the STDs considered in this chapter and find that, for cost ranges relevant to developing countries, screening is rarely more cost-effective than treating without a test. Furthermore in those cases in which screening is cost-effective, clinical diagnosis is almost always more cost-effective than laboratory tests (see appendix 20C for details.)

One use of screening not analyzed in appendix 20C is for the prevention of congenital syphilis by screening pregnant women for serological markers for syphilis. By treating infected women, congenital syphilis is prevented in the newborn. Case finding is also used for gonorrhea control in populations where the prevalence of this infection is reasonably high. It has been used with success in STD control programs in prostitutes in various parts of the world (Tuliza and others 1991).

EFFECTIVE THERAPY. Because of the development of antimicrobial resistance of N. gonorrhoeae strains, mainly in Southeast Asia and Sub-Saharan Africa, treatment of gonorrhea has become more complicated and more expensive. Treatment guidelines for STDs and adequate training of health care workers in STD management are not available in most developing countries.

Although not as such part of individual therapy, treatment of primary (the source contact) and secondary sexual contacts (individuals exposed to the patient) through partner notification is an essential part of case management, aiming at reducing the reinfection rate in the patient, limiting the spread of the infection in the population, and decreasing the rate of complications and sequelae in these contacts. This requires considerable resources in time and personnel and is heavily influenced by the cultural-behavioral environment. Its cost-effectiveness remains to be explored in a developing country context.

COUNSELING. Finally, because STD patients may put themselves again at risk for STD—and because a small group of core transmitters is directly and indirectly responsible for the majority of cases of STD—counseling aiming at behavioral change should also be part of the STD case management.

HIV INFECTION. Case management of patients with HIV infection includes treatment of the associated opportunistic infections in patients with AIDS, therapy for HIV infection itself, and appropriate social and psychological support. Whereas several opportunistic infections can be reasonably effectively treated (such as tuberculosis, candidiasis, herpes simplex virus infections), others are either difficult to diagnose (such as cerebral toxoplasmosis, cytomegalovirus infection), requiring sophisticated imaging or laboratory technology, or very difficult to treat (such as crytosporidiosis, infection with atypical mycobacteria). Relapses after the end of therapy are frequent for all opportunistic infections, and treatment is often purely palliative. Estimates of the costs of treating opportunistic infections in AIDS patients in Zambia are shown in appendix 20C.

Treatment of AIDS patients with AZT results in an average prolongation of life of at least two years and a considerable improvement in the quality of life. Still, side effects (mainly hematological, necessitating blood transfusions and interruption of therapy) are common. Resistant strains of HIV appear to emerge under therapy, and the drug costs as much as $750–$1,000 per month.

Costs of Case Management

This section considers issues in the cost of case management of both HIV and STD.

COSTS OF AN STD TREATMENT PROGRAM. Operation of an STD treatment program in a developing country involves both domestic and foreign resources. In most developing countries, the foreign resources include the cost of drugs and of diagnostic materials. Domestic resources include the personnel who deliver the services and the buildings in which they work. In appendix 20C we assemble the available information on the cost of STD treatment in order to arrive at an estimate of the cost per effectively treated case of STD. In table 20C-3 we present sensitivity analysis of the cost per effectively treated case with respect to two key parameters, the cost per clinic-hour and the prevalence rate of the STD in the population. The first of these parameters varies with the GNP of the country—relatively rich countries will have more highly paid medical workers and more expensive rental rates for their buildings. Contrarily, a high prevalence rate decreases the cost per effectively treated case by ensuring that few resources are wasted on people who are not really sick.

Two strategies can be defined. The first is the one usually recommended by medical experts: the health care provider applies a diagnostic procedure. He or she might take a specimen and examine it with a microscope or culture it in a laboratory in an attempt to diagnose the etiologic agent accurately. Or the provider might simply examine the patient, take a medical history, and apply a decision rule or "health care algorithm" to decide whether, and how, to treat. Each of these three diagnostic procedures has a different degree of precision and a different cost. We call a strategy that applies one of these procedures a "test-before-treatment" strategy.

The second strategy is an extreme form of presumptive treatment. In this method, the provider prescribes a broad-spectrum antibiotic to everyone in some defined population, without taking the time to do a careful examination or history. Such a method might be especially worth considering at small health posts, in which the health provider is not trained to follow accurately a diagnostic algorithm. The population treated might consist of all patients who present to the clinic complaining of STD symptoms. A more radical strategy would be to provide this broad-spectrum treatment to everyone in a community, whether or not they are currently experiencing STD symptoms or have presented for treatment. The cost-effectiveness of this "treat everyone" strategy compared with a test-before-treatment strategy will vary, depending on the cost of drugs and diagnostic tests, the prevalence rate of STDs in the reference population, and the sensitivity and specificity of the diagnostic procedure being considered.[57]

COST OF AIDS TREATMENT IN DEVELOPING COUNTRIES. Estimates of the treatment costs of persons with AIDS in developing countries have been constructed by applying use patterns (based, in the absence of data, on expert opinion) to imperfectly known inpatient and outpatient average costs (Over and others 1988). Such AIDS treatment cost estimates, therefore, should be considered preliminary. Nevertheless, the results provided in table 20-26 are indicative of the range of values to be expected in developing countries.

A principal finding of the studies which generated these estimates is that the cost per patient varies considerably, both across countries and within a country. Most cross-country

Table 20-26. *Treatment Costs of* AIDS *in Selected Developing Countries*
(U.S. dollars)

Country	GNP per capita	Treatment cost		Treatment cost as percentage of GNP per capita	
		Low	High	Low	High
Brazil	2,160	6,000	12,000	278	556
Mexico	2,080	3,286	7,344	158	353
Tanzania	290	104	631	36	218
Zaire	170	132	1,585	78	932

Note: Brazil, estimates are 1988 U.S. dollars; Mexico, 1985 U.S. dollars; Tanzania and Zaire, 1986 U.S. dollars. All estimates include both inpatient and outpatient treatment costs. The low and high estimates correspond, respectively, to the most modest and the most comprehensive health care options available in the country. The average cost will typically be closer to the low than to the high end of this range.
Source: Over and others 1988; Tapia and Martin 1990; authors' calculations.

variation in costs is caused by differences in wage rates paid to providers, which tend to vary with levels of per capita GNP. Treatment costs per case exhibit a range within a country for two principal reasons: variation in the clinical symptoms which manifest themselves and variation in the socioeconomic characteristics of the patient and the medical and institutional characteristics of the available health care options (Over and Kutzin 1990). On a percentage basis, the poorest countries tend to exhibit greater cost variation because only a small proportion of all illness episodes are treated in a relatively high-cost hospital setting (Scitovsky and Over 1988). Cost variation exists in industrial countries but to a lesser degree because widespread insurance coverage provides better access to hospital care for a greater proportion of the population and standard treatment protocols are used on a wider basis.

Cost-Effective Case Management Strategies

As various options exist for case management, it is important to examine the cost-effectiveness of each approach to optimize resource allocation.

COST-EFFECTIVE CSTD TREATMENT AND SECONDARY PREVENTION. How cost-effective is STD control in a developing country in the presence of an HIV epidemic? First, consider the cost-effectiveness of CSTD treatment in the absence of HIV. In this scenario, the measure of effectiveness would be the static and dynamic DALYs saved per case from the averted CSTD only, which are presented in the last two columns of table 20-16. Dividing the minimum cost of an effectively treated case of a CSTD from table 20C-3 by these effects yields estimates of the cost-effectiveness of CSTD treatment in the absence of HIV. These estimates are presented in table 20-27.

In the presence of an HIV epidemic, the effective treatment of a CSTD has the dynamic effect of averting cases of HIV infection. The total DALYs saved in this scenario are presented in the last two columns of table 20-18 and depicted graphically in figure 20-15. By again dividing the minimum effective treatment cost estimates by these greater effects, cost-effectiveness estimates of CSTD treatment in the presence of an HIV epidemic are generated. In table 20-28 we present these esti-

mates, which reveal the increased cost-effectiveness of CSTD treatment where an HIV epidemic exists.

Because they are derived from the estimates in tables 20-16, 20-18, and 20C-3, the cost-effectiveness estimates in tables 20-27 and 20-28 share a sensitivity to the level of sexual activity of the treated person, the prevalence rate of the STD, and the average cost per clinic-hour. The magnitude of the difference in cost-effectiveness strongly suggests targeting treatment programs at the highly sexually active core group. In a region experiencing an HIV epidemic, for example, curing or preventing a CSTD where it has a prevalence rate of 25 percent and the cost per clinic-hour is $2.00 will buy disability-adjusted life-years for between $0.02 and $0.11 each.[58] If the cost per clinic-hour was $10.00, a disability-adjusted life-year could be saved for between $0.04 and $0.25 by curing a CSTD. After interventions targeted at the core have been successfully implemented, a country can purchase additional life-years with programs aimed at noncore groups with low prevalence rates for less than $30.00 each (assuming $2.00 per clinic-hour) to less than $87.00 each (assuming $10.00 per clinic-hour). This higher range still compares favorably with the cost of saving life-years among adults with other health care interventions.

COST-EFFECTIVE MANAGEMENT OF AIDS CASES. Case management of HIV or AIDS through the prophylactic administration of an antiviral agent like AZT is clearly not a cost-effective option for purchasing DALYs in developing countries. This situation could change dramatically, however, if the price of antiviral therapy drops dramatically. In the absence of antivirals, treatment of the opportunistic illnesses of an AIDS patient can buy disability-adjusted life-years at the substantial but feasible cost of $235 to $384 when clinic time costs $10 per hour. This sum is approximately equal to the GNP per capita of many of the heavily affected countries and is substantially less than the annual income of prime age urban adults in those countries. There is a strong argument to ensure the provision of the basic drugs required to manage these opportunistic infections in order to buy an extra year or two of life for the person with AIDS and to protect the drug supplies needed to treat other patients who are not infected with HIV.

Table 20-27. Cost per Discounted Disability-Adjusted Life-Year Saved by STD Treatment in Absence of an HIV Epidemic: Sensitivity to Prevalence Rate and Core vs. Noncore Strategy
(1990 U.S. dollars)

Disease	Disability-adjusted life-years saved per effectively treated case	$2 per clinic hour			$10 per clinic hour			$30 per clinic hour		
		1 percent prevalence	5 percent prevalence	25 percent prevalence	1 percent prevalence	5 percent prevalence	25 percent prevalence	1 percent prevalence	5 percent prevalence	25 percent prevalence
Chancroid										
Minimum treatment cost	n.a.	73	15	3	333	67	14	983	199	42
Core group	1.8	40.56	8.33	1.67	185.00	37.22	7.78	546.11	110.56	23.33
Noncore group	0.4	182.50	37.50	7.50	832.50	167.50	35.00	2,457.50	497.50	105.00
Chlamydia, female										
Minimum treatment cost	n.a.	322	64	13	544	109	22	1,100	220	44
Core group	44.1	7.30	1.45	0.29	12.34	2.47	0.50	24.94	4.99	1.00
Noncore group	5.5	58.55	11.64	2.36	98.91	19.82	4.00	200.00	40.00	8.00
Chlamydia, male										
Minimum treatment cost	n.a.	63	13	3	286	59	13	822	164	33
Core group	44.1	1.43	0.29	0.07	6.49	1.34	0.29	18.64	3.72	0.75
Noncore group	5.5	11.45	2.36	0.55	52.00	10.73	2.36	149.45	29.82	6.00
Gonorrhea, female										
Minimum treatment cost	n.a.	295	59	12	463	93	19	884	177	35
Core group	37.3	7.91	1.58	0.32	12.41	2.49	0.51	23.70	4.75	0.94
Noncore group	4.5	65.56	13.11	2.67	102.89	20.67	4.22	196.44	39.33	7.78
Gonorrhea, male										
Minimum treatment cost	n.a.	62	13	4	245	51	12	678	141	31
Core group	37.3	1.66	0.35	0.11	6.57	1.37	0.32	18.18	3.78	0.83
Noncore group	4.5	13.78	2.89	0.89	54.44	11.33	2.67	150.67	31.33	6.89
Syphilis										
Minimum treatment cost	n.a.	185	38	9	269	56	14	477	102	27
Core group	160.8	1.15	0.24	0.06	1.67	0.35	0.09	2.97	0.63	0.17
Noncore group	19.8	9.34	1.92	0.45	13.59	2.83	0.71	24.09	5.15	1.36

n.a. Not applicable.
Source: Authors.

Table 20-28. Cost per Discounted Disability-Adjusted Life-Year Saved by STD Treatment in Presence of an HIV Epidemic: Sensitivity to Prevalence Rate and Core vs. Noncore Strategy
(1990 U.S. dollars)

Disease	Disability-adjusted life-years saved per effectively treated case	$2 per clinic hour			$10 per clinic hour			$30 per clinic hour		
		1 percent prevalence	5 percent prevalence	25 percent prevalence	1 percent prevalence	5 percent prevalence	25 percent prevalence	1 percent prevalence	5 percent prevalence	25 percent prevalence
Chancroid										
Minimum treatment cost	n.a.	73	15	3	333	67	14	983	199	42
Core group	55.6	1.31	0.27	0.05	5.99	1.21	0.25	17.68	3.58	0.76
Noncore group	3.8	19.21	3.95	0.79	87.63	17.63	3.68	258.68	52.37	11.05
Chlamydia, female										
Minimum treatment cost	n.a.	322	64	13	544	109	22	1,100	220	44
Core group	113.5	2.84	0.56	0.11	4.79	0.96	0.19	9.69	1.94	0.39
Noncore group	11.4	28.25	5.61	1.14	47.72	9.56	1.93	96.49	19.30	3.86
Chlamydia, male										
Minimum treatment cost	n.a.	63	13	3	286	59	13	822	164	33
Core group	113.5	0.56	0.11	0.03	2.52	0.52	0.11	7.24	1.44	0.29
Noncore group	11.4	5.53	1.14	0.26	25.09	5.18	1.14	72.11	14.39	2.89
Gonorrhea, female										
Minimum treatment cost	n.a.	295	59	12	463	93	19	884	177	35
Core group	120.2	2.45	0.49	0.10	3.85	0.77	0.16	7.35	1.47	0.29
Noncore group	11.6	25.43	5.09	1.03	39.91	8.02	1.64	76.21	15.26	3.02
Gonorrhea, male										
Minimum treatment cost	n.a.	62	13	4	245	51	12	678	141	31
Core group	120.2	0.52	0.11	0.03	2.04	0.42	0.10	5.64	1.17	0.26
Noncore group	11.6	5.34	1.12	0.34	21.12	4.40	1.03	58.45	12.16	2.67
Syphilis										
Minimum treatment cost	n.a.	185	38	9	269	56	14	477	102	27
Core group	396.3	0.47	0.10	0.02	0.68	0.14	0.04	1.20	0.26	0.07
Noncore group	41.1	4.50	0.92	0.22	6.55	1.36	0.34	11.61	2.48	0.66

n.a. Not applicable.
Source: Authors.

Greater expenditure per AIDS case does not improve the probability of survival. Palliative care in the home and community may not be as effective at prolonging life as is the use of antivirals, but the data in table 20C-1 suggest that palliative care is almost certainly more cost-effective. Assuming that clinic time costs $10 per hour, palliative care alone (second row in the table) buys one year of healthy life, and antivirals (first row in the table) buy two years of healthy life, a disability-adjusted life-year is purchased much more inexpensively with palliative care ($235 for one year by treating AIDS without AZT) than with antiviral treatment ($1,200 for each of two years by treating AIDS with AZT). More evidence of the opportunity for considerable improvement in the cost-effectiveness of AIDS treatment is provided in table 20-26, where the ranges of estimates for each country suggest the feasibility of reducing the cost per case.

Developments in Case Management in the Next Decade

It is anticipated that major advances will be seen in case management, particularly of AIDS, in the near future.

DIAGNOSTICS. The most promising area for innovation in case management is probably the development of simple diagnostic tests for most STDs. The basic technology (mainly enzyme immunoassays) is already available, and research is currently focusing on improving test performance. This will allow on-the-spot simple and rapid specific diagnosis of CSTDs such as gonorrhea, chlamydial infection, and chancroid—an important, if not essential, element in the control of gonococcal and chlamydial infections in women. The cost of such tests is presently still high ($4 to $7), but it is expected that prices will decrease because many companies are becoming active in this field. It is not clear, however, how and if these new diagnostic tools will be used in developing countries.

DRUGS. New antibiotics are being continuously developed, including agents active against bacterial STDs. Inexpensive oral antibiotics able to cure gonorrhea caused by multiresistant strains when given as a single dose are urgently needed and may become available. Numerous antiviral compounds have recently been developed and are being or will be evaluated for their clinical effectiveness in HIV infection, both in asymptomatic carriers of HIV and in AIDS patients. It is expected that more effective and less toxic therapy for HIV infection will become available in the 1990s. It will probably consist of lifelong treatment with a combination of antiviral drugs. This would have a significant effect on the prevention of HIV infection, because secondary prevention would then become an important additional strategy for the control of HIV infection.

For these new pharmaceutical developments to be relevant to developing countries, prices must be low. Yet low prices remove the incentive for continued research and development by private firms. International political collaboration, perhaps coordinated by WHO, could help to negotiate lower prices for de-veloping countries while keeping prices higher in the industrial countries. Care must be taken, however, on three fronts.

First, WHO must be protected from the fate that has befallen most regulatory bodies throughout the history of regulation—capture by the regulated industry. Only if mechanisms can be arranged to ensure that WHO can remain an independent, flexible regulatory body responsive to the health needs of the poorer countries, should it be mandated to play that role.

Second, there must be allowance for competition among private firms, which implies that several produce the same product. A regulatory decision to allocate the production of each drug to only one firm would remove the benefits of competition and prevent the lower prices and higher quality that competition would eventually entail.

Finally, despite the currently high prices of antivirals, developing countries should prepare now for the day when their prices will fall. We predict that, as a combined result of patent expiration, technical change, increased competition, and political pressure on pharmaceutical companies, prices for antivirals will fall rapidly—perhaps by a factor of 100 in the next three years. How much AZT should Uganda buy and how should it be distributed if a year's dose costs $700? How much if $70? How much if $7? Rather than responding to this price drop in an ad hoc manner, governments of developing countries should prepare now by developing guidelines for the purchase and equitable allocation of antivirals under every possible set of future prices.

Priorities

It is clear from the above that AIDS and STD programs have not prioritized enough, and also that rational prioritization is possible on the basis of available data and modeling exercises.

Priorities for Resource Allocation

As extensively pointed out above, STDs in general and HIV infection, chlamydial infection, and syphilis in particular are a considerable source of morbidity and mortality in many parts of the developing world, ranking them first among the top fifteen causes of disability-adjusted life-years lost in the most heavily affected urban populations. Even in low-prevalence urban populations, HIV infection and CSTDs rank eleventh among the causes of health lost, ahead of tuberculosis, adult pneumonia, and neonatal tetanus, for example. The growing urbanization and the increasing population share of young adults in most parts of the developing world can only make things worse.

Still, our analysis has shown that prevention of HIV infection, and to a lesser extent of some CSTDs, can result in considerable health gain, as compared with other common health problems in the developing world. In addition, sex education, use of condoms, and prompt treatment of STDs all contribute to reproductive health, which includes the ability to bear and raise healthy children.

It is truly remarkable that this high rank both in burden and potential health gain is not reflected in higher specific expenditure for the control of HIV infection and CSTDs. Neglected training, poor diagnostic and therapeutic capabilities, high rates of quasi-irreversible sequelae, and insufficient research and development efforts (at least for CSTDs) are all symptoms of this inadequate response. We can only guess why this situation has arisen.

Given the complex mosaic of areas of high and low prevalence, even within a single county, rational allocation of resources for care and prevention of HIV infection and CSTDs is even more difficult to plan in the developing world than in North America or Europe. This is also the case, however, for other health problems that are increasingly important in urban populations of the developing world, such as cardiovascular diseases. The continuing strong urbanization in all developing countries and the growing proportion of the population in the sexually active age range indicate that the global population potentially at risk for sexually acquired infections will continue to increase.

Priorities for the Control of STDs and HIV Infection

An argument for allocation away from other diseases and toward STD control must be based on the costs and the effects of relevant options. In this chapter we have made a strong case for the important health benefits both statically and dynamically of preventing STDs. Although we have not been able to assign costs to all the interventions that would produce these effects, alternatives for which we have quantified results in table 20-29 include three important preventive interventions and a variety of treatment options. The results reflect the sensitivity of alternative interventions to assumptions regarding targeting strategy, CSTD prevalence, the presence of an HIV epidemic, and clinic costs. Extreme assumptions are used to define the unfavorable and favorable cost-effectiveness scenarios.

An important conclusion that can be drawn from table 20-29 is that certain STD interventions are extraordinarily cost-effective under favorable assumptions. If the highly sexually active population is targeted, STD prevalence is high, and inexpensive strategies are used, blood screening, condom subsidies, and IEC interventions can save a DALY for less than $0.15. Using similar assumptions in the presence of an HIV epidemic, we find that STD treatment is also remarkably cost-effective. Even under unfavorable assumptions, however, some of the interventions, such as condom subsidies and STD treatment, remain cost-effective in relation to other adult health interventions or to the level of per capita GNP. But some interventions, such as the use of antivirals to treat persons with AIDS or blood screening of the general population in an environment of low STD prevalence, should be pursued only after other health investments are made.

TARGETING. A general finding made earlier in the chapter is that the cost-effectiveness of programs to prevent and control STDs can be extremely high when the program, whether preventive or curative, is tightly targeted. The cost per discounted disability-adjusted life-year saved can be as low as $0.15 for a blood-screening program and $0.56 for a CSTD treatment program, when such programs are aimed at a high-prevalence core group of transmitters. Blood screening or case management in the rural noncore or in a segment of the population in which

Table 20-29. Cost per Discounted Disability-Adjusted Life-Year Saved for Alternative STD Interventions

Intervention	Parameter	Unfavorable assumptions	Favorable assumptions
Prevention			
Condom subsidies and IEC	Cost	High	Low
	Target group	Noncore	Core
	Target disease	Chancroid and HIV	Syphilis and HIV
	Cost per DALY	$40.91	$0.13
Blood screening	Cost of test	Expensive	Inexpensive
	Target group	Noncore	Core
	Prevalence	< 0.1 percent	> 5 percent
	Cost per DALY	> $244	$0.15
Gonococcal ophthalmia neonatorum	Prevalence	< 0.1 percent	> 1 percent
	Cost per DALY	>$111	<$5.32
Treatment			
CSTDs	Hourly clinic cost	$10	$2
	Target group	Noncore	Core
	HIV epidemic	No	Yes
	Prevalence	< 1 percent	> 5 percent
	Cost per DALY	> $50	< $0.56
AIDS	Hourly clinic cost	$10	$2
	Treatment	Antivirals	Palliative and home care only
	DALYs gained	2	1
	Cost per DALY	$1,200	$75

Source: Authors' calculations.

there is no HIV epidemic, however, can be a much more expensive way to save DALYs. Blood screening can cost $300 or more per DALY saved, and treatment of chlamydia in the noncore when there is no HIV epidemic saves DALYs at a cost of $2,457 each. Hence, our main recommendation is that all national health programs should at a minimum include a few STD clinics and control programs targeted at urban core groups. Furthermore, in view of the fact that much of the benefit of these programs will accrue to individuals other than those directly contacted, the economic theory of externalities argues that these services to the core group should be highly subsidized.

The degree of extension of STD treatment and control beyond the core groups and the most cost-effective disease interventions should vary across countries according to their STD epidemiology and their access to resources to fund these programs. Assume that countries might seek to equate the cost-effectiveness of interventions on all diseases to approximately their level of per capita GNP. Then a country with a per capita GNP of $300 and a cost per clinic-hour of $10 would be guided to consider STD treatment of syphilis, gonorrhea, chlamydia, and AIDS opportunistic illnesses in the core groups. Blood-screening and safe-sex programs would also be conducted there. The only case management option which can save DALYs at less than $300 in the noncore group, however, is syphilis treatment, which would be robust even if the resource cost of the program per patient contact (the cost per clinic-hour) triples to $30 per hour.

In contrast, a middle-income country might have a GNP per capita of $4,000 and a cost per clinic-hour of $30. Such a country should implement all the programs described above. In addition, syphilis, chlamydia, and gonorrhea could be attacked in the noncore for less than $4,000 per DALY saved. Provided antiviral therapy can be obtained for as low as $2,000 per year, even AZT treatment of AIDS and HIV-infected people would be cost-effective in both the core and the noncore in such a country. Universal blood screening would be cost-effective provided the prevalence rate of infection is greater than one in 76,800 in the core or greater than one in 6,800 in the noncore.

Because our estimates of the cost-effectiveness of prevention programs are less solidly based than are our estimates of treatment costs, our recommendations regarding the allocation of resources between prevention and treatment programs are less certain. The qualitative conclusions arrived at earlier, however, point in the same direction as the more quantitative ones described above: targeted programs will typically be more cost-effective. Our estimates in table 20-24, summarized in the first row of table 20-29, suggest that focusing an IEC program on the core group will be from four to eight times more cost-effective in saving DALYs than if the program is targeted at the noncore. Of course, countries should include the costs of preventing or reducing any undesirable social and epidemiological side effects when they estimate the costs of targeted programs. Assuming such side effects can be avoided or reduced, we recommend that AIDS prevention programs first exhaust the possibilities for campaigns targeted at high-risk groups via an access group which provides both high coverage of the risk group and high concentration of the message as defined in table 20-23 and the accompanying discussion above. Only later and after thorough analysis should those campaigns be extended to noncore groups.

EMPLOYMENT OPPORTUNITIES FOR URBAN WOMEN. In view of the findings reported in earlier sections of the chapter, we are persuaded that STDs play a particularly noxious role in the lives of women in developing countries. Especially in countries with low female-to-male ratios in urban areas, STDs are both the cause and the consequence of the entrapment of women in a position of low socioeconomic status. We recommend that "women-in-development" (WID) programs join forces with STD control programs to break this vicious circle. More especially, in order to maximize this development effect in countries with small female-to-male ratios in urban areas, WID programs should request help from STD control programs in targeting job training and employment opportunity programs. Resources for WID programs targeted at women at high risk of STDs should come from both WID and STD programs, to serve both their goals.

INTEGRATION OF STD CONTROL INTO EXISTING STRUCTURE. The existing health care structure should be strengthened in its components for the diagnosis and treatment of CSTDs and AIDS and for health promotion. This requires manpower training; availability of diagnosis, drugs, and educational materials; and programmatic coordination and supervision. Improving the access of women to health services is particularly important for STD control. In areas of high or medium prevalence, STD and HIV services should be integrated into primary health care, mother and child health services, antenatal and, especially, family planning clinics.

Because of fundamentally identical strategies, STD and AIDS control programs should be developed in close coordination. National medium-term plans with clear and achievable objectives should also be formulated for STD control.

PATIENT CARE AND SUPPORT. More emphasis should be given to support activities as part of AIDS control programs. Such activities include not only etiologic and palliative therapy but also psychological and social support of the patient and his or her family. Where resources are scarce, such support should be targeted to the families of high-risk individuals so that the support efforts have the side benefit of minimizing subsequent infection. Secondary prevention of STD complications through early diagnosis and treatment remains a cornerstone in the control of bacterial STDs.

Research and Development

While writing this document, we became aware that many essential data on CSTDs and HIV infection are lacking and that both operational and basic research on STDs continue to be neglected. This is undoubtedly a handicap for control and prevention programs.

TECHNICAL RESEARCH AND DEVELOPMENT. Simple, rapid, and inexpensive diagnostic methods are a prerequisite for the successful implementation of both individual case management and screening and case detection programs for treatable STDs. Such tests are not available, however, particularly for the detection of genital infections in women. Priority diseases include gonorrhea, chlamydial infection, congenital syphilis, and chancroid. In addition, further development of simple serological tests for HIV antibody is necessary, ideally leading to a cheap way of confirmatory testing.

The necessary technology is available, and important developments are anticipated in the near future. Special consideration should be given to make these tests affordable for developing countries and to make them available through the health care system.

Priority should be given to prevention technologies that are fully controllable by women, such as mechanical and chemical barriers. Products not traditionally used as contraceptives should be screened for both bactericidal and virucidal activity against HIV and the full range of STD agents. Innocuous and acceptable vehicles for these products should be developed and evaluated. The possibility of the production of reusable condoms should be investigated.

The availability of vaccines against CSTDs and HIV infection would obviously revolutionize the control of these diseases. For infections such as gonorrhea and genital chlamydial infection in women, even a vaccine which would not completely prevent infection but would prevent the development of complications and sequelae may be acceptable. Insufficient knowledge of the immunobiology of many STDs, complex mechanisms by microorganisms to escape the immune response in humans, and poor commercial interest (at least for the CSTDs) have all been significant obstacles to vaccine development. Guidelines and methods should be developed for phase III vaccine trials (which evaluate protective efficacy).

EPIDEMIOLOGICAL AND BEHAVIORAL RESEARCH. Epidemiological research priorities include the collection of baseline data on STDs and their complications; the development of methods for disease surveillance; further investigations on the natural history and risk factors for STDs; the effect of HIV infection on the natural history and response to treatment of other diseases; the dynamics of core groups; and factors determining diverse epidemiologic patterns. The relative and population-attributable risks for transmission of HIV should be better quantified.

Behavioral sciences have been particularly neglected in STD research, though their importance in the prevention of AIDS and in the assessment of its effect is increasingly recognized. Data on sexual, health, and substance use behaviors, with emphasis on risk behaviors, should be collected in various societies and groups to lead to a rational strategy of prevention and control. The study of societal patterns as determinants of STDs and of the social effect of STDs should be helpful to define the limitations of interventions directed only at the level of individuals' risk behaviors.

INTERVENTIONS. There is an urgent need to develop and evaluate innovative behavioral and medical interventions against HIV infection and CSTD in different societies. Such development and evaluation would include trials and feasibility studies, demonstration projects, and community-wide interventions. This research is relevant for both primary and secondary prevention. Examples of such research include the effect and sustainability of campaigns for safe sex and condom use in various groups (adolescents, prostitutes, and so on); screening of pregnant women for syphilis to prevent congenital syphilis; eye prophylaxis at birth by traditional birth attenders to prevent gonococcal ophthalmia neonatorum; evaluation of syndrome-oriented algorithms for STDs to prevent complications; evaluation of various mechanical and chemical barrier methods for the prevention of HIV infection; use of rapid tests for the screening of blood donations; evaluation of the effectiveness and cost benefit of partner notification; and different methods of counseling. The identification of appropriate target populations for interventions has traditionally been a problem and deserves more research. More attention should be given to the development and evaluation of methods for the evaluation of interventions, with emphasis on simple indicators usable in developing countries.

HEALTH SERVICES RESEARCH AND IEC. Service delivery plays an important role in CSTD and AIDS control. Yet both the costs and the effects of alternative STD prevention and case management are almost completely unknown. Crucial questions are how, whether, and at what cost STD control can be integrated into existing health systems, including primary health care structures, family planning services, mother and child programs, and drug abuse programs. This issue involves not only case detection and management, but also some of the weakest components of the health care system, such as information, counseling, and education. Possibilities of involvement of the community, for instance, through home care, should be explored and evaluated.

CASE MANAGEMENT. Because of the increasing number of patients with AIDS and AIDS-related complex, there is an urgent need to develop simple and inexpensive strategies of case management for adults and children, making use of essential drugs, home remedies, and community members. Effective antiviral therapy will probably become widely available in the near future, but it is not clear how this will affect case management in developing countries. Individual countries should commission studies to determine the recommended treatment protocols for AIDS under today's set of prices. These studies should also recommend criteria for the government to use in determining at what price it will begin to buy and allocate antiviral drugs. Clinical trials of high priority include the effectiveness of syndrome-oriented algorithms for the management of STDs; innovative treatments of resistant gonorrhea and of acute PID to reduce postinfectious infertility; and evaluation of the validity of simple tests for the diagnosis of HIV, gonorrhea, chlamydial infection, genital ulcer disease, and PID.

ECONOMIC EFFECT ON HOUSEHOLDS. Information on the magnitude of the effect on the surviving household members of fatal illness from AIDS and other causes would serve three important purposes. First and most immediately, such information could guide the design of carefully targeted programs to assist temporarily certain surviving household members after an AIDS death. Although government-financed life-insurance policies will clearly be beyond the financial reach of the most severely affected African countries for some time, many African countries are currently considering the implementation of poverty alleviation programs. To the extent that research could discover indicators which predict which surviving households were most likely to be plunged into poverty by the AIDS death, poverty alleviation programs would be able to add these households to their beneficiaries, thereby mitigating some of the worst effects of the AIDS epidemic.

Second, information on the relative effects of STDs and other diseases would guide policy choices on the allocation of resources among alternative disease programs. By an extension of the logic of this collection, a disease is important not only for its effect on the infected individual, but also for its effect on other household members. If it is determined, for example, that an adult with an STD has a more negative effect on the health of other family members than an adult sick with other diseases, then this would strengthen the argument for reallocating resources to STDs.

Third, and finally, information on the magnitude of the economic effects of STDs on households would move the allocation of resources away from other sectors and toward the health sector.

Appendix 20A. The Medical Consequences of Sexually Transmitted Diseases

First we describe the medical consequences of each sexually transmitted disease discussed in the text, and then we summarize this information in quantitative form. We end the appendix with the presentation of estimated discounted disability-adjusted life-years lost from a single typical case of each STD and a comparison of these figures with those for other important diseases. As explained in the text, these figures can be interpreted as the benefit of averting a case of each disease: for example, of the disability-adjusted life-years saved per case prevented or cured.

Gonorrhea

Gonorrhea is caused by *Neisseria gonorrhoeae*, a fastidious gram-negative diplococcus, which displays antigenic variation. Strain type specific, temporary protective immunity has been documented. In general, however, protective immunity does not appear significantly to affect the spread of gonococcal infection, probably because of a multitude of antigenic types and because most infections may not induce protective antibody when they are limited to the genital mucosa. The risk of acquiring *N. gonorrhoeae* during heterosexual vaginal intercourse is 30 to 40 percent for the uninfected male partner and 50 to 80 percent for the uninfected female partner (Hooper and others 1978).

Gonorrhea is the main cause of urethritis among male clinic attenders in the developing world (Meheus and others 1980; Antal 1987). Urethral stricture is the most severe complication of gonococcal urethritis in males and may make up the majority of cases seen by urologists in some parts of Africa (Bewes 1973). Still, it is in women that gonococcal infection leads most often to severe complications and sequelae.

Women with gonorrhea mostly have genital manifestations, although these may be nonspecific (McCormack and others 1977). If untreated, between 5 and 10 percent of women with gonococcal infection develop salpingitis—a potentially life-threatening condition if peritonitis develops. The risk of involuntary infertility is about 15 percent after one episode of salpingitis, 30 percent after two episodes, and over 50 percent after three or more episodes (Weström 1980).

The proportion of women who are infertile because of *N. gonorrhoeae* has not been defined, but in Uganda there was an inverse correlation between the fertility rate and the incidence of gonorrhea by district (Arya, Taber, and Nsanze 1980). In addition, the risk of ectopic pregnancy—one of the leading causes of maternal death—is increased tenfold after one episode of PID (Weström 1980).

N. gonorrhoeae is also an important cause of morbidity in mother and neonate. Maternal gonococcal infection is a risk factor for premature delivery, and it may be a cause of chorioamnionitis. Furthermore, it is a significant cause of postpartum endometritis and salpingitis, a complication that occurred in up to 20 percent of all parturient women in studies in eastern Africa (Plummer, Laga, and others 1987; Temmerman and others 1988). The risk of transmission of *N. gonorrhoeae* from an infected mother to her infant's eyes is 30 to 40 percent if ophthalmic prophylaxis at birth is not used (Galega, Heyman, and Nash 1984; Laga and others 1986a and 1986b). Depending on the prevalence of gonococcal infection in pregnant women, the incidence of gonococcal ophthalmia neonatorum is up to 3.5 percent of all live births in some African populations (Laga, Meheus, and Piot 1989). Gonococcal ophthalmia is associated with keratitis in 10 to 20 percent of cases (Fransen and others 1986), and an unknown but probably small proportion of cases will become blind. *N. gonorrhoeae* is also an important cause of keratoconjunctivitis in adults in the tropics (Kesteleyn, Bogaert, and Meheus 1987).

Genital Infection with Chlamydia trachomatis

Chlamydia trachomatis is an intracellular parasitic bacterium with a complex replication cycle that takes forty-eight to seventy-two hours. It is susceptible to several groups of antimicrobial agents, including the tetracyclines and macrolides. Fourteen serotypes have been described. Of these serotypes L1, L2, and L3, which have distinct biologic features, cause lymphogranuloma venereum, a fairly uncommon cause of inguinal and femoral lymphadenitis in the tropics. Three serotypes (A, B, C) are mainly, but not exclusively, associated with trachoma, a potentially blinding eye disease endemic in many developing countries. The remaining types cause basically the same clinical syndromes as *N. gonorrhoeae* (table 20-1). Generally, genital chlamydial infections and their complications, such as PID, are associated with milder, and even subclinical, disease—although their complications and sequelae may be equally severe. This implies that many infections go unnoticed or do not come to medical attention.

The risk of heterosexual transmission of *C. trachomatis* is probably somewhat lower than for *N. gonorrhoeae*, but the risk of developing PID for women with cervical chlamydial infection is also of the order of 5 to 10 percent (Weström 1980). The agent has been identified in 15 to 20 percent of women with acute salpingitis in Africa, and there is strong serological evidence of a role played by *C. trachomatis* in ectopic pregnancy and infertility, particularly in women with evidence of tubal disease (Meheus, Remeis, and Collet 1986; Plummer and others 1987; De Muylder and others 1990).

C. trachomatis is the main identifiable cause of ophthalmia neonatorum in Africa (Maybey and Whittle 1982; Meheus and others 1982; Laga and others 1986a and 1986b; Buisman and others 1988). It is also a cause of neonatal pneumonia, but it is unknown what proportion of cases in the developing world is due to *C. trachomatis*. The negative effect of *C. trachomatis* on pregnancy outcome is controversial, though it seems plausible that the agent is a significant cause of postpartum endometritis in the tropics (Gravett and others 1986; Plummer and others 1987; Temmerman and others 1989).

There is as yet no evidence for protective immunity in genital chlamydial infections. In two studies in Africa, genital chlamydial infection was found to be a risk factor for the acquisition of HIV in female prostitutes (Plummer and others 1991; Laga and others 1989).

Syphilis

Syphilis is caused by a fastidious, slowly replicating spirochete, *Treponema pallidum*, which is still not cultivable in vitro. *T. pallidum* is highly sensitive to penicillin, and no in vitro resistance to this antibiotic has as yet been reported. The risk of acquiring syphilis through heterosexual intercourse is thought to be less than 30 percent, but receptive anal intercourse significantly increases this risk (Sparling 1990).

The disease is characterized by distinct clinical phases and a long latency period between the initial manifestations (primary chancre and secondary syphilis) and the severe systemic complications of tertiary syphilis, including neurosyphilis and cardiovascular syphilis, which occur five to twenty years after infection. Primary syphilis in 20 to 40 percent of those who did not have therapy progressed to symptomatic tertiary

syphilis in two cohort studies in Norway and the United States (Sparling 1990). The case-fatality rate in these studies was approximately 20 percent. Pregnant women with untreated syphilis of under two years' duration transmit the infection to their fetus in almost all cases. The proportion of affected fetuses decreases in women who have had syphilis longer than two years. Approximately 50 percent of the pregnancies in mothers with primary or secondary syphilis result in abortion, stillbirth, perinatal death, or premature delivery. Clinical manifestations usually appear between two and eight weeks in infected neonates and resemble those of secondary and tertiary syphilis (Hira and Hira 1987). Irreversible sequelae and death due to syphilis occur in 50 to 75 percent of the infants.

Genital Ulcer Disease

Genital ulcer disease has a diverse etiology, including primary syphilis, chancroid, genital herpes, donovanosis, and lymphogranuloma venereum (Piot and Meheus 1986). It is relatively more common in many parts of the developing world than in Europe or North America. There is growing evidence that genital ulcers increase both the susceptibility to HIV during sexual intercourse with an HIV-infected partner and the infectiousness of an HIV-infected person for uninfected partners (WHO 1989a; Piot and others 1988). Only chancroid will be discussed here, because it is the most common cause of GUD in the tropics. Chancroid is caused by *Haemophilus ducreyi*, a small gram-negative rod with fastidious growth requirements. There is geographic variation in antigenic properties, and protective immunity has not been reported. *H. ducreyi* strains show increasing resistance to antimicrobial agents.

The hallmark of chancroid is multiple, painful, purulent genital ulcers, accompanied in more than half of the cases by a painful inguinal lymphadenopathy. The incubation period is short, three to ten days. Unlike syphilis, chancroid yields no long-term or systemic complications. Without effective therapy, lesions last for an average of two months.

In Sub-Saharan African and Southeast Asia, *H. ducreyi* can be isolated from 20 to 60 percent of patients with genital ulcerations. In most countries, patients with GUD belong to low socioeconomic strata. Chancroid seems to be associated with prostitutes in several parts of the world, including North America, and is more common in uncircumcised men.

AIDS and HIV Infection

Human immunodeficiency virus is a retrovirus that preferentially infects CD4 bearing cells, including T lymphocytes and macrophages. Though other cell types may also become infected, there are at least two types of HIV, named HIV-1 and HIV-2, which share some antigenic properties (mainly at the level of core proteins) but which are clearly distinct in their genome. In addition, individual HIV isolates exhibit significant genetic variability (Clavel 1988). Once infected, an individual remains infected (and infectious) throughout his or her life.

At six to sixteen weeks after infection, approximately one-third of those infected develop a benign acute viral syndrome which resolves spontaneously after a few weeks. Subsequently, infected individuals go through an asymptomatic latent phase which may last for ten years or longer, after which they develop AIDS and AIDS-related complex (ARC). By definition, AIDS is characterized by the occurrence of life-threatening opportunistic infections and tumors, whereas ARC may be considered as a non-life-threatening symptomatic HIV disease. Approximately one-third of the patients suffer from subacute encephalopathy, characterized by progressive behavioral changes associated with dementia (the AIDS dementia complex). The case-fatality rate of AIDS is virtually 100 percent, with an average time of two to three years between diagnosis and death. Because of inadequate means of diagnosis and treatment, this period is probably much shorter in developing countries.

In the United States, individuals with HIV infection progress to AIDS at an average rate of 3 to 6 percent per year, and the median time from infection to progression to AIDS has been estimated at seven to ten years (Moss and Bacchetti 1989). There is evidence that the rate of progression to AIDS is related directly to age, at least among hemophiliacs residing in North America (Goedert and others 1989). In addition, HIV-seropositive persons who have not progressed to AIDS show steadily increasing impairment, with two-thirds of the subjects having some clinical problem after three years of infection. It appears that in the absence of treatment, most, if not all, infected persons will progress to AIDS. Epidemiologists hypothesize that the rate of progression to AIDS is faster in a developing country because of greater stress on the immune system due to frequent exposure to infectious diseases, but no data to test this hypothesis are yet available.

Table 20A-1. *Outcome Probabilities for* STD *and Other Major Diseases*

| Disease | Prevalence[a] | Sex | Case-fatality rates, by age (per 1,000) | | | | | | Probability of permanent disablement |
			0–1	1–4	5–14	15–49	50–64	65+	
Sexually transmitted disease									
Chancroid	High	Both	...	...	...	...	...	...	0.5
	Low	Both	...	...	...	...	...	...	0.5
Chlamydia	High	Female	0.05	...	...	1	...	...	5
	High	Male	0.05	...	...	0.05	...	...	5
	Low	Female	...	...	...	...	...	...	5
	Low	Male	...	...	...	...	...	...	5
Gonorrhea	High	Female	...	...	0.1	0.2	...	...	5
	High	Male	...	...	...	...	...	...	5
	Low	Female	...	...	0.1	0.2	...	...	5
	Low	Male	...	...	...	...	...	...	5
HIV	High	Both	100	100	100	100	100	100	n.a.
	Low	Both	100	100	100	100	100	100	n.a.
Syphilis	High	Female	60	...	...	1	...	...	1.5
	High	Male	60	...	...	1	...	...	1.5
	Low	Female	25	...	...	0.35	...	...	1.5
	Low	Male	25	...	...	0.35	...	...	1.5
Other diseases									
Birth injury	n.a.	Both	67	...	...	...	...	...	33
Cerebrovascular disease	n.a.	Both	...	...	...	35	35	35	35
Cirrhosis	n.a.	Both	80	80	80	80	80	80	20
Congenital malformations	n.a.	Both	15	15	15	15	15	15	85
Gastroenteritis	n.a.	Both	7	3	0.2	0.2	0.2	0.4	...
Injuries (i.e., accidents)	n.a.	Both	10	10	10	10	10	10	5
Malaria	n.a.	Both	14	6	1	1	1	1	86
Measles	n.a.	Both	18	17	1	...	...	...	...
Pneumonia, adult	n.a.	Both	n.a.	n.a.	n.a.	10	10	10	...
Pneumonia, child	n.a.	Both	40	40	40	n.a.	n.a.	n.a.	...
Prematurity	n.a.	Both	10.2	n.a.	n.a.	n.a.	n.a.	n.a.	...
Severe malnutrition	n.a.	Both	70	65	10	10	10	20	...
Sickle cell	n.a.	Both	80	...	...	...	...	...	20
Tetanus (neonatal)	n.a.	Both	80	n.a.	n.a.	n.a.	n.a.	n.a.	...
Tuberculosis	n.a.	Both	35	35	35	35	35	35	...

n.a. Not applicable.
... Negligible.
a. Urban areas of high or low prevalence, as defined by table 20-7.
Source: Authors; Ghana Health Assessment Project Team 1981.

Quantification of the STD Sequelae for Comparison

The method introduced in the main text of this chapter for quantifying the static burden of disease requires that the sequelae be described in terms that can be roughly compared across diseases. For simplicity the method divides the possible outcomes of contracting a case of each disease into three classes: death, permanent disablement, and recovery. In table 20A-1 we summarize the assumptions made regarding the probability of each of these outcomes for each of the diseases included in the analysis. (Note that, for simplicity, only the case-fatality rate is assumed to vary across age groups.) In table 20A-2 we summarize our assumptions regarding the duration and degree of disablement due to the sequelae of the STDs and the other main diseases.

Finally, in table 20A-3 we present estimated disability-adjusted life-years lost per case, or saved per case averted,

for each of these diseases, ranked in order of the discounted disability-adjusted life-years saved. We assumed that individuals would have otherwise lived to the age of sixty-five years, and we applied a discount rate of 3 percent to all future years. The second column of the table presents the results of first weighing each lost year by a productivity weight before discounting and adding the years to arrive at the discounted productivity-weighted disability-adjusted life-years saved per case averted. As in Barnum 1987; Over and others 1988; and Over, Bertozzi, and Chin 1989, productivity weights are attached to future disability-adjusted life-years before they are discounted to the time the disease is contracted. Age ranges and the weights attached to the years that would have been lived at those ages are: ages 0–1, 0; ages 1–5, 0; ages 5–15, 0.2; ages 15–50, 1.0; ages 50–65, 0.85; age 65+, 0.25. These weights roughly follow the age profile of hourly wages in a developing country (for exam-

Table 20A-2. Death and Disablement from Sequelae of STDs and Other Major Diseases

Disease	Prevalence[a]	Sex	Years until death	Disablement until death[b]	Chronic disablement[b]	Disablement until recovery[b]	Days until recovery
Sexually transmitted disease							
Chancroid	High	Both	n.a.	n.a.	20	20	73
	Low	Both	n.a.	n.a.	20	20	73
Chlamydia	High	Female	1	30	30	20	292
	High	Male	5	10	50	10	91
	Low	Female	1	30	30	20	292
	Low	Male	5	10	50	10	91
Gonorrhea	High	Female	1	50	50	20	146
	High	Male	n.a.	n.a.	50	10	55
	Low	Female	1	50	50	20	146
	Low	Male	n.a.	n.a.	50	10	55
HIV	High	Both	8	18	n.a.	n.a.	n.a.
	Low	Both	8	18	n.a.	n.a.	n.a.
Syphilis	High	Female	20	50	50	0	730
	High	Male	20	50	50	0	730
	Low	Female	20	50	50	0	730
	Low	Male	20	50	50	0	730
Other diseases							
Birth injury	n.a.	Both	0	...	20	...	...
Cerebrovascular disease	n.a.	Both	0	...	75	...	120
Cirrhosis	n.a.	Both	5	50	25	...	...
Congenital malformations	n.a.	Both	0	...	25	...	...
Gastroenteritis	n.a.	Both	0	...	n.a.	...	14
Injuries (i.e., accidents)	n.a.	Both	0	...	25	...	30
Malaria	n.a.	Both	0	...	2	...	...
Measles	n.a.	Both	0	...	...	...	21
Pneumonia, adult	n.a.	Both	0	...	...	...	30
Pneumonia, child	n.a.	Both	0	...	...	...	30
Prematurity	n.a.	Both	0	...	...	...	...
Severe malnutrition	n.a.	Both	0	...	...	...	180
Sickle cell	n.a.	Both	5	50	30	...	...
Tetanus (neonatal)	n.a.	Both	0	...	...	...	...
Tuberculosis	n.a.	Both	5	25	200	...	...

n.a. Not applicable.
... Not significant.
a. Urban areas of high or low prevalence, as defined in table 20-7.
b. Disablement expressed as a percentage of full health. A year at 100 percent disablement is weighted the same as a year lost to death.
Source: Authors; Ghana Health Assessment Project Team 1981.

Table 20A-3. Health Gains From Preventing One Case of STD or Other Diseases

Disease	Discounted disability-adjusted life-years saved		Discounted productive disability-adjusted life-years saved	
	Years	Rank	Years	Rank
Sickle cell	24.5	1	14.2	3
Tetanus (neonatal)	22.7	2	14.2	2
Birth injury	20.9	3	13.1	4
HIVa	19.5	4	15.5	1
Severe malnutrition	17.0	5	11.2	6
Cirrhosis	15.6	6	12.8	5
Pneumonia, child	11.2	7	8.1	7
Congenital malformations	10.3	8	6.4	9
Cerebrovascular disease	9.4	9	7.8	8
Tuberculosis	7.1	10	5.6	10
Measles	5.0	11	3.3	11
Syphilis,[a] female[b]	3.9	12	2.3	13
Syphilis,[a] male[c]	3.7	13	2.1	14
Malaria	3.7	14	2.4	12
Prematurity	2.9	15	1.8	16
Injuries (i.e., accidents)	2.7	16	2.1	15
Pneumonia, adult	2.0	17	1.6	17
Gastroenteritis	1.4	18	0.9	18
Chlamydia,[a] female[b]	1.3	19	0.9	19
Gonorrhea,[a] female[b]	1.0	20	0.7	20
Chlamydia,[a] male[c]	0.8	21	0.6	21
Gonorrhea,[a] male[c]	0.7	22	0.5	22
Chancroid[a]	0.2	23	0.1	23

a. Sexually transmitted disease.
b. Benefit of a program targeted at females, per case averted or prevented.
c. Benefit of a program targeted at males, per case averted or prevented.
Source: Ghana Health Assessment Project Team 1981 and authors' calculations.

ple, Lucas 1985). The results are discussed in the main part of the text.

Appendix 20B. A Simulation Model of an STD Epidemic

The basic model used here is drawn from Hethcote and Yorke 1984 (for example, their equation 3.1). It consists of two differential equations, one for the core group (group 1) and one for the noncore group (group 2). In a given group, the equation describes the net effect of two flows, one from the pool of susceptibles into the pool of infectives (the incidence of new infections) and one in the reverse direction as infectives are cured of their disease and again become susceptibles. Note that the model ignores the possibility that an individual's sexual behavior might change so that he or she moves from the core group to the noncore group, or vice versa. Such behavioral changes must be imposed on the model from the outside.

Let I_i represent the proportion of group i that is infected on a given day, where ($i = 1$) is the core group and ($i = 2$) is the noncore group. Suppose that the number of individuals in group i is N_i. Then the sizes of the pools of infectives and susceptibles on any day are, respectively, I_iN_i and $(1 - I_i)N_i$.

The basic differential equation for group i is an equation for the rate of change of I_iN_i, or, because N_i is constant, for

I_i. The equation can be written as the difference between the newly infected people and the newly cured people during the day, or

$$(1) \quad \frac{d I_i N_i}{d t} = \left[\begin{array}{c} Newly\ infected \\ group\ i \end{array} \right] - \left[\begin{array}{c} Newly\ cured \\ group\ i \end{array} \right].$$

The rate of new cures is simply given by the total number of infected people divided by the number of days each is infected or

$$(2) \quad \left[\begin{array}{c} Newly\ cured \\ group\ i \end{array} \right] = \frac{I_i N_i}{D},$$

where D is the average duration of infectivity in days.

The rate of new infection is more complex and requires assumptions about the following: a_i = the probability of a new sexual contact on a given day by a group i person; G = selectivity of partner choice; Q = probability of infection on a single contact. From these assumptions can be computed:[59]

the reproductive rate for group i:

$$R_i = Q \cdot D \cdot a_i,$$

the proportion of new partners in group i:

the "mixing" coefficients:[60]

$$b_i = \frac{N_i\, a_i}{N_1\, a_1 + N_2\, a_2},$$

$$M_{ij} = \begin{cases} (1 - G)\, b_i + G & \text{if } i = j \\ (1 - G)\, b_j & \text{if } i \neq j \end{cases}$$

Finally, a set of parameters, C_{ij}, are defined as follows as functions of those defined above:

$$(3) \qquad C_{ij} = M_{ij} \cdot \frac{R_i}{D} = M_{ij} \cdot Q \cdot a_i.$$

These parameters allow us to write the expression for the rate of new infections per day as:

$$(4) \quad \begin{bmatrix} Newly \\ infected \\ group\ i \end{bmatrix} = \Big[C_{ii}\, I_i + C_{ij}\, I_j \Big] \cdot (1 - I_i) \cdot N_i \quad \forall\ i \neq j$$

Thus the two equations of motion for our simulation model are:

$$(5) \qquad \frac{d\,I_1}{d_t} = \Big(C_{11}\, I_1 + C_{12}\, I_2 \Big) \cdot (1 - I_1) - \frac{I_1}{D};$$

$$(6) \qquad \frac{d\,I_2}{d_t} = \Big(C_{22}\, I_2 + C_{21}\, I_1 \Big) \cdot (1 - I_2) - \frac{I_2}{D}.$$

Sensitivity with Respect to Selectivity

One special case of the model is worth examining. Suppose that members of each group are so selective in their choice of partner that they always choose members of their own group, so that $G = 1.0$. Then by the definitions of M_{ij} and C_{ij}, the two equations of motion simplify to:

$$(7) \qquad \frac{d\,I_i}{d_t} = I_i \cdot (1 - I_i) \cdot \frac{R_i}{D} - \frac{I_i}{D}.$$

By setting this equation to zero we solve for the equilibrium value (denoted by an asterisk) of the prevalence rate I_i:

$$(8) \qquad I_i^* = \frac{(R_i - 1)}{R_i}.$$

When G is not equal to 100 percent, no analytical solution exists for the two simultaneous quadratic equations in the unknowns I_1^* and I_2^*. Lajmanovich and Yorke (1976), however, have proved that the numerical solution of the two

equations tends toward equilibrium values of the two prevalence rates under general conditions.

The simulations in the text constitute sensitivity analysis with respect to the disease parameters, because those vary substantially across the six simulated diseases. Also reported in the text and in table 20-15 is a sensitivity analysis of the main result on targeting with respect to two dimensions of sexual behavior, selectivity and rate of partner change. Because selectivity is a particularly interesting parameter of sexual activity, and because it could itself be the object of policy, we report here on sensitivity analysis of the main results with respect to the entire range of possible selectivity coefficients.

Consider the effects of increasing the selectivity coefficient above the value of zero assumed in the text. It is clear (and confirmed by the simulations) that there is a monotonic increasing relationship between the value of the selectivity coefficient and the speed with which the core group attains its equilibrium prevalence rate. Furthermore, the level of the core's equilibrium prevalence rate increases as G increases. By symmetry, one might expect that both the speed with which the noncore approaches equilibrium and the level of that equilibrium would decrease monotonically with increases in G. Only the second of these two expectations is confirmed.

It is shown in figure 20B-1 that, although the long-run equilibrium prevalence in the noncore is lower at G = 30 percent than at G = 0 percent, the equilibrium rate is approached more quickly. How could this be the case if the relatively uninfected noncore (starting at a prevalence rate of only 1 percent) is now selecting a smaller proportion of its

Figure 20B-1. Effect on Evolution of Epidemic in Noncore Group from Increasing Selectivity: Gonorrhea and Syphilis

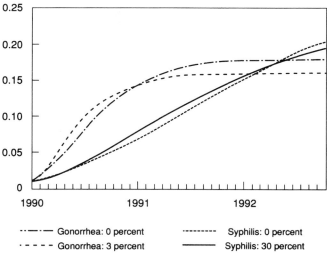

Proportion infected

·—·— Gonorrhea: 0 percent   -------- Syphilis: 0 percent
- - - - Gonorrhea: 3 percent   ——— Syphilis: 30 percent

Source: Authors.

Figure 20B-2. *Effect of Selectivity Coefficient on Present Value of Averted Case-Years in Noncore Group*

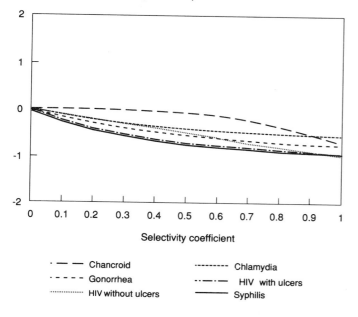

Discounted years of illness (thousands)

Selectivity coefficient

- — Chancroid
- - - Gonorrhea
········· HIV without ulcers
-------- Chlamydia
-··-··- HIV with ulcers
——— Syphilis

Source: Authors.

partners from the more heavily infected core (starting prevalence of 20 percent)?

The explanation is in the dynamic behavior of the seroprevalence rate in the core group. In the early stages of a gonorrhea or syphilis epidemic, a higher selectivity makes the prevalence rate of the core group increase much more rapidly. As a result, even though fewer persons in the noncore are contacting core individuals, this effect is more than offset by the fact that more of the core individuals are infected. Thus the prevalence rate of the noncore climbs faster than it would if G were 0 percent.

Figures 20B-2 and 20B-3 display the effect on the core and noncore, respectively, of alternative selectivity coefficients from 0 to 100 percent. Both figures display on the vertical axis the present value of the case-years of illness that would be averted in each group by changing the selectivity coefficient at the beginning of the epidemic from 0 percent to the level indicated on the horizontal axis. Note from figure 20B-2 that increasing G increases the burden on the core group for all diseases, the effect being greater at higher selectivity coefficients. Now examine figure 20B-3.

For small increases in selectivity, the burden of illness of four of the diseases is greater on the noncore than it would be with a zero selectivity. Because of the more rapid early increase in the epidemic demonstrated in figure 20B-1, the three-year burden on the noncore actually gets worse when selectivity is slightly increased above zero. Within this three-year horizon

the worst selectivity value for syphilis and HIV with ulcers is 20 percent. Selectivity must be increased to 40 percent before the three-year burden on the noncore of these two diseases would be reduced.

Interaction of STD and HIV Epidemics

The model presented in equations (1) through (6) above represents the dynamic of a single STD, in the absence of any risk factors other than sexual activity. As reviewed in the text, however, there is substantial evidence that infection with several of the CSTDs increases the transmission probability of HIV infection. When both diseases exist in a sexually active population, preventing or curing an STD will avert cases of HIV infection even in the absence of an intervention aimed directly at HIV. To estimate the magnitude of this effect requires that the HIV epidemic be simulated simultaneously with the epidemic of one of the CSTDs. In such a simulation, the probability that a contact between an HIV-infected person and an HIV-susceptible person will result in an infection will depend on the probability that one or both of these individuals is suffering from the STD on the day of the contact.

We assume that HIV infection has no effect on the simultaneous epidemic of a CSTD. Thus, simultaneous modeling of the two epidemics affects the value of Q in equation (3) and therefore the values of the C_{ij} in equations (4) through (6) for the HIV epidemic only. Let V_1 be the instantaneous prevalence rate of the STD in the core group and V_2 be the rate in the noncore group. Then, the probability of a new HIV infection

Figure 20B-3. *Effect of Selectivity Coefficient on Present Value of Averted Case-Years in Core Group*

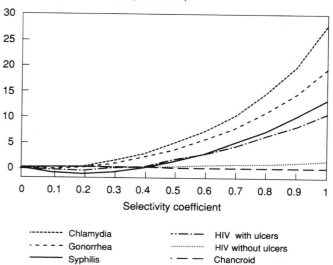

Discounted years of illness (thousands)

Selectivity coefficient

-------- Chlamydia
- - - Gonorrhea
——— Syphilis
-··-··- HIV with ulcers
········· HIV without ulcers
-··-··- Chancroid

Source: Authors.

on a given sexual contact, H_{ij}, varies over time with the STD prevalence rate according to:

$$(9) \qquad H_{ij} = (1 - V_i) \cdot (1 - V_j) \cdot h$$

$$+ \ (1 - V_i) \cdot V_j \cdot \alpha \cdot h$$

$$+ \ V_i \cdot (1 - V_j) \cdot \alpha \cdot h$$

$$+ \ V_i \cdot V_j \cdot \alpha^2 \cdot h,$$

where h is the probability of HIV infection without concomitant STD and α is the multiple by which h is increased when either of the two partners is infected. Note that we assume a multiple of ^{2} when both partners have the STD.

Using equation (9), the coefficients of the equations of motion for the HIV epidemic are modified to become:

$$(10) \qquad C_{ij} = M_{ij} \cdot H_{ij} \cdot a_i.$$

Substitution of equation (10) into equations (5) and (6) yields equations of motion for HIV infection which are sensitive to a simultaneous STD epidemic.

Reduced Transmission Probability

In the main part of the text, we presented simulation results for an intervention which consists of assuring that all sex contacts by 100 individuals in one of the two groups are protected for a year. To model this intervention, let U_1 be the proportion of individuals who are unprotected in the core group and U_2 be the proportion unprotected in the noncore. Then the modified versions of equations (5) and (6) above can be written:

$$(11) \quad \frac{d\,I_1}{d\,t} = \Big(C_{11}\,U_1\,I_1 + C_{12}\,U_2\,I_2 \Big) \cdot U_1 \cdot (1 - I_1) - \frac{I_1}{D};$$

$$(12) \quad \frac{d\,I_2}{d\,t} = \Big(C_{22}\,U_2\,I_2 + C_{21}\,U_1\,I_1 \Big) \cdot U_2 \cdot (1 - I_2) - \frac{I_2}{D}.$$

The base simulation is run with both U_1 and U_2 set to 1.0. To run the simulation of 100 protected individuals in the core, we set U_1 to 0.9 and maintain the value of U_2 at 1.0. To run the simulation of 100 protected individuals in the noncore, we return U_1 to 1.0 and set U_2 to 0.998. In both cases we use equations (11) and (12) to track the epidemic for one year and then continue the simulation for nine more years with both U parameters reset to 1.0.

We model each CSTD jointly with HIV infection by using equation (10) to modify the transmission probability of the simultaneous HIV epidemic. We assume that the protected individuals are simultaneously protected from both concomitant epidemics by introducing the U_1 and U_2 parameters in the same way in the equations for both epidemics. In addition, we

maintain the link between the CSTD epidemic and the HIV epidemic by maintaining the substitution of equation (10) for the C_{ij} parameters. The result is that an intervention which protects 100 individuals has three beneficial effects: (a) it directly prevents cases of the CSTD being modeled, (b) it directly prevents transmission of the concomitant HIV epidemic, and (c) it indirectly prevents HIV infection through the mechanism modeled in equations (9) and (10) above.

Appendix 20C. Management of Selected Classic Syndromes

Effective therapy is available for all bacterial CSTDs. The main issues are discussed below.[61]

Management of Gonorrhea and Chlamydial Infection

Isolation of the etiologic agent is the optimal method of diagnosis but is technically demanding and expensive. Though nonculture methods for the diagnosis of both genital infections are now available, they are as yet rarely used in the developing world. A decrease in their cost may increase their use and have a significant effect on the diagnostic capacity for STDs.

Oral tetracycline taken for seven to fourteen days is the treatment of choice for chlamydial infection and has a cure rate of 85 to 90 percent. Oral erythromycin at the appropriate dosage should be given to pregnant women and infants and children.

In those areas in which gonococci are still susceptible to penicillin, procaine penicillin as a single intramuscular injection together with oral probenecid has a cure rate of 90 to 95 percent, as has oral amoxicillin. In most areas in Sub-Saharan Africa and in Southeast Asia, however, more than 50 percent of gonococcal strains are highly resistant to penicillin, as well as to the tetracyclines in 20 to 30 percent of cases. Single-dose intramuscular injections with third-generation cephalosporins, such as ceftriaxone sodium or cefotaxime sodium, or oral therapy with the new quinolones, such as norfloxacin and ciprofloxacin, have virtually a 100 percent cure rate. Spectinomycin cures 95 percent of cases of gonorrhea, including those caused by penicillin-resistant strains. These are presently the recommended drugs for treatment of gonorrhea, but less-effective alternatives (cure rate below 95 percent, depending on the antimicrobial susceptibility of local strains) are being used because they are less expensive, including thiamphenicol, sulfamethoxazole trimethoprim, and kanamycin (WHO 1989b).

Urethritis in Men

Because basically only two etiological entities have to be considered for urethral discharge in men, a simplified method of management has been used widely. In figure 20C-1 we present such an algorithm and include figures on its effectiveness (WHO 1991). The selection of the antibiotic should ideally be based on the sensitivity of local strains of *N. gonorrhoeae*,

Figure 20C-1. Algorithm: Urethral Discharge (in the Absence of Laboratory Support)

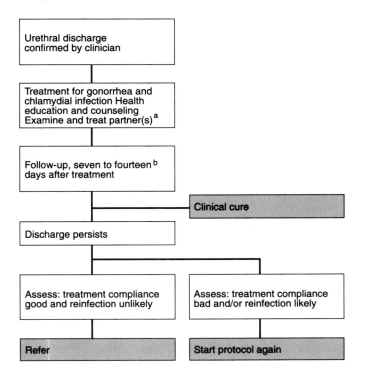

a. Notification and treatment of female partners of men with urethritis are of the highest priority as one of the best ways of identifying women at high risk of having asymptomatic gonococcal and chlamydial infections.
b. Patient may be advised to return only if symptoms persist.
Source: WHO 1991b.

besides such other considerations as cost, availability, and mode of administration. In addition, the relative frequency of gonococcal and nongonococcal urethritis in the patient population should be taken into account. Microscopy of a Gram's stained smear of the discharge represents the minimal standard of laboratory examination.

Vaginal Discharge

Because the etiology, and consequently the therapy, of cervico-vaginal discharge is complex, clinical algorithms have not been successful for the management of this syndrome. The primary objective of case management of this problem should be the diagnosis and treatment of gonococcal and chlamydial cervical infection and the identification of women with an associated PID. Though a simple "swab test" had an acceptable sensitivity and specificity for the diagnosis of mucopurulent cervicitis—mainly caused by *C. trachomatis* and *N. gonorrhoeae*—in one study in Seattle, Washington, its validity was limited in field studies in Africa with a sensitivity and specificity for chlamydial and gonococcal infection combined of less than 50 percent, respectively (Brunham and others 1984; Braddick and others 1990).

A simplified clinical algorithm using a clinical examination with visualization of cervix but no microscopy is shown in figure 20C-2. Several other algorithms have been proposed, but evaluations of them have not been published and their effectiveness is unknown (WHO 1991b).

Pelvic Inflammatory Disease

The objectives of PID management are twofold: cure of PID and prevention of tubal infertility and ectopic pregnancy. Pelvic inflammatory disease has a polymicrobial etiology and its clinical expression includes a variety of fairly non-

Figure 20C-2. Algorithm: Vaginal Discharge (Speculum Examination Possible, but no Laboratory Support)

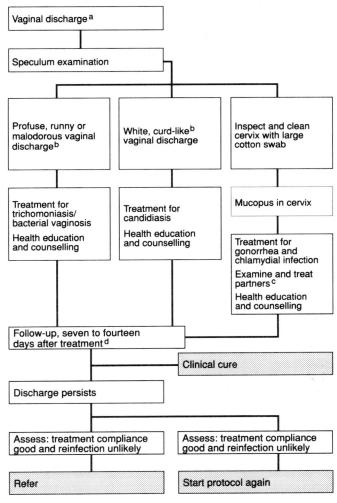

a. If vaginal discharge is accompanied by lower abdominal pain or pain on moving the cervix, use the appropriate "lower abdominal pain" algorithm.
b. In addition, the pH paper test can be used: if pH lower than 4.5, treat for candidiasis; if pH higher than 4.5, treat for trichomoniasis/bacterial vaginosis.
c. In the absence of a confirmed diagnosis, the decision to notify partner(s) should take into account local cultural and epidemiological factors.
d. Patient may be advised to return only if symptomatic.
Source: WHO 1991b.

specific signs and symptoms, such as lower abdominal pain and tenderness, malaise, fever, and adnexal tenderness. When validated by laparoscopy, the sensitivity and specificity of a clinical diagnosis of PID, particularly cases caused by *C. trachomatis*, are found to be in the range of 65 to 85 percent (Jacobson and Weström 1969; De Muylder 1986). Valid diagnostic criteria for postpartum endometritis and PID remain to be developed. Because of the serious outcome, sequelae, and mortality, early recognition and treatment are essential, and sensitive criteria for diagnosis should be set even if overtreatment is the result.

Treatment should be directed against infection with *N. gonorrhoeae*, *C. trachomatis*, and anaerobes and may consist of a regimen of spectinomycin single-dose plus tetracycline and metronidazole taken for two weeks. Cheaper regimens, such as thiamphenicol, have also been used (De Muylder 1986). The cure rate with these regimens is not precisely known, but it is presently estimated that 15 percent of women with acute PID fail to respond to initial antimicrobial treatment and 20 percent have at least one recurrence (Brunham 1984). The effect of antimicrobial therapy on long-term tubal function is unclear, but several studies have shown that women treated within two days of the onset of symptoms have a lower incidence of tubal occlusion than do women treated later in the disease (Weström and others 1979).

Hospitalization is required in a substantial but ill-defined proportion of women with PID in developing countries. Up to 25 percent of PID patients were hospitalized in Zimbabwe in 1986 (X. De Muylder, personal communication 1989). Peritonitis, a pelvic mass, and a tubo ovarian abscess are the main reasons for hospitalization and require intravenous therapy and often surgery as well.

Neonatal Infection with N. gonorrhoeae and C. trachomatis

The objectives of the management of ophthalmia neonatorum are the identification of cases of gonococcal infection; the clinical cure of conjunctivitis; the prevention of visual impairment and blindness (a complication of infection with *N. gonorrhoeae* and, to a lesser extent, *C. trachomatis*); and the treatment of STDs in the parent. The proportion of cases of neonatal conjunctivitis caused by *N. gonorrhoeae* depends mainly on the use of effective eye prophylaxis at birth. Treatment for both gonococcal and chlamydial (nongonococcal) ophthalmia should include a systemic antibiotic, because extraocular infection and disease (pneumonia) are common.

The accuracy of a stained conjunctival smear is high for the differentiation between gonococcal and nongonococcal ophthalmia (Fransen and others 1986), and this method should be used for every case of purulent conjunctivitis in the first week of life, because these have a high probability of being gonococcal. Single-dose ceftriaxone administered intramuscularly ($5 for 125 milligrams) has a 100 percent cure rate for gonococcal conjunctivitis but is not available everywhere (Laga and others 1986a and 1986b). Other recommended treatment regimens for this indication in areas with penicillin-resistant strains

include tetracycline ointment for ten days plus kanamycin or cefotaxime as a single injection, the cure rates of which are 90 to 95 percent (Fransen and others 1984; WHO 1985a and 1985b). A regimen of tetracycline ointment plus erythromycin syrup for ten days is the recommended treatment of nongonococcal ophthalmia neonatorum, but in practice only topical therapy is given. As for other respiratory infections, the diagnosis of chlamydial infant pneumonia is extremely complex and is possible only in sophisticated medical centers.

Infertility and Ectopic Pregnancy

Tubal infertility is an irreversible sequela of PID and may be repaired with microsurgery at a low (<10 percent) rate of success. In vitro fertilization (rate of success 10 to 20 percent) is also used to achieve pregnancy. Both techniques are expensive and rarely available in developing countries. Hospitalization with surgery, often with removal of the tuba, is virtually always required for ectopic pregnancy.

Genital Ulcer Disease

Though the etiology of genital ulcer disease is diverse, clinical algorithms for management have been used with success in

Figure 20C-3. Algorithm: Genital Ulcer (without Laboratory Support)

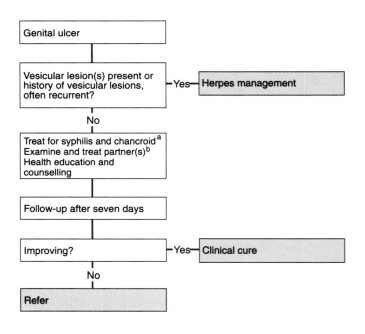

a. Combined treatment for both syphilis and chancroid is recommended, except in areas where chancroid is very uncommon. Where granuloma inguinale occurs, treatment for this condition should also be considered.
b. In the absence of a confirmed diagnosis, the decision to notify partner(s) should take into account local cultural and epidemiological factors.
Source: WHO 1991b.

several settings. The basic objectives of these algorithms are cure of chancroid, the most common cause of GUD; and treatment of syphilis, the most severe cause with respect to systemic complications and sequelae. Though genital herpes is a common cause of GUD throughout the world, specific therapy is not considered in these algorithms because the high cost of antiviral treatment with acyclovir makes it rarely available. Early diagnosis and treatment of GUD has become critical in populations with HIV infection, because genital ulcers have been shown to increase the rate of transmission of HIV (WHO 1989a).

A management algorithm for GUD is shown in figure 20C-3 and includes probabilities for the different outcomes. The simultaneous presence of HIV infection, however, may significantly decrease the cure rate of both chancroid and primary syphilis when the recommended single-dose treatment regimens are used (Lukehart and others 1988; Cameron and others 1989).

Syphilis

Whereas the treatment of the various stages of syphilis is fairly simple and well standardized and has cure rates approaching 100 percent for primary, secondary, and latent syphilis, its diagnosis is more problematic, requiring the use of laboratory tests. Nevertheless, assays such as the rapid plasma reagin tests are inexpensive (+ $0.40 per test) and easy to perform, and they should be available as a minimum laboratory support for the management of STD and the screening of pregnant women. Their sensitivity for infectious syphilis beyond the primary stage (where the algorithm for genital ulcer disease can be applied in most instances) is virtually 100 percent.

Treatment of syphilis of less than two years' duration and of neonates born to mothers with a positive serological test for syphilis consists of one or two injections of benzathine penicillin G. Therapy of neurosyphilis and cardiovascular syphilis consists of a course of penicillin, in addition to palliative measures often requiring hospitalization.

Cost-Effective Treatment Strategies

In order to devise recommendations for a cost-effective approach to controlling STDs, it is necessary to estimate the approximate average cost and the approximate effectiveness of treating a case of each STD (Washington, Browner, and Korenbrot 1987). In a developing country, where diagnostic materials are difficult to obtain and the diagnostic test may cost five to fifty times the cost of the drug treatment, part of the choice of treatment is the decision whether or not to condition treatment on a positive test for the disease. Here we consider two alternatives. The first alternative is simply to treat everyone in a given population regardless of whether they have symptoms and without attempting to diagnose the disease. The second alternative is to screen the population and then treat only those who test positive. For some diseases, the option of screening only by clinical examination is compared with the option of using microscopy or of using a culture.

In table 20C-1 we present basic comparative cost data on the various diseases. In the costs for treating a given disease we include the drug cost per treatment episode and the number of minutes of clinic time per treatment episode. For the classic STDs, the latter cost typically is the duration of a single encounter between patient and medical practice. For AIDS and HIV infection, however, the number of minutes is an estimate of the total number of minutes in all encounters with a medical practice in a period of twelve months. In the last three columns, we give three different estimates of the cost per treatment for each of the classic STDs. If we denote the drug cost by Rx, the number of minutes by T, and the proportion of cures that are effective by E, the figures in these columns can be calculated from the relationship:

$$(13) \qquad C_i = \frac{Rx + \left(\dfrac{T}{60}\right) \cdot H_i}{E},$$

where H_i is the assumed cost per hour of clinic time, which varies from $2 to $10 to $30 across the three columns.

Table 20C-1. Average Cost per Treatment of Case of STD by Disease and Cost per Clinic Hour

Disease	Sex	Drug cost (U.S. dollars per episode)	Clinic time (minutes per episode)	Treatment by cost per clinic hour		
				$2	$10	$30
AIDS with AZT	Both	2,000	2,400	2,080.00	2,400.00	3,200.00
AIDS without AZT	Both	35	1,200	75.00	235.00	635.00
Chancroid	Both	0.15	10	0.48	1.82	5.15
Chlamydia	Both	0.25	15	0.75	2.75	7.75
Gonorrhea	Female	1.00	12	1.40	3.00	7.00
	Male	1.20	10	1.53	2.87	6.20
HIV with AZT	Both	2,000	120	2,004.00	2,020.00	2,060.00
Syphilis	Both	0.80	15	1.30	3.30	8.30

Source: Estimates by authors.

Table 20C-2. Alternative Diagnostic Approaches for STDs: Costs, Time, and Positive Predictive Value

Disease	Sex	Diagnostic method	Cost of test (U.S. dollars per test)	Lab or clinic time (minutes per test)	Sensitivity	Specificity	Positive predictive value		
							1 percent prevalence	5 percent prevalence	25 percent prevalence
AIDS with AZT	Both	Serology	2.00	10	98	98	0.33	0.72	0.94
AIDS without AZT	Both	Serology	2.00	10	98	98	0.33	0.72	0.94
Chancroid	Both	Clinical	0.00	10	80	60	0.02	0.10	0.40
	Both	Culture	5.00	5	70	100	1.00	1.00	1.00
Chlamydia	Female	Clinical	0.00	10	20	20	0.00	0.01	0.08
	Female	Culture	12.00	5	80	99	0.45	0.81	0.96
	Female	Antigen	5.00	5	70	95	0.12	0.42	0.82
	Male	Clinical	0.00	10	80	80	0.04	0.17	0.57
	Male	Culture	12.00	5	85	99	0.46	0.82	0.97
Gonorrhea	Female	Clinical	0.00	10	25	25	0.00	0.02	0.10
	Female	Culture	5.00	5	85	100	1.00	1.00	1.00
	Female	Microscopy	1.00	10	50	80	0.02	0.12	0.45
	Male	Clinical	0.00	10	85	90	0.08	0.31	0.74
	Male	Culture	5.00	5	95	100	1.00	1.00	1.00
	Male	Microscopy	1.00	10	95	99	0.49	0.83	0.97
HIV with AZT	Both	Serology	2.00	10	98	98	0.33	0.72	0.94
Syphilis	Female	Serology	1.50	5	95	95	0.16	0.50	0.86
	Male	Serology	1.50	5	95	95	0.16	0.50	0.86
Average			—	—	n.a.	n.a.	0.34	0.54	0.73

— Data not available.
n.a. Not applicable.
Source: Authors' estimates.

518

Table 20C-3. Minimum Cost per Effectively Treated Case of STD: Sensitivity to Prevalence and Cost per Clinic Hour

Disease	Sex	Diagnostic method	$2 per clinic hour			$10 per clinic hour			$30 per clinic hour		
			1 percent prevalence	5 percent prevalence	25 percent prevalence	1 percent prevalence	5 percent prevalence	25 percent prevalence	1 percent prevalence	5 percent prevalence	25 percent prevalence
AIDS with AZT	Both	Serology	6,521	2,934	2,217	7,623	3,405	2,562	10,380	4,584	3,424
AIDS without AZT	Both	Serology	465	152	89	1,084	401	264	2,632	1,024	702
Chancroid	Both	Clinical	73	15	3	333	67	14	983	199	42
	Both	Culture	821	165	33	928	187	39	1,196	244	53
	Both	Presumptive treatment[a]	304	61	12	452	90	18	822	164	33
Chlamydia	Female	Clinical	516	101	18	2,139	420	77	6,196	1,219	223
	Female	Culture	1,692	339	68	1,789	360	74	2,033	413	89
	Female	Antigen	827	166	34	951	192	41	1,260	258	58
	Female	Presumptive treatment[a]	322	64	13	544	109	22	1,100	220	44
	Male	Clinical	63	13	3	286	59	13	845	172	38
	Male	Culture	1,592	319	64	1,682	338	69	1,908	386	82
	Male	Presumptive treatment[a]	304	61	12	452	90	18	822	164	33
Gonorrhea	Female	Clinical	580	114	20	1,643	324	60	4,301	848	158
	Female	Culture	641	129	27	726	148	32	936	193	45
	Female	Microscopy	341	69	14	690	139	29	1,562	316	67
	Female	Presumptive treatament[a]	295	59	12	463	93	19	884	177	35
	Male	Clinical	62	13	4	245	51	12	702	145	34
	Male	Culture	574	116	25	649	132	29	838	173	40
	Male	Microscopy	151	31	8	302	63	15	678	141	33
	Male	Presumptive treatment[a]	288	50	12	428	86	17	779	156	31
HIV with AZT	Both	Serology	6,291	2,829	2,136	6,475	2,878	2,159	6,936	3,002	2,215
Syphilis	Both	Serology	185	38	9	269	56	14	477	102	27
	Both	Presumptive treatment[a]	293	59	12	495	99	20	1,000	200	40

Note: Cost-effectiveness values are those that would obtain if 100 percent of patients had the specific disease in question. Treatment effectiveness is 99 percent for syphilis, 95 percent for gonorrhea, and 90 percent for chancroid and chlamydia. For AIDS treatment is assumed 100 percent effective at prolonging life one year without AZT or two years with AZT.

a. Treatment of all patients with the drugs for all four STDs, at an estimated cost of $2.40 per visit.

Source: Authors' estimates.

In table 20C-2 we present the estimated cost of the laboratory test for each disease, the estimated sensitivity and specificity of each test and, in the last three columns, the positive predictive value of the given test for three different prevalence rates. Let x represent the sensitivity of the test (that is, the proportion of truly positive cases which the test finds positive) and y represent the specificity of the test (that is, the proportion of truly negative cases which the test finds negative). Then the positive predictive value of a test is defined for prevalence rate I to be:

$$(14) \qquad PPV = \frac{x \cdot I}{[x \cdot I + (1 - y)(1 - I)]} .$$

To compare the "treat all" strategy with the "screen" strategy, we calculate the estimated cost per cure using each strategy for each of the classic STDs. For AIDS and HIV infection we simply calculate the cost of treatment. Let N be the number of individuals in a given population and I be the proportion of individuals infected at a given moment, that is, the point prevalence rate of the infection. Then the cost of treating all N individuals will be $C \cdot N$. Because a proportion I is infected, and the treatment is effective on a proportion E of these, the number cured will be $E \cdot I \cdot N$. Hence, the cost per cure for the treat-all strategy is $C/(E \cdot I)$.

The cost of testing all N individuals and treating those who are positive on the test is the sum of these two cost components. At a cost of T dollars per test, the testing cost for N individuals is $T \cdot N$. Let T be defined analogously to C except that the cost per hour of laboratory or clinic time is set to half the value used to compute the treatment cost. The test will be positive for x proportion of the $I \cdot N$ who are truly positive and for $(1 - y)$ proportion of the $(1 - I) \cdot N$ who are truly negative, so the total cost of treatment will be $C[x \cdot I \cdot N + (1 - y)(1 - I) N]$. Of the $x \cdot I \cdot N$-infected people who are treated, a proportion E will be cured. Thus the cost per cure from the screen strategy is given by:

$$(15) \quad \begin{array}{c} \text{Cost per cure} \\ \text{of the screen} \\ \text{strategy} \end{array} = \frac{C[x \cdot I + (1 - y)(1 - I)] + T}{E \cdot x \cdot I}$$

$$= \frac{C}{E \cdot PPV} + \frac{T}{E \cdot x \cdot I} .$$

A comparison of the cost per cure of the two strategies then reveals the preferred strategy for any given disease and for given assumptions regarding the hourly cost of clinic time, H, and the prevalence rate in the population in question, I. Other things being equal, a higher cost of clinic time in relation to testing cost, T, increases the relative cost advantage of the screen strategy. Conversely a higher prevalence rate, other things being equal, reduces the relative cost advantage of screening. The specific assumptions determine whether one

strategy will dominate the entire domain of reasonable parameter values.

In table 20C-3 we present the lowest cost solution for each disease and, for those diseases which vary by sex, for each sex. Two remarkable findings stand out from this table. First, over a large range of parameter values the "treat without testing" option dominates the "screen, then treat" option. Second, in those few situations in which screening is more cost-effective than treating everyone, the clinician's judgment produces a lower cost per effectively treated case than do the alternatives, which in the case of gonorrhea include microscopy and a culture.

Notes

All dollars in this chapter are 1989 U.S. dollars.

1. In his seminal work on the benefits of a syphilis control program, Klarman (1965) was unable to estimate these dynamic benefits.

2. Hethcote and Yorke (1984, pp. 16 and 17) use the terms "contact number" and "infectee number" to refer to different versions of this concept.

3. The concept can be extended further by including tertiary, quaternary, and other cases. This extension presents problems because some of the individuals not infected by the prevented case will instead be infected by a case that has not been prevented. The greater the number of rounds considered, the more serious is this problem, which can be avoided only by addressing the problem more generally in the context of an explicit mathematical epidemiological model. Prevented cases that would have occurred more than twelve months in the future must be discounted by an appropriate rate.

4. The new equation for R becomes $R = QD[m + s^2/m]$, where m is the mean of the a_i and s^2 is their variance. Note that as the heterogeneity disappears, s^2 approaches zero and this equation approaches the one given earlier. This result depends on the assumption of proportionate mixing of sexual partners. See appendix 20B for a discussion of alternative models of mixing.

5. The "prevalence" of an infection refers to a point in time and is defined as the proportion of a given population infected at that moment. The "incidence" of infection refers to a specific period of time and is defined as the number of new cases of infection during that period. Economists will note that the former is a "stock" and the latter a "flow."

6. See Heymann (1990) for sensitivity analyses with respect to several parameters not considered by Kennedy and others (1990).

7. None of the three studies reported in table 20-6 breaks out the results by sex. This is more of a problem for the Rwandan and Zambian studies than for the Zairian one, because the latter is based on a group of employees which is almost entirely male.

8. Rural women are much less likely to attend secondary school in Africa than are urban women.

9. Data on urban sex ratios of adults age twenty through thirty-nine are available only for these eighteen Sub-Saharan African countries in Larson (1989, table 1).

10. The number of females enrolled per 100 enrolled males is drawn from World Bank 1989 (table 32). Secondary education is likely to be concentrated in urban women.

11. The regression equation is:

$$\text{HIV}\% = -4.3 - 0.10 \cdot \text{FENR} + 1,240 \cdot \frac{1}{\text{FURB}}$$
$$\quad (-0.8) \quad (-2.3) \qquad\qquad (3.1)$$

$$n = 18 \quad R^2 = 0.48 \quad F_{2,15} = 7.03 \quad \text{Prob} > \text{F } 0.007$$

where FENR is the number of girls enrolled in secondary school for every 100 boys, FURB is the number of females age twenty through thirty-nine resident in urban areas for every 100 males. Numbers in parentheses are t-statistics. Dropping Rwanda from the regression reduces the significance of the coefficients but does not change their sign or magnitude. Grossbard-Schechtman, DuCharme, and Loomin (1989) also obtain significant coefficients on the young adult female-to-male ratio in their study of gonorrhea and syphilis prevalence in a cross-section of thirty-seven U.S. cities. They did not attempt to control for female education but did control for the prevalence of male homosexuality.

12. The magnitudes of the estimated coefficients suggest that a five-point reduction in the adult prevalence of HIV could be achieved either by increasing FURB by 35 per 100 men or by increasing FENR by 50 girls per 100 boys.

13. Sometimes it will be more convenient to refer to a disability-adjusted life-day (DALD) than a disability-adjusted life-year. There are 365 DALDs in one DALY. GHAP originally used the term healthy life-year, which we have changed for conformity with usage in this volume.

14. This is the parameter referred to as *a* previously and in table 20-10 below.

15. This is referred to in the literature as the assumption of proportionate mixing and is defined by setting a "selectivity parameter" equal to zero. When this parameter, G, is set to 100 percent, each group prefers members of its own group to the complete exclusion of members of the other, so that there is no interaction between the two groups. Although proportional mixing probably does not exactly describe actual behavioral patterns (Anderson 1989), Rothenberg and Potterat (1988, table 3) provide evidence from a Colorado Springs cohort of a remarkably large degree of mixing, especially by core men, for whom only 74 of 251 sexual contacts were with core women. The actual degree of mixing in pattern II countries is currently unknown.

16. Although the parameters of table 20-10 are not currently known for any African population, the guesses here are roughly consistent in order of magnitude with the estimates of doubling time of the infection presented by Anderson and McLean (1988).

17. The case-fatality rates of the other CSTDs, although important for the static burden calculations presented above, are too small and too long after infection to have an appreciable influence on this short-term model and thus are assumed to be zero. For HIV we set D equal to ten years, the average time until death, at which point we assume that a new susceptible is recruited through migration on maturation to replace the dead individual.

18. New biomedical findings on the variation of infectivity during the period of infection may affect these results.

19. For other values of the selectivity coefficient G, the two equilibrium prevalence levels are the solutions to two simultaneous quadratic equations, which are solved numerically by the simulations reported below. For G = 0 the solutions are given in the last two rows of table 20-11.

20. Furthermore there is some evidence that other STDs, such as chlamydial infection and trichomoniasis, also increase the efficiency of HIV transmission (Laga and others 1989, 1990; Pepin and others 1989).

21. A further question is whether HIV and other STDs discriminate between the poor and the rich in urban areas. Limited evidence indicates that HIV prevalence rates may be positively correlated with income levels among urban males and negatively correlated with income levels among urban females. This may, however, be only a temporary feature, because the epidemic has not yet reached stable levels in most populations.

22. Indeed the authors later state that "Our parameter values . . . may well lead to conclusions more representative of say Kinshasa and Nairobi than of Zaire and Kenya as a whole" (p. 233).

23. The last two columns of table 20-12 show that the health gain in preventing a single case of STD in a woman is 19 percent larger on average than preventing a single case in a man.

24. Although anthropologists have focused on describing the range and meaning of cultural practices, they have not typically attempted to estimate valid population-based frequencies of those practices.

25. For example, *Forbes* magazine recently reprinted and endorsed the oxymoronic request by the American activist group ACT UP for the public to "demand . . . [e]ffective prevention education programs that target *all* people in *all* cultural groups" (AIDS Coalition to Unleash Power 1989).

26. The youth group entitled "Les jeunes contre les MST" has been organized in Lubumbashi, Zaire, to combat STDs within the peer group.

27. To the extent that different measures of health gained result in different decisions, the decisionmaker will also have to select a preferred measure. The possibilities include discounted disability-adjusted life-days saved, discounted productive disability-adjusted life-days saved, and money-valued discounted disability-adjusted life-days saved.

28. For most diseases, we use relative incidence rates to average the effects over the six age groups. Following GHAP (1981), we distinguish adult from child pneumonia. At the expense of greater complexity, it would be possible to perform a separate analysis for each age group.

29. In the absence of dynamic analyses of the health benefits of preventing the other communicable diseases in figure 20-10 and table 20A-3 (for example, measles, pneumonia), dynamic benefits of STDs cannot be compared with those of other diseases.

30. In 1981 the country of Burkina Faso introduced the activist expression "commando program" for a one-time vaccination campaign.

31. For a full description of the model and sensitivity analyses with respect to its key parameters, see appendix 20B.

32. The net effect of the intervention, however, remains strongly positive, because the averted cases early in the period more than outweigh the small number of additional cases later. The effect of future additional cases is reduced even further because they are discounted at 3 percent.

33. Effectiveness is not the whole story. Cost-effectiveness is discussed in the rest of the chapter.

34. An intervention which produces sustained behavioral change would yield additional benefits from the permanent reduction in the prevalence rate.

35. When both partners are infected with one of these four CSTDs, we assume that infectivity is multiplied by the square of the factor operating when only one is infected. See appendix 20B for a formal statement.

36. These sums are represented graphically by the areas under the two curves in the bottom panel of figure 20-14.

37. For simplicity we model the condom user as absolutely protected, although in fact some condoms break or are incorrectly used and thus do not protect absolutely. Given the (unknown) frequency of condom failure, the cost-effectiveness figures can be inflated by that amount.

38. The others are frequency of sexual partner change (*a*), selectivity (*G*), and the CSTD's duration of infectivity (*D*). The costs of changing the frequency and duration are much harder to calculate. Theoretically an IEC program could also slow the epidemic in the noncore (and accelerate it in the core) by encouraging increased selectivity of sexual partners. Sensitivity analysis reported elsewhere in this chapter, however, reveals that even a substantial increase in selectivity has a relatively small effect on the speed of the epidemic's spread. Furthermore, IEC programs to encourage selectivity would inevitably also lead to increased stigmatization of people who seem to fit the program's stereotype of "partners to avoid." In addition to creating deep and harmful social divisions and scapegoating, such stigmatization would drive the epidemic further underground, where it would be even harder to combat. For these reasons we do not consider this behavioral parameter to be the legitimate target of an IEC program.

39. Bertozzi (1991) presents two more complex models and sensitivity analyses to show that they differ little from one another.

40. This is the prevalence rate recently reported among blood donors in Delhi, India, by Singh and others (1990).

41. In those countries in which donor assistance has provided virtually unlimited financial assistance, the binding constraint is trained, competent manpower to manage those resources.

42. This is a consensus estimate by a WHO/GPA panel of experts reported in Chin, Sato, and Mann (1989).

43. This is the same Elliot Ness who earlier conducted such a vigorous and unsuccessful war against bootleg liquor.

44. Brandt goes on to point out the illogic of placing the blame for STDs uniquely on women. "The fact that controlling prostitution did not control sexuality forced many to confront the change in American sexual mores" (p. 168).

45. By placing HIV-infected persons in quarantine, Cuba is the only country in which a full-scale mandatory program for the whole population is in effect. There the regulators are presumably closely supervised (Bayer and Healton 1989). Although the program's effectiveness is undoubtedly increased by the

absence of civil rights and by the surrounding ocean barrier at the borders, its actual effectiveness is unknown.

46. An average of 1.9 partners were named per cooperating index case. Interestingly, when asked to choose whether personally to notify their own partners (patient referral) or to have the public health staff perform the notification (provider referral), index cases chose the relatively anonymous provider referral for 75 percent of all named contacts (Spencer, Raevsky and, Wolf 1989).

47. One hundred dollars is 0.5 percent of the U.S. 1987 per capita GNP.

48. In a poor country it may be difficult to persuade the public that any allocation mechanism which distributes treatment to only five or ten of several thousand enrolled HIV-positive candidates is fair. One possible mechanism would be a community review board similar to those used in the United States and Great Britain to allocate scarce kidneys to transplant candidates. Another possibility is simply to use a lottery.

49. Because no population-based studies yet exist which estimate the proportion of adults with multiple sexual partners, these figures must be viewed as hypotheses which require confirmation. The population-based figures, such as proportion of adolescents or of health care providers, can be adjusted to the data of an individual country as they become available.

50. As an analogy with the epidemiology of screening, think of the communication as a screening test. Then the coverage of the target group by the communication is analogous to the proportion of all positives identified by the test, that is, the sensitivity of the test.

51. In accord with the preceding note, the "concentration" of a message on a target group is analogous to the positive predictive value of a screening test for a specific disease.

52. If the delivery of an IEC or training message to the wrong group has political or social costs (for example, by inflaming political antagonism to the AIDS prevention program or by stigmatizing prostitutes), then the "specificity" of the access group for the target group is also a desirable attribute.

53. Behrman (1989) discusses the economics of social marketing programs in a family planning context.

54. For example, Mposo and others (1989) found that HIV-infected infants in Zaire incurred annual health care costs that were 60 percent higher than control infants.

55. The estimate of one DALY saved per case averted is derived by applying the appendix A methodology to gonorrhea after setting to zero all incidence rates for age greater than zero.

56. This policy is cost-effective in comparison with treating later cases, even in populations that have prevalence rates of syphilis as low as 0.005 percent in pregnant women (Stray-Pedersen 1983).

57. The presumptive treatment of syndromes has the additional disadvantage of exposing more people to antibiotics and thereby increasing resistance to those antibiotics in the population of disease agents and potentially causing mild to severe side effects in individuals taking antimicrobials. Consideration of these drawbacks is beyond the scope of this chapter.

58. According to World Bank sources, the cost per clinic-hour in one poor Sub-Saharan African country is $2.20 (1990 U.S. dollars).

59. See Hethcote and Yorke 1984, pp. 25–31, for details.

60. For a more general specification of mixing in a one-sex mixing model, see Blythe and Castillo-Chavez 1988 and the references therein.

61. For a more detailed discussion, the reader is referred to the STD treatment guidelines issued by WHO (1989).

References

Ades, A. E., M. L. Newell, C. S. Peckham. 1991. "Children Born to Women with HIV-1 Infection: Natural History and Risk of Transmission." *Lancet* 337:253–60.

AIDS Coalition to Unleash Power (ACT-UP). 1989. "Statement." *Forbes* 144(1): 20–21.

Aladesanmi, A. F. K., G. Mumtaz, D. C. W. Mabey. 1989. "Prevalence of Cervical Chlamydial Infection in Antenatal Clinic Attenders in Lagos, Nigeria." *Genitourinary Medicine* 65:130.

Anderson, R. M. 1989. "Mathematical and Statistical Studies of the Epidemiology of AIDS." *AIDS* 3:333–46.

Anderson, R. M., and A. R. McLean. 1988. "Possible Demographic Consequences of AIDS in Developing Countries." *Nature* 332:228–34.

Anderson, R. M., and R. M. May. 1988. "Epidemiological Parameters of HIV Transmission." *Nature* 333:514–19.

Anderson, R. M., G. F. Medley, R. M. May, and A. M. Johnson. 1986. "A Preliminary Study of the Transmission Dynamics of the Human Immunodeficiency Virus (HIV), the Causative Agent of AIDS." *IMA Journal of Mathematics Applied in Medicine and Biology* 3:229–63.

Antal, G. M. 1987. "The Epidemiology of Sexually Transmitted Diseases in the Tropics." In A. O. Osoba ed., *Sexually Transmitted Diseases in the Tropics*. 2(1) of *Baillière's Clinical and Tropical Medicine and Communicable Diseaes*. London: Baillière-Tindall.

Arnal, S. O., and K. K. Holmes. 1990. "Sexually Transmitted Diseases in the AIDS Era." *Scientific American* 264(February):62–69.

Arya, O. P., A. O. Osoba, and F. J. Bennett. 1988. *Tropical Venereology*. 2d ed. Edinburgh: Churchill Livingstone.

Arya, O. P., S. R. Taber, and H. Nsanze. 1980. "Gonorrhea and Female Infertility in Rural Uganda." *American Journal of Obstetrics and Gynecology* 138:929–32.

Austin, H., W. C. Louv, and W. J. Alexander. 1984. "A Case-Control Study of Spermicides and Gonorrhea." *JAMA* 251:2822–24.

Ballard, R. C., H. G. Fehler, and P. Piot. 1986. "Chlamydial Infections of the Eye and Genital Tract in Developing Societies." In J. D. Oriel, Geoffrey Ridgeway, Julius Schachter, David Taylor-Richardson, and Michael Ward, eds., *Chlamydial Infections: Proceedings of the Sixth International Symposium on Human Chlamydial Infections*, Cambridge: Cambridge University Press.

Barnum, H. 1987. "Evaluating Healthy Days of Life Gained from Health Projects." *Social Science and Medicine* 24:833–41.

Bayer, Ronald. 1990. *Private Acts and Social Consequences: AIDS and the Politics of Public Health*. New Brunswick, N.J.: Rugers University Press.

Bayer, R., and C. Healton. 1989. "Controlling AIDS in Cuba: The Logic of Quarantine." *New England Journal of Medicine* 320:1022–24.

Behrman, J. R. 1989. "The Simple Analytics of Contraceptive Social Marketing." *World Development* 17(10):1499–1521.

Bentsi, C., C. A. Klufio, P. L. Perine, T. A. Bell, L. D. Cles, C. M. Koester, and S.-P. Wang. 1985. "Genital Infections with *Chlamydia trachomatis* and *Neisseria gonorrhoeae* in Ghanaian Women." *Genitourinary Medicine* 61: 48–50.

Berkley, S. 1991. "Parental Transmission of HIV in Africa." *AIDS*. 5:S87–S92.

Bertozzi, Stefano. 1990. "The Economics of HIV Screening of Blood for Transfusion." Abstract. Fifth International Conference on AIDS in Africa, Kinshasa, Zaire. October.

———. 1991. "Combating HIV in Africa: A Role for Economic Research." *AIDS* 5:S45–S54.

Bewes, P. C. 1973. "Urethral Stricture." *Tropical Doctor* 3:77–81.

Blythe, S. P., and C. Castillo-Chavez. 1988. "Like with Like Preference and Sexual Mixing Models." Cornell University, Department of City and Regional Planning, Cornell University, Ithaca, N.Y.

Bongaarts, J. 1988. "Modeling the Spread of HIV Infection and the Demographic Impact of AIDS in Africa." Working Paper 140. The Population Council, New York.

———. 1989. "A Model of the Spread of HIV Infection and the Demographic Impact of AIDS." *Statistics in Medicine* 8:103–20.

Bongaarts, J., P. Reining, P. Way, and F. Conant. 1989. "The Relationship between Male Circumcision and HIV Infection in African Populations." *AIDS* 3:373–77.

Bongaarts, J., and P. O. Way. 1989. "Geographic Variation in the HIV Epidemic and the Mortality Impact of AIDS in Africa." Working Paper 1. Population Council, New York.

Braddick, M., and J. Kreiss. 1988. "Mother-to-Child Transmission of HIV." In P. Piot and J. M. Mann, eds., *AIDS and HIV infection in the Tropics*. London: Baillière-Tyndall.

Braddick, M., J. O. Ndinya-Achola, N. B. Mirza, F. A. Plummer, G. Irungu, S. K. A. Sinei, and P. Piot. 1990. "Towards Developing a Diagnostic Algorithm for *Chlamydia trachomatis* and *Neisseria gonorrhoeae* Cervicitis in Pregnancy." *Genitourinary Medicine* 66:62–65.

Brandt, Allan M. 1987. *No Magic Bullet*. New York: Oxford University Press.

Brown, S., F. Zacarias, and S. Aral. 1985. "STD Control in Less Developed Countries: The Time Is Now." *International Journal of Epidemiology* 14:505–10.

Brunham, R. C. 1984. "Therapy for Acute Pelvic Inflammatory Disease: A Critique of Recent Treatment Trials." *American Journal of Obstetrics and Gynecology* 148:235–40.

Brunham, R. C., K. K. Holmes, and J. Embree. 1989. "Sexually Transmitted Diseases in Pregnancy." In K. K. Holmes, P. A. Mårdh, P. J. Wiesner, and P. F. Sparling, eds., *Sexually Transmitted Diseases*, 2nd ed., New York: McGraw-Hill.

Bugingo, G., A. Ntilivamunda, D. Nzaramba, P. Van de Perre, A. Ndikuyeze, S. Munyantore, A. Mutwewingabo, and C. Bizimungu. 1988. "Etude sur la séropositivité liée à l'infection au virus de l'immunodéficience humaine au Rwanda." *Revue Médicale Rwandaise* 20:37–42.

Buisman, N. J. F., T. Abong Mwemba, G. Garrigue, J. P. Durand, J. S. Stilma, and T. M. Van Balen. 1988. "Chlamydia Ophthalmia Neonatorum in Cameroon." *Documenta Ophthalmologica* 70:257–64.

Bulatao, R. A. 1985. "Expenditures on Population Programs in Developing Regions: Current Levels and Future Requirements." Working Paper 679, Population and Development 4. World Bank, Washington, D.C.

Caldwell, J. C., P. Caldwell, and P. Quiggin. 1989. "The Social Context of AIDS in Sub-Saharan Africa." *Population and Development Review* 15(2):185–235.

Cameron, D. W., J. N. Simonsen, L. D'Costa, A. R. Ronald, G. M. Maitha, M. N. Gakinya, M. Cheang, J. O. Ndinya-Achola, P. Piot, R. C. Brunham, and F. A. Plummer. 1989. "Female to Male Transmission of Human Immunodeficiency Virus Type 1: Risk Factors for Seroconversion in Men." *Lancet* 2:403–7.

Cates, W., T. M. M. Farley, and P. J. Rowe. 1985. "Worldwide Patterns of Infertility: Is Africa Different?" *Lancet* 2:596–98.

Centers for Disease Control (CDC). 1986. "Classification System for Human T-Lymphotropic Virus Type III/Lymphadenopathy Associated Virus Infections." *Morbidity and Mortality Weekly Report* 35:334–39.

———. 1988. "Continuing Increase in Infectious Syphilis." *Morbidity and Mortality Weekly Report* 37:35–38.

———. 1989. "Tuberculosis and Human Immunodeficiency Virus Infection: Recommendations of the Advisory Committee for the Elimination of Tuberculosis." *Morbidity and Mortality Weekly Report* 38:236–50.

Chin, J., P. Sato, and J. Mann. 1989. "Estimates and Projections of HIV/AIDS to the Year 2000." Paper presented at the Achieving Health for All Symposium, September 3, Seattle, Wash.

Clavel, F., D. Guétard, F. Brun-Vézinet, S. Chamaret, M. A. Rey, M. O. Santos-Ferreira, A. G. Laurent, C. Dauget, C. Katlama, C. Rouzioux, D. Klatzmann, J. L. Champalimaud, and L. Montagnier. 1986. "Isolation of a New Human Retrovirus from West-African Patient with AIDS." *Science* 233:343–46.

Clumeck, N., H. Taelman, P. Hermans, P. Piot, M. Schoumacher, and S. De Wit. 1989. "A Cluster of HIV Infection among Heterosexual People without Apparent Risk Factors." *New England Journal of Medicine* 321:1460–63.

Cole, C. H., T. G. Lacher, J. C. Bailey, and D. L. Fairclough. 1980. "Vaginal Chemoprophylaxis in the Reduction of Reinfection in Women with Gonorrhoea." *British Journal of Venereal Diseases* 56:314–18.

Colebunders, R. L., B. Kapita, W. Nekwei, U. Y. Bahwe, I. Lebughe, M. Oxtoby, and R. W. Ryder. 1988. "Breastfeeding and Transmission of HIV." *Lancet* 2:1487.

Colebunders, R. L., R. W. Ryder, N. Nzila, D. Kalunga, J. C. Willame, M. Kaboto, B. Nkoko, J. Jeugmans, M. Kalala, H. L. Francis, J. M. Mann, T. C. Quinn, and P. Piot. 1989. "HIV Infection in Patients with Tuberculosis in Kinshasa, Zaire." *American Review of Respiratory Diseases* 139:1082–85.

Cooper-Poole, B. 1986. "Prevalence of Syphilis in Mbeya, Tanzania: The Validity of the VDRL as a Screening Test." *East African Medicine Journal* 63:646–50.

Coutinho, R. A., P. van Griensven, and A. Moss. 1989. "Effects of Preventive Efforts among Homosexual Men." *AIDS* 3(Supplement 1):S53–S56.

Curran, J. W. 1980. "Economic Consequences of Pelvic Inflammatory Disease in the United States." *American Journal of Obstetrics and Gynecology* 138:848–51.

Datta, P., M. Laga, F. A. Plummer, J. O. Ndinya-Achola, P. Piot, G. Maitha, A. R. Ronald, and R. C. Brunham. 1988. "Infection and Disease after Perinatal Exposure to *Chlamydia trachomatis* in Nairobi, Kenya." *Journal of Infectious Diseases* 158:524–28.

D'Costa, L. J., F. A. Plummer, I. Bowmer, L. Fransen, P. Piot, A. R. Ronald, and H. Nzanze. 1985. "Prostitutes Are a Major Reservoir of Sexually Transmitted Diseases in Nairobi, Kenya." *Sexually Transmitted Diseases* 12:64–67.

De Cock, K. M., A. Pozter, K. Odehouri. 1989. "Rapid Emergence of AIDS in Abidjan, Ivory Coast." *Lancet* 2:408–10.

De Muylder, X. 1986. "Clinical Diagnosis of Pelvic Inflammatory Disease in a Developing Country." *Annales de la Société belge de Médecine Tropicale* 66:339–42.

De Schampheleire, I., L. Van De Velden, E. Van Dyck, S. Guindo, W. Quint, and L. Fransen. 1990. "Maladies sexuellement transmissibles dans la population féminine à Pikine, Sénégal." *Annales de la Société belge de Médecine Tropicale* 70:227–35.

Fakeya, R., B. Onile, and T. Odugbemi. 1986. "Antitreponemal Antibodies among Antenatal Patients at the University of Ilorin Teaching Hospital." *African Journal of Sexually Transmitted Diseases* 2:9–10.

Fleming, A. F. 1988. "Prevention of Transmission of HIV by Blood Transfusion in Developing Countries." In A. F. Fleming and others, eds., *The Global Impact of AIDS*. New York: Alan R. Liss.

Frank, Odile. 1983. "Infertility in Sub-Saharan Africa: Estimates and Implications." *Population and Development Review* 9(1):137–44.

Fransen, L., H. Nsanze, L. D'Costa, R. C. Brunham, A. R. Ronald, and P. Piot. 1984. "Single-Dose Kanamycin Therapy of Gonococcal Ophthalmia Neonatorum." *Lancet* 2:1234–37.

Fransen, L., H. Nsanze, V. Klauss, P. van der Stuyft, L. D'Costa, R. C. Brunham, and P. Piot. 1986. "Ophthalmia Neonatorum in Nairobi, Kenya: The Roles of *Neisseria gonorrhoeae* and *Chlamydia trachomatis*." *Journal of Infectious Diseases* 153:862–69.

Galega, F. P., D. L. Heyman, and B. T. Nasah. 1984. "Gonococcal Ophthalmia Neonatorum: The Case of Prophylaxis in Tropical Africa." *Bulletin of the World Health Organization* 61:85–88.

George, W. F. 1974. "An Approach to VD Control Based on a Study in Kingston, Jamaica." *British Journal of Venereal Diseases* 50:222–27.

Ghana Health Assessment Project Team (GHAP). 1981. "Quantitative Method of Assessing the Health Impact of Different Diseases in Less Developed Countries." *International Journal of Epidemiology* 10:73–80.

Goedert, J. J., C. M. Kessler, L. M. Aledort, R. J. Biggar, W. R. Andes, G. C. White, J. E. Drummond, K. Vaidya, D. L. Mann, and M. E. Eyster. 1989. "A Prospective Study of Human Immunodeficiency Virus Type 1 Infection and the Development of AIDS in Subjects with Hemophilia." *New England Journal of Medicine* 321:1141–48.

Gravett, M. G., H. P. Nelson, T. De Rouen, C. Critchlow, D. Eschenbach, and K. K. Holmes. 1986. "Independent Association of Bacterial Vaginosis and *Chlamydia trachomatis* Infection with Adverse Pregnancy Outcome." *JAMA* 256:1899–1903.

Greenberg, A. E., P. Nguyen-Dinh, J. M. Mann, N. Kabote, R. L. Colebunders, H. Francis, T. C. Quinn, P. Baudoux, B. Lyamba, F. Darachi, and others. 1988. "The Association between Malaria, Blood Transfusions, and HIV

Seropositivity in a Pediatric Population in Kinshasa, Zaire." *JAMA* 259: 545–49.

Grimes, D. A. 1986. "Deaths Due to Sexually Transmitted Diseases: The Forgotten Component of Reproductive Mortality." *JAMA* 255:1727–29.

Grossbard-Schechtman, Soshana, F. DuCharme, and M. Loomin, 1989. "Sex-Ratio Effects on the Incidence of Sexually Transmitted Diseases," *Population Association of America 1989 Annual Meetings: Program Abstracts.* 52:94.

Guiness, L. F., S. Sibandze, E. McGrath, and A. L. Cornelis. 1988. "Influence of Antenatal Screening on Perinatal Mortality Caused by Syphilis in Swaziland." *Genitourinary Medicine* 64:294–97.

Hammerschlag, M. R., C. Cummings, P. M. Roblin, T. H. Williams, and I. Delke. 1989. "Efficacy of Neonatal Ocular Prophylaxis for the Prevention of Chlamydial and Gonococcal Conjunctivitis." *New England Journal of Medicine* 320:769–72.

Hethcote, H. H., and J. A. Yorke. 1984. *Gonorrhea Transmission Dynamics and Control.* Lecture Notes in Biomathematics 56. New York: Springer-Verlag.

———. 1990. "Modeling the Impact of Breastfeeding by HIV-Infected Women on Child Survival." *American Journal of Public Health* 80:1305–1309.

Heyman, S. J. 1990. "Modeling the Impact of Breastfeeding by HIV-Infected Women on Child Survival." *American Journal of Public Health* 80:1305–9.

Hira, S. K., and R. S. Hira. 1987. "Congenital Syphilis." In A. O. Osoba, ed., *Sexually Transmitted Diseases in the Tropics.* Baillière's Tindall, London.

Hira, S. K., J. Kamanga, and G. J. Bhat. 1989. "Perinatal Transmission of HIV-1 in Zambia." *British Medical Journal* 299:1250–52.

Holmes, K. K., P.-A. Mårdh, P. F. Sparling, and P. J. Wiesner, eds., 1989. *Sexually Transmitted Diseases.* 2d ed. New York: McGraw-Hill.

Hooper, R. R., G. H. Reynolds, O. G. Jones, and K. K. Holmes. 1978. "Cohort Study of Venereal Diseases 1. The Risk of Gonorrhea Transmission from Infected Women to Men." *American Journal of Epidemiology* 108:136–44.

Hornik, R. 1988. "The Knowledge-Behavior Gap in Public Information Campaigns: A Development Communication View." Working Paper 110. University of Pennsylvania, Annenberg School of Communications, State College, Penn.

———. 1989a. "Channel Effectiveness in Development Communication Programs." Working Paper 111. University of Pennsylvania, Annenberg School of Communications, State College, Penn.

———. 1989b. "General AIDS Education: Cross-National Evidence of Effects." Working Paper 117. University of Pennsylvania, Annenberg School of Communications, State College, Penn.

Jacobson, L. L., and L. Weström. 1969. "Objectivized Diagnosis of Acute Pelvic Inflammatory Disease." *American Journal of Obstetrics and Gynecology* 105:1088–98.

Jama, H., B. Heberstedt, S. Osman, K. Omar, A. Isse, and S. Bygdeman. 1987. "Syphilis in Women of Reproductive Age in Mogadishu, Somalia: Serological Survey." *Genitourinary Medicine* 63:326–28.

Janowitz, B. S., J. H. Bratt, and D. B. Fried. 1990. "Investing in the Future: A Report on the Cost of Family Planning in the Year 2000." Discussion paper. Family Health International, Research Triangle Park, N.C.

Johnson, A., and M. Laga. 1988. "Heterosexual Transmission of HIV." *AIDS* 2(Supplement 1):S49–S56.

Kaptue, L., L. Zekeng, R. Salla, A. Trabucq, J. P. Lewis, Andele, A. Ndonmore, Yanga, P. Lamptey, and S. Mitchell. 1990. "Setting Up a Sentinel Surveillance System for HIV Infection in Cameroon." Paper presented at the 6th International Conference on AIDS, June 20–23, San Francisco.

Kennedy, K. I., J. A. Fortney, M. G. Bonhomme, M. Potts, P. Lamptey, and W. Carswell. 1990. "Do the Benefits of Breastfeeding Outweigh the Risk of Postnatal Transmission of HIV via Breast Milk?" *Tropical Doctor* 20:25–29.

Kesteleyn, P., J. Bogaerts, and A. Z. Meheus. 1987. "Gonorrheal Keratoconjunctivitis in African Adults." *Sexually Transmitted Diseases* 14:191–94.

Klarman, H. E. 1965. "Syphilis Control Programs." In R. Dorfman, ed., *Measuring Benefits of Government Investment.* Washington, D.C.: Brookings Institution.

Kreiss, J. K., D. Koech, F. A. Plummer, K. K. Holmes, M. Lightfoote, P. Piot, A. R. Ronald, J. O. Ndinya-Achola, L. J. D'Costa, P. Roberts, E. N. Ngugi, T. C. Quinn. 1986. "AIDS Virus Infection in Nairobi Prostitutes: Spread of the Epidemic to East Africa." *New England Journal of Medicine* 314:414–18.

Laga, M., A. Z. Meheus, and P. Piot. 1989. "Epidemiology and Control of Gonococcal Ophthalmia Neonatorum." *Bulletin of the World Health Organization* 67:471–77.

Laga, M., W. Namaara, R. C. Brunham, L. J. D'Costa, H. Nsanze, P. Piot, D. Kunimoto, J. O. Ndinya-Achola, L. Slaney, A. R. Ronald, and F. A. Plummer. 1986a. "Single Dose Therapy of Gonococcal Ophthalmia Neonatorum with Ceftriaxone." *New England Journal of Medicine* 315:1382–85.

Laga, M., H. Nsanze, F. A. Plummer, W. Namaara, G. Maitha, R. C. Brunham, J. O. Ndinya-Achola, J. K. Mati, A. R. Ronald, and P. Piot. 1986b. "Epidemiology of Ophthalmia Neonatorum in Kenya." *Lancet* 2: 1145–48.

Laga, M., N. Nzila, A. T. Manoka, M. Kivuvu, F. Behets, B. Edidi, P. Piot, and R. Ryder. 1989. "High Prevalence and Incidence of HIV and Other Sexually Transmitted Diseases (STD) among 801 Kinshasa Prostitutes." Paper presented at the 5th International Conference on AIDS, June 4–9, Montreal.

Laga, M., N. Nzila, A. T. Manoka, M. Malele, M. Tuliza, T. Bush, P. Piot, F. Behets, W. L. Heyward, and R. Ryder. 1990. "Non Ulcerative Sexually Transmitted Diseases as Risk Factors for HIV Infection." Paper presented at the 6th International Conference on AIDS, June 20–23, San Francisco.

Laga, M., and P. Piot. 1988. "HIV Infection after Plasma Donation in Valencia: Yet Another Case." *Lancet* 2:905.

Laga, M., F. A. Plummer, P. Piot, P. Datta, W. Namaara, J. O. Ndinya-Achola, H. Nsanze, G. Maitha, A. R. Ronald, H. O. Pamba, and R. C. Brunham. 1988. "Prophylaxis of Ophthalmia Neonatorum: Silver Nitrate versus Tetracycline." *New England Journal of Medicine* 318:653–57.

Lajmanovich, A. and J. A. Yorke. 1971. "A Deterministic Model for Gonorrhea in a Nonhomogeneous Population," *Mathematical Bioscience,* 28:221–36.

Laleman, G., K. Magazani, N. Badibanga, N. Kapila, M. Konde, V. Salemani, and P. Piot. 1992. "Prevention of Blood Acquired HIV Transmission through a Decentralized Approach and Using a Rapid HIV Test in Shaba Province, Zaire." *AIDS* 6: in press.

Lallemant, M., S. Lallemant-Le Coeur, D. Cheynier, J. Nzingoula, G. Jourdain, M. Sinet, M. C. Dazza, and B. Larouzé. 1989. "Mother-Child Transmission of HIV-1 and Infant Survival in Brazzaville, Congo." *AIDS* 3:643–46.

Lamptey, P., and G. A. W. Goodridge. 1991. "Condom Issues in AIDS Prevention in Africa." *AIDS* 5:S183–S91.

Lamptey, P., A. Neequay, S. Weir, and M. Potts. 1988. "A Model Program to Reduce HIV Infection among Prostitutes in Africa." Paper presented at the 4th International Conference on AIDS, June, Stockholm.

Lamptey, P., and M. Potts. 1990. "Targeting of Prevention Programs in Africa." In P. Lamptey and P. Piot, eds., *Handbook on AIDS Prevention in Africa.* Durham, S.C.: Family Health International.

Larson, A. 1989. "Social Context of HIV Transmission in Africa: Historical and Cultural Bases of East and Central African Sexual Relations." *Reviews of Infectious Diseases* 11:716–31.

Leclerc, A., E. Frost, M. Collet, J. Goeman, and L. Bedjabaga. 1988. "Urogenital *Chlamydia trachomatis* in Gabon: An Unrecognized Epidemic." *Genitourinary Medicine* 64:308–11.

Louv, W. C., H. Austin, W. J. Alexander, S. Stagno, and J. Cheeks. 1988. "A Clinical Trial of Nonoxynol-9 for Preventing Gonococcal and Chlamydial Infections." *Journal of Infectious Diseases* 158:518–23.

Lucas, R. E. B. 1985. "The Distribution of Wages and Employment in Rural Botswana." In Dov Chernichovsky, R. E. B. Lucas, and Eva Mueller, eds., *The Household Economy of Rural Botswana.* Staff Working Paper 715. World Bank, Washington, D.C.

Lukehart, S. A., E. W. Hook, III, S. A. Baker-Zander, A. C. Collier, C. W. Critchlow, and H. H. Handsfield. 1988. "Invasion of the Central Nervous System by *Treponema pallidum*: Implications for Diagnosis and Treatment." *Annals of Internal Medicine* 109:855–62.

Luyeye, M., M. Gerniers, N. Lebughe, F. Behets, N. Nzila, B. Edidi, and M. Laga. 1990. "Prévalence et facteurs de risque pour les MST chez les femmes enceintes dans les soins de santé primaires à Kinshasa." Paper presented at the 5th International Conference on AIDS in Africa. 10–12 October, Kinshasa, Zaire.

Mabey, D. C. W., N. E. Lloyd-Evans, S. Conteh, and T. Forsey. 1984. "Sexually Transmitted Diseases among Randomly Selected Attenders at an Antenatal Clinic in the Gambia." *British Journal of Venereal Diseases* 60:331–36.

Mabey, D. C. W., and H. C. Whittle. 1982. "Genital and Neonatal Chlamydial Infection in a Trachoma Endemic Area." *Lancet* 2:301–2.

McCormack, W. M., R. J. Stumacher, K. Johnson, A. Donner, and R. Rychwalski. 1977. "Clinical Spectrum of Gonococcal Infection in Women." *Lancet* 1:1182–85.

Meheus, A. Z., R. Ballard, M. Dlamini, J. P. Ursi, E. Van Dyck, and P. Piot. 1980. "Epidemiology and Etiology of Urethritis in Swaziland." *International Journal of Epidemiology* 9:239–45.

Meheus, A. Z., R. Delgadillo, R. Widy-Wirsky, and P. Piot. 1982. "Chlamydial Ophthalmia Neonatorum in Central Africa." *Lancet* 2:882.

Meheus, A. Z., and A. Deschryver. 1989. "Syphilis and Safe Blood." WHO/DVT/89.444. World Health Organization, Geneva.

Meheus, A. Z., F. Friedman, E. Van Dyck, and T. Guyver. 1980. "Genital Infections in Prenatal and Family Planning Attendants in Swaziland." *East African Medical Journal* 57:212–17.

Melbye, M., E. K. Nselesani, and A. Bayley, 1986. "Evidence for Heterosexual Transmission and Clinical Manifestations of Human Immunodeficiency Virus Infection and Related Conditions in Lusaka, Zambia." *Lancet* 2:1113–15.

Monny-Lobe, M., D. Nichols, R. Zekeng, R. Solda, L. Kaptue. 1989. "Prostitutes as Health Educators for Their Peers in Yaoundé: Changes in Knowledge, Attitudes and Practices." Paper presented at the 5th International Conference on AIDS, June 4–9, Montreal.

Moses, S., F. A. Plummer, A. R. Ronald, J. O. Ndinya-Achola. 1989. "Male Circumcision in Eastern and Southern Africa: Association with HIV Seroprevalence." Abstract (Th.G.0.27) of paper presented at the 5th International Conference on AIDS, June 4–9, Montreal.

Moss, A. R., and P. Bacchetti. 1989. "Natural History of HIV Infection." *AIDS* 3:55–62.

Mposo, N., B. Engele, S. Bertozzi, S. Hassig, and R. Ryder. 1989. "Prospective Quantification of the Economic and Morbid Impact of Perinatal HIV Infection in a Cohort of 245 Zairian Infants Born to HIV(+) Mothers." Paper presented at the 5th International Conference on AIDS, June, 4–9, Montreal.

Mvula, M., R. Ryder, and T. Manzila. 1989. "Response to Childhood Vaccinations in African Children with HIV Infection." Paper presented at the 5th International Conference on AIDS, June 4–9, Montreal.

Nasah, B. T., R. Nguematcha, M. Eyong, and S. Godwin. 1980. "Gonorrhea, Trichomonas, and Candida among Gravid and Nongravid Women in Cameroon." *International Journal of Gynaecology and Obstetrics* 18:48–52.

Ndilu, Mibandumba, D. Sequeira, S. Hassig, R. Kambale, R. Colebunders, M. Kashamuka,, and R. Ryder. 1988. "Medical, Social, and Economic Impact of HIV Infection in a Large African Factory." Paper presented at the 4th International Conference on AIDS, Stockholm.

N'Galy, B., R. W. Ryder, B. Kapita, M. Kashamuka, R. L. Colebunders, H. Francis, J. M. Mann, and T. C. Quinn. 1988. "Human Immunodeficiency Virus Infection among Employees in an African Hospital." *New England Journal of Medicine* 319:1123–27.

Ngugi, E. N., J. N. Simonsen, M. Bosire, A. R. Ronald, and F. A. Plummer. 1988. "Prevention of HIV Transmission in Africa: The Effectiveness of Condom Promotion and Health Education among High Risk Prostitutes." *Lancet* 2:887–90.

Nzila, N., K. M. De Cock, D. Forthal, M. Laga, P. Piot, and J. B. McCormick. 1988. "The Prevalence of Infection with Human Immunodeficiency Virus over a 10-year Period in Rural Zaire." *New England Journal of Medicine* 318:276–79.

Office of Technology Assessment. 1988. *How effective is AIDS Education?* Congress of the United States, OTA Staff Paper 3, June.

Okpere, E. E., E. E. Obaseiki-Ebor, and G. M. Oyaide. 1987. "Type of Intra-Uterine Contraceptive Device (IUCD) Used and the Incidence of Asymptomatic *Neisseria gonorrhoeae*." *African Journal of Sexually Transmitted Diseases* 3:7–8.

Osegbe, D. N., and E. O. Amaku. 1981. "Gonococcal Strictures in Young Patients." *Urology* 18(1):37–41.

Osoba, A. O., ed. 1987. "Sexually Transmitted Diseases in the Tropics." 2(1) of *Baillière's Clinical and Tropical Medicine and Communicable Diseases*. London: Baillière-Tyndall.

Over, Mead, S. Bertozzi, J. Chin, B. N'Galy, and K. Nyamuryekunge. 1988. "The Direct and Indirect Cost of HIV Infection in Developing Countries: The Cases of Zaire and Tanzania." In A. F. Fleming, et al, eds., *The Global Impact of AIDS*. New York: Alan R. Liss.

Over, Mead, S. Bertozzi, and J. Chin. 1989. "Guidelines for Rapid Estimation of the Direct and Indirect Costs of HIV Infection in a Developing Country." *Health Policy* 11:169–86.

Over, Mead, and J. Kutzin. 1990. "The Direct and Indirect Costs of HIV Infection: Two African Case Studies." *Postgraduate Doctor Middle East* 13(11):632–38.

Pepin, J., F. A. Plummer, R. C. Brunham, P. Piot, D. W. Cameron, and A. R. Ronald. 1989. "The Interaction between HIV Infection and Other Sexually Transmitted Diseases: An Opportunity for Intervention." *AIDS* 3:3–9.

Perriens, J., Y. Mukadi, D. Nunn. 1991. "Tuberculosis and HIV Infection: Implications for Africa." *AIDS* 5.

Phanuphak, P., Y. Poshychinda, T. Un-eklabh, and W. Rojanapithayakron. 1989. "HIV Transmission among Intravenous Drug Users." Paper presented at the 5th International Conference on AIDS, June 4–9, Montreal.

Piot, P., and M. Caraël. 1988. "Epidemiological and Sociological Aspects of HIV-Infection in Developing Countries." *British Medical Bulletin* 44:68–88.

Piot, P., and K. K. Holmes. 1989. "Sexually Transmitted Diseases." In K. Warren and A. Mahmoud, eds., *Tropical and Geographical Medicine*. New York: McGraw-Hill.

Piot, P., J. K. Kreiss, J. O. Ndinya-Achola, E. N. Ngugi, J. N. Simonsen, D. W. Cameron, H. Taelman, and F. A. Plummer. 1987. "Heterosexual Transmission of HIV." *AIDS* 1:199–206.

Piot, P., M. Laga, R. Ryder, J. Perriens, M. Temmerman, W. Heward, and J. W. Curran. 1990. "The Global Epidemiology of HIV Infection: Continuity, Heterogeneity, and Change." *Journal of AIDS* 3:403–11.

Piot, P., and A. Z. Meheus. 1983. "Epidémiologie des maladies sexuellement transmissibles dans les pays en développement." *Annales de la Société belge de Médecine Tropicale* 63:87–110.

Piot, P., F. A. Plummer, F. S. Mhalu, J. L. Lamboray, J. Chin, and J. M. Mann. 1988. "AIDS: An International Perspective." *Science* 239:573–79.

Plummer, F. A., M. Laga, R. C. Brunham, P. Piot, A. R. Ronald, V. Bhullar, J. Y. Mati, J. O. Achola, M. Cheang, and H. Nzanze. 1987. "Postpartum Upper Genital Tract Infections in Nairobi, Kenya: Epidemiology, Etiology, and Risk Factors." *Journal of Infectious Diseases* 156:92–97.

Plummer, F. A., H. Nsanze, P. Karasina, L. J. D'Costa, J. Dylewski, and A. R. Ronald. 1983. "Epidemiology of Chancroid and *Haemophilus ducreyi* in Nairobi." *Lancet* 2:1293–95.

Plummer, F. A., J. N. Simonsen, D. W. Cameron, J. O. Ndinya-Achola, J. K. Kreiss, M. N. Galeinya, P. Waiyaki, M. Cheang, P. Piot, A. R. Ronald, and E. N. Ngugi. 1991. "Co-factors in Male-Female Sexual Transmission of Human Immunodeficiency Virus Type 1." *Journal of Infectious Diseases* 163:233–39.

Pokrovski, V. V., I. Eramova, V. Arzamastsev, V. Nikonova, and G. Mozharova. 1990. "Epidemiological Surveillance for HIV-Infection in the USSR in 1987–1989." Paper presented at the 6th International Conference on AIDS, June 20–23, San Francisco.

Population Information Program. 1983. "Infertility and Sexually Transmitted Diseases: A Public Health Challenge." *Population Reports* 4.

Rajan, V. S. 1978. "Sexually Transmitted Diseases on a Tropical Island." *British Journal of Venereal Diseases* 54:141–43.

Ratnam, A. V., S. N. Din, S. K. Hira, G. J. Bhat, D. S. Wacha, A. Rukmini, and R. C. Mulenga. 1982. "Syphilis in Pregnant Women in Zambia." *British Journal of Venereal Diseases* 58:355–58.

Reeves, W. C., L. A. Brinton, and M. M. Brenes. 1985. "Case Control Study of Cervical Cancer in Herrera Province, Republic of Panama." *International Journal of Cancer* 36:55–60.

Reeves, W. C., W. E. Rawls, and L. A. Brinton. 1989. "Epidemiology of Genital Papilloma Viruses and Cervical Cancer." *Reviews of Infectious Diseases* 11:426–39.

Reining, P. 1972. "Haya Kinship Terminology: An Explanation and Some Comparison." In P. Reining, ed., *Kinship Studies in the Morgan Centennial Year*. Washington, D.C.: Anthropological Society of Washington.

Rosenberg, M. J., K. F. Schultz, and N. Burton. 1986. "Sexually Transmitted Diseases in Sub-Saharan Africa." *Lancet* 2:152–53.

Rothenberg, R. B. 1983. "The Geography of Gonorrhea: Empirical Demonstration of Core Group Transmission," *American Journal of Epidemiology* 117:688–94.

Rothenberg, R. B., and J. J. Potterat. 1988. "Temporal and Social Aspects of Gonorrhea Transmission: The Force of Infectivity." *Sexually Transmitted Diseases* 15:88–92.

Rwandan Seroprevalence Study Group. 1989. "Nationwide Community-Based Survey of HIV-1 and Other Human Retrovirus Infections in a Central African Country." *Lancet* 1:947–49.

Ryder, R. W., and F. S. Mhalu. 1988. "Blood Transfusion and AIDS in the Tropics." In P. Piot and J. M. Mann, eds., *AIDS and HIV Infection in the Tropics*. London: Baillière-Tyndall.

Ryder, R. W., M. Ndilu, S. E. Hassig, M. Kamenga, D. Sequeira, M. Kashamuka, H. Francis, F. Behets, R. L. Colebunders, A. Dopagne, R. Kambale, and W. L. Heyward. 1990. "Heterosexual Transmission of HIV-1 among Employees and Their Spouses at Two Large Businesses in Zaire." *AIDS* 4:725–32.

Ryder, R. W., W. Nsa, S. Hassig, M. Rayfield, B. Ekungola, A. M. Nelson, U. Mulenda, H. Francis, and K. Mwangagalirur. 1989. "Perinatal Transmission of HIV-1 to Infant of Seropositive Women in Zaire." *New England Journal of Medicine* 320:1637–42.

Ryder, R. W., and P. Piot. 1988. "Epidemiology of HIV Infection in Africa." In P. Piot and J. M. Mann, eds., *AIDS and HIV Infection in the Tropics*. London: Baillière-Tyndall.

Scitovsky, A., and Mead Over. 1988. "AIDS: Costs of Care in the Developed and the Developing World." *AIDS* 2(supplement 1):S71–S81.

Senyonyi, F. 1987. "Prévalence des infections gynécologiques à *Chlamydia trachomatis* et à *Neisseria gonorrhoeae* chez 199 femmes examinées en consultations prénatales ou en consultations pour planning familial à Kigali et à Kabgayi." *Revue Médicale Rwandaise* 19:85–89.

Simonsen, J. N., D. W. Cameron, M. N. Gakinya, J. O. Ndinya-Achola, L. J. D'Costa, P. Karasira, M. Cheang, A. R. Ronald, P. Piot, and F. A. Plummer. 1988. "Human Immunodeficiency Virus Infection among Men with Sexually Transmitted Diseases." *New England Journal of Medicine* 319:274–78.

Singh, Y. N., A. N. Malaviya, S. P. Tripathy, K. Chaudhuri, S. D. Khare, A. Nanu, and R. Bhasin. 1990. "Human Immunodeficiency Virus Infection in the Blood Donors of Delhi, India." *Journal of Acquired Immune Deficiency Syndrome* 3(2):152–54.

Sittitrai, W. 1990. "Outreach to Bar Workers in Bangkok." *Hygie* 9(4):25–28.

Sparling, P. F. 1990. "Natural History of Syphilis." In K. K. Holmes, P.-A. Mårdh, P. F. Sparling, and P. J. Wiesner, eds., *Sexually transmitted diseases*. McGraw-Hill, New York.

Spencer, Nancy, C. Raevsky, and F. Wolf. 1989. "Results and Benefit-Cost Analysis of Provider-Assisted HIV Partner Notification and Referral." Abstract WAO21 in International Development Research Centre, 5 *International Conference on AIDS: The Scientific and Social Challenge*. Montreal, Canada. June:6–7.

Standaert, B., F. Niragira, P. Kadende, and P. Piot. 1989. "The Association of Tuberculosis and HIV Infection in Burundi." *AIDS Research and Human Retroviruses* 5:247–51.

Stanley, E. A., S. T. Seity, P. O. Way, P. D. Johnson, and T. F. Curry. 1989. "The Iwg AIDS Model for the Heterosexual Spread of HIV and the Demographic Impact of the AIDS Epidemic." Paper prepared for the UN/WHO Workshop on Modeling the Demographic Impact of the AIDS Epidemic in Pattern II Countries, Los Alamos National Laboratories, December, Los Alamos, N.M.

Stray-Pedersen, B. 1983. "Economic Evaluation of Maternal Screening to Prevent Congenital Syphilis." *Sexually Transmitted Diseases* 10:167–72.

Tapia, R., and A. Martin. 1990. "The Cost of AIDS in Mexico." Paper presented at the 6th International Conference on AIDS, June 20–23, San Francisco.

Temmerman, M., M. Laga, J. O. Ndinya-Achola, M. Paraskevas, R. C. Brunham, F. A. Plummer, and P. Piot. 1988. "Aetiology of Postpartum Endometritis in Nairobi, Kenya." *Genitourinary Medicine* 64:172–75.

Temmerman, M., N. Mirza, F. Plummer, J. O. Ndinya-Achola, I. Wamola, and P. Piot. 1989. "HIV Infection as a Risk Factor for Poor Obstetrical Outcome." Paper presented at the 5th International Conference on AIDS, June 4–9, Montreal.

Temmerman, M., S. Moses, D. Kiragu, S. Fussallah, I. Wamola, and P. Piot. 1990. "Impact of Single Session Postpartum Counseling of HIV Infected Women on Their Subsequent Reproductive Behavior." *AIDS Care* 2:247–52.

Temmerman, M., F. A. Plummer, N. B. Mirza, J. O. Ndinya-Achola, I. A. Wamola, N. Nagelkerke, R. C. Brunham, and P. Piot. 1990. "Infection with Human Immunodeficiency Virus as a Risk Factor for Adverse Obstetrical Outcome." *AIDS* 4:1087–93.

Toomey, K. E., and W. Cates, Jr. 1989. "Partner Notification for the Prevention of HIV Infection." *AIDS* 3(Supplement 1):S57–S62.

Tuliza, M., A. T. Manoka, N. Nzila, W. Way, M. St. Louis, P. Piot, and M. Laga. 1991. "The Impact of STD Control and Condom Promotion on the Incidence of HIV in Kinshasa Prostitutes." Paper presented at the 7th International Conference on AIDS, June 16–21, Florence.

United Kingdom, National Health Service. 1988. "AIDS Prevention through Health Promotion: The U.K. Experience at National Level." Health Education Authority, London.

U.S. Bureau of the Census. 1991. "Recent HIV Seroprevalence Levels by Country: February 1991." Washington, D.C.: Research Notes 3, Health Studies Branch, Center for International Research.

Urquhart, J. 1979. "Effect of the Venereal Disease Epidemic on the Incidence of Ectopic Pregnancy—Implications for the Evaluation of Contraceptives." *Contraception* 19:455–80.

Ursi, J. P., E. Van Dyck, C. Van Houtte, P. Piot, J. Colaert, M. Dlamini, and A. Z. Meheus. 1981. "Syphilis in Swaziland: A Serological Survey." *British Journal of Venereal Diseases* 57:95–99.

Valleroy, L. A., J. R. Harris, and P. O. Way. 1990. "The Impact of HIV-1 Infection on Child Survival in the Developing World." *AIDS* 4:667–72.

Van de Perre, P., M. Caraël, D. Nzaramba, G. Zissis, J. Kayihigi, and J.-P. Butzler. 1987. "Risk Factors for HIV Seropositivity in Selected Urban-Based Rwandese Adults." *AIDS* 1:207–11.

van Griensven, G. J. P., E. M. M. de Vnoome, J. Goudsmit, and R. A. Coutinho. 1989. "Changes in Sexual Behavior and the Fall in Incidence of HIV Infection among Homosexual Men." *British Medical Journal* 298:218–21.

Warner, K. E. 1983. "Bags, Buckles, and Belts: The Debate over Mandatory Passive Restraints in Automobiles." *Journal of Health Politics, Policy, and Law* 8(1):44–75.

Washington, A. E., P. S. Arno, and M. A. Brooks. 1986. "The Economic Cost of Pelvic Inflammatory Disease." *JAMA* 255:1735–38.

Washington, A. E., W. S. Browner, and C. C. Korenbrot. 1987. "Cost-Effectiveness of Combined Treatment for Endocervical Gonorrhea Considering Co-infection with *Chlamydia trachomatis*." *JAMA* 257:2056–60.

Washington, A. E., R. E. Johnson, and L. H. Sanders. 1987. "*Chlamydia trachomatis* Infections in the United States. What Are They Costing Us?" *JAMA* 257:2070–72.

Wasserheit, J. N. 1989. "The Significance and Scope of Reproductive Tract Infections among Third World Women." *International Journal of Gynecology and Obstetrics* 3(supplement):145–68.

Way, Peter W., and K. Stanecki. 1991. "The Demographic Impact of an AIDS Epidemic on an African Country: Application of the Iwg AIDS Model." CIR Staff Paper 58. U.S. Bureau of Census, Center for International Research, Washington, D.C.

Weström, L. 1975. "Effect of Acute Pelvic Inflammatory Disease on Infertility." *American Journal of Obstetrics and Gynecology* 121:707–13.

———. 1980. "Incidence, Prevalence, and Trends of Acute Pelvic Inflammatory Disease and Its Consequences in Industrialized Countries." *American Journal of Obstetrics and Gynecology* 138:880–92.

Weström, L., I. Serafim, L. Svensson, and P-.A. Mårdh. 1979. "Infertility after Acute Salpingitis: Results of Treatment with Different Antibiotics." *Current Therapeutic Research*, 26:752–59.

Williams, Eka, N. Hearst, and O. Ndofia. 1989. "Sexual Practices and HIV Infection of Female Prostitutes in Nigeria," Abstract WAO 24 in International Development Researach Centre, 5 *International Conference on AIDS: The Scientific and Social Challenge*. Montreal, Canada. June 1985, 985.

Wilson, David and Amir Mehryar. 1981. "The Role of AIDS Knowledge, Attitudes, Beliefs and Practices Research in Sub-Saharan Africa." *AIDS* 5:S177–S81.

WHO (World Health Organization). 1978. "*Neisseria gonorrhoeae* and Gonococcal Infections." Technical Report 616. Geneva.

———. 1985a. "Control of Sexually Transmitted Diseases." Geneva.

———. 1985b. "Simplified Approaches for Sexually Transmitted Diseases (STD) Control at the Primary Health Care (PHC) Level." WHO/VDT/85.437. Geneva.

———. 1989a. "Consensus Statement on STDs as Risk Factors for HIV Transmission." WHO/GPA/1989-1. Geneva.

———. 1989b. "STD Treatment Strategies." WHO/VDT/89.447. Geneva.

———. 1991a. "Global Programme on AIDS Update, AIDS Cases Reported to Surveillance Forecasting and Impact Assessment Unit." Mimeo. Geneva.

———. 1991b. "Management of Patients with Sexually Transmitted Diseases." WHO Technical Report 810, World Health Organization, Geneva.

World Bank. 1989. *World Development Report*. Baltimore: Johns Hopkins University Press.

Yorke, J. A., H. W. Hethcote, and A. Nold. 1978. "Dynamics and Control of the Transmission of Gonorrhea." *Sexually Transmitted Diseases* 5:51–56.

Yvert, F., J. Y. Riou, E. Frost, and B. Ivanoff. 1984. "Les infections gonococciques au Gabon (Haut Ogooué)." *Pathologie Biologie* 32:80–84.

Zachariah, K. C., and M. T. Vu. 1988. *World Population Projections*. World Bank, Washington, D.C.

Ziegler, J. B., D. A. Cooper, R. D. Johnson, and J. Gold. 1985. "Postnatal Transmission of AIDS-Associated Retrovirus from Mother to Infant." *Lancet* 1:896.

21

Cancers

Howard Barnum and E. Robert Greenberg

Human cancer consists of more than 100 distinct diseases, each defined by its anatomic site of origin and microscopic features (cell type). The two characteristics shared by all cancers are the uncontrolled proliferation of cells and their invasion into other tissues. Cancers differ, however, in their clinical features. Some, such as esophageal cancer, progress rapidly, are relatively intractable to treatment, and are almost uniformly fatal. Others, chronic lymphocytic leukemia, for example, usually follow an indolent course and may persist for decades with little morbidity.

Cancers differ also in their etiology. As a consequence, individual cancer types tend to have distinct epidemiological features, preferentially affecting particular populations as defined by geography, culture, and personal habits. For example, cervical cancer occurs more often in the developing world and among women with low income and a history of many pregnancies. In contrast, breast cancer tends to strike more affluent women who live in industrial countries and have a history of fewer or no pregnancies (Kelsey and Hildreth 1983).

An analysis of the health policy implications of cancer can therefore not proceed very far using an aggregate concept of cancer because aggregation obscures important details of cause and potential interventions. Two countries can have the same aggregate rate of occurrence of cancer but need to employ very different types of intervention. The discussion that follows uses a level of disaggregation that distinguishes the ten most important cancers in the developing world and considers their individual etiological and clinical characteristics.

The focus of this chapter is the implications of cancer epidemiology for health policy in developing countries. A common notion is that cancer is primarily a disease of industrial countries, occurring late in life as a consequence of affluent lifestyle. It thus is felt to be not important in developing countries, where the focus should be on infectious diseases and childhood. There are good reasons why cancer deserves attention, however. First, several important cancers, including stomach and liver cancer, occur most often in poorer countries (Stjernsward and others 1985; Parkin, Laara, and Muir 1988). Second, some low-income and middle-income countries, such as China, Sri Lanka, Malaysia, and Brazil, have reduced fertility and causes of infant and childhood death, and the relative

importance of cancer has increased as the age structure of the population has changed (see, for example, Bumgarner 1992). Third, once an individual is past the hurdle of childhood diseases, cancer looms as one of the three largest causes of death (the other two being accidents and cardiovascular diseases) even in the lowest-income countries of Africa and Asia (Stjernsward and others 1985). Last, changing demographics and increasing tobacco consumption virtually ensure that an epidemic of lung cancer will occur in many developing countries during the next century (Stanley 1986). It is important to act now to prevent tobacco use rather than to wait until the epidemic is manifest.

Despite its importance in adult mortality, cancer has not been considered in shaping health policy in most developing countries. The discussion that follows provides a brief survey of the epidemiology of cancer and gives suggestions for incorporating cancer planning in health policy. The appendix provides a review of the salient characteristics of ten of the most important cancers and the environmental, behavioral, physiological, and occupational circumstances—collectively referred to as risk factors—that have been associated with their occurrence.

Public Health Importance

Accurate information on cancer occurrence (mortality and incidence rates) and on the prevalence of risk factors is essential in assessing the public health importance of cancer and in planning control strategies.

Data Sources

Determination of cancer mortality rates primarily requires a reliable system of death registration and accurate demographic data and thus can be accomplished within the context of mortality measurement for other diseases. Determination of cancer incidence is best achieved through specialized tumor registries (Waterhouse and others 1976). These require an effort directed toward cancer, and in their absence cancer incidence may be approximated by applying estimated case-fatality rates to cancer mortality data (Parkin, Laara, and Muir

1988). The prevalence of risk factors is measured by surveys employing questionnaires or by direct measurement of physical and biochemical characteristics.

Countries vary greatly in the availability and reliability of their cancer data (Muir and Nectoux 1982). This fact largely reflects the limited resources devoted to the measurement of vital statistics by many governments in the developing world. Also, the reliability of cancer data depends on coding practices (Percy and Muir 1989), on the level of medical care, and on the availability and quality of diagnostic procedures. Cancer incidence and mortality rates are likely to be underestimated in countries in which people have little access to high-technology medical care. Although some excellent tumor registries have been established in several low-income countries (Muir and others 1988), they cover cancer incidence in only a minor fraction of the developing world. There also are large gaps in the international data on cancer mortality rates (Kurihara, Aoki, and Tominaga 1984). Thus, the incidence and mortality rates quoted here must be interpreted with the realization that there are severe deficiencies in cancer data.

Global Epidemiology

Cancer accounts for approximately 8.5 percent of the 51 million deaths occurring in the world each year (Hakulinen and others 1986). Of the estimated 4.3 million cancer deaths, more than half (2.5 million) occur in developing countries. In relation to other causes of death, however, cancer seems less important in these countries, in which it accounts for approximately 5.5 percent of all deaths, well below those due to infections (40 percent), circulatory diseases (19 percent), and perinatal events (8 percent). In most industrial countries cancer accounts for approximately 20 percent of deaths, second only to circulatory diseases (about 50 to 55 percent).

There are four principal reasons for the relatively lower importance of cancer as a cause of death in developing countries. One is the continued high death toll from infectious and parasitic conditions that have been largely eliminated as causes of death in the industrial countries. A second reason is that the age structure of the populations of most developing countries is heavily weighted toward young children. Cancer occurs most frequently among older adults, and this group accounts for a small percentage of the populations of these countries. The third reason is that aggregate cancer risks are truly lower in many (though not all) developing countries. Among countries such as Cuba and Costa Rica, age-adjusted cancer mortality rates are approximately one-third to two-thirds less than in typical heavily industrialized countries (Kurihara, Aoki, and Tominaga 1984). Many of these differences, however, are accounted for by lower rates of lung cancer and other tobacco-associated cancers, and the picture is complicated considerably when we consider other cancers, such as those of the stomach and liver. Last, cancers are more likely to be unrecognized in populations with less access to advanced diagnostic facilities, so the actual effect of cancer is underestimated.

In the near future, cancer will become increasingly important in developing countries. Improved sanitation and im-

munization should lead to better control of infectious diseases, decreasing deaths from these causes. Declining fertility and reduced infant and childhood mortality will eventually shift population age structures from a pyramidal to a more columnar pattern (with a greater proportion of older adults, whose risk of cancer is higher). In addition, tobacco use is increasing in many developing countries, and increases in cancer will undoubtedly follow (Crofton 1984; Stanley 1986).

The pattern of cancer occurrence now differs greatly between developing and industrial countries. In industrial countries, most cancer deaths are due to tumors of the lung, colorectum, breast, prostate, and pancreas. In developing countries the main causes of cancer death are tumors of the stomach, esophagus, lung, liver, and cervix (Parkin, Laara, and Muir 1988). In table 21-1 we provide estimates of numbers of deaths and new cases for the ten most frequent cancers in developing countries.[1] Note that the relative importance of these cancers differs depending on whether one focuses on deaths or new cases. This is because cancers of the lung, stomach, and esophagus are almost invariably fatal, whereas prolonged survival and cure are common for breast, oral, and cervical cancer cases.

The degree of industrial development is an unreliable guide to the pattern of cancer occurrence in a given country. For example, although esophageal cancer is generally more frequent in developing countries, its incidence is also high in northwestern France and parts of eastern Europe (Ghadirian, Thouez, and Simard 1988). Similarly, stomach cancer is common not only in developing countries but also in Japan, where it is the leading cause of cancer death (Kurihara, Aoki, and Tominaga 1984). The occurrence of most cancers actually appears to be determined by factors (such as tobacco consumption, diet, and reproductive practices) that are related only indirectly to industrial development (Doll and Peto 1981).

Accordingly, statements about the cause and prevention of cancer in the developing world (considered as a whole) may not be applicable to all developing countries. Policies to address the cancer problem must be formulated on a country-by-

Table 21-1. Estimated Annual Deaths and New Cases of Ten Most Important Cancers in the Developing World, 1980
(thousands)

Site or type of cancer	Deaths	New cases
Stomach	280	336
Esophagus	231	254
Lung	187	206
Liver	174	192
Cervix	154	370
Colon/rectum	108	183
Mouth/pharynx	101	272
Breast	97	224
Lymphoma	81	122
Leukemia	81	106

Note: Excludes skin cancers.
Source: Parkin, Laara, and Muir 1988.

country basis, taking into account particular features of cancer occurrence and the prevalence of particular risk factors in each population. Clearly, reliable country-specific data will be crucial to this process.

Time Trends in Cancer Occurrence

There is relatively little information on cancer trends in developing countries themselves, and one must try to draw parallels from industrial countries that have a longer history of collecting cancer incidence and mortality data. Over the past fifty years, the most striking changes in cancer occurrence in many of these countries have been increasing rates of lung cancer and falling rates of cancers of the stomach and uterine cervix (Kurihara, Aoki, and Tominaga 1984; Stanley, Stjernsward, and Koroltchouk 1988). The profound increase in lung cancer is almost entirely attributable to tobacco use, which became prevalent (in the United States and western Europe) early in this century (Doll and Peto 1981). There has also been a smaller increase in other tumors, such as bladder cancer, that are related to tobacco use but not as strongly as is lung cancer. The fall in uterine cervical cancer deaths is not fully understood (Knox 1982). Possible contributing factors, besides Pap testing, include changes in sexual practices, improved genital hygiene, and increased frequency of hysterectomy (removing the uterus removes the risk of cervical cancer). Reasons for declines in stomach cancer mortality in developing countries are uncertain (Stanley, Stjernsward, and Koroltchouk 1988). A plausible explanation is that diets have improved and consumption of spoiled or mold-contaminated food (due to better food storage and refrigeration) is thus lower (Bjelke 1982). Also, increased consumption of antioxidants (as food additives and vitamin C) may have contributed to the decline. Lastly, reduced rates of infection with *Helicobacter pylori*, a pathogenic bacterium implicated in gastric carcinogenesis, may have resulted from better sanitation in industrial countries (Correa 1992).

Within the industrial countries there has been little change during the last several decades in deaths due to cancers of the breast (Stanley, Stjernsward, and Koroltchouk 1988) and colon (Boyle, Zaridze, and Smans 1985). Reported increases in some countries of breast cancer and pancreatic cancer are difficult to interpret because there have been improvements in diagnostic capabilities and greater efforts to find cancer, particularly among the elderly. A modest decline in large bowel cancer mortality in some industrial countries also cannot be easily explained, although dietary changes (Boyle, Zaridze, and Smans 1985) or earlier diagnosis and improved treatment may be partly responsible.

In North America and western Europe, mortality from childhood leukemia and lymphoma has fallen dramatically. This observation is attributable to improved treatment methods developed during the past thirty years through a massive investment in cancer research (Miller and Mckay 1984). In countries such as the United States, however, decreases in cancer deaths achieved by improved treatment of leukemia, lymphoma, and other, uncommon, cancers have been offset by

increases in deaths from tobacco-associated cancers (Bailar and Smith 1986). These latter cancer deaths are occurring as a result of tobacco smoking initiated decades in the past.

Will these changes be repeated in the developing countries? Tobacco-associated cancers are certain to increase in countries where tobacco use has risen. Cancers of the breast and colorectum are also likely to increase in populations that adopt the reproductive patterns and diet of more industrialized countries. A drop in the occurrence of stomach cancer seems likely in countries in which diets have come to include more fresh fruits and vegetables and fewer spoiled foods. Changes in sexual practices may lead to declines in cervical cancer. Changes in health care and hygienic practices could lead to a reduction in hepatitis and, hence, liver cancer. In the absence of direct intervention, however, these favorable changes are apt to occur gradually, and increases in lung, colorectal, and breast cancer may offset declines in stomach, liver, and cervical cancer.

The Current Burden of Cancer

The total economic cost of cancer to society can be conveniently partitioned into indirect and direct costs. The indirect cost is the cost to society from the loss of productive life, and the direct cost is the value of the resources (including those used for health sector services) required by cancer. The proportional split of total cost between these two categories varies considerably by disease. In a study by Rice, Hodgson, and Kopstein (1985) of the cost of disease in the United States for 1980, direct costs for cancer were only 26 percent of total cost, and the remainder was composed of the indirect costs of morbidity (11 percent) and mortality (63 percent). Only injuries, at 23 percent, had direct costs that were a lower percentage of the total. For comparison, the direct costs of diseases of the genitourinary system were 80 percent. The importance of indirect costs of cancer is attributable to the high case-fatality rates for cancers and the fact that in the developing countries cancer primarily affects people during their productive years (albeit often relatively late in life).

Although morbidity and mortality rates, and therefore the total costs of cancer, vary considerably on a global basis, with a few exceptions, the parameters determining the proportional importance of indirect cost per case do not vary markedly between countries. In figures 21-1, 21-2, and 21-3, respectively, we show the age-specific mortality rates for lung cancer, liver cancer, and stomach cancer in China and the United States. As for most cancer, the force of mortality is highest late in life. Leukemia (shown in figure 21-4) is a notable exception, with appreciable mortality occurring earlier in life.

A general measure of the burden of specific cancers is given by calculation of years of life lost (YLL), measured as the difference between the age of death for victims of the disease in comparison with life expectancy. In table 21-2 we give the average YLL per case and the total number of years lost out of a population of 1 million for eight main cancers in a prototypical developing country. In order of total burden, cervical, breast, and stomach cancers are the most important for women, and

Figure 21-1. Age-Specific Mortality for Cancer in China and the United States

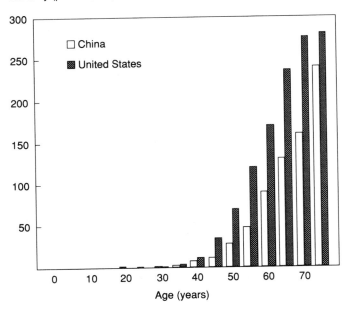

Source: China: unpublished Disease Surveillance Point data 1986; U.S.: National Institutes of Health 1988.

Figure 21-2. Age-Specific Mortality for Liver Cancer in China and the United States

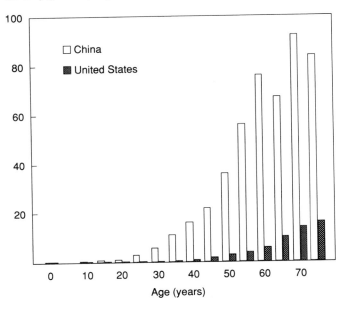

Source: China: unpublished Disease Surveillance Point data 1986; U.S.: National Institutes of Health 1988.

Figure 21-3. Age-Specific Mortality for Stomach Cancer in China and the United States

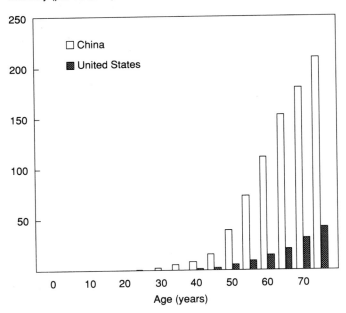

Source: China: unpublished Disease Surveillance Point data 1986; U.S.: National Institutes of Health 1988.

Figure 21-4. Age-Specific Mortality for Leukemia in China and the United States

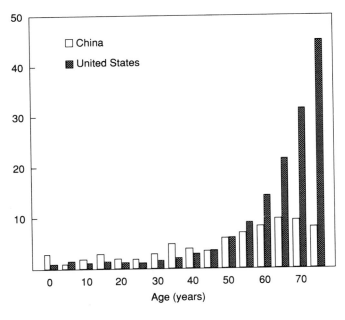

Source: China: unpublished Disease Surveillance Point data 1986; U.S.: National Institutes of Health 1988.

Table 21-2. Average Years of Life Lost from Premature Mortality from Cancer in Developing Countries

Site or type of cancer	Average age at death		Average years of life lost per death		Years of life lost per million population[a]		Total
	Male	Female	Male	Female	Male	Female	
Stomach	64	62	16	18	853	561	1,414
Liver	56	57	22	22	814	312	1,126
Esophagus	65	65	16	16	714	402	1,116
Leukemia	32	34	42	41	599	418	1,016
Lung	63	66	17	15	721	210	931
Cervix	n.a.	61	n.a.	18	n.a.	837	837
Colon/rectum	61	60	18	20	313	304	617
Breast	n.a.	57	n.a.	22	n.a.	645	645
Total	59	58	20	21	6,611	5,906	12,517

n.a. Not applicable.
a. Based on population distribution, incidence, and case-fatality rates.
Source: Parkin, Laara, and Muir 1988.

stomach, liver, lung, and esophageal cancers are of primary concern for men.

Prevention

A large number of primary and secondary prevention activities have been proposed for control of cancer mortality. These activities vary greatly, however, in their cost and potential effectiveness as part of a national cancer strategy. A considerable literature has emerged that discusses causes of cancer and the effectiveness, hazards, and (to a regrettably lesser extent) the costs of preventive activities. Most of this literature has been oriented toward industrial countries, but some general conclusions apply in the developing world. In the next two subsections we discuss the implications of current knowledge of cancer risks for primary and secondary prevention programs in developing countries.

Primary Prevention

Primary preventive activities are designed to lessen exposure to risk factors. The main potential risk factors identified for intervention include tobacco consumption, food, alcohol, infections, environmental and occupational chemicals, and radiation (Doll and Peto 1981). Evaluation of the potential usefulness of alternative interventions has several components: (a) the importance of targeted cancers and the prevalence of targeted risk factors in individual countries must be established by surveillance; (b) the technical effectiveness of specific interventions is being explored in experiments in industrial countries, but little is known about the ease of transferring the results of these experiments to other countries; (c) the feasibility of preventive activities, even though they may be technically effective, is impeded by the practical difficulty of altering underlying behavior and customs, interfering in production or consumption processes, and managing large-scale preventive campaigns; and (d) prevention activities must compete with other resource uses, and the cost of the activities

is an important determinant of their competitiveness. Thus, the relative potential of preventive interventions is dependent on the ranking of the targeted cancer as a cause of lost life and economic productivity, the technical effectiveness of the intervention, the feasibility of implementing the primary prevention activity, and the cost per person covered by the activity. These factors are considered in the specific interventions discussed below.

PROGRAMS TO REDUCE TOBACCO CONSUMPTION. A clear causal relationship is established between tobacco consumption and many cancers, including tumors of the lung, mouth, upper respiratory and digestive tracts, kidney and urinary tract, and other sites, with the most important link being to lung cancer (USDHHS 1982; IARC 1986). The many cancer deaths attributable to tobacco consumption mark antitobacco programs for special consideration among cancer prevention activities. In Europe and North America the dramatic increase in lung cancer in the last thirty years has made it the leading cause of cancer mortality and one of the main causes of death. The increase has been firmly linked to earlier changes in smoking behavior. Because of formerly low levels of cigarette consumption, lung cancer has been a relatively less important cause of death in developing countries, but as life expectancy and smoking prevalence increase, lung cancer and other smoking-related causes of death are becoming more important. Additionally, chewing tobacco, especially betel nut chewing in India, has long been an important cause of oral cancer (WHO 1984).

Studies of the hazards of tobacco consumption have included examinations of the difference in risk for alternative forms of consumption (cigarettes, pipes, cigar), dose (daily number of cigarettes, tar and nicotine content, and method of ingestion), and duration (age started or years of habit [Peto 1986]). The risk of lung cancer for those who smoke approximately one to ten cigarettes per day is three to five times greater than for nonsmokers; for those who smoke one pack (twenty cigarettes) the relative risk is seven to nine times greater; and for two packs, nine to twenty-five times greater. Smokers who report that they do not inhale nevertheless have a risk four to eight times that of nonsmokers.

A striking aspect of the link between smoking and cancer is that duration of smoking appears to be more important than daily dose in determining lung cancer risk. For example, in one summary of the literature the author concludes that "a three-fold increase in the daily dose-rate may produce only about a three-fold increase in effect, while a three-fold increase in duration might produce about a 100-fold increase in effect" (Peto 1986 p. 23). The effect of duration of the smoking habit on lung cancer is crucial in assessing past trends of cancer in industrial countries and in projecting the future effect of cancer in developing countries. Current high rates of lung cancer in industrial countries result from a high percentage of the population that started smoking at an early age and continued to smoke for several decades. Cultural and social changes in developing countries are lowering the starting age for smoking, increasing the duration of smoking, and increasing the percentage of the population that smokes.

Tobacco consumption is increasing in developing countries at the same time that it is leveling off or decreasing in the industrial world (Crofton 1984). Between 1980 and 1986, consumption increased at an average of 5.4 percent per year in developing countries. The percentage of the population that smokes is higher in many developing countries, but per capita consumption tends to be greater in higher-income countries (IARC 1986). Rising per capita income, however, is expected to increase per capita tobacco consumption, and this effect is greater for lower-income countries. A 10 percent increase in per capita income can be expected to create a 7 percent increase in tobacco consumption in middle-income countries and more than a 13 percent increase in lower-income countries.[2] Thus, it is clear that, unless preventive measures are taken, tobacco consumption will continue to increase as development proceeds in developing countries.

Although the current pool of smokers will inevitably generate more lung cancer in the future, even greater increases can be avoided by preventing starts. Possible components for prevention programs include prohibiting cigarette advertising, requiring warning labels on cigarette packages, using anti-smoking advertising, instituting educational programs in schools and in work groups, banning tobacco smoke from workplaces and public areas, increasing the price of tobacco products through special taxes, and finally (with limited effectiveness) decreasing the carcinogenic content of cigarette smoke through tobacco processing and filters.

Most of these program components involve behavioral change, so their feasibility is highly dependent on the cultural context in which they are carried out. In addition, the numerous elements in a smoking prevention program require national coordination, monitoring, and motivation (Mackay 1989). The feasibility of an effective program is thus apt to vary considerably across developing countries. Some encouragement can be taken from the moderate success in reducing smoking in the United States during the last twenty years,

despite the relatively loose social structure and limited government ability to produce behavioral change. The United States effort has benefited from effective national coordination provided by the Surgeon General's office and the Office of Smoking and Health in the Department of Health and Human Services. Progress has been retarded, however, by agricultural and commercial interests within and outside government. Thus, a full national program to contain tobacco consumption in a given country would also likely involve several ministries directly, notably the education and health ministries, and would need to be coordinated through a special agency or committee to ensure interagency cooperation.

The cost of an antismoking program is difficult to estimate but is probably not great; implementation is more a matter of political and social will than specific costly activities. The primary cost of a basic antismoking education program is that of organizing and supplying an informational effort. An information campaign could include warnings of the adverse health consequences of smoking on cigarette packets; antismoking messages in posters, billboards, newspapers, and on the radio; information dissemination through the health system; and school programs. Cost items would include advertising expense; short-term training courses and seminars for health professionals, teachers, and local leaders; and supervision and management. The cost would be dependent on the available infrastructure for information and education dissemination and on the scale of the program. Some estimate of the cost can be made from examination of other programs that use informational campaigns to bring about behavioral change. On the basis of the cost of training programs and information and education activities in several World Bank projects, the cost per capita could vary between 0.005 and 0.025 percent of the annual gross national product per capita (GNPN) in a typical low-income country.[3]

A particularly important problem for antitobacco programs is that tobacco, because of its nicotine content, produces a strong consumption dependence that must be recognized in prevention strategies. For this reason it seems more feasible, and less costly, to prevent new starts than to convert those who have already developed a dependence.[4] The beneficial effects of an antismoking campaign would be to prevent new smokers from starting, to convert previous smokers to nonsmoking status, to convert some smokers to the use of low-tar cigarettes, and to reduce passive smoking. It is possible to use a few plausible and simple assumptions from available information to demonstrate the low cost per unit of effect in preventing new starters and encouraging smoking cessation in a hypothetical low-mortality population of 1 million.

Out of 1 million people with a smoking prevalence of 0.5 among the adult male population and 0.2 among adult females, the annual number of new starters is estimated to be 8,307 (6,390 men and 1,917 women). Of these, approximately 25 percent will die from causes attributable to smoking, and the average age of death will be fifty-five years, resulting in a premature loss of thirteen years of life for each smoking-induced male death and sixteen years for each female death. The total

Table 21-3. Cost per Year of Life Gained from an Antismoking Campaign, as a Function of Smoking Starts Averted

(percent of per capita GNP)

Program cost per capita (percent GNPN)	Proportion of new smoking starts averted		
	0.10	0.25	0.50
0.005	1.8	0.7	0.4
0.010	3.5	1.4	0.7
0.015	5.3	2.1	1.1
0.020	7.0	2.8	1.4

Note: For a hypothetical program. Information for the United States indicates that 25 percent of smokers will die from smoking-attributed causes (50 percent from coronary, 20 percent from cancer, and 15 percent each from cerebrovascular and pulmonary diseases. When weighted across YLL per death by cause, there is an average of thirteen YLL for men and sixteen YLL for women. The total years of life lost from all smoking starts is 28,435 per million persons in the absence of any intervention program.

Source: Authors.

years of life lost will be 28,000. If a national smoking campaign, costing 0.01 percent GNPN per person could have prevented 50 percent of new starts, the cost per year of life gained (YLG) would have been 0.7 percent GNPN. Obviously, this is a low cost for such a significant benefit.

The cost of an antismoking campaign per YLG is sensitive to the program cost per capita and the efficiency of the program measured as the proportion of new starts averted. In table 21-3 we give the cost-effectiveness of an antismoking campaign under several alternative assumptions. Even under adverse assumptions—a cost per capita of 0.02 percent GNPN and an efficiency of only 0.10 of new starts averted—the program remains relatively inexpensive at only 7 percent GNPN per year of life gained.

It might be argued that, because most effects of the smoking campaign expenditure would not occur until many years after the program expenditure, some adjustment is needed to take account of time. Discounting provides a method of comparing events that occur at different points in time. If we use a discount rate of 3 percent and use the difference between the average age of starting smoking (twenty-one years) and the average age of a smoking death (fifty-five years) as the discount period, the cost per discounted unit of effect is still only 1.9 percent GNPN (table 21-4).[5]

The cost-effectiveness calculations above were made on the assumption that the total effect of the program would be to prevent new starts. There will also be effects in bringing about cessation in response to the basic informational and educational campaign, and these effects, added to prevention of new starts, will increase the cost-effectiveness of the program. Cessation is difficult to achieve but can be cost-effective. Over a ten-year period of sustained informational effort, without any special programs targeted specifically at selected smoker groups, a 10 percent quit rate would be possible in the industrial countries (Altman and others 1987; Warner 1987), and a well-designed program conceivably would be more successful in some developing countries. Compared with preventing new starts, the effects of quitting would be less, however. The relative risk (RR) of mortality from all causes for smokers as opposed to nonsmokers is about 2 on average, and a smoker's chance of dying from a cause attributable to smoking is roughly 0.25. About ten years after cessation the RR falls to about 1.25 and a former smoker's chance of dying from a smoking-related cause falls to about 0.0625. With a program cost of 0.01 percent GNPN and a quit rate of 10 percent over ten program years, the cost per YLG is 0.5 percent GNPN undiscounted or 1.6 discounted at 3 percent.

PRIMARY PREVENTION OF VIRUS-ASSOCIATED CANCERS. Several cancers are associated with viral infections. These include liver cancer, which is an outcome of infection with the hepatitis B

Table 21-4. Cost-Effectiveness of Antismoking Programs

Study	Percent of GNPN per death prevented [a]		Percent of GNPN per year of life gained [a]	
	ra – 0	ra – 0.03	ra – 0	ra – 0.03
Hypothetical example in text				
New starters only	9.6	26.3	0.7	1.9
Quitters included	7.5	17.6	0.5	1.6
United States cessation programs [b]				
Smoking cessation classes	11.8	18.4	0.8	1.2
Incentive-based contest	6.5	10.1	0.4	0.6
Self-help antismoking kit	2.1	3.2	0.2	0.3
Eddy [c] cessation program	12.0	18.0	0.8	1.0

Notes: Effects include prevention of excess mortality from lung cancer, other cancers, cardiovascular disease, chronic obstructive lung disease, and other causes; it is not practical to identify cancer as a sole objective.

a. Discount rate.

b. Altman and others 1987 present cost per quitter, which has been converted to deaths prevented using an excess mortality rate of 0.1875 and to years of life gained assuming fourteen years of life lost per smoking-associated death. Discounting assumes that the mean age of quitters is forty-two and the mean age at death is fifty-seven. The figures given are based on the additional cost of the special programs and do not include the cost of the national information program.

c. Based on Eddy 1981. Converted to percent GNPN using U.S. GNPN of $12,800.

Source: Eddy 1981; Altman and others 1987.

virus (HBV); cervical cancer, which is related to the human papilloma virus; and nasopharyngeal cancer and Burkitt's lymphoma, which are both related to the Epstein-Barr virus. Of these, the most immediate interest is in the link between HBV and liver cancer because of the strength of the evidence indicating causality and because of development, during the last fifteen years, of an effective vaccine (WHO 1983; Beasley 1988).

The etiology of HBV infection is complex. The virus is transmitted through close contact with serum-derived fluids, including blood, dental exudates, skin exudates, and semen. Of those who develop infection, the proportion dying within a few months is approximately 0.00125, although a much higher proportion have symptoms of hepatitis. Longer-term consequences of the infection are much more frequent and are associated with development of a chronic carrier state of the virus. From twenty to forty years following HBV infection those with the carrier state are at much greater risk of mortality from both primary liver cancer (PLC) and cirrhosis. The percentage of persons who become chronic virus carriers is closely related to the age of infection; most infected infants develop the carrier state, but fewer than 10 percent of those infected in adulthood become carriers. A study of HBV carriers in Taiwan found that the incidence of PLC among carriers was about 200 times greater than among noncarriers (Beasley and others 1981). Other studies indicate that aflatoxin consumption acts with the HBV carrier state to increase risks of PLC and cirrhosis (Bulatao-Jayme and others 1982; Van Rensburg and others 1985; Yeh and others 1989). The long-term excess risk of mortality from HBV-linked causes is about 15 to 30 per 1,000 cases (ITFH 1988).

There is no standard treatment for HBV infection. Prevention strategies include immunization, better sanitation, and improved sterilization of medical instruments, needles, and syringes. During the last ten years, development of both plasma-derived and recombinant DNA types of vaccine against HBV virus has made it technically possible to prevent infection (Szmuness and others 1981; Francis and others 1982; Wainwright and others 1989). Both types of vaccine are safe and 75 to 95 percent effective, depending on delivery conditions. Until recently the price of vaccine was high (more than $100 for a full course of three shots using the recombinant DNA type of vaccine), but a fall in the price of HBV vaccine to below $1 per injection has increased the possibility of large-scale programs for the control of hepatitis.

The International Task Force on Hepatitis B Immunization (ITFH) distinguishes between areas of low, intermediate, and high HBV prevalence. In areas of low prevalence (western Europe, Australia, North America, and southern South America), 4 to 6 percent of the population show HBV antibodies and only 0.2 to 0.5 percent are carriers; neonatal infection is infrequent. In areas of intermediate prevalence (eastern Europe, countries of the former U.S.S.R., the Mediterranean and the Middle East, Central and South America, and North Africa), 20 to 55 percent of the population show HBV antibodies and 2 to 7 percent are carriers; neonatal infection is frequent. In areas of high prevalence (China, southern Asia,

tropical Africa, and the Amazon region of South America), 70 to 95 percent of the population show HBV antibodies and 7 percent to 20 percent are carriers; neonatal infection is frequent. Three-fourths of the world's population live in areas of intermediate or high prevalence. In areas of low prevalence the ITFH recommends that only high-risk groups (such as medical and dental workers) be immunized. In areas of intermediate or high prevalence the most effective preventive strategy is immunization of neonates as part of immediate postnatal care because of the large proportion of infections that are acquired at birth or perinatally.

The feasibility of immunization programs closely parallels that of WHO's Expanded Programme on Immunization (EPI) in general. In countries with a low quality of maternal child health services the obstacles to a correctly timed delivery of the first of the three doses required must be overcome to ensure coverage of the neonatal population. In countries such as China and Indonesia, where development of preventive health services is more advanced, the feasibility of an effective HBV program is high.

Hepatitis immunization can be added to existing EPI programs (The Gambia Hepatitis Study Group 1989), with the additional requirement that, to interrupt transmission, newborn children of infected mothers must be inoculated as soon as possible after birth (usually within seven days). Subsequently, a second dose is to be delivered with EPI vaccines as convenient from four to twelve weeks later, and then a third dose two to twelve months following the second. Two strategies are possible. The first is to immunize all newborns. The second is to screen mothers for hepatitis B surface antigen positivity and immunize only the infants of mothers who were positive (that is, carriers). Because of the cost and current low production of the vaccine, the second strategy is tempting. In low-income countries with high endemicity, however, the first strategy appears preferable. Epidemiological modeling by the ITFH indicates that the screening strategy would not reduce the HBV carrier state by more than 30 to 50 percent compared with a long-run reduction of at least 90 percent for a continued strategy of total newborn vaccination. The capacity for screening and effective follow-up may also be difficult to develop.

Immunization against the hepatitis B virus is a relatively new technology, and the cost has only recently fallen to levels that make it a possible strategy. There are no existing large-scale programs that can be examined for cost-effectiveness. Tentative projections, however, have been made of the cost-effectiveness of immunization strategies for China and Indonesia, where programs for HBV vaccination are under active consideration or in the early stages of implementation. In addition, the ITFH has made estimates for a prototypical program in a high-prevalence country.

Recast in annual percentage of per capita GNP, the costs for the three nonscreening programs lie within a range of 19 to 88 per undiscounted death prevented and 1 to 6 per undiscounted year of life gained (table 21-5). These costs, although greater than those for tobacco prevention programs, make HBV immunization an attractive candidate for inclusion in a cancer

Table 21-5. Cost-Effectiveness of Hepatitis B Vaccine in Various Settings

Setting	Percent GNPN per death prevented [a]		Percent GNPN per year of life gained [a]	
	ra – 0	ra – 0.03	ra – 0	ra – 0.03
Indonesia[b]				
Immunize all newborns	87	404	6	25
Screen mothers and vaccinate newborns at risk	151	700	9	44
China[c]				
Immunize all newborns	74	340	5	22
Screen mothers and immunize newborns at risk	77	356	5	23
Hypothetical example[d]				
Low-cost estimate	19	87	1	6
High-cost estimate	88	408	6	26

Notes: Effects include prevention of excess mortality from hepatitis B, liver cancer, and cirrhosis; it is not practical to identify liver cancer as the sole objective. The discounted values assume that intervention occurs at age 0 and the average HBV-caused death occurs at age fifty-two. The GNPN is estimated at 810 yuan.

a. Discount rate.

b. Widjaya (1988) calculated the cost per carrier prevented. This has been converted to deaths prevented and years of life gained using an excess mortality rate of 0.25 and sixteen years of life lost per HBV-associated death. Widjaya assumed vaccine cost of US$15 (does not include delivery cost). The program costs have been recalculated using vaccine cost of US$1.50 per dose and estimated delivery cost of US$1.20 per dose. Calculated for 1985, the GNPN is estimated to be 588,000 rupiah.

c. Circa 1986.

d. Assumes no screening. The ITFH 1988 estimates, which are given in U.S. dollars, have been converted to percent GNPN. Assumes per capita GNP of US$400.

Source: Widjaya 1988; Barnum 1988; ITFH 1988.

prevention strategy. Discounting affects the estimated cost-effectiveness of HBV programs more than many other interventions because of the long lag between delivery of the intervention (which occurs at birth) and prevented death (which, for liver cancer or cirrhosis occurs at an average age of about fifty-five years). Using a 3 percent discount rate, we find that the cost per death prevented ranges from 87 to 408 and the cost per YLG ranges from 6 to 26. Even after discounting, HBV vaccine remains an attractive program possibility.

The cost-effectiveness of a maternal screening program is equal to the newborn program in the China example but is much less cost-effective than the newborn program in the Indonesia example (table 21-5). In both examples, however, cost-effectiveness calculations include only the deaths directly prevented in the newborn cohort. Additional deaths will be prevented from reduced transmission of hepatitis to other cohorts in the future. This indirect effect will be substantial for the total immunization strategy but only modest for the screening strategy. Thus the total immunization strategy is superior, because it holds out the possibility of a dramatic containment of hepatitis B in the future, instead of continued endemicity that would result from the screening strategy.

FOOD AND ALCOHOL. Abundant epidemiological evidence links dietary habits to occurrence of cancer. There is still considerable uncertainty, however, both about the actual dietary constituents that influence risk and about the proportion of cancer occurrence that can be explained by diet. Alcohol consumption clearly increases risk of cancers of the oral cavity and esophagus. Alcohol has been implicated as a cause of breast cancer and large bowel cancer, although the epidemio-

logical evidence is not conclusive. Consumption of foods contaminated with aflatoxin (produced by *Aspergillus flavus* fungal growth on stored peanuts and grains) is likely to be a cause of primary liver cancer. With the exception of these substances, however, no single component of diet has been conclusively shown either to cause or to prevent cancer (Doll and Peto 1981; Willett and MacMahon 1984; Byers 1988). Nevertheless a number of intriguing relationships between diet and cancer have emerged from epidemiological studies. These include positive associations between poorly preserved or pickled foods and stomach cancer, traditionally prepared salted fish and nasopharyngeal cancer (among southern Chinese), and total fats (or perhaps saturated fats) and large bowel cancer. Interesting negative (protective) associations have been observed between vegetable or fruit consumption (or their constituents such as beta-carotene and fiber) and a variety of epithelial cancers, most notably lung and colorectal cancer.

Estimates of the proportion of cancers attributable to diet in the industrial world range widely from about 10 percent to more than 70 percent. Given this uncertainty, and the lack of firm conclusions about most postulated dietary causes of cancer, it is not possible to predict the benefits (in reduced cancer) that may accrue from dietary interventions. An assessment of the costs and value of dietary interventions must await the results of further studies, which may likely include randomized controlled trials. Several relationships between diet and cancer, however, are particularly relevant in the developing world, and these may well figure in a natural cancer control program. Especially noteworthy are the relation between aflatoxin-contaminated food and liver cancer and between traditional Chinese salted fish and nasopharyngeal cancer. Other aspects of diet that merit attention in the developing world include consumption of alcohol (related to esophageal and oral cancers), poorly preserved foods (related to stomach cancer), and obesity.

In countries with high rates of liver cancer, a program to reduce aflatoxin intake (by better storage of grains and peanuts and by monitoring the aflatoxin content of commercial foods) may be justifiable as an adjunct to hepatitis B virus immunization. At present, one cannot precisely estimate the amount of liver cancer that could be avoided through reduction of aflatoxin. Although hepatitis B immunization programs may eventually prove to be the most cost-effective method for preventing liver cancer, they will not benefit people who are already infected with HBV and thus at risk for developing liver cancer. Aflatoxin appears to be an important cofactor leading to liver cancer development in HBV carriers (Bulatao-Jayme and others 1982; Yeh and others 1989); thus reduction of aflatoxin consumption offers promise for reducing liver cancer mortality in the near future, whereas immunization programs are unlikely to show a substantial benefit for forty or more years. Consumption of traditionally prepared salted fish in southern China (and in areas settled by migrants from southern China, such as Singapore) is strongly related to nasopharyngeal cancer (Yu and others 1986). Educational programs to discourage the practice of feeding salted fish to infants, weanlings, and children may be justifiable in these populations. It also seems reasonable to discourage consumption of other traditionally prepared foods that are high in volatile nitrosamines in countries where nasopharyngeal cancer is common (Poirier and others 1987).

In certain countries the possibility of reducing cancer occurrence may provide additional justification for implementing programs to decrease alcohol consumption, although the primary value of these programs is to reduce injuries and other ills. The cancer prevention benefits of reduced alcohol consumption (historically, difficult to achieve through government policy) cannot be reliably assessed, however, because the proportion of oral and esophageal cancers caused by alcohol is uncertain. The contribution of tobacco use to these cancers appears to be greater than that of alcohol.

Many other foods and nutrients are strongly suspected of influencing cancer occurrence, and these have figured in national dietary policies in the industrial world. For example, Americans are advised to eat a diet containing less fat and more fiber and to consume larger amounts of fresh fruits and vegetables. There is no conclusive information from scientific studies that these recommendations will lower cancer risks. Nevertheless, several expert review groups have concluded that one or more of these recommendations should be presented to the public as prudent advice for dietary change.

The justification for advising people to eat more fruits and vegetables is that epidemiological studies have shown decreased risks for many types of cancer in people whose diet is high in these foods (National Research Council 1982). Also fruits and vegetables may displace other, less desirable, foods from the diet. The evidence linking lowered risk of cancer with consumption of fresh fruits and vegetables should be carefully considered in discussions of national food policy. At the minimum, it would be prudent to avoid strategies that discourage production and consumption of these foods.

Obesity itself, apart from constituents of diet, is also associated with cancer mortality (Lew and Garfinkel 1979; Simopoulos 1987). The association is particularly notable for female breast and endometrial cancers. Of course, obesity is a complex phenomenon, and its occurrence is determined by genetic factors and physical activity as well as by caloric intake. Still, obesity often appears to accompany other features of economic development, and it is associated with diabetes, cardiovascular diseases, and other conditions in addition to cancer. It therefore merits consideration for public health preventive programs.

Diet affects many diseases besides cancer, and it would be unwise to alter diet without considering all the potential health consequences. Also, dietary change has economic and social implications. Planning and application of dietary strategies to prevent cancer should therefore occur only within the context of an overall national policy on diet. The relative importance of nutritional deficiency diseases, obesity, cardiovascular disease, diabetes, cancer, and other diet-related conditions must be considered country by country. Likewise, the expected economic consequences, in changing agriculture and food marketing, must be considered if a successful dietary intervention is to be accomplished.

ENVIRONMENTAL AND OCCUPATIONAL PROGRAMS. Exposure to environmental and occupational factors accounts for an undetermined but probably small number of cancers in the developing world. In the industrial world the actual contribution of such factors to cancer occurrence has been the subject of considerable debate (Doll and Peto 1981). Much confusion has arisen about the definition of "environmental" causes of cancer. If "environmental factors" are taken to mean only agents in the ambient environment (excluding diet and habits such as smoking, chewing, and so on), then only a small proportion (probably less than 10 percent) of cancers can be attributed to these causes. Nevertheless, in certain highly exposed groups, usually defined by occupation, environmental agents are more important.

Several environmental agents have been identified as possible causes of lung cancer. These include both ambient and occupational exposure to industrial chemicals and radon. These causes are important in selected subpopulations in which exposure is intense. For example, workers involved in the manufacture of asbestos, chromates, and ion exchange resins (involving chloromethylethers) are all at elevated risk of lung cancer. Likewise, underground miners exposed to high levels of radon have an increased risk of lung cancer.

Cigarette smoking acts with environmental factors to increase greatly the risk of lung cancer. Before implementation of protective measures for asbestos workers in the United States, asbestos workers who smoked cigarettes had approximately five times the risk of lung cancer as smokers who did not work with asbestos and more than fifty times the risk of people who neither smoked nor worked with asbestos. Similarly, the risk for uranium miners who smoke cigarettes is four times the risk of smokers who are not miners. Nonetheless, within the United States population as a whole, these other environmental factors are of little significance when compared with the effect of tobacco smoking. After taking account of the effects of other known causes of lung cancer, tobacco smoking still appears to account for at least 80 to 90 percent of lung cancer deaths in North America (Doll and Peto 1981).

Present information does not appear to warrant a general recommendation regarding environmental and occupational interventions to control cancer. For limited exposed populations these types of intervention may be cost-effective or necessary on moral grounds. Asbestos merits particular concern in this regard for two principal reasons. First, it is widely used in many developing countries in applications for which there are no cheap substitutes. Second, the rising prevalence of cigarette smoking greatly magnifies the potential for asbestos-related lung cancer. Programs to reduce workers' exposure and to use safer forms of asbestos will likely be worthwhile for many countries. For much of the developing world, however, control of environmental and occupational carcinogens appears to deserve a lower priority than other, proven cancer prevention activities.

CANCER PREVENTION BENEFITS AND OTHER HEALTH MEASURES. Programs directed toward other important diseases may, as an ancillary benefit, also help to control cancer. For example, schistosomiasis is clearly associated with urinary tract cancer (in the case of Schistosomiasis hematobium) and possibly related to bowel cancer (in the case of S. japonicam and S. mansoni). An evaluation of the cost-effectiveness of a mass treatment program to control S. hematobium, for example, should take account of the expected reduction in urinary cancers that would result. Likewise, control of Clonorchis and Opisthorchis infection, besides reducing acute morbidity, will lessen the risk of biliary tract cancer. Last, programs to decrease spread of sexually transmitted diseases seem likely to diminish cervical cancer occurrence. In all these examples the reduction of cancer occurrence would be a secondary benefit that would be realized only years (or decades) after an effective program was implemented.

Secondary Prevention

The cost-effectiveness of secondary prevention (that is, screening and early detection) programs is dependent on the incidence of the disease in question, the technical feasibility of screening and treatment at early stages in the cancer's development, the possibility of targeting to reduce costs by covering groups at highest risk, and the availability and cost of appropriate health infrastructure so that the screening can be carried out with accuracy and the findings followed with an effective intervention. Among the ten primary cancers, on the basis of the experience in industrial countries, cervix and

breast cancer hold greatest promise as candidates for national-level screening programs. These are discussed in detail later.

Large bowel cancer and oral cancer are also of interest, although evidence supporting the value of screening for these two tumors is inconclusive. Several procedures for colorectal cancer screening have been proposed, but none has yet been shown clearly to reduce the risk of death from this condition (Chamberlain and others 1986; Clayman 1989; Fleischer and others 1989; Knight, Fielding, and Battista 1989). Institution of screening programs cannot now be recommended as a public policy, but further tests of screening efficacy and controlled clinical trials are clearly worth undertaking. Examination by flexible sigmoidoscopy appears particularly promising as a procedure, although not in countries with limited health resources. Screening for oral cancer in conjunction with other medical procedures, such as dental care or general care, theoretically should prevent deaths from this disease. The expected low cost of screening (by simple inspection), and the possibility of identifying premalignant changes (leukoplakia), make oral cancer a good prospect for intervention (McMichael 1984). Also, high-risk individuals (those who chew or smoke tobacco) are readily identifiable. There have not, however, been any published studies showing the effectiveness of oral cancer screening. In countries, such as India, with high mortality rates for oral cancer, screening programs may now be worth undertaking but only within a research context.

Most other cancers such as lung, liver, esophageal, and stomach cancer are not suitable targets for a screening program in a developing country.[6] Although they can be detected in a presymptomatic phase, no controlled studies have shown that screening reduces the risk of death from these tumors. Also, these tumors tend to progress rapidly to a clinically symptomatic phase, so there is only a brief period during which the cancer is screen detectable but not symptomatic.

CERVICAL CANCER SCREENING (PAP SMEAR). Because of its high incidence in many lower-income countries, screening for cervical cancer is among the most promising of the secondary prevention possibilities. The objective of cervical cancer screening is to detect neoplastic cells at an early stage when a relatively low-cost and low-risk surgical procedure can be used to remove the cells and prevent occurrence or spread of invasive cancer. The cost-effectiveness of cervical cancer screening has been debated in the literature, but evidence in support of screening has become compelling (Cramer 1982; Lynge, Madsen, and Engholm 1989), and cervical cancer screening is an important component in the World Health Organization's strategy for combating cancer (WHO 1988b). The cost-effectiveness of screening, however, varies greatly with the setting in which a program is carried out. Important factors determining the advisability of the test include incidence and mortality rates (and therefore the prevalence of occult disease), type of program (mass screening or integrated medical examination), availability of adequate facilities for following the test findings, accuracy of laboratory facilities, and cost of the test and follow-up procedures.

The World Health Organization (1986b) has recommended that in low-income countries every woman should be screened once in her lifetime between the ages of thirty-five and forty years. If additional resources are available, screening should take place at intervals of ten years for women between the ages of thirty-five and fifty-five. In middle-income countries the interval should be increased to five years. The cost-effectiveness of tests falls off rapidly as the frequency of testing goes much above three to five years and as the age of testing falls below thirty-five.

Estimates of the cost-effectiveness of cervical cancer screening, in percentage of per capita GNP per year of life gained, range from about 70 to 300 percent per undiscounted death prevented, or 4 to 18 percent per year of life gained (table 21-6). Because of the brief time between the start of screening and the average age of death, the effect of discounting is not great. Using a discount rate of 3 percent, we find that the cost per year of life gained ranges from 5 to 26 percent GNPN. At the upper extreme, cervical cancer screening is not competitive with other health interventions, whereas at the lower extreme the program would be an attractive component of a chronic disease strategy. Clarification of the epidemiological basis and cost-effectiveness of program design should be made in individual countries before embarking on a program of secondary cervical cancer prevention. Cost-effectiveness will be greater in countries with higher rates of cervical cancer and in those with clearly identifiable high-risk groups. It will be lower where cultural norms prevent women from having pelvic examinations and where the quality of cytology laboratory work is low.

BREAST CANCER SCREENING. Breast cancer screening can be carried out through a physical examination by a health care worker (Baines, Miller, and Bassett 1989) or a combination of a physical examination and mammography. Controlled clinical studies with long-term follow-up have demonstrated that a physical examination combined with mammography can reduce breast cancer mortality by about 20 to 30 percent (Shapiro and others 1982; Tabar and others 1985; Day and others 1986). Breast self-examination has also been promoted as a secondary prevention policy, but evidence for its effectiveness in reducing mortality is weak (Day and others 1986).

The cost-effectiveness of breast examination using mammography is much less than that of cervical cancer screening in the examples we considered. The estimated cost per YLG from mammography ranges from about 100 to 200 percent GNPN using a discount rate of 3 percent. The estimated cost per YLG from the physical examination alone is, however, competitive with other prevention activities. Using only a physical examination and discounting costs and effects at 3 percent, the cost per YLG was 12 percent GNPN as recalculated from the results reported in a study by D. Eddy (1981; see table 21-7).

Treatment

The three primary modalities for treating cancer are surgery, radiation therapy, and chemotherapy (including hormonal manipulation). Surgery alone offers a chance of cure for cancers of the breast, uterine cervix, colorectum, and oral cavity. Although some cancers of the stomach, lung, liver, and esophagus are also curable by surgery, their number is very small. The surgical treatment required for early stage cancers of the breast, cervix, colorectum, and oral cavity does not require highly technological facilities, nor does it require training beyond that ordinarily received by surgical specialists. The procedures generally take approximately two to four hours to complete and are associated with a hospital stay of seven to fourteen days. Accurate assessment of the degree of cancer spread (staging) is important so that performing surgery is avoided on patients in whom the procedure cannot be curative, and it necessitates reliable diagnostic imaging facilities.

Table 21-6. Cost-Effectiveness of Screening for Cervical Cancer

	Percent GNPN per death prevented [a]		Percent GNPN per year of life gained [a]	
Study	*ra – 0*	*ra – 0.03*	*ra – 0*	*ra – 0.03*
Parkin and Moss (United Kingdom)[b]				
Five-year interval, age 35–64	66	94	4	5
Five-year interval, age 25–64	154	220	7	11
Barnum (China)[c]				
Five-year interval, age 35–59	310	390	18	26
Luce (United States)[d]				
Five-year interval, age 30–39	138	250	13	25
Three-year interval, age 30–39	145	290	12	23

a. Discount rate.

b. Based on model identified as "H3C" in Parkin and Moss 1986. Their results are scaled in terms of unit costs representing the cost for a routine screening. To convert their results to percent GNPN, 1 unit of input was evaluated as 4.6£ (1982 prices), using a price index for medical services in the United Kingdom, and then rescaled using a 1982 GNPN of 4,907£. Discounting assumes an average of twelve years from the age of screening to the averted cancer mortality.

c. Estimates are not based on as complete a model as other two studies. For example, false positives and false negatives are not included.

d. Luce results reported in terms of 1979 U.S. dollars per death prevented and year of life gained from using a 10 percent discount rate. These have been converted by interpolating from Luce's discount rate sensitivity table and using a 1979 GNPN of US$10,810. Luce's "Low cost" public provider model has been used.

Source: Luce 1980; Parkin and Moss 1986; Barnum 1988.

Table 21-7. Cost-Effectiveness of Screening for Breast Cancer

Study	Percent GNPN per death prevented [a]		Percent GNPN per year of life gained [a]	
	ra – 0	ra – 0.03	ra – 0	ra – 0.03
Eddy [b]				
Physical exam only	—	—	—	12
Physical exam and mammography, one-year interval, age 50 and older [c]	—	—	—	97–210
Schwartz, three-year interval, age 40–70 [d]	—	—	15	135

— Data not available.

a. Discount rate.

b. Assumes U.S. GNPN of $12,800.

c. The costs and effects are incremental with the addition of mammography to a routine annual physical examination. Based on U.S. GNPN of $10,600 (1979). Based on present value of total incremental cost ranging from $482 to $1,042.

Based on the increase in life expectancy from age forty. Assumes a cost of US$100 per screening and eleven screenings between age forty and seventy. Based on U.S. GNPN of $10,600 (1979).

Source: Schwartz 1978; Eddy 1981.

Radiation therapy involves administration of high-energy radiation in an effort to kill tumor cells. The technique requires sophisticated equipment and skilled therapists, who are likely to be found only in technologically advanced tertiary care centers. Radiation therapy is capable of curing lymphoma (particularly Hodgkin's lymphoma) and cancer of the cervix. Radiation therapy is useful for control of breast cancer and lung cancer, although it only rarely cures lung cancer. Most courses of radiation therapy must be administered over a prolonged period (usually several weeks), but the patient may not have to be kept in the hospital.

Chemotherapy is administration of drugs that kill cells or inhibit their growth. Chemotherapy is potentially curative in leukemia and certain lymphomas. It also contributes to length of survival and possibility of cure in breast cancer. Chemotherapy provides palliation in certain forms of lung cancer. Intensive chemotherapy such as that given for most lymphomas and leukemias requires highly trained physicians who have substantial experience with administration of these toxic agents. Less toxic chemotherapy for relief of symptoms often can be carried out in primary medical settings, providing that consultant guidance is readily available. Many of the drugs used for chemotherapy are expensive, and they require close monitoring of laboratory tests and intense skilled nursing support because of side effects. An exception is the antiestrogen drug Tamoxifen. It clearly reduces risk of recurrence and death in breast cancer yet is relatively free of toxic side effects, is simple to administer in oral form, and should be available at low cost in most countries (WHO 1985).

More recent advances in cancer treatment have shown the importance of multidisciplinary management, involving more than one treatment modality. This strategy requires the combined efforts of highly trained professionals and is possible only in the context of a technologically sophisticated tertiary care center. Many of the gains noted in the probability of survival of patients with certain cancers (particularly leukemias and lymphomas) are attributable to use of multimodal therapy.

Application of the most advanced therapy can be vastly expensive. For some cancers, for example, childhood lympho-cytic leukemia, treatment may continue for a prolonged period and require repeated hospitalization, intensive chemotherapy, and radiation therapy. During the course of treatment the child may require sixty to ninety days in the hospital.

A policy decision to provide access to this type of technologically advanced treatment has implications beyond the immediate cost of the procedure. First, a facility must be developed that has the technological capacity to support advanced therapies. This involves diagnostic imaging capabilities, advanced laboratory facilities, and radiation therapy devices. Second, highly trained and experienced personnel are needed from both the medical and nursing professions to carry out the therapy. Third, the patients who are likely to benefit from advanced multimodal therapy are relatively few in number, so referral to a few specialized treatment facilities will be necessary. To provide ready access to advanced cancer treatment will require the development of a system of central treatment facilities with an outlying referral network. This implies a heavy investment in facilities located in urban areas and will further concentrate resources away from rural populations.

Cost-Effectiveness of Treatment

Given the resource intensity of cancer treatment, evaluation of its cost-effectiveness is particularly important to make informed planning decisions. Cancers differ greatly in severity and potential for treatment or prevention, and, for the most part, it is necessary to consider the effects and costs for separate types of cancer. In the remainder of this section we provide a cost-effective analysis of cancer treatment using United States data to model effectiveness and general information to model costs in a prototypical country. The results are acknowledged to be highly approximate, and our intention is to allow rough comparisons of the cost-effectiveness of treatment and prevention. For certain cancers, notably cervix and breast, and perhaps colorectal and oral cancer, the close link between secondary prevention and treatment prevents a clear assignment of gains in survival to treatment per se. For these cancers screening and treatment need to be considered as joint interventions if the full cost-effectiveness of treatment is to be achieved. In fact, the cost-effectiveness of treatment of cancers for which screening is feasible exceeds the estimates in this section (which are based on an average for all stages), because the effect of treatment on early stage cancer is greater and, in some instances, the cost of treatment is less.

EFFECTS. We approximate the effectiveness of treatment using data on the change in survival rates for cancer in the United States from the period 1945–50 through the years 1955–60 to 1975–80. Conceptually, the objective is to estimate the benefits in developing countries of treatment in a higher-level hospital with relatively modern technology in comparison with treatment at an entry-level hospital or with no treatment or only palliative care. As an approximation, the higher-level hospital is equated with the level of care in the United States in the period 1975–80, and the low-level care alternative is equated with the level of treatment in the United States during 1945–50. Baseline, minimal treatment survival rates are specified arbitrarily after a literature search of technical improvements in cancer prior to 1940.

Equating institutional care at various levels with chronological change in cancer care in the United States is obviously only an oversimplification because, on the one hand, there are a few modern techniques that can be delivered with effect and at low cost at smaller, low-level institutions and, on the other hand, there were some effective treatments used in large, technically advanced hospitals in the United States in the years 1945–50. During the last forty years, however, there have been substantial advances in radiation, chemotherapy, and surgery. Radiation therapy has advanced through development of new sources of radiation and techniques that allow better control of the intensity and the focus of radiation. Chemotherapy has advanced with the development of new drugs and their use in combined therapies. Surgery has improved in safety and precision. Another change during the thirty-year period has been in the accuracy of diagnostics, which has made it possible to identify cancers at an earlier stage.

All these factors are likely contributors to the changes that can be seen in relative survival in table 21-8.[7] It would be a mistake to view the apparent improvements in survival as entirely attributable to improved therapy. Part of the recorded increase may also be due both to earlier diagnosis and to detection of less aggressive tumors, factors which give an illusion of improved survival without any true change in the underlying risk of death. The size of these effects is debated in the literature and unknown, but in any case, the apparent increase in survival almost certainly overestimates the effect of new therapy techniques.

The data show very little improvement in survival for esophageal, stomach, and liver cancer. Lung cancer improvements that are shown are small and difficult to attribute to technical improvements. Although there have been modest gains in treating small cell carcinoma, this cell type represents less than 20 percent of all lung cancer. Much of the increase that is shown is likely an artifact resulting from earlier diagnosis. Improved survival for leukemia (and perhaps for breast cancer) is more reflective of the effects of new therapies. In the analysis below we lack the quantitative information to make an adjustment for the effects of earlier diagnosis and different spectra of tumor aggressiveness, but these sources of error should be borne in mind when one interprets the results.

The effectiveness of treatment is estimated by calculating the implied gain in years of life in going from the baseline fatality rates that would exist with only minimal treatment to the fatality rates after treatment equivalent to the United States level in the period 1975–80. The fatality rates implied by the published survival data and the baseline fatality rate used in the analysis are summarized in table 21-9.

COSTS. Surprisingly few studies have been done on the total direct costs incurred over the course of specific cancers. Costing cancer is particularly difficult because for given cancers there may be a number of treatment options at each stage of the disease, and the duration of treatment may last several years. Also, treatment procedures and therefore the costs of treatment vary considerably for the different types of cancer.

Table 21-8. Five-Year Relative Survival for Cancer in the United States, by Year

Site or type of cancer	1950	1960	1970	1980
Mouth/pharynx	0.45	0.45	0.43	0.53
Esophagus	0.04	0.04	0.04	0.06
Stomach	0.12	0.11	0.13	0.16
Colon/rectum	0.41	0.44	0.46	0.53
Liver	0.01	0.02	0.03	0.03
Lung	0.06	0.08	0.10	0.13
Breast	0.60	0.63	0.68	0.75
Cervix	0.59	0.58	0.64	0.67
Leukemia	0.10	0.14	0.22	0.33

Source: Axtell, Asire, and Myers 1976; American Cancer Society 1987.

Table 21-9. Estimated Five-Year Fatality for Cancer, by Year

Site or type of cancer	Baseline minimal treatment[a]	1950	1960	1970	1980
Mouth/pharynx	0.82	0.58	0.58	0.60	0.50
Esophagus	0.97	0.97	0.97	0.97	0.95
Stomach	0.90	0.90	0.91	0.89	0.86
Colon/rectum	0.75	0.64	0.61	0.59	0.52
Liver	0.99	0.99	0.98	0.97	0.97
Lung	0.95	0.95	0.93	0.91	0.89
Breast	0.75	0.47	0.43	0.38	0.31
Cervix	0.80	0.50	0.50	0.45	0.41
Leukemia	0.90	0.90	0.86	0.78	0.67

Note: Five-year fatality computed as $F = 1 - R * S$, where R is the relative survival given in table 21-8 and S is overall survival (for all stages) from United States life tables for 1950–80.

a. Either 1950 fatality or higher rate implied from literature search.

Source: Axtell, Asire, and Myers 1976; American Cancer Society 1987.

For the purposes of this study, we approximated the costs of treatment using information on the relative costs of treatment for different cancers in the United States (Cromwell and Gertman 1979; Rice, Hodgson, and Kopstein 1985). These costs were then scaled to the cost of tertiary treatment and expressed as a percentage of per capita GNP for a lower-middle-income developing country. Although this procedure is inexact, it is probably sufficient for the comparisons between cancers and between prevention and treatment that are sought here. In table 21-10 we present the estimates of total costs per case, varying from a low of about 175 percent GNPN for cervical cancer to 780 percent GNPN for lung cancer.

COST-EFFECTIVENESS. The costs and effects derived in the two preceding sections can be compared to give the costs per year of life gained from treatment. Looking first at the cost per YLG for the average of cancer in all stages (table 21-11), we find that the results suggest that it is relatively cost-ineffective to treat esophageal, stomach, liver, and lung cancer and more cost-effective to treat colorectal, cervical, and breast cancer. To compare extremes, the cost per year of life gained from treatment for esophageal cancer is more than 100 times that for cancers of the breast, mouth, and cervix. The results also suggest that it is much more cost-effective to treat cancers at younger ages; in particular, the cost per year of life gained for treatments at age fifty and over are very high.

The analysis above underestimates the true costs and overestimates the effects and therefore must be interpreted cautiously. First, only the direct costs of health services are included. Costs to patients and their families in travel to the hospital and provision of supplementary care or food are not included. Second, for several cancers, especially of a certain type and in advanced stages, the number of years of additional life is very small and may be largely an artifact of earlier detection, diagnosis of less malignant tumors, and staging changes (Feinstein, Sosin, and Wells 1985). Third, there is no adjustment for quality of life. This omission can be especially important for the marginal gains (in extended life) for treatment of later stage cancer and for treatment of esophageal, stomach, lung, or other cancers for which the gain in fractional years of life follows debilitating treatments that usually result in only short periods of remission.

The analysis is also based on improvements in survival rates in the United States, where there has been an increased emphasis on early detection during the last forty years and where there is substantial training and treatment capacity. This link between detection and treatment is especially important as an underlying factor in the cost-effectiveness of treatment for cancers of the mouth, cervix, breast, and colon. It is important to emphasize the link between detection and treatment because it is not useful to develop treatment capacity in the absence of improved detection; nor is it useful to develop detection programs in the absence of treatment capacity. This link has been underlined by the World Health Organization, which stresses the importance of linking the development of therapy with early referral (WHO uses the term "down staging") and improved training for cancer detection among primary health care workers (Stjernsward 1990).

PAIN RELIEF. An important component of palliative care for cancer patients is adequate treatment of pain (Portenoy 1988). More than 80 percent of cancer is not detected until an advanced stage at which treatment other than palliation is not effective (Stjernsward 1988). A WHO document setting out guidelines on cancer pain relief estimates that 50 to 70 percent of cancer patients experience pain (WHO 1986a). Of these, pain is moderate to severe in about 50 percent and very severe in 30 percent. The World Health Organization recommends a three-stage analgesic program going from nonopioids (such as aspirin or paracetamol) for mild pain, through weak opioids (such as codeine plus paracetamol) for moderate pain, to strong opioids (morphine) for intense pain. They note that these agents, possibly supplemented by adjuvant drugs (see the details in WHO 1986a and Stjernsward 1988), can provide relief in 90 percent of cancer patients with pain.

Past inadequacy of cancer pain control is attributable to a lack of recognition by health care professionals that effective methods existed for cancer pain management, a lack of availability of the required drugs, unreasonable fears concerning addiction, and poor education of health professionals on can-

Table 21-10. Cost per Case Treated
(percent GNPN)

Site or type of cancer	Costs relative to average for US [a]	Costs per case in high-income country [b]	Cost per case in lower-middle-income country [c]
Mouth/pharynx	0.76	79	243
Esophagus	1.11	115	709
Stomach	1.07	112	687
Colon/rectum	1.05	110	336
Liver	1.13	118	727
Lung	1.22	127	782
Breast	0.65	67	206
Cervix	0.54	57	174
Leukemia	1.09	114	700
Average	1.00	104	641

a. Based on 1969–71 average direct costs for cancer treatments as reported in Cromwell and Gertman 1979.

b. The number of bed-day equivalents for the cost of the average cancer in the United States was multiplied by the cost of a bed-day (expressed as percent GNPN) to obtain the cost of an average case of cancer. This average was, in turn, multiplied by the relative costs in the first column to obtain the costs for individual cancers. In 1980 the average direct cost of cancer in the United States was fifty-three times the cost of the average bed-day based on a reanalysis of data in Rice, Hodgson, and Kopstein 1985 and thirty-seven times based on 1969–71 data in Cromwell and Gertman 1979; 40 is used for these calculations. The percentage GNPN per bed-day in a large urban hospital remains relatively stable over a sample of countries, 2.6 was used for these calculations.

c. Because the technical hospital procedures involved in cancer therapy can have a high foreign exchange content when cost is determined by international prices, the estimated cost is a weighted sum of a foreign exchange component (including specialized training, equipment, and pharmaceuticals) and a local component. The calculations are made for a lower-middle-income country with a per capita GNP of US$1,500. As an approximation, it is assumed that the foreign exchange content is 0.2 for early stages of oral, cervical, breast, and rectal cancer treatment and 0.5 for all other cancers.

Source: Cromwell and Gertman 1979; Rice, Hodgson, and Kopstein 1985.

Table 21-11. Cost per YLG Gained from Tertiary-Level Treatment in a Lower-Middle-Income Country, by Age at Diagnosis
(percent GNPN)

Site	Average age	65 years	60 years	55 years	50 years	45 years	40 years
Undiscounted							
Mouth/pharynx	44	179	80	51	38	30	25
Esophagus	3,574	8,755	3,891	2,502	1,843	1,459	1,208
Stomach	2,462	6,525	2,900	1,864	1,374	1,087	900
Colon/rectum	126	472	210	135	99	79	65
Liver	3,315	13,011	5,783	3,717	2,739	2,168	1,795
Lung	1,183	3,075	1,367	879	647	512	424
Breast	26	93	46	31	23	19	16
Cervix	27	69	35	23	17	14	12
Discounted at 3 percent							
Mouth/pharynx	55	187	89	62	49	41	36
Esophagus	4,056	9,147	4,367	3,010	2,374	2,008	1,772
Stomach	2,826	6,817	3,254	2,243	1,769	1,496	1,320
Colon/rectum	154	493	235	162	128	108	96
Liver	4,083	13,593	6,489	4,473	3,528	2,984	2,633
Lung	1,354	3,213	1,534	1,057	834	705	622
Breast	33	122	58	40	32	27	24
Cervix	32	90	43	30	23	20	18

Note: Costs are averaged over all stages. Costs per YLG gained from tertiary level treatment of leukemia diagnosed in a ten-year-old are 48 percent of GNP undiscounted and 100 percent discounted at 3 percent.
Source: Authors.

cer pain management. Legislative reform, better pharmaceutical management, and improved training can remove these blocks to better pain therapy.

Adequate treatment of pain could alleviate much suffering while placing fewer demands on medical resources than ineffective attempts at higher-level curative treatment. For example, for an average duration of pain therapy of ninety days, the cost of drugs and outpatient delivery in a lower-middle-income developing country would be about $18 to $65 per case, or 1 to 4 percent GNPN, for, respectively, mild to severe pain management.[8] This would represent less than 1 percent of the cost of inpatient tertiary treatment of, say, lung or esophageal cancer.

COST-EFFECTIVE TREATMENT POLICY. The results of the cost-effectiveness analysis can be helpful in fashioning a policy to increase dramatically the effective use of secondary and tertiary hospital resources in place of available space to treat all cancer on the basis of random referral or first come, first serve. Applying a criteria of no more than 50 percent GNPN per year of life saved and bearing in mind the cautionary comments noted in the preceding paragraph, a possible policy would be the following:

- Use existing referral capacity to treat younger patients with early stage cancers amenable to curative treatment, especially breast, mouth, cervical, and possibly colorectal cancer.
- Use existing tertiary-level referral capacity to treat children with leukemia and lymphoma.

- Provide for decentralized supportive care and symptom relief for the vast majority of other cancer patients using community-based alternatives for palliative care. For patients with breast cancer, Tamoxifen therapy could also be accomplished at this level.

Such alternatives include community-staffed nursing homes, health center outpatient care and hospices for the terminally ill, and home beds managed from lower-level hospitals. Almost all patients with stomach, liver, and lung cancer would receive care at this level. Older patients and those with advanced disease would not be referred for curative therapy, but reasonable efforts would be made to alleviate pain and suffering through use of palliative medications.

Developing a Strategy for Cancer

The World Health Organization has recommended the development of national cancer strategies based on surveillance and prevention programs tailored to local needs (Stjernsward and others 1985; WHO 1988b). The recommendations of WHO for the development of a national cancer strategy are especially important in countries in which infectious diseases have been reduced and life expectancies are lengthening. It is not effective to allow the resources devoted to combating cancer to be allocated without plan on an ad hoc basis depending on local interests. Instead, a national cancer strategy needs to be developed formally. Such a strategy would recognize local variations in cancer occurrence and risk factor prevalence. It would also allow setting an overall national strategy to combat cancer and

Table 21-12. Subjective Potential for Primary Preventive Activities for Cancer

Activity	Potential reduction of YLL	Feasibility[a]	Potential technical effect[b]	Persons covered per unit cost	Priority
Antismoking measures	High	Medium	High	High	Highest
Hepatitis immunization	Medium	High	High	Medium	High
Control of carcinogens in food[c]	Low	Medium	Medium	High	Medium
Reduced fat and increased fiber in diet	Unknown	Low	Unknown	High	Low
Occupational hazards					
Agriculture: pesticides, fertilizers, equipment	Low	Medium	High	Low	Low
Mining (dust exposure)	Low	High	Medium	Medium	Medium
Industrial safety	Low	High	High	Medium	Medium
Air pollution control	Low	Low	Low	Low	Low
Home environment: heating	Medium	Low	Medium	Low	Medium
Genetic screening and counseling	Low	Low	Medium	Low	Low

a. As demonstrated, for example, from implementation in other countries.
b. Related to prevalence of diseases affected, age and social characteristics of people affected, and effectiveness of program. A possible measure of effectiveness is healthy days of life saved.
c. Including aflatoxin.
Source: Authors.

mobilization of national resources to reduce cancer morbidity and mortality. This can be accomplished by setting priorities based on epidemiological information, demonstrating the value of specific cancer control activities, and anticipating changes in cancer incidence and resource needs. Several countries have developed national cancer control strategies on the basis of WHO recommendations. (Examples are Chile [WHO 1988a]; Indonesia [WHO/Indonesia, Ministry of Health 1989]; India [India, Ministry of Health and Family Welfare 1984; Nair 1988; and Bhargava, n.d.]; and Sri Lanka [Warnakulasuriya and others 1984].)

The cost-effectiveness analysis in the preceding sections is suggestive of appropriate priorities and does not take the place of the analysis of country-specific situations. The analysis does, however, provide an indication of the main components of a general cancer strategy. This section recommends a four-component general strategy for cancer consisting of primary prevention, secondary prevention, case management, and surveillance. The strategy is in direct contrast to the current picture in Europe and the United States in that it places less emphasis on centralized higher-level technology and acute care and greater emphasis on diffused basic institutional care and prevention. The strategy is based on the superior cost-effectiveness of prevention and lower-level case management.

Primary Prevention

Primary prevention programs are the key element in a strategy for cancer. Cancers targeted by the strategy and the program design need to be consistent with the pattern of cancers and risk factors in individual countries. The analysis above suggests that antismoking programs are of utmost priority and ought to be implemented as soon as possible. An antismoking campaign would be the single most cost-effective preventive activity and

would likely be at least several times less costly per year of life saved than any other anticancer program. Smoking prevention and cessation programs could reduce lung and other cancers as well as provide benefits in reduced mortality from cardiovascular and nonmalignant respiratory diseases. Programs to reduce tobacco chewing are needed in countries in which oral cancer is prevalent. Hepatitis immunization is also likely to be cost-effective and should be a part of national strategies in countries in which HBV incidence is high, perhaps in conjunction with efforts to reduce aflatoxin exposure. These findings are consistent with a subjective evaluation of alternative primary prevention possibilities in the context of the limited resources of developing countries. A list of potential primary prevention activities is given in table 21-12. The activities are rated as to the importance of the associated disease as a cause of years of life lost, feasibility (including ease of behavioral modification), potential technical effectiveness, and cost per person covered.

Secondary Prevention

Analysis of the cost-effectiveness of individual secondary prevention programs is needed in specific country situations before they can be adopted as components of a national cancer strategy. Of all secondary prevention possibilities, cervical cancer screening through periodic pelvic examinations and Pap tests shows the most potential as a universal strategy component. In table 21-13 we list secondary prevention activities and give an evaluation of their potential as components of a national strategy. Again, as with the primary prevention activities, the list is subjective and only meant to be used as a basis for discussion. A salient aspect of the table, confirmed in several studies of specific secondary prevention activities, is the high cost of vertical secondary prevention programs in relation to benefits.

The high cost is a result of the fact that often thousands of people must be screened to identify one case of the disease and that most people who test positive in a screening program are found (on definitive testing) not to have cancer. Thus, the cost of screening per new case can be very high. Generally, secondary prevention is more attractive if the screening and early treatment costs are low, early therapy is effective, and the cost of late treatment is high (Kristein, Arnold, and Wynder 1977).

Secondary prevention generally appears less cost-effective than smoking prevention and HBV immunization. Still, well-planned and executed programs of cervical and (perhaps) breast cancer screening (using physical examination without mammography) directed at high-risk women may be cost-effective in areas of high incidence. Other screening programs are either of unproven benefit or do not seem highly cost-effective in most situations. But as the health sector develops and evidence of effectiveness accumulates, additional screening strategies may become cost-effective. Especially strong candidate programs for future evaluation are screening for oral and large bowel cancer.

Studies in the United States and Canada indicate that many secondary prevention programs are not cost-effective individually but may be important components of an integrated program. For example, pelvic examinations carried out as a result of mass vertical campaigns have been shown to be expensive per year of additional life gained among U.S. women, but when carried out as an integrated part of other activities, such as a periodic check-up or for contraceptive visits, the cost-effectiveness increases. Targeting also increases the cost-effectiveness of secondary prevention activities.

Case Management

Given the inadequacy of existing and projected resources to cope with chronic disease through conventional tertiary-level care, alternative modes of case management must be developed. Expansion of treatment care to cope with all cancer at the secondary or tertiary level would far exceed projected resources during the next twenty years in developing countries, and in any case it is not advisable, given the practicality of lower-level case management. Criteria need to be defined for developing and using upper-level and specialized facilities. To facilitate development of treatment policies, an evaluation of the effectiveness of treatment in extending the life of cancer

patients must be made on a disease-by-disease basis and with differentiation by stage of disease and other prognostic factors.

Limited centralized facilities for treatment of selected referred cancer patients may be appropriate as discussed in the section on treatment, above, especially if improved treatment capacity is coordinated with earlier referral and diagnosis. Criteria for referral to treatment in higher levels of the health care system would make it possible to achieve longer and higher-quality lives for more people with existing and projected levels of resources. For most cancers, however, treatment with higher-level tertiary care is not cost-effective, and the investment by low-income countries in the special capacity for cancer treatment is not warranted. The small gains in life expectancy that may be achieved are often associated with a poor quality of existence, great discomfort, and stress. Use of scarce technical medical resources to treat cancer reduces their availability for other diseases for which there is greater probability of a favorable outcome from treatment and a higher quality of the years of life saved. Instead, development of less centralized, lower-level, treatment or case management alternatives, including adequate pain relief, would not only save resources but would also allow more humane care for the terminally ill.

Alternative lower-level and community-based care that could be developed includes substitution of outpatient for inpatient care; use of nonphysician professionals; use of home beds, community nursing care, and hospices; and an emphasis on palliative care rather than cure. Such care is not only of lower cost but may also be more humane.

Surveillance and Research

Rational planning of health resource allocation requires a continuous flow of information on disease occurrence, prevalence of etiological factors, and the cost and effectiveness of health interventions. This information can be used to set health investment priorities, to develop guidelines or triage rules for the use of health services, and to examine the cost-effectiveness of health activities from broad aspects of program strategy down to the assessment of specific technologies.

Ongoing data collection and research programs in most developing countries do not provide a good basis for building the capacity to analyze health program effectiveness in the future. These programs need to be strengthened and use made

Table 21-13. Subjective Potential for Secondary Preventive Activities for Cancer

Activity	Potential reduction of YLL	Feasibility[a]	Potential technical effect	Persons covered per unit cost	Priority
Pelvic exam	Medium	High	Medium	Low	Medium
Rectum, colon, prostate exam	Medium	High	Unknown	Medium	Low
Breast exam (mammography)	Low	Medium	Medium	Low	Low
Lung, stomach, esophagus cytology	High	Medium	Low	Low	Low
Oral exam	Medium	High	Unknown	Medium	Medium

a. As demonstrated, for example, from implementation in other countries.
Source: Authors.

of the analytical findings in cancer planning. For example, in China the Disease Surveillance Points System is providing crucial mortality information for setting health priorities on a disease-specific basis. This information, supplemented with cost data, will make it possible to analyze the cost-effectiveness of specific preventive and curative care interventions. It will also help to improve program efficiency by formulating criteria for prevention programs and triage rules for the use of curative care.

In-country capacity for research on questions of operational prevention programs needs to be developed. Particularly important are questions on the cost-effectiveness of health care technology. Cancer treatments and diagnostic procedures, perhaps more than those for other diseases, have led to adoption of high-cost technology with little established effectiveness. The contrast between the benefits of prevention and cure is acute for cancer. This contrast needs to be effectively and continually questioned using local analytical capacity.

Prototypical models for longitudinal operational research programs to reduce mortality and morbidity related to cancer and other chronic diseases need to be developed. Such programs would encompass a surveillance system for chronic diseases, an experimental framework for testing community-based interventions, and collaboration with the existing disease prevention and health care system in testing new programs. Activities that might come under examination include alternative antismoking measures, early detection of breast and cervical cancer, and a program of case management that employs home care and attempts to coordinate the capacity of different levels of care to provide cost-effective palliation. Establishment of such models in several regions with diverse epidemiological and socioeconomic environments would make it possible to test alternative primary and secondary prevention programs in specific local conditions.

Appendix 21A: The Ten Most Important Cancers in the Developing World

We consider each of the cancers individually, including a brief description of its biological characteristics, pattern of occurrence, important risk factors, effectiveness of treatment, possibility for screening, and potential for primary prevention. The descriptions, of necessity, are brief. Our purpose is to provide a background to the discussion in the text. More complete information can be obtained from any of several references, although Schottenfeld and Fraumeni 1982 is particularly recommended. Tables 21A-1 and 21A-2 provide rates and percentages of cancer incidence, respectively.

Stomach Cancer

Stomach cancer arises within the glandular cells that line the inside of the stomach. Almost all these tumors are adenocarcinomas. They may show varying degrees of differentiation and may take several forms; a polyp projecting into the lumen of the stomach, a superficially spreading mass on the stomach mucosa, or an infiltrating process in the stomach wall. In its early stages stomach cancer usually causes no symptoms. With more advanced disease patients experience lack of appetite, weight loss, abdominal pain, and other nonspecific digestive symptoms. Diagnosis is usually made by barium x-ray studies or gastroscopy. Within the United States more than 85 percent of patients have advanced disease at the time of diagnosis, and only 10 to 15 percent survive five years.

OCCURRENCE. About 670,000 cases of stomach cancer occur in the world each year, the cases being about equally divided between the industrial and developing countries. Mortality rates are particularly high (above 30 per 100,000 for males) in Japan, Chile, Hungary, and Poland. They are much lower in United States whites (about 6 per 100,000), reflecting the dramatic decline during this century in the occurrence of stomach cancer. Stomach cancer incidence among Japanese immigrants to the United States falls in succeeding generations. Incidence tends to be 1.5 to 2 times higher in men than in women. There is a progressive increase in incidence with increasing age.

ETIOLOGY. International variations and results of migrant studies strongly support a role of nongenetic factors in stomach cancer etiology. The actual causative factors, however, remain uncertain. The most promising explanation is that the diet may contain both carcinogenic and anticarcinogenic substances that influence stomach cells. Likely candidates for dietary carcinogens are (a) nitrosamines and (b) toxins produced by molds and bacteria in the course of food spoilage or pickling. Highly salted foods also appear to increase risk. Candidates for protective substances in the diet include vitamin C and beta-carotene, a vitamin A precursor. Nitrosamines are present in preserved or smoked foods and can be formed in the stomach through metabolism of naturally occurring nitrates and nitrites in food and water. Antioxidants, such as vitamin C, appear to inhibit nitrosamine formation. Although nitrosamines are potent carcinogens, their hypothesized role in the etiology of human stomach cancer remains unproven. Infection with *Helicobacter pylori* is a cause of gastritis and may predispose individuals to the carcinogenic effects of dietary nitrosamines.

TREATMENT. When detected early, stomach cancer may be treated by removal of all or part of the stomach. The great majority of patients are not candidates for this surgery either because the tumor has spread beyond the stomach or because they are too ill to withstand a major operative procedure. Other forms of cancer therapy such as radiation or drugs are not curative and have little palliative effect.

SCREENING. There is evidence, principally from Japan, that screening by barium x-ray studies, gastroscopy, or gastric cytology may detect stomach cancer at a stage when surgical cure is more likely. None of these techniques has had a rigorous

Table 21A-1. Estimated Crude Rates of Cancer by Site, Sex, and Region, 1980
(per 100,000 people)

Site or type of cancer	Africa		Latin America		China		Other Asia		All developing countries		All industrial countries	
	Male	Female	Male	Female	Male	Female	Male	Female	Male	Female	Male	Female
Mouth/pharynx	6.2	3.7	8.7	3.3	6.1	4.4	15.2	8.3	10.5	5.9	14.7	4.4
Esophagus	3.0	1.1	5.8	2.2	21.0	12.3	4.9	3.5	9.6	5.6	7.3	2.9
Stomach	3.2	2.0	17.7	10.2	24.6	15.6	6.2	3.5	12.6	7.6	35.8	23.2
Colon/rectum	2.9	2.5	9.1	10.1	8.3	7.7	4.2	3.3	5.8	5.2	34.4	34.1
Liver	7.5	2.9	2.9	2.0	15.2	7.1	4.4	1.6	8.0	3.5	6.7	3.9
Lung	3.1	0.8	17.7	5.0	8.5	4.7	9.5	2.4	9.2	3.1	65.3	16.3
Breast	n.a.	12.3	n.a.	30.8	n.a.	6.4	n.a.	15.0	n.a.	13.8	n.a.	59.2
Cervix	n.a.	18.1	n.a.	27.0	n.a.	27.4	n.a.	20.0	n.a.	22.7	n.a.	16.4
Lymphoma	8.8	4.9	6.3	4.6	2.2	1.7	4.4	2.3	4.6	2.7	11.4	9.1
Leukemia	2.3	2.0	4.7	4.0	4.7	3.4	3.1	2.1	3.6	2.7	8.3	6.3
Other	31.7	26.3	57.4	48.1	35.4	18.3	27.0	22.1	33.5	24.5	108.8	83.0
Total	68.6	76.7	130.4	147.3	126.0	109.0	78.9	84.2	97.3	97.4	292.6	258.9

n.a. Not applicable.
Source: Parkin, Laara, and Muir 1988.

scientific evaluation (through a controlled clinical trial), so their actual value remains uncertain. In countries with high incidence and mortality from stomach cancer, the effectiveness of screening programs may be worth investigating. Stomach cancer does not occur with sufficient frequency in most populations, however, to justify mass screening activities. In these populations more selective screening of high-risk individuals may be practical if any screening measure is eventually proven to be effective in preventing stomach cancer death.

PREVENTION. Knowledge of risk factors is insufficient to recommend specific primary preventive strategies. In the industrial countries, particularly in North America, time trends in stomach cancer suggest a benefit from increased consumption of fresh fruits and vegetables and decreased consumption

of spoiled foods or those preserved by pickling. Epidemiological data linking lowered risk to consumption of fresh fruits and vegetables (particularly those containing large amounts of vitamin C and beta-carotene) should be considered in discussions of national food policy. For example, it seems prudent to avoid strategies that discourage production and consumption of these foods.

Esophageal Cancer

Esophageal cancer arises from the cells lining the inside of the esophagus. The tumors may be either squamous cell or adenocarcinoma in histological appearance. Usual presenting symptoms are difficulty swallowing and steady chest pain. Diagnosis is made by barium x-ray studies or endoscopy. At diagnosis

Table 21A-2. New Cancer Incidence, by Site, Sex, and Region
(percent)

Site or type of cancer	Africa		Latin America		China		Other Asia		All developing countries		All industrial countries	
	Male	Female	Male	Female	Male	Female	Male	Female	Male	Female	Male	Female
Mouth/pharynx	9.0	4.8	6.7	2.2	4.8	4.0	19.2	9.8	10.7	6.0	5.0	1.7
Esophagus	4.4	1.4	4.4	1.5	16.7	11.3	6.2	4.2	9.9	5.8	2.5	1.1
Stomach	4.6	2.6	13.6	6.9	19.5	14.3	7.8	4.2	12.9	7.8	12.2	9.0
Colon/rectum	4.2	3.2	7.0	6.9	6.6	7.1	5.3	3.9	5.9	5.4	11.7	13.2
Liver	11.0	3.7	2.2	1.3	12.1	6.5	5.6	1.9	8.2	3.6	2.3	1.5
Lung	4.5	1.0	13.6	3.4	6.7	4.3	12.1	2.9	9.4	3.2	22.3	6.3
Breast	n.a.	16.0	n.a.	20.9	n.a.	5.9	n.a.	17.8	n.a.	14.1	n.a.	22.9
Cervix	n.a.	23.7	n.a.	18.3	n.a.	25.1	n.a.	23.8	n.a.	23.3	n.a.	6.3
Lymphoma	12.8	6.4	4.9	3.1	1.7	1.6	5.6	2.7	4.7	2.8	3.9	3.5
Leukemia	3.3	2.6	3.6	2.7	3.7	3.1	3.9	2.5	3.7	2.8	2.8	2.4
Other	46.1	34.3	44.0	32.6	28.1	16.8	34.2	26.2	34.4	25.1	37.2	32.1

n.a. Not applicable.
Note: Figures reflect percentage of each cancer in the region.
Source: Parkin, Laara, and Muir 1988.

most esophageal cancers have spread into adjacent tissues. The prognosis is dismal, and fewer than 5 percent of patients survive for five years.

OCCURRENCE. Esophageal cancer accounts for approximately 310,000 new cases of cancer per year, four-fifths of which occur in the developing world. Esophageal cancer incidence and mortality rates vary greatly in different parts of the world. In the areas of Iran and the former Soviet Union which surround the Caspian Sea, mortality rates of more than 100 per 100,000 per year pertain for both men and women. Within North America the rate is less than 5 per 100,000 per year. The occurrence of esophageal cancer increases progressively with age. Rates tend to be about twice as high among men as women in most parts of the world, although in some areas of high incidence the male-female differences are less, whereas in others they are much greater. In the United States, esophageal cancer rates are higher among blacks than whites, and there appears to be a socioeconomic gradient, the disease being more frequent among the poor. Mortality rates for esophageal cancer, unlike those for stomach cancer, have not declined much in recent years in industrial countries.

ETIOLOGY. Tobacco and alcohol are the principal risk factors for esophageal cancer in industrial countries. The joint effect of these two substances in increasing risk appears to be greater than the sum of their individual effects. There is no clear explanation for the extremely high rates of esophageal cancer in areas such as the Caspian littoral and parts of northern China. Dietary characteristics have been implicated, but no particular component or habit has yet been proven to account for the highly elevated risk. Factors of interest include toxins in pickled foods and fermented drinks, carcinogens from burning tobacco or opium, and deficiencies in nutrients such as vitamin A, zinc, or selenium.

TREATMENT. Surgical resection offers the only chance of cure in localized disease, and surgery is also useful for relief of symptoms in more advanced cases. Radiation therapy may also relieve symptoms, particularly the inability to swallow.

SCREENING. The feasibility of screening for esophageal cancer has been considered in high-risk populations of northern China. Thus far, screening by endoscopy or cytology has not been shown to reduce mortality. This topic merits further study in areas of extremely high risk.

PREVENTION. In countries in which there is relatively low risk of esophageal cancer, the most reasonable primary preventive strategies are avoidance of tobacco and reduced consumption of alcoholic beverages. In countries with extraordinarily high rates of esophageal cancer, the actual risk factors have yet to be identified, so there is little information on which to base a primary prevention program. Studies of dietary supplementation with vitamins now being conducted in northern China may provide a better scientific basis for intervention.

Lung Cancer

Cancers of the lung may arise at any site in the respiratory tree beyond the trachea, but most of these tumors occur in small airways within the lung itself. There are four main histological subtypes: adenocarcinoma, squamous cell, small cell undifferentiated, and large cell undifferentiated. The relative frequency of these different histological types varies according to sex and exposure to cigarette smoking. Among nonsmokers, adenocarcinoma is most common. In smokers, squamous cell tumors are most common, although women smokers also have a high frequency of small cell undifferentiated cancers. The principal importance of histological type is that small cell undifferentiated tumors behave differently from the others. They are virtually always metastatic when diagnosed, and they are more responsive to combined chemotherapy and radiation. Initial symptoms of lung cancer are cough, bloody sputum, chest pain, or systemic symptoms of weight loss and fatigue. At least two-thirds of lung cancers have spread beyond the local site by the time of diagnosis. These tumors progress both by regional extension and distant metastases to the brain and other organs (this is particularly true for small cell undifferentiated tumors). About 90 percent of patients die within two years of diagnosis.

OCCURRENCE. Lung cancer accounts for approximately 660,000 new cases of cancer per year; just over 200,000 of these occur in developing countries. Countries with the highest mortality rates (for males) include the United Kingdom (about 115 deaths per 100,000 per year) and other countries of northern Europe and North America (about 75 deaths per 100,000 per year). Rates are lower in countries in which smoking is less common, such as Costa Rica (6 per 100,000) and Israel (25 per 100,000). In most countries mortality rates for females are approximately one-fifth to one-third those of males. Lung cancer incidence rates increase progressively with age except where cigarette smoking has been taken up more recently; in such countries relatively few older adults have smoked, so lung cancer rates are lower among the elderly. Incidence and mortality rates from lung cancer have increased dramatically in the past fifty years in many countries, and lung cancer has become the largest cause of cancer death in the world as a whole. The increases parallel (with a delay of at least twenty years) the uptake of tobacco smoking.

ETIOLOGY. The most important risk factor for lung cancer is cigarette smoking. Numerous studies have shown that smokers have ten to fifteen times the risk of lung cancer as nonsmokers. Among heavy smokers the risk is approximately twenty-five times that of nonsmokers. Risk is most closely related to the number of years a person has smoked. Filtered and low-tar cigarettes appear to be less risky than other types with regard to causing lung cancer (although they are not clearly less hazardous with respect to cardiovascular disease). In certain limited populations other risk factors are also important in lung cancer etiology. These include asbestos (related to mining and industrial exposure), radon (principally related to underground mining but perhaps related to household exposures), and industrial exposure to substances such as bischloromethylether (BCME), nickel, and chromates. Dietary and serum studies show a decreased risk in persons eating large amounts of foods containing beta-carotene and in those with higher blood levels of this substance. The importance of these findings is uncertain.

TREATMENT. Surgical resection of lung cancer offers the only real chance of cure. Fewer than one-third of patients are candidates for this surgery, either because the tumor is no longer localized or because the patient is too unwell to withstand a major operation. Radiation therapy can palliate symptoms of lung cancer and, in some patients, may extend survival. A small fraction of patients with small cell undifferentiated tumors appear to have prolonged survival following intensive radiation or chemotherapy.

SCREENING. Various methods of early detection of lung cancer have been tested, but none has been shown to be effective. Methods tried include periodic chest radiographs and examination of sputum cytology. The principal problem with screening is that lung cancer progresses rapidly from the time when it is first detectable by screening methods to when it is no longer curable by surgery. Screening programs designed to increase this "window of opportunity" are under consideration and may eventually prove beneficial in selected groups of very high risk individuals.

PREVENTION. The principal preventive efforts are discouraging uptake of cigarette smoking and encouraging its discontinuance among those who already smoke. There is evidence that adult and teenage education can decrease use of cigarettes. More effective programs, however, will likely be aimed at restricting cigarette marketing (through prohibition of advertising) or sales (by heavy taxation). Efforts to portray cigarette smoking as antisocial behavior also may be effective in groups which are responsive to these social pressures. Reduction of occupational exposures to asbestos and other lung carcinogens is also warranted.

Liver Cancer

Most primary liver cancers are hepatocellular carcinomas (HCCs) and arise from hepatic parenchymal cells. Another important cell type is cholangiocarcinoma, which arises from the bile ducts. It accounts for fewer than 25 percent of all primary liver cancers in low-incidence areas and probably fewer than 10 percent in areas with high primary liver cancer incidence. Risk for cholangiocarcinoma appears to be increased in persons infected with *Clonorchis* and *Opisthorchis*, which are liver fluke infections prevalent in Southeast Asia and are acquired by eating uncooked fish. Within the developing world the great majority of liver cancers are HCCs, and the remainder of this discussion primarily focuses on that

histological category. These tumors develop within the liver and cause localized destruction and enlargement of that organ. Presenting symptoms are abdominal mass, pain, and weight loss. The tumor tends to progress rapidly by local growth and extension. Distant metastases may occur but usually are not an important feature. Fewer than one person in twenty survives five years following diagnosis.

OCCURRENCE. Primary liver cancer accounts for 250,000 new cases of cancer per year; more than 190,000 of these occur in developing countries. Areas of highest incidence and mortality are in Sub-Saharan Africa and southern Asia. Rates tend to be lower in North America and western Europe. In Hong Kong, mortality rates for males are roughly 39 per 100,000; in the United States, they are less than 2 per 100,000. Mortality rates for females are generally one-half to one-quarter of the male rates. Substantial differences in rates occur for different ethnic groups within countries; for example, in the United States, ethnic Chinese have liver cancer rates approximately five to eight times those for whites. In countries of high incidence, liver cancer rates appear to plateau in middle adulthood, whereas in areas of low incidence they continue to rise progressively with age.

ETIOLOGY. There is compelling evidence from epidemiological and laboratory studies that hepatitis B virus can cause hepatocellular carcinoma. Liver cancer is most common in countries with high rates of HBV infection; the vast majority of patients with HCC have serological evidence of HBV infection, particularly the carrier state; and laboratory studies have shown viral DNA within hepatocellular carcinoma cells. In areas with high liver cancer incidence and mortality, HBV infection occurs early in life, probably during the perinatal period, and is spread from carrier mothers to their children. Other likely etiological factors include alcohol consumption and aflatoxin. In areas of low incidence, alcohol use and cirrhosis are usually (though not always) identified as risk factors in epidemiological studies; but in high incidence areas, alcohol is probably of minimal importance. In tropical Africa and Asia, food preservation is difficult, and growth of a mold (*Aspergillus flavus*) can contaminate foods with aflatoxins, which are strongly carcinogenic in laboratory animals. Epidemiological data support a higher risk of liver cancer in persons who consume relatively larger amounts of foods (particularly peanuts and grains) likely to be contaminated with aflatoxins. This factor appears to act jointly with hepatitis B virus in explaining much of the worldwide distribution of primary liver cancer. Other exposures (such as smoking) and hereditary disorders (such as hemochromatosis) are also associated with the risk of liver cancer, but these factors could only account for a small proportion of primary liver cancers in the developing countries.

TREATMENT. If detected very early, liver cancers can be surgically resected, although the procedure is a lengthy one and requires great surgical skill. Some patients have been treated successfully with total resection of the liver and transplantation. Other treatment modalities, such as radiation and chemotherapy, are of little or no benefit for this condition.

SCREENING. Hepatocellular carcinomas produce alpha-fetoprotein, which can be detected by assay of peripheral blood. There are reports from uncontrolled studies in very high risk groups that alpha-fetoprotein screening detects asymptomatic persons who may be cured by surgical resection. The screening procedure has not, however, been the focus of any rigorous scientific study.

PREVENTION. In high-risk areas, preventive efforts are directed toward neonatal immunization with HBV vaccine. The effectiveness of this vaccine in preventing liver cancer has not been established, although current studies in China and the Gambia should eventually provide a better basis for assessing its value. Because of the strong evidence linking HBV infection to primary liver cancer, and because of the apparent safety of the vaccine, widespread programs of immunization are a prudent course of action until vaccine field trials have been completed. Other preventive efforts should focus on maintaining food stores, such as peanuts, under conditions that minimize growth of molds. Testing commercial food stores for aflatoxin is also a reasonable strategy. In areas endemic for liver fluke infection, control of these parasites may reduce cholangiocarcinoma occurrence.

Cervical Cancer

Cervical cancer arises in cells covering the lower, vaginal portion of the uterus. Progression from normal cells to cancerous ones appears to occur through phases of dysplasia, carcinoma in situ, and, finally, invasive cancer. Some terminology breaks down the preinvasive phases into three categories: cervical intraepithelial neoplasia I, II, and III. In most women, the transformation from normal cells to invasive carcinoma occurs over a long period (probably fifteen to thirty years), so there is long time when the condition can be detected at an early, noninvasive stage. In some women, however, the process appears to progress much more rapidly. Once cervical cancer becomes invasive it tends to spread by direct extension to the adjacent tissues of the pelvis and by metastases to distant sites such as the lung and liver. In the United States approximately 50 percent of invasive cervical cancers are still localized when detected. Approximately 80 percent of patients survive for five years if tumors are still localized and approximately 60 percent survive for five years through all stages. Most cervical cancers are found by screening examinations; however, symptoms of vaginal bleeding and pelvic pain occur if the disease progresses beyond the initial stage.

OCCURRENCE. Cancer of the cervix accounts for 470,000 new cases of cancer per year in the world. Approximately 80 percent of these occur in developing countries, where they cause about 155,000 deaths annually. Areas of highest incidence include Colombia (50 per 100,000) and Brazil (40 per 100,000); very low incidence is found among Israeli Jews (5 per 100,000). There is a strong socioeconomic gradient, the poorer countries and poorer groups of women within countries having the highest risk. Peak incidence of invasive cervical cancer occurs in late adulthood, and lower rates are observed in the elderly. In North America, cervical cancer mortality rates have declined dramatically during the past fifty years. This decline began before institution of Pap testing. Nevertheless, there is strong evidence from studies in the United States, Canada, and northern Europe that widespread use of the Pap test has contributed to the decline in mortality from this condition. In some countries of western Europe there has been a recent reversal of the trend toward falling rates, and cervical cancer appears to be increasing among younger women.

ETIOLOGY. Cervical cancer has many features of a sexually transmitted disease. Risks are highest among women who have had multiple sexual partners (or whose husbands have had multiple partners), who began sexual intercourse early in life, and who have sexual partners of lower socioeconomic status. Barrier methods of contraception appear protective; oral contraceptives increase risk moderately. Intensive efforts to identify an infectious cause of cervical cancer initially focused on herpes simplex virus 2 (HSV2). Indeed, cervical cancer risk is strongly associated with evidence of HSV2 infection, and laboratory studies have found HSV2 genetic material in cervical cancer cells. Nevertheless, more recent studies strongly suggest an etiological role for human papilloma virus (HPV), particularly types 16 and 18. This virus is more strongly associated with cervical cancer risk than is HSV2. Human papilloma virus causes benign growths (genital warts), and HPV DNA has been found intercalated in the human DNA of cervical cancer cells. Another risk factor is cigarette smoking. In most studies smokers have cervical cancer risks 1.5 to 2 times higher than nonsmokers. Although this association might be noncausal and due to the relationship between smoking and early sexual activity, the weight of evidence appears to favor a causal role for smoking in cervical cancer.

TREATMENT. Treatment of cervical neoplasia varies according to stage. For noninvasive lesions, initial destruction of the affected tissue by incision or laser and periodic follow-up may be all that is necessary to achieve a cure. As an alternative, hysterectomy removes the affected tissue and obviates any need for further surveillance. In more advanced disease the treatment options depend on the extent of tumor spread and the preferences of the patient. Extensive pelvic surgery and radiation are capable of curing disease which has spread beyond the cervix, although success in more advanced stages is less likely.

SCREENING. Pap testing involves cytological examination of cells scraped from the cervix and is the established screening method for cervical cancer. Properly performed, the Pap test is capable of detecting the vast majority of cervical neoplasms before they become invasive. Positive tests require follow-up by repeat testing, biopsy, and, perhaps, culdoscopic examination to establish the diagnosis. Although annual Pap tests are recommended for high-risk women, less frequent testing (even as rarely as every five years) should be highly effective in reducing mortality. The principal obstacle in Pap test programs is that the women at highest risk are hard to reach because they are poor and avoid doctors. Failure to follow up positive or suspicious tests and unreliable cytology readings have also been problems in some programs. In most settings, highest priority should be assigned to achieving widespread acceptance of the Pap test program and to providing adequate definitive care. More frequent testing of already screened women is usually less important.

PREVENTION. No primary prevention programs have proven effective. The fact that cervical cancer is amenable to early detection and the lack of certainty about its etiology have directed public health efforts to screening. Some authors propose development and implementation of HPV vaccines, but these suggestions (like earlier suggestions for an HSV2 vaccine) appear to be premature.

Nasopharyngeal Cancer

Cancers of the oral cavity and pharynx fall into two relatively separate epidemiological categories. The first is nasopharyngeal cancer, which occurs principally among the populations of southern China and Southeast Asia. The second category, discussed separately below, includes other tumors of the mouth and pharynx, which occur with greatest frequency in people who habitually chew tobacco, betel, or similar substances.

Nasopharyngeal cancer arises in epithelial cells lining the surface of the nasopharynx. Usual presenting symptoms are lymph nodes in the neck; nasal bleeding and obstruction; symptoms of nerve compression, including headache; and earache or hearing loss. The five-year survival rate after treatment (radiotherapy) is approximately 22 to 35 percent.

OCCURRENCE. Although rare in most of the world, nasopharyngeal cancer is the most common cause of cancer death in some southern Chinese populations. Rates are high in areas with large groups of Chinese origin, as in Singapore and Malaysia. Nasopharyngeal cancer occurs with peak frequency among adults between the ages of thirty-five and sixty-five, but it also occurs relatively often in children and adolescents. Risk is somewhat higher in males than in females. The condition is associated with lower socioeconomic class in China and perhaps in other countries.

ETIOLOGY. The principal identified risk factors for nasopharyngeal cancer are Epstein-Barr virus infection and the consumption during infancy of traditionally prepared Chinese salted fish. The role of Epstein-Barr virus in this condition is unclear, because Epstein-Barr virus infection occurs throughout the world but nasopharyngeal cancer is seen principally in the Orient. Traditionally prepared Chinese salted fish contains carcinogens (perhaps volatile nitrosamines) which can produce nasopharyngeal tumors in rats. Volatile nitrosamines exist in other traditionally prepared foods in endemic areas, and further study of this issue may lead to an effective preventive strategy.

TREATMENT. Treatment of nasopharyngeal cancer involves high-dose radiation therapy. The tumor is generally responsive. Most patients achieve palliation and approximately one-quarter are cured.

SCREENING. There are no proven effective screening mechanisms for nasopharyngeal cancer.

PREVENTION. Primary prevention methods are speculative. Development of an Epstein-Barr virus vaccine has been proposed as a possible preventive method, but none has yet been developed, and the value of this method is uncertain. Changes in infant feeding practices (should the initial findings regarding salted fish and other foods be confirmed) appear to offer more promise for prevention.

Oral and Other Pharyngeal Cancers

Other cancers of the oral cavity and pharynx principally arise in the lining of the mouth and throat. Most of these tumors have a squamous cell histology. They typically present either as an oral ulcer or as enlarged lymph nodes in the neck, and they progress through local and regional extension rather than distant metastases. The usual outcome varies according to where the tumor arises within the mouth or pharynx. Cancers of the lip are generally found early and are cured by surgery. Those of the tongue or pharynx are approximately 70 percent fatal within five years.

OCCURRENCE. Worldwide, cancers of the mouth and pharynx account for more than 300,000 new cases of cancer per year, about two-thirds of which occur in developing economies. Incidence and mortality rates are highest in India, Hong Kong, Puerto Rico, Brazil, France, and Singapore. In most parts of the world, incidence rates are many times higher for males than for females. Rates increase progressively with age, and there is a strong socioeconomic gradient, the poorer people having higher rates.

ETIOLOGY. The principal risk factor for oral and pharyngeal cancers is tobacco smoking and chewing. In countries such as India, tobacco is often mixed with betel leaves, lime, and other substances. Chewing betel, or areca, nut may be a risk factor even in the absence of tobacco use. Cigarette smoking (especially reverse smoking) is also associated with risk. Other risk factors include alcohol consumption and lower intake of fruits and vegetables (which contain beta-carotene as well as other possible anticarcinogens). Cancers of the lip are strongly related to sunlight exposure.

TREATMENT. Treatment of these tumors principally involves surgery and radiation therapy. Surgery can be curative if tumors are found early, but it often results in substantial loss of function and requires intense rehabilitative efforts. Radiation therapy is used in conjunction with surgery and may contribute to survival. Radiation also may palliate patients with nonresectable tumors.

SCREENING. Although no screening programs have been proven to be effective, they appear likely to be beneficial. Examination of the mouth and pharynx of high-risk persons (perhaps linked to dental examinations) can detect many tumors before they have advanced to an untreatable stage. Oral examination also detects leukoplakia (white patches), a premalignant condition which requires close observation to monitor development of invasive cancer.

PREVENTION. Primary prevention should focus on reduced use of tobacco, either for chewing or smoking. Currently researchers are also investigating whether dietary supplementation, particularly with beta-carotene, can prevent oral and pharyngeal cancers. This notion remains to be proven.

Large Bowel Cancer

Cancers of the large bowel usually arise from the glandular epithelium and are classified histologically as adenocarcinomas. Most of these tumors appear to result from malignant transformation of benign adenomatous polyps. Tumors may arise anywhere in the large bowel; in the United States about three-quarters occur in the colon and one-quarter in the rectum. Although rectal and colonic cancers differ somewhat in their epidemiology and clinical behavior, they are considered together in this discussion. Large bowel cancers typically present as rectal bleeding, anemia, or signs of partial bowel obstruction. They tend to metastasize to regional lymph nodes and the liver, and about two-thirds have spread beyond the local stage by the time of diagnosis. About 50 percent of patients survive five years.

OCCURRENCE. Large bowel cancers cause more than 570,000 new cases of cancer in the world per year; about 30 percent of these occur in developing countries. Areas of greatest occurrence are the more westernized and industrialized countries. Mortality rates for males in New Zealand, Denmark, England, and Hungary range between 20 and 25 per 100,000. Typical areas of intermediate mortality are Greece (6 per 100,000) and Spain (11 per 100,000). The lowest rates are reported from less industrialized countries, such as Costa Rica (5 per 100,000) and Nigeria (probably below 2 per 100,000). Within areas of high incidence there are often populations with lower incidence. For example, in New Zealand, incidence rates in the Maori are approximately one-third those of the non-Maori. Incidence and mortality rates in women are generally about 20 percent lower than those in men. Risk increases progressively with age.

ETIOLOGY. The causes of large bowel cancer are unknown. International comparisons and migrant studies implicate dietary habits in the etiology of this disease. Dietary fat consumption is a strong candidate for a causal role, but the epidemiological data are inconclusive. Relative deficiency of vegetable fiber is also implicated in large bowel cancer etiology, particularly in persons with a high dietary fat intake. The risk of large bowel cancer is lower in people who consume large amounts of vegetables and fruit. Possible protective substances from these sources include vitamins C and E, beta-carotene, indoles, and the like. Adenomatous polyps and bowel cancers also appear to be at least partly determined genetically.

TREATMENT. Surgical resection of tumor and adjacent large bowel is curative if the cancer is detected early. For rectal cancer, radiation therapy may also contribute to the chance of cure and palliation. Chemotherapy of advanced lesions does not prolong survival materially, although some patients are improved by this treatment. Patients with rectal cancer often require a colostomy and need postoperative rehabilitation.

SCREENING. Although several screening practices have been broadly recommended for early detection of large bowel cancer, none has been conclusively shown to reduce mortality from this condition. Screening methods fall into three categories: stool occult blood testing, digital rectal examination, and sigmoidoscopic examination. Occult blood screening involves testing a small specimen of stool for the presence of hemoglobin. The test is easy to perform, inexpensive, and generally acceptable to patients. The principal problems with the test are that it results in a high number of false-positive findings, which require subsequent and (often costly) definitive diagnostic studies, and it has a relatively low sensitivity in the detection of small polyps and very early cancers (because these generally do not bleed). Large clinical trials of occult blood screening, despite involving tens of thousands of patients, have thus far failed to show a statistically significant reduction in large bowel cancer mortality associated with use of the test. It appears, therefore, that even if occult blood testing is effective, the magnitude of benefit is not large. A second method of screening is finger examination of the distal rectum; this can be performed at the time of a complete physical examination. Advantages of this screening method are simplicity and low cost. The primary disadvantage is that only a small proportion of large bowel cancers are potentially detectable in this way. The third screening method is visual examination of the rectum and sigmoid colon; this is best accomplished with a flexible sigmoidoscope. The procedure reliably detects early cancers and adenomatous polyps in the distal large bowel (usually the last 60 centimeters). Advantages of this procedure are that it appears to identify as many as 80 percent of persons who harbor polyps (although identification of all polyps in these people will require examination of the remainder of the large bowel by colonoscopy or contrast x-rays). Because polyp formers are the group at greatest risk of later developing bowel cancer, they should be kept under surveillance after being identified by sigmoidoscopic examination. Disadvantages of the procedure are that it requires a skilled examiner (usually a physician, although trained nurses and paramedical personnel have been used successfully), the equipment is expensive, and the procedure entails more time and discomfort than other screening methods. Although flexible sigmoidoscopic screening has not yet been tested in a controlled clinical trial, on present evidence it appears to offer the best prospect for reducing colon cancer mortality.

PREVENTION. Uncertainty about the cause of large bowel cancer has largely prevented implementation of primary prevention programs. Dietary changes that include reduced fat and increased fiber intake have been recommended on the basis of epidemiological and laboratory data. The value of these interventions is largely a matter of conjecture, but it would be prudent for developing countries to resist dramatic changes away from their current high-fiber and low-fat diets.

Breast Cancer

The great majority (80 to 90 percent) of breast cancers arise from epithelial ductal cells; perhaps 10 percent are of lobular origin. The disease usually presents as a nodule or mass in the breast. Metastatic spread is common and may affect sites throughout the body. Involvement of the axillary lymph nodes is a usual feature of larger tumors. Other common sites of metastatic spread are the bones, liver, lung, and brain. Most breast cancers progress relatively slowly, and prolonged survival (several years) with active disease is common. After initial treatment the patients often follow a path of remission and relapse. In the United States approximately 70 percent of breast cancer patients survive five years. An important feature of breast cancer, unlike most other tumors, is that recurrence is common after a prolonged survival free of disease.

OCCURRENCE. There are approximately 575,000 new cases of breast cancer in the world each year; about 40 percent occur in developing countries. Areas of highest incidence include North America and western Europe (between 50 and 80 per 100,000), whereas incidence is lowest in Japan (about 20 per 100,000). Breast cancer incidence rates have been increasing in nearly all countries that have reliable data. The proportional increase has been greatest in areas of previously low incidence, such as Japan. Some of the increase in incidence in the United States, and perhaps elsewhere, is due to better detection of tumors. Breast cancer mortality rates in the United States have been relatively constant in the past fifty years. Mortality and incidence rates increase progressively with age until the time of menopause, after which point the rate of increase is less.

ETIOLOGY. Ionizing radiation is the only exogenous exposure that has been clearly shown to cause breast cancer. Nevertheless, several dietary and reproductive practices are related to breast cancer occurrence. Risk is increased in nulliparous women, and multiparity is associated with lower risk. Among women who have been pregnant, risk is highest in those who

delayed pregnancy into their fourth decade. In most studies, earlier menarche and later menopause are associated with higher risk. A positive family history of breast cancer is also a risk factor. Increased consumption of dietary fat and calories is implicated in breast cancer etiology, but the epidemiological data are inconclusive. In general, women who are more obese have higher death rates from breast cancer, although it is not clear whether this is due to a greater risk of developing the disease or a greater risk of dying once it has occurred. Alcohol consumption also is implicated as a risk factor, particularly for high levels of consumption.

TREATMENT. Surgical resection of the tumor is the standard initial therapy for breast cancer. Surgery may remove only the tumor or, more commonly, the entire breast and associated axillary lymph nodes. Radiation therapy is often given to the breast and adjacent lymph nodes of women treated with simple excision. For an increasing proportion of women, primary treatment of breast cancer has come to include chemotherapy and hormonal therapy with Tamoxifen. There is strong evidence that these additional therapies lessen recurrence following surgery. Metastatic disease is treated with radiation or chemotherapy and hormonal therapy to reduce local symptoms and to induce remission. Many women with metastatic breast cancer respond well to treatment and have prolonged periods of normal function. In both industrial and developing countries Tamoxifen offers safe, inexpensive, and effective treatment.

SCREENING. There is conclusive evidence from randomized clinical trials that screening programs, consisting of mammography and physician examination of the breast, reduce breast cancer mortality by about 30 percent. The value of mammography alone is less certain. Hazards of screening are a small risk of cancer from radiation exposure and a risk of needless surgery generated by false-positive results. Of all cancers, however, evidence is strongest for a beneficial effect of screening in breast cancer.

PREVENTION. Epidemiological information on breast cancer is insufficient to support institution of any primary prevention program. The clearest risk factors relate to reproductive practices which are not readily amenable to preventive intervention. In fact, policies in developing countries are likely to emphasize reduced parity and delayed childbearing as ways to reduce population growth. These policies, if implemented successfully, are likely to increase breast cancer occurrence. Although several groups have recommended reduced dietary fat intake to control breast cancer, the epidemiological data do not consistently support this course of action. Most efforts at breast cancer control are now correctly directed toward earlier detection and improved treatment.

Lymphoma

These tumors arise from cells of the immune system, including lymphocytes, histiocytes, and their precursor cells. Lymphomas are a heterogeneous group of neoplasms which differ greatly in their epidemiology and clinical course. The reasons for including them in this chapter are (a) the Burkitt's lymphoma type occurs with great frequency in young children in parts of East Africa, (b) the Hodgkin's type tends to occur in children and in young adults during their productive years, and (c) both varieties are often cured by intensive therapy. Lymphoma usually presents as enlarged lymph nodes. Concomitant features include fever, weakness, loss of appetite, itching, and other symptoms of general illness. As it progresses it involves multiple sites in the body. Accordingly, lymphoma can produce a variety of complicating problems and usually causes death unless quickly treated.

OCCURRENCE. Lymphomas, considered as a group, account for approximately 135,000 new cases of cancer per year in the world; just over half of these occur in developing countries. Occurrence of different varieties of lymphoma varies from country to country. Burkitt's lymphoma occurs with highest frequency in parts of East Africa and New Guinea, where malaria is endemic. International patterns of Hodgkin's disease vary according to age group. Childhood Hodgkin's disease occurs most often in developing countries, whereas the disease in young adults is more common in northern Europe and North America. Both Hodgkin's disease and Burkitt's lymphoma affect males more often than females.

ETIOLOGY. Burkitt's lymphoma is strongly associated with Epstein-Barr virus infection in epidemiological and laboratory studies. The exact role of Epstein-Barr virus in causing Burkitt's lymphoma is uncertain, however. Areas with highest rates of Burkitt's lymphoma also have endemic malaria, and this geographic relationship has not been fully explained. Why should Epstein-Barr virus infection be associated with Burkitt's lymphoma in Africa and with nasopharyngeal cancer in China? Also, Epstein-Barr virus is a ubiquitous virus (it is the cause of infectious mononucleosis). What circumstances of infection or other factors are necessary for Burkitt's lymphoma, and how can they explain the dramatic geographic variations? These questions remain to be answered.

The cause of Hodgkin's disease is unknown, although some epidemiological data support an infectious etiology. The pattern of occurrence is in many ways consistent with the late effects of an early childhood infection. Thus far, however, no infectious agent has been identified. The causes of lymphomas other than Burkitt's lymphoma and Hodgkin's disease also are unknown. Patients on immunosuppressive therapy (for example, following organ transplantation) are at higher risk of lymphomas in the brain, but this is of relatively little importance to developing countries.

TREATMENT. Both Hodgkin's disease and Burkitt's lymphoma are highly responsive to therapy with radiation and chemotherapy. Many patients can be cured of Hodgkin's disease even if they have advanced disease. In early disease, cure may be achieved by radiation alone. More advanced disease requires intensive chemotherapy. African Burkitt's lymphoma also responds dramatically to chemotherapy, and more than 90 percent of patients achieve complete remission of their tumors. Perhaps 50 percent or more of them can be cured with currently available therapy.

SCREENING. There are no practical screening programs for lymphoma.

PREVENTION. Programs to control or eradicate malaria conceivably will decrease Burkitt's lymphoma. There is no good evidence, to date, that this occurs, however. Development of an Epstein-Barr virus vaccine has also been suggested as a preventive strategy for Burkitt's lymphoma. If an effective Epstein-Barr virus vaccine is developed, it logically should be tested in controlled trials for effectiveness in preventing Burkitt's lymphoma.

Leukemia

Leukemias are malignancies of the blood-forming cells. They are generally categorized according to the cell of origin and to whether the disease is chronic or acute in onset. The clinical behavior and treatment requirements differ for the various types of leukemia. We consider all leukemias together here because they often respond to treatment, and because the technological requirements for their treatment are similar. Leukemias are characterized by an overproduction of either mature (chronic leukemias) or immature (acute leukemias) bone marrow cells. Consequences of leukemia relate to deficiencies of normally functioning red cells, white cells, and platelets (necessary for control of bleeding). Accordingly, presenting symptoms of leukemia are anemia, loss of resistance to infection, or bruising and bleeding. Untreated, acute leukemias are rapidly fatal. Chronic leukemias may persist for years without causing debilitating symptoms. Alternatively, chronic myelogenous leukemia may enter an accelerated phase which mimics an acute leukemia and is rapidly fatal.

OCCURRENCE. Leukemias account for approximately 190,000 new cases of cancer per year worldwide. About 105,000 of these cases occur in developing countries. Leukemia incidence rates peak first in early childhood, decline, and then progressively rise again with age. Much of the childhood peak in leukemia is due to acute lymphocytic cell type, which is also highly responsive to intensive therapy. The adult leukemias are more often of the acute or chronic myelogenous varieties. International variations in leukemia incidence and mortality are not as pronounced as those for most other cancers, except that chronic lymphocytic leukemia is rarely seen in the Far East. Leukemia occurs more often in males than in females and in whites than in blacks or Asians.

ETIOLOGY. There is clear evidence from atomic bomb survivors in Japan and from other exposed groups that radiation causes acute leukemia. Increased leukemia rates are detectable within three years following acute radiation exposure, and the excess persists for decades. The increased risk is principally for the myelocytic types. Other environmental exposures, including exposure to chemicals (particularly benzene), have been implicated as causes of leukemia. Alkylating drugs such as melphalan and busulfan, which are used in cancer chemotherapy, also can cause leukemia. For the vast majority of cases, however, there is no history of exposure to a known leukemogen other than normal background levels of radiation.

TREATMENT. Treatment of acute leukemias, particularly acute lymphocytic leukemia of childhood, has advanced dramatically in the past three decades. Intensive chemotherapy of acute lymphocytic leukemia appears capable of curing 50 percent of affected children. Treatment requires intensive medical support with close monitoring of chemotherapy side effects. Infectious complications are common. After an initial phase of induction therapy, children require prolonged periods of maintenance with intermittent chemotherapy. Adults with acute myelogenous leukemia require even more intensive therapy, but there is now the possibility of curing some of these patients. The chemotherapy regimens are intensely toxic to the normal bone marrow and other organs, and patients require close monitoring and support to treat complications of infection, bleeding, and anemia. Newer techniques of bone marrow transplantation, using either a closely matched donor or treated marrow cells from the patient, offer prospects for curing more leukemia patients. This therapy requires great technological sophistication and intense supportive care by medical and nursing personnel.

SCREENING. Acute leukemias progress very rapidly from the time at which they might be detectable by screening to the time of symptoms. There is no known value in treating chronic leukemias before they are symptomatic. For these two reasons, screening has no role in the management of these conditions.

PREVENTION. Avoiding unnecessary exposure to medical radiation is probably the most feasible approach to leukemia prevention. Other strategies include reduced occupational exposure to known leukemogens (such as benzene), and avoiding environmental contamination with these substances. These preventive strategies, even if effectively implemented, are unlikely to produce a measurable decrease in leukemia occurrence, because few cases are directly related to these factors.

Notes

We are indebted to Richard Doll, Kenneth Stanley, and Jan Stjernsward for their careful comments on earlier drafts. We have also benefited from discussions of this material at the World Health Organization and the United States Centers for Disease Control. The authors remain responsible for errors and conclusions. In particular, the conclusions do not necessarily reflect the views of the World Bank.

1. The use of aggregate numbers may obscure important differences between men and women. For most cancers, site specific incidence for men is about double that for women. Rates of cervical and breast cancer are sufficiently high

in most of the developing world, however, that they nearly compensate for sex differences in other cancers and the overall rate of cancer in women is nearly equal to that of men. In tables 21A-1 and 21A-2 we give rates for men and women by main developing country region. Also refer to Parkin, Laara, and Muir (1988) for an excellent discussion of detailed rates.

2. Without any adjustment for price or cultural differences, an estimated relationship between 1982 manufactured cigarette consumption and income based on a cross-section sample of eighty-four countries is

$$cig/pop = 361 + 0.25 \, NNP/pop - 0.000009 \, (NNP/pop)^2 \quad R^2 = .56$$
$$(4.4) \quad (5.9) \quad (3.4)$$

At the mean per capita income ($3,500) for the sample the estimated income elasticity is 0.7. At incomes below $1,000 the income elasticity of cigarette consumption is above 1.3. The t-statistics are in parentheses (World Bank 1988; IARC 1986).

3. The purpose of using the percentage of per capita GNP, or %GNPN, rather than monetary units is to reduce measures of program costs across countries to approximately comparable units. The measure is deficient in that it primarily adjusts for labor cost differences between countries but does not account well for differences in foreign supply costs or in productivity. The deficiencies are offset, however, by the convenience of the measure.

4. The effect of increasing tobacco prices, for example, is greater in reducing consumption by the young than in reducing consumption among the currently addicted. Similarly, the costs of programs to convert present smokers to nonsmoking status can be high (Altman and others 1987).

5. After correcting nominal rates of interest for inflation, the real rate of interest has been in the vicinity of 3 percent in much of the world during the last twenty years.

6. Under exceptional circumstances and at very high cost, screening procedures appear to detect esophageal, stomach, or liver cancer at a stage at which early surgery may be successful. Research in Japan is under way on the practicality of endoscopy programs in areas of high stomach and esophageal cancer incidence.

7. Relative cancer survival is the survival probability for cancer patients in relation to that expected for persons of similar age in the general population.

8. Assuming an outpatient visit every fourteen days at $1.50 per visit, the cost of aspirin or paracetamol is $0.10 per day, the cost of codeine is $1.00 per day and the cost of morphine is $0.20 per day. For severe symptoms it is assumed that there would be forty-five days during which codeine and paracetamol were required and forty-five days during which morphine was needed.

References

Altman, D. G., J. A. Flora, S. P. Fortman, and J. W. Farquhar. 1987. "The Cost Effectiveness of Three Smoking Cessation Programs." *American Journal of Public Health* 77(2):162–65.

American Cancer Society. 1987. "Cancer: Basic Data." In *Cancer Facts and Figures—1987*. American Cancer Society: Atlanta, Ga.

Axtell, L. M., A. J. Asire, and M. H. Myers. 1976. *Cancer Patient Survival*. Report 5. U.S. Department of Health, Education, and Welfare; National Cancer Institute, Washington, D.C.

Bailar, John, III, and Elaine M. Smith. 1986. "Progress against Cancer?" *New England Journal of Medicine* 314:1226–32.

Baines C. J., A. B. Miller, and A. A. Bassett. 1989. "Physical Examination: Its Role as a Single Screening Modality in the Canadian National Breast Screening Study." *Cancer* 63:1816–22.

Barnum, H. 1988. "Economic Issues in Planning the Use of Health Resources for Chronic Diseases in China." Background Document for World Bank Sector Review, Population, Health, and Nutrition Department. Washington, D.C.

Beasley, R. Palmer. 1988. "Hepatitis B Immunization Strategies." WHO/EPI/GEN/88.5. World Health Organization/Expanded Programme on Immunization, Geneva.

Beasley, R. Palmer, Chia-Chin Lin, Lu-Yu Hwang, and Chia-Siang Chien. 1981. "Hepatocellular Carcinoma and Hepatitis B Virus." *Lancet* November 21, 1129–33.

Bhargava, M. Krishna. N.d. *Karnataka State Cancer Control Programme.* Kidwai Memorial Institute of Oncology, Bangalore.

Bjelke, E. 1982. "The Recession of Stomach Cancer: Selected Aspects." In K. Magnus, ed., *Trends in Cancer Incidence.* Washington, D.C.: Hemisphere Publishing.

Boyle, P., D. G. Zaridze, and M. Smans. 1985. "Descriptive Epidemiology of Colorectal Cancer." *International Journal of Cancer* 36:9–18.

Bulatao-Jayme, J., E. M. Almero, C. A. Castro, T. R. Jardeleza, and L. A. Salamat. 1982. "A Case-Control Dietary Study of Primary Liver Cancer Risk from Aflatoxin Exposure." *International Journal of Epidemiology* 11:112–19.

Bumgarner, J. Richard, ed. 1992. *China: Long-Term Issues and Options in the Health Transition.* A World Bank Country Study. Washington, D.C.

Byers, T. 1988. "Diet and Cancer. Any Progress in the Interim?" *Cancer* 62:1713–24.

Chamberlain, J., N. E. Day, M. Hakama, A. B. Miller, and P. Prorok. 1986. "UICC (Union International Contre le Cancer [International Union against Cancer]) Workshop on Evaluation of Screening Programmes for Gastrointestinal Cancer." *International Journal of Cancer* 37:329–34.

Clayman, C. B. 1989. "Mass Screening for Colorectal Cancer: Are We Ready?" *JAMA* 261(4):609.

Correa, P. 1992. "Human Gastric Carcinogenesis: A Multistep and Multifunctional Process." *Cancer Research* 52:6735–40.

Cramer, D. W. 1982. "Uterine Cervix." In Schottenfeld and Fraumeni, Jr., eds., *Cancer Epidemiology and Prevention.* Philadelphia: W. B. Saunders.

Crofton, J. 1984. "The Gathering Smoke Clouds: A Worldwide Challenge." *International Journal of Epidemiology* 13:269–70.

Cromwell, J., and P. Gertman. 1979. "The Cost of Cancer." *Laryngoscope* 89:393–409.

Dahl, June, and David Joranson. 1987. "Relieving Cancer Pain." *World Health* 11:28–29.

Day, N. E., C. J. Baines, J. Chamberlain, M. Hakama, A. B. Miller, and P. Prorok. 1986. "UICC (Union International Contre le Cancer [International Union against Cancer]) Project on Screening for Cancer: Report of the Workshop on Screening for Breast Cancer." *International Journal of Cancer* 38:303–8.

Doll, Richard, and Richard Peto. 1981. *The Causes of Cancer: Quantitative Estimates of Avoidable Risks of Cancer in the United States Today.* Oxford: Oxford University Press.

Eddy, David M. 1981. "The Economics of Cancer Prevention and Detection." *Cancer* 47:1200–09.

———. 1986a. *A Computer-Based Model for Designing Cancer Control Strategies.* NCI Monographs 64(2):74–82.

———. 1986b. "Secondary Prevention of Cancer: An Overview." *Bulletin of the World Health Organization* 64(3):421–29.

Eddy, David M., and Michael Schwartz. 1982. "Mathematical Models in Screening." In David Schottenfeld and Joseph Fraumeni, Jr., eds., *Cancer Epidemiology and Prevention.* London: W. B. Saunders Company.

Editorial Committee for the Atlas of Cancer Mortality, eds. 1976. *Atlas of Cancer Mortality in the People's Republic of China.* Beijing National Cancer Control Office of the Ministry of Health.

Feinstein, A. R., D. M. Sosin, and C. K. Wells. 1985. "The Will Rogers Phenomenon: Stage Migration and New Diagnostic Techniques as a Source of Misleading Statistics for Survival in Cancer." *New England Journal of Medicine* 312:1604–8.

Fleischer, D. E., S. B. Goldberg, T. H. Browning, J. N. Cooper, E. Friedman, F. H. Goldner, E. B. Keeffe, and L. E. Smith. 1989. "Detection and Surveillance of Colorectal Cancer." *JAMA* 261:580–85.

Francis D. P., S. C. Hadler, S. E. Thompson, J. C. Maynard, D. G. Ostrow, N.

Altman, E. H. Braff, P. O'Malley, D. Hawkins, F. N. Judson, K. Penley, T. Nylund, G. Christie, F. Meyers, J. N. Moore, Jr., A. Gardner, I. L. Doto, J. H. Miller, G. H. Reynolds, B. L. Murphy, C. A. Schable, B. T. Clark, J. W. Curran, and A. G. Redeker. 1982. "The Prevention of Hepatitis B with Vaccine: Report of the Centers for Disease Control Multi-Center Efficacy Trial among Homosexual Men." *Annals of Internal Medicine* 97(3):362–66.

Gambia Hepatitis Study Group. 1989. "Hepatitis B Vaccine in the Expanded Programme of Immunization: The Gambian Experience." *Lancet* May 13:1057–60.

Ghadirian, P., J. P. Thouez, and A. Simard. 1988. "La géographie du cancer de l'oesophage." *Social Science and Medicine* 27:971–85.

Gray, Nigel. 1985. "Cancer Risks and Cancer Prevention in the Third World." In M. P. Vessey and M. Gray, eds., *Cancer Risks and Prevention.* Oxford: Oxford University Press.

Greenwald, P., and E. J. Sondik, eds. 1986. "Cancer Control Objectives for the Nation: 1985–2000." NCI Monographs 2. National Cancer Institute, Washington, D.C.

Hakulinen, T., H. Hansluwka, A. D. Lopez, and T. Nakada. 1986. "Global and Regional Mortality Patterns by Cause of Death in 1980." *International Journal of Epidemiology* 15:227–33.

Hanley, James A. 1986. "Evaluating Primary Prevention Programmes Against Cancer." *Bulletin of the World Health Organization* 64(2):311–20.

Hartunian, Nelson, Charles N. Smart, and Mark Thompson. 1980. "The Incidence of Economic Costs of Cancer, Motor Vehicle Injuries, Coronary Heart Disease, and Stroke: A Comparative Analysis." *Public Health* 70(12):1249–60.

Hodgson, Thomas. 1988. "Annual Costs of Illness Versus Lifetime Costs of Illness and Implications of Structural Change." *Drug Information Journal* 22:323–41.

Hsu, Hsu-Mei, Ding-Shinn Chen, Cheng-Hua Chuang, Joseph Chih-Feng Lu, De-Min Jebo, Chin-Chang Lee, Hsing-Chi Lu, Shih-Hsiung Chen, Yue-Fen Wang, Chinying Chen Wang, Kwang-Juei Lo, Chun-Jen Shih, and Juei-Low Sung. 1988. "Efficacy of a Mass Hepatitis B Vaccination Program in Taiwan." *JAMA* 260:2231–35.

IARC (International Agency for Research on Cancer). 1986. *Tobacco Smoking.* Monographs on the Evaluation of the Carcinogenic Risk of Chemicals to Humans 38. Lyons.

IARC (International Agency for Research on Cancer) Working Group on Evaluation of Cervical Cancer Screening Programmes. 1986. "Screening for Squamous Cervical Cancer: Duration of Low Risk after Negative Results of Cervical Cytology and Its Implication for Screening Policies." *British Medical Journal* 293:659–64.

India, Ministry of Health and Family Welfare. 1984. *National Cancer Control Programme for India.* Directorate General of Health Services, New Delhi.

ITFH (International Task Force on Hepatitis B Immunization). 1988. *Notes on Hepatitis B and Its Control.* PATH (Program for Appropriate Technology in Health.) Seattle, Wash. Published report.

Kelsey, J. L., and N. G. Hildreth. 1983. *Breast and Gynecologic Cancer Epidemiology.* Boca Raton, Fla.: CRC Press.

Knight, K. K., J. E. Fielding, and R. N. Battista. 1989. "Occult Blood Screening for Colorectal Cancer." *JAMA* 261:587–93.

Knox, E. G. 1982. "Cancer of the Uterine Cervix." In K. Magnus, ed., *Trends in Cancer Incidence.* Washington, D.C.: Hemisphere Publishing.

Kristein, M. M., C. B. Arnold, and E. L. Wynder. 1977. "Health Economics and Preventive Care." *Science* 195(4277):457–62.

Kurihara, Minoru, Kunio Aoki, and Suketami Tominaga. 1984. *Cancer Mortality Statistics in the World.* Nagoya, Japan: University of Nagoya Press.

Lew, E. A., and L. Garfinkel. 1979. "Variations in Mortality by Weight among 750,000 Men and Women." *Journal of Chronic Diseases* 32(8):563–76.

Luce, B. R. 1980. "Allocating Costs and Benefits in Disease Prevention Programs: An Application to Cervical Cancer Screening." Case Study 7. U.S. Congress, Office of Technology Assessment, Washington, D.C.

Lynge, E., M. Madsen, and G. Engholm. 1989. "Effect of Organized Screening on Incidence and Mortality of Cervical Cancer in Denmark." *Cancer Research* 49:2157–60.

Mackay, Judith. 1989. "Battlefield for the Tobacco War." JAMA 261:28–29.

McMichael, A. J. 1984. "Oral Cancer in the Third World: Time for Preventive Intervention?" *International Journal of Epidemiology* 13:403–5.

Maynard, J. E., M. A. Kane, M. J. Alter, and S. C. Hadler. 1988. "Control of Hepatitis B by Immunization." *Viral Hepatitis and Liver Disease*. New York: Alan R. Liss.

Miller, R. W., and F. W. McKay. 1984. "Decline in the U.S. Childhood Cancer Mortality: 1950 through 1980." JAMA 251:1567–70.

Muir, C. S., and J. Nectoux. 1982. "International Patterns of Cancer." In D. Schottenfeld and J. F. Fraumeni, Jr., eds.,*Cancer Epidemiology and Prevention*. Pennsylvania: W. B. Saunders.

Muir, C. S., J. Waterhouse, R. Mack, J. Powell, and S. Whelan. 1988. *Cancer Incidence in Five Continents*. Scientific Publication 88. Lyons: International Agency for Research on Cancer.

Nair, M. Krishnan. 1988. *Ten-Year Action Plan for Cancer Control in Kerala*. Printed at St. Joseph's Press, Trivandrum. Approved by the State Cancer Control Advisory Board of Kerala. Jointly published by the Regional Cancer Centre, Trivandrum and the Cancer Unit, World Health Organization, Geneva.

National Research Council, Committee on Diet, Nutrition, and Cancer. 1982. *Diet, Nutrition, and Cancer*. Washington, D.C.: National Academy Press.

NIH (National Institutes of Health). 1988. *1987 Annual Cancer Statistics Review*. NIH Publication 88-2789, National Cancer Institute, Division of Cancer Prevention and Control. U.S. Department of Health and Human Services. Bethesda, Md.

Parkin, D. M. 1985. "A Computer Simulation Model for the Practical Planning of Cervical Cancer Screening Programmes." *British Journal of Cancer* 51:551–68.

———, ed. *Cancer Occurrence in Developing Countries*. Scientific Publication 75. Lyons: International Agency for Research on Cancer.

Parkin, D. M., E. Laara, and C. S. Muir. 1988. "Estimates of the Worldwide Frequency of Sixteen Major Cancers in 1980." *International Journal of Cancer* 41:184–97.

Parkin, D. M., and S. M. Moss. 1986. "An Evaluation of Screening Policies for Cervical Cancer in England and Wales Using a Computer Simulation Model." *Journal of Epidemiological and Community Health* 40(2):143–53.

Percy, C., and C. S. Muir. 1989. "The International Comparability of Cancer Mortality Data: Results of an International Death Certificate Study." *American Journal of Epidemiology* 129:934–46.

Peto, Richard. 1986. "Influence of Dose and Duration of Smoking on Lung Cancer Rates." In D. G. Zaridze and Richard Peto, eds., *Tobacco: A Major International Health Hazard*. Scientific Publication 74. Lyons: International Agency for Research on Cancer.

Poirier, S., H. Ohshima, G. De-The, A. Hubert, M. C. Bourgade, and H. Bartsch. 1987. "Volatile Nitrosamine Levels in Common Foods from Tunisia, South China, and Greenland: High-Risk Areas for Nasopharyngeal Carcinoma (NPC)." *International Journal of Cancer* 39:293–96.

Portenoy, Russell K. 1988. "Practical Aspects of Pain Control in the Patient with Cancer." *Ca-A Cancer Journal for Clinicians* 38(6):327–52.

Rice, D. P., and T. A. Hodgson. 1981. *Social and Economic Implications of Cancer in the United States of America*. Publication (PHS) 81-1404. U.S. Department of Health and Human Services, Washington, D.C.

Rice, D. P., T. A. Hodgson, and A. N. Kopstein. 1985. "The Economic Costs of Illness: A Replication and Update." *Health Care Financing Review* 7(1):61–80.

Schottenfeld, D., and J. F. Fraumeni, Jr. 1982. *Cancer Epidemiology and Prevention*. Philadelphia: W. B. Saunders.

Schwartz, M. 1978. "An Analysis of the Benefits of Serial Screening for Breast Cancer Based on a Mathematical Model of the Disease." *Cancer* 51:1550–64.

Schweitzer, Stuart. 1977. "Cost Effectiveness of Early Detection of Disease." *Health Services Research* 9(1):22–32.

Scotto, Joseph, and Leonard Chiazze. 1976. "Third National Cancer Survey: Hospitalizations and Payments to Hospitals." DHEW Publication 76-1094. Department of Health, Education, and Welfare, Washington, D.C.

Segi, Mitsuo, Suketami Tominaga, Kunio Aoki, and Isaburo Fujimoto, eds. 1981. *Cancer Mortality and Morbidity Statistics: Japan and the World*. GANN Monograph on Cancer Research 26. Tokyo: Japan Scientific Societies Press. Published report.

Shapiro, S., W. Venet, P. Strax, L. Venet, and R. Roeser. 1982. "Ten to Fourteen Year Effect of Screening on Breast Cancer Mortality." *Journal of the National Cancer Institute* 69(2):349–55.

Silverberg, E. and J. Lubera. 1987. "Cancer Statistics 1987." *Ca-A Cancer Journal for Clinicians*. 37(1)2–19.

Simopoulos, A. P. 1987. "Obesity and Carcinogenesis: Historical Perspective." *American Journal of Clinical Nutrition* 45:271–76.

Stanley, K. 1986. "Lung Cancer and Tobacco—A Global Problem." *Cancer Detection and Prevention* 9:83–89.

Stanley, K., J. Stjernsward, and V. Koroltchouk. 1988. "Cancers of the Stomach, Lung, and Breast: Mortality Trends and Control Strategies." *World Health Statistics Quarterly* 41:107–14.

Stjernsward, J. 1988. "WHO Cancer Pain Relief Programme." *Cancer Surveys* 7(1):195–208.

———. 1990. "National Training of Radiotherapists in Sri Lanka and Zimbabwe: Priorities and Strategies for Cancer Control in Developing Countries." *International Journal of Radiation Oncology and Biological Physics* 19(5):001–4.

Stjernsward, J., K. Stanley, David M. Eddy, M. Tschkovski, L. Sobin, I. Koza, and K. H. Notaney. 1985. "Cancer Control: Strategies and Priorities." *World Health Forum* 6:160–64.

Sun Tsung-Tang, Chu Yuan-Rong, Ni Zhi-Quan, Lu Jian-Hua, Huang Fei, Ni Zheng-Ping, Pei Xu-Fang, Yu Zhi-Ian, and Liu Guo-Ting. 1986. "A Pilot Study on Universal Immunization of Newborn Infants in an Area of Hepatitis B Virus and Primary Hepatocellular Carcinoma Prevalence with a Low Dose of Hepatitis B Vaccine." *Journal of Cellular Physiology* 4(supplement):83–90.

Szmuness, W., C. E. Stevens, E. A. Zang, E. J. Harley, and A. Kellner. 1981. "A Controlled Clinical Trial of the Efficacy of the Hepatitis B Vaccine (Heptavax B): A Final Report." *Hepatology* 1:377–85.

Tabar, L., C. J. Fagerberg, A. Gad, L. Baldetorp, L. H. Holmberg, O. Grontoft, U. Ljungquist, B. Lundstrom, J. C. Manson, and G. Eklund. 1985. "Reduction in Mortality from Breast Cancer after Mass Screening with Mammography." *Lancet* 1(8433):829–32.

Takenaga, Nobuyuki, Ichiro Kai, and Gen Ohi. 1985. "Evaluation of Three Cervical Cancer Detection Programs in Japan with Special Reference to Cost-Benefit Analysis." *Cancer* 55(10):2514–19.

Thorn, Jennifer B., J. Elizabeth MacGregor, Elizabeth M. Russell, and Kathleen Swanson. 1975. "Costs of Detecting and Treating Cancer of the Uterine Cervix in North-East Scotland in 1971." *Lancet* March 22 674–76.

USDHHS (U.S. Department of Health and Human Services). 1977. *Cancer Patient Survival*. Report 5. DHEW Publication NIH (National Institutes of Health) 77–992. Department of Health, Education, and Welfare; Washington, D.C.

———. 1982. *The Health Consequences of Smoking: CANCER*. Report of the Surgeon General. Public Health Service, Office of Smoking and Health, Washington, D.C.

———. 1988. *1987 Annual Cancer Statistics Review, Including Cancer Trends: 1950–1985*. NIH (National Institutes of Health) Publication 88-2789. National Cancer Institute, Washington, D.C.

Van Rensburg, S. J., P. Cook-Mozaffari, D. J. Van Schalkwyk, J. J. Van Der Watt, T. J. Vincent, and I. F. Purchase. 1985. "Hepatocellular Carcinoma and Dietary Aflatoxin in Mozambique and Transkei." *British Journal of Cancer* 51:713–26.

Wainwright, R. B., B. J. McMahon, L. R. Bulkow, D. B. Hall, M. A. Fitzgerald, A. P. Harpster, S. C. Hadler, A. P. Lanier, and W. L. Heyward. 1989. "Duration of Immunogenicity and Efficacy of Hepatitis B Vaccine in a Yupik Eskimo Population." *JAMA* 261:2362–66.

Warnakulasuriya, K. A. A. S., A. N. I. Ekanayake, S. Sivayoham, J. Stjernsward, J. J. Pindborg, L. H. Sobin, and K. S. G. P. Perera. 1984. "Utilization of Primary Health Care Workers for Early Detection of Oral Cancer and Precancer Cases in Sri Lanka." *Bulletin of the World Health Organization* 62(2):243–50.

Warner, Kenneth. 1987. "Health and Economic Implications of a Tobacco Free Society." *JAMA* 258:2080–86.

Waterhouse, J., C. S. Muir, P. Correa, and J. Powell, eds. 1976. *Cancer Incidence in Five Continents*. Vol. 3. Scientific Publication 15. Lyons: International Agency for Research on Cancer.

Waterhouse, J., C. S. Muir, K. Shanmugaratnam, and J. Powell, eds. 1982. *Cancer Incidence in Five Continents*. Vol. 4. Scientific Publication 42. Lyons: International Agency for Research on Cancer.

Widjaya, A. 1988. "Cost Effective Analysis in Various Hepatitis B Virus Control Programs in Indonesia." Department of Health, Centre for Laboratory Services, Jakarta.

Willett, W. S., and B. MacMahon. 1984. "Diet and Cancer—An Overview (Parts 1 and 2)." *New England Journal of Medicine* 310:633–38.

World Bank. 1988. *World Development Report 1988*. Washington, D.C.: Oxford University Press.

WHO (World Health Organization). 1983. "Prevention of Liver Cancer." Technical Report 691. Geneva.

———. 1984. "Control of Oral Cancer in Developing Countries." *Bulletin of the World Health Organization* 62(6):817–30.

———. 1985. "Essential Drugs for Cancer Chemotherapy: Memorandum from a WHO Meeting." *Bulletin of the World Health Organization* 63(6): 999–1002.

———. 1986a. *Cancer Pain Relief*. WHO Monograph. Geneva.

———. 1986b. "Control of Cancer of the Cervix: A WHO Meeting." *Bulletin of the World Health Organization* 64(4):607–18.

———. 1986c. "The Use of Quantitative Methods in Planning National Cancer Control Programmes." *Bulletin of the World Health Organization* 64(5):683–93.

———. 1988a. "General Strategies and Provisions for Cancer Control in Chile." CAN/88.1. Geneva.

———. 1988b. "Global Medium-Term Programme for the WHO Cancer Control Programme during the Period 1990–1995." CAN/MTP/88.1. Geneva.

———. 1990. "Diet, Nutrition, and Prevention of Chronic Diseases." Technical Report. Geneva.

WHO (World Health Organization)/Indonesia, Ministry of Health. 1989. *National Cancer Control Program in Indonesia*. Geneva.

Yeh, F.-S., M. C. Yu, C.-C. Mo, S. Luo, M. J. Tong, and B. E. Henderson. 1989. "Hepatitis B Virus, Aflatoxins, and Hepatocellular Carcinoma in Southern Guangxi, China." *Cancer Research* 49:2506–9.

Yu, M. C., J. H. C. Ho, S.-H. Lai, and B. E. Henderson. 1986. "Cantonese-Style Salted Fish as a Cause of Nasopharyngeal Carcinoma: Report of a Case-Control Study in Hong Kong." *Cancer Research* 46:956–61.

22

Diabetes

J. Patrick Vaughan, Lucy Gilson, and Anne Mills

In recent years there has been growing concern that diabetes mellitus is becoming more common, mainly in the more urbanized and industrialized countries, where the prevalence rates of the disease in the total population are often 1 to 3 percent or more. In these countries it is widely agreed that diabetes is a significant public health problem, particularly among people in the older age groups. There are also well-documented populations in developing countries in which diabetes has become much more frequent in the past ten to twenty years. Given the changing age structures and health patterns of the populations of developing countries, what public health priority should be given to diabetes, now and for the next twenty years or so?

In order to answer this question, we summarize in this chapter the information on the frequency and time trends for diabetes in developing countries and on the indirect and direct costs of the disease. We consider the evidence for prevention and case management strategies and assess the feasibility and cost of these strategies. Until recently little consistent information was available on diabetes in developing countries, but under the leadership of the International Diabetes Federation and the World Health Organization (WHO), interest in the subject has grown steadily during the past ten to fifteen years. A great deal of this information has been well summarized in a World Health Organization Technical Report (WHO 1985).

Diabetes mellitus is a chronic and noncommunicable disease which is largely irreversible. Although it can occur at any age, its onset is most frequent among the young and older persons. Diagnosis is based on finding an abnormally high level of glucose in the blood, a condition caused by poorly functioning beta cells in the pancreas gland and an insufficient output of the hormone insulin. The actual underlying etiological mechanisms that lead to this pathological state, however, are still largely unknown.

Despite the fact that all diabetes cases have been classified and reported under one code (number 250) in the *International Statistical Classification of Diseases, Injuries, and Causes of Death* (WHO 1975), it is now generally accepted that epidemiologically there are two main types of the illness, and this is to be acknowledged in the forthcoming revision. The onset of insulin-dependent diabetes mellitus (IDDM) generally occurs among younger age groups (with 25 to 50 percent of patients presenting before the age of fifteen years), and it is nearly always acute in onset. Sufferers require regular doses of insulin, by injection or a similar process at least once per day, in order to sustain life and to avoid acute and more long-term complications. Those with non-insulin-dependent diabetes mellitus (NIDDM) usually suffer from a less severe illness, which has a slower onset and is most common in the older age groups (older than forty years). People with NIDDM, however, may suffer from the same long-term complications as those with IDDM, such as retinopathy, nephropathy, neuropathy, and ischemic heart disease. In this review we will focus on these two types of diabetes and will largely consider their epidemiology separately.

With regard to diabetes incidence by sex, IDDM appears to be about equal in males and females (Rewers and others 1988), but NIDDM may be more frequent in females. A third type of diabetes, now frequently called malnutrition-related diabetes mellitus (MRDM), has been reported from many developing countries. The patients are usually young and have a history of nutritional deficiency. This disease is believed to be clinically distinct, and therefore the separate grouping has been proposed (WHO 1985). It has been extensively reviewed (Abu-Bakare and others 1986), but the incidence rate of MRDM is still largely unknown. Although the etiology is not understood, it is possibly caused by toxins in cassava, other food toxins, or protein-energy malnutrition. The case management is similar to that for IDDM. We will not consider this form of diabetes separately here because there is inadequate epidemiological evidence and the subject clearly needs further research.

Some healthy individuals have lesser degrees of tolerance to glucose, and when challenged with a dose of 75 grams of glucose taken by mouth (WHO 1985) they cannot be classified as diabetics, but they are, nevertheless, at increased risk of coronary heart and peripheral and cerebrovascular diseases. About one-third of these individuals with impaired glucose tolerance will revert spontaneously to a normal state but, as a group, people with impaired tolerance are at higher risk of subsequently developing diabetes mellitus and are believed to make a significant contribution to total mortality (Bennett 1985; Grabauskas 1988).

Gestational diabetes usually presents as NIDDM and only rarely is insulin required. There is poor epidemiological data on this condition in developing countries, and, although its importance is not denied, criteria for its diagnosis remain controversial ("Glucose Tolerance in Pregnancy" 1988).

The classification of diabetes into three main types and the criteria for diagnosing impaired glucose tolerance have gained wide acceptance only during the past five to ten years. This causes considerable difficulty in interpreting much of the older published literature and in comparing newer with older data. The new internationally accepted criteria for diagnosing diabetes and impaired glucose tolerance are shown in appendix 22A.

The Significance of Diabetes to Public Health

Before considering the distribution and time trends for diabetes in various parts of the world, it is important to understand the problems encountered in interpreting the available information, particularly that on incidence.

Limitations of the Morbidity and Mortality Information

The diagnosis of new cases of diabetes depends both on clinical symptoms and signs and on the detection of an elevated blood glucose level, or, where this is not possible, on the persistent presence of glucose in the urine and a satisfactory response to the appropriate treatment. The detection and reporting of new cases, therefore, depends heavily on the availability and use of health services, or on the results of large-scale population-based surveys. Access to, and use of, health facilities is poor in many developing countries, and so the reported figures for the frequency of cases (both for incidence and prevalence) of IDDM and NIDDM must be highly suspect. The results of many of the older surveys are also suspect because of the use of non-standardized diagnostic criteria, different screening methods, and inadequate sample sizes. Such surveys were undertaken before the present classification and diagnostic criteria were internationally accepted. This cautionary note is equally if not more important for mortality data. The International Classification of Disease (ICD) statistics, now used by most national death registration and certification systems, is based on naming the "underlying" pathological process, but the ICD data do not distinguish between the epidemiologically different forms of diabetes (that is, between IDDM and NIDDM). Moreover, it is well recognized that in most developing countries the registration of deaths is grossly inadequate, and even the certification of the pathological causes of the registered deaths is often incorrect. In addition, diabetes mellitus is frequently not included by the certifying doctor on death certificates, and coding rules preferentially select cardiovascular diseases and cancers in favor of diabetes (WHO 1985). Studies in the United Kingdom and the United States suggest that up to 75 percent of diabetics may not be counted in the internationally published mortality data (Fuller and others 1983). This situation has led to the following crude, but general, rule. In populations in which diabetes is relatively common, there is probably another case

of undiagnosed NIDDM for every one or two diagnosed diabetics in the community.

When interpreting information on the frequency of a chronic and irreversible disease such as diabetes, it is crucial to be clear what the incidence and prevalence estimates may mean. For example, IDDM is a relatively rare disease with regard to incidence, but the prevalence rate can reach 0.5 percent, or 1 in 200 people, because of the long duration of survival with good case management and medical care. Therefore, as the case management for individual cases improves in developing countries, the prevalence rates may rise without any significant change in the real incidence. This has implications in the assessment of alternative strategies for addressing IDDM. Where the incidence is low the costs per new case averted by a preventive strategy may seem relatively high. With regard to case management, however, IDDM may become a relatively common disease, and the cumulative costs per diabetic treated are considerable; thus, substantial savings on treatment could result from an effective preventive strategy. It is, therefore, important to take account not only of control costs but also of treatment savings when assessing preventive strategies. Since the duration of survival varies, it is important when making comparisons of the cost-effectiveness of treating chronic diseases such as IDDM to standardize for illness duration, by using a unit such as cost per year of life saved.

In general, industrial countries have good information on the epidemiology of IDDM and NIDDM, but for many developing countries the national data are very scanty or do not exist. This is well illustrated by map 22-1, which represents data collected by the World Health Organization up to the early 1980s (WHO 1985) and shows unrealistic and low prevalence levels for many areas, especially in Latin America and Africa.

Current Trends for Insulin-Dependent Diabetes

There is considerable discussion about the etiology of IDDM, but it is clear that both genetic and environmental factors are involved (Krolewski and others 1987). Studies of identical twins show an overall concordance rate for developing diabetes of over 50 percent, rising to about 70 percent if certain genetic markers are also included. These rates contrast with the fact that 85 percent of newly diagnosed diabetics have no close relative with the same condition (Bennett 1985). Other evidence also suggests that although the clinical onset is acute and severe, there is probably a long latent period before the illness becomes apparent (Tarn and others 1988).

The incidence of new cases of IDDM has been found to vary considerably with the seasons, more new cases presenting during the winter months (DERI 1988). This variation has been linked to the possibility that IDDM may be caused by a viral infection, but a number of extensive reviews have concluded that, apart from a few instances, no good epidemiological evidence exists for this hypothesis (Gamble 1980; Barratt-Connor 1985). It should also be remembered, however, that a viral infection occurring early in a person's life may not be detected and hence not associated with the later onset of IDDM.

Map 22-1. Prevalence of Diabetes Mellitus in Some Countries

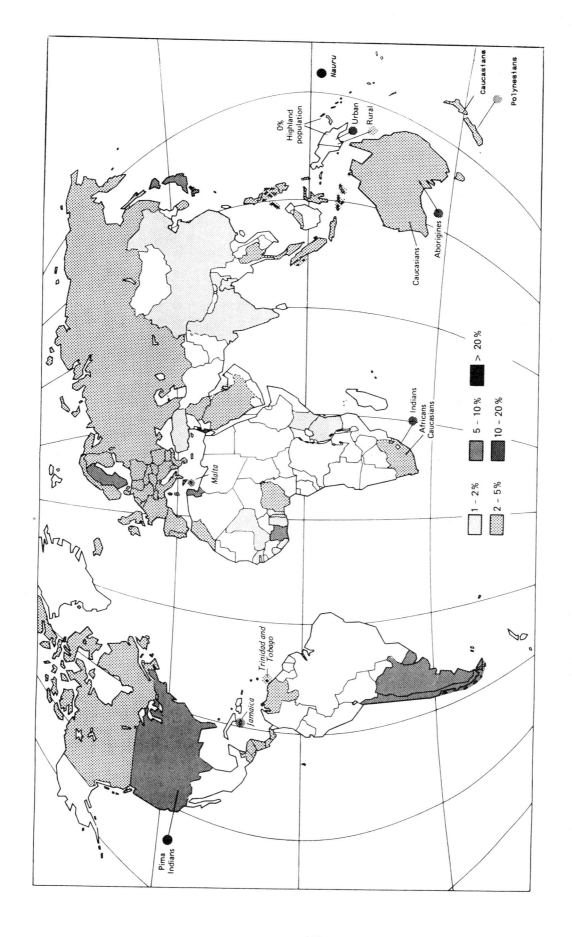

Note: The rates shown include both NIDDM and IDDM, though the latter represents a small proportion of the total. Rates are derived from many sources, principally national and regional surveys but also hospital statistics in some developing countries. In most cases WHO standardized diagnostic criteria have not been used.

Source: Reproduced by permission of the World Health Organization, Geneva from *Diabetes mellitus: Report of a WHO Study Group* (Technical Report Series no. 727, 1985).

In addition, the incidence of IDDM does not appear to have fallen with the much wider use of childhood vaccines. On the basis that an infective process may be involved in triggering off the onset of diabetes, it has been suggested that large-scale immunization may even lead to an increase in IDDM in developing countries (King 1987).

The incidence of IDDM appears to vary greatly between different ethnic groups, being commonest in white people and in the northern temperate zone. Indeed, there may be as much as a tenfold increase in incidence rates from southern Europe to Finland, which has one of the highest rates worldwide, and there is a thirty-four-fold difference in the childhood incidence of the disease between the highest in Finland and Japan (DERI 1987). The Finnish incidence of diabetes in children between the ages of zero to fourteen (in which about half of the new IDDM cases would be expected to occur) is estimated at 29 per 100,000 persons per year. Assuming an average duration of survival of fifteen to twenty years, the prevalence of IDDM in Finland in the total population would be about 0.5 percent.

In many developing countries, particularly in Africa, IDDM is considered to be a rare disease, but no reliable estimates are available. If, for the sake of illustration, we assume an incidence rate for a developing country of between 1 and 5 new cases per 100,000 children age zero to fourteen years per year (and that those children are 40 percent of the developing country population), we might expect between 4 and 20 new cases of IDDM per year in children in a population of 1 million people, or approximately twice this number (that is, 10 to 40 new cases) among all age groups per year. Assuming an average duration of survival for IDDM cases in developing countries of five years, we might expect the population prevalence to be 0.005 to 0.02 percent. Even at such low prevalence levels the widespread lack of diagnostic and treatment facilities could lead to a high case-fatality rate within the year following the onset of the disease. Moreover, a high case-fatality rate means that even if the incidence rate were higher than predicted the disease would appear to be very uncommon.

Limited contact with the health system, scarcity of specialist staff, and the lack of regular supplies of insulin and the necessary equipment are bound to lower the prognosis for patients with IDDM in developing countries. A report from a specialist clinic at a large teaching hospital in a capital city in Sub-Saharan Africa put the case-fatality rate at 30 to 40 percent during the first four to six years following diagnosis (Lutalo and Mabonga 1985). Even with appropriate care, patients undergoing insulin therapy may suffer from hypo- (low) or hyperglycemia (elevated blood glucose). They are also especially vulnerable to the potential complications resulting from injections—such as sepsis, hepatitis, and acquired immunodeficiency syndrome (AIDS)—if they do not strictly adhere to sterilization procedures. Education programs need to stress the importance of preventing or immediately combating such problems.

There is an unresolved question about whether the incidence of IDDM is stable or rising, particularly in Europe and the United States. Although incidence appears to be relatively steady, there is some evidence to suggest that recently it has been rising, particularly in Finland (Reunanen and others 1982), Scotland (Patterson and others 1983), and Poland (Rewers and others 1987). The authors of another analysis of standardized epidemiological data from sixteen population-based IDDM case registries (all in industrial countries) have concluded that there has been a linear increase in incidence during the past two decades in Europe and the western Pacific but not in North America (Diabetes Epidemiology Research International [DERI] 1990). The situation in developing countries is inconclusive because of the very poor data base. Even if the incidence is rising, IDDM is still, in general, considered to be a rare disease in most developing countries.

Current Trends for Non-Insulin-Dependent Diabetes

When considering the balance between genetic and environmental factors in the etiology of NIDDM, we find that the evidence for a genetic susceptibility appears in some ways to be stronger than that for IDDM. The concordance rate in identical twins is higher for NIDDM, but so far no genetic markers have been discovered. There is good evidence that the incidence of NIDDM does vary considerably between different ethnic and racial groups, such as Indians and Chinese (Zimmet 1982). It is also generally agreed that the prevalence (and probably incidence) of NIDDM can rise in the relatively short period of one to two decades as more people, such as the population of Nauru (Schooneveldt and others 1988) and Australian aborigines (Cameron, Moffitt, and Williams 1986), become urbanized and "westernized." Studies have shown that increased food intake, obesity, and lack of exercise can all be associated with NIDDM. Considerable discussion still exists, however, as to whether these are causal factors operating in susceptible individuals or ethnic groups and whether reversing these trends in populations would lead to a reduction in the incidence of NIDDM.

Eighty-five to 90 percent of all diabetics in industrial countries suffer from NIDDM, and the rapid rise in the prevalence of diabetes in the United States from just under 1 percent of the general population in 1960 to over 2.5 percent by the late 1970s was largely due to an increase in NIDDM (Zimmet 1982). Although some of this increase may have been the result of improved diagnosis and prognosis, there is good evidence that the incidence of NIDDM has also risen. In 1936 the incidence of diabetes in the United States was reported as 5 per 10,000 population per year and by 1973 it was 29.7 per 10,000, a sixfold increase. Worldwide, the most spectacular rise in the incidence of NIDDM has been clearly documented in the Pima Indians of North America (Godhes 1986) and in certain Melanesian, Micronesian, and Polynesian island populations in the Pacific (King and others 1984; King and Zimmet 1988).

Such data from "special" populations has strengthened the belief that genetic susceptibility to NIDDM is unmasked as such people undergo urbanization and modernization (Zimmet 1982; Zimmet and others 1986). For example, studies comparing Indian immigrants and indigenous people living in countries as diverse as Fiji (Zimmet 1982), Singapore (Cheah and Tan 1979), South Africa (Marine and others 1969), and Trinidad and Tobago (Poon-King and others 1968) have shown prevalence rates for diabetes in Indians of 14.0, 6.1, 10.4, and 4.5 percent, respectively, all of which were higher rates than for the indigenous peoples. Both forms of diabetes were previously thought to be uncommon in India, but a recent survey of known diabetics showed a higher prevalence among residents in a wealthy suburb of Delhi than in Indians living in London. The crude prevalence of diabetes in Delhi was found to be 3.1 percent, and as many as 16 percent were being treated with insulin (Mather and Keen 1985; Mather and others 1987). Another community-based survey in Coventry, United Kingdom, found age-adjusted prevalence rates for diabetes of 11.2 percent in Asian men and 8.9 percent in Asian women in contrast to 2.8 percent and 4.3 percent in white men and women, respectively. The difference was not explained by differences in body mass (Simmons and others 1989).

A rise in the prevalence of NIDDM has been fairly widely reported from other migrant groups. For instance, diabetes was thought to be uncommon in mainland China (Shanghai Diabetes Research Cooperative Group 1980), but surveys in Singaporean Chinese revealed that prevalence had risen from 1.6 percent in 1975 to 4.0 percent ten years later (Thai and others 1987). A survey of people age forty years and older in urban and rural Taiwan (China), carried out during 1985–86, revealed age-adjusted prevalence rates of 7.6 percent and 4.7 percent, respectively, and by 1984, diabetes, mainly NIDDM, ranked fifth as a cause of death in Taipei, Taiwan (Tong-Yuan Tai and others 1987). Two other recent surveys are worth noting because they demonstrated surprisingly high prevalence rates. In a rural population in Saudi Arabia a crude prevalence for all ages and both sexes of 4.3 percent was found, but the proportion rose to 13.4 percent for both sexes age fifty-five years or older and to 18.7 percent for the females in this group (Fatani and others 1987). In Tunisia, surveys of an urban and a rural population showed the age-standardized rate to be twice as high or higher in the urban population (4.6 percent as opposed to 2.3 percent in men and 3.5 percent in contrast to 0.6 percent in women). Within the urban sample the prevalence rate was similar for those people born in the urban area as compared with those born elsewhere in the country (Papoz and others 1988).

Some evidence from Sub-Saharan Africa suggests that NIDDM may be increasing in some urban populations. For instance, in a report from a chronic disease register compiled in Zimbabwe it was shown that diabetes was responsible for 12.4 percent of the cases (Lutalo and Mabonga 1985), and in population-based estimates from Tanzania the prevalence in adults was between 0.2 percent and 1.1 percent (Ahren and Corrigan 1985; McLarty and others 1989). Such estimates, however, contrast with a report from rural Nigeria, where no one with diabetes was found in a survey of more than 1,300 villagers (Teuscher and others 1987).

The authors of a most useful review of the world situation on trends in the incidence and prevalence of NIDDM conclude

that the information available for Africa and Latin America is incomplete and that very little up-to-date information is available in which the new international guidelines for the diagnosis of NIDDM have been used (King and Zimmet 1988). Most of the available information is for prevalence estimates, and very little data exists on incidence. The information for Latin America is sparse and poorly standardized (Seneday and Masti 1987).

Economic Costs of Diabetes

Using epidemiological and financial data, the economic costs of an illness to society can be calculated by its indirect and direct costs. The former reflect the cost of morbidity and mortality to the community as a whole, and the latter, the costs to the health sector of prevention, diagnosis, and treatment.

Unfortunately, virtually no published economic study has differentiated between the two forms of diabetes. The few studies of the economic burden that are available assess indirect costs with respect to lost production. Only one study for a developing economy has been found (Guam). A review of studies in industrial countries, however, can point to the potential burden diabetes may represent for developing countries and the potential benefits to be gained from prevention and case management programs. In table 22-1 we summarize the main studies that are currently available. These studies inevitably suffer from the weaknesses of the epidemiological and economic data on which they are based and the fact that IDDM and NIDDM are combined as one disease in the analysis.

Two particular problems with using estimates from industrial countries and projecting them for developing countries are that it is unclear what level of disability or death results from illnesses to which diabetes contributes and what the likelihood is that either IDDM or NIDDM patients will develop complications. In general, the only apparent pattern is that the longer a patient survives with either form of diabetes, the more likely it is that such complications will develop (WHO 1985). A WHO study group reports that in industrial countries diabetic kidney disease, for example, is present in one in six diabetics and directly causes or contributes to premature death in 50 percent of those in whom IDDM began in youth (WHO 1985). Nearly all IDDM patients and many NIDDM patients will eventually develop some form of eye disease, but only some of them appear to be at risk of developing the severe life-threatening complications. The risk of coronary heart disease is two to three times higher in both IDDM and NIDDM patients older than forty years in industrial countries. In these countries the outlook for stabilized IDDM patients is good and there is some evidence that good control of the disease can delay (and may even prevent) the onset of long-term pathological complications (WHO 1985; Ward 1988). Indeed, after stabilization, patients with diabetes in industrial countries may live for fifteen or more years before the onset of complications—although life expectancy is generally reduced by up to one-third (WHO 1985). This is true for nephropathy and probably also for the other complications of diabetes, and individual

Table 22-1. Studies on the Economic Burden of Diabetes

Country	Year	Total economic burden	Indirect/direct cost (percent of total cost)	Source
Guam	1976	US$3 million	80/20[a]	Kuberski and Bennet 1979
Sweden	1979	1,317 million Skr	57/43	Jonsson 1983
United Kingdom	1979–80	£144.3 million[b]	42/58	Laing 1981
United States	1969	US$2.6 billion	62/38	SBMLIC c
United States	1973	US$4.0 billion	59/41	SBMLIC c
United States	1975	US$5.3 billion	53/47	SBMLIC c
United States	1979	US$15.7 billion	64/36	Platt and Sudovar[d]
United States	1980	US$9.7 billion	51/49	SBMLIC c
United States	1984	US$13.8 billion	46/54	SBMLIC c
United States	1987	US$20.4 billion	53/47	American Diabetes Association 1988

a. Approximate.
b. Excludes cost of 64,047 years lost through premature death.
c. Statistical Bureau of the Metropolitan Life Insurance Company. Discussed in Songer, in press.
d. Discussed in Songer, in press.
Source: See last column.

susceptibility interacts with levels of diabetes control to determine the tissue response, rate of damage, and ultimate severity in the organ concerned. Early recognition and treatment of retinopathy and foot problems, for example, can reduce disability and prolong life. Correction of hypertension and hyperlipidemia are also important to prolong survival.

INDIRECT COSTS. The broad trends shown by the studies suggest that indirect costs are of decreasing importance within the overall economic burden of diabetes (for example, in the United States they fell from about 62 percent in 1969 to 46 percent in 1984). In most studies indirect costs are dominated by the cost of the disability caused by the disease, although the most recent U.S. study (American Diabetes Association 1988) suggests that mortality costs are more important. This finding, however, probably results from the inclusion in the study of deaths in which diabetes was a contributory cause rather than only those deaths directly due to the disease. Unfortunately this study did not also consider the potentially important costs of disability in which diabetes was a contributory factor, instead focusing only on the costs of disability directly caused by diabetes. Taken together, the total of these disability costs would probably exceed mortality costs and dominate indirect costs, even in this study.

The only figures from developing economies that shed light on indirect costs are those reported from Guam (Kuberski and Bennet 1979) and Ghana (Ghana Health Assessment Project Team 1981). Of the total costs attributable to diabetes in Guam, about 80 percent were indirect costs, but it is not clear whether mortality or morbidity costs were dominant. In Ghana, the average age at onset of the disease was estimated to be forty years (suggesting that only NIDDM was considered), with a 50 percent case-fatality rate after fifteen years (average age at death being fifty-five) and 30 percent disablement before death. The total days of life lost were calculated as 217 per 1,000 persons per year; 52 percent of these days were lost

because of premature death. This picture of the balance of indirect costs differs from that in most industrial country studies, in which morbidity costs are dominant. The difference may reflect the younger average age at death of diabetics in Ghana; many of the deaths could occur before the onset of complications and other disabilities. It may also reflect technical differences between the studies: the monetary valuation of the costs in industrial country studies and the use of undiscounted days of life lost in the Ghana study.

Overall it is difficult to suggest the likely level of the indirect costs associated with diabetes in developing countries because of poor epidemiological data and the failure to separate the two forms of the disease in the available cost data. Indirect costs will also depend on the level and quality of the health care available. Because IDDM is a rarer disease worldwide, it might be expected that NIDDM would dominate the indirect costs attributable to diabetes in developing countries. The former disease, however, occurs in younger age groups and is likely to cause death, so years of life lost as a result of the disease may be substantial even though it is an uncommon disease. In contrast, NIDDM is more common, occurs in older people, and is less likely to cause death if untreated; but it may lead to substantial disability as a result of the complications associated with diabetes. As the prevalence of NIDDM rises and the age of onset falls (as some evidence appears to indicate is likely), these disability costs will increase. Both forms of diabetes, therefore, have serious but not directly comparable consequences with regard to indirect costs.

DIRECT COSTS. Only Kuberski and Bennet (1979), in their study in Guam, discuss the direct costs of diabetes in developing economies. Direct hospital costs alone exceeded $600,000 in 1976, including 5,352 disability days from 435 patients admitted to the hospital (an average of 12.3 days per person admitted).[1] These costs, however, will probably not be representative of all developing economies but will reflect the relatively high level of care offered within Guam's health system.

Similarly, the evidence of direct costs from industrial countries reflects their more sophisticated health systems and so cannot be directly transferred to situations in developing countries. Industrial country studies do, however, indicate the main influences on these costs and may suggest future cost levels for developing countries.

The studies that are available show that the cost of diabetes treatment programs is substantial and is increasing in industrial countries (for example, rising from $1.65 billion in the United States in 1973 to $7.4 billion in 1984). This trend reflects the inflation of medical care prices, the increased prevalence of diabetes, the increased use of medical care among diabetics, and the development of new treatment technologies (Songer, in press). Direct costs are now equally important to, if not more important than, indirect costs within the overall economic burden of the disease. A high portion of direct costs (usually not estimated) are likely to be the result of the complications of, and illnesses associated with, diabetes rather than of diabetes itself. Indeed, one study demonstrated that patients with chronic complications of diabetes incurred health care costs fourteen times as high as diabetic patients without any record of complications (Gambert and others 1988). Prevention and case management programs, therefore, have the potential both to reduce the indirect costs of the disease and to reduce the costs of caring for complications. Still, the cost of such programs is itself dependent on the nature of the strategy adopted, and careful consideration of the cost and effectiveness of treatment options is important in seeking to contain costs. Songer (in press) suggests, for example, that economic evaluations techniques should be used in evaluating screening programs, insulin treatment programs (multiple as opposed to single injections as opposed to insulin pump therapy), complications treatment programs (laser surgery, dialysis, transplants, and so on), and home blood glucose monitoring programs.

In most developing countries the existing level of direct costs associated with diabetes is likely to be low. Although the true incidence of IDDM is not known, it is clear that many such patients probably do not survive long after the onset of illness and so do not obtain medical care. Those people with diabetes who do survive receive only such care as is available, which for many of these countries will be limited, leading to high case fatality in the first few years following diagnosis. The costs in Guam may suggest the upper end of the cost range for developing economies, and the lower end is probably suggested by the hypothetical costing for diabetes case management presented later in the chapter.

Lowering or Postponing Diabetes Incidence

A reduction in the incidence of new cases of diabetes will only be achieved by primary prevention strategies, whereas the incidence of diabetes complications may be reduced by improvements in case management and through earlier case detection.

Primary Prevention

Beliefs concerning the cause or causes of diabetes have recently moved away from genetic and immunological explanations to a much greater emphasis on environmental factors, thus increasing the relevance of primary preventive strategies. An eminent international study group claimed in 1987 "that at least 60 percent of IDDM worldwide, and perhaps over 95 percent, is environmentally determined and thus potentially avoidable" (DERI 1987). Even if this is true, however, the causal factors in the environment have not been clearly defined, and although it may be possible to identify some high-risk individuals, the costs and technical difficulties would prohibit this option, even in most industrial countries (Zimmet 1987). As a consequence, it is not possible to make specific recommendations for the prevention of IDDM in industrial, let alone developing, countries, and given the apparently low incidence rates in the latter, a preventive strategy would not appear to be a high priority for them. A far greater priority for diabetes in developing countries lies with further international collaborative research to establish the true incidence and the determinants of IDDM through the use of population-based studies. Although diabetes has been studied using such registers in numerous industrial countries, no successful such register yet exists in Africa or Latin America (DERI 1987).

At present there are also no proven intervention strategies that reduce the incidence of NIDDM. Still, many authorities believe there is now sufficient evidence that experimental community or population intervention studies should be made of lowered dietary intake of carbohydrates (including reductions in fat and sugar intakes), reduced obesity, and increased physical exercise and activity (Zimmet 1987). Considerable attention would have to be given to establishing sound methods for measuring both the successful implementation of the interventions and for evaluating the possible changes in incidence of NIDDM over time.

The links between diabetes, coronary heart disease, hypertension, and other noncommunicable diseases have led the World Health Organization to propose an integrated program for the prevention and control of noncommunicable diseases (for example, by stressing good nutrition, avoidance of obesity, increased physical activity, and reductions in smoking and alcohol consumption). A parallel has been drawn with intervention projects for coronary heart disease (WHO 1985; Zimmet and others 1986). Because no specific and modifiable causes are known to account clearly for the rise in diabetes, a broad strategy that tackles a wider range of emerging health problems makes sense for many developing countries. The strategy would need to rely heavily on modifying individual human behavior, improvements in the health services, mass health education, and government regulation and legislation.

Costs and Consequences of Preventing Diabetes

In assessing whether or not to undertake a primary preventive strategy for diabetes, it is useful to consider the possible costs and consequences of such a program. Both costs and consequences will be influenced by the nature of the preventive strategy adopted. In particular, costs are influenced by the scale of the educational program (and by the nature of other preventive activities); the consequences, by the effectiveness of potential educational strategies.

Given the existing inadequacy of the epidemiological understanding of IDDM, such a preventive strategy is currently only a possibility for NIDDM. Prevention of NIDDM would involve mass health education in order to change the behavioral patterns that increase the risk of diabetes. Unfortunately, little is known about either the costs or the effectiveness of such education programs. Phillips, Feachem, and Mills (1987) report that the total costs of mass media campaigns have varied substantially—from less than $20,000 for a Kenyan childcare program to more than $500,000 for programs involving foreign expertise, careful audience research, and prime-time broadcasting (for example, the Tanzanian "Man Is Health" program costs about $600,000). It would appear difficult to justify similar programs for diabetes alone, because the relatively low incidence results in a small potential target population and so would generate high costs per capita of this population. The promotion of healthy lifestyles through mass media programs aimed at the entire population would be more justifiable and would, in part, seek to prevent the development of diabetes. On the basis of Phillips, Feachem, and Mills's hypothetical costings for five possible education programs (varying from cheap to "luxury"), the cost per capita might be between $0.04 and $0.96 for a population of 500,000, or between $0.02 and $0.54 for a population of 1 million.

A number of factors clearly influence the effectiveness of such programs—in particular, their coverage and the subsequent use of their messages by the general or targeted population. The author of a review of fifteen mass media health and nutrition projects in developing countries concluded that although mass media programs can quickly reach large numbers of people and up to half of those reached by the message remember it in the short term, there is only limited evidence that people actually adopt new behavioral patterns (Leslie 1987). Other studies (for example, Foote 1985 on the promotion of oral rehydration therapy in the Gambia) present a more optimistic picture of the influence of broad educational programs on some health-related behavioral patterns. The success of programs aimed at the control of cardiovascular disease and hypertension in a number of industrial countries may suggest that changes in lifestyle can be effective means of preventing noncommunicable diseases, including diabetes. Yet studies have not clearly shown that patient knowledge and patient behavior in diabetes care are correlated (Marquis and Ware 1979). In general, the evidence on the effectiveness of educational programs remains limited and contradictory, and the costs per case prevented of such programs are at present impossible to evaluate.

Alternatively, or in conjunction with healthy lifestyle promotion, educational messages could be targeted at the groups known to be at high risk of developing NIDDM. Zimmet (1987), however, suggests that a population strategy is preferable for primary prevention purposes because a high-risk strategy would affect only a small proportion of all people who would subsequently develop diabetes. Targeting educational messages at specific people might, however, reduce costs and improve effectiveness (by permitting more precise messages to be delivered). Such a high-risk strategy might also go hand-in-hand with a screening program for these vulnerable groups. The World Health Organization (WHO 1985) suggests that screening programs provide the opportunity for creating public awareness and educating health professionals. Target groups should include those at high risk of glucose intolerance (for example, the obese) and those in whom even mild glucose intolerance might be a risk factor (for example, pregnant women). The costs and effectiveness of these programs are not currently known but will be influenced by the sensitivity and specificity of screening methods, the definition and size of target populations, and the level of care provided for those found to have diabetes.

The potential negative consequences of a preventive strategy that are suggested in table 22-2 could be forestalled by greater investment in existing health services, but in the short term such investment is rarely forthcoming in developing countries. It is, therefore, important to consider the total amount of resources that can be harnessed to provide health care in developing countries, how these resources should be allocated among the health needs of a country, and how to allocate responsibilities for the provision of health care among different providers. This approach will ensure more efficient use of currently available resources and will provide the basis for efficient use of investment funds available in the long term.

Table 22-2. Costs and Consequences of Undertaking a Preventive Diabetes Strategy

Bearer of costs	Examples	Consequences
Government	Education program, required strengthening of health infrastructure, screening program	Reduction in morbidity and mortality from diabetes and its complications; indirect and direct cost savings
Household	Increased visits, more medications, better diet	Household savings (for example, reduced time and monetary costs because less treatment and less loss of earnings)

Note: In addition, positive spin-offs include reduction in associated diseases, leading to indirect and direct cost savings (such as improved general knowledge and behavior). Negative spin-offs include lower quantity and quality of care for other conditions because of emphasis on diabetes.
Source: Authors.

Case Management

The case management of IDDM and NIDDM are very different and are, therefore, considered separately here.

Insulin-Dependent Patients

Case management varies between IDDM and NIDDM. For IDDM, the main requirements are the establishment of the diagnosis, stabilization of patients on daily insulin therapy, and the training of these patients to inject their own insulin and to monitor their own control on a regular basis. Patients using insulin must also lower their dietary carbohydrates and sugar intake, eat regular meals, and increase their physical activity. Good control of diabetes requires the regular monitoring of blood glucose or urinary glucose levels, or both, and the early detection of the long-term clinical complications. Because of the high incidence of diabetic complications, it is essential to maintain good case follow-up and monitoring procedures for all patients with diabetes. This follow-up can be the responsibility of primary-level care but shared appropriately with secondary and tertiary levels.

It is important to point out that insulin has been available for the treatment of diabetes for more than fifty years and that it is a highly effective treatment in saving and prolonging the lives of patients with IDDM. It is ironical, therefore, that the control of IDDM can be so difficult for patients and health workers in many developing countries (Serantes 1985). In particular, the regular supply of a suitable insulin preparation and appropriate syringes may be difficult to ensure, despite their obvious importance to survival (WHO 1985). Most of the world's insulin is produced by a few manufacturers based in industrial countries, and although there is a move to standardize both the insulin (to 100 international units per milliliter) and the syringe, there are many different strengths and types available (Bloom 1985; WHO 1985). In addition, insulin is a biological product with a limited storage life that requires appropriate cold-chain conditions. It is also an expensive drug, which is not available through the United Nations Children's Fund (UNIPAC) in Copenhagen, although it is included in the World Health Organization's list of essential drugs (WHO 1988). Because insulin availability is such a problem in many developing countries, particularly in Africa, the International Diabetes Federation has been organizing the collection and international transportation of unwanted insulin vials (IDF 1987).

Non-Insulin-Dependent Patients

People with NIDDM suffer from a less severe illness day to day and so, if the necessary equipment and specialist advice is available, can largely be cared for by general medical practitioners and trained nurses in industrial countries (Howe and Walford 1984; Burrows and others 1987). Because of the insidious onset of NIDDM, patients are commonly diagnosed only incidentally by screening procedures, such as the testing of a urine sample for glucose, or during the investigation of another illness or diabetic complication. Once diagnosed, most NIDDM patients can be stabilized as outpatients and do not require more than brief treatment with insulin. Their blood glucose or urine glucose needs to be monitored less frequently than that of IDDM patients, and they often respond well, at least initially, to a modified diet, weight reduction, and increased exercise and physical activity.

Only if these methods fail are drugs that lower oral blood glucose (hypoglycemic drugs) required. Such drugs have been available for the treatment of NIDDM for nearly thirty years. Data from a twenty-two-year analysis (1964–86) of the use of such drugs in the United States showed that chlorpropamide (a sulfonylurea) was then the most widely used, two new preparations introduced in 1984 gaining 41 percent of the market by 1986. Patients age sixty years and older received oral hypoglycemic drug prescriptions at the rate of 478 per 1,000 visits in 1986, and 35 percent of all diabetic patients were taking such drugs (Kennedy and others 1988). The inadequacy of primary-level services, poor dietary and general advice, and the lack of patient supervision in developing countries is likely to result in greater use of these drugs. For instance, evidence from a number of Pacific countries suggested that about 80 percent of NIDDM patients were using oral hypoglycemic drugs (South Pacific Commission 1978). If oral hypoglycemic drugs fail to control the diabetes, insulin is required and is costly for the health services and for patients. In industrial countries the number of NIDDM patients who finally require insulin therapy may be more than the number of IDDM patients regularly using insulin.

It appears, therefore, that providing adequate case management in developing countries is a much more feasible option for NIDDM than IDDM patients, particularly if planned primary-level health care strategies are adopted. It is important to note, however, that even though patients are classified as IDDM and NIDDM, insulin is important in the treatment of both groups.

Costs and Consequences of Diabetes Case Management

The case management strategies presented in the previous two sections have implications for the care ideally available at all levels of the health care system. The World Health Organization (1985) recommends that at the primary level the components of diabetes care offered should include self-care, home care, basic care, screening for complications, and health education (WHO 1985). Support for families should be provided by a primary care physician, a nurse, and other health professionals. Health workers must know the diagnostic, therapeutic, and preventive aspects of care. A list of essential items required for IDDM and NIDDM management, as recommended by the World Health Organization, is shown in table 22A-3. Referral from the primary level to the secondary or tertiary level will be necessary when specialized assistance is required in the management of the disease or its complications. Laboratory services will also be needed. At the tertiary level special clinics should be organized to provide diagnostic and management skills for

Table 22-3. Costs and Consequences of Diabetes Case Management Strategies

Bearer of costs	Examples	Consequences
Government	Case management (diagnosis, monitoring, treatment), patient education	Reduction in morbidity and mortality from diabetes and its complications as result of improved treatment; indirect and direct cost savings
Household	Increased visits, more medications, better diet	Household savings of time and money from improved treatment

Note: In addition, positive spin-offs include strengthened health services. Negative spin-offs include clinical side effects (for example, AIDS and hepatitis, effects of inappropriate use of hypoglycemic drugs and insulin), impact on existing health services.
Source: Authors.

the treatment of diabetic retinopathy, end-stage renal disease, and vascular disease.

Case management must include a patient-oriented educational strategy, focusing on face-to-face education of known diabetic patients concerning the dietary and behavioral changes necessary to maintain optimal metabolic control and to prevent and reduce the severity of diabetic complications.

As with preventive strategies, it is useful in decisionmaking to outline the costs and consequences of case management strategies (see table 22-3). Given the potentially large costs and unknown effectiveness of preventive strategies, the first option should be for improved case management. Developing countries will need to improve case management to ensure appropriate and cost-effective care and to reduce the likelihood of acute and chronic complications.

In broad terms, diabetes management aims to preserve the life of the diabetic patient, to relieve the symptoms of the disease, and to avoid its associated complications. The studies of direct costs indicate that there is substantial variation between countries in the treatment patterns adopted and that these differences also influence costs. The technology used is an especially important influence, and the trend toward more expensive care within industrial countries is one that developing countries can ill afford. Developing countries must assess the cost-effectiveness of standard case management practices. For example, the authors of a study in the United Kingdom stress the need for a structured clinic recall system for diabetics in order to improve clinical surveillance (Burrows and others 1987). There is, however, considerable uncertainty about appropriate practices—some patients are monitored frequently and others infrequently. In another study in the United Kingdom, Jones and Hedley (1986) showed that if follow-up times were increased by 30 percent (for example, from six to eight months) an additional 2,000 known nonattenders could be seen for a cost increase of less than 5 percent of the existing annual cost. Recommended practices must aim to be as cost-effective as possible in order to ensure that best use is made of limited available resources.

More is known about the effectiveness of patient education as a part of case management than the effectiveness of other educational strategies, but the evidence is not conclusive. In one hospital, patient education led to a reduction in occupancy by diabetic patients from 5.6 days per year to 1.4 days (Miller and Goldstein 1972). Similarly, patient education in self-care led to a 78 percent decrease in hyperglycemic coma (Davidson

1983) and a 75 percent decrease in below-knee amputations (Assal and others 1982). In contrast, the long-term (more than one year) effect of nutrition education on weight loss was disappointing (Foreyt and others 1981; Wing and others 1985). Studies show that education provided in the outpatient setting can be effective for diabetes (for example, intensive outpatient education was associated with lowered plasma glucose levels [Mazzuca and others 1986]), but it is also often undermined by attrition rates. A review of such studies showed that in the five in which attrition rates were reported, up to 90 percent of the patients failed to complete the educational program (Kaplan and Davis 1986). This emphasizes the importance of motivation and of linking education to follow-up visits.

The key resource required for such an education program is appropriately trained personnel, although literature, equipment, and facilities are also necessary (WHO 1985). Education can take place in the hospital or in the outpatient setting; unfortunately there is little cost data for either strategy. The authors of a study in Australia in which the outpatient initiation of insulin therapy was assessed showed that this strategy is feasible where the facilities for education about diabetes exist; they also showed that it is safe, achieves satisfactory metabolic control, is acceptable to most patients, and, compared with inpatient care, reduces costs by Aus$1,857 per new patient stabilized (Bruce and others 1987).

In order to estimate the annual costs of treating IDDM and NIDDM patients in a low-income developing country, data from Malawi on inpatient and outpatient costs and from international essential drugs lists (WHO and the nongovernment Dutch organization [IDA]) were used. In the absence of developing country data on hospitalization rates for diabetes patients, the analysis used estimates based on data from the United States. Despite the limitations of the available data, it is clear that the cost of treating IDDM patients will be dominated by their need for insulin and the equipment for its administration, at an estimated cost of $191 per diabetic per year (1987 prices), approximately 90 percent of total costs. The finding reflects the high cost of insulin in developing countries in relation to that of hospitalization, and the relatively low probability of hospitalization. It is more difficult to estimate the costs associated with NIDDM patients, but it seems likely that the biggest cost is for oral hypoglycemic drugs at an estimated $20 per diabetic per year. If we assume no hospitalizations, this represents nearly 90 percent of the total cost per patient.

It is possible that as case management improves and case fatality is reduced, the cost of hospitalizations for complications will rise and eventually dominate the total cost of institutional care for diabetic patients. These rising treatment costs theoretically increase the potential benefits (with respect to cost savings) of primary and secondary preventive strategies and also stress the importance of improved case management of the complications of diabetes to reduction of the direct costs associated with them.

In practice, diabetes case management (and preventive) strategies must balance what is feasible in each developing country situation against the potential benefits. Feasibility is related to the cost of the strategy, to the coverage and quality of care achieved, to the availability of trained health workers in existing health systems, to the pool of available health resources, and to the range of other compelling health needs that exist. For example, although recall systems are a relatively cheap and very cost-effective method of protecting the health of diabetics, existing recall systems (for example, those for tuberculosis patients) often do not function effectively: health staff have too many other "priority activities" to give adequate attention to patient monitoring, and patients either do not understand the benefits of monitoring systems or judge that the costs of regular check-ups outweigh the potential benefits. In addition, record systems are frequently poorly maintained in health facilities, and health cards are not always kept by patients. Remedying this situation requires patient and provider education and additional resources (additional health or clerical personnel, card index systems, and so on).

The broad case management strategy presented here must therefore be adapted to the country-specific situation through consideration of the needs of existing diabetic patients and the level of available resources. Important issues will include whether basic care can be offered at health centers or only at local hospitals on an outpatient basis and whether drugs or insulin can be made widely available, possibly dispensed through the private sector. A growing trend is to recommend district diabetes centers, which can offer routine care and education and ensure the adequacy of supplies and drugs.

In many developing countries, a diabetes case management strategy will be based on primary care facilities, the regular supply of essential drugs and equipment, and the setting of appropriate clinical priorities, such as standard diagnosis and treatment protocols. After these have been achieved, consideration should then be given to the additional resources needed for the development of secondary and tertiary levels of care.

The cost of treating an IDDM patient can be used to estimate the cost per disability-adjusted life-year gained by a case management strategy. A similar estimate is not made for NIDDM patients because of the uncertainty about the number of years of life saved by treatment.

Treatment of an IDDM patient is lifesaving; thus each year's treatment saves a year of life. There is marginal reduction in the quality of life because of the inconvenience of treatment and lifestyle limitations. Assuming that 0.9 of a disability-adjusted year of life is obtained for the $213 annual cost of treatment, then the cost per disability-adjusted life-year gained is $237.

Priorities

In any consideration of future priorities, there is an inevitable trade-off between investing resources in primary prevention and in better management of patients. In addition, there are major equity and ethical questions to be considered.

Priorities for Resource Allocation

Resource allocation plans need to take into account questions of public health policy and equity.

PUBLIC HEALTH CONSIDERATIONS. The current evidence about the public health significance of diabetes worldwide is limited. It would seem that IDDM is numerically the lesser problem, but its recognition and management requires the use of relatively specialized and more costly techniques. By contrast, NIDDM is relatively more common and with changing conditions is of growing significance, particularly in the Pacific, China, Asia, and the Middle East. This is probably also true for Latin American and African countries, although there is less clear evidence for these two continents. In the United States more deaths are attributed to diabetes than to lung cancer, breast cancer, motor vehicle accidents, cirrhosis of the liver, or infant mortality (WHO 1985). Improved case recognition and management is, therefore, important and can be justified for industrial countries simply on the grounds of its potential to reduce both the future indirect (morbidity and mortality) costs of the complications associated with the disease and the future direct costs of caring for patients suffering with such complications. It is also probable that emphasizing the preventive strategy could reduce the costs of the disease and its complications. Given this situation and the changing health patterns of developing countries, it seems clear that the burden of diabetes and the predictable potential costs of the disease for developing countries cannot be ignored as they undergo development.

The position faced by developing countries concerning the broad policy options of primary prevention and case management is as follows:

- In general, primary prevention has the potential to reduce both the indirect and direct costs of diabetes but only at substantial expense

- Primary prevention is not, currently, a realistic option for IDDM

- Primary prevention has more potential for NIDDM, but prevention would need to rely on interventions and educational programs of unknown effectiveness

- In general, case management has the possibility of reducing the potentially large indirect and direct costs of the complications of diabetes, except in its most developed forms, when medical care may be beyond the level affordable by many developing countries

- Only a small number of IDDM patients will require case management, but it will be potentially expensive because such patients need regular insulin throughout their lives and most patients eventually suffer from at least one complication. Still, because treatment postpones death for many years, it may well be cost-effective in comparison with interventions for some other chronic diseases

- Case management is very important for NIDDM patients and should be based on patient education, behavior modification, and appropriate use of oral hypoglycemic drugs.

The diversity of manifestations of diabetes makes it difficult to suggest universally appropriate policy strategies. Each country needs to determine for itself how it will tackle the potential problems of the disease, within the primary care framework proposed by WHO (1985). In table 22-4 we summarize some policy options for discussion and indicate that the options differ between developing countries as a result of the differing income levels, the differing health infrastructure, and the differing relative significance of diabetes as a health problem. Within policies, the differences between IDDM and NIDDM must also be recognized. In the table we assume the incidence of both forms of diabetes taken together is either high or low. The distributional issues discussed next must also be considered and should feed into policy discussions about how to finance diabetes case management activities and what levels of care can be afforded.

EQUITY CONSIDERATIONS. Considerations of distribution and equity can have an important influence on investment priorities. Discussion of the equity implications of diabetes prevention and case management programs must be based on who suffers from the disease and therefore who will gain from prevention and treatment, as well as on the sources of finance for the programs.

Non-insulin-dependent diabetes mellitus is often characterized as a disease of the rich, because it is clearly associated with environmental changes reflecting increased wealth. Within developing countries, for example, the urbanized population is generally deemed to be more affluent than the rural population and may be more at risk of developing NIDDM. Insulin-dependent diabetes mellitus, however, is less clearly associated with such environmental factors, and so patients suffering from this type of diabetes may be of high or low income. The country-specific situation must obviously be assessed before the relative status of diabetics can be judged.

What would these characterizations suggest about the effect on equity of diabetes prevention and case management programs? One argument might be that late-onset NIDDM patients are not only more wealthy but probably in the productive years of life, possibly in responsible and influential jobs, and that they are an important economic asset which must be protected. It can also be argued that the existing bias of many developing country health systems is already set against lower socioeconomic groups and in favor of wealthier patients and further state expenditure on upper-income groups cannot be justified.

This latter argument does not imply that little or no provision should be made for diabetes but rather that it cannot be viewed as a priority for state health services alone. It might be possible to consider, for example, the provision of drugs and insulin on a means-tested basis in the public sector or on a fee-for-service basis in the private sector. Such a strategy has many practical difficulties, however, and the possible benefits may exceed the costs of implementation. For example, it would promote the development of dual health standards: high-quality private care for the more wealthy diabetics and low-quality or inadequate public care for the less wealthy. This strategy would also probably conflict with ethical considerations. Since insulin has been available for more than fifty years and it is an essential, life-sustaining drug for IDDM patients, many people would consider it unethical to adopt a health policy which fails to guarantee adequate supplies of insulin. This is the implicit policy in many countries, however; because they cannot afford to provide the drug, the way is left open to the private sector to supply unregulated care for those who can afford to pay. Inequities already exist, and countries must consider the effect on them of possible policy changes.

Resolution of distributional problems is not easy, especially when resources are scarce and policy choices often have unwanted consequences. Future health care investments in developing countries, however, must seek to reflect both existing resource constraints and such distributional concerns. The production and distribution of insulin as a life-preserving drug is an important part of the broader considerations involving its usage, such as patient monitoring and health education.

Table 22-4. *Policy Options for Control of Diabetes Mellitus*

Incidence of DM	*Higher-income developing countries*	*Lower-income developing countries*
Low	Focus on primary and secondary care only, especially face-to-face education of known diabetics Develop standard case management protocols for IDDM and NIDDM Have appropriate drugs available	Do nothing Consider minimum case management requirements
High	Consider tertiary provision Screen high-risk patients Strengthen preventive and case management efforts (for example, through broader education programs) Secure regular supplies of insulin and oral hypoglycemic drugs, and ensure delivery to patients Stimulate epidemiologic, clinical, and laboratory research	Focus on primary and secondary care only, especially for NIDMM Face-to-face education of known diabetics Develop standard protocols Make insulin and oral hypoglycemic drugs available on demand only Form links with international research efforts

Source: Authors.

There is a clear need to bring together the interested parties worldwide, including the manufacturers, the International Diabetes Federation, the World Health Organization, and other international agencies, to develop more effective and acceptable strategies for developing countries.

Priorities for Operational Research

Specific international actions can assist the development of appropriate strategies, and the International Diabetes Federation and the World Health Organization are active in these areas (King and Mitrofanov 1988). For example, there is an urgent need for operational research to find ways of facilitating the purchase of insulin and oral hypoglycemics at reasonable prices (for example, through UNIPAC) and to guarantee their availability in developing countries in order to improve case management strategies and to reduce the cost per case. Moreover, international support for diabetes research is necessary, and more international collaborative research centers are needed in the developing world. Such research should aim to clarify the importance of diabetes and the options available for its prevention and case management. The following are the preliminary research priorities that we have identified in this chapter for national and international action:

- Assessment of the incidence and prevalence of both IDDM and NIDDM in developing countries, particularly in Asia, Sub-Saharan Africa, and Latin America, through a greater support to epidemiological studies

- Large-scale evaluation studies of possible interventions and strategies to prevent NIDDM, including studies of the cost and effectiveness of a broad strategy of noncommunicable disease control

- Assessment of the costs and effectiveness of alternative case management procedures (IDDM/NIDDM)

- Case studies to assess what resources are currently consumed by IDDM and NIDDM

- Operational research to improve the quality of case management within existing health services, such as the development of standard treatment protocols for primary care

- Consideration of appropriate financing mechanisms for expanding the management of diabetes patients, particularly within secondary and tertiary health care facilities.

Appendix 22A. Diagnosis and Self-Care of Diabetes

The tables that follow show the blood glucose levels of both diabetics and nondiabetics and the glucose concentrations they produce during the glucose tolerance test, as well as the equipment essential to self-care for diabetics.

Table 22A-1. Blood Glucose Levels for Diagnosis of Diabetes Mellitus

	DM *likely*		DM *uncertain*		DM *unlikely*	
Sample	*mmol/l*	*mg/dl*	*mmol/l*	*mg/dl*	*mmol/l*	*mg/dl*
Whole blood						
Venous	> 10.0	> 180	4.4–10.0	80–180	< 4.4	< 80
Capillary	> 11.1	> 200	4.4–11.1	80–200	< 4.4	< 80
Plasma						
Venous	> 11.1	> 200	5.5–11.1	100–200	< 5.5	< 100
Capillary	> 12.2	> 220	5.5–12.2	100–220	< 5.5	< 100

Note: Unstandardized (casual, random) blood glucose values.
Source: WHO 1985.

Table 22A-2. Diagnostic Glucose Concentration Values in the Oral Glucose Tolerance Test
[mmol/l (mg/dl)]

	Diabetes mellitus		*Impaired glucose tolerance*	
Sample	*Fasting*	*Two hours after glucose load*	*Fasting*	*Two hours after glucose load*
Whole blood				
Venous	≥ 6.7 (120)	≥ 10.0 (180)	< 6.7 (<120)	6.7–10.0 (120–180)
Capillary	≥ 6.7 (120)	≥ 11.1 (200)	< 6.7 (< 120)	7.8–11.1 (140–200)
Plasma				
Venous	≥ 7.8 (140)	≥ 11.1 (200)	< 7.8 (< 140)	7.8–11.1 (140–200)
Capillary	≥ 7.8 (140)	≥ 12.2 (200)	< 7.8 (< 140)	8.9–12.2 (160–220)

Note: For epidemiologic or population screening purposes, the two-hour value after 75g oral glucose may be used alone or with the fasting value. The fasting value alone is considered less reliable because true fasting cannot be assured.
Source: WHO 1985.

Table 22A-3. Basic Equipment for Self-Care of Diabetics

Self-management of IDDM	Self-management of NIDDM	Primary health care center
Urine testing materials for glucose and ketone bodies and/or blood glucose testing materials	Urine testing materials for glucose and ketone bodies and/or blood glucose testing materials	Urine testing materials for glucose and ketone bodies and/or blood glucose testing materials
Book or chart and pencil for recording results	Book or chart and pencil for recording test results and body weight	Book or chart and pencil for recording results
Insulin as prescribed and cool place for storage	Oral hypoglycemic agents, when applicable	Insulin, plus cool place for storage
Syringe, needles, and carrying case	Sugar lumps or other readily absorbed carbohydrates	Syringe and needles
Sterilization facilities		Sterilization facilites
Cotton wool		Cotton wool
Sugar lumps or readily absorbed carbohydrates		Cleansing agent
		Sugar lumps or readily absorbed carbohydrates
		Oral hypoglycemic agents
		Materials for testing the presence of protein in urine
		Weighing machine
		Blood glucose monitors or meters and test-strips
		Glucose for intravenous use (glucagon, if available)
		Simple printed education materials and teaching aids
		Place for storing patients' records

Source: WHO 1985.

Notes

This chapter has benefited greatly from all the most helpful comments and criticisms that we received on early drafts, but we would particularly like to thank the following: Dr. H. Keen, Guy's Hospital, London; Dr. H. King, World Health Organization, Geneva; Dean Jamison, University of California at Los Angeles; Dr. R. E. LaPorte and Dr. T. J. Songer, Diabetes Epidemiological Research International, Pittsburgh; Dr. R. Williams, Department of Community Medicine, Cambridge; and Dr. P. Zimmet, Lions International Diabetes Institute, Melbourne. In addition, our colleagues within the Department of Public Health and Policy at the London School of Hygiene and Tropical Medicine gave us many new insights and happily commented on our ideas.

1. All dollar amounts are current U.S. dollars unless otherwise indicated.

References

Abu-Bakare, A., R. Taylor, G. V. Gill, and K. G. M. M. Alberti. 1986. "Tropical or Malnutrition-Related Diabetes: A Real Syndrome?" *Lancet* 1:1135–38.

Ahren, B., and C. B. Corrigan. 1985. "Prevalence of Diabetes Mellitus in North-Western Tanzania." *Diabetologia* 26:333–36.

American Diabetes Association. 1988. *Direct and Indirect Costs of Diabetes in the United States in 1987.* Alexandria, Va.

Assal, J. P., R. Gseller, and J.-M. Ekoe. 1982. "Patient Education in Diabetes." In H. Bostrom, ed., *Recent Trends in Diabetes Research.* Stockholm: Almqvst and Wicksell.

Barratt-Connor, E. 1985. "Is Insulin Dependent Diabetes Mellitus Caused by Coxsackie Virus B Infection? A Review of the Epidemiological Evidence." *Reviews of Infectious Diseases* 7:207–15.

Bennett, P. H. 1985. "Changing Concepts of the Epidemiology of Insulin Dependent Diabetes" *Diabetes Care* 8:29–33.

Bloom, A. 1985. "Syringes for Diabetics." *British Medical Journal* 290:727–28.

Bruce, D. G., E. M. Clark, G. A. Danesi, C. V. Campbell, and D. J. Chisholm. 1987. "Outpatient Initiation of Insulin Therapy in Patients with Diabetes Mellitus." *Medical Journal of Australia* 146:19–22.

Burrows, P. J., P. J. Gray, A.-L. Kinmouth, D. J. Payton, G. A. Walpole, R. J. Walton, D. Wilson, and G. Woodbine. 1987. "Who Cares for the Patient with Diabetes? Presentation and Follow-Up in Seven Southampton Practices." *Journal of the Royal College of General Practitioners* 37:65–69.

Cameron, W. I., P. S. Moffitt, and D. R. R. Williams. 1986. "Diabetes Mellitus in the Australian Aborigines of Bourke, New South Wales." *Diabetes Research and Clinical Practice* 2:307–14.

Cheah, J. S., and B. Y. Tan. 1979. "Diabetes amongst Different Races in a Similar Environment." In I. W. Waldhouse, ed., *Diabetes.* Amsterdam: Excerpta Medica.

Davidson, J. K. 1983. "The Grady Memorial Hospital Diabetes Programme." In J. Mann, K. Pyorala, and A. Teuscher, eds., *Diabetes in Epidemiological Perspective.* London: Churchill Livingstone.

Diabetes Epidemiological Research International (DERI). 1987. "Preventing Insulin Dependent Diabetes Mellitus: The Environmental Challenge." *British Medical Journal* 295:479–81.

———. 1988. "Geographic Patterns of Childhood Insulin-Dependent Diabetes Mellitus." *Diabetes* 37:1113–19.

———. 1990. "Secular Trends in Incidence of IDDM in 10 Countries." *Diabetes* 39:858–64.

Fatani, H. H., S. A. Mira, and A. G. El-Zubier. 1987. "Prevalence of Diabetes Mellitus in Rural Saudi Arabia." *Diabetes Care* 10:180–83.

Foote, D. R. 1985. *The Mass Media and Health Practices Evaluation in The Gambia: A Report of Major Findings.* Stanford University, Stanford, Calif.

Foreyt, J. P., D. G. Goodrick, and A. M. Gotto. 1981. "Limitations of Behavioural Treatments of Obesity: Review and Analysis." *Journal of Behavioural Medicine* 4:159–74.

Fuller, J. H., J. Elford, P. Goldblatt, and A. Adelstein. 1983. "Diabetes Mortality: New Light on an Underestimated Public Health Problem." *Diabetologia* 24:336–41.

Gambert, S., N. Fox, and J. Jacobs. 1988. "Oral Hypoglycaemic Therapy and Rates of Health Care Utilisation in Type 2 Diabetes (NIDDM)." In *Direct and Indirect Costs of Diabetes in the United States in 1987*. American Diabetes Association Inc. Alexandria, Va.

Gamble, D. R. 1980. "The Epidemiology of Insulin Dependant Diabetes, with Particular Reference to the Relationship of Virus Infection to Its Etiology." *Epidemiologic Reviews* 2:49–70.

Ghana Health Assessment Project Team. 1981. "A Quantitative Method of Assessing the Health Impact of Different Diseases in Less Developed Countries." *International Journal of Epidemiology* 10:73–80.

"Glucose Tolerance in Pregnancy—The Who and How of Testing." 1988. *Lancet* (editorial) 2:1173.

Godhes, D. M. 1986. "Diabetes in American Indians: A Growing Problem." *Diabetes Care* 9:609–13.

Grabauskas, V. J. 1988. "Glucose Intolerance as a Contributor to Non-communicable Disease Morbidity and Mortality." *Diabetes Care* 11:253–57.

Howe, P., and S. Walford. 1984. "Diabetes Care: Whose Responsibility?" *British Medical Journal* 289:713–14.

IDF (International Diabetes Federation). 1987. "Finland Begins Insulin-Redistribution Program." *International Diabetes Federation Bulletin* 32:193.

Jones, R. B., and A. J. Hedley. 1986. "Adjusting Follow-Up Intervals in a Diabetic Clinic: Implications for Costs and Quality of Care." *Journal of the Royal College of Physicians of London* 20:36–39.

Jonssen, B. 1983. "Diabetes—The Cost of Illness and Control: An Estimate for Sweden, 1978." *Acta Medica Scandinavica* 671(supplement):19–27.

Kaplan, R. M., and W. K. Davis. 1986. "Evaluating the Costs and Benefits of Outpatient Diabetes Education and Nutrition Counselling." *Diabetes Care* 9:81–86.

Kennedy, D. L., J. M. Piper, and C. Bawm. 1988. "Trends in the Use of Oral Hypoglycaemic Drugs, 1964–1986." *Diabetes Care* 11:558–62.

King, H. 1987. "Preventing Insulin Dependent Diabetes Mellitus: The Environmental Challenge." *British Medical Journal* 295:923.

King, H., and M. P. Mitrofanov. 1988. "World Health Organization Activities in the Field of Diabetes Mellitus." *World Health Statistical Quarterly* 41:197–99.

King, H., and P. Zimmet. 1988. "Trends in the Incidence and Prevalence of Diabetes: 11. Non-insulin Dependent Diabetes Mellitus." *World Health Statistical Quarterly* 41:190–96.

King, H., P. Zimmet, K. Pargeter, L. R. Raper, and V. Collins. 1984. "Ethnic Differences in Susceptibility to Non-insulin Dependent Diabetes: A Comparative Study of Two Urbanised Micronesian Populations." *Diabetes* 33:1002–7.

Krolewski, A. S., J. H. Warrem, I. R. Lawrence, and C. R. Kahn. 1987. "Epidemiologic Approach to the Etiology of Type 1 Diabetes Mellitus and Its Complications." *New England Journal of Medicine* 317:1390–98.

Kuberski, T., and P. Bennet. 1979. *The Status of Diabetes Mellitus in the Territory of Guam*. South Pacific Commission Information Document 47. Sura, Fiji.

Laing, W. 1981. "The Cost of Diet-Related Disease." In M. Turner, ed., *Preventative Nutrition and Society*. London: Academic Press.

Leslie, J. 1987. "The Use of Health Statistics as an Effectiveness Measure in Certain Development Communications Projects in UNESCO." In *The Economics of New Education Media*. Vol. 2, *Costs and Effectiveness*. Paris: UNESCO.

Lutalo, S. K., and N. Mabonga. 1985. "Some Clinical and Epidemiological Aspects of Diabetes Mellitus on an Endemic Register in Zimbabwe." *East African Medical Journal* 26:433–45.

McLarty, D. G., H. M. Kitange, B. L. Mtinangi, W. J. Makene, A. B. M. Swai, G. Masuki, P. M. Kilima, L. M. Chawa, and K. G. M. M. Alberti. 1989. "Prevalence of Diabetes and Impaired Glucose Tolerance in Rural Tanzania." *Lancet* 1:871–75.

Marine, N., O. Edelstein, W. P. W. Jackson, and A. I. Yinik. 1969. "Diabetes Hyperglycaemic and Glycosuria among Indians, Malays, and Africans (Bantu) in Cape Town, South Africa." *Diabetes* 18:433–45.

Marquis, K., and J. E. Ware. 1979. *New Measures of Diabetic Patient Knowledge, Behaviour, and Attitude*. Santa Monica, Calif.: Rand.

Mather, H. M., and H. Keen. 1985. "The Southall Diabetes Survey: Prevalence of Known Diabetes in Asians and Europeans." *British Medical Journal* 291:1081–84.

Mather, H. M., N. P. S. Verna, S. P. Mehta, S. Madhu, and H. Keen. 1987. "The Prevalence of Known Diabetes in New Delhi and London." *Journal of the Medical Association of Thailand* 70(supplement 2):54–58.

Mazzuca, S. A., N. H. Moorman, M. L. Wheeler, J. A. Norton, N. S. Fineberg, F. Vinicor, S. J. Cohen, and C. M. Clark, Jr. 1986. "The Diabetes Education Study: A Controlled Trial of the Effects of Diabetes Education." *Diabetes Care* 9:1–10.

Miller, L. V., and G. Goldstein. 1972. "More Efficient Care of Diabetic Patients in a Country-Hospital Setting." *New England Medical Journal* 286:1388–94.

Papoz, L., F. Ben Khalifa, E. Eschwege, and H. Ben Ayed. 1988. "Diabetes Mellitus in Tunisia: Description in Urban and Rural Populations." *International Journal of Epidemiology* 17:419–22.

Patterson, C. C., M. Thorogood, P. G. Smith, M. A. Heasman, J. A. Clarke, and J. I. Mann. 1983. "Epidemiology of Type 1 (Insulin-Dependent) Diabetes in Scotland, 1968–1976: Evidence of an Increasing Incidence." *Diabetologia* 24:238–43.

Phillips, M., R. G. Feachem, and A. Mills. 1987. *Options for Diarrhoeal Diseases Control: The Cost and Effectiveness of Selected Interventions for the Prevention of Diarrhoea*. Evaluation and Planning Centre. Publication 13. London School of Hygiene and Tropical Medicine.

Poon-King, T., M. V. Henry, and F. Rampersad. 1968. "Prevalence and Natural History of Diabetes in Trinidad." *Lancet* 1:155–60.

Reunanen, A., H. K. Akerblom, and M. L. Kaar. 1982. "Prevalence and Ten Year (1970–1979) Incidence of Insulin Dependent Diabetes Mellitus in Children and Adolescents in Finland." *Acta Paediatrica Scandinavia* 71:893–99.

Rewers, M., R. E. LaPorte, H. King, and J. Tuornilehto. 1988. "Trends in the Prevalence and Incidence of Diabetes: Insulin-Dependent Diabetes Mellitus in Childhood." *World Health Statistical Quarterly* 41:179–89.

Rewers, M., R. E. LaPorte, M. Walczak. K. Dmochowski, and E. Bogaczynska. 1987. "An Apparent 'Epidemic' of Youth Onset, Insulin Dependent Diabetes Mellitus in Midwestern Poland." *Diabetes* 36:106–13.

Schooneveldt, M., T. Songer, P. Zimmet, and K. Thoma. 1988. "Changing Mortality Patterns in Nauruans: An Example of Epidemiological Transition." *Journal of Epidemiology and Community Health* 42:89–95.

Seneday, M., and M. L. Masti. 1987. "Diabetes in Latin America." *Journal of the Medical Association of Thailand* 70(supplement 2):77–78.

Serantes, N. A. 1985. "The Problem of the Diabetic Patient in Developing Countries." *Diabetologia* 28:597–601.

Shanghai Diabetes Research Cooperation Group. 1980. "Diabetes Mellitus Survey in Shanghai." *Chinese Medical Journal* 93:663–70.

Simmons, D., D. R. R. Williams, and M. J. Powell. 1989. "Prevalence of Diabetes in a Predominantly Asian Community: Preliminary Findings of the Coventry Diabetes Study." *British Medical Journal* 298:18–21.

Songer, T. J. In press. "The Economics of Diabetes Care." In K. G. G. M. Alberti, R. A. de Fronzo, H. Keene, and P. Zimmet, eds., *International Textbook of Diabetes Mellitus*. London: John Wiley and Sons.

South Pacific Commission. 1978. *Diabetes, Gout, and Hypertension in the Pacific Islands*. Information Document 43. Sura, Fiji.

Tarn, A. C., J. M. Thomas, B. M. Dean, D. Ingram, G. Schwarz, G. F. Bottazzo, and E. A. M. Gale. 1988. "Predicting Insulin-Dependent Diabetes." *Lancet* 1:845–50.

Teuscher, T., P. Baillol, J. B. Rosman, and A. Teuscher. 1987. "Absence of Diabetes in a Rural West African Population with a High Carbohydrate/Cassava Diet." *Lancet* 1:765–68.

Thai, A. C., P. Yeo, K. Lun, K. Hughes, K. Waugh, S. Sothy, K. Luni, W. Ng, J. Cheah, W. Phoon, and P. Lim. 1987. "Changing Prevalence of Diabetes

Mellitus in Singapore over a Ten Year Period." *Journal of the Medical Association of Thailand* 70(supplement 2):63–67.

Tong-yuan, Tai, Chih-liang Yang, Chih-jen Cgang, Shu-meilha, Yuh-huey Chen, Boniface Juisiang Lin, Kiang-Shi Ko, Muy-Shy Chen, and Chien-Jen Chen. 1987. "Epidemiology of Diabetes Mellitus in Taiwan, R.O.C.—Comparison between Urban and Rural Areas." *Journal of the Medical Association of Thailand* 70(supplement 2):49–53.

Ward, J. D. 1988. "Preventing the Longterm Complications of Diabetes." *Proceedings of the Royal College of Physicians of Edinburgh* 18:146–53.

WHO (World Health Organization). 1975. *International Statistical Classification of Diseases, Injuries, and Causes of Death.* 9th rev. Geneva.

———. 1985. *Diabetes Mellitus: Report of a WHO Study Group.* Technical Report Series 727. Geneva.

———. 1988. *Essential Drugs List.* Geneva.

Williams, D. R. R. 1985. "Hospital Admissions of Diabetic Patients: Information from Hospital Activity Analysis." *Diabetic Medicine* 2:27–32.

Wing, R. R., L. H. Epstein, M. P. Norwalk, R. Koeske, and S. Hagg. 1985. "Behaviour Change, Weight Loss, and Physiological Improvements in Type 2 Diabetic Patients." *Journal of Consultant Clinical Psychologists* 53:111–22.

Zimmet, P. 1982. "Type 2 (Non-insulin-dependent) Diabetes—An Epidemiological Overview." *Diabetologia* 22:399–411.

———. 1987. "The Prevention and Control of Diabetes—An Epidemiological Perspective." *Journal of the Medical Association of Thailand* 70 (supplement 2):30–35.

Zimmet, P., H. King, and S. Bjorntorp. 1986. "Obesity, Hypertension, Carbohydrate Disorders, and the Risk of Chronic Diseases: Is There Any Epidemiological Evidence for Integrated Prevention Programmes?" *Medical Journal of Australia* 145:256–62.

23

Cardiovascular Disease

Thomas A. Pearson, Dean T. Jamison, and Jorge Trejo-Gutierrez

Disorders of the circulatory system cover a broad range. We focus in this chapter on four chronic vascular diseases for which atherosclerosis and/or hypertension are the defining characteristics. These are coronary heart disease (CHD), stroke, peripheral vascular disease, and hypertensive heart disease. The reasons for this are several. First, these conditions are the most important cardiovascular diseases (CVDs) in industrial countries, accounting for half of mortality in North America and Europe. Second, they are already quite prevalent in developing countries, contributing approximately 16 percent of deaths (WHO MONICA Project 1989). Indeed, it has been observed that the majority of the world's cases of cardiovascular disease no longer occur in industrial nations but, rather, in developing countries (figure 23-1); demographic analyses, summarized in this chapter (table 23-3), confirm this view. Third, they have some risk factors in common and, thus, share preventive strategies. Indeed, in those industrial countries experiencing declining cardiovascular mortality rates, most of the declines in total mortality could be attributed to declines in CVD. Fourth, a great deal is known about the pathogenesis, risk factors, prevention, and treatment of these conditions, allowing priorities to be set regarding preventive and therapeutic interventions.

Several important cardiovascular diseases have not been included in this chapter. These include rheumatic heart disease, cor pulmonale, congenital heart diseases, and cardiomyopathies. Rheumatic heart disease remains a worldwide problem, especially in developing nations; Chapter 10 of this collection (Rheumatic Heart Disease) provides a review of the main issues concerning this condition. Cor pulmonale results principally from chronic obstructive pulmonary disease and is, therefore, discussed in the chapter on that subject by Bumgarner and Speizer (chapter 24, this collection). Little is known about the causes and preventability of congenital heart disease, with the exception of rubella-related disease, and, therefore, these conditions are not dealt with in this collection. Finally, cardiomyopathies are regionally, rather than globally, important (for example, Keshan disease in China, Chagas' disease in South America, West African cardiomyopathy). These conditions are beyond the scope of the chapters in this collection. Hutt (1991) provides an overview, with extensive references, of these more traditional patterns of cardiovascular diseases in Africa.

Atherosclerosis and Hypertension

We begin this chapter with a brief discussion of the etiology and pathogenesis of atherosclerotic and hypertensive cardiovascular disease, emphasizing the role of modifiable risk factors as targets for preventive strategies. We then review trends in these diseases, making projections into the twenty-first century. Finally, we discuss preventive and case management strategies as appropriate to countries with limited health care resources.

Etiology and Pathogenesis of Atherosclerosis

Atherosclerosis is a chronic vascular condition characterized by focal accumulations of smooth muscle cells, collagen, and lipids in medium and large arteries. The condition may begin as early as childhood, initiated by injury to the endothelial lining of these major arteries, exposing the subintimal smooth muscle cells and macrophages to serum lipoproteins, platelets, and other constituents (Ross 1986). These in turn stimulate the proliferation of the smooth muscle cells and the focal accumulation of lipids. Initially, small, flat fatty streaks are observed. Previous studies have noted rather high prevalence of these lesions in autopsy studies even in developing countries (McGill 1968). If cellular proliferation continues, there may be growth into the lumen of the artery, forming the lesion pathognomonic of atherosclerosis, the fibrous-capped plaque. Tracey and Toca (1975) found that, at least in the 1960s, these lesions were much less prevalent in developing than industrial countries. Evidence has long suggested that fatty streaks can undergo regression; some recent evidence has suggested that even fibrous-capped plaques can regress, though this point is controversial (Blankenhorn and others 1987).

CLINICAL SYNDROMES RELATED TO ATHEROSCLEROSIS. Angina pectoris, myocardial infarction, sudden death, transient ischemic attacks, atherothrombotic stroke, aortic aneurysm, and intermittent claudication are all related to atherosclerosis and

Figure 23-1. Estimated Distribution of Causes of Death, 1980

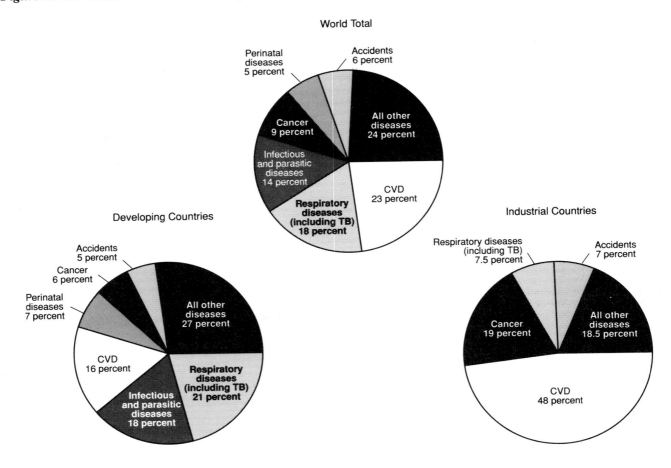

TB = Tuberculosis
Note: Of the total deaths, 78 percent are in developing countries.
Source: Authors' compilation; WHO MONICA Project, 1989.

its complications. When the atherosclerotic plaque occludes the lumen to the extent that blood flow is impaired, any increased demand for blood flow (such as that brought about by exertion) will lead to deficiency of oxygen and nutrients to the organ supplied. When the coronary arteries are narrowed, chest pain (angina pectoris) occurs; when the peripheral arteries are narrowed, intermittent claudication occurs. Plaques may undergo complication when the fibrous cap ulcerates, ruptures, or forms a clot. Subacutely, this can result in unstable angina in the coronary circulation or transient ischemic attacks in the cerebral circulation. Complete occlusion of the coronary artery with thrombosis then leads to myocardial infarction; occlusion or embolism in the cerebral circulation leads to atherothrombotic stroke. Myocardial oxygen deprivation from arterial stenosis or occlusion can also cause a variety of cardiac arrhythmias, including those causing cardiovascular collapse and sudden death. Myocardium damaged by infarction may be unable to maintain cardiac output, leading to congestive heart failure. Atherosclerotic involvement of the aorta can lead to a weakening of the arterial wall, resulting in aortic aneurysm and aortic dissection.

Hypertension-Related Diseases: Etiology and Pathogenesis

The end organs affected most by elevated blood pressure include the arteries, the heart, and the kidneys. Hypertension is a risk factor for atherosclerosis. Furthermore, hypertension is thought to play a significant role in weakening the arterial wall in the cerebral circulation, leading to cerebral hemorrhage. Though the sequence of events is controversial, cardiac hypertrophy is strongly associated with hypertension. Severe cardiac hypertrophy impairs the heart's ability to fill with blood, resulting in congestive heart failure. The increased myocardial mass interacts with atherosclerotic disease to predispose to infarction and arrhythmia. The arteries of the kidneys are susceptible to medial and intimal hypertrophy, known as nephrosclerosis, a common cause of chronic renal failure.

The Role of Risk Factors

The pathogenesis of vascular disease is summarized in figure 23-2. These so-called risk factors have been associated with the clinical cardiovascular syndromes, usually in epidemiologic

Figure 23-2. *The Pathogenesis of Atherosclerotic Vascular Diseases*

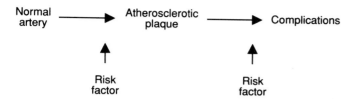

Source: Authors' compilation.

studies. The other point illustrated in figure 23-2 is that some risk factors act to cause atherosclerosis, whereas others act after the formation of the atherosclerotic plaques to cause the complications (thrombosis, hemorrhage, and so on) which present as clinical syndromes.

There are several practical implications of these roles for risk factors. First, risk factors causing the formation of atherosclerotic plaques would be logical targets for primary prevention efforts. Those risk factors acting after the formation of atherosclerosis should be modified in secondary prevention efforts. Second, it is conceivable that in certain populations which do not develop atherosclerotic plaques, certain risk factors may not be as important as in other atherosclerosis-prone groups.

As demonstrated in table 23-1, most of the important cardiovascular diseases share important risk factors. An example of this is the powerful effect of elevated blood pressure in increasing relative risk for both stroke and coronary heart disease, as is illustrated in figure 23-3. (Notice that risk for both conditions rises over the range of even "normal" values of diastolic blood pressure [DBP], suggesting, thereby, the limited usefulness of specific cutoff values to define "hypertension.") Thus, reduction in one or more risk factors may prevent several cardiovascular diseases. Several general comments are in order. First, the multifactorial nature of the etiology of cardiovascular disease makes complex the development and evaluation of preventive strategies; multifactorial interventions may be necessary to maximize the effect of preventive efforts. Second, the relative strength of association differs between diseases such that control of a risk factor may be more important for the control of one vascular disease than another. This may also be true for specific cardiovascular diseases within different racial and ethnic groups. For example, the relative risk of hypertension as in cases of stroke appeared higher in American blacks than American whites. Third, some of the risk factors are modifiable, whereas others are not. The physiological risk factors are only indirectly modifiable, through change in the behavioral ones; they thus serve principally as indicators to spur behavior change (or medical intervention) and as measures of progress. Fourth, in contrast to many other conditions, there appear to be no important environmental or infectious

Table 23-1. *Association between Risk Factors and Cardiovascular Diseases*

	Degree of association				
Risk factor	Coronary heart disease	Atherothrombotic stroke	Peripheral vascular disease	Hemorrhagic stroke	Hypertensive heart disease
Nonmodifiable					
Age	++++	++++	++++	++++	++++
Male sex	++++	++++	++++	++++	+
Black race	+	+ +	?	+++	+++
Family history	++++	+ +	+ +	+ +	+ +
Modifiable physiological					
Elevated LDL (low-density lipoprotein)	++++	+ +	+++	−	0
Decreased HDL (high-density lipoprotein)	++++	+	+ +	0	0
Hypertension	+++	+ +	+ +	++++	++++
Diabetes	+++	+++	++++	0	0
Obesity	+ +	?	?	?	+
Behavioral					
Smoking	+++	+ +	++++	0	0
Dietary cholesterol and saturated fat	+ +	+	+ +	−	−
Salt consumption	0	+	0	−	−
Alcohol consumption	−	+	0	+ +	+ +
Sedentary lifestyle	+ +	?	?	+	+

Key: ++++ Strong association between disease and risk factor.
+++ Moderately strong association between disease and risk factor.
++ Moderate association between disease and risk factor.
+ Weak association between disease and risk factor.
0 No association between disease and risk factor.
+/− Association varies with the level of the risk factor.
? Unclear association between disease and risk factor.
− Inverse association between disease and risk factor.
Source: Authors.

Figure 23-3. Diastolic Blood Pressure and the Risk for Stroke and Coronary Heart Disease

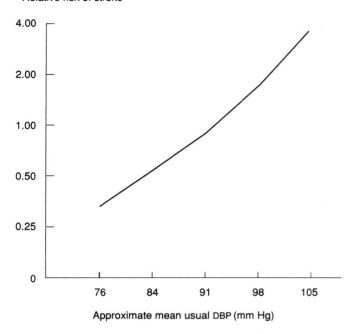

Relative risk of stroke

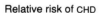

Approximate mean usual DBP (mm Hg)

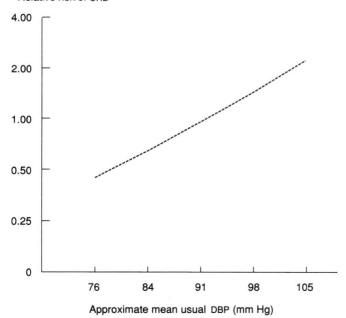

Relative risk of CHD

Approximate mean usual DBP (mm Hg)

Note: Stroke risk based on seven prospective observational studies with 843 events. CHD risk based on nine prospective observational studies with 4,856 events. The five baseline DBP categories are estimated from remeasurements in the Framingham study.
Source: MacMahon and others 1990.

risk factors, with the possible exceptions of water hardness (WHO 1982, p. 33) and cytomegalovirus infection (Melnick, Adam, and DeBakey, 1990). Fifth, males are at substantially higher risk than females, although to different extents for different diseases. In table 23A-1 we summarize MONICA (Monitoring Trends and Determinants in Cardiovascular Disease Project) mortality data that suggest a very strong effect for ischemic heart disease and a much weaker one for stroke; indeed, as a proportion of overall mortality, males appear less affected by stroke than females. Although race, sex, and age are obviously unmodifiable, their importance suggests the need for specific modeling of other risk factor effects for these characteristics.

THE ORIGIN OF RISK FACTORS. A useful concept is that of the "proximal" risk factor; that is, the factor which causes the development of the risk factors (table 23-2). Several points deserve emphasis. First, age is related to most risk factors. Second, several risk factors are transmitted genetically, rendering a subgroup of the population at high risk regardless of their lifestyles. Third, other risk factors may cause the development of certain risk factors (for example, smoking is related to low high-density lipoprotein [HDL] cholesterol), and some of the effect of one risk factor may be mediated through another risk factor. Fourth, as reflected in table 23-1, a number of the risk factors are physiologic, which, in turn, appear to be related to behavioral or lifestyle factors (for example, smoking and sedentary lifestyle are related to low HDL cholesterol). Thus, alteration of these behaviors may control the risk factor, even if it has never been clinically identified. Finally, risk factors tend to cluster within individuals as a result of behavioral or genetic mechanisms. Thus, the treatment of risk factors must often take these coexisting risk factors into account.

The multifactorial nature of etiology of cardiovascular disease and the interrelated nature of the most important risk factors makes for a rich and complex range of possibilities in the development of preventive strategies. In practical application, both the alteration of human behaviors leading to the risk factors (the population-based strategy) and the clinical treatment of those with high-risk factor levels (the high-risk strategy) may be more straightforward strategies to reduce cardiovascular risk. When the population-based strategy is implemented before risk factors become highly prevalent in a population, it is called primordial prevention (Dodu 1984, 1988).

The preceding discussion can, perhaps, best be summarized in a diagram (figure 23-4) that shows a (simplified) scheme of the relationships among groups of risk factors and end points. Policy instruments per se are not shown in the figure, but they divide naturally into those that operate through the behavioral risk factors (for example, antismoking campaigns and taxes on fatty meat products) and medical interventions that operate directly on physiological risk factors (such as medication that lowers cholesterol). Emphasis on one policy or the other may differ between population subgroups, depending on the prevalence and relative risk of the risk factors.

Table 23-2. Association between Nonmodifiable and Behavioral Risk Factors and Development of Physiological Risk Factors

Nonmodifiable and behavioral risk factors	Degree of association				
	Elevated LDL	Decreased HDL	Hypertension	Diabetes	Obesity
Nonmodifiable					
Age	+ +	–	+	+	+
Male sex	–	+ +	–	+	+
Black race	–	P	+ + + +	+ +[a]	–
Family history	+ + + +	+ +	+ + +	+	+ +
Behavioral					
Smoking	–	+ +	–	–	–
Dietary saturated fat	+ + +	–	+	–	+
Dietary calories	+	+ +	+ +	+ +	+ + + +
Salt consumption	–	–	+ + +	–	–
Alcohol consumption	–	P	+ +	–	+
Sedentary lifestyle	–	+ +	+ +	+ +	+ + +

a. Women only.
Key: +++ Strong association.
    +++ Moderately strong association.
    ++ Moderate association.
    + Weak association.
    – No association.
    P Protective association.
Source: Authors' compilation.

The breadth and sophistication of current epidemiologic knowledge of the etiology of cardiovascular disease is a scientific triumph of the past two decades. This knowledge provides the tools for prevention that have been applied, with remarkable success, in several high-income countries. Applying this knowledge in a developing country remains a central challenge.

Clinical Presentation and Mortality Rates

This section reviews the available data for the specific diseases.

CORONARY HEART DISEASE. As mentioned previously, coronary heart disease can present as angina pectoris, myocardial infarction, or sudden cardiac death. If worldwide proportions are similar to those in the United States, approximately 40 percent of coronary disease presents as angina pectoris, 40 percent as myocardial infarction, and 20 percent results in sudden cardiac death (death within one hour of onset of symptoms [Kannel and Feinleib 1972]). Because as many as 20 percent of the myocardial infarction victims will die in the hospital (in addition to the victims of sudden death) and a significant portion will remain disabled after infarction, primary prevention is an obviously important objective. The reduction in case-fatality rates following infarction and the prevention of infarction or sudden death in angina patients would be important goals in secondary prevention. It should be pointed out that any reduction in case-fatality rates for myocardial infarction would yield prevalent cases of coronary disease, requiring great expenditure of health resources. This again emphasizes the need for primary prevention strategies.

Coronary heart disease mortality rates increased in North America and Western Europe until the late 1960s and early 1970s, since which time they declined—a trend continuing today. The data are much different for Eastern Europe, where cardiovascular disease rates have increased steadily without evidence of stabilization or decline (Feinleib 1984; Thom and others 1985; Uemura and Pisa, 1988; Thom 1989; see table 23-3).

Rates in the developing world are much less well documented. Urban China, for example, appears to be experiencing a similar rise in coronary heart disease (Wu and others 1984; Tao and others 1989). Other developing countries appear to have similar rises in coronary heart disease rates (the reasons are discussed later). A significant exception is the recently documented experience of the city of São Paulo, Brazil, which, during the period 1970–83, experienced a 28 percent decline in mortality from ischemic heart disease and a 16 percent decline in deaths from stroke for the age group forty through sixty-nine (de Lolio and others 1986). These reductions were from quite high initial levels, so the pattern is like that of many of the industrial market economies.

STROKE. Because the presentation of hemorrhagic and atherothrombotic stroke appears similar clinically and developing countries may not have the technology to estimate their occurrence separately, their importance will be discussed together. In the United States, approximately 70 percent of strokes are atherothrombotic, with an additional 12 percent hemorrhagic (Schoenberg 1979). An additional 10 percent are made up of subarachnoid hemorrhage and other stroke syndromes. In Asia, the occurrence of intracranial hemorrhage is higher, with 50 percent of strokes being atherothrombotic and 40 percent being hemorrhagic.

The type of stroke is an important distinction, in that the mortality and prognoses differ (Marquardsen 1986). No more

Figure 23-4. Relationships among Risk Factors for Cardiovascular Disease

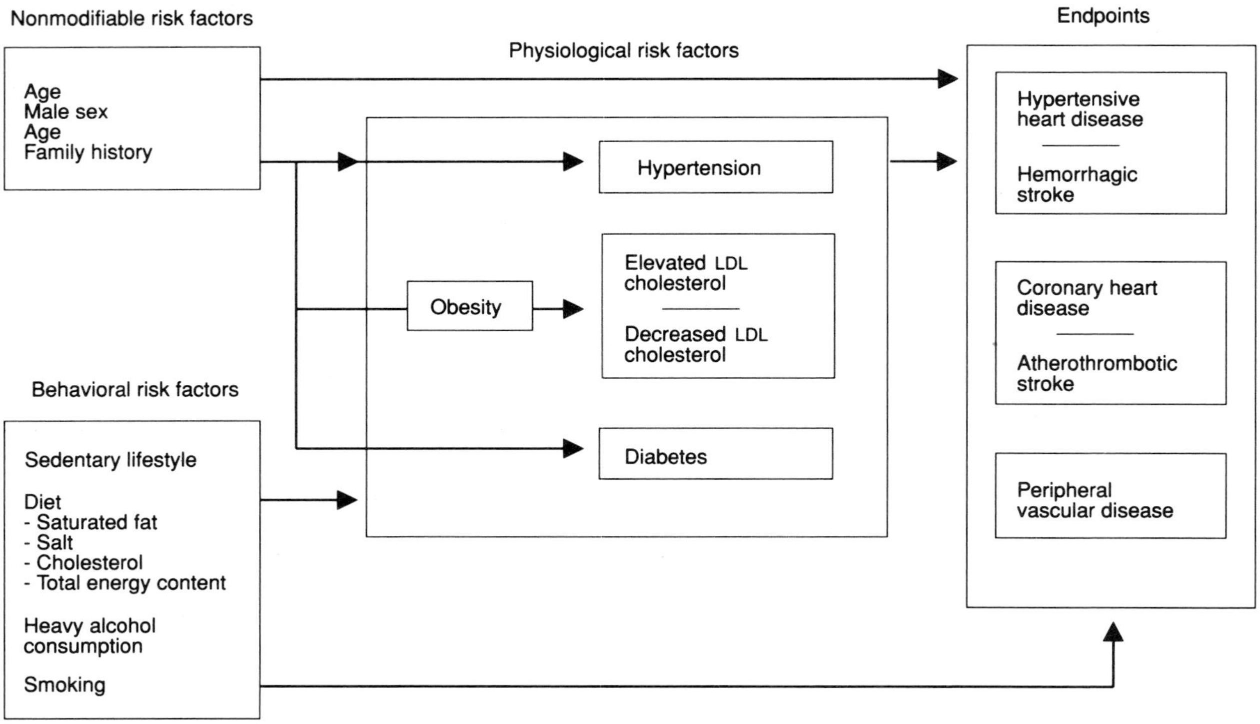

Source: Authors' compilation.

than 30 percent of those who suffer atherothrombotic stroke will die in the following three weeks; the prognosis for those with hemorrhagic stroke is worse, with case-fatality rates of 60 to 85 percent. Overall, 20 to 30 percent of stroke victims suffer major disability; only 50 percent to 75 percent are able to walk unaided. Again, primary prevention appears to be the logical target for intervention.

HYPERTENSIVE HEART DISEASE. Estimates of the prevalence of hypertensive heart disease have been difficult because of the aggregation of hypertensive heart disease with coronary heart disease in the International Classification of Disease. Because congestive heart failure and sudden death can be due to a variety of causes, including coronary heart disease, estimates of this condition are imprecise. Yet, in some countries, especially those with low atherosclerotic prevalence (for example, China), this condition appears to be an important cause of morbidity and mortality (Nissinen and others 1988, Hutt and Burkitt 1986). Blacks residing either in Africa, North America, or Europe consistently appear to have earlier onset, higher levels, and more severe cardiac sequelae than do whites ("Hypertension in Blacks and Whites" 1980; Falase 1987). Blood pressure control appears to be the main thrust of primary prevention; growing evidence suggests potential for regression of left ventricular hypertrophy with control of blood pressure.

The Burden of Cardiovascular Disease

This section reviews the effects of increased incidences of cardiovascular disease on current mortality levels.

Current Levels of Mortality

In table 23-4 we show rough demographic estimates, globally and by region, of the burden of mortality, in 1985, due to vascular diseases. In the table in appendix 23A we provide more detailed information on sex differences. It is evident from table 23-4 that death rates, and even proportion of deaths, due to circulatory disease are already very high indeed in Africa and Latin America and quite significant in Asia. Although the demographic assessments in table 23-4 are strongly suggestive of current levels of the mortality burden from CVD in different regions of the world, it is essential to bear in mind the substantial uncertainty surrounding the numbers in that table. They rely, for most of the developing countries, not on good national cause-of-death data but, rather, on extrapolations to the developing countries today of the experience of other countries, mostly European, from a time when their mortality levels were lower. It is therefore useful to supplement those extrapolations with examples from developing countries for which data do exist, and in table 23-5 we summarize such data from a number of sources.

Table 23-3. Change in Death Rates from Coronary Heart Disease, Selected Countries, 1969–78 and 1979–85
(percent)

Country	Men 1969–78	Men 1979–85	Women 1969–78	Women 1979–85
Australia	−24	−25	−25	−26
Austria	4	−11[a]	−6	−14[a]
Belgium	−13	−16[b]	−24	−7[b]
Canada	−14	−24	−21	−22
Czechoslovakia	8	12	2	16
Denmark	14	−14	1	−16
England and Wales	5	−12	9	−6
Finland	−8	−16	−18	−23
France	4	−4	−21	−2
Former Fed. Rep. of Germany	3	−10	−3	1
Hungary	37	27	21	23
Ireland	12	−7[b]	−10	3[b]
Israel	−22	−20	−19	−28
Italy	13	−10[c]	−7	−11[c]
Japan	−22	−20	−37	−27
Netherlands	1	−3	−2	−9
New Zealand	−13	−20	−16	−21
Norway	−5	−16	−11	−6
Northern Ireland	18	−18	28	−16
Poland	77[d]	21[a]	71[d]	26[a]
Portugal	2	−15[a]	−11	−5[a]
Scotland	3	−14	2	−7
Spain	53	—	29	—
Sweden	19	−12	−12	−19
Switzerland	10	−13	−7	−17
United States	−25	−22	−24	−15
Yugoslavia	32	15[c]	11	−2[c]

— Not available.

Note: Death rates are for men and women aged 45–64.
a. 1980–86.
b. 1979–84.
c. 1979–83.
d. 1971–78.

Trends to 2015

It is likely that all the important cardiovascular diseases will increase sharply in their morbidity and mortality between now and the years 2000 and 2015. Assumed in these conclusions is the control of major childhood and infectious diseases, with concomitant increase in population, life expectancy, and standard of living. The epidemiologic transition from infections to degenerative diseases as the main causes of death may be divided into at least four stages (table 23-6). A progressive change in risk factors and concurrent change in cardiovascular diseases is suggested by international comparisons of risk-factor prevalence and cardiovascular mortality in industrial countries (see table 23-3 and Knuiman and others 1980; Masironi and Rothwell 1988; Nissinen and others 1988; Uemura and Pisa 1988; WHO MONICA Project 1988). It is predicted that coronary disease, stroke, or hypertensive heart disease will be the leading cause of death for many developing countries by the year 2000.

This will very likely be true even where age-specific death rates from CVD are declining, as they already are in parts of the developing world (for example, São Paulo [see de Lolio and others 1986]); where age-specific rates are rising—as they are for ischemic heart disease in Mexico (Lozano-Ascencio and others 1990)—the increasing prominence of CVD will be more pronounced. This will be particularly true of the managerial and professional classes in those countries. The trend toward the increasing importance of these diseases is dramatically illustrated in table 23-7.

EFFECT OF INCREASE IN LIFE EXPECTANCY. The crude incidence and prevalence of cardiovascular diseases must increase as life expectancy increases. This so-called "epidemiologic conversion" predicts such a rise in chronic disease rates as a function of life expectancy (Dodu 1988). Because coronary disease occurs even in people in their forties, it could represent significant burdens from those who are younger.

Another effect of increased age will be an increased prevalence of risk factors which may require control. Hypertension and elevated cholesterol are both examples of risk factors that become increasingly prevalent as age increases in most industrial countries, although these age-related increases may not be inevitable.

EFFECT OF INCREASE IN STANDARD OF LIVING. An increased affluence of population, if it were to occur, would have several possible effects on cardiovascular disease rates. First, an improved diet may also increase saturated fat, dietary cholesterol,

Table 23-4. Estimated Mortality from Circulatory System Diseases, by Region, 1985

Region	Deaths (thousands)	Total deaths (percent)	Age-standardized death rate (per 100,000 population)[a] Total	Ischemic disease	Cerebro-vascular disease
Industrial market economies	3,355	46	235	99	59
Industrial nonmarket economies	2,220	47	357	164	106
Latin America and the Caribbean	691	22	222	69	57
Sub-Saharan Africa	756	10	273	85	74
Middle East and North Africa	602	14	250	82	68
Asia	3,841	17	195	46	91
Total	11,466	23	243	84	81

Note: Constructed from the figures used by Bulatao and Stephens in tables 3 and 4 for "ischemic heart disease," "cerebrovascular disease," and "other cardiovascular." The total deaths in this table refer to the sum of these three categories, not to Bulatao and Stephens' "circulatory" category.
a. Rates are standardized using the 1985 world age structure.
Source: Bulatao and Stephens 1990.

Table 23-5. Age-Standardized Mortality from Vascular Diseases in Men in Selected Industrial and Developing Countries

| Country | Annual mortality rate (per 100,000 population) | | Ratio of ischemic heart disease to stroke |
	Ischemic heart disease	Cerebro-vascular disease	
Industrial			
Canada	276	61	4.5:1
Japan	53	122	0.43:1
Portugal	108	240	0.45:1
United States	274	59	4.6:1
Former U.S.S.R.	486	245	2.0:1
Developing			
Brazil (São Paulo)[a]	310	198	1.6:1
China (Beijing)[b]	124	—	1:5[c]
China (Guangzhou)[b]	42	—	1:5[c]
Mauritius	123	94	1.3:1
Costa Rica	65	26	2.5:1
Cuba	168	65	2.6:1

— Not available.

a. Age group forty through sixty-nine.
b. Age group thirty-five through seventy-four.
c. For China as a whole.
Source: WHO 1988b, 1989; Tao and others 1989; de Lolio and others 1986.

calories, sodium, and alcohol, leading to increases in blood cholesterol, body weight, and blood pressure. For example, increases over time in dietary cholesterol, dietary fat, meat consumption, and cigarettes smoked per adult all correlated with increases in coronary heart disease in industrial countries (Byington and others 1979; Blackburn 1989; Epstein 1989). Sodium consumption correlates significantly with blood pressure levels in a recent study of fifty-two centers worldwide (Intersalt Cooperative Research Group 1988). Second, increased use of transportation and increased mechanization of industry may increase the prevalence of sedentary lifestyles. Third, increased affluence may increase cigarette consumption; indeed, in the companion piece on cancer in this collec-

tion (chapter 21), Barnum and Greenberg report enormously high income elasticities of consumption of tobacco products, particularly among the countries with the lowest incomes. Another, but favorable, effect of increased standard of living may be the improved cold storage of food, which has been suggested as the cause for the decline in strokes since 1900. The reduced requirement for smoked and salted foods may reduce the sodium content, resulting in reduced hypertension.

An increase in medical care services may also provide opportunity for reduction in cardiovascular disease rates. The disbursement of funds for preventive as opposed to acute care services, however, may determine the extent to which morbidity and mortality are reduced.

The Economic Burden of Cardiovascular Disease

Analyses of the economic burden of disease in developing countries are currently unavailable. It may, however, be suggestive to summarize findings on the burden of circulatory system disease in the United States based on one recent analysis (Rice, Hodgson, and Kopstein 1985). The authors of this analysis found that the direct cost of illness (that is, the cost of providing care) was $211 billion in 1980; given a gross national product (GNP) of approximately $2.6 trillion, this amounted to 8.1 percent of GNP. Of direct costs, about 15.4 percent were for circulatory diseases, so the cost of caring for these diseases was about 1.25 percent of GNP. The indirect costs of all disease (productivity loss due to morbidity and premature mortality) were slightly more, about 9.4 percent of GNP; for circulatory disease, the indirect costs were about 2 percent of GNP. Two points are notable: first, at a cost of more than 3 percent of GNP, circulatory disease imposes an enormous economic burden. Second, because deaths due to circulatory system disease were about 47 percent of total deaths, and its cost was less than 20 percent of the total costs of illness, the burden of circulatory illness is relatively much less measured in economic terms than mortality ones.

Analyses of this sort are sensitive to alternative assumptions and methodologies, and transfer of results from the U.S. situ-

Table 23-6. Circulatory System Disease at Phases of the Epidemiologic Transition

Phase of epidemiologic transition	Deaths from circulatory disease (percent)	Circulatory problems	Risk factors
Age of pestilence and famine	5–10	Rheumatic heart disease; infectious and deficiency-induced cardiomyopathies	Uncontrolled infection; deficiency conditions
Age of receding pandemics	10–35	As above, plus hypertensive heart disease and hemorrhagic stroke	High-salt diet leading to hypertension; increased smoking
Age of degenerative and man-made diseases	35–55	All forms of stroke; ischemic heart disease	Atherosclerosis from fatty diets; sedentary lifestyle; smoking
Age of delayed degenerative diseases	Probably under 50	Stroke and ischemic heart disease[a]	Education and behavioral changes leading to lower levels of risk factors

Note: Omran 1971 introduced the concept of epidemiologic transition with discussion of phases 1, 2, and 3. Olshansky and Ault 1986 added the concept of a fourth phase.
a. At older ages. Represents a smaller proportion of deaths.
Source: Omran 1971; Olshansky and Ault 1986.

Table 23-7. Ratio of Deaths from Circulatory System Diseases to Deaths from Infectious and Parasitic Diseases, by Region and Year

Region	1970	1985	2000	2015
Industrial market countries	5.63	6.64	9.61	11.88
Industrial nonmarket countries	2.44	4.72	5.24	4.41
Latin America and the Caribbean	0.68	1.09	2.46	4.74
Asia	0.42	0.60	1.55	2.75
Middle East and North Africa	0.37	0.41	0.81	1.26
Sub-Saharan Africa	0.23	0.27	0.38	0.54
Total	0.69	0.89	1.62	2.39

Source: Bulatao and Stephens 1990.

ation can, at best, be suggestive. That said, until country-specific analyses from developing countries are available, these estimates do probably serve as a reasonable first approximation of the cost of CVD (in percentage of GNP) for middle-income developing countries.

Strategies for Preventing Cardiovascular Disease

The preventive strategies, along with their cost in manpower, technology, and drugs, are listed for coronary heart disease, stroke, and hypertension in table 23-8. The preventive strategies are divided into public health (community-based) and high-risk (clinic-based) strategies. Several conclusions can be reached. First, several of the public health interventions are effective, including smoking cessation. The recent reviews by Warner (1989, 1990a) and the Surgeon General ("Reducing the Health Consequences of Smoking" 1989) of antismoking campaign effectiveness in the United States are encouraging in this regard. The Surgeon General's report, for example, summarizes evidence on the potent effect of taxes on tobacco products, particularly in the young and particularly with respect to initiation of use. The estimated price elasticity of demand is a substantial –0.42 for adults and a dramatic –1.2 for twelve- to seventeen-year-olds. In what is perhaps the first study of the price (actually, tax level) elasticity of tobacco consumption from a developing country, Chapman and Richardson (1990) found stronger elasticities in Papua New Guinea than in the United States. Efforts to promote low-fat diets and active lifestyles are also probably effective. Second, the public health interventions are often not costly. Much of the cost for community-based cardiovascular interventions may constitute the use of manpower, depending on the nature of the intervention. Many developing countries have a relative abundance of workers, including those with some training, which can be applied to these tasks. The technology and drug requirements for these strategies are low. Third, the ability to shift the risk of an entire population is calculated to have more promise in the prevention of the majority of deaths than does the treat-

ment of high-risk individuals (Kottke and others 1985; Fries, Green, and Levine 1989; Gunning-Schepers and others 1989), although arguments to the contrary have been presented (Oliver 1984; Lewis and others 1986; McCormick and Skrabanek 1988). The current policy of the World Health Organization, which is to emphasize primordial prevention in developing countries, is predicated on a broad consensus among experts that a community-based strategy is feasible (WHO 1982). Finally, all the community-based strategies might be carried out in clinical settings, so that the community-based and clinic-based strategies are overlapping, rather than exclusive.

The high-risk, or clinic-based, strategy does include several effective interventions, however. Lipid-lowering drugs, for coronary disease and peripheral vascular disease, and antihypertensive drugs, for stroke, hypertension, and coronary disease, are clearly effective (MacMahon and others 1990). With the exception of antihypertensive therapies, it has been difficult to attribute recent declines in coronary disease in industrial countries to the medical management of risk factors (Pearson 1989). These strategies will often require large numbers of well-trained workers, however, as well as technology in the form of laboratories to monitor effects and side effects of therapy (for example, lipid laboratories to monitor serum potassium levels). Drugs can also be relatively expensive, although there are a number of important antiplatelet, antidysrhythmic, and antihypertensive drugs (for example, verapamil, propranolol, and hydrochlorothiazide) available through the World Health Organization/United Nations Children's Fund (WHO/UNICEF) Essential Drugs program at costs of under $5 per patient per year (UNICEF 1989). It should be emphasized, however, that a wide range of costs exists for drugs, from inexpensive lipid-lowering (for example, nicotinic acid) and antihypertensive agents (for example, reserpine) to expensive drugs (HMG-CO-A [3-hydroxy-3 methylglutaryl coenzyme A] reductase inhibitors, angiotensin converting enzyme inhibitors). Aspirin, which is extremely inexpensive and widely available, plays a potentially central role through its antiplatelet effects. Antiplatelet drugs may be effective in the primary prevention of coronary disease but not stroke (Hennekens and others 1989).

It should be pointed out that the relationship between the population-based and high-risk strategies remains to be assessed; nonetheless, the European Atherosclerotic Society (1987) has noted that it seems highly probable that the two strategies would be mutually supportive. Along these lines, Rothenberg, Ford, and Vartiainen (1990) have undertaken a multirisk-factor modeling exercise that suggests that overall preventive strategy may well focus on high-risk groups for some risk factors and whole populations (probably age targeted) for others, depending on specific characteristics of available interventions.

It is not likely that new technologies available for public health interventions will become available. Knowledge regarding the beneficial effects of lipid-lowering diets, exercise,

Table 23-8. Efficacy and Cost of Preventive Strategies for Major Cardiovascular Diseases

Preventive strategy	Effectiveness		Costs		
	Compliance	Clinical efficacy	Manpower	Technology	Drugs
Coronary heart disease					
Community-based					
Smoking cessation	+	++++	+/–	0	0
Low-salt diet	+	?	+/–	0	0
Modified fat diet	+	+++	+/–	0	0
Exercise	+	+++	+/–	0	0
Diabetic diet	+	—	+/–	0	0
Obesity control	–	?	+/–	0	0
Clinic-based					
Antihypertensive drugs	+	+ +	+ +	+	+ +
Lipid-lowering drugs	+/–	++++	+ +	+ +	+ +
Diabetic drugs	+	—	++++	+ +	++++
Antiplatelet drugs	+ +	+ +	+	+	+
Stroke					
Community-based					
Smoking cessation	+	+++	+/–	0	0
Low-salt diet	+	+	+/–	0	0
Obesity control	–	+	+/–	0	0
Clinic-based					
Antihypertensive drugs	+	++++	+ +	+	+ +
Antiplatelet drugs	+ +	++++	+	+	+
Hypertension					
Community-based					
Low-salt diet	+	+	+/–	0	0
Exercise	+ +	+ +	+	0	0
Obesity control	–	+++	+/–	0	0
Alcohol restriction	?	+	0	0	0
Clinic-based					
Antihypertensive drugs	+/++	++++	+ +	+	+ +

Key: ++++ Highly favorable.
+++ Moderately favorable.
++ Favorable.
+ Minimal.
+/– Variable.
– Poor.
— Not effective.
0 Not required.
? Unknown.
Source: Authors' compilation.

and sodium restriction, however, should continue to increase. For example, results are now being published from the study undertaken by the Intersalt Cooperative Research Group (1988) in thirty-two countries, including twelve developing countries, of the prevalence of hypertension and its association with sodium, potassium, and alcohol intake. Community intervention strategies that will probably be generalizable to developing countries are now being implemented in the United States and Europe (Blackburn 1983).

A number of changes will likely occur with physician-based preventive strategies (Pearson 1989). New antihypertensive drugs with better treatment schedules and fewer side effects are constantly being developed. It is hoped that inexpensive, low side-effect, and once-a-day dosing drugs will become available. New techniques for detection of high blood cholesterol are being implemented but are probably too costly for most developing countries at present prices (Weinstein and Stason 1985). Diabetic drugs, including new insulin delivery systems, are being evaluated for efficacy. Again, these are high-technology instruments, usually with high unit costs.

The Gap between Good Practice and Actual Practice

Many, or perhaps most, countries, industrial or developing, have not enacted national policies intended to prevent the use of tobacco products. Further, few countries encourage low-fat, low-cholesterol, low-salt diets; indeed, few countries have a national nutrition policy of any kind. Exercise and fitness are variably encouraged in schools and work sites. Thus, a number of public health or regulatory policies need to be implemented.

Physicians in industrial countries remain oriented toward acute care, rather than preventive care. Many health messages are therefore not delivered at the time of the acute care visit (for example, an antismoking message). Thus, risk factors in the high-risk patient are often not detected or treated.

In judging the potential for improving practice, assessments of the cost-effectiveness of alternative strategies for prevention provide potentially useful guides. Weinstein and Stason (1985) provide a valuable introduction to the relevant literature that was available at the time of their writing; that literature is limited, unfortunately, to studies from high-income countries. Further, we have been unable to find any studies assessing community-based interventions; the closest was a study of screening of hypertensives followed by their treatment in North Karelia, Finland. The authors of the North Karelia assessment estimated the cost per (disability-adjusted) year of life gained to be about $3,600 (Nissinen and others 1986). Weinstein and Stason reported that in earlier studies on hypertension control rather more costly, although not markedly higher, results had been found. Naturally, the cost per year of life gained falls as the cutoff level for treatment of blood pressure rises—but with concomitant loss of some lives that would have been saved were the cutoff level lower. In a recent study, Hatziandreu and others (1988) assessed the cost-effectiveness of exercise as a preventive measure for ischemic heart disease, finding costs of about $11,000 per disability-adjusted year of life saved. The main cost is that of the time taken for exercise and that "cost" is itself highly dependent on whether exercise is a pleasure; the authors assumed that, on average, it was not.

Much of the work on the cost-effectiveness of prevention has addressed the attractiveness of efforts to reduce serum cholesterol. Taylor and others (1987) put forward an often-refuted model linking changes in cholesterol levels to changes in life expectancies for varying initial ages and cholesterol levels; the results provide the effectiveness measures that can be used in cost-effectiveness analyses and suggest very little benefit (several months' gain in life expectancy) for lifelong programs to lower cholesterol by typical dietary means. More substantial gains result from the potent effect of cholesterol-lowering drugs, but an early analysis of the cost per year of life gained from the use of cholestyramine resulted in high estimates, in the region of $125,000 (Weinstein and Stason 1985). In a still earlier assessment of a pediatric screening program followed by dietary management, Berwick, Cretin, and Keeler (1980) found much more modest costs—in the region of $10,000. Kinosian and Eisenberg (1988) assessed several agents in their investigation into the medical management of cholesterol. Their findings on cholestryamine were similar to those of Weinstein and Stason, but they found that the use of oat bran resulted in much lower costs—about $18,000 per year of life saved, which is still expensive in relation to the hypertension control efforts assessed.

The purpose of these assessments is to help guide resources toward uses that buy the greatest possible gain in disability-adjusted life-years for the money available. They do not, in this case, point more sharply in one direction than another; rather, they suggest adjustments of treatment cutoff points (hypertension cutoffs down, cholesterol cutoffs up) to maximize health gains. Further, for developing countries, these costs are high; later we suggest that care taken in implementation could lower costs in developing countries.

Suggested Intervention in a Standardized Population

A concerted effort through public education, including that in the schools, work sites, and media, should be carried out to reduce the prevalence of smoking. Regulations to restrict smoking from work sites, public places, and the like might be enacted. The sale of cigarettes might be heavily taxed. Nutritional programs to provide low-fat, low-cholesterol sources of protein should be enacted. The use of nonsaturated fat in cooking oils should be encouraged. Facilities and encouragement for exercise should be made policy at schools, work sites, and public places. The use of personal transportation might emphasize expenditure of calories for the nonpoor population subgroups.

As health care strategies, all adults might have their blood pressure taken, and those in whom it is found to be elevated might begin a weight loss, salt-restricted diet with appropriate physician follow-up, including the use of inexpensive antihypertensive agents. Cholesterol screening might be restricted to persons with relatives who have developed cardiovascular disease at age fifty years or less. Follow-up and treatment would require dietary restrictions of fats and cholesterol, and possibly low-cost medicines to lower cholesterol.

We have made several tentative calculations to estimate probable cost and effect, in the hypothetical population of 1 million, of several preventive interventions—a general public preventive package (education, screening, counseling, referral), a program to control hypertension, a program to control hyperlipidemia, and a 20 percent tax on tobacco products. Our preliminary estimates, which assume low-cost medications (such as propranolol purchased at prices on the *Essential Drug List* [UNICEF 1989]), are as follows:

- For hypertension control, perhaps 90 deaths per year could be averted at a cost of about $2,000 per year of life gained

- For hypercholesterolemia control, somewhat fewer deaths could be averted at a cost of about $4,000 per year of life gained

- Assuming that a public preventive package could be implemented for about half the cost as in the United States (that is, for about $0.75 per capita per year) perhaps 250 lives per year could be saved at a cost of about $150 per year of life gained

- A 20 percent tobacco tax would reduce consumption by about 20 percent and free resources for other uses. Assuming that there were 200,000 smokers in the population of 1 million and that the health effect was as though 40,000 people stopped smoking and others did not change behavior, perhaps 40 deaths per year from coronary artery disease would be averted.

Calculations of this sort will, obviously, give quite different results in different epidemiological and health service environments; and even these estimates for a hypothetical population should be viewed as tentative. Nonetheless, these estimates do give a rough sense of the cost-effectiveness that might be expected for several key interventions.

Case Management of Cardiovascular Conditions

The potential elements of case management strategies are listed in table 23-9 and are separated into acute and chronic interventions. Several conclusions can be drawn. First, the acute interventions are often not extremely effective when tested in clinical trials (for example, antiarrhythmic drugs such as lidocaine, coronary care units, cardiopulmonary resuscitation, calcium channel blockers; see MacMahon and others 1988; Yusuf, Wittes, and Friedman 1988a; Held, Yusuf, and Finberg 1989). Second, these acute interventions are costly with regard to manpower, technology, and drugs. Third, the effectiveness of some chronic interventions is perhaps better, with more widespread application feasible. Again, several interventions such as angioplasty and bypass surgery are costly; even so, targeted interventions (for example, coronary artery bypass surgery [CABS] for left main coronary artery disease only) can be cost-effective, at least in industrial countries (Williams 1985). Certain interventions, such as smoking cessation, lowering of serum cholesterol, and exercise in cardiac rehabilitation, show promise of being effective at low cost (Oldridge and others 1988; Yusuf, Wittes, and Friedman 1988b; "The Surgeon General's 1990 Report on the Health Benefits of Smoking Cessation" 1990). It is further logical that chronic risk factor intervention may be more effective in populations also in community-based programs.

It is further predicted that the classes with greater education and income may demand this high-technology care, obtained in their home countries or by traveling to an industrial country. Because it is these classes that will develop cardiovascular disease first in a country, extreme pressures will likely be exerted to develop high-technology health care. It is probable that for this reason a small amount of this high technology will be needed in all countries. Nonetheless, a key element of overall strategy will be to make low-cost but effective alternative interventions regularly available. In many cases, these options do exist.

The field of interventional cardiology is rapidly changing, with the advent of new therapies for the patient with angina pectoris, myocardial infarction, stroke, or peripheral vascular disease. Most invasive strategies (for example, laser angioplasty) and those involving new drugs (new thrombolytic agents, free radical scavengers, and so on) are likely to be costly in manpower, technology, and drugs. A full description of potential advances is beyond the scope of this review.

Gaps between Good Practice and Actual Practice

It appears likely that some of the new technology will improve case-fatality rates. Many institutions, however, even in the industrial countries, cannot afford its implementation. There also appears to be a lack of attention to some of the rather simple chronic interventions (smoking cessation, cardiac rehabilitation, beta-blocker therapy) which have been shown to be related to improved chance of survival in patients with CHD. Thus, an improved use of these interventions may increase survival rates. Cost-effectiveness studies for several of these strategies have been attempted, including bypass surgery, use of beta blockers after myocardial infarction (MI), coronary care units, and cardiopulmonary resuscitation programs (Weinstein and Stason 1985). More recently, Steinberg and others (1988) examined the use of thrombolytic therapy in treating acute MI. Most of these strategies are expensive (upward of $30,000 per year of life saved), although CABS for left main coronary artery disease and three-vessel coronary artery disease is a relatively cost-effective treatment in high-income countries, at costs well under $10,000. Risk stratification appears able to identify patients who have especially attractive cost-benefit ratios; Goldman and others (1988) estimate beta-blocker therapy to cost from $23,400 per year of life saved in low-risk patients to $3,600 per year of life saved in high-risk patients.

Suggested Intervention in a Standardized Population

Four interventions appear worthy of serious consideration— risk reduction in post-MI patients, risk management in post-stroke patients, angina control, and low-cost management of acute MI. These are discussed below.

For both the post-MI and poststroke patients, emphasis on the modification of risk factors should be made, including the control of hypertension in the stroke victim; the cessation of smoking in the coronary, cerebrovascular, and peripheral vascular patient; and the lowering of blood cholesterol by diet or inexpensive drugs. For the patient with chronic cardiovascular disease, rather inexpensive drugs might be used for the treatment of angina or following myocardial infarction (for example, beta blockers; see Julian 1989). Antiplatelet agents, particularly aspirin, may be helpful in patients with coronary artery disease, and atherothrombotic but not hemorrhagic stroke. These low-cost secondary preventive measures for this high-risk group might cost $3 per patient per year, if carefully implemented. They might be expected to reduce the annual probability of death by 0.01 or 0.02 for an age group in which a death would result in loss of, perhaps, fifteen discounted (at 3 percent) life-years for the post-MI patient and ten years for the poststroke patient. This would result in a cost per disability-adjusted life-year gained of $155 for intervention in the post-MI group and $230 in the poststroke group.

Of particular importance in case management is the cost-effectiveness of angina control medication, which is inexpensively available from the WHO/UNICEF Essential Drugs program. It is estimated that the standard population would have about

Table 23-9. Effectiveness and Cost of Case Management Strategies for Cardiovascular Disease

Case management strategy	Efficacy	Costs		
		Manpower	Technology	Drugs
Coronary heart disease				
Acute MI/unstable angina				
Cardiopulmonary resuscitation	+/–	+++	+++	+++
Coronary care units	+	++++	++++	+++
Antiarrhythmic drugs	–	+ +	+ +	+++
Thrombolysis	+ +	++++	++++	++++
Nitrates	+ +	+/+++	+	+/+++
Antiplatelet/anticoagulant drugs	+ +	+	+	+
Chronic angina/stable post-MI				
Beta-blocking agents	+++	+++	+	++++
Calcium channel blockers	0	+++	+	++++
Angioplasty	?	++++	++++	+ +
Coronary artery bypass surgery	+	++++	++++	+ +
Antiarrhythmic drugs	–	+++	+ +	++++
Cardiac rehabilitation (including smoking cessation)	+++	+++	+	0
Antiplatelet agents	+ +	+	0	+
Cholesterol-lowering drugs	+ +	+ +	+++	++++
Congestive heart failure				
Drug therapy	+	++++	+++	++++
Heart transplantation	+ +	++++	++++	++++
Stroke				
Acute stroke				
General support	?	+++	+ +	0
Stable poststroke/transient ischemic attack				
Antiplatelet agents	+ +	+	0	+
Antihypertensive drugs	+++	+ +	+	+++
Carotid surgery	?	+++	++++	+
Peripheral vascular disease				
Acute				
Surgery	+ +	+++	++++	+ +
Chronic				
Surgery/angioplasty	+ +	++++	++++	+ +
Smoking cessation	+++	+	0	0
Hypertensive disease				
Congestive heart failure				
Drug therapy	+/–	++++	+++	++++
Hypertensive renal disease				
Dialysis	+ +	++++	++++	+ +

Key: ++++ Very high.
    +++ High.
    ++ Moderate.
    + Minimal.
    – Not effective.
    +/– Variable.
    0 Not required.
    ? Unknown.
Source: Authors' compilation.

6,000 cases of moderate to severe angina at any given time, which could be medically controlled for perhaps $150,000 to $200,000 per year. If, consistent with Weinstein and Stason, we use a Q factor of 0.7 to 0.9 for angina (that is, between 0.1 and 0.3 years of healthy life are assumed to be lost per angina-affected person per year), the cost per disability-adjusted year of life gained from angina control would be only $100 to $200.

Table 23-9 contains a range of options for management of acute MI and unstable angina. Many of these are highly costly, and some are of limited or unproven effectiveness. One strategy of medical intervention, however, would be relatively easily managed and involve only very low cost drugs—nitroglycerin and aspirin (as an antiplatelet agent). Pitt (1989) suggested that at least some of the reduced case-fatality rates for MI observed in industrial countries during the past two decades may be attributed to these agents. Patients presenting with acute MI would be provided these medications (and supportive care) on an inpatient basis for several days. The drug cost would be close to negligible; depending on local circumstances, the cost of hospital stay and physician time might be in the range of $100 to $250. Intervention of this sort might reduce the short-term mortality risk from 20 to 15 percent, resulting in a gain of 0.75 disability-adjusted life-years (again assuming that a death averted at about this age will result in a gain of fifteen disability-adjusted life-years). The resulting cost-effectiveness would, then, be in the range from $135 to $335 per disability-adjusted life-year gained.

The above cost-effectiveness estimates can be considered only approximate; much more careful analyses could (and should) be done in country-specific circumstances. The estimates of cost and effectiveness are, nonetheless, within reasonable ranges; the resulting cost-effectiveness estimates serve to give a realistic (if approximate) sense of what is possible.

In table 23-10 we summarize the range of case management options for vascular disease with regard to their objectives (secondary prevention or rehabilitation) and the sophistication of the probable venue for the intervention. Priority interventions tend to be those that can be delivered in less sophisticated environments, such as those described in more detail in the preceding paragraphs.

Conclusions and Priorities

We have attempted to summarize available data and analyses concerning the epidemiology of cardiovascular diseases in developing countries, strategies of prevention, and methods of case management. Imbalances in the available literature are striking: there is a vast medical and epidemiological literature on cardiovascular disease, but almost none of it deals with problems of developing countries, where well over half of

cardiovascular mortality occurs. Likewise, although cardiovascular disease already accounts for 10 to 35 percent of all deaths in developing countries (and, soon, will account for a much higher percentage), the substantial literature on epidemiology and health planning for developing countries concentrates almost exclusively on communicable diseases, particularly the communicable diseases of childhood. Nonetheless, for a few developing countries, and in a preliminary way, explicit consideration has begun of the implications for health policy of the increasing prominence of chronic diseases; for example, for China (Jamison and others 1984), for Malaysia (Harlan and others 1984), for Mexico (chapter 3, this collection), and for Brazil (de Lolio and others 1986, and ongoing World Bank work). Our purpose in this chapter has been to take stock of what literature does exist concerning cardiovascular diseases in developing countries as a starting point for further work.

The appropriate range of policy instruments to consider, as well as research priorities, will vary, of course, depending on the epidemiological and economic conditions in a particular country. Although many of those conditions are quite country specific, we have nonetheless found it useful to characterize the evolving nature of circulatory problems in a way that parallels the epidemiological transition; in table 23-6 we summarized this characterization. During the pretransition phase of high mortality, circulatory problems are of modest relative importance (although, perhaps, of substantial absolute importance); they are, in this phase, dominantly conditions of infectious origin, which we have not discussed in this chapter. As mortality declines, there appear to be, first, rising problems associated with the hypertension-related circulatory diseases; this stage is followed, perhaps substantially later, by diseases that are principally atherosclerotic in origin. (Indeed, the low levels of atherosclerotically related diseases in Japan today suggests the general possibility that a major epidemic of these diseases could be avoided in other parts of the world.) This phasing has important implications for the timing of the introduction of both preventive and case management interventions.

Table 23-10. Objectives and Venue for Case Management of Cardiovascular Disease

Objective	Venue			
	Household	Primary facility	Secondary facility	Tertiary facility
Secondary prevention				
Angina pectoris	Behavioral change: risk	Simple diagnosis:	Complex diagnosis;[b]	Invasive diagnosis; surgical
Myocardial infarction	factor management;	prescription of first-	second-line drugs[c]	therapy; complex drugs and
Stroke	drug compliance	line drugs[a]		technologies
Rehabilitation				
Myocardial infarction	Habits of daily living;	Monitored outpatient	Supervised inpatient	Specialized rehabilitative
Stroke	long-term, unsupervised	program	program; physical and	occupational therapy;
	exercise program		occupational therapy	prostheses, patient-assist devices

a. Propranolol, verapamil, aspirin.
b. Established through exercise electrocardiogram, echo-doppler examination, and similar technologies.
c. For example, long-acting nitrates, anti-arrhythmic drugs.
Source: Authors' compilation.

Operational Priorities for Developing Countries

The following steps might be appropriately emphasized as ones that developing countries might take to forestall (primordial prevention) or reduce the forthcoming epidemic of cardiovascular disease and to deal with its consequences. These interventions tend also to be appropriate for other chronic diseases, and the suggestions here are generally consistent with those of WHO's "Interhealth" program (Integrated Programme for Noncommunicable Disease Prevention and Control, Shigan 1988). The interventions are listed in order of priority for implementation.

PREVENTION. The range of appropriate preventive interventions in developing countries is similar to that for industrial ones and includes the following:

- Regulation, taxation, and education to reduce the production and use of tobacco products. These form perhaps the single most important cluster of preventive interventions. The potential benefits of this strategy are reviewed in more detail in appendix A of this collection, and Warner (1990b) emphasizes the particularly important role that taxation policy can play in limiting tobacco use in developing countries.

- National nutrition policies, including substantial use of taxes, to improve nutrition without the use of excess saturated fat, dietary cholesterol, salt, calories, and alcohol. These policies should be targeted at those segments of a society in whom malnutrition (that is, undernutrition) is not a problem. The prevention of obesity should be a major target of these programs.

- Screening for (probably in the context of other screening) and nonpharmacologic treatment of hypertension. Use of even relatively inexpensive antihypertensive drugs in those high-risk patients not responding to nonpharmacologic therapy is probably not cost-effective, except for individuals at very high risk. The drugs themselves are now quite inexpensive (UNICEF 1989); the cost issue is that of monitoring of response, side effects, and the compliance of patients with their treatment regimens. The large number of compliant individuals required per death averted is the limiting factor on cost-effectiveness.

- National fitness programs. Such programs should be emphasized for those segments of the population that have occupations or lifestyles which reduce their levels of physical activity, or those subgroups prone to obesity.

- Toward later stages of the epidemiologic transition, limited introduction of inexpensive antihyperlipidemics. These might be considered for individuals with very adverse lipid profiles; the WHO/UNICEF *Essential Drug List* should, therefore, be expanded to include an effective, inexpensive lipid-lowering agent (such as nicotinic acid). As with control of hypertension, however, but even more so, the large number of compliant individuals required to avert a death sharply constrains cost-effectiveness.

CASE MANAGEMENT. The range of cost-effective case management interventions is much narrower in developing countries than in industrial ones. They include the following:

- Post-MI and poststroke care. Improvement is needed in such care, with emphasis on modification of risk factors (for example, smoking) and inexpensive drug treatment (for example, beta blockers, aspirin).

- Low-cost drugs (propranolol, aspirin) and modification of risk factors for treatment of angina. Risk factor modification should include lipid-lowering diet or drugs, smoking cessation, and the like. Treatment of angina appears particularly cost-effective.

- An inexpensive (and cost-effective) protocol to treat acute MI and unstable angina. Such a protocol should emphasize the use of aspirin and nitroglycerin.

- Strict limitations on provision for (locally or abroad) invasive diagnostic (coronary arteriography) and treatment (coronary care units, coronary bypass surgery) facilities, with their use limited to the young, highest-risk subgroups of patients, and then only after the more cost-effective strategies just described have already been tried.

Operations Research in Developing Countries

The following are areas of priority for operations research, along the lines that Tanzania has initiated with the assistance of WHO (WHO 1986). Given the public health significance of cardiovascular disease in developing countries, and its rising absolute and relative importance, the current neglect of applied research is striking.

EPIDEMIOLOGY. Additional data on the distribution, causes, and national history of CVD is needed in the following areas:

- Better data must be sought on the incidence, prevalence, case-fatality rates, and prognosis of cardiovascular diseases to determine the circumstances under which development and increasing affluence result in increased age-specific cardiovascular disease rates.

- Better data must be sought on the prevalence of modifiable risk factors, especially in those countries with increasing cardiovascular disease rates.

- Better data must be sought on the relative risk and the attributable risk of risk factors in developing countries.

- Developing country participation must be greatly expanded in international programs of cardiovascular epidemiologic investigations and surveillance, such as MONICA, to provide standardized measurement techniques and numerous industrial countries for comparison.

RISK MODIFICATIONS. Little information is available on the effectiveness of interventions to lower the risk of CVD. Additional research is needed in the following areas:

- Research must be undertaken in community-specific and culture-specific strategies to use mass media, community resources, and other modifiers of human behavior to alter the level of risk factors.

- The effectiveness of price and taxation policies in modifying the distribution of risk factors must be studied.
- Studies must be undertaken of the relative effectiveness and cost-effectiveness of both nonpharmacologic and drug interventions to reduce risk factors in individuals of that particular culture.

CASE MANAGEMENT. The management of established CVD also needs further investigation.

- Studies must be conducted of the relative effectiveness and cost-effectiveness of both nonpharmacologic and drug interventions to reduce case-fatality rates and to improve prognosis in patients with cardiovascular disease.
- Given that only very small numbers of expensive invasive procedures will be undertaken, research must be carried out concerning the economics of referral for these procedures and optimal location for them (including at centers abroad).

In this chapter we have assembled evidence that points to the large and growing significance of cardiovascular disease in developing countries; we have reviewed the range of available options for prevention and case management; and we have assessed the cost-effectiveness of a range of the most attractive intervention options. A number of broadly relevant interventions have been identified that, potentially, have cost-effectiveness measures from $150 to $350 per disability-adjusted life-year gained; although these figures are not the most attractive that Jamison (chapter 1 of this collection) has summarized for interventions addressing health problems of adults, they do fall at the low end of the range and should become integral to the range of services most countries provide. Interventions to reduce smoking are even more attractive, in part because they simultaneously reduce the risk of lung cancer and other conditions. Finally, it is worth stressing that many interventions of very low cost-effectiveness have also been identified; considerations of both efficiency and equity suggest that their use should be curtailed.

Appendix 23A. Cardiovascular Mortality Differentiated by Sex

MONICA data suggest a very strong effect for ischemic heart disease and a much weaker one for stroke among males.

Table 23A-1.   Sex Differences in Age-Standardized Cardiovascular Mortality, Selected Populations, 1984

	Cerebrovascular disease				Ischemic heart disease			
Location	Male mortality rate (10^{-5})	Female mortality rate (10^{-5})	Male/female ratio	Male/female ratio of proportional mortality[a]	Male mortality rate (10^{-5})	Female mortality rate (10^{-5})	Male/female ratio	Male/female ratio of proportional mortality[a]
Perth, Australia	26	24	1.1	0.57	161	38	4.2	2.1
Bejing, China	98	82	1.2	0.96	40	28	1.4	1.3
Finland	60	42	1.4	0.46	374	57	6.6	2.1
Italy: Latina area	68	33	2.1	0.92	96	20	4.8	2.3
California	25	20	1.3	0.59	221	40	5.5	2.7

Note: Mortality rates are annual, for a population of 100,000 age thirty-five through sixty-four.
a. Obtained by dividing the percent of total mortality in males by the same percentage in females.
Source: MONICA Principal Investigators 1987.

Notes

The authors wish to acknowledge their gratitude to Robert Beaglehole, Jeanne Bertolli, John Briscoe, Elaine Eaker, Jon Eisenberg, John Evans, Richard Feachem, William Harlan, Millicent Higgins, Tord Kjellstrom, Jeffrey Koplan, Matthew Longnecker, Adetokunbo O. Lucas, Anthony R. Measham, Richard Morrow, P. Nordt, Kenneth Powell, and P. Tatsanavivat for their assistance and comments on earlier drafts of this chapter. Richard Peto provided particularly detailed and valuable critical comments.

References

Berwick, D. M., S. Cretin, and E. B. Keeler. 1980. *Cholesterol, Children, and Heart Disease: An Analysis of Alternatives.* Oxford: Oxford University Press.

Blackburn, H. W. 1983. "Research and Demonstration Projects in Community Cardiovascular Disease Prevention." *Journal of Public Health Policy* 4:398–421.

———. 1989. "Trends and Determinants of CHD Mortality: Changes in Risk Factors and Their Effects." *International Journal of Epidemiology* 18(supplement 1):S210–S215.

Blankenhorn, D. H., S. A. Nessim, R. L. Johnson, M. E. San Marco, S. P. Azen, and L. Cashin-Hemphill. 1987. "Beneficial Effects of Combined Colestipol-Niacin Therapy on Coronary Atherosclerosis and Coronary Venous Bypass Grafts." *JAMA* 257:3233–40.

Bulatao, R., and P. Stephens. 1992. "Global Estimates and Projections of Mortality by Cause, 1970–2015." PRE Working Paper 1007. Population, Health, and Nutrition Department, World Bank. Washington, D.C.

Byington, R., A. R. Dyer, D. Garside, and others. 1979. "Recent Trends of Major Coronary Risk Factors and CHD in the United States and Other

Industrialized Countries." In R. J. Havlik and M. Feinleib, eds., *Proceedings of the Conference on the Decline in Coronary Heart Disease Mortality.* NIH 79-1610. U.S. Department of Health, Education, and Welfare, Public Health Service, National Institutes of Health, Washington, D.C.

Chapman, Simon, and Jeff Richardson. 1990. "Tobacco Excise and Declining Tobacco Consumption: The Case of Papua New Guinea." *American Journal of Public Health* 80:537–40.

Dodu, S. R. A. 1984. "Coronary Heart Disease in Developing Countries: The Threat Can Be Averted." *World Health Organization Chronicle* 38:3–7.

———. 1988. "Emergence of Cardiovascular Diseases in Developing Countries." *Cardiology* 75:56–64.

Epstein, F. H. 1989. "The Relationship of Lifestyle to International Trends in CHD." *International Journal of Epidemiology* 18(supplement 1):S203–S209.

European Atherosclerosis Society Study Group. 1987. "Strategies for the Prevention of Coronary Heart Disease: A Policy Statement of the European Atherosclerosis Society." *European Heart Journal* 8:77–88.

Falase, A. O. 1987. "Are There Differences in the Clinical Pattern of Hypertension between Africans and Caucasians?" *Tropical Cardiology* 13:141–51.

Feinleib, Manning. 1984. "The Magnitude and Nature of the Decrease in Coronary Heart Disease Mortality Rate." *American Journal of Cardiology* 54:2c–8c.

Fries, James F., Lawrence W. Green, and Sol Levine. 1989. "Health Promotion and the Compression of Morbidity." *Lancet* 1:481–82.

Goldman, L., S. T. B. Sia, E. F. Cook, J. D. Rutherford, and M. C. Weinstein. 1988. "Costs and Effectiveness of Routine Therapy with Long-Term Beta-Adrenergic Antagonists after Acute Myocardial Infarction." *New England Journal of Medicine* 319:152–57.

Gunning-Schepers, L. J., J. J. Barendregt, and P. J. van der Maas. 1989. "Population Interventions Reassessed." *Lancet* 1:479–80.

Harlan, W. R, L. C. Harlan, and W. L. Oii. 1984. "Changing Disease Patterns in Developing Countries: The Case of Malaysia." In P. Leaverton and L. Massi, eds., *Health Information Systems.* New York: Praeger Scientific.

Hatziandreu, E. I., J. P. Koplan, M. C. Weinstein, C. J. Caspersen, and K. E. Warner. 1988. "A Cost-Effectiveness Analysis of Exercise as a Health Promotion Activity." *American Journal of Public Health* 78:1417–21.

Held, P. H., S. Yusuf, and C. D. Furberg. 1989. "Calcium Channel Blockers in Acute Myocardial Infarction and Unstable Angina: An Overview." *British Medical Journal* 299:1187–89.

Hennekens, C. H., J. E. Buring, Peter Sandercock, Rory Collins, and Richard Peto. 1989. "Aspirin and Other Antiplatelet Agents in the Secondary and Primary Prevention of Cardiovascular Disease." *Circulation* 80:749–56.

Hutt, M. S. R. 1991. "Cancer and Cardiovascular Disease." In R. G. Feachem and D. T. Jamison, eds., *Disease and Mortality in Sub-Saharan Africa.* New York: Oxford University Press.

Hutt, M. S. R., and D. P. Burkitt. 1986. *The Geography of Non-infectious Disease.* New York: Oxford University Press.

"Hypertension in Blacks and Whites." 1980. *Lancet* (editorial) 2:73–74.

Intersalt Cooperative Research Group. 1988. "Intersalt: An International Study of Electrolyte Excretion and Blood Pressure: Results for 24 Hour Urinary Sodium and Potassium Excretion." *British Medical Journal* 297:319–28.

Jamison, D. T., J. R. Evans, T. King, I. Porter, N. Prescott, and A. Prost. 1984. *China: The Health Sector. A World Bank Country Study.* Washington, D.C.: The World Bank.

Julian, D. 1989. "Treatment for Chronic CHD." *International Journal of Epidemiology* 18(supplement 1):S228–S230.

Kannel, W. B., and Manning Feinleib. 1972. "Natural History of Angina Pectoris in the Framingham Study." *American Journal of Cardiology* 29:154–63.

Knuiman, J. T., R. J. J. Hermus, and J. G. A. J. Hautvast. 1980. "Serum Total and High-Density Lipoprotein (HDL) Cholesterol Concentrations in Rural and Urban Boys from 16 Countries." *Atherosclerosis* 36:529–37.

Kottke, T. E., P. Puska, J. T. Salonen, J. Tuomilehto, and A. Nissinen. 1985. "Projected Effects of High-Risk versus Population-Based Presentation Strategies in Coronary Heart Disease." *American Journal of Epidemiology* 121:697–704.

Lewis, B., J. I. Mann, and M. Mancini. 1986. "Reducing the Risks of Coronary Heart Disease in Individuals and in the Population." *Lancet* 1:956–59.

de Lolio, C. A., J. M. P. de Souza, and R. Laurent. 1986. "Decline in Cardiovascular Disease Mortality in the City of S. Paulo, Brazil, 1970 to 1983." *Revista de Saude Publica* 20:454–64.

Lozano-Ascencio, R., and others. 1990. "Tendencia de la mortalidad por cardiopatia insquemica en México, de 1950 a 1985." *Salúd Pública de México* 32:405–20.

McCormick, James, and Petr Skrabanek. 1988. "Coronary Heart Disease Is Not Preventable by Population Interventions." *Lancet* 2:839–41.

McGill, Henry. 1968. "Fatty Streaks in the Coronary Arteries and Aorta." *Laboratory Investigation* 18:560–64.

MacMahon, S., R. Collins, R. Peto, R. W. Koster, and S. Yusuf. 1988. "Effects of Prophylactic Lidocaine in Suspected Acute Myocardial Infarction: An Overview from the Randomized, Controlled Trials." *JAMA* 260:1910–16.

MacMahon, S., R. Peto, J. Cutler, R. Collins, P. Sorlie, J. Neaton, R. Abbott, J. Godwin, A. Dyer, and J. Stamler. 1990. "Blood Pressure, Stroke, and Coronary Heart Disease. Part 1—Prolonged Differences in Blood Pressure: Prospective Observational Studies Corrected for the Regression Dilution Bias." *Lancet* 335:765–74.

Marquardsen, J. 1986. "Epidemiology of Strokes in Europe." In H. J. M. Barnett, B. M. Stein, J. P. Mohr, and F. M. Yatsu, eds., *Stroke: Pathophysiology, Diagnosis, and Management.* London: Churchill Livingstone.

Masironi, R., and K. Rothwell. 1988. "Tendances et effects du tabagisme dans le monde." *World Health Statistical Quarterly* 41:228–41.

Melnick, J. L., Evin Adam, and Michael E. DeBakey. 1990. "Possible Role of Cytomegalovirus in Atherogenesis." *JAMA* 263:2204–7.

MONICA (Monitoring Trends and Determinants in Cardiovascular Disease) Principal Investigators. 1987. "WHO MONICA Project: Geographic Variation in Mortality from Cardiovascular Disease." *World Health Statistics Quarterly* 40:171–84.

Nissinen, A., S. Bothig, H. Granroth, and A. D. Lopez. 1988. "Hypertension in Developing Countries." *World Health Statistical Quarterly* 41:141–54.

Nissinen, A., J. Toumilehto, T. E. Kottke, and P. Puska. 1986. "Cost-Effectiveness of the North Karelia Hypertension Program, 1972–1977." *Medical Care* 24:767–80.

Oldridge, N. B., G. H. Guyatt, M. E. Fischer, and A. A. Rimm. 1988. "Cardiac Rehabilitation after Myocardial Infarction: Combined Experience of Randomized Clinical Trials." *JAMA* 260:945–50.

Oliver, Michael. 1984. "Coronary Risk Factors: Should We Not Forget about Mass Control?" *World Health Forum* 5:5–18.

Olshansky, S. J., and A. B. Ault. 1986. "The Fourth Stage of the Epidemiologic Transition: The Age of Delayed Degenerative Diseases." *Milbank Memorial Fund Quarterly* 64:355–91.

Omram, A. R. 1971. "The Epidemiological Transition: A Theory of the Epidemiology of Population Change." *Milbank Memorial Fund Quarterly* 49:509–38.

Pearson, T. A. 1989. "Influences on CHD Incidence and Case Fatality: Medical Management of Risk Factors." *International Journal of Epidemiology* 18(supplement 1):S217–S222.

Pitt, Bertram. 1989. "Therapy for Myocardial Infarction: Effect on Trends in Coronary Disease Mortality." *International Journal of Epidemiology* 18(supplement 1):S223–S227.

Reducing the Health Consequences of Smoking: Thirty-five Years of Progress: A Report of the Surgeon General. 1989. CDC-89-8411. Washington D.C: U.S. Department of Health and Human Services.

Rice, D. P., T. A. Hodgson, and A. N. Kopstein. 1985. "The Economic Costs of Illness: A Replication and Update." *Health Care Finance Review* 7:61–80.

594 *Thomas A. Pearson, Dean T. Jamison, and Jorge Trejo-Gutierrez*

Ross, Russell. 1986. "The Pathogenesis of Atherosclerosis: An Update." *New England Journal of Medicine* 314:488–500.

Rothenberg, R., E. Ford, and E. Vartiainen. 1990. "Cardiovascular Disease Prevention: Estimating the Impact of Interventions." Paper presented at the International Symposium on Health, Environment, and Social Change, July, Taipei, Taiwan.

Schoenberg, B. S. 1979. "Epidemiology of Cerebrovascular Disease." *Southern Medical Journal* 72:331–37.

Shigan, E. N. 1988. "Integrated Programme for Noncommunicable Diseases Prevention and Control." *World Health Statistical Quarterly* 41:267–73.

Steinberg, E. P., E. J. Topol, J. W. Sakin, S. N. Kahane, L. J. Appel, N. R. Powe, G. F. Anderson, J. E. Erickson, and A. D. Guerci. 1988. "Cost and Procedure Implications of Thrombolytic Therapy for Acute Myocardial Infarction." *Journal of the American College of Cardiology* 12:58A–68A.

"The Surgeon General's 1990 Report on the Health Benefits of Smoking Cessation." *Morbidity and Mortality Weekly Report* 39(RR-12), pi-xv, 1–12.

Tao, Shouchi, Zhendong Huang, Xigui Wu, Beifan Zhou, Zhikui Xiao, Jiansheng Hao, Yihe Li, Runchao Cen, and Xuxu Rao. 1989. "CHD and Its Risk Factors in the People's Republic of China." *International Journal of Epidemiology* 18(supplement 1):Sl59–S163.

Taylor, W. C., T. M. Pass, D. S. Shepard, and A. L. Komoroff. 1987. "Cholesterol Reduction and Life Expectancy." *Annals of Internal Medicine* 106:605–14.

Thom, T. J. 1989. "International Mortality from Heart Disease: Rates and Trends." *International Journal of Epidemiology* 18(supplement 1):S20–S28.

Thom, T. S., F. H. Epstein, J. J. Feldman, and P. E. Leaverton. 1985. "Trends in Total Morbidity and Mortality from Heart Disease in 26 Countries from 1950 to 1978." *International Journal of Epidemiology* 14:510–20.

Tracy, R. E., and V. Toca. 1975. "Relationship of Raised Atherosclerotic Lesions to Fatty Streaks in 19 Location-Race Groups." *Atherosclerosis* 21:21–36.

Uemura, K., and Z. Pisa. 1988. "Trends in Cardiovascular Disease Mortality in Industrialized Countries since 1950." *World Health Statistical Quarterly* 41:155–78.

UNICEF (United Nations Children's Fund). 1989. "Essential Drugs Price List." UNICEF Supply Division, Copenhagen.

Vaughan, J. P., and W. E. Miall. 1979. "A Comparison of Cardiovascular Measurements in The Gambia, Jamaica, and the United Republic of Tanzania." *Bulletin of the World Health Organization* 57:281–89.

Warner, K. E. 1990a. "Behavioral and Health Effects of the Antismoking Campaign in the U.S." Paper presented at the International Symposium on Health, Environment, and Social Change. July, Taipei, Taiwan.

———. 1990b. "Tobacco Taxation as Health Policy in the Third World." *American Journal of Public Health* 80:529–31.

Weinstein, M. C., and W. B. Stason. 1985. "Cost-Effectiveness of Interventions to Prevent or Treat Coronary Heart Disease." *Annual Review of Public Health* 6:41–63.

WHO (World Health Organization). 1982. *Prevention of Coronary Heart Disease*. Technical Report 678. Geneva.

———. 1986. "The WHO Programme on Cardiovascular Diseases, 1985–1986." Division of Noncommunicable Diseases. Geneva.

———. 1988a. *Appropriate Diagnostic Technology in the Management of Cardiovascular Diseases*. Technical Report 772. Geneva.

———. 1988b. *1988 World Health Statistics Annual*. Geneva.

———. 1989. "Mortality in Developed Countries." *Weekly Epidemiological Record* 14:103–7.

WHO (World Health Organization) MONICA (Monitoring Trends and Determinants in Cardiovascular Disease) Project. 1988. "Geographical Variation in the Major Risk Factors of Coronary Heart Disease in Men and Women Aged 35–64 Years." *World Health Statistical Quarterly* 41:115–40.

———. 1989. "WHO MONICA Project: Objectives and Design." *International Journal of Epidemiology* 18(Supplement 1):S29–S37.

Williams, Alan. 1985. "Economics of Coronary Artery Bypass Grafting." *British Medical Journal* 291:326–29.

Yusuf, Salim, Janet Wittes, and Lawrence Friedman. 1988a. "Overview of Results of Randomized Clinical Trials in Heart Disease. 1. Treatment Following Myocardial Infarction." *JAMA* 260:2088–93.

———. 1988b. "Overview of Results of Randomized Clinical Trials in Heart Disease. 2. Unstable Angina, Heart Failure, Primary Precautions with Aspirin, and Risk Factor Modification." *JAMA* 260:2259–64.

24

Chronic Obstructive Pulmonary Disease

J. Richard Bumgarner and Frank E. Speizer

Chronic obstructive lung (pulmonary) disease refers to several disease manifestations and is known by many names—cor pulmonale (heart disease with an underlying pulmonary deficiency), right-sided heart disease, asthma, emphysema, chronic bronchitis, and peripheral airways disease are among the most common. Often these names refer to one or another of the pathological manifestations which are here grouped as chronic obstructive pulmonary disease (COPD) and its allied conditions. The many and varied names indicate in part the uncertainty in the clinical diagnoses of these conditions as well as the fact that the respiratory tract has a limited number of ways to respond to injury: the obstructive pattern is the unifying manifestation of these conditions.

Description of the Diseases

Because all the conditions of COPD are characterized by airways obstruction, the clinical manifestations and definitions overlap considerably, and diagnosis and measurement of their progression have not in the past, unfortunately, been obtained in a uniform manner.[1] For example, *chronic bronchitis* involves inflammation and narrowing of the large bronchial passageways to the lung. It is accompanied by severe coughing caused by the hypersecretion of mucus in the inflamed passages. The cough sounds terrible and is discomforting to the patient, but in itself it is seldom seriously disabling. The condition is not normally fatal, providing there is good access to medical care to control primary inflammation and to avoid the consequences of secondary infection. Usually the condition abates when the cause of the inflammation is removed. Clinical information about this condition is usually obtained from a standard set of questions about cough and sputum production. *Emphysema* is best characterized by a history of shortness of breath resulting from progressive destruction of lung tissue. In sequence there is a loss of elastic structure followed by the destruction of alveolar walls and the collapse of smaller airways. This eventually results in the loss of ability to transport oxygen from the airways to the blood and the reduced rate of exchange of carbon dioxide from the blood to the airways. This change in diffusion may eventually affect the heart, leading to right-sided heart failure. There is no cure for emphysema—once tissues have been degraded the loss of ventilatory function is irreversible. Diagnosis is normally accomplished through measurements of abnormally premature and permanent declines in lung function, but clinical confirmation has been dependent upon the pathologic examination of lung tissue, generally obtained by autopsy. Newer, but expensive, imaging techniques—computerized tomography (CT) scanning—now make it possible to confirm diagnosis of emphysema while the patient is alive. *Cor pulmonale* is characterized by clinical evidence of right-sided heart failure with edema (fluid retention in the limbs). This condition is generally superimposed on severe obstructive airways disease and long-standing respiratory insufficiency with hypoxia and hypercapnia. *Chronic obstructive lung disease not otherwise specified*, more recently reported in many health systems, generally means irreversible obstructive disease by physiologic testing but does not specify the type of disease. A great deal of this disease category is probably chronic bronchitis with obstruction or emphysema. Collectively, these diseases are referred to here as COPD.

Persons suffering from one or more manifestations of COPD have abnormally rapid rates of decline in lung function to levels which are severely disabling by middle life and fatal in severe cases. In addition, COPD contributes to the severity and eventual fatal outcome of cardiovascular diseases, including coronary and rheumatic heart disease, and other respiratory diseases, such as pneumonia and pulmonary tuberculosis.

Other diseases affect and can also complicate declines in respiratory function. *Asthma* is induced by a wide variety of allergic and nonallergic agents and produces widespread inflammation and narrowing of the airways. It is characterized by a history of recurrent episodes of wheeze, with or without shortness of breath, but with reversible airways obstruction. Its onset can be sudden and severe. Treatment with bronchodilators or anti-inflammatory agents can provide rapid return of normal lung function. In many patients lifestyle and productivity remains normal until the next episode. Other pulmonary conditions, such as pneumonia, pneumoconiosis, silicosis, and byssinosis can complicate or exacerbate underlying COPD. These diseases, however, are distinct from COPD.

Etiology of COPD

The pathogenesis of COPD is not yet fully understood. Two main mechanisms have been postulated (airflow obstruction and mucus hypersecretion), and these are believed to be independent but overlapping disease processes (Peto and others 1983). First, airflow obstruction can be caused by the presence of excessive amounts of elastase, an enzyme that is responsible for degrading elastin in the lung and destroying alveolar walls, resulting in emphysema. The absence of alpha₁-antiprotease, a protein that acts as an elastase inhibitor, is one genetic model for the occurrence of emphysema. In addition, it is known that the inhalation of particulates in smoke results in an inflammatory response in the lung, which increases production of elastase. At the same time, it has been shown that cigarette smoke acts by oxidizing alpha₁-antiprotease, resulting in the removal of the natural control on elastase production (U.S. Surgeon General 1984). These processes and other unknown enzymatic processes may interact and lead to the resulting destruction of lung tissue and the condition of emphysema.

Second, the muco-ciliary apparatus of the respiratory tract is a natural defense against particulate matter which may be inhaled. The cilia, tiny hairlike projections, are coated with a thin layer of mucus that envelops entering foreign particles. The cilia beat in waves about 1,000 to 1,500 times each minute, propelling foreign particles upward to the trachea. Many pollutants, including cigarette smoke, cause transient paralysis of the cilia. Over a long period, the cilia may be permanently injured by such pollutants. In addition, chronic irritation increases production of mucus by the bronchial mucus glands. The thick, excess mucus not only overwhelms the cilia but may also plug the bronchioles, resulting in the development of chronic bronchitis with recurrent lower respiratory tract infections and increased morbidity from airways obstruction (Carnow and others 1970). Protection of the alveoli from the particular matter and pollutants is consequently reduced, and production of elastase and greater oxidization of alpha₁-antiprotease is likely to be increased.

Lung Function and the Development of COPD

Lung function can be clinically measured and recorded as various indexes of the ability of the lungs to take in and expel air. A simple physiologic test is performed by having patients take as big a breath as they can and blow out as fast and as hard as they can into a recording device (a spirometer) that measures the volume of air expelled in a specified time. The forced expiratory volume in 1 second (FEV₁) is a common measure. By comparing the FEV1 of individuals with standards measured in large population groups and adjusting for body size (height or height squared) and age for each individual, one can calculate a percent-predicted (percentage of norm) value for FEV1. Because no single study has been able to follow a population from early adult life on into the development of COPD in mid-life to late mid-life, investigators have relied upon relatively short-term prospective studies of several years to piece together the approximate natural history of lung function in a healthy individual. They have found that it increases with age until about the mid-twenties, when it begins a slow, natural decline. The lungs have a large ventilatory reserve, and the decline does not normally become evident as a significant limit on lifestyle or work capacity (curve A; see figure 24-1). Most persons who fall between 35 percent and 50 percent of the predicted value of FEV1 become short of breath on minimal exertion, and to a variable degree this may lead to a complaint to their health care provider. Because decreases of function to this level generally occur only gradually, the definition of the onset of disease, when such a complaint is made, is also variable. This is in sharp contrast to the definition of onset of a myocardial infarction or the diagnosis of a cancer. For COPD it is thus difficult to define the transition between health and disease.

Only a relatively small group (approximately 20 percent) of the population (mostly, but not all, smokers) reach a level of lung function associated with disability. The remaining non-smokers and smokers simply do not live long enough to become disabled from lowered levels of lung function. Smokers whose rate of decline of lung function is rapid and who stop smoking in early mid-life do not regain a substantial amount of lung function, but their rate of loss becomes more like that of a nonsmoker (curve D and/or curve E in figure 24-1); if they stop smoking soon enough they may not reach the disabling level of lung function in a normal lifetime. This does not mean that such a smoker will be protected from the other ravages of smoking.

Figure 24-1. *Theoretical Curve Representing Varying Rates of Change in FEV by Age*

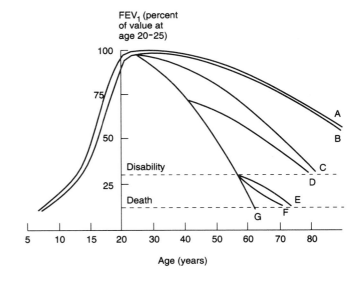

Note: Curve A represents normal decline in FEV₁. Curve B shows less than optimal development of normal lung function. Often, the disability-related decline continues as a variable rate curve (C). Curve D shows effect of smoking cessation; also seen in disabled individuals (curve E). Curve F is a disability-related decline continuing at variable rate. Curve G represents the accelerating decline in FEV₁ with cigarette smoking and continuing rapid decline until death as a consequence of respiratory failure.
Source: Speizer and Tager 1979.

For those patients who do become disabled and do not give up smoking, COPD is a devastating disease that often kills in less than five years. Death from respiratory insufficiency would occur at about FEV1 at 15–25 percent of predicted value. Even before being disabled those subjects with lower levels of lung function at approximately age forty-five have almost a fifty-fold higher risk of mortality in a twenty-year period (Peto and others 1983) than subjects whose level of function is better than average.

Maximal lung capacity is different for each individual. One question of current research interest in the industrial world is how to identify which persons, and in particular which smokers, are at greatest risk of developing COPD. Authors of longitudinal studies in children have observed a high degree of tracking of lung function, leading to the suggestion that risk factors that put children on tracks of lower growth rate of lung function, such that these children never quite reach their maximum predicted level of lung function in early adult life, may explain those persons with more decline in lung function. Factors that reduce the rate of lung growth in children are discussed below.

Risk Factors

The main risk factors for COPD are several and diverse.

Cigarette Smoking

The best-documented cause-and-effect relationship in the etiology of COPD is cigarette smoking (Palmer 1954; U.S. Surgeon General 1984). Numerous studies have confirmed cigarette smoking as a primary cause of COPD. There is a clear dose-response relationship between the prevalence of chronic mucus hypersecretion and obstructive airways disease and the quantity of cigarettes smoked (Anderson, Ferris, and Zickmantel 1964; Ferris 1973). Prospective studies in a number of countries show much higher COPD mortality in smokers than in nonsmokers. The onset of symptoms associated with COPD may occur at an early age and at relatively low levels of cigarette smoking (Peters and Ferris 1967).

Individual Susceptibility

Individual susceptibility must play a role and the multiple factors involved are not yet fully understood. A hereditary cause of emphysema was first described by Eriksson (1965). A deficiency in alpha$_1$-antiprotease is a recessive genetic trait that in its severest form predisposes subjects to the development of emphysema even without exposure to cigarette smoke.[2] Those who are heterozygote for the putative gene appear to be more susceptible to cigarette smoke. Fortunately the gene frequency of this condition is relatively low, and the condition cannot account for more than a few percentage points of the total number of cases of emphysema. Other familial factors include increased frequency of allergies, possibly associated with increased airways responsiveness, and pos-

sibly with common indoor environmental exposures. The roles and importance of these factors are unknown at present.

Air Pollution

Both indoor and outdoor air pollution have long been recognized to be potentially exacerbating factors for COPD. Illness in patients with preexisting disease symptoms clearly worsened in association with daily changes in peak levels of smoke (Lawther 1970), and overall levels of air pollution have been recognized to have a short-term acute effect on persons with the disease. During dramatic episodes of air stagnation and pollution in London, New York, Japan, and Dublin, substantial excess mortality occurred among the elderly and in those with preexisting disease who were exposed to the high concentrations of smoke and sulfur dioxide (Holland 1983). The morbidity resulting from short-term exposure could not distinctly be attributed to pollution rather than adverse meteorological (cold temperature and high moisture) conditions.

The causal role of air pollution in COPD has been examined in several British studies done in the 1950s and 1960s (such as Holland and Reid 1965; Holland and others 1965). Both these and American studies (Reid and others 1964; Deane, Goldsmith, and Quma 1965; Wynder, Lemon, and Mantel 1965; Densen and others 1967) have to date failed to demonstrate conclusively a causal link between air pollution and the onset of COPD. Conversely, smoking behavior alone has not been sufficient to explain the geographic differences in the prevalence of symptoms in England (Lambert and Reid 1970). Prevalence rates for symptoms were found to increase with increasing levels of air pollution independently of cigarette consumption, indicating that atmospheric and indoor smoke pollution may account for the urban-rural differences in the data on respiratory morbidity in Britain (Reid and Fairbairn 1958).

In developing countries also COPD appears to be unexplainable solely by cigarette smoking, because mortality and prevalence rates often appear to be much higher than in industrial countries and to have more equal sex ratios. For example, the frequency of chronic bronchitis in northern India would appear to be explainable by tobacco use among men, but its prevalence in women may be indicative of the effect of chronic exposure to fumes produced during cooking with cow dung, wood, and coal (Malik 1977). In a study of nonspecific lung disease in Delhi in which similar studies in London and Chicago were compared, Saha and Jain (1970) found that 16 percent of Delhi patients were nonsmokers, whereas nearly all patients in the other two studies were smokers. In addition, cigarette smoking and occupational air pollution (including exposure to steel, coal, cotton, and other dust) act additively in causing chronic lung disease (Commission of the European Communities 1975). Exposure to multiple risk factors in developing countries may be much higher than in industrial countries, and the effect of these multiple exposures has not been fully evaluated.

Childhood Respiratory Tract Infections

Samet, Tager, and Speizer (1983) reviewed suggestive but not conclusive evidence on the relationship between lower respiratory tract infections in childhood and the subsequent development of COPD. Respiratory illness in early childhood has been shown to be associated with lower levels of lung function in children six to ten years old (Tager 1983; Gold 1989). Among Chinese children, passive exposure to cigarette smoke from fathers who smoked nearly doubled the relative risk of severe respiratory infection in the first eighteen months of life (Chen 1986). Studies in Papua New Guinea, where from birth people are exposed to wood smoke in unventilated huts, show high rates of respiratory infection and chronic bronchitis (Colley and Reid 1970). Other studies support the notion that respiratory disorders in children predispose them to later disease (Cooreman and others 1990); and in general, children's lung function tracks uniformly from early childhood (Dockery 1983). As shown on curves A and B in figure 24-1, lower lung function in early adult life would be anticipated to result from impaired respiratory functions in childhood. The effect of this reduced maximally attained lung function may determine the plateau from which further declines during adulthood can be expected. This hypothesis remains unconfirmed, however, because no studies have yet followed individuals long enough to determine whether it is the effects of cigarette smoking or other factors that put those who have slightly lower lung function by early adulthood at greater risk of developing COPD in later life.

Occupational Dust Exposure

Becklake (1988) and other researchers have documented an association between other specific and nonspecific occupational dust exposure and excess chronic mucus hypersecretion and obstructive airways disease. Dust exposure appears to exacerbate (but not cause) COPD, and the effects can often be managed by improved ventilation or protective respirator equipment use at work.

Socioeconomic Status

Low socioeconomic status may be a surrogate factor for a number of less fully understood risk factors for the development of COPD and has been investigated in a number of studies (Colley and Reid [1970] list many studies). Factors may include higher prevalence of cigarette smoking, poorer nutrition, higher levels of indoor smoke exposure, and poor housing conditions, all associated with increases in the frequency of other respiratory illnesses, occupational exposure, difficulties in reaching health care services, and less contact with health education. Rapidly changing external and domestic factors have made long-term cohort studies among such groups difficult and expensive to conduct. Firm conclusions related to these associations remain few even after more than two decades of work relating to these questions.

The Public Health Significance of the Condition

From an epidemiological perspective COPD must rank as a major public health problem.

Mortality and Morbidity

Death from COPD as the primary cause can occur directly because of respiratory failure or because of right-sided heart failure. Mortality rates from COPD in many industrial countries have consistently been higher for men than for women because of the longer and heavier smoking experience among men.

Figure 24-2. Age-Specific Mortality Rates for COPD in United States and China, by Sex

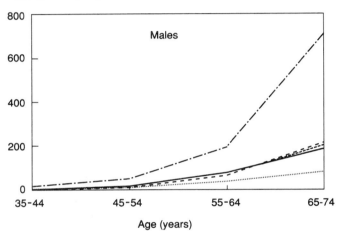

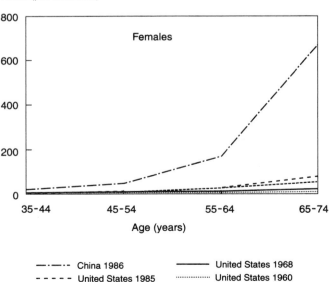

Rates (per 100,000)

Rates (per thousand)

————·—— China 1986   ——————— United States 1968
— — — — United States 1985   ·················· United States 1960
———————— United States 1977

Source: National Center for Health Statistics for United States; Disease Surveillance Points, Ministry of Public Health, for China.

Death rates from COPD for women are increasing more rapidly than for men in the United States as the effect of more widespread cigarette smoking among women is becoming evident. This trend is substantiated by changes in female mortality from lung cancer, now the leading cause of cancer death among U.S. women. Total deaths in the United States from COPD have more than doubled from 30,000 in 1970 to more than 71,000 in 1986, with increases for each age group (figure 24-2). The corresponding male-to-female ratio declined from 4.3:1 to 1.8:1. Indirectly, COPD contributes to death from a wide variety of other conditions, including most particularly cardiovascular diseases and infectious pulmonary diseases. In many places death reports do not specify contributory causes reliably, and it is very difficult to estimate the true overall mortality contribution of COPD. In the United States, COPD is estimated to be a contributing cause of death about 1.7 times as often as it is a primary cause (U.S. Surgeon General 1984). Because of the silent, progressive nature of the disease, much underlying morbidity is never discovered or reported. In the United States, COPD morbidity is estimated at about 10 times direct COPD mortality, and many patients suffer illness and disability for many years before death (U.S. Surgeon General 1984). This hidden morbidity burden may be even larger in developing countries in which health care contacts are few.

Availability of good prevalence and incidence data for COPD in most countries is seriously hampered by a lack of consistency in reporting. The disease has been redefined and reclassified frequently under the international classification systems. Inconsistency and weaknesses in recording of underlying causes of death in most countries further mask COPD's contributory effect and the disability burden which the disease poses. In the developing world COPD has been little studied and does not rank high on the public health agenda. Yet both relatively and absolutely, it is certainly a more important cause of death and illness in the developing countries than in industrial nations.

Current Levels and Trends in the Developing World

Data on COPD for the developing world is scarce. Cor pulmonale accounted for 20 percent of hospital admissions, evenly distributed between the sexes, for heart disease in Delhi, India (Pahmavati 1958). Studies in India have shown chronic bronchitis prevalence to be between 1.5 and 12 percent, and similar figures have been reported for other parts of the world. In Nepal, prevalence rates for chronic bronchitis (about 18 percent male; 19 percent female) are close to parity, and a hospital survey found prevalence of emphysema and cor pulmonale to be 3 percent and 1.5 percent, respectively (Pandey 1984a and 1984b). Nepalese data also indicate significant morbidity burdens. Among 39,000 inpatient admissions, COPD-type diseases accounted for 5.4 percent in 1984. Among 127,000 health post visits by patients (fifteen posts, Kaski district), 3.4 percent of the illnesses were bronchitis, emphysema, and asthma. In the 210,000 population served by these health posts, these diseases, at a rate of 60 per 100,000, were the third leading cause of death in 1985 (Nepal: His Majesty's Government/WHO

1987). Very limited data from the annual health survey of Pakistan show nonspecific respiratory disease accounting for about 5 percent of total morbidity. Jamaica reported death rates from bronchitis, asthma, and emphysema of only 8 to 9 per 100,000 in the early 1980s (USAID 1987). In Bangladesh in 1975–78, these disease categories accounted for 2 percent of total mortality. In Indonesia, COPD was the third ranked cause of death in the age group forty-five through fifty-four, and the main killer in the age group over fifty-five (Indonesia 1984). Review of epidemiological information from a number of African countries also points to relatively high prevalence of COPD and to the primary need for prevalence surveys with consistent criteria and methodology to establish better baseline data (Chaulet 1989).

Detailed data from China on cause of death provide the best perspective of COPD epidemiology from a developing country.[3] These data indicate that progressively higher age-specific rates prevail just as they do in the industrial nations (figure 24-3) and at rates which are much higher than even in the United States (figure 24-2). Other data reported by China in 1989 to the World Health Organization (WHO) on death among a population of 100 million corroborate this and add evidence that COPD may be a much more serious problem for the developing world than generally recognized. In China many large-scale surveys of respiratory disease document three common manifestations of COPD (cor pulmonale, chronic bronchitis, and emphysema). Cigarette smoking is an identified primary cause in most studies, but nearly equal sex ratios, a poverty-linked gradient, and dust and smoke exposure show that other

Figure 24-3. Rates and Deaths from COPD in China, by Age, Sex, and Residences, 1986

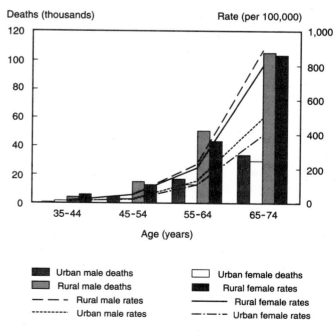

Source: Disease Surveillance Points, Ministry of Public Health, China.

factors are at work (Yan 1989). Smoking of traditional forms of tobacco may be part of the explanation. Although no detailed data on traditional tobacco use in China are available, it is common in rural areas and among middle-aged women as well as men.[4] More detailed examination of the cause of death data from China also reveals that the high COPD rates are not simply misdiagnosed rheumatic heart disease or misclassified respiratory disease.

Whatever their cause, the high rural rates in China may signal a potentially serious development for China and perhaps for other developing countries. The prevalence of cigarette smoking in China is increasing, and the age of initiation is falling. The epidemiological effect of the spread of cigarette smoking in the last decade cannot yet be fully reflected in the data shown in the charts, and large increases in smoking-induced COPD must therefore inevitably lie ahead. Declines in chronic nonspecific respiratory illness, which China and other countries might be expected to achieve as a result of reduction of poverty, fewer respiratory infections in childhood, cleaner indoor air, and improved living standards generally, could be offset, even overwhelmed, with increased morbidity and mortality attributable to a group of smoking-related diseases, including much higher incidence of COPD.

Much of the present burden must be related to indoor and outdoor smoke exposure, poor living and nutritional conditions for some children, and childhood respiratory infections, even though today we cannot conclusively document the causal role and interaction of these factors. Indoor air pollution from soft coal, wood, and dung used for household heating and cooking has been demonstrated to cause high levels of indoor smoke pollution in the absence of adequate ventilation and chimneys and can add substantially to the level of outdoor smoke. Clifford (1972), in his study in the Kenyan highlands, estimated the exposure to (mainly indoor) airborne total suspended particulates at 25,000 milligrams per year. Similarly, Smith and others (1983) showed that women in kitchens in Gujarat, India, were inhaling levels of benzopyrene, a potent carcinogen present in cigarette smoke, equivalent to smoking twenty cigarettes a day. Although the carcinogenic effects of this smoke level may have no direct link to COPD, they are indicative of the levels of smoke which must be present in such "micro" environments. Overall, these examples strongly indicate that COPD is a much heavier burden on the poor in developing countries, and on poor women and girls in particular, than the literature has thus far generally recognized.

The Progression of COPD in Developing Countries

The prevalence of COPD in most developing countries is today only roughly known, despite the evidence summarized above that COPD is a significant cause of morbidity and death in many parts of the developing world. Data on the prevalence of COPD and its risk factors and on COPD deaths are not adequate for most countries to permit even crude quantitative estimates of the overall economic effect of COPD and the benefits of its prevention. Too little is yet known about the mix of both

traditional and modern risk factors and their relative roles, other than cigarette smoking. Trends in developing countries for traditional risk factors are largely unknown. Prevalence of cigarette smoking and per capita consumption are following upward trends, sometimes sharply, as is the initiation of smoking at younger average ages.

Costs and the attributable benefit of programs for COPD prevention must remain educated guesses at best, given the absence of much better data on risk factors, disease prevalence, and case treatment. Three factors will, however, inevitably make COPD a much more important disease in the future:

- COPD is a disease which mainly strikes in middle and old age. As populations in the developing world age, the absolute number of COPD cases and deaths will increase. With regard to absolute demand for care, and in comparison with infectious and childhood diseases, COPD will become more important.

- Factors which are not well understood cause high rates of COPD in many developing countries. The longer the exposure that aging populations have to risk factors, the greater probability they have of developing disease. Conversely, prospects for reductions in these risks are uncertain at best.

- Cigarette smoking continues to increase in all parts of the developing world and probably will add to the existing age-specific rates, perhaps rapidly and substantially.

These three factors allow at least a very rough estimation of the future course and seriousness of COPD. In table 24-1 we provide an estimate of COPD mortality by major region of the world for 1985. We also show the increases by region in the number of COPD deaths which can be expected if age-specific rates remain as they are today. These increases are the result of the demographic shift that is taking place as more people live to middle and old age because they are no longer dying from infectious diseases at younger ages. This increase in COPD

Table 24-1. Estimated and Projected COPD Mortality by Region, Considering Prospective Demographic Changes Only
(thousands)

Region	Year		
	1985	2000	2015
Industrial market economies	205	255	316
Industrial nonmarket economies	109	150	175
Latin America and the Caribbean	18	28	43
Sub-Saharan Africa	57	90	145
Middle East and North Africa	21	33	51
Asia and the Pacific	510	788	1,155
World	926	1,328	1,954

Source: 1985 data from paper prepared for World Bank Health Priorities Review 1989; future deaths derived by using 1985 age-specific rates applied to population cohorts presented in World Bank Population Projections 1987–88.

deaths (and morbidity) that is induced by age structure will, of course, be more pronounced in those areas of the world where present-day societies are mainly young and the number of middle-aged and old persons will grow sharply in the next thirty 30 years. The industrial countries are least affected by changes in age structure as these have already largely taken place. Overall there may be more than a doubling of COPD mortality in the developing world.

The second factor which will influence future COPD incidence and mortality is exposure to risk factors. It is clear that there are multiple risk factors for COPD in the developing countries, which can be only poorly documented or explained. These include early childhood respiratory infection, exposure to indoor smoke, air pollution, occupational dust exposure, and others. It is at least a plausible hypothesis that some of these risks will decline in time with general economic improvement, better access to primary health care, improved housing and living conditions, better nutrition, and other changes. Factors such as these may underlie the substantial decline in COPD prevalence in Britain among nonsmokers in the first three-quarters of this century. It is equally plausible, however, that persistent poverty, malnutrition, inadequate health services, poor housing, and rigid social systems in poor countries will preclude early development of a declining trend in COPD prevalence.

Increased cigarette smoking in developing countries will substantially affect COPD rates, particularly among the young in Asia, who in many places are becoming early and heavy smokers. In table 24-2 we show an estimate of COPD mortality which may occur from the combined effects of an aging population and increasing age-specific death rates resulting from cigarette smoking. It is assumed in these estimates that risks associated with other (traditional) factors remain constant and do not multiply cigarette-associated risk. The estimated growth in age-specific mortality rates used to derive these numbers is similar to that experienced by smokers in the same age groups in the United States from the mid-1950s to the mid-1980s. It entails the simple assumption that similar etiological effects will be evident among large populations elsewhere who smoke.

In developing countries it is possible that age-specific rates will rise even more rapidly than they did in the United States for three reasons. First, during the latter half of the period used to derive these data, there were sizable reductions in the United States in the number of cigarettes smoked and in smoking prevalence. Similar trends may not occur in developing countries. In fact, many poor countries are experiencing rapid growth in both per capita consumption and in overall smoking prevalence. Second, the effect of increased cigarette smoking in a population with lung function already impaired by other long-standing risk factors is likely to be more severe than smoking among a relatively unimpaired population such as that of the United States. Third, to the extent that potentially offsetting improvements in living standards, health care, and so on are achieved in the developing countries during the next thirty years, the beneficial effect on COPD mortality will be limited. The irreversible nature of most COPD and the effects of impaired respiratory development and of earlier lifetime exposure mean that for most of those between the ages of fifteen and fifty today, prospective risk of COPD mortality will not diminish rapidly. The effect of reduced risk exposure to factors other than cigarettes would mainly be realized among the young and only during later periods of time, after 2015. If risk factors other than smoking do not decline in importance, or if the synergistic interaction of these risks and smoking is greater than the sum of their individual effects, then possible COPD mortality may be considerably higher than indicated in table 24-2.

The conclusion is that very early, aggressive, publicly funded programs of smoking cessation provide the only significant hope of reducing this burden for the developing world. Efforts to address the other possible risk factors may contribute to reducing future morbidity and mortality from COPD, but the strategic mix of actions and their effect is much less clear. Exactly the opposite is true for smoking—the steps and their probable effect on future COPD is quite clear.

Data to estimate present or prospective costs of the COPD illness and mortality burden for different parts of the world do not exist. In industrial countries, efforts to quantify the effect of the disease have shown its large cost. In Britain, COPD accounted for a rate of 3.7 percent of the working-age population being incapacitated for work, or about 25 percent of the total inception rate for work incapacity (Alderson 1967). A total of 300 million working days were lost annually in that country as a result of incapacitating illness lasting four or more days; this directly cost the National Insurance Fund more than £220 million (in 1965; approximately £2 billion in 1991 prices).[5] Of the total, 40 million days lost (13 percent) were attributable to COPD ("Incapacity for Work" 1966).

In the United States in 1979, COPD was estimated to cost the economy about $6.5 billion (USDHHS 1982). Of this total, about a third each was accounted for by direct treatment costs,

Table 24-2. Estimated and Projected COPD
Mortality by Region, Considering both Prospective Demographic Changes and Epidemiologic Changes
(thousands)

Region	Year		
	1985	2000	2015
Industrial market economies	205	417	529
Industrial nonmarket economies	109	231	293
Latin America and the Caribbean	18	57	72
Sub-Saharan Africa	57	191	243
Middle East and North Africa	21	68	86
Asia and the Pacific	510	1,524	1,934
World	926	2,446	3,104

Note: Projections based on table 24-1 but with deaths in 2000 and 2015 adjusted to account for age-specific COPD rate increases as experienced in the United States from 1960–85.
Source: See table 17-1; World Bank Population Projections 1987–88.

indirect morbidity costs (for example, lost wages), and indirect mortality costs (premature loss of life).

In hospital studies in China, patients with cor pulmonale had one of the highest average lengths of stay (thirty-six days in a middle-size hospital; forty-six days in a large hospital), and the disease ranked in the middle of all diseases in costliness to treat per episode (535 Chinese yuan, or about US$150, in a middle-size hospital; 795 yuan, or about US$210, in a large hospital), equivalent to 48 percent and 72 percent of gross national product per capita, respectively, for each patient's hospitalization episode (Chen Jie 1986). With regard to direct costs attributable to treatment, COPD seems sure to present a large burden on already underfinanced health systems in many developing countries. The indirect economic losses due to incapacity for work and premature death are almost certain to be higher. In China, COPD is estimated to account for about 2.5 million premature years of life lost annually (3.2 percent of the total premature years of life lost). Undiscounted, this would be roughly equivalent to losses of US$750 million annually, conservatively valuing each year of life lost at average per capita gross national product (World Bank staff estimates). Much further work in health economics and accounting needs to be done to quantify better the effect and costs of COPD, particularly losses and costs resulting from morbidity, to give public health leaders the facts they need to devise and defend an effective strategy for COPD prevention and case management. It seems clear, however, that both the present and prospective costs of COPD for developing countries are much higher than commonly realized.

Lowering or Postponing Disease Incidence

Clinical studies have shown that, once lung damage has occurred, cessation of smoking can only arrest the rate of further decline. Changes in ventilatory function that have occurred to that point are essentially irreversible. There are no known studies to show whether removal of risk from indoor (non-cigarette) smoke exposure or from outdoor smoke pollution has a similar, immediate, salutary effect, but it seems reasonable to assume so. Avoidance of exposure to smoke and other respiratory insults by patients suffering from ventilatory decline has been shown to reduce acute attacks, complications, and premature death.

Elements of a Preventive Strategy

The long incubation period of COPD and its silent, progressive, and irreversible nature require that prevention strategy be founded on very early, continuous primary prevention efforts. Prevention strategy must have two broad population targets: persons who do not yet have detectable signs of excess deterioration of lung function and persons who show early and moderate clinical signs of disease. Most persons in the former group will be children, young adults, and those adults who have not been long exposed to known risk. Persons in the second group will almost all be adults, most probably already in middle age (older than forty); their needs are discussed in the section entitled Case Management, below.

For the first group the strategy must aim at preventing or reducing the exposure to known and suspected risk factors. Elements of this strategy would appear to be four, in order of priority: broad and comprehensive tobacco smoking control programs; early and widespread health education programs for both the community and for primary-level health workers; a variety of investments and programs to reduce severe indoor air pollution, particularly in the home and among the poor; and limited, focused programs to reduce severe exposure to workplace or industrial air pollution. Good case management of other diseases may provide good primary prevention of COPD by the identification of children at increased risk. This can be determined by identifying children who suffer from frequent respiratory illness and who are failing in some way to grow and develop normally. Efforts need to be directed not only to caring for their respiratory illnesses but also, at a social level, to improving nutrition and reducing indoor smoke exposure—for example, by providing means to vent cooking stoves in the child's household. As the children get older and are in school, an integrated program of health education that emphasizes not smoking needs to be instituted.

Primary Prevention Strategy Elements

Because of the nature of these strategy elements, multiple agencies of government and of the community would need to be involved. In order of priority these would include the following:

- *Financial, planning, health, agriculture, industry, and commerce authorities*, who can provide the most important elements of a prevention strategy for COPD by adopting and implementing a cohesive tobacco smoking control program, probably consisting of at least the elements indicated in the next paragraph.

- *Community, religious, and other citizen groups*, which need to stimulate and cooperate with public health authorities to target women and their children who are subject to frequent respiratory infections. The range of their activities should include school, maternal and child health, family planning, and nongovernmental programs to improve childhood nutrition. Such action will build resistance to infection, a likely risk factor for impaired lung growth.

- *Urban and rural development and housing authorities*, who are responsible for, or who can influence, the design of homes and apartments to reduce indoor smoke.

- *Health authorities*, who must provide the epidemiological and professional inputs for targeting of risk groups, for continuing operational research into causes and effective interventions, and for the technical content of health education efforts.

- *Education authorities*, who must develop means and programs to ensure broad and early introduction of appropriate health education content as the influences of "modern," especially "prosmoking," images grow.

TOBACCO SMOKING. The main risk factor for development of COPD, tobacco smoking, is common to many of the other chronic noncommunicable diseases that are important causes of mortality and morbidity in the developing world. Neither the etiology of these diseases nor the basis for a preventive strategy are well understood in many government circles. Moreover, cigarettes are often associated with governmental revenue, powerful individuals in trade and commerce, and popular images of development and sophistication and are backed by sophisticated methods of propaganda to encourage the initiation of smoking. International experience with tobacco control shows the necessity for a comprehensive, prioritized approach of tax (price) increases and legislation and regulation of access to tobacco and of its advertising. Good epidemiologic surveillance, analysis, and effective forms of health education and publicity need to be aimed at creating a social environment supportive of cessation of smoking by individuals. The overall scope of these strategy elements goes far beyond the responsibility of any single government agency in any country and requires the informed attention and action of the highest political and community leadership in each country. Tobacco control efforts also will provide one of the only country-effective primary prevention strategies for lung, larynx, oral, esophageal, bladder, pancreatic, and kidney cancers. It will substantially reduce risks of coronary heart disease, stroke, fetal mortality and spontaneous abortion, prematurity, subsequent respiratory distress syndrome death, low birth weight, and subsequent infant morbidity. The implications of tobacco control mean that this difficult topic needs to be near the top of the health policy agenda in most countries.

INDOOR SMOKE EXPOSURE. Indoor smoke exposure is related both to fuels and their price and to housing styles and familial customs and expectations. Poor persons will generally be those most necessarily reliant on the cheapest and potentially most toxic fuels (wood, soft coal briquettes, and animal dung). They will also be those who are limited to the most simple housing designs and among whom social practices may dictate additional risk—for example, lack of ventilation, attributable to beliefs that windows may allow evil spirits to enter or to efforts to ward off insects, and customs requiring that women and young children, especially girls, spend considerable time indoors, often in the rooms in which cooking or heating fires are located. Substitution of cooking gas and kerosene for powdered charcoal briquettes, dung, and wood could help to reduce indoor air pollution, but problems of expense, distribution, and adaptation of customs will surely impede widespread implementation in many countries. Simpler, and likely cheaper solutions, such as reduction of indoor smoke exposure through better ventilation, seem likely to have a more significant effect on illness and premature death in the short and medium term.

Free access of girls to primary education may offer the best hope of strengthening their position in society and their capacity to bring about eventual change in social practices which put them at risk not only of respiratory illness but of other diseases and injuries as well.

OUTDOOR AIR POLLUTANTS. The less-than-clear causal link of outdoor air pollutants to chronic lung disease mediates against aggressive, expensive strategies solely on health grounds. Considerations of other aspects of environmental degradation and of other benefits from reductions in the levels of pollution will provide additional justification and perhaps contribute to better overall strategy formulation than if only COPD prevention aspects are considered. This expanded view would call for a coordinated strategy by economic, urban, housing, agricultural, forestry, educational, social, and health authorities to ensure that well-considered programs of better fuel utilization and atmospheric pollution reduction are developed. The prospects of these programs having salutary health effects are good, but the many other considerations call for a broad, multisectoral strategy.

Government programs to affect potential indoor and outdoor air pollution as a risk factor will be difficult to implement and may be costly if "alternative fuels" and housing reconstruction programs are given high priority. In conditions of poverty and restricted opportunity, resources needed for such programs may be more effectively used in other ways. Realistic strategies would seem to include concentrated antismoking efforts, coupled with well-financed health education programs to counsel nutritional, social, and behavioral changes which reduce the risk to the poor without adding to their economic burden. Social and health returns from this strategy are likely to be higher.

These efforts call for strong social and political leadership on the importance of tobacco control in the developing world together with substantial, sustained, and targeted public funding for health and social education for the poor—a goal which has proved virtually unattainable in even the richest of societies unless a national consensus is reached on the definition of problems and strong leadership effectively directs the focus of intervention. Examples are provided by earlier success in China, Sri Lanka, Kerala State in India, and in parts of Latin America with control of some endemic and infectious diseases, by the worldwide eradication of smallpox, and by the impending eradication of polio.

Case Management

The management of patients with COPD is complicated by the difficulties in defining when a subject becomes a patient. Most patients seek medical attention when they have sufficient difficulty from shortness of breath that it interferes with their activities of daily living. Persons with sedentary jobs may perceive themselves to be less affected by the disease than those who work at manual labor and may seek help later in the development of the disease. At present the only objective measure of disease is the degree of reduction of air flow and volume from the values expected by age, sex, and stature.

Case Management Strategies

Unfortunately, by the time lung function shows excessively rapid declines, the disease generally has progressed to a point at which most of the loss of lung function is permanent and will not be recovered with treatment. This is not to say, however, that treatment is not warranted. Treatment may shorten the duration of an exacerbation of symptoms and may prevent mortality. If the patients survive, however, they are returned only to their pre-exacerbation state, and then continue on an unrelenting downward course unless the putative risk factor (most often cigarette smoking) is removed.

Because little can be offered to patients with established disease, the most cost-effective method of case management requires the finding of and intervening in the natural history of the disease at a preclinical stage with simple and relatively inexpensive procedures that require neither highly trained technical personnel nor equipment (table 24-3).

Secondary Prevention

Secondary prevention requires health care providers to begin routinely to question patients about respiratory symptoms in a standardized manner and carry out simple measures of pulmonary function to identify those subjects at greatest risk of developing disabling lung disease. Antismoking efforts and reduced occupational dust exposure must be emphasized, particularly among those subjects identified as being at risk. Medical treatment of exacerbations requires smoking cessation on the part of the patient, the forcing of fluids, and the use of a broad spectrum of antibiotics. Only if symptoms persist or worsen does the patient need to go beyond the primary provider to a facility staffed by physicians, where the same treatments with the added opportunity for bed rest and fluid administration would be available.

Rehabilitation: Management of Exacerbations

Ideally, treatment of exacerbations of COPD depend both on severity of symptoms and clinical findings and level and severity of the obstructive components of the disease. For patients

Table 24-3. Case Management, Primary and Secondary Care

| Objective | Primary care | | Secondary care | |
	Diagnosis	Management	Diagnosis	Management
Secondary prevention	Positive findings of respiratory symptom questionnaire	Stop smoking	n.a.	n.a.
	Abnormally reduced lung function on simple pulmonary function testing (such as spirometry)	Reduce occupational dust exposure. Improve indoor ventilation.	n.a.	n.a.
Cure	n.a.	Cure not possible	n.a.	Cure not possible
Rehabilitation and treatment of exacerbations	Changes in symptoms (increased mucus secretion, breathlessness)	Stop smoking Administer fluids Use broad-spectrum antibiotics	Severe respiratory distress n.a.	Stop smoking Administer fluids
Maintenance care for chronic condition	Monitoring symptoms	Stop smoking	Response to bronchodilators	Trial of corticosteroids
		Improve indoor ventilation	n.a.	n.a.
	Rapid loss of pulmonary function	Breathing exercises	n.a.	n.a.
	Reduced activities of daily living			
Palliation	n.a.	None possible	Fluid retention	Home oxygen
			Severe shortness of breath	Ventilatory support in hospital only if patient has respiratory reserve
			Blood gases determination	

n.a. Not applicable.
Source: Authors.

with mild cases, removal of the inciting agent (cigarette smoking), hydration, and being kept warm may be sufficient to reduce morbidity from a given exacerbation. Antibiotics often are added to such a regime; however, the evidence is weak that they contribute substantially to shortening the duration of the exacerbation. In those patients with more severe disease, hospitalization and ventilatory support may be necessary for treatment of acute episodes. At some time during the course of severe disease patients should be given a trial of corticosteroids or at least a test of the degree of reversibility of their airways obstruction.

Because treatment has such little effect on the course of the disease the most important strategy in first dealing with patients with established disease is to remove existing risk factors. This would most certainly include requiring that the patient stop smoking; reducing or providing ventilatory protection from occupational dust and fume exposure, where possible; and reducing indoor smoke exposure.

Maintenance Care

Maintenance care is required for those patients with increasing development of disability. This can be monitored by the primary provider through evidence of increasing symptoms—"rapid" loss of pulmonary function and decreased activity in daily living. Again the treatment is to have the patient stop smoking and to teach the patient self-care strategies with breathing exercises and graded exercise training. Because a modest percentage of these patients will have or may develop a reversible component to their disease, an evaluation for reversibility should be carried out. This can be a relatively simple test of response to a bronchodilator with simple measures of pulmonary function before and after the test drug. A more formal test of response to a therapeutic trial of bronchodilator or corticosteroid lasting several weeks may be appropriate in some settings. The latter requires that the health care worker see the patient on several occasions and measure pulmonary function repeatedly.

Palliation

Palliation requires specialized treatment which in general has not been shown to have a significant effect on the course of the disease. Patients with severe fluid retention (cor pulmonale), severe shortness of breath, hypoxemia, and hypercapnia are at risk of immediate death. There are no cost-effective measures to deal with these conditions. Only life-saving treatment can be rendered, and it is only temporarily effective. Unless the prior physiologic state of lung function is known to have been at a level compatible with independent functioning, ventilatory support (up to and including assisted ventilation) is not warranted. On rare occasions in which blood gas determinations have been carried out and when local geography (for example, altitude) dictates, home use of oxygen may be required to support specific patients and may be affordable to some individuals (it cannot cost-effectively be included in

public programs as long as primary and secondary prevention efforts remain underfunded). It must be stressed that these measures have no effect on the natural history of the disease but serve to keep patients comfortable and functioning for whatever time they have.

These considerations, the costs of treatment, and the long period of disablement which often accompanies COPD before death strongly mediate in favor of effective primary prevention programs with substantial public funding. In most countries it has been extremely difficult to achieve a consensus in this regard. This seems to be at least partly attributable to the complex history and characteristics and multifactorial causes of the disease. The diffuse pattern of the disease burden in the community, the socioeconomic classes most affected, and the slow progression of symptoms have added to the problem of achieving a consensus of COPD as a disease priority. With better understanding in the last decade of the causes, diagnosis, appropriate classification, and importance and effectiveness of prevention in relation to treatment alternatives, this situation may begin to change.

Chronic obstructive pulmonary disease seems to be one of the chronic diseases for which broad, well-funded, targeted, primary prevention programs and health education should be adopted by government agencies. The efforts that seem likely to be most cost-effective are those provided in the context of regular primary health care and the frequent use of widespread, nonhealth mass media (for example, newspapers, television, and radio).

Priorities

A structured approach to progress in reducing the future burden of COPD morbidity and mortality requires prioritization in several key dimensions.

Priorities for Resource Allocation

The priorities of primary prevention programs, mainly smoking control but also low-technology, low-cost interventions to reduce exposure to suspected risks, especially among the poor, should be clear from the previous discussions. The limited effectiveness and high cost of attempts at secondary prevention and treatment and cure mean that these strategies will in most countries be options only for those who are relatively well off. Public financing to deal with COPD illness will be unaffordable for most countries and, if pursued, might only increase inequities of health service provision and detract from spending which should be allocated to primary prevention.

A number of priority research activities are suggested by the current state of knowledge about COPD and its effect in the developing world. Basic research should include both epidemiology and a number of clinical and biological questions. Collection of consistent age- and sex-specific morbidity and mortality data on COPD and its course in the developing world is needed to provide a better assessment of the magnitude and trend of the problem. In addition, given the uniqueness of some of the risks of respiratory disease to which people in developing countries are exposed, there are some questions which should be explored to investigate respiratory infection or illness as predisposing factors:

- How does nutritional status interact with the frequency, duration, and severity of acute respiratory infection in the first two years of life?
- Does the immune status (both passive and active) affect an infant's (less than two years old) or child's (age two to five) response to a viral or bacterial respiratory infection?
- What is the relation between these early life infections and eventual development of COPD?

Similar questions can be applied to other unique environmental settings—for example, in the villages in Nepal, where cold and high altitude interact with soft coal and biomass fuels to produce high levels of indoor air pollution, or in Mexico City, where altitude, weather, and high temperature interact with auto exhaust to produce high levels of ozone.

Sociobehavioral Research

Sociobehavioral research on the determinants of effective COPD health education programs (social marketing) that are focused specifically on the young, on women, and on rural populations provide another area in which research may yield important findings. Subject matter to be covered by health education could include both disease-specific information and primary prevention messages. The importance of early secondary prevention efforts can be conveyed to family members to encourage them to help those who are already at risk to take steps to stop progression of the disease. Smoking control policies provide a second important topic of research in the sociobehavioral field.

Educational Research

Educational research in both pedagogy and effectiveness of curricula for in-service training of health workers, and medical education curricula for new doctors and health workers, could include specific emphasis on the epidemiology and importance of COPD to developing countries, and on the importance of primary prevention as the basis for health care strategy. Primary school health education programs need to develop and test programs which stress healthy lifestyle practices that children can relate to in a positive way.

Priorities for Operational Research

Priorities would appear to include at least the following topics:

- Determination of the COPD risk attributable to both indoor and outdoor air pollution in developing countries

- Approximation of the attributable risk of the synergistic interaction of exposure to general smoke and to tobacco smoke, for both the smoker and the nonsmoker
- Determination of effective modes and health education messages to convey the risks and causes of COPD to different social groups in developing countries
- Cross-national epidemiologic studies to confirm and quantify better the burden which COPD poses for the poor and for women in particular

In addition, because the exposure to risk factors seems to be so high in rural areas and the population at risk is so large, it may be that the greatest marginal return to national expenditure on air pollution control will be with low-technology strategies in rural areas rather than, for example, through the purchase of high-technology emission controls for fossil-fueled power plants. In the near term, the most cost-effective means of achieving a reduction in human exposure may well be a concentration on the traditional rather than the modern sectors of the economy. Research to understand better the priorities and advantages of this strategy may yield useful insights.

These conclusions must remain speculative until further work is done, however, and this points to the overall need for much better operational research on the cost-effectiveness and cost-benefits of COPD prevention and treatment. Today we should, but cannot yet, analyze quantitatively the cost-effectiveness of alternative interventions to prevent and treat COPD. Neither can we quantify how expenditure on COPD prevention and the outcomes of it compare with the costs and effects of other health interventions. Data to permit detailed analyses of these kinds do not yet exist. We can only broadly assess some of the main factors which would determine the results of such analyses.

From an overall cost and benefit perspective, the distribution of COPD mortality among relatively older people will mean that many future potential years of life saved by COPD prevention are retirement years or the years close to them, even in developing countries. The long periods of disability preceding death which characterize COPD would mean that effective prevention and case management efforts could preserve productivity, minimize dependency, and postpone or avoid completely the expensive phases of treatment of COPD.

From a public health perspective, efforts to treat COPD seem likely to be hopelessly cost-ineffective compared with primary prevention aimed at the main known risk factors. Rehabilitation, maintenance, and palliative care for individual patients have no public health benefits. Because morbidity will already be substantial in most patients when they first seek medical attention, loss of some productivity will have already occurred, and economic benefits will thus also be limited. In comparison, early secondary prevention can arrest further morbidity, preserve productivity, and reduce or at least postpone expenditure for treatment. If conducted in a primary health care setting, opportunistic screening through simple questioning of those suspected of having COPD, followed by spirometry, should allow rapid, low-cost finding of suitable candidates for intensive counseling, job change, house or work ventilation improvement, or bronchodilator therapy (listed in descending order of their probable cost-effectiveness).

It is less clear, however, that the cost-effectiveness of early secondary prevention would compare favorably with that of primary prevention. It seems probable that priority should be given to primary prevention for three reasons. First, most primary prevention efforts for COPD will have an effect on other chronic and communicable diseases. Second, the main risk for COPD in the future appears certain to be cigarette smoking. School and public educational campaigns and workplace and regulatory programs are known to be low cost and many have proved effective. Third, among the most effective tools for smoking reduction are taxes and fees attached to the sale of tobacco to help reduce demand for cigarettes, particularly among vulnerable low-income groups and youth. It would not be unreasonable to expect that all primary prevention efforts for smoking-related diseases could be fully funded from tobacco taxes and thus be highly cost-effective, even profitable, from a public health perspective.

Operational research in these areas to quantify better the characteristics and patterns of the costs of COPD morbidity and mortality, and the benefits of avoiding or minimizing these costs, is clearly needed and would help to establish and underpin effective programs to deal with the disease.

Notes

During his experience as a Hubert H. Humphrey North-South Fellow at Johns Hopkins University, Sanjoy Ghose of the Urmul Rural Health Research and Development Trust (Bikaner, Rajasthan), participated in the early stages of research and conceptualization of this chapter. His contributions, enthusiasm, and dedication are gratefully acknowledged.

1. The classification of these conditions has changed several times with revisions of the *International Classification of Diseases*. These changes reflect better understanding of the disease and its forms but make cross-national and longitudinal data analysis very difficult. Good analysis of COPD mortality and morbidity has probably been adversely affected by the classification changes and their subsequent, gradual, adoption in various national cause-of-death reporting systems.

2. The mechanism appears to be an inability to neutralize the activity of protease normally occurring in the respiratory tract.

3. The China data reported are for a 9 million population sample widely distributed across the country and are only for cor pulmonale, death from right-sided heart disease, which in the normal cause-of-death reporting for China would include most patients with long-standing respiratory insufficiency which had culminated in deterioration of the circulatory system. This category excludes tuberculosis, pneumonia, pneumoconiosis, byssinosis, and silicosis. It also excludes deaths diagnosed as respiratory disease for unspecified causes. Inclusion of these deaths would raise the reported rates by about 75 percent in most age groups.

4. Traditional tobacco smokers elsewhere are known to be at risk. In a study in rural India, "reverse chutta" smokers experienced high rates of COPD. "Reverse chutta" smoking involves consuming home-grown tobacco rolled in a semidried leaf with the lighted end inside the mouth during inhalation. Chronic bronchitis was diagnosed in 33 percent of the chutta smokers; a high, 24 percent, prevalence was found in those age thirty-one through forty years; and of those older than forty-one, a remarkable 49 percent prevalence of

bronchitis was observed. Chronic airways obstruction also was found to be frequent with significant reductions in FEV1 values (Malik, Behera, and Jindal 1983).

5. A billion is 1,000 million.

References

Alderson, M. R. 1967. "Data on Sickness Absence in Some Recent Publications of the Ministry of Pensions and National Insurance." *British Journal of Preventive Social Medicine* 21:1–6.

Anderson, D. O., B. G. Ferris, and R. Zickmantel. 1964. "Levels of Air Pollution and Respiratory Diseases in Berlin, New Hampshire." *American Review of Respiratory Diseases* 90:877–87.

Becklake, M. R., J. Bourbeau, R. Menzies, and P. Ernst. 1988. "The Relationship between Acute and Chronic Responses to Occupational Exposures." In *Current Pulmonology*, Vol. 9, Chapter 2. London: Year Book Medical Publishers, Inc.

Carnow, Bertram W., Robert M. Senior, Robert Karsh, Stanford Wessler, and Louis V. Avioli. 1970. "The Role of Air Pollution in Chronic Obstructive Pulmonary Disease." *JAMA* 214(5):894–99.

Chaulet, P. 1989. "Asthma and Chronic Bronchitis in Africa: Evidence from Epidemiologic Studies." *Chest* 96(Supplement 3):334s–39s.

Chen Jie. 1986. Paper prepared for the World Bank by Shanghai Medical University, Department of Health Management and Economics.

Clifford, Peter. 1972. "Carcinogen in the Nose and Throat: Nasopharyngeal Carcinoma in Kenya." *Proceedings of the Royal Society of Medicine* 65(8): 682–86.

Colley, J. R. T., and D. D. Reid. 1970. "Urban and Social Origins of Childhood Bronchitis in England and Wales." *British Medical Journal* 2:213–17.

Commission of the European Communities. 1975. "Researchers on Chronic Respiratory Disease." Medical Symposium 18. Luxembourg.

Cooreman, J., S. Redon, M. Levallois, R. Liard, and S. Perdrizet. 1990. "Respiratory History during Infancy and Childhood, and Respiratory Conditions in Adulthood." *International Journal of Epidemiology* 19(3):621–27.

Deane, M., J. R. Goldsmith, and D. Quma. 1965. "Respiratory Conditions in Outside Workers." *Archives of Environmental Health* 10:232–331.

Densen, P. M., E. W. Jones, H. E. Bass, and others. 1967. "A Survey of Respiratory Disease among New York City Postal and Transit Workers." *Environmental Research* 1:265–86.

Dockery, D. W., C. S. Berkey, J. H. Ware, F. E. Speizer, and B. G. Ferris, Jr. 1983. "Distribution of Forced Expiratory Volume in One Second in Children 6 to 11 Years of Age." *American Review of Expiratory Disease* 128: 405–12.

Eriksson, S. 1965. "Studies in Alpha 1-Antitrysin Deficiency." *Acta Medica Scandinavica* 177 (Supplement 432):1–85.

Ferris, Benjamin, Jr. 1973. "Chronic Bronchitis and Emphysema: Classification and Epidemiology." *Medical Clinics of North America* 57(3):637–49.

Gold, Diane, I. B. Tager, S. T. Weiss, T. Tosteson, and F. E. Speizer. 1989. "Acute Lower Respiratory Illness in Childhood as a Predictor of Lung Function and Chronic Respiratory Symptoms." *American Review of Respiratory Disease* 140:877–84.

Holland, Walter W. 1983. "Evidence for the Implication of Environmental Factors in the Aetiology of Chronic Bronchitis." *Zeitschrift Erkrank. Atm. Org.* 161:130–37.

Holland, Walter W., and D. D. Reid. 1965. "The Urban Factor in Chronic Bronchitis." *Lancet* 2:445–48.

Holland, Walter W., D. D. Reid, R. Seltser, and others. 1965. "Respiratory Disease in England and the United States." *Archives of Environmental Health* 10:338–43.

"Incapacity for Work." 1966. *British Medical Journal* 8:61–62.

Indonesia, Ministry of Health Statistics. 1984. Jakarta.

Lambert, P. M., and D. D. Reid. 1970. "Smoking, Air Pollution, and Bronchitis in Britain." *Lancet.*

Lawther, P. J., R. E. Waller, and M. Henderson. 1970. "Air Pollution and Exacerbations of Bronchitis." *Thorax* 25:525–39.

Malik, S. K., D. Behera, and S. K. Jindal. 1983. "Reverse Smoking and Chronic Obstructive Lung Disease." *British Journal of Diseases of the Chest* 77:199–201.

Nepal: His Majesty's Government/WHO (World Health Organization). 1987. Geneva: Management Group Report.

Palmer, K.N.V. 1954. "The Role of Smoking in Bronchitis." *British Medical Journal*, 1473–74.

Pandey, Mrigendra Raj. 1984a. "Domestic Smoke Pollution and Chronic Bronchitis in a Rural Community of the Hill Region of Nepal." *Thorax* 39:337–39.

———. 1984b. "Prevalence of Chronic Bronchitis in a Rural Community of the Hill Region of Nepal." *Thorax* 39:331–36.

Peters, J. M., and B. G. Ferris. 1967. "Smoking and Morbidity in a College-Age Group." *American Review of Respiratory Diseases* 95:783–89.

Peto, Richard, F. E. Speizer, A. L. Cochrane, F. Moore, C. M. Fletcher, C. M. Tinker, I. T. T. Higgins, R. G. Gray, S. M. Richards, J. Gilliland, and B. Norman-Smith. 1983. "The Relevance in Adults of Air-Flow Obstruction, But Not of Mucus Hypersecretion, to Mortality from Chronic Lung Disease." *American Review of Respiratory Diseases* 128:491–500.

Reid, D. D., D. O. Anderson, B. G. Ferris, and others. 1964. "An Anglo-American Comparison of the Prevalence of Bronchitis." *British Medical Journal* 2:1487–91.

Reid, D. D., and A. S. Fairbairn. 1958. "Air Pollution and Other Local Factors in Respiratory Disease." *British Journal of Preventive Social Medicine* 12:94–103.

Rogan, J. M., M. D. Attfield, M. Jacobsen, S. Rae, D. D. Walker, and W. H. Walton. 1973. "Role of Dust in the Working Environment in Development of Chronic Bronchitis in British Coal Miners." *British Journal of Industrial Medicine* 30:217–26.

Saha, N. C., and S. K. Jain. 1970. "Chronic Obstructive Lung Disease in Delhi: A Comparative Study." *Indian Journal of Chest Diseases* 12(1/2):40–51.

Samet, M., I. B. Tager, and F. E. Speizer. 1983. "The Relationship Between Respiratory Illness in Childhood and Chronic Air-Flow Obstruction in Adulthood." *American Review of Respiratory Diseases* 127:508–23.

Smith, Kirk R., A. L. Aggarwal, and R. M. Dave. 1983. "Air Pollution and Rural Biomass Fuels in Developing Countries: A Pilot Village Study in India and Implications of Research and Policy." *Atmospheric Environment* 17(11): 2343–62.

Speizer, F. E., and I. B. Tager. 1979. "Epidemiology of Chronic Mucous Hypersecretion and Obstructive Airways Disease." *Epidemiologic Review* 1: 124–42.

Tager, I. B., S. T. Weiss, A. Muñoz, B. Rosner, and F. E. Speizer. 1983. "Longitudinal Study of Maternal Smoking on Pulmonary Function in Children." *New England Journal of Medicine* 309:8699–703.

USAID (U.S. Agency for International Development). 1987. Review of Jamaica Health Sector.

USDHHS (U.S. Department of Health and Human Services). 1982. *Tenth Report of the Director, Ten-Year Review and Five-Year Plan.* Vol. 3, *Lung Diseases.* NIH Report 84-2358. National Heart, Lung, and Blood Institute, Washington, D.C.

U.S. Surgeon General. 1984. *The Health Consequences of Smoking: Chronic Obstructive Lung Disease.* U.S. Department of Health and Human Services, Washington, D.C.

Yan, Bi-ya. 1989. "Epidemiologic Studies of Chronic Respiratory Diseases in Some Regions of China." *Chest* 96 (Supplement 3):339s–43s.

Wynder, E. L., F. R. Lemon, and N. Mantel. 1965. "Epidemiology of Persistent Cough." *American Review of Respiratory Diseases* 92:679–700.

25

Injury

Sally K. Stansfield, Gordon S. Smith, and William P. McGreevey

Injuries are too often referred to as "accidents," suggesting that such events are random and have causes not within our control. On the contrary, injuries occur with definable patterns which help to identify risk factors and thereby imply strategies for prevention. Injury control, including reduction of the frequency, severity, and consequences of injury, can reduce the growing burden of injury in the developing world (Smith and Barss 1991). Already one of every four to nine persons suffers a disabling injury each year in developing countries, and it is estimated that 2 percent of the world's population is currently disabled as a result of injury (WHO 1986).

In developing countries, injury is frequently viewed as an inevitable consequence of technological change and economic development. In the view of both business and the community, short-term economic gains often outweigh the cost of death and disability from injury. Because they are socioeconomically and politically disadvantaged, people in developing countries live daily with a risk of injury which would be unacceptable in industrial nations. As emphasized in the recently adopted "Manifesto for Safe Communities," this "inequality in the safety status of an individual in developing and developed countries is of concern to all countries" (WHO 1989a, p. 7).

The heterogeneity of the mechanisms and effects of injury has interfered with awareness of its public health importance and thereby hampered the development of comprehensive programs to address this important health problem. Yet as injury emerges as the leading cause of death in more and more countries, there is a growing demand for the development of national and international programs for injury control.

Definitions

Physical injury is caused by an acute exposure to damaging energy (mechanical, electrical, thermal, or chemical) or by the sudden absence of essentials (such as the lack of oxygen in drowning, or heat in hypothermic injury). The study of injury focuses on the acute effects and long-term disability resulting from the acute injury; therefore it does not include delayed or indirect effects of chronic exposure, such as those from carcinogenic chemicals (Waller 1985; Robertson 1992). Important,

though often neglected, are the "adverse psychological and social consequences" (WHO 1989a, p. 5) of such injurious events as rape or child abuse.

It is important to distinguish the "pathological outcome" of an injurious event from its mechanism, or "external cause." Figure 25-1 is a schematic drawing of the chain of events of injuries; the drawing also emphasizes that opportunities for *prevention* of injury depend on (a) reduction of the probability of an injurious event (through risk reduction) and (b) reduction of the severity of injury (through alteration of the nature of the event). In contrast, *case management* depends on (c) reduction of the consequences of the injury (through altering the pathological outcome) once that injury has occurred. Haddon (1980) referred to these three "phases" of injury control as "pre-event," "event," and "post-event."

Injuries are categorized by both their *external cause* (E-codes, which describe the injurious event) and by their *pathological outcome* (N-codes, which describe the nature of the injury) in the WHO *International Classification of Diseases* (WHO 1977). In table 25-1 we list the pathological outcomes most commonly associated with selected injurious events (external causes).

Figure 25-1. *Chain of Injury Events and Opportunities for Injury Control*

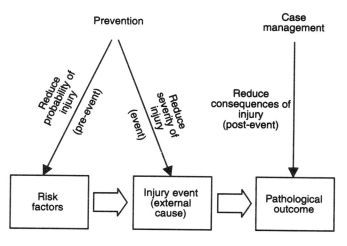

Source: Authors' data.

Table 25-1. Pathological Outcomes Commonly Associated with Injury Events in the Developing World

Injury event	Type of injury	Infectious complications
Fire	Burn and thermal injury	Yes
	Anoxic injury	Yes
Electric shock	Burn and thermal injury	Yes
Collision	Crush and deceleration injury	Yes
	Abrasion and laceration	
	Dislocation and fracture	
Fall	Crush and deceleration injury	Yes
	Abrasion and laceration	
	Dislocation and fracture	
Assault	Abrasion and laceration	Yes
	Dislocation and fracture	
	Anoxic injury	
Submersion (drowning)	Anoxic injury	Yes
Poisoning	Toxic injury	No

Source: Authors' data.

Different preventive strategies are also implied by the further categorization of the external cause of injury as *unintentional* or *intentional* (homicide, other assaults, and suicide). Reflecting the increasing recognition of the preventability of injury, the term "unintentional injury" has been preferred to "accidents" (Langley 1988).

Risk Factors

Just as specific pathological outcomes are seen more commonly with certain injurious events, each injurious event is commonly associated with specific risk factors. Some of the main risk factors for the injurious events prevalent in developing countries are shown in table 25-2. The importance of each of these risk factors varies, however, for each external cause of

injury and according to local patterns of transport and of domestic and occupational activities.

Demographic characteristics which are determinants of exposure to risk of injury include gender, age, occupation, and socioeconomic status. The behavior patterns of males place them at higher risk for most injuries (burns are one of the exceptions; see Taket 1986), and there is a trend of increasing difference between males and females with increasing age. Infanticidal deaths are, however, more common among female children.

Adolescents and younger adults, who already sustain more injuries than others, further increase that risk with alcohol use. For example, persons between the ages of sixteen and twenty-four drive approximately 20 percent of the total vehicle miles traveled in the United States, yet they account for 42 percent of the alcohol-related fatalities (NHTSA 1988). Although there is less such information from developing countries, it appears that the patterns are similar (Wyatt 1980; Sinha, Sengupta, and Purohit 1981). Age also affects the case-fatality ratio, or the risk of mortality once an injury has been sustained, with increased mortality observed among both the very young and the very old (Waller 1985; Baker and others 1992).

The poor suffer disproportionately from homicide, assault, pedestrian fatality, and burn injury fatality. The death rate from unintentional injury is also twice as high in low-income areas as in high-income areas of the United States (NRC/IOM 1985). Similar patterns are evident in developing countries, especially in poor urban areas. The demands of economically and politically underprivileged groups for safe products, working environments, and communities are less likely to meet with success. Psychologic disorders, such as substance abuse, violence (toward both self and others), isolation or withdrawal, and depression, are also more commonly found among populations marginalized by poverty. These disorders, along with the risky behaviors associated with lack of safety education, all predispose people to injury.

In addition to affecting people's exposure to risk of injury, socioeconomic status often alters the case-fatality ratio once the injury occurs (Baker, O'Neill, and Karpe 1984), in part because of variation in access to definitive surgical care. In

Table 25-2. Selected Risk Factors Associated with Events in the Developing World

Risk factor	Injury event						
	Fire	Electric shock	Collision	Fall	Assault	Submersion (drowning)	Poisoning
Male sex	No	Yes	Yes	Yes	Yes	Yes	No
Age							
Under 15	Yes	No	No	Yes	No	Yes	Yes
15–64	No	Yes	Yes	No	Yes	No	Yes
65 or older	No	No	No	Yes	No	No	No
Low socioeconomic status	Yes	No	No	No	Yes	No	No
Hazardous products	Yes	Yes	Yes	Yes	Yes	Yes	Yes
Alcohol use	Yes	No	Yes	Yes	Yes	Yes	Yes
Psychologic disorders	Yes	No	No	Yes	Yes	Yes	Yes
Poor safety education	Yes	Yes	Yes	Yes	No	Yes	Yes

Source: Authors' data.

lower socioeconomic groups both the children (who are often poorly supervised) and their parents (who must often take greater occupational risks) have a higher frequency of both fatal and nonfatal injury. In their study of an urban slum in Rio de Janeiro, Reichanheim and Harpham (1989) found an association between children's injury and maternal marital status, maternal stress or depression, and mothers' work outside the home.

Among the substance abuse disorders, alcohol consumption represents the main avoidable risk for injury. In the United States, alcohol-related mortality (ARM) accounts for 4.5 percent of deaths from all causes (CDC 1990). Unintentional injury accounts for 28.7 percent of all ARM and more than half of all years of potential life lost (YPLL) before age sixty-five. Intentional injury accounts for 16.8 percent of all ARM and 29.1 percent of all YPLL before age sixty-five. Of fatally injured motor vehicle drivers in 1987, 38 percent were intoxicated (blood alcohol concentration greater than 0.10 percent), a decline from 44 percent in 1982 (NHTSA 1988).

Like the other lifestyle features which accompany economic development, alcohol abuse and its adverse health effects are beginning to be recognized for their importance in developing countries (Edwards 1979). Although the per capita consumption of alcohol in industrial countries has decreased or at least remained stable, it is clearly on the increase in most of the developing world. The total availability of alcoholic beverages in developing countries has increased by 146 percent since the early 1960s (Kortteinen 1988). Per capita consumption and the fraction of annual income spent on alcohol have both increased each year since 1978 in Singapore (Curry 1989).

Even more dramatic are the data from the rural Kisii District of Kenya, where Bittah, Owola, and Oduor (1979) documented that up to 27 percent of randomly selected males and 24 percent of females met the WHO criteria (WHO 1952) for alcoholism. Nearly half of male and one-quarter of female heads of households in a Nairobi slum have been categorized as alcoholics (Nielsen, Resnick, and Acuda 1989). In addition to predisposition to alcohol-related disease and mortality, including that from injury, these families are characterized by worsening economic status, higher rates of separation and divorce, other psychiatric disorders, and premature mortality among both the adults and their children.

The role of alcohol and other drug use in predisposing people to injury in the developing world is also only beginning to be documented (Patel and Bhagwatt 1977; Jacobs and Sayer 1983). In addition to limited awareness among health and law enforcement professionals of alcohol as a risk factor, the lack of technology for blood or breath alcohol measurements is a constraint to further definition of the problem (Ryan 1990). In Papua New Guinea, where a few studies have been conducted, one-third to more than half of fatally injured drivers were found to be legally intoxicated, and 69 to 90 percent of fatally injured pedestrians were found to have blood alcohol levels above 80 milligrams per 100 milliliters (Wyatt 1980; Sinha, Sengupta, and Purohit 1981).

Although there are few studies even in industrial countries, alcohol is also a risk factor for nonvehicular injuries (Wechsler, Kasey, and Thum 1969; Dietz and Baker 1974; Davis and Smith 1982; Mierley and Baker 1983; CDC 1984; Pleuckhahn 1984; Smith and Kraus 1988). For example, alcohol abuse underlies more than one-fifth of nonvehicular trauma deaths in urban areas of Papua New Guinea (Sinha, Sengupta, and Purohit 1981; Attah Johnson 1989). Alcohol and other drug abuse is known to be a growing problem which has undoubtedly been widely underestimated in developing countries (Edwards 1979; Wyatt 1980; Weddell and McDougall 1981), and its importance needs to be further characterized by epidemiologic research.

Injurious Events

The severity of injuries and the case-fatality rate from them depend largely on their cause. Specific external causes and groups at risk for injury vary widely among countries by level of industrialization and by occupational and cultural practices. Because of the lack of surveillance systems or population-based studies, there is limited information available about injury frequency, risk groups, mechanism, and outcome. Much of the information that has been developed regarding the epidemiology of injury has been descriptive, based on hospital data rather than more reliable community-based studies.

Unintentional Injuries

Fatal injuries in the developing world most often result from motor vehicle collisions, burns, poisonings, drownings, and falls (Manciaux and Romer 1986; Taket 1986; Smith and Barss 1991). As in the industrial countries (Barancik and others 1983), the leading causes of injury deaths are usually not the same as the most prevalent causes of nonfatal injuries. For example, drowning is a frequent cause of death but an infrequent cause of nonfatal injury due to its high case-fatality ratio. The main causes of nonfatal injuries include laceration by cutting and piercing instruments and interaction with animals, in addition to minor motor vehicle collisions and falls. Each of the most important mechanisms of injury are discussed below; data are included from developing countries regarding risk factors as they may pertain to the selection of intervention strategies.

MOTOR VEHICLE COLLISIONS. Among injuries resulting in death, those due to motor vehicle crashes are emerging as the most important for people between the ages of five and forty-five in many developing countries (Jacobs and Sayer 1983; Lourie and Sinha 1983; Mohan and Bawa 1985; Ezenwa 1986a, 1986b). In some countries, particularly the oil-producing countries in which the number of vehicles and roads are rapidly expanding, motor vehicle collisions rank first among causes of death for all ages (Bayoumi 1981). Mixed traffic, which may include trucks, buses, automobiles, motorcycles, mopeds, rickshaws, bicycles, and pedestrians, all moving at different speeds, clearly predisposes people to collision and injury. Pedestrians and drivers of two-wheeled vehicles are at especially high risk in developing countries, accounting for more than half of all fatalities (WHO 1987b).

Mortality rates per vehicle in Ethiopia and Nigeria in 1978, for example, were fifty times higher than in the United States or United Kingdom (Jacobs and Sayer 1983). Where the use of motor vehicles is rapidly increasing, mortality related to them is also increasing, as has been observed in Thailand, Papua New Guinea (a fourfold increase from 1969 to 1978) (Wyatt 1980), and Malaysia (a fourfold increase in the five years preceding 1975) (Silva 1978). Similar trends have been noted in Latin America and Africa. As development increases further and safety improves, the mortality per vehicle or per mile traveled typically decreases, although the rate per 100,000 population may continue to increase because of increasing exposure.

BURNS AND FIRES. Burns are most prevalent among women and children, with the great majority occuring in domestic environments (Sowemimo 1983; Bang and Saif 1989; Jamal and others 1989). In Lagos, for example, more than half (56.2 percent) of the burn injuries occurred among children less than fifteen years of age. Mortality ranges from 6.7 percent to 35 percent among patients admitted to hospitals (Datey, Murthy, and Taskar 1981; Sowemimo 1983; Bang and Saif 1989; Jamal and others 1989). Burns caused from 15 to 45 percent of all injury deaths seen in three hospital centers in India (Datey, Murthy, and Taskar 1981), where fatality rates among hospitalized patients range up to 35 percent.

In many countries, burns are most commonly sustained by women who work over open stoves or cookfires (Saleh and others 1986; Gupta and Srivastava 1988) and are a significant cause of death for women of childbearing age. Fatal burns in Kanpur, India, occur primarily among young Hindu housewives, whose unintentional burns are frequently attributed to open cookfires or overturning stoves and their loose, highly inflammable clothing. Approximately half of the women who suffer fatal burns, however, are intentionally burned or forced to commit suicide, most often in association with marital disharmony (Gupta and Srivastava 1988). Untreated epilepsy has also been shown to be a risk factor for burns in several studies (Subianto, Tumada, and Margono 1978; Barss and Wallace 1983).

Cigarette smoking, a frequent cause of house fires and death due to burn injuries in the United States (Mierley and Baker 1983; Technical Study Group 1987), needs to be investigated for its role in developing countries as a risk for burn injury and death (Smith and Barss 1991). The prevalence of cigarette smoking, currently on the increase in the developing world, will likely continue to increase as cigarette manufacturers face contracting markets in many industrial countries.

POISONING. In many developing countries, poisoning has emerged as a significant cause of death (Smith and Barss 1991). Local industry and agricultural practices often determine the epidemiology and causes of poisoning. Traditional healing practices also account for the patterns of acute poisoning in some countries (Joubert and Mathibe 1989). The majority of cases occur among children (Gaind, Mohan, and Ghosh 1977; Banerjee and Bhattachariya 1978) and agricultural workers (Hayes 1980; Jeyaratam, Senevirante, and Copplestone 1982); however, suicide accounts for many of the deaths among adults.

In Sri Lanka in 1978, for example, the more than 1,000 deaths from pesticide poisoning alone greatly exceeded the 572 deaths from polio, diphtheria, tetanus, and pertussis combined (Jeyaratam, Senevirante, and Copplestone 1982). The United Nations Children's Fund estimates that up to 2 million pesticide poisonings and 10,000 deaths from such poisonings occur annually (UNICEF 1989); however, recent reports from the Philippines suggest that these figures may represent a substantial underestimate (Loevinsohn 1987). Recent evidence also suggests that subacute poisoning and chronic disability may result from continuous low-level exposure. Eighty to 90 percent of pesticide poisonings are caused by highly toxic preparations which account for only 4 to 5 percent of pesticide use (Xue 1987). That developing countries account for more than half of all acute pesticide poisonings and 80 to 99 percent of all deaths from such poisonings, despite their using only 20 percent of the world's pesticide (WHO 1987a; Xue 1987), also indicates that this is an area for intervention.

Accidental ingestion of kerosene is a prominent cause of poisoning among children (Ramesh, Srikanth, and Parvathy 1987; Joubert and Mathibe 1989), most typically when it has been stored in soft drink bottles or other inappropriate containers. An important cause of death in a number of countries is carbon monoxide poisoning, often from motor vehicle exhaust or heating systems, such as those used in Korea, in which hot combustion gases circulated under floors may leak into homes (Lee and others 1971).

Inappropriate use of medications is emerging as an important cause of toxic ingestions, particularly in urban areas. For example, in a recent report from Pakistan, Bhutta and Tahir (1990) describe nineteen cases of loperamide hydrochloride (Imodium) poisoning, of which at least six deaths were a result of inappropriate marketing and use of this antimotility agent for childhood diarrhea.

DROWNING. Ponds, irrigation ditches, and wells in developing countries represent the danger of drowning for young children. In Brazil, drowning occurs most often among children between ten and fourteen years of age and is second only to motor vehicle collisions as a cause of death among these children (de Mello and Bernardes-Marques 1985). In many countries in Asia, drowning is the primary cause of injury death (Ng, Chao, and How 1978; Meade 1980; Selya 1980; Gu and Chen 1982; Kleevens 1982). Many of the deaths among young adults aged fifteen through twenty-four may represent suicide, drowning being a preferred method in Asian countries (Ng, Chao, and How 1978). Drowning is probably underestimated as a cause of death in many countries because so few cases ever reach the hospital or are reported to police (Smith and Barss 1991).

FALLS. Injury from falls is most prevalent in occupational settings, among young boys, and, where larger such populations exist, among the elderly. Falls from roofs and trees, especially during the harvesting of fruit, are among the most important causes of fatal and nonfatal injury (Barss, Dakulala, and Doolan 1984). The burden to society of these injuries is substantial, particularly in view of the high incidence of paraplegia resulting from spinal cord injury. In Hong Kong, falls accounted for 32 percent of all trauma patients who were discharged from the hospital, and hospitalized patients alone accounted for a reported rate of 416 cases of fall injuries per 100,000 per year prior to 1979, a figure even greater than that for motor vehicle accidents (Kleevens 1982).

OTHER UNINTENTIONAL INJURIES. Animals, bicycles, and cutting tools are additional important instruments of injury in most developing as well as industrial countries (Smith and Barss 1986, 1991), imposing a considerable burden on the health system. Gordon, Gulati, and Wyon (1962) found that 13 percent of injury deaths in rural India were linked to infectious complications of such minor injuries, suggesting that many deaths could be prevented by simple interventions such as proper wound care and tetanus immunization. Permanent disability resulting from ocular trauma, which is responsible for 2.4 percent of all bilateral blindness in Nepal (Schwab 1990), represents another important preventable loss of productivity.

Manmade disasters, such as the chemical leak in Bhopal and the meltdown at the nuclear plant at Chernobyl, underline the importance of chemical agents and nuclear energy in human injury (Bertazzi 1989). These and the natural disasters, such as droughts, earthquakes, and floods, frequently crystallize local and international response more effectively than the less catastrophic but more common causes of injury death. Yet the more than 5,000 reported disasters in the last two decades have affected more than 2.3 billion lives and resulted in more than 4 million deaths (CRED 1991), most of which are due to injury. These episodic calamities remind us periodically of the greater toll of injury in settings where capacity is limited to predict, prepare for, and respond to such events.

OCCUPATIONAL INJURY. Injuries sustained in the workplace, primarily impact and overexertion injuries, are more frequent and perhaps more severe in the developing world. The death rate for factory workers in India, for example, is 50 percent higher than that in the United States (Mohan 1982). The injury rate among coal miners in Nigeria is seven times that for the same occupational group in Britain (Asogwa 1980). In Brazil during 1970, nearly 18 percent of industrial workers were injured (Pupo Nogueira 1987). More than a quarter of industrial workers in Mexico experience a disabling injury each year (Cuellar 1980). The injury of workers in Sri Lanka occurs at a rate of 1,000 per 1,000 or one for every worker per year and

results in permanent disability in 25 percent of cases (Krishnarajah 1972).

Intentional Injury

Distinction among injuries by motive has little import for case management; however, it has clear implications in the selection of preventive strategies. Suicide, homicide, and genocide (including war) are important causes of injury for which preventive strategies must be identified. Terrorism and torture are threats or acts designed to coerce individuals or groups, often resulting in long-term social and psychological injury. Rape and child abuse also inflict psychological injury which can be considerably more disabling than any associated physical injury. More dramatically than in any other cause of injury, males are most commonly the actors in such interpersonal and intergroup violence. Women and children are frequently the victims (Chelala 1990). Locally important factors predisposing people to intentional injuries, such as poverty, racism, social isolation, and drug and alcohol abuse, should be investigated as risk factors (Rosenberg and others 1987).

Criminal homicide represents a significant proportion of injury deaths in many parts of the world. For example, homicide rates of 8.2 per 100,000 population are observed in Latin America; comparable figures are 6.7 for the Caribbean, 4.7 in North Africa and the Middle East, and 2.3 per 100,000 in Asia. Such intentional interpersonal injury is most prevalent in urban areas throughout the world. In the area surrounding Bangkok, for example, homicides are the leading cause of death due to injury, accounting for 27 percent of injury mortality (WHO 1987a). The mortality rate associated with firearms was less than 1 per 100,000 in the United States in 1980; it was nearly 30 per 100,000 in São Paulo, Brazil, in 1984. In neighboring Colombia, the homicide rate per 100,000 inhabitants rose from about 20 in the early 1970s, before drug trafficking became such an important problem, to more than 50 in 1987 (Losada Lora and Velez Bustillo 1988).

Suicide is also probably more important than is suggested by currently available statistics. In Sri Lanka, for example, suicide is the most common cause of injury death, with organophosphate pesticide poisoning a frequent method of choice (Sri Lanka Psychiatric Association 1982; Berger 1988).

The importance of armed combat as a cause of injury morbidity and mortality cannot be ignored. Since 1980, forty-five countries have been involved in forty wars with more than 4 million soldiers globally. More recent wars are tragically distinguished by the occurrence of the majority of the mortality (80 to 90 percent) among civilians, most of whom were women and children. More than 1 million people have perished in Uganda alone during the last twenty years of political unrest. For every death, three times as many people sustain a nonfatal injury (Werner 1987). The more indirect effect of such strife on health status—diversion of national resources to defense from health care—has been pointed out by Ogba (1989) in Nigeria and Chelala (1990) in Central America.

The Public Health Significance of Injury

Worldwide, injury ranks fifth among the leading causes of death, accounting for 5.2 percent of the total mortality (Manciaux and Romer 1986) and 10 to 30 percent of all hospital admissions (WHO 1988). One review of global survey data has suggested that one child in every five to ten sustains an injury each year (Manciaux 1984). A summary of global age-specific patterns of mortality from injury and poisoning is presented as table 25-3. We developed these estimates and projections using the methodology outlined by Alan D. Lopez in chapter 2 of this collection.

Current Levels and Trends in the Developing World

Injury morbidity in developing countries is more difficult to ascertain, because of the lack of adequate community-based studies of injury (Smith and Barss 1991). Data collection regarding the incidence of milder injury is further hampered by the absence of a consistent case definition for injury or disability. In the United States, it is estimated that 1 in 4 people suffer injuries requiring medical attention each year, and 1 in 3 have a day of restricted activity or required medical attention (Collins 1985). The definition of the severity of injuries as either requiring hospitalization or outpatient medical attention is useful for defining the burden to the health system in industrial countries. Such case definitions, however, will clearly record many fewer cases of similar severity in countries in which medical care is less available.

MORBIDITY AND MORTALITY LEVELS, ABOUT 1985. Nearly 3 million deaths are reported from injury and poisoning annually; two-thirds of these occur in the developing countries (WHO 1989c). In many industrial countries, injuries are now the leading cause of death during the first half of the human life span (Baker, O'Neill, and Karpe 1984), and they are becoming one of the leading causes of death and disability in developing countries (Wintemute and others 1985). Because of the greater toll taken by injuries among the work force and younger age groups, however, their importance to the public health is best recognized when measured as years of potential life lost, a reflection of premature mortality.

Although prospective, population-based studies of injuries in developing countries are rare, Gordon, Gulati, and Wyon (1962) demonstrated a low incidence of disabling (that is, causing disruption of normal activity) injury of 111 per 1,000 people per year in eleven very rural Indian villages in 1959. Gordon, Gulati, and Wyon's definition of "injury" as that resulting in short- or long-term disability will be a less sensitive measure of injury morbidity, although this is probably the best definition where medical care is not universally available. In a community-based survey of children in an urban slum of Rio de Janeiro, Reichanheim and Harpham (1989) documented that 30 percent of the children had been injured within the last fifteen days; 85 percent of them were treated at home.

The rates of nonfatal injury in developing countries are probably as high as or higher than those observed in the industrial world. Data from the United States suggest that for every fatal injury there are 16 hospitalizations and almost 400 injuries serious enough to restrict activity or require medical treatment (Rice and others 1989). It is likely that there are also several hundred nonfatal injuries for every fatal injury in developing countries. Because of the lack of available survey methods for identifying and quantifying disability, the real economic and social effect of these injuries is unknown.

TRENDS IN THE PERIOD 1970 TO 1985. Observation of trends in the epidemiology of injury in developing countries raises the question of the relationship between development and injury. Omran (1971) pointed out that developing countries move through an "epidemiologic transition," from a disease profile dominated by infectious diseases to one characterized by the "posttransition" noncommunicable health problems, including injury. This transition is brought about through development-associated evolution in three important determinants of the pattern of disease: (a) changes in demographics due to changes in fertility and mortality rates, (b) changes in the prevalence of infectious disease resulting from improved control and reduced incidence, and (c) changes in risk factors resulting from technological and social change.

Demographic changes (such as the shift in age structure and urbanization) have had an effect on the epidemiology of injury primarily through an increase in the incidence of injuries which are more prevalent among the elderly (such as falls) and in urban environments (such as motor vehicle collisions). Reduction in the prevalence of infectious diseases during the past fifteen years has resulted in a growth in the relative importance of injury because it has typically emerged as the most important cause of death for ages one to forty-four.

In many rapidly industrializing countries of the developing world, the absolute injury mortality rates have also grown rapidly. With development have come technological and social changes which alter the risk of injury. These changes have the potential to affect the incidence of injury either adversely (such as through increased hazards or increased risk-taking behaviors) or beneficially (such as through safer products and behaviors). In most developing countries to date, however, these changes in environment and lifestyle have exacerbated rather than ameliorated the problem of injury.

For example, Selya (1980) describes this trend in Taiwan (China), where from 1960 to 1977 unintentional injuries rose from the seventh to the third leading cause of death, and the absolute injury mortality rate increased from 38.9 to 57.2 per 100,000 population. In Shanghai County, China, injuries have already emerged as the leading cause of death for people between the ages of one and forty-five (Gu and Chen 1982).

The increased motorization of transportation in developing countries is perhaps the best-documented example of the unintended negative consequences of technological change. The explosion in the number of roads and vehicles

Table 25-3. *Estimated Global Mortality from Injury and Poisoning (by Region, Age, Sex, and Year)*
(per 100,000)

Population	1970 Male	1970 Female	1985 Male	1985 Female	2000 Male	2000 Female	2015 Male	2015 Female
World								
Under 1	96	84	95	78	78	62	68	50
1–4	99	85	67	57	47	35	43	30
5–14	31	14	28	13	26	11	23	10
15–44	100	22	92	22	86	20	79	19
45–64	124	32	115	31	111	28	107	27
65 and older	216	153	201	140	202	144	205	151
Industrial countries								
Under 1	78	30	63	24	44	19	38	16
1–4	363	312	112	109	28	26	19	20
5–14	24	3	17	2	13	2	11	1
15–44	63	11	53	11	47	8	39	6
45–64	88	28	74	25	84	21	81	20
65 and older	224	188	191	151	209	167	208	168
Nonmarket countries								
Under 1	81	45	86	45	62	36	58	28
1–4	64	49	52	43	45	22	44	25
5–14	32	11	27	10	23	6	22	4
15–44	105	20	88	18	84	14	74	11
45–64	137	33	116	31	116	29	114	27
65 and older	230	155	217	156	208	157	213	155
Latin America and the Caribbean								
Under 1	68	52	101	67	68	47	61	39
1–4	67	44	87	61	45	32	44	23
5–14	32	13	32	14	23	10	22	8
15–44	119	24	105	25	86	21	80	18
45–64	157	35	147	36	114	30	110	29
65 and older	258	133	263	152	206	144	204	151
Sub-Saharan Africa								
Under 1	141	126	118	103	99	84	83	66
1–4	74	60	71	56	55	41	50	35
5–14	50	22	42	19	35	15	28	13
15–44	133	26	120	25	108	24	97	23
45–64	149	33	138	32	129	32	123	31
65 and older	210	118	204	120	200	121	199	121
Middle East and North Africa								
Under 1	110	105	103	93	88	74	76	59
1–4	54	47	60	52	48	37	43	31
5–14	36	19	30	14	27	13	23	10
15–44	113	30	103	24	96	23	85	21
45–64	135	34	133	32	124	32	114	30
65 and older	197	110	208	130	202	129	195	127
Asia								
Under 1	94	91	91	82	75	63	66	50
1–4	65	59	58	49	46	36	43	31
5–14	29	15	27	13	25	12	23	11
15–44	104	24	96	24	90	23	81	20
45–64	131	32	124	32	117	30	110	29

Source: Lopez, chapter 2, this collection..

in Saudi Arabia has been associated with an increase in both morbidity and mortality (nearly 600 percent) due to motor vehicle crashes (Ergun 1987; Ofosu 1988). In Thailand, where the motor vehicle mortality rate has increased almost 30 percent each year (Punyahotra 1982), injuries have risen from sixth to first among all causes of death since 1947 (Choovoravech 1980). Motor vehicles alone were responsible for more years of potential life lost than tuberculosis and malaria combined.

The social changes which accompany development have also generally led to an increase in the frequency of injury in developing countries. With the rapid introduction and diffusion of new technologies, they are frequently used without concern for their safety. For example, in India the grain mills were mechanized without appropriate protective shields over drive belts, resulting in an increase in the incidence of severe injury (Gupta, Bhasin, and Khanka 1982). The economic benefits of mechanization of industry or transportation are seen as greater than the cost of injury or death that may result from the inappropriate use of these technologies. The large underclasses found in developing countries, who are virtually denied access to the wealth of the dominant group, have little to lose by high-risk behavior. Hopelessness in the face of poverty, racism, social isolation, and drug and alcohol abuse does not encourage the investments necessary to improve safety or health.

Possible Morbidity and Mortality Patterns: 2000 and 2015

Still, development may be accompanied by technological and social changes that raise income and improve the equity of its distribution. Studies have confirmed that safety is considered a normal good, the demand for which rises with income (Peltzman 1975). The development of a complex institutional structure (including legislation, enforcement, insurance and litigation services, and complex capital markets) helps to reduce the incidence of injury by forcing implementation of safety measures. Such social organization also applies disincentives to the creation or maintenance of hazards by forcing those who do so to compensate the victims of resulting injuries. Individuals and industry may thereby be coerced to reduce injury risks to the larger community if there is public support for such social change.

Mechanization associated with development may reduce the incidence of injury if it reduces the interaction between people and machines or replaces more hazardous methods. In Nigeria, for example, mechanization of a coal mine was associated with a 60 percent reduction in mining injuries as well as a reduced severity of those injuries (Asogwa 1988). In São Paulo, Brazil, in 1970, nearly 18 percent of industrial workers suffered a work-related accident; with increasing mechanization the incidence was reduced to 3.8 percent by 1984 (Pupo Nogueira 1987). Improved traffic safety and occupational injury control measures in the United States resulted in reductions in injury mortality on the road and in the workplace after industrialization had initially brought about increases

(Chesnais 1985). Rising then declining injury rates from motor vehicles, such as those seen in São Paulo, Brazil, during the quarter century beginning in the 1960s (Haight 1980), will likely be observed. Similar trends may be expected in other developing countries as the demand for safety increases.

Growing prominence of alcohol and drug abuse often accompanies economic development. So few developing nations have begun to recognize or address this problem that it will likely worsen before abuse control measures are instituted. The relative lack of mechanisms to implement legislation, taxation, or treatment and rehabilitation for the control of alcohol and drug abuse will also probably hamper efforts to control the associated injuries.

The increasing availability of firearms is likely to increase intentional injuries throughout the world. Global expenditure for arms continues to rise, already exceeding $1 trillion dollars annually. Arms transfers to developing countries exceeded $52.7 billion from the United States alone in 1987. There will be, however, tremendous resistance to any international action to halt this lucrative trade in an effort to contain intergroup and international violence.

The currently increasing use of pesticides in agriculture will be associated with an increased risk of poisonings unless the higher exposure can be offset by stringent safety controls and replacement of the more hazardous agents with safer alternatives. Successful implementation of other injury control measures would be expected to interrupt the worsening trends in injury incidence on the road, in the workplace, and in the home. In those countries which have begun to address the potential hazards associated with technological and social development, such as in Europe and North America, the absolute rates of injury mortality have already begun to fall (Baker and others 1992).

Economic Costs of Injury

The annual medical and social costs of injury are estimated to exceed $500 billion worldwide (WHO 1989a). Injuries are responsible for up to one-third of all hospital admissions (WHO 1989a). In addition to costs for emergency services, tremendous costs are incurred in continuing care, rehabilitation, and lost productivity due to both death and disability. It is estimated that the cost of injury treatment in the United States in 1985 was approximately $317,000 for each fatality, $34,000 for each hospitalization, and $500 for each injury not requiring hospitalization (Rice and others 1989). It has been estimated that the cost of injuries from motor vehicle collisions alone amounts to nearly 1 percent of the gross national product of many developing countries. Thailand, however, estimates that the cost of these injuries is more nearly 2 percent of the gross national product, not including the costs of the long-term disabilities (WHO 1987b).

Because of its high toll among the younger age groups, injury is the main cause of years of potential life lost in industrial countries. In the United States, for example, injury accounts for 40.8 percent of YPLL, at an estimated cost of $158 billion per year for both fatal and nonfatal injury (Rice and others 1989). The relative economic importance of injury in developing countries such as Egypt is even greater, where it accounts for 78 percent of YPLL and 10 to 30 percent of all hospital admissions (WHO 1988).

Disability, both temporary and permanent, resulting from nonfatal injury is perhaps the most important, yet often overlooked, cost of injury. There are few studies which quantify such disability in developing countries. In the United States, disability from injury results in a loss of normal activity for an estimated 3 days per person per year (Smith and Kraus 1988). In a study in Sri Lanka, Krishnarajah (1972) showed that the disability which resulted from industrial injuries accounted for annual losses of 1.6 million working days. The World Health Organization (WHO 1986) estimates that 13 percent of the world's population is disabled and that at least 15 percent of these disabilities result from injury. These data suggest that of 78 million persons (2 percent of the world's population) disabled because of injury, most live in developing countries, where disabilities frequently become handicaps because of the lack of appropriate rehabilitation services.

Although little such cost data are available from the developing world, in a study in northeast Brazil, DeCodes, Baker, and Schumann (1988) assessed the direct and indirect costs of various categories of illness. Although injuries accounted for only 11.8 percent of all direct costs of disease or injury, they accounted for 27.5 percent of indirect and 25.5 percent of total costs. Most (68.7 percent) of the total injury costs accrue from disability-related losses in productivity, whereas approximately a quarter (25.3 percent) of the costs are from loss of life. In figure 25-2 we compare these findings by DeCodes, Baker, and Schumann to the analogous figures for respiratory diseases.

The costs of lost productivity and medical care for injury are often exceeded by costs of property damage, insurance, and other nonmedical items. Researchers who conducted a survey of five developing countries (Turkey, Thailand, and three African countries) between 1961 and 1971 found that damage to vehicles and property accounted for 60 to 87 percent of the costs resulting from vehicle crashes (Jacobs and Sayer 1983; Baudouy 1989). In no case did medical costs exceed 9 percent of the cost of crashes. Medical attention and subsequent disability payments account for only one-fifteenth of an estimated $1.5 billion in annual traffic-accident costs in Brazil (Airton Fischmann, personal communication, 1988).

Lowering the Incidence and Severity of Injury

As emphasized in figure 25-1, the opportunities for prevention of injury lie in alteration of the risk factors (to reduce the probability of injury) and of the injurious events (to reduce the severity of injury). The strategies designed to reduce the consequences of injury are discussed later, in the section on case management.

Figure 25-2. Direct and Indirect Costs of Injuries and Respiratory Diseases

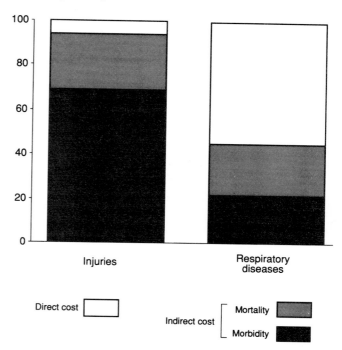

Source: DeCodes, Baker, and Schumann 1988.

Elements of Preventive Strategy

Of the risk factors for injury incidence and severity included in table 25-2, those most amenable to change include alcohol use, unsafe behaviors due to poor safety education, and poor product design. For each of the interventions designed to reduce these risks, we summarize in table 25-4 calculations of expected disability-adjusted life-years (DALYs) gained by the prevention of injuries from motor vehicles, falls, burns, and toxic substances. The derivations of the estimates and calculations in table 25-4 are described in appendix 25A.

Candidate preventive interventions should be assessed for their expected cost and effectiveness prior to implementation. Proposed interventions may then be assigned a priority by a multidisciplinary body of community members and experts in injury control, which must include persons familiar with local sociocultural constraints. For example, Calonge (1987) has identified six factors for consideration in selecting an intervention strategy for injury control: (a) demonstrated efficacy in reducing injuries; (b) demonstrated effectiveness when implemented; (c) public acceptance; (d) ease of implementation considering political, economic, and logistic barriers; (e) level of personal commitment required; and (f) cost-effectiveness. A sample semiquantitative framework for assigning priorities to interventions for reduction of injury from motor vehicle collisions is provided in table 25-5.

The strategies for implementing preventive interventions include: engineering; legislation, regulation, and litigation;

Table 25-4. Effectiveness of Interventions for Injury Control in Developing Countries

Demographic and intervention parameters	Transportation injury	Fall injury	Burn/fire	Poisoning
Demographics				
Incidence (per 100,000)	665	2,000	600	100
Case-fatality ratio (percent)	1.7	0.2	1.0	6.0
Average age at onset	30	30	10	10
Morbidity (life-years lost) per injury	0.22	0.03	0.86	0.01
DALYS lost	3,098	1,278	13,438	180
Preventive interventions				
Alcohol taxation				
Reduction in incidence (percent)	30	26	34	8
DALYS gained	929	332	4,569	14
Product/environmental improvements				
Reduction in incidence (percent)	70	50	70	80
DALYS gained	2,169	639	9,407	144
Behavioral change				
Reduction in incidence (percent)	40	40	50	40
DALYS gained	1,239	511	6,719	72
Case Management interventions				
Acute care improvement				
Reduction in case-fatality ratio (percent)	50	50	60	60
Reduction in disability (percent)	50	50	86	60
DALYS gained	1,549	639	11,557	108
Rehabilitation care				
Reduction in disability (percent)	70	70	70	70
DALYS gained	2,169	909	9,407	126

Source: Authors' data.

taxation and other economic incentives; and education. The effectiveness of an injury control program will depend not only on the effectiveness of the intervention (seat-belt use *does* reduce injuries), but also on the effectiveness of the mechanisms used to promote or implement that intervention (health education in the absence of supportive legislation and enforcement, for example, has not been effective in changing patterns of seat-belt use; see Robertson and others 1974).

ENGINEERING. Perhaps the most effective injury control strategies are those that alter the design of environmental features (such as roads) or equipment to reduce or eliminate the risk of injury. Such passive interventions, which do not rely on changes in volitional behavior, are generally more likely to be effective than those that require the active participation of the individual to reduce injury risk. Air bags, for example, which inflate automatically in a motor vehicle crash will provide passive protection even of occupants who fail to wear seat belts.

Manufacturers seeking to limit costs of improving product safety frequently argue that customers should be given the freedom to choose less expensive products without added safety features. This issue is raised in both industrial and developing countries. The difficulty, however, of ensuring individual "informed consent" to the risks of using unsafe products and the costs to the society that are imposed by injuries must be considered by governments in establishing policy.

LEGISLATION, REGULATION, LITIGATION. Because of the failure of corporations and industry to regulate themselves in matters of product safety, it becomes incumbent upon governments to provide requirements or incentives to protect their citizens. Powerful industry lobbies are often formed to resist such efforts. For example, U.S. legislators concerned with safety have been unable to ban the use of additives in cigarettes that enhance their burning, although such a ban would help to prevent the house fires which claim more than 2,300 lives annually in the United States (Smith and Barss 1986; Technical Study Group 1987). Some legal and regulatory strategies have been more effective in altering injury frequency and severity. Legislation or regulation in the mid-1970s to improve automobile safety (for example, through design standards for brakes, door locks, restraints, fuel systems) is credited with saving 9,000 lives annually (Robertson 1981). Most of these interventions were actually developed by industry itself but were not implemented initially because of short-term cost considerations.

In industrial countries, litigation or the fear of it has led to increasing corporate responsibility for providing safer workplaces and products (Teret and Jacobs 1989). In the United States, for example, some states have strict product liability laws that impose penalties if injuries occur that could have been prevented through use of state-of-the-art safety designs (Robertson 1983). Although litigation may be an important means of injury control in the United States, its applicability in developing countries is likely to be limited for the near future.

Table 25-5. Sample Programs for Control of Injury from Motor Vehicle Collisions

Phase	Intervention	Expected impact	Acceptability	Feasibility/ Enforceability	Low cost	Priority
Pre-event	Adopt the 1975 UN guidelines for issue and validity of driving permits, with periodic visual screening of drivers	+ +	+ +	+ +	+ +	3
	Initiate vehicle registration requirements, with periodic inspection for safety features	+ +	+ +	+++	+ +	3
	Limit dangerous vehicles (such as motorcycles over 250 c.c.) through taxation or import restrictions	+++	+++	++++	++++	2
	Require imported vehicles to have padded dashboards, anti-lacerative windshields	++++	++++	++++	++++	1
Event	Establish and enforce speed limits	++++	+ +	+++	+ +	2
	Identify and improve "black spots" or hazards; divide highways	++++	++++	++++	+ +	1
	Create pedestrian and bicycle-segregated traffic areas	++++	+ +	+ +	+++	3
	Modify roadways through towns to ensure slowing of traffic	++++	+ +	+++	+ +	3
	Improve roadside lighting	+ +	++++	+	+	4
	Mandate and enforce use of seatbelts and child restraint systems in passenger vehicles	++++	+++	+ +	+++	2
	Mandate and enforce use of crash helmets and daytime headlights for motorcycles	++++	+++	+++	+++	2
	Provide basic emergency care training for police, public transport drivers, and others likely to be first at scene	++++	+++	++++	+++	2
Post-event	Train primary health care workers in injury diagnosis and primary management, including use of local materials for collars, splints, and stretchers	++++	++++	++++	+++	1
	Coordinate local communications and transport resources to provide emergency transport to trauma centers	+++	+++	+++	+++	2
	Regionalize and upgrade trauma care in urban centers	+++	++++	+++	+	2
	Improve or develop community-based rehabilitation services, including training and referral resources at regional trauma centers	++++	++++	+++	+++	2

+ Low, ++ moderate, +++ high, ++++ very high.
Source: Authors' data.

TAXATION AND SUBSIDY. Taxes and other economic incentives have been used creatively to reduce injury frequency and severity. Reductions in insurance rates for vehicles equipped with airbags, for example, have been used to promote their selection by consumers and thereby reduce the severity of injury in motor vehicle crashes. Taxes on the use of private vehicles combined with subsidies of safer modes of transportation (such as trains and buses) can help to shift transportation preferences and reduce injury because all forms of mass transportation experience much lower death rates than do private vehicles for the same number of miles traveled (Baker and others 1992).

Taxation has been particularly effective in modulating behaviors such as alcohol use. Alcohol sales and consumption have been shown to be elastic such that price increases through taxation effectively reduce consumption (Cook 1981). A recent study estimated that a tax of approximately 35 percent on the retail price of beer in the United States would eliminate half the alcohol-related fatalities, and a 50 percent tax would eliminate approximately 75 percent of these deaths (Phelps 1988). There is evidence to suggest that consumers in developing countries may be even more responsive to price changes (Warner 1990), and excise taxes have already been successful in reducing cigarette consumption in Papua New Guinea (Chapman and Richardson 1990).

Because most of the alcohol consumed in developing countries is produced indigenously, it is frequently argued that state monopoly systems should be instrumental in preventing alcohol abuse. Although the feasibility of control over traditional, noncommercial alcohol production and consumption must be considered, the potential profit (as well as public health benefits) of state taxation and control of alcohol should provide incentives for adopting national preventive policies. Successful state control cannot be implemented, however, without public support and stable political conditions. If national alcohol policy is not viewed as a reflection of the society's attitudes, black market trade in alcohol quickly emerges, undermining national control and revenues.

Successes have been achieved in the Gambia, for example, where 90 percent of alcohol is consumed as palm wine (made from the sap of the trees); fees are collected for the license to tap the palm trees and for distribution to the local markets

(Kortteinen 1989). The economic significance of trade in palm wine in rural areas is immense and represents an opportunity for governments to provide disincentives for alcohol abuse through taxation and to finance other costs of alcohol abuse prevention or treatment with the revenue generated.

The availability of highly dangerous products may also be shaped by economic incentives through the use of import duties. Although duties on the import of every potentially dangerous product may raise the cost of doing business and retard economic growth, a more targeted strategy could limit injury frequency and severity without hampering development. For example, commercial interest in the importation of more dangerous technologies might be altered in favor of safer products by imposing a tax on imports which is proportional to the risk of injury. The structure of duties could be adjusted to encourage import, for example, of less toxic pesticides or safer cookstoves. Control or even elimination of the importation of many products (such as handguns or other firearms), could probably be more effective in developing countries than it is in industrial countries because local production is more limited.

EDUCATION. Education is frequently advocated to effect changes in environmental and behavioral factors which alter risk of injury, yet there is little evidence to support the effectiveness of such interventions, even in the industrial world. The most promising results have been achieved with educational interventions which are intended to prompt a single behavior (such as installation of smoke detectors) rather than sustained behavior change (such as seat-belt use or reduction in alcohol use; see Robertson and others 1974; Miller and others 1982). Training workers in safe work habits has been shown to reduce the risk of injury, although the behavior changes were not sustained for long periods after that training (Margolis and Kroes 1975). It may be pointed out that the generally lower level of knowledge about safety in many developing countries may leave more room for gains to be made through education. Educational interventions have been most effective, however, when used in support of legislative, taxation, or engineering interventions, to increase their acceptability (National Committee for Injury Prevention and Control 1989).

Good Practice and Actual Practice: Are There Gaps?

Injury has not been recognized as a preventable public health problem worthy of allocation of resources proportionate to its importance. It is demonstrated in figure 25-3, for example, that research funding for cancer in the United States is more than twenty-one times that for injury when compared on the basis of preretirement years of life lost (NRC/IOM 1985). Moreover, the research information vacuum created by the historical lack of resources has been used to explain continuing neglect of the injury problem. In recent years, however, in both industrial and developing countries, injury control has been given higher priority than it had previously.

An additional obstacle to the development of comprehensive preventive programs has been the inherent need for interdisciplinary and multisectoral action for injury control. Although the health sector might best take the lead, health ministries rarely have had the inclination or power to coordinate the multiple disparate groups necessary to plan and implement the necessary environmental, policy, and behavioral changes. Agencies responsible for public health; curative and rehabilitative health care; legislative affairs; public policy; criminal justice; sociologic, psychiatric, and anthropologic investigation; occupational hazards (including agricultural pesticides); regulation of alcohol and drug use; education; and transportation safety must all be coordinated to ensure a comprehensive preventive strategy.

Despite these obstacles, many developing countries have made significant progress in strengthening injury prevention. Eleven of thirty-two developing countries in a recent survey (WHO 1989c) have established a coordinating body for injury prevention or traffic safety. Many have also established strategies for planning and financing research and injury control activities. The World Health Organization's Injury Prevention Programme provides assistance to member countries in the planning and implementation of national injury control programs.

For example, countries such as Nigeria have begun to recognize the need for national policy to address the growing problem of alcohol-related injury. Odejide, Ohaeri, and Ikuesan (1989, p. 235) have called for policy reform, including "legislation on age limit for purchasing or drinking alcohol in public places; legislation on drunk driving behavior; control of alcohol advertising and period of sale; provision of breathalizer equipment in hospitals; provisional law enforcement agents; and massive education on the issue."

Although many preventive technologies have been developed in industrial countries, there is no reason to believe that most would not be applicable in developing countries. Many proven preventive measures are not costly, yet they have not been adequately exploited to reduce injury frequency and severity in the developing world.

For example, the 27 percent reduction in passenger car deaths observed in the United States from 1965 to 1985 (despite a near doubling of mileage exposure) would probably be reproducible in many developing countries (Ezenwa 1986b). This success was attributed to improved roads (National Safety Council 1986) and progress in making passenger vehicles more crash-worthy (Campbell 1987). The decline in motor vehicle mortality observed in São Paulo, Brazil, since 1980 has also been ascribed to multiple preventive interventions, including better control of driving speeds, greater police surveillance, improved traffic engineering, and placement of more footbridges over principal thoroughfares (de Mello and Bernardes-Marques 1985).

Seat belts are infrequently used in most developing countries, although they might be expected to reduce the risk of fatality by 43 percent (Evans 1986) and serious injury by 40 to 70 percent in motor vehicle crashes (SAE 1984) on the basis of

Figure 25-3. Preretirement Years of Life Lost Annually and Federal Research Expenditures for Major Causes of Death, United States

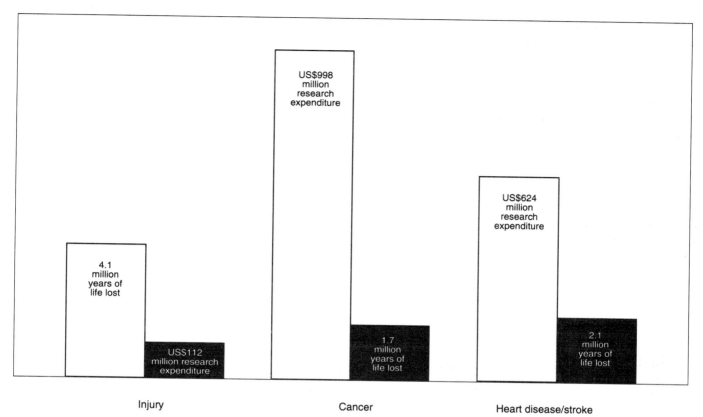

Source: NRC/IOM 1985.

the experience in the United States. In Singapore, a seat-belt law accompanied by education and law enforcement efforts have already successfully reduced motor vehicle injuries (Chao, Khoo, and Poon 1984).

Other legislative interventions which have been effective in industrial countries and would be of benefit in developing countries include laws requiring motorcyclists to use helmets and to have their headlights on at all times (Muller 1982; Zador 1983). The repeal of a mandatory helmet law in Texas was followed by a 73 percent increase in fatalities and 20 percent increase in injuries associated with motorcycle accidents. The high incidence of crash injury and mortality among motorcycle riders in developing countries also suggests that such laws concerning helmet and headlight use may be effective. Even in India, where cultural traditions restrict helmet use, studies showed that turbans offer partial protection from head injury (Sood 1988).

Evidence suggests that reducing the flammability of clothing (such as by using a borax rinse) and its looseness may be expected to reduce morbidity and mortality from burn injury (Durrani 1974; Durrani and Raza 1975; McLoughlin and others 1977). Improved design and safer use of stoves and lamps would also be expected to reduce burn injury (Auchincloss and Grave 1976; Lee 1982; Wintemute and others 1985). Epilepsy

is frequently associated with burns and drownings, suggesting that better treatment could reduce the incidence of injuries in persons with poorly controlled seizure disorders (Buchanan 1972; Pearn, Bart, and Yamaoka 1978; Subianto, Tumada, and Margono 1978; Sonnen 1980; Barss and Wallace 1983).

There is an urgent need to apply already existing preventive strategies, such as reducing availability of dangerous drugs, use of childproof caps, and proper storage of toxic substances, to reduce poisonings in developing countries (Oliver and Hetzel 1972; Baker, O'Neill, and Karpe 1984). Information from developing countries suggests that regulation and education to reduce inappropriate use of medications and other poisonings by better packaging and labeling, addition of emetics or stenchants, and restriction of the availability of highly toxic preparations would also be expected to reduce morbidity and mortality (Mowbrey 1986; Choudry and others 1987).

In Zimbabwe, for example, 34 percent of agricultural workers working with dangerous pesticides reported they had received no safety instruction, and 38 percent believed that pesticide containers could be reused for other purposes, such as storing food or drinking water (Bwititi and others 1987). A program to reduce pesticide poisonings in China through regulation, education, and other preventive measures resulted in a reduction in incidence of more than 98 percent, despite a nearly thirteenfold increase in the use of pesticides during the same period (Shih and others 1985).

Studies from industrial countries show that legislation mandating adequate fencing, together with self-closing, self-locking gates, around swimming and other pools of water can prevent most toddler drowning deaths (Milliner, Pearn, and Guard 1980). Improved supervision and enclosure of small ponds, wells, and drainage canals in residential areas in developing countries would also be expected to reduce drowning deaths among children (Gordon, Gulati, and Wyon 1962; Nixon, Pearn, and Dugdale 1979; Thapa 1984).

Other examples of proven technologies which are underused include safety guards to prevent hair or clothes from being caught in drive belts (Gupta, Bhasin, and Khanka 1982). The important problem of injury due to falls must be addressed using locally appropriate strategies. For example, use of the new, shorter hybrid varieties of tropical trees such as mango and oil or coconut palms would undoubtedly prevent many serious injuries in areas where these products are prominent. Falls from rooftops, windows, or into wells can clearly be prevented by appropriate design modifications or barriers.

Regulations for safe workplace conditions and regular inspections can clearly reduce injuries. In Brazil, a 79 percent reduction in the proportion of industrial workers suffering accidents between 1970 and 1984 has been ascribed to legislation regarding the protection of workers (Pupo Nogueira 1987).

For criminal assault, homicide, and suicide, limiting access to the means, such as firearms and medications, is likely to be the most effective means of prevention. The evidence from the United States and Canada suggests that the reduction of the availability of weapons which inflict fatal injury would be effective in reducing the incidence of homicide and suicide (Sloan and others 1988). Elimination of carbon monoxide from the coal gas in Birmingham, England, resulted in a 50 percent reduction in suicide deaths (Hassall and Trethowan 1972). Selection of effective strategies to prevent homicide, suicide, and genocide (including war) must also clearly take cultural factors into account.

The prevention of arms sales to countries at war is one strategy that would be effective if international cooperation could be achieved. Yet the barriers to rational public health policy for the prevention of war are great. Werner (1989) poses the key question: Has the huge arms industry been created in the service of national security, or has the national security paranoia been created in the service of the arms industry? Industry's pressures upon governments and governments' pressures upon international agencies may explain the otherwise incredible neglect of this important public health problem.

Case Management

Although preventive strategies to control injury primarily seek to alter the external causes of injury, case management interventions act to limit or reverse the pathological outcome of injuries. It is the extent or character of the pathological out-

come which generally guides case management decisions. Decisions in the transport or care of the injured must also consider the mechanism or external cause of injury, however, because this clinical history may be the sole clue to serious injury which is occult or late in manifestation.

Elements of the Case Management Strategy

Deaths due to trauma in the industrial world have been described by Trunkey (1983) as occurring in three periods after the injury. "Immediate" death, occurring within an hour of the injury, is generally the result of massive injury. "Early" deaths are defined as those occurring one to three hours after the injury, are generally from internal or other bleeding, and are regarded as being preventable through early, good quality, medical and surgical care. The "late" deaths occur days to weeks after the injury and are generally due to infectious complications or multiple organ failure. Trunkey estimates that more than half of the trauma deaths in the United States are immediate, and approximately 30 percent are early. In the developing world, however, it appears that many more deaths occur in the early and late periods, suggesting that considerable death and disability might be prevented through improvement in the quality of care and transport.

Five major factors are linked to the outcome of care for the injured: the severity of the injury, the age of the injured individual, the preexisting health status of the injured individual, the time elapsed from injury to definitive care, and the quality of care. Therefore, once an injury is sustained, the strategies available to reduce morbidity and mortality through improved case management are improvement in the quality of care, improvement in the emergency transport system, or both.

IMPROVED QUALITY OF CARE. The overall excess case-fatality ratio of injuries sustained in the developing world also suggests room for intervention through improved case management (WHO 1988). There is evidence that modern treatment techniques can reduce mortality rates of burn victims (Demling 1985) and that early and effective rehabilitation of such victims can reduce disability (Sinha 1984). Many needless deaths are caused by preventable complications of minor injuries, such as bleeding and infection. Gordon, Gulati, and Wyon (1962) found, for example, that three of twenty-three (13 percent) deaths from injury were from infections following the injury. There is little information on the cost-effectiveness of improving the quality of care. Because these interventions would depend largely on training existing health professionals, however, the expense would likely be minimal.

Even at the community level, appropriate first aid may reduce the consequences of injury. Although there are few prospective studies of the effectiveness of such basic care, not many people would doubt the beneficial effect of controlling hemorrhage, cleansing wounds, or stabilizing fractures. One study in India demonstrated the effectiveness of cooling burns with cold water (Mohan and Varghese 1990). Yet in some developing countries few community members are familiar with such first-aid principles.

At the primary health care level, workers may provide the care above in addition to managing minor trauma, including simple fractures and minor open wounds and burns. Appropriate immediate stabilization of suspected fractures prior to transport of the injured person, especially in neck injuries, often prevents subsequent paralysis or other disability. Simple removal of toxins and prompt use of emetics at this level may significantly limit the extent of injury due to poisoning. Routine rehabilitation care, such as that after bone fracture, amputation, or burns, is also best conducted at the primary health care level to optimize the function of injured persons within their own community.

More sophisticated care is required at the secondary and tertiary levels for appropriate surgical treatment, such as for thoracoabdominal trauma, and for inpatient care of injury or poisoning. Data from Trinidad and Tobago (Ali and Naraynsingh 1987) suggest that once the injury victim arrives at the hospital, the twofold higher death-to-injury ratio observed there than in North American hospitals might be reduced by improved in-hospital care. In another study, in Natal, Bullock and others (1988) estimated that one-third of deaths due to head injury could have been prevented with adequate medical treatment at referral sites. Adala (1983) found that, in developing countries, treatment of eye injuries in tertiary care centers is often delayed, resulting in extensive infection and loss of sight.

Rehabilitation, although, ideally, community-based, also requires the backup and referral services of secondary and tertiary care centers for specialized problems (Smith and Barss 1991). To limit disability due to injury effectively, rehabilitation requires long-term, multidisciplinary, and comprehensive service delivery. The goal of rehabilitation is the optimal return of function—physical, psychological, social, and vocational—to the injured individual. Rehabilitation is accomplished both through changes in the functional capacity of the disabled person (for example, development of compensatory muscle strength or the use of prosthetics) and through changes in the physical and social environment. Simple rehabilitative practices, such as range-of-motion exercises to reduce contractures after burns, may have tremendous effect in improving function. Strategies which have been outlined for community-based rehabilitation of the disabled with the limited resources available in developing countries (Miles 1985; Werner 1987) can considerably reduce the economic and sociopsychological costs of injury-related disabilities.

In an evaluation of a rehabilitation program for patients with spinal cord injuries in Taiwan, Wong, Chen, and Lien (1981) suggested that significant reduction of disability could be achieved with rehabilitation interventions. After rehabilitation 75 percent of the patients were able to walk unassisted, and 68 percent were able to resume activities of daily living. Of the rehabilitated group, 17.6 percent were able to resume working at their previous occupations, whereas only 5.2 percent of those who received routine treatment were able to do

so, a difference of 70 percent. These observations are supported by the estimates of those concerned with rehabilitation in developing countries that one-half to three-quarters of those rehabilitated can subsequently return to income-generating activities (David Werner, personal communication, 1990).

IMPROVED TRIAGE AND TRANSPORT SYSTEMS. A significant challenge of emergency care of the injured is the process of "triage," which ensures that injury is managed with the appropriate priority and at the appropriate level in the health care system. In multiple injury and disaster settings, it is of paramount importance that case management activities be prioritized and tasks allocated to optimize use of health care resources. Each community must take responsibility for disaster preparedness by ensuring that local resources (for communications, transport, and health care) are assessed, priorities established, and tasks assigned in advance or as promptly as possible.

The model from industrial countries for the case management of injuries includes an elaborate system of emergency medical services (EMS), including communications, transport, and prehospital and hospital care. Although this strategy of case management of the injured is of interest to many developing countries, the cost of such a system is often prohibitive. Even in the United States, EMS systems are generally available only in large urban areas (West, Williams, and Trunkey 1988). The benefits of improved communications and transport systems, however, would be observed in improved case management of other medical and surgical problems, most notably obstetrical emergencies. Among patients transported by EMS systems in the United States, for example, only about one in six has sustained an injury (Meador, Cook, and Larkin 1989).

At least four essential elements should be included in EMS systems: (a) detection and assessment of emergencies; (b) notification and coordination of transport and definitive care services; (c) organization, training, and performance evaluation of key participants in the EMS system; and (d) stabilization and provision of definitive emergency care. If these four elements are developed, integrated, and strengthened appropriately, the EMS system will also be capable of coordinating the medical response to natural or other disasters.

Ali and Naraynsingh (1987), in their study of Trinidad and Tobago, document that excess numbers of injury victims who are alive after the injury event are dying before they reach the hospital, suggesting that mortality could be reduced by basic improvements to transport and prehospital care. Bhatnagar and Smith (1989) point out the increased fatalities associated with lack of transport among soldiers injured in the Afghan war. Compared with their counterparts in wars in which there was prompt access to good medical care, few patients with thoracoabdominal injuries survived long enough to make it to the only hospitals available, which were on the Pakistan border.

Although studies before and after development of improved prehospital care and transport have shown large differences in survival rates (West, Williams, and Trunkey 1988), such systems should be developed only where good quality definitive care is reliably available. Where such secondary and tertiary care is adequately developed, simple emergency communications and transport systems may effectively reduce injury morbidity and mortality. In their study of one such system in Papua New Guinea, based on radio linkages and intermittent charter use of local aircraft, Barss and Blackford (1983) documented an annual cost per capita of $0.20 for all medical, surgical, and obstetric conditions, with a cost per life saved of $450.00.

A telephone-based EMS for prehospital care and transport has been established in five cities and surrounding areas on the three most populated islands in Indonesia (Pusponegoro 1989). This system has been successful in providing prompt triage, treatment, and transport during several disasters as well as more than 5,000 routine ambulance responses in Jakarta alone. Similar systems in the Dominican Republic (Eaton and Perez Mera 1989), Egypt (Sarn 1989), and Nigeria (Owosina 1989) have been planned or implemented with creative methods of community participation, financing, and use of currently available resources.

The estimated effectiveness of simple improvements in the acute care and rehabilitation of the injured for four common sources of injury is presented in table 25-4. Effectiveness estimates are stated as DALYs gained as a result of appropriate acute care and rehabilitation. The derivations of the estimates and calculations in the table are described in appendix 25A.

Good Practice and Actual Practice: Are There Gaps?

Efforts to design strategies to reduce injury morbidity and mortality through improved case management are hampered by the lack of data on the effectiveness of such interventions in the developing world. In the absence of such information, many countries' first efforts are focused on emulating the elaborate EMS systems for emergency prehospital care and transport which are such a dramatic element of case management strategies in industrial countries. Many moderately industrial countries might profit from improved triage, regionalization of medical services, communications, and transport systems; however, there is no benefit to saving minutes or even hours of transport time if referral centers are not adequately staffed and equipped to provide definitive trauma care.

Another important obstacle to the development of appropriate primary care for the injured has been the emphasis in developing countries on vertical programs addressing the traditional infectious disease causes of mortality. Few programs emphasizing such a selective strategy incorporate the basic principles of management of minor injuries into the curriculum for training community health workers. Although the additional cost of training workers in basic first-aid practice would be minimal, this opportunity to reduce injury mortality has generally been neglected. Incorporation of first aid into the curriculum in primary schools in developing countries, for example, is an inexpensive intervention which would be effective in reducing the consequences of injury.

Training of currently available personnel at secondary and tertiary care centers in basic trauma care also represents an inexpensive intervention to reduce morbidity and mortality which would probably be effective. For example, existing communications and transport resources (such as police, fire, or military systems) might be used to improve triage and prehospital care, avoiding duplication and limiting costs. In industrial countries, however, creation of separate EMS systems and development of regional trauma centers may represent the most cost-effective next step to reduce injury mortality and disability.

Priorities for Injury Control

Enough is already known to establish the importance of injury as a public health problem in developing countries. Proven interventions exist to begin to address key injury problems. Although more work is needed to define locally specific injury problems further, the need for more information to refine strategies continuously should be addressed in the design of injury control programs but should not delay prompt action.

The First World Conference on Accident and Injury Prevention was held in "response to the urgent need for promoting accident and injury prevention and to mitigate their consequences on the health of people" (WHO 1989a). Policymakers from fifty countries developed a "Manifesto for Safe Communities," elaborating recommendations for action to (a) formulate public policy for safety, (b) create supportive environments, (c) strengthen community action, and (d) broaden public services. They emphasized the need to encourage politicians and decisionmakers to recognize the importance of injury and to identify injury prevention as a priority goal.

Recognizing and addressing the importance of injury will require integrated efforts at the international, national, and community levels. The tasks of highest priority at each of these levels are outlined below.

Priorities for Action by International and Donor Agencies

The focus of the "Manifesto" on the need for injury control action at the national and community levels in developing countries is appropriate. The governments of some of the more economically powerful nations, however, currently defend the profits of their national and multinational industries at the expense of the health and safety of the people of developing countries. Because injurious products, including alcohol, tobacco, pesticides, pharmaceuticals, and arms, are often pressed upon developing countries, little progress can be made in injury control until such marketing tactics have been proscribed.

Yet these industries, which together yield $619 billion per year (Werner 1989), will not easily be encouraged to be more responsible in their exploitation of the markets of developing countries. They have already successfully blocked legislation designed to restrict or control the export or import of such hazardous products (Hill 1988; Werner 1989). The first priority for injury control, therefore, is immediate legislative reform in the industrial nations and prompt policy reform both in the industrial countries and in international agencies.

Donor agencies concerned with bilateral development assistance should take responsibility for educating lawmakers and politicians in their own countries to encourage such policy reform. As a first step to restriction of "dumping" of hazardous products, donor agency regulations must ensure that products imported with donor assistance should be made to the same or similar safety standards as those in the donor country and country of origin.

International and donor agencies should assist governments in recognizing that the minimal short-term cost savings in buying such hazardous products is likely outweighed by the social and medical costs of the resulting injuries. The cost savings resulting from the prevention of injury are societal, whereas the costs of specific interventions are often borne by individuals or special interest groups. In order to protect their profit margins, industry can be expected to provide organized resistance to injury prevention. International and donor agencies should support injury control efforts, recognizing that long-term national economic growth will be hampered if safety is sacrificed to spare the short-term profits of these special interest groups.

Donors should complete an assessment of the injury effects prior to funding nonhealth sectors to ensure that hazards, such as those created by the construction of roads or the development of industry or trade, are recognized and minimized. Funding should also be made contingent upon compliance with international standards for worker, roadway, and product safety. Countries may be encouraged to address the public health importance of injury responsibly by earmarking a percentage of the funding for each project to be allocated to injury prevention activities. Donor agencies should also allocate development assistance resources for core funding to support the development of injury control programs and research.

International agencies, such as WHO, should continue to provide information and guidance regarding policy and research priorities of international significance. Other United Nations agencies, including the United Nations Environment Programme and the United Nations Disaster Relief Office, represent global resources which assist nations in achieving disaster preparedness or provide assistance to them during a disastrous event.

International organizations concerned with health, human rights, and security must take courageous action, sometimes against the will of powerful member states, to halt intergovernmental and intergroup violence. Some responsibility also rests with these agencies to coerce the governments of industrial nations to halt the dumping of their unsafe products in developing countries. Many major donor countries, however, which often control the international agencies, will resist such pressure because of the huge financial profits to be made in the sale of hazardous products such as arms.

Priorities for National Action in Developing Countries

Enough is presently known about the importance of injury in developing countries to justify action on a national level in every country. The "Manifesto for Safe Communities" (WHO 1989a, p. 8) states, "As part of its national health plan, each government should formulate a national policy and plan of action to create and sustain safe communities."

Formulation of a national policy and plan of action would best be preceded by a review of the available national data regarding locally important injury problems (Smith and Barss 1991). The first step would be to conduct an assessment of the injury situation, using existing data sources to characterize injury epidemiology, cost and effectiveness of interventions, and needs for additional information. Frequently the data that are already available have not been analyzed or used to develop strategies of injury control. Information available from police or hospital records, for example, should be exploited before additional data needs are identified and new information systems developed.

A national injury control program must establish a mechanism for intersectoral and multidisciplinary collaboration for policy planning and coordination of program implementation. A national injury control program cannot, in view of the need for multisectoral action, be designed as a vertical program to be fully contained within a ministry of health. Central coordination might best be achieved, therefore, through establishment of a task force or coordinating committee which reports directly to senior-level government officials (WHO 1987a). Such an administrative arrangement would also reflect the necessary national political commitment to ensure the cooperation of sectors responsible for education, transportation, industry and trade, housing, legislation, and enforcement.

The central coordinating body should then act to provide the necessary political and technical support for the injury control activities at intermediate (for example, regional or district) and community levels. It is at these levels that specific hazards will most often be recognized and dealt with to prevent injury. The political and technical support will include strengthening education, communication, research, and training for injury control. In establishing priorities and providing support, governments must be mindful of their special responsibility for addressing injury problems among politically and socially disadvantaged groups, such as children, women, and minorities.

Ongoing monitoring or periodic evaluation should be conducted to document the economic effect of injury problems and the cost and effectiveness of interventions. These information systems, once established, will be instrumental in refining strategies for implementation of any successful injury control program. Pilot projects may be established and evaluated prior to the widespread implementation of unproven interventions for injury control.

Governments of developing countries should supervise trading partners and collaborate with donors to ascertain that their countries are not dumping grounds for hazardous products which have been banned or become less marketable in their country of origin (Navarro 1984). Import policies and duties and national taxes or subsidies should be designed to increase product and environmental safety. Other national legislation should also be reviewed to ensure that it addresses the environmental and behavioral hazards associated with locally important injury problems.

Although no single list of interventions can be appropriate to every developing country, several injury control measures may be identified which address problems common to most countries. The following low-cost interventions are likely to have the greatest cost-effectiveness in most countries and should be considered as first priority actions:

- Import policy and product and environmental improvements to address burn, fall, and poisoning injuries
- Legislation, regulation, and enforcement to improve occupational and transportation safety
- Alcohol abuse control, especially through taxation
- The strengthening of education for first aid and acute care of the injured at the community and primary health care levels
- Maintenance of trained personnel, basic treatment facilities, and essential drugs for secondary-level management and prevention of complications due to injury
- Coordination of existing transport and communications resources to speed access to emergency care at secondary- and tertiary-level health centers
- The strengthening of rehabilitation services at the community level and referral resources at secondary and tertiary levels

Priorities for Action at the Community Level

The impetus for injury control programs comes most appropriately and effectively from the community level. As development permits individuals and communities to take control of the economic and political forces which affect their lives, industry and governments can be pressed to address the public health problem of injury. Grassroots advocacy groups have accomplished much where governments have failed in the industrial world—for example, to change environmental factors (such as product design for safety) and behavioral risk factors (such as alcohol use).

Unfortunately, however, such spontaneous community organization to demand social change is less likely to occur in the politically disadvantaged communities in many developing countries. Communities are unlikely to demand increased personal security when more basic needs are unmet. A larger share of the responsibility for ensuring adequate protection of its citizens will therefore fall to governments until injuries are seen as unacceptable by an organized community.

Meanwhile, however, communities should begin to work with their governments to increase public knowledge of injury problems and demand for safer communities. Organized com-

Table 25-6. Initial Injury Research Priorities

Action	Examples
Develop and test injury surveillance and survey techniques	Identification and quantification of disability; sensitivity and specificity of case definitions
Elucidate local role of specific factors as risk for injury	Alcohol and drugs
Investigate cost, effectiveness, and impact of specific interventions for injury control	Preventive measures (especially those known to be effective in industrial countries); case management at primary health care level; EMS systems; regionalization of care (including trauma and poison control centers); rehabilitation technologies and programs

Source: Authors' data.

munities are best able to recognize local hazards and pressure local and national governments to improve the prevention and treatment of injury. Effective communications to communities regarding injury problems, through both the press and the government, will help ensure community support for injury control efforts.

Collaboration with the private sector may be an important contribution to the success of national injury control programs. Education and communications efforts might best be targeted for private sector decisionmakers, managers, and educators who are in positions to affect preventive practices. Industries may already have well-developed concerns regarding injury prevention and provide a ready source of support for program design and implementation. Many international nongovernmental organizations have stated an interest in injury prevention (WHO 1986), and their local chapters may also help to organize critical support.

Priorities for Injury Control Research

The continuing need for evidence of the effectiveness of specific interventions to aid in program design must be addressed by incorporating strong evaluation or operational research components into every injury control program. Development of the capacity for conducting such operational research must be a high priority for resource allocation. There are many examples of interventions which have had the opposite effect intended, emphasizing the need to assess the effectiveness of every intervention for injury control.

The World Health Organization (1989c) has identified nine areas of injury research: epidemiological and vital statistical, behavioral and psychological, mechanical and biomechanical, therapeutic, rehabilitative, environmental design standards, economic and legislative policy, toxicological and pharmacological, and health systems research. Several research topics which should be of the highest priority because of their importance for program design are listed in table 25-6. Initiatives in each of these research areas will be most cost-effective if undertaken as operational research, in conjunction with the design, implementation, and evaluation of national, regional, or community programs.

Appendix 25A. Sources of Data for Effectiveness Calculations

Even for industrial countries, the effectiveness of specific injury control strategies has been poorly documented, except for certain motor vehicle injury prevention efforts (Rice and others 1989). The data from developing countries are even more limited, but estimates of the effectiveness of injury control strategies may be made by using the available information and generalizing from the industrial world if these figures are poor or not available. Although the effectiveness of injury control interventions would likely vary considerably from one country to another, figures have been selected which might best represent global averages. The lack of information on the cost of implementing these injury control interventions in developing countries currently precludes calculation of any cost-effectiveness estimates.

The effectiveness estimations presented in table 25-4 are calculated for four of the most frequent causes of injury mortality and disability in developing countries (Manciaux and Romer 1986; Taket 1986). It must be realized, therefore, that because these injuries represent perhaps only 35 to 40 percent of injury disability and mortality, the opportunity for effect on health is much greater than suggested by these four model intervention programs. Estimates are calculated as disability-adjusted life-years gained.

Estimates of percentage reductions in incidence or disability to be achieved with multiple interventions may exceed 100 percent, because there may be considerable overlap in the effect of specific interventions. For example, the same motor vehicle collision injury of an intoxicated driver might be prevented (or reduced in severity) through prevention of alcohol abuse, improved design of the vehicle, or by changing the driver's behavior to incorporate seat-belt use.

For each injury problem, the expected effectiveness of alcohol taxation in the prevention of injury is calculated by multiplying the expected reduction in alcohol-related injury times the proportion of that injury problem which has been attributed to alcohol (CDC 1990), or the "alcohol attributable fraction" (AAF). On the basis of the work of Phelps (1988) and recent suggestions that price elasticity may be even higher in developing countries than that observed in the United States (Chapman and Richardson 1990; Warner 1990), a 75 percent expected effectiveness in reducing alcohol-related injury through taxation has been assumed.

Because data from developing countries regarding the effectiveness of rehabilitation in reducing disability are so limited, the same estimate is used for all four of the injuries. An analysis of a rehabilitation program for patients with spinal cord inju-

ries in Taiwan (China) is detailed earlier in this chapter as an illustration of data contained in table 25-4.

Transportation Injury

The incidence of motor vehicle injury in the United States is 2,266 per 100,000 people; of those injured, 9.7 percent are hospitalized and 0.86 percent (19.4/100,000) are fatally injured (Rice and others 1989). The incidence of all injuries due to motor vehicle collision in developing countries is likely to be at least 665 per 100,000. This estimate is based on the average reported mortality rates for twenty-one developing countries of 11.3 per 100,000 (PAHO 1986) and the injury-to-fatality ratio, or case-fatality ratio (CFR), of 1.7 percent, double that of industrial nations (Ali and Naraynsingh 1987). The CFR for motor vehicle injury of 1.7 percent is consistent with the observed fatalities of 18 to 21 per 100,000 in Argentina, El Salvador, Costa Rica, and Thailand (although a higher rate [34 per 100,000] is found in Mexico, for example, and a lower rate [6 per 100,000] is found in the Philippines).

The average age of thirty at the time of injury reflects the fact that persons injured in motor vehicle collisions in developing countries are older than their counterparts in the industrial world (PAHO 1986; Ali and Naraynsingh 1987; Salgado and Clombage 1988). For those not fatally injured, the morbidity (in life-years lost) per injury is assumed to be the same as the 0.22 calculated by Rice and others (1989) for these injuries.

The likely effectiveness of alcohol taxation as a preventive measure for motor vehicle injury is based on an AAF of approximately 40 percent, as is observed in both the United States (CDC 1990) and Papua New Guinea (Wyatt 1980; Sinha, Sengupta, and Purohit 1981). With the expected 75 percent effectiveness in reduction of alcohol-related fatalities through taxation and other such economic incentives (Phelps 1988), an estimated reduction of injury incidence of 30 percent is calculated.

Environmental and vehicle improvements might be expected to result in at least a 70 percent reduction in incidence or severity of injury due to motor vehicle collisions. Support for this estimate is provided by the 40 percent reduction in mortality observed in the United States resulting only from vehicular improvements (Robertson 1984). It has also been estimated (Smith and Falk 1987; Rice and others 1989) that 75 percent of motor vehicle fatalities could be prevented through the use of currently available vehicular and environmental safety standards (including vehicle modifications, provision of airbags, and reduction of roadside hazards). Behavior change through education and appropriate enforcement of seat-belt use might reduce injury incidence and severity of these injuries by 40 percent (Evans 1986; Rice and others 1989).

Data from Trinidad and Tobago (Ali and Naraynsingh 1987) and similar observations in the United States indicate that improvement of trauma care for victims of motor vehicle injury would result in an estimated 50 percent reduction in the CFR. A similar reduction in the disability of those not fatally injured is assumed to be achievable with these interventions.

Falls

The incidence of injury due to falls in the United States is 5,184 per 100,000 people; of those injured, 0.1 percent are fatally injured and 6.4 percent require hospitalization (Rice and others 1989). The incidence of injury from falls in developing countries is probably at least 2,000 per 100,000, in view of the observed death rate of 4 per 100,000 and an assumed injury-to-fatality ratio of 0.2 percent (double that observed in the industrial world, as is the case for other traumatic injuries; see Ali and Naraynsingh 1987). The average age of thirty at the time of injury reflects the higher incidence among the elderly and the occupational nature of many of these injuries. For those not fatally injured, the morbidity (in life-years lost) per injury is assumed to be the same as the 0.03 calculated by Rice and others (1989) for these injuries.

The probable effectiveness of alcohol taxation as a preventive measure for injury due to falls is based on an AAF of 35 percent , as is observed in the United States (CDC 1990), and an expected 75 percent effectiveness in reduction of alcohol-related fatalities from falls (Phelps 1988). These figures suggest that a 26 percent reduction in injury incidence and severity may be achieved with high alcohol taxes.

Environmental improvements might be expected to result in approximately a 50 percent reduction in incidence or severity of injury due to falls. Asogwa (1988) observed, for example, a 60 percent reduction in mining injuries (primarily falls) when environmental improvements were made in the workplace in Nigeria. Education designed to improve safety behavior has been observed to reduce the incidence or severity of fall injuries among children by 40 percent (Kravitz 1973). That these estimates are realistic (or even low) is suggested by the 92 percent reduction in injury from falls among children which was reported in New York City following initiation of a program including both environmental regulation and education (Bergner, Mayer, and Harris 1971; Bergner 1982).

Data on excess deaths among trauma victims in Trinidad and Tobago (Ali and Naraynsingh 1987) indicates that improvement of trauma care for victims of injuries from falls would likely result in a 50 percent reduction in the CFR. Although it is likely to be conservative, a similar estimate can be made of the reduction in the disability of those not fatally injured.

Fires and Burns

The incidence of moderate to severe burn injury is probably at least 600 per 100,000 people in developing countries. In support of this estimate, a similar incidence is implied if 2 to 3 percent of such burn victims require hospitalization in Saudi Arabia (3.7 percent in United States), because the observed hospitalization rate is 16 per 100,000 (Jamal and others 1989). The incidence of burn injury in the United States, for comparison, is 617 per 100,000 (Rice and others 1989).

The average age of ten at the time of injury reflects the higher incidence among children. For example, Sowemimo (1983) and Haberal and others (1987) reported that well over half of burn victims admitted in Lagos (56.2 percent) and Turkey (69.7 percent) were less than fifteen years of age. In each case, most of these were less than six years of age. Similar age distributions for burn injuries have been observed in India (Gupta and Srivastava 1988).

Data from India (Gupta and Srivastava 1988) and Saudi Arabia (Jamal and others 1989) indicate that the CFR for moderate to severe burn injuries is about 1 percent, although mortality rates for hospitalized patients are generally much higher. For comparison, the case-fatality ratio among burn injuries in the United States is 0.4 percent. For those not fatally burned, the morbidity (in life-years lost) per injury is assumed to be the same as the 0.86 calculated by Rice and others (1989) for these injuries.

The likely effectiveness of alcohol taxation as a preventive measure for injury due to fires and burns is based on an AAF of 45 percent, as is observed in the United States (CDC 1990), and an expected 75 percent effectiveness in reduction in alcohol-related fatalities (Phelps 1988). These figures suggest that a 34 percent reduction in the incidence and severity of these injuries might be achieved at a tax rate of 50 percent.

Product improvements such as safer stoves and less flammable clothing might be expected to result in a substantial reduction in incidence and severity of burn injury. Sixty-three percent of burn deaths in Minuflya, Egypt, are of women and are ascribed to overturned portable stoves (Saleh and others 1986); this epidemiology of burns is typical of that in many developing countries. In addition, more than 30 percent of burns are related to clothing ignition (Durrani 1974; Barss and Wallace 1983). In the United States the introduction of improved flammability standards for children's sleepwear reduced these burn deaths among children by more than 98 percent between 1968 and 1980 (Baker, O'Neill, and Karpe 1984). It is therefore estimated that improved stoves and less flammable fabrics in developing countries would achieve approximately a 70 percent reduction in injury incidence.

Educational interventions might also be used to reduce the frequency of overturned stoves. It has been estimated that 90 percent of burns to children in Central Africa might be prevented with simple barriers around open fires and cookstoves (Auchincloss and Grave 1976). Education designed to improve safety behavior is rarely fully effective in altering the target behaviors, however, so the expected reduction in the incidence or severity of these injuries is estimated to be 50 percent (Barss and Wallace 1983; Schelp 1987).

Improvement of trauma care for burn victims would result in an estimated 60 percent reduction in the CFR, if the CFR is reduced to that observed in industrial nations. The observed reduction in the proportion of burn victims requiring skin grafts when cold water was immediately applied to a burn suggests that this intervention could reduce the disability of those not fatally injured by an estimated 86 percent (Mathews and Radakrishnan 1987). Improved rehabilitation of burn victims would likely contribute an estimated 70 percent reduction in disability, because simple range-of-motion exercises greatly reduce the formation of disabling contractures after burn injury.

Toxic Injury

The incidence of organophosphate poisoning alone is estimated to be 100 per 100,000 people (Xue 1987) in China's largely agricultural society. In Sri Lanka, however, the incidence is probably much greater, because pesticide poisonings severe enough to hospitalize the victim occur in 90 per 100,000 people. Organophosphates account for 20 to 50 percent of poisoning injury, so it can be estimated that the overall incidence of poisoning in developing countries is approximately 300 per 100,000 people. The incidence of injury from poisoning in the United States, for comparison, is 718 per 100,000 (Rice and others 1989). The higher incidence in the United States might be expected in view of the higher prevalence of toxic substance use and the higher likelihood that mild toxicity would be detected.

The average age of ten years at the time of toxic injury reflects the higher incidence among children (Joubert and Mathibe 1989), although many poisonings occur in the workplace. On the basis of the ninefold excess fatality rate among cases of organophosphate poisoning in China (Xue 1987), we estimate the CFR for poisonings to be approximately nine times the 0.7 percent case-fatality ratio in the United States (Rice and others 1989), or 6 percent. This percentage is consistent with average CFRs observed for other toxic ingestions (Shih and others 1985; Joubert and Mathibe 1989; Bhutta and Tahir 1990). For those not fatally injured, the morbidity (in life-years lost) per injury is assumed to be the same as the 0.01 calculated by Rice and others (1989) for these injuries. Although most poisoning victims who survive will recover without disability, the high disability ratio observed, for example, in Bhopal (where 3 to 5 persons were permanently disabled for each of the estimated 10,000 fatalities) suggests that this is probably a conservative estimate.

Alcohol abuse is associated with poisonings from other toxins, especially in suicides. The likely effectiveness of alcohol taxation as a preventive measure for poisoning is based on an AAF of 10 percent, as is observed in toxic ingestions in Sri Lanka (Hettiarachchi and Kodituwakku 1989), and an expected 75 percent effectiveness in reduction of alcohol-related fatalities (Phelps 1988). These figures suggest that alcohol taxation (at a rate of 50 percent) might be expected to result in an 8 percent reduction in toxic ingestions.

Product improvements (that is, use of less toxic preparations of pesticides, child-proof caps, and so on) might be expected

to result in an 80 percent reduction in the incidence and severity of poisoning. A 95 percent reduction in poisonings was observed, for example, with the elimination of carbon monoxide from coal gas in Birmingham, England. Because organophosphates account for nearly half of poisonings, and 80 to 90 percent of pesticide poisonings are caused by highly toxic preparations which account for only 4 to 5 percent of pesticide use (Xue 1987), one could expect nearly a 50 percent reduction in overall poisoning incidence with use of less toxic organophosphate preparations. Educational interventions and safer use of toxic substances might also be expected to contribute a 40 percent reduction in the incidence of poisoning (Shih and others 1985).

Improvement of emergency care for poisoning victims might be expected to result in an estimated 60 percent reduction in the CFR, if fatality rates are reduced to near those observed in industrial countries. Although the disability rate is small, improved rehabilitation for poisoning victims might result in an estimated 70 percent reduction in the severity or duration of disability.

Notes

The authors gratefully acknowledge the support and comments of Susan Baker, Peter Barss, Lawrence Berger, Carlos F. C. Dora, Philip Graitcer, Dean Jamison, Claude Romer, M. C. Thuriaux, and David Werner.

References

Adala, H. S. 1983. "Ocular Injuries in Africa." *Social Science and Medicine* 17:1729–53.

Ali, Jameel, and Vijay Naraynsingh. 1987. "Potential Impact of Advanced Trauma Life Support (ATLS) Program in a Third World Country." *International Surgery* 72(3):179–84.

Armstrong, K., R. Sfeir, J. Rice, and M. Kerstein. 1988. "Popliteal Vascular Injuries and War: Are Beirut and New Orleans Similar?" *Journal of Trauma* 28(6):836–39.

Asogwa, S. E. 1980. "A Review of Coal-Mining Accidents in Nigeria over a 10-Year Period." *Journal of Social and Occupational Medicine* 30:(2)69–73.

———. 1988. "The Health Benefits of Mechanization at the Nigerian Coal Corporation." *Accident Analysis and Prevention* 20:103–8.

Attah Johnson, F. Y. 1989. "Prevention and Management of Problems Related to Alcohol Abuse in Papua New Guinea through Primary Health Care." *Medicine and Law* 8:175–89.

Auchincloss, J. M., and G. F. Grave. 1976. "The Problem of Burns in Central Africa." *Tropical Doctor* 6:114–17.

Baker, S. P., B. O'Neill, M. J. Ginsbury, and G. Li. 1992. *The Injury Fact Book.* 2d ed. New York: Oxford University Press.

Baker, S. P., B. O'Neill, and R. S. Karpe. 1984. *The Injury Fact Book.* Lexington, Mass.: Lexington Books.

Banerjee, P., and S. Bhattachariya. 1978. "Changing Pattern of Poisoning in Children in a Developing Country." *Tropical Pediatrics and Environmental Child Health* 24:136–39.

Bang, R. L., and J. K. Saif. 1989. "Mortality from Burns in Kuwait." *Burns* 15:315–21.

Barancik, J. I., B. F. Chatterjee, Y. C. Greene, E. M. Michenzi, and D. Fife. 1983. "Northeastern Ohio Trauma Study: 1. Magnitude of the Problem." *American Journal of Public Health* 73:746–51.

Barss, P. G., and C. Blackford. 1983. "Medical Emergency Flights in Remote Areas: Experience in Milne Bay Province, Papua New Guinea." *Papua New Guinea Medical Journal* 26:198–202.

Barss, P. G., P. Dakulala, M. Doolan. 1984. "Falls from Trees and Tree Associated Injuries in Rural Melanesians." *British Medical Journal (Clinical Research)* 289:1717–20.

Barss, P. G., and K. Wallace. 1983. "Grass Skirt Burns in Papua New Guinea." *Lancet* 1:733–34.

Baudouy, J. 1989. "Road Accidents: An Emerging Epidemic in Developing Countries." Harvard School of Public Health, Boston, Mass.

Bayoumi, A. 1981. "The Epidemiology of Fatal Motor Vehicle Accidents in Kuwait." *Accident Analysis and Prevention* 13:339–48.

Berger, Lawrence R. 1988. "Suicides and Pesticides in Sri Lanka." *American Journal of Public Health* 78:826–28.

Bergner, L. 1982. "Environmental Factors in Injury Control: Preventing Falls from Heights." In A. Bergman, ed., *Preventing Childhood Injuries. Report of the Twelfth Ross Roundtable on Critical Approaches to Common Pediatric Problems*. Ross Laboratories, Columbus, Oh.

Bergner, L., S. Mayer, and D. Harris. 1971. "Falls from Heights: A Childhood Epidemic in an Urban Area." *American Journal of Public Health* 61:90–96.

Bertazzi, P. A. 1989. "Industrial Disasters and Epidemiology: A Review of Recent Experiences." *Scandinavian Journal of Work and Environmental Health* 15:85–100.

Bhatnager, M. K., and G. S. Smith. 1989. "Trauma in the Afghan Guerilla War: Effect of Lack of Access to Care." *Surgery* 105:699–705.

Bhutta, Tariq Iqbal, and Khalid Iqbal Tahir. 1990. "Loperamide Poisoning in Children." *Lancet* 335:363.

Bittah, O., J. A. Owola, and P. Oduor. 1979. "A Study of Alcoholism in a Rural Setting in Kenya." *East African Medical Journal* 56:665–70.

Buchanan, R. C. 1972. "The Causes and Prevention of Burns in Malawi." *Central African Journal of Medicine* 18:55–56.

Bullock, M. R., M. D. du Trevou, J. R. van Dellen, J. P. Nel, and C. P. McKeown. 1988. "Prevention of Death from Head Injury in Natal." *South African Medical Journal* 73:523–27.

Bwititi, T., O. Chikuni, R. Loewenson, W. Murambiwa, C. Nhachi, and N. Nyazema. 1987. "Health Hazards in Organophosphate Use among Farm Workers in the Large-Scale Farming Sector." *Central African Journal of Medicine* 33:120–26.

Calonge, N. 1987. "Objectives for Injury Control Intervention—The Department of Health and Human Services Model." *Public Health Reports* 102:602–5.

Campbell, B. J. 1987. "Research Trends in Injury Prevention." *Public Health Reports* 102:592–93.

CDC (Centers for Disease Control). 1984. "Alcohol and Violent Death: Erie County, New York, 1973–1983." *Morbidity and Mortality Weekly Report* 33:226–27.

———. 1990. "Alcohol-Related Mortality and Years of Potential Life Lost—United States, 1987." *Morbidity and Mortality Weekly Report* 39:173–79.

Chao, T. C., J. H. Khoo, and W. N. Poon. 1984. "Road Traffic Accident Casualities in Singapore (with Special Reference to Drivers and Front Seat Passengers)." *Annals of the Academcy of Medicine of Singapore* 13(1):96–101.

Chapman, S., and J. Richardson. 1990. "Tobacco Excise and Declining Tobacco Consumption: The Case of Papua New Guinea." *American Journal of Public Health* 1990; 80:537–40.

Chelala, Cesar A. 1990. "Central America: The Cost of War." *Lancet* 335:153–54.

Chesnais, J. C. 1985. "The Prevention of Deaths from Violence." In J. Vallin and A. D. Lopez, eds., *Health Policy, Social Policy, and Mortality Prospects.*

Institut National d'Etudes Démographiques (INED) and International Union for the Scientific Study of Population (IUSSP), Ordina Editions.

Choovoravech, P. 1980. "Motor Vehicle Accident in Childhood." *Journal of the Medical Association of Thailand* 63:304–9.

Choudhry, V. P., A. J. Jalali, G. Haider, and M. A. Qureshi. 1987. "Spectrum of Accidental Poisonings among Children in Afghanistan." *Annals of Tropical Pediatrics* 7:278–81.

Collins, J. G. 1985. *Persons Injured and Disability Days Due To Injuries, United States, 1980–81*. Vital and Health Statistics Series 10, 149. DHHS Publication (PHS) 85-1577. Public Health Service, National Center for Health Statistics, Washington, D.C.

Cook, P. 1981. "The Effect of Liquor Taxes on Drinking, Cirrhosis, and Auto Accidents." In M. H. Moore and D. R. Gersteion, eds., *Alcohol and Public Policy: Beyond the Shadow of Prohibition*. Washington, D.C.: National Academy Press.

CRED (Center for Research on the Epidemiology of Disasters). 1991. *Disasters in the World: Statistical Update from CRED Disasters Events Database*. University of Louvain School of Public Health, Brussells.

Cuellar, A. 1980. "Occupational Health and Safety in the Smelting and Foundry Industries in Mexico." *American Journal of Industrial Medicine* 1:261–63.

Curry, Robert L. 1989. "Beverage Alcohol Spending in Singapore: A Potential Development Constraint?" *International Journal of the Addictions* 24(8):821–28.

Datey, S., N. S. Murthy, and A. D. Taskar. 1981. "A Study of Burn Injury Cases from Three Hospitals." *Indian Journal of Public Health* 15(3):117–24.

Davis, S., and L. S. Smith. 1982. "Alcohol and Drowning in Cape Town: A Preliminary Report." *South African Medical Journal* 62:931–33.

DeCodes, J., T. D. Baker, and D. Schumann. 1988. "The Hidden Costs of Illness in Developing Countries." *Research in Human Capital Development* 5:127–45.

de Mello, M. H. Jorge, and M. Bernardes-Marques. 1985. "Violent Childhood Deaths in Brazil." *Bulletin of the Pan-American Health Organization* 19(3):288–99.

Demling, R. H. 1985. "Burns (Medical Progress)." *New England Journal of Medicine* 313:1389–98.

De Wind, Christina M. 1987. "War Injuries Treated under Primitive Circumstances: Experiences in an Ugandan Mission Hospital." *Annals of the Royal College of Surgeons of England* 69:193–95.

Dietz, P. E., and S. P. Baker. 1974. "Drowning: Epidemiology and Prevention." *American Journal of Public Health* 64:303–12.

Durrani, K. M. 1974. *The Epidemiology of Burn Injuries*. Burns Research Project, Civil Hospital, Dow Medical College, Karachi, Pakistan.

Durrani, K. M., and S. K. Raza. 1975. "Studies on Flammability of Clothing of Burn Victims, Changes Therein, and Their Wearability after a Borax Rinse." *Journal of the Pakistan Medical Association* 25(5):99–102.

Eaton, D., and A. Perez Mera. 1989. "The Rise and Fall of EMS Innovation: A Cautionary Tale from the Dominican Republic." Paper presented at the International Conference on Emergency Health Care Development, Crystal City, Va.

Edwards, G. 1979. "Drinking Problems: Putting the Third World on the Map." *Lancet* 2:402–4.

Ergun, G. 1987. "Condition of Vehicles in Saudi Arabia." *Accident Analysis and Prevention* 19:343–58.

Evans, L. 1986. "The Effectiveness of Safety Belts in Preventing Fatalities." *Accident Analysis and Prevention* 18:229–41.

Ezenwa, A. D. 1986a. "Prevention and Control of Road Traffic Accidents in Nigeria." *Journal of the Royal Society of Health* 106(1):25–26.

———. 1986b "Trends and Characteristics of Road Traffic Accidents in Nigeria." *Journal of the Royal Society of Health* 106(1):27–29.

Fox, D. K., B. L. Hopkins, and W. K. Anger. 1987. "The Long Term Effects of a Token Economy on Safety Performance in Open-Pit Mining." *Journal of Applied Behavior Analysis* 20(3):215–24.

Gaind, B. N., M. Mohan, and S. Ghosh. 1977. "Changing Pattern of Poisoning in Children." *Indian Pediatrics* 14(4):295–301.

Gordon, J. E., P. V. Gulati, and J. Wyon. 1962. "Traumatic Accidents in Rural Tropical Regions: An Epidemiological Field Study in Punjab, India." *American Journal of Medical Science* 243(3):158–78.

Gu, X. Y., and M. L. Chen. 1982. "Vital Statistics (of Shanghai County)." *American Journal of Public Health* 72(supplement):19–23.

Gupta, R. C., S. K. Bhasin, and B. S. Khanka. 1982. "Drive-Belt or Patta Injuries." *Injury* 13(6):495–99.

Gupta, R. K., and A. K. Srivastava. 1988. "Study of Fatal Burn Cases in Kanpur (India)." *Forensic Science International* 37(2):81–89.

Haberal, M., Z. Oner, U. Bayraktar, and N. Bilgin. 1987. "Epidemiology of Adults' and Children's Burns in a Turkish Burn Center." *Burns Including Thermal Injuries* 13(2):136–40.

Haddon, W., Jr. 1970. "On the Escape of Tigers: An Ecologic Note." *American Journal of Public Health* 60:2229–34.

———. 1980. "Options for Prevention of Motor Vehicle Injury." *Israel Journal of Medical Science* 16:45–65.

Haight, F. A. 1980. "Traffic Safety in Developing Countries." *Journal of Safety Research* 12:50–58.

Hassall, C., and W. H. Trethowan. 1972. "Suicide in Birmingham." *British Medical Journal* 1:717–18.

Hayes, W. J. 1980. "Factors Limiting Injury from Pesticides." *Journal of Environmental Science and Health* B15(6):1005–21.

Hettiarachchi, J., and G. C. S. Kodituwakku. 1989. "Self Poisoning in Sri Lanka: Motivational Aspects." *International Journal of Social Psychiatry* 35(2):204–8.

Hill, R. 1988. "Problems and Policy for Pesticide Exports to Less Developed Countries." *Natural Resources Journal* 28(4):699–720.

Jacobs, G. B., and I. Sayer. 1983. "Road Accidents in Developing Countries." *Accident Analysis and Prevention* 15:337–53.

Jamal, Y. S., M. S. M. Ardawi, A. A. Ashy, H. Merdad, and S. A. Shaik. 1989. "Burn Injuries in the Jeddah Area of Saudi Arabia: A Study of 319 Cases." *Burns* 15:295–98.

Jeyaratam, J., R. S. de Alwis Senevirante, and J. F. Copplestone. 1982. "Survey of Pesticide Poisonings in Sri Lanka." *Bulletin of the World Health Organization* 0(4):615–19.

Joubert, P. H., and L. Mathibe. 1989. "Acute Poisoning in Developing Countries." *Adverse Drug Reactions and Acute Poisoning Reviews* 8(3):165–78.

Kleevens, J. W. 1982. "Accidents in Hong Kong." *Public Health, London* 96(5):297–304.

Kortteinen, Timo 1988. "International Trade and Availability of Alcoholic Beverages in Developing Countries." *British Journal of Addiction* 83:669–76.

———. 1989. "State Monopoly Systems and Alcoholism Prevention in Developing Countries: Report on a Collaborative International Study." *British Journal of Addiction* 84:413–25.

Kravitz, H. 1973. "Prevention of Falls in Infancy by Counseling Mothers." *Illinois Medical Journal* 144:570–73.

Krishnarajah, V. 1972. "Industrial Accidents—A Survey." *Ceylon Medical Journal* 18–27.

Landemann Szarcwald, C., and E. Ayres de Castilho. 1986. "Mortalidade por causas externas no estado de Rio de Janeiro no periodo de 1976 a 1980." *Cadernos de Salude Publica, R.J.* 1:19–41.

Langley, J. D. 1988. "The Need to Discontinue the Use of the Term 'Accident' when Referring to Unintentional Injury Events." *Accident Analysis and Prevention* 20:1–8.

Lee, K. N., Y. O. Choi, C. H. Kim, and D. R. Yun. 1971. "An Epidemiological Study on the Incidence of Carbon Monoxide Poisoning in Korea." *Journal of the Korea Preventive Medicine Society* 4:95–106.

Lee, S. T. 1982. "Two Decades of Specialized Burns Care in Singapore." *Annals of the Academy of Medicine of Singapore* 11(3):358–65.

Loevinoshn, M. E. 1987. "Insecticide Use and Increased Mortality in Rural Central Luzon, Philipinnes." *Lancet* 1:359–62.

Losada Lora, R., and E. Velez Bustillo. 1988. "Muertas violentas en Colombia, 1979–1986." Instituto SER de Investigación, Bogotá, Colombia.

Lourie, J., and S. Sinha. 1983. "Port Moresby Road Traffic Accident Survey." *Papua New Guinea Medical Journal* 26:186–89.

McLoughlin, E., N. Clarke, K. Stahl, and J. D. Crawford. 1977. "One Pediatric Burn Unit's Experience with Sleepwear-Related Injuries." *Pediatrics* 60:405–9.

Manciaux, M. 1984. "Accidental Injuries in the Young: From Epidemiology to Prevention." *Effective Health Care* 2(1):21–28.

Manciaux, M., and C. J. Romer. 1986. "Accidents in Children, Adolescents, and Young Adults: A Major Public Health Problem." *World Health Statistical Quarterly* 39:227–31.

Margolis, B., and W. Kroes. 1975. *The Human Side of Accident Prevention.* Springfield, Ill.: Charles C. Thomas.

Mathews, R. N., and T. Radakrishnan. 1987. "First Aid for Burns." *Lancet* 1:1371.

Meade, M. S. 1980. "Potential Years of Life Lost in Countries of Southeast Asia." *Social Science and Medicine* 14D:277–81.

Meador, S., R. T. Cook, and G. L. Larkin. 1989. "Advanced Life Support Medical Care Distribution in a Rural/Urban Population." Paper presented at the International Conference on Emergency Health Care Development, Crystal City, Va.

Mierley, M. C., and S. P. Baker. 1983. "Fatal Housefires in an Urban Population." *JAMA* 249:1466–68.

Miles, M. 1984. *Where There is No Rehab Plan.* Mental Health Centre, Peshawar, India.

Miller, R. E., K. S. Reisinger, M. M. Blatter, F. Wucher. 1982. "Pediatric Counseling and Subsequent Use of Smoke Detectors." *American Journal of Public Health* 72:392–93.

Milliner, N., J. Pearn, and R. Guard. 1980. "Will Fenced Pools Save Lives? A 10-Year Study from Mulgrave Shire, Queensland." *Medical Journal of Australia* 2:510–11.

Mohan, D. 1982. "Accidental Death and Disability in India—A Case of Criminal Neglect." *Industrial Safety Chronicle* 24–43.

Mohan, D., and P. S. Bawa. 1985. "An Analysis of Road Traffic Fatalities in Delhi, India." *Accident Analysis and Prevention* 17:33–45.

Mohan, D., and M. Varghese. 1990. "Fireworks Cast a Shadow on India's Festival of Lights." *World Health Forum* 11:323–26.

Mowbrey, D. L. 1986. "Pesticide Poisoning in Papua New Guinea and the South Pacific." *Papua New Guinea Medical Journal* 29:131–41.

Muller, A. 1982. "An Evaluation of the Effectiveness of Motorcycle Headlight Use Laws." *American Journal of Public Health* 72:1136–41.

National Committee for Injury Prevention and Control. 1989. "Injury Prevention: Meeting the Challenge." *American Journal of Preventive Medicine* 5(supplement):1–303.

NHTSA (National Highway Traffic Safety Administration). 1988. *Fatal Accident Reporting System, 1987.* U.S. Department of Transportation, Washington, D.C.

NRC/IOM (National Research Council/Institute of Medicine), Committee on Trauma Research, Commission on Life Sciences. 1985. *Injury in America: A Continuing Public Health Problem.* Washington, D.C.: National Academy Press.

National Safety Council. 1986. *Accident Facts.* Chicago, Ill.

Navarro, V. 1984. "Policies on Exportation of Hazardous Substances in Western Developed Countries." *New England Journal of Medicine* 311:546–48.

Ng, S. C., T. C. Chao, and J. How. 1978. "Deaths by Accidental Drowning in Singapore, 1973–76." *Singapore Medical Journal* 19:14–19.

Nielsen, M. F. J., C. A. Resnick, and S. W. Acuda. 1989. "Alcoholism among Outpatients of a Rural District General Hospital in Kenya." *British Journal of Addiction* 84:1343–51.

Nixon, J. W., J. H. Pearn, and A. E. Dugdale. 1979. "Swimming Ability of Children: A Survey of 4000 Queensland Children in a High Drowning Region." *Medical Journal of Australia* 6:271–72.

Odejide, A. O., J. U. Ohaeri, and B. A. Ikuesan. 1989. "Alcohol Use among Nigerian Youths: The Need for Drug Education and Alcohol Policy." *Drug and Alcohol Dependence* 23:231–35.

Ofosu, J. B., A. M. Abouammoh, and A. Bener. 1988. "A Study of Road Traffic Accidents in Saudi Arabia." *Accident Analysis and Prevention* 20:95–101.

Ogba, Leo Oko. 1989. "Violence and Health in Nigeria." *Health Policy and Planning* 4(1):82–84.

Okonkwo, C. A. 1988. "Spinal Cord Injuries in Enugu, Nigeria—Preventable Accidents." *Paraplegia* 26(1):12–18.

Oliver, R. G., and B. S. Hetzel. 1972. "Rise and Fall of Suicide Rates in Australia: Relationship to Sedative Availability." *Medical Journal of Australia* 2:919–23.

Omran, A. R. 1971. "The Epidemiologic Transition: A Theory of the Epidemiology of Population Change." *Milbank Memorial Fund Quarterly* 49:509–38.

Owosina, F. A. O. 1989. "National Policy on Injury Control and Emergency Medical Services." Paper presented at the International Conference on Emergency Health Care Development, Crystal City, Va.

PAHO (Pan-American Health Organization). 1986. *Health Conditions in the Americas, 1981–1984.* Vol. 1. Scientific Publication 500. Washington, D.C.

Patel, N. S., and G. P. Bhagwatt. 1977. "Road Traffic Accidents in Lusaka and Blood Alcohol." *Medical Journal of Zambia* 11(2):46–49.

Pearn, J. H., R. Bart, and R. Yamaoka. 1978. "Drowning Risks to Epileptic Children: A Study from Hawaii." *British Medical Journal* 2:1284–85.

Peltzman, S. 1975. "The Effects of Automobile Safety Regulation." *Journal of Political Economy* 83(4):677–725.

Phelps, C. E. 1988. "Death and Taxes: An Opportunity for Substitution." *Journal of Health Economics* 7:1–24.

Pleuckhahn, V. D. 1984. "Alcohol and Accidental Drowning: A 25-Year Study." *Medical Journal of Australia* 141:22–25.

Punyahotra, V. 1982. *Epidemiology of Road Traffic Accident in Thailand.* National Safety Council, National Accident Research Center, Bangkok, Thailand.

Pupo Nogueira, C. 1987. "Prevention of Accidents and Injuries in Brazil." *Ergonomics* 30(2):387–93.

Pusponegoro, A. D. 1989. "Pre-hospital Emergency Care in Indonesia: Concepts and Problems." Paper presented at the International Conference on Emergency Health Care Development, Crystal City, Va.

Ramesh, S., S. Srikanth, and V. R. Parvathy. 1987. "Poisoning in Children." *Indian Journal of Pediatrics* 54:769–73.

Reichanheim, M. E., and T. Harpham. 1989. "Child Accidents and Associated Risk Factors in a Brazilian Squatter Settlement." *Health Policy and Planning* 4(2):162–67.

Rice, D. P., E. J. MacKenzie, and others. 1989. *Cost of Injury in the United States: A Report to Congress.* Institute for Health and Aging, University of California and Injury Prevention Center (San Francisco) and Johns Hopkins University.

Robertson, Leon S. 1981. "Automobile Safety Regulations and Death Reductions in the States." *American Journal of Public Health* 71:818–22.

———. 1983. *Injuries: Causes, Control Strategies, and Public Policy.* Lexington, Mass.: Lexington Books.

———. 1984. "Automobile Safety Regulation: Rebuttal and New Data." *American Journal of Public Health* 74:1390–94.

———. 1990. "Car Design and the Risk of Pedestrian Deaths." *American Journal of Public Health* 80:609–10.

———. 1992. *Injury Epidemiology.* New York: Oxford University Press.

Robertson, L. S., A. B. Kelley, B. O'Neill, C. W. Wixom, R. S. Eiswirth, W. Haddon, Jr. 1974. "A Controlled Study of the Effect of Television Messages on Safety Belt Use." *American Journal of Public Health* 64:1071–80.

Rosenberg, M. L., R. J. Gelles, P. C. Hollinger, M. A. Zahn, and others. 1987. "Violence: Homicide, Assault, and Suicide." *American Journal of Preventive Medicine* 3(5 supplement):164–78.

Ryan, G. Anthony. 1990. Assignment report, for Prevention and Control of Road Traffic Accidents Project. (WP)MNH/ICP/APR/001-E. World Health Organization, Geneva.

SAE (Society of Automotive Engineers). 1984. *Advances in Belt Restraint Systems: Design, Performance, and Usage.* Special Publication P-141. Warrandale, PA.

Saleh, S., S. Gadalla, J. A. Fortney, S. M. Rogers, and D. M. Potts. 1986. "Accidental Burn Deaths to Egyptian Women of Reproductive Age." *Burns* 12:241–45.

Salgado, M. S., and S. M. Clombage. 1988. "Analysis of Fatalities in Road Accidents." *Forensic Science International* 36(1/2):91–96.

Sarn, J. 1989. "International Donor Aid to EMS Development." Paper presented at the International Conference on Emergency Health Care Development, Crystal City, Va.

Schelp, Lothar. 1987. "Community Intervention and Changes in Accident Pattern in a Rural Swedish Municipality." *Health Promotion* 2(2):109–25.

Schwab, Larry. 1990. "Blindness from Trauma in Developing Nations." *International Ophthalmology Clinics* 30(1):28–29.

Selya, R. M. 1980. "Deaths Due To Accidents in Taiwan: A Possible Indicator of Development." *Social Science and Medicine* 14D:361–67.

Shanmugasundaram, T. K. 1988. "The Care of SCI Patients in the Developing Nations—Can We Stem the Rot?" *Paraplegia* 26(1):10–11.

Shepherd, A. 1980. "Road Traffic Accidents: A View from the Highlands." *Papua New Guinea Medical Journal* 23:57–58.

Shih, J. H., Z. Q. Wu, Y. L. Wang, Y. X. Zhang, S. Z. Xue, and X. Q. Gu. 1985. "Prevention of Acute Parathion and Demeton Poisoning in Farmers around Shanghai." *Scandinavian Journal of Workers' and Environmental Health* 11 (Supplement 4):49–54.

Silva, J. F. 1978. "A Comparative Study of Road Traffic Accidents in West Malaysia." *Annals of the Royal College of Surgery of England* 60:457–63.

Sinha, R. N. 1984. "Burns in Tropical Countries." *Clinics in Plastic Surgery* 1(1):121–27.

Sinha, S. N., S. K. Sengupta, and R. C. Purohit. 1981. "A Five Year Review of Deaths Following Trauma." *Papua New Guinea Medical Journal* 24: 222–28.

Sloan, J. H., A. L. Kellerman, D. T. Reay, J. A. Ferris, T. Koepsell, F. P. Rivara, C. Rice, L. Gray, and J. LoGerfo. 1988. "Handgun Regulations, Crime, Assaults, and Homicide: A Tale of Two Cities." *New England Journal of Medicine* 319:1256–62.

Smith, G. S., and P. G. Barss. 1986. "Beyond the Motor Vehicle: The Importance of Other Unintentional Injuries as a Preventable Cause of Ill Health in Developing Countries." Paper presented at Risks Old and New: A Global Consultation on Health, April 27–May 1, Emory University, Atlanta, Ga.

———. 1991. "Unintentional Injuries in Developing Countries: The Epidemiology of a Neglected Problem." *Epidemiologic Reviews* 13:228–66.

Smith, G. S., and H. Falk. 1987. "Unintentional Injuries." *American Journal of Preventive Medicine* 5(supplement):143–63.

Smith, G. S., and J. F. Kraus. 1988. "Alcohol and Residential, Recreational, and Occupational Injuries: A Review of the Epidemiologic Evidence." *Annual Review of Public Health* 9:99–121.

Smith, R. S. 1974. "The Feasibility of an Injury Tax Approach to Safety." *Law and Contemporary Problems* 38(4):730–44.

Sonnen, A. E. H. 1980. "Epilepsy and Swimming." In *Epilepsy: A Clinical and Experimental Research*. Monographs in Neural Science 42. Basel: Karger.

Sood, S. 1988. "Survey of Factors Influencing Injury among Riders Involved in Motorized Two-Wheeler Accidents in India: A Prospective Study of 302 Cases." *Journal of Trauma* 28(4):530–34.

Sowemimo, G. O. 1983. "Burn Injuries in Lagos." *Burns Including Thermal Injuries* 9(4):280–83.

Sri Lanka Psychiatric Association. 1982. *National Plan on Mental Health for Sri Lanka*.

Subianto, D. B., L. R. Tumada, and S. S. Margono. 1978. "Burns and Epileptic Fits Associated with Cysticercosis in Mountain People of Irian Jaya." *Tropical Geography and Medicine* 30(3):275–78.

Taket, A. 1986. "Accident Mortality in Children, Adolescents, and Young Adults." *World Health Statistical Quarterly* 39:232–56.

Technical Study Group. 1987. *Toward a Less Fire-Prone Cigarette: Final Report of the Technical Study Group on Cigarette and Little Cigar Fire Safety*. U.S. Consumer Product Safety Commission, Washington, D.C.

Teret, S. P., and M. Jacobs. 1989. "Prevention and Torts: The Role of Litigation in Injury Control." *Law, Medicine, and Health Care* 17:17–22.

Thapa, N. B. 1984. "Injury Prevention in Nepal." *Souvenir Napas Journal* 3(1):136–39.

Trunkey, D. D. 1983. "Trauma." *Scientific American* 249:28–36.

UNICEF (United Nations Children's Fund). 1989. *State of the World's Children*. New York: Oxford University Press.

Waller, J. A. 1985. *Injury Control: A Guide to the Causes and Prevention of Trauma*. Lexington, Mass.: D. C. Heath.

Warner, K. E. 1990. "Tobacco Taxation as Health Policy in the Third World." *American Journal of Public Health* 80:529–31.

Wechsler, H., E. H. Kasey, D. Thum, H. W. Demone, Jr. 1969. "Alcohol Level and Home Accidents." *Public Health Reports* 84:1043–50.

Weddell, J. M., and A. McDougall. 1981. "Road Traffic Injuries in Sharjah." *International Journal of Epidemiology* 10:155–59.

Werner, David. 1987. *Disabled Village Children*. Palo Alto, Calif.: Hesperian Foundation.

———. 1989. "Health for No One by the Year 2000: The High Cost of Placing 'National Security' before Global Justice." Paper presented to the 16th Annual International Health Conference, National Council on International Health, June, Arlington, Va.

West, J. G., M. J. Williams, and D. D. Trunkey. 1988. "Trauma Systems: Current Status, Future Challenges." *JAMA* 259:3597–600.

WHO (World Health Organization). 1952. Technical Report 48. Geneva.

———. 1977. *International Classification of Diseases. Manual of the International Statistical Classification of Diseases, Injuries, and Causes of Death*. 9th rev. Geneva.

———. 1986. *Report of the Second Global Liaison Meeting on Accident and Injury Prevention*. IRP/APR 218 m21A. Geneva.

———. 1987a. *Accident and Injury Prevention at the Primary Health Care Level*. IPR/APR 218 H. Inter-Regional Consultation on Research Development for Injury Prevention, Pattaya, Thailand.

———. 1987b. *Report of the Asian Seminar on Road Safety*. IPR/APR 218 G. WHO Regional Office for Europe, Geneva.

———. 1988. *Global Medium-Term Programme: Accident Prevention*. APR/MTP/88.1. Geneva.

———. 1989a. "Manifesto for Safe Communities: Safety—A Universal Concern and Responsibility for All." Resolution adopted at the First World Conference on Accident and Injury Prevention, September 20, Stockholm.

———. 1989b. *New Approaches to Improve Road Safety*. Technical Report 781. Geneva.

———. 1989c. *Research Development for Accident and Injury Prevention*. IPR/APR 216 m31R, 8923E. Geneva.

Wintemute, G. J., S. P. Baker, D. Mohan, S. P. Teret, and C. J. Romer, eds. 1985. *Principles for Injury Prevention in Developing Countries*. IPR/ADR 217-40. World Health Organization, Geneva.

Wong, M. K., C. F. Chen, and I. N. Lien. 1981. "Evaluation of the Results of a Rehabilitation for Spinal Cord Injury over a Recent Ten Year Period." *Journal of the Formosan Medical Association* 80:433–41.

Wyatt, G. B. 1980. "The Epidemiology of Road Accidents in Papua New Guinea." *Papua New Guinea Medical Journal* 23:60–65.

Xue, Shou-Zhen. 1987. "Health Effects of Pesticides: A Review of Epidemiologic Research from the Perspective of Developing Nations." *American Journal of Industrial Medicine* 12:269–79.

Zador, P. 1983. "How Effective are Daytime Motorcycle Headlight Use Laws?" *American Journal of Public Health* 73:808–10.

26

Cataract

Jonathan C. Javitt

"Cataract" refers to an opacity in the natural, crystalline lens of the eye. Although cataract surgery has been performed for more than 2,000 years, cataract remains the most common cause of blindness in the world today (Dawson and Schwab 1981; Whitfield and others 1983; Al Salem and Ismail 1987; Schwab 1987). The World Health Organization (WHO) estimates suggest that 17 million people are currently blinded by cataract (Wilson 1980) worldwide. New data show that in China alone there are 5.4 million cases of cataract blindness, suggesting that the world total may be higher than previously thought (CDC 1983). As of 1983, incident cases of cataract-related blindness exceeded 1.25 million annually (CDC 1983). Because of increasing life span and an expanding elderly population in the developing world, the prevalence of blinding cataract is expected to double by the year 2010.

The crystalline lens of the eye is normally transparent and, together with the cornea, focuses light on the retina. Although a small degree of opacity may interfere minimally with vision, cataract can and frequently does cause severe vision loss. Cataract blindness, according to the definition of the World Health Organization, results when the degree of opacity reduces vision to less than 3/60 (i.e., inability to recognize the largest letter) on the standard eye chart.

Cataract progression is characterized by painless, progressive loss of vision. In general, vision loss induced by cataract is entirely reversible upon removal of the opacified lens. Only occasionally can cataract-induced lens swelling or leakage cause permanent damage to the eye.

Like many degenerative and disabling conditions associated with age, blindness from cataract is associated with complete disability, an increased need for support from family members, loss of social status and authority within the family and community, and early demise. Unlike many degenerative and disabling conditions, however, cataract blindness is entirely curable. The current cost of restoring sight in a mass-surgery program ranges from $15 for cataract extraction in an Indian eye camp (temporary mass surgical facility) to $22 in an African mobile surgical facility to $33 in an urban Latin American public hospital (HKI 1986). The limited studies conducted to date suggest that restoration of sight by cataract surgery produces economic and social benefits to the individual, the family, and the community that far outweigh the investment in surgery. A study in rural India found that individuals undergoing cataract surgery demonstrated increased productivity amounting to a 1,500 percent annual return on the cost of the surgery (Javitt, Venkataswamy, and Sommer 1983).

Public Health Significance of Cataract

The current backlog of curable blindness from cataract is the result of an interplay between disease incidence, surgical rates, and mortality. As illustrated in figure 26-1, most individuals in the developing world who are blind from cataract are likely to be so for the rest of their lives. Only the minority are likely to have sight restored. Decreasing the backlog of cataract blindness can be achieved both by increasing the volume of curative surgery and decreasing risk factors for cataract wherever possible. These strategies must include not only increased provision of care but also operations research to determine methods for increasing individual participation in care.

Current Levels and Trends in the Developing World

Enormous variation exists in the prevalence of cataract blindness worldwide. As can be seen from figure 26-1, rates range from 14 per 100,000 people (0.014 percent) in Scandinavia to 1,525 per 100,000 (1.525 percent) in Asia (WHO Programme for the Prevention of Blindness 1987). The prevalence of a disease in the population is a function of its incidence in that population, the duration of disease in those affected, and the likelihood that the disease will resolve on its own, be cured, or result in an increased risk of mortality. Variations in any one of these factors may lead to variation in observed prevalence. There are several possible explanations when the prevalence of cataract blindness is higher in one region than another:

- An increased incidence of cataract by age group
- An increased longevity of those with cataract or of older persons in general
- A decreased likelihood that individuals with cataract will have sight-restoring surgery

Figure 26-1. Prevalence of Cataract Blindness, by Region

Cataract blindness per 100,000 population

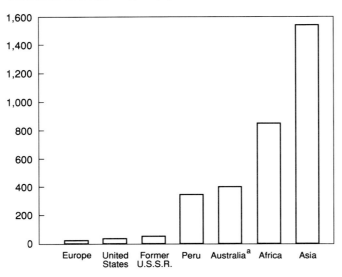

a. Aboriginal population.
Source: Wilson 1980.

• Errors and biases in data collection that may affect data validity

In considering the epidemiology of cataract blindness, one must study variations in the incidence of cataractous change, in the rate of progression to cataract blindness, in the likelihood that an individual will receive cataract surgery, and in the longevity of individuals who are blind from cataract.

The prevalence of cataract blindness varies substantially, not only from continent to continent but within smaller regions as well. The prevalence of blindness reported from survey data published by the World Health Organization is shown in table 26-1. The data presented are all drawn from government-sponsored blindness surveys that specifically addressed the rate of cataract-related blindness in relation to other causes of blindness. A critical consideration of the sampling techniques and survey methodology employed in each country is beyond the scope of this chapter. The reader must evaluate the reliability of the underlying data, however, before drawing conclusions based upon small variations in cataract rates from one region to another.

Even within a country, rates of cataract blindness obtained from survey data may vary considerably. In table 26-2 the rates from nine provinces of China are shown (WHO 1987). In comparing Hunan and Sichuan, it is important to note that, although the overall prevalence of blindness is the same, the prevalence of cataract blindness in Sichuan is double that of Hunan. Because of the large number of people examined, the reliability of these data is unusually high and, assuming that unbiased samples were obtained, the likelihood that the ob-

served difference could have been observed if chance alone was operating is less than 1 percent ($p < .01$).

Cataract Surgery in Developing Countries

Approximately 1 million cataract extractions were performed in 1988 in both India (Venkataswamy, 1987) and the United States (HCFA 1986), although the population of India is more than triple that of the United States. Even if the prevalence of cataract were equal in the two countries, the lower rate of surgery might account for a good portion of the excess in cataract blindness. Fewer than 10 percent of blinding cataracts are extracted annually in developing countries (HKI 1986). Although cataract has recently been shown to be the leading cause of blindness in an American urban population, the overall prevalence of cataract blindness is an order of magnitude lower than in the developing world (Sommer and others 1991).

One way to estimate the effect of variations in rates of cataract surgery on overall prevalence of cataract blindness is to examine the prevalence of cataractous change by age. If individuals with cataract and those who have had cataract extraction are combined, such a survey should yield a reliable indication of the overall prevalence of cataract by age in the population.

Few surveys of this type have been conducted because the survey methodology to detect any clinically significant degree of cataract is far more complex than that required to detect blinding cataract. In the United States, researchers for the Framingham Eye Study examined a representative sample of residents of Framingham, Massachusetts, a primarily white, middle-class community (Sperduto and Hiller 1984). Researchers for a second American study, the National Health and Nutrition Examination Survey, drew a random sample of all Americans, based upon census data (Ederer, Hiller, and Taylor 1981; Hiller, Sperduto, and Ederer 1983). In figure 26-2 the U.S. data are compared with those obtained in the Nepal Blindness Survey, a random cluster sample of the entire kingdom of Nepal (Brilliant and others 1988). This is the only epidemiologic survey in developing countries in which the entire population of a country has been sampled and studied for eye disease.

As is readily apparent from figure 26-2, even when cataractous and aphakic individuals are combined, the prevalence of cataract is substantially higher in Nepal than in the United States in each age group. Thus, the difference in surgical rate alone does not account for the higher rate of cataract blindness observed in at least one developing nation. Because some degree of lens change inevitably accompanies aging, these data may also be interpreted to suggest that individuals in Nepal develop cataract at a younger age than their counterparts in the United States.

If the prevalence of cataract itself is truly greater in the developing world, there are only two possible explanations. Either the incidence of cataract by age is greater in developing countries, or persons with cataract in such countries live longer

Table 26-1. Prevalence of Cataract Blindness, by Country

Country	Prevalence of blindness	Percent of blindness from cataract	Prevalence of cataract blindness	Population (millions)	Population with cataract blindness (millions)
Africa					
Botswana	1.4	0.45	0.63	1.01	0.01
Chad	2.3	0.48	1.104	4.79	0.50
Egypt	3.3	0.32	1.056	44.50	0.47
Ethiopia	1.3	0.46	0.598	33.68	0.20
The Gambia	0.7	0.55	0.385	0.80	0.00
Kenya	1.1	0.67	0.737	18.78	0.14
Liberia	2.1	0.45	0.945	2.06	0.02
Malawi	1.3	0.40	0.52	6.43	0.03
Mali	1.3	0.32	0.416	7.53	0.03
Nigeria	1.5	0.41	0.615	89.02	0.55
Sudan	6.4	0.30	1.92	20.36	0.39
Togo	1.3	0.45	0.585	2.76	0.02
Tunisia	3.9	0.52	2.028	6.89	0.14
Zimbabwe	1.2	0.40	0.48	7.14	0.03
Americas					
Brazil	0.3	0.10	0.03	129.70	0.04
Peru	1.0	0.34	0.34	18.70	0.06
United States	0.2	0.13	0.026	233.70	0.06
Asia					
Afghanistan	2.0	0.31	0.62	17.22	0.11
Bangladesh	0.9	0.33	0.30	94.65	0.28
China[a]	0.875	0.22	0.14	1040.00	1.41
Hong Kong	0.2	0.34	0.07	5.31	0.01
India	0.5	0.55	0.27	732.00	2.01
Indonesia	1.2	0.67	0.80	159.00	1.28
Japan	0.3	0.23	0.07	119.00	0.08
Korea	0.1	0.361	0.04	40.00	0.01
Nepal	0.8	0.67	0.54	15.74	0.08
Pakistan	2.3	0.60	1.38	89.00	1.23
Saudi Arabia	1.5	0.55	0.82	10.40	0.09
Sri Lanka	2.0	0.46	0.92	15.00	0.14
Syrian Arab Rep.	0.3	0.35	0.10	9.60	0.01
Thailand	1.1	0.57	0.62	49.00	0.31
Viet Nam	0.8	0.39	0.31	57.00	0.18
Yemen, Rep. of	3.6	0.34	1.22	2.16	0.03
Europe					
Germany	0.1	0.04	0.004	61.42	0.002
Norway	0.2	0.07	0.014	4.13	0.001
Sweden	0.3	0.05	0.015	8.00	0.001
U.S.S.R.[b]	0.27	0.16	0.0432	272.50	0.12

a. Average.
b. Entire country (European and Asian parts).
Source: WHO Programme for the Prevention of Blindness 1987.

than those in the industrial world. Because the rate of mortality from all causes of those between the ages of forty-five and sixty-five in Asia is 1.65 times that of the industrial world and the mortality rate of those over sixty-five 1.25 times greater, increased longevity is an unlikely explanation for the increased prevalence of cataract. Increased incidence of cataract in developing countries must play a significant role.

Although the evidence strongly suggests an increased incidence of cataract in the developing world, few actual studies of cataract incidence have ever been conducted. Whereas prevalence surveys require that a large population be randomly sampled, recruited for study, and examined, incidence surveys require that those same individuals be located and reexamined after a defined time interval. The logistics and expense of conducting a longitudinal study of this nature are orders of magnitude greater than for a prevalence study.

Possible Explanations for Increased Cataract Incidence

One cannot rule out genetic differences as an explanation for increased cataract incidence in developing countries, but these factors are least amenable to modification. During the past

Figure 26-2. Prevalence of Cataract by Age, United States and Nepal

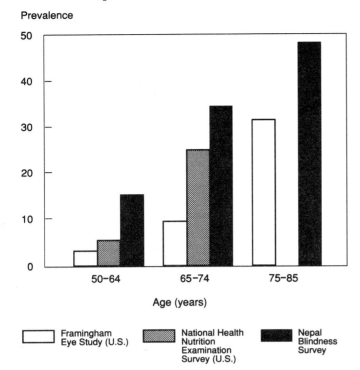

Note: No data for population age 78–85 in the National Health Nutrition Examination Survey.
Source: Framingham Eye Study (Sperduto and Hiller 1984); National Health Nutrition Examination Survey (Hiller, Sperduto, and Ederer 1983); Nepal Blindness Survey (Brilliant 1988).

decade, epidemiologists and lens biochemists have worked to gain a better understanding of the process of cataract formation and the role played by nutritional and environmental factors.

Although "age-related" or "senile" cataract is the most prevalent form, cataracts may be metabolic, traumatic, nutritional, or toxic in etiology. In general, cataract results from a denaturation of natural proteins within the lens of the eye. Just as the

Table 26-2. Prevalence of Cataract Blindness in Nine Provinces of China

Province	Prevalence of blindness	Percent of blindness from cataract	Prevalence of cataract blindness	Population examined
Fujian	0.2	0.35	0.07	50,620
Sichuan	0.3	0.4	0.12	21,869
Hunan	0.3	0.2	0.06	94,222
Anhui	0.7	0.36	0.25	13,852
Tianjin City	0.3	0.39	0.12	74,348
Guangdong	0.4	0.571	0.23	10,180
Guangxi	0.5	0.37	0.19	26,210
Heilonjiang	0.2	0.39	0.08	40,097
Huairon County	0.5	0.16	0.08	10,063

Note: Based on government-sponsored surveys.
Source: WHO Programme for the Prevention of Blindness 1987.

clear albumin of an egg white congeals, opacifies, and turns white with heat, the natural crystalline proteins of the lens are known to coalesce and discolor in response to certain stimuli.

Cross-linking and denaturation of lens proteins have been produced in laboratory settings by ultraviolet light and chemical oxidants. Thus, "oxidative-stress" from a variety of causes may be a common mechanism in the formation of cataract. The human lens is constantly exposed to oxidant stress, both from environmental light and from naturally occurring free radicals that are ubiquitous in the human body. Highly efficient enzyme systems are present within the eye to prevent damage from these agents. Inquiry into the etiology of cataract has therefore focused upon the environmental and nutritional exposures of individuals with cataract as well as any deficiencies that may exist in their antioxidant enzyme systems.

ASSOCIATION WITH DIABETES. Diabetes has been associated with an increased risk of cataract in Americans under fifty-five years of age (Hiller, Sperduto, and Ederer 1983) as well as with an increased rate of cataract surgery (Hiller and Kahn 1976). However, diabetes-related cataracts account for only 6 percent of all cases in the United States and an even lower proportion of cases worldwide. Despite this, cataract formation in diabetics is of substantial research interest, because of evidence that the underlying biochemical mechanism may involve the abnormal formation of sugar alcohols (sorbitol) in the lens, resulting in subsequent lens swelling and opacification. Human studies are now under way to determine if inhibition of this biochemical pathway is feasible and if such inhibition reduces the rate of cataractogenesis in humans. The longevity of diabetics in the developing world is substantially lower than elsewhere, and thus diabetes is unlikely to account for the excess cataract rate.

ASSOCIATION WITH SUNLIGHT. The association of cataract and sunlight has long been suspected on the basis of case-control studies. Hiller and colleagues found a higher cataract-to-control ratio for persons age sixty-five or older in areas with longer duration of sunlight (Hiller, Giacometti, and Yuen 1977; Hiller, Sperduto, and Ederer 1983). Taylor (1980a) reported an association of cataract with increased ultraviolet light, latitude, and average hours of sunlight. Other investigators have noted higher prevalence of cataract among Tibetans living at altitudes of 4,000 meters than those living at altitudes of 2,000 meters (Wen-shi 1979). Although a survey of 29,683 residents of the Punjab revealed a lower prevalence of cataract among those who lived in mountain regions than among those on the plains (Chatterjee, Milton, and Thyle 1982), this study did not control for the effect of cloud cover on the actual hours of sunlight exposure in each region. Researchers in the Nepal Blindness Survey calculated mean sunlight exposure for each village sampled on the basis of altitude, skyline obstructions, and cloud cover. As can be seen from table 26-3, there was a strong association between average daily sunlight hours and cataract prevalence (Brilliant and others 1983, 1988). Even so, this study controlled only for the sunlight exposure of the

Table 26-3. Cataract Prevalence by Average Daily Hours of Sunlight

Sunlight[a]	Population examined	Cataract cases	Prevalence (per 100)	Odds ratio
Low (7–9 hours)	7,236	133	1.84	1.0
Medium (10–11 hours)	10,263	221	2.15	1.2
High (12 hours)	10,286	476	4.63	2.6

a. Based on sunlight exposure for lifelong residents of ninety-seven rural villages.
Source: Brilliant and others 1988.

village and did not take into account the exposure of individuals based upon their occupations and use of such protective clothing as hats.

Taylor and co-workers (1988) addressed the issue of individual exposure to sunlight and ultraviolet radiation in their survey of 838 Maryland watermen who earn their living by fishing on the Chesapeake Bay. Using dosimeters, the researchers correlated the watermen's actual ocular exposure to ultraviolet radiation (UVR) with working hours, sheltered vs. unsheltered work sites, and protective devices worn. They found a clear association between increased exposure to UVR and the presence of cortical cataract. As reported in a related paper by Bochow and others (1989), the outdoor worker wearing sunglasses and a hat has only twice the exposure to UVR of the indoor worker. When no eye protection is worn, however, the exposure of the outdoor worker to UVR is eighteen times that of the indoor worker. The authors of this related study compared patients suffering from posterior subcapsular cataract who were exposed to UVR during sunlight hours with normal controls who were similarly exposed. A strong association ($p < .001$) was detected between ocular sunlight exposure and cataract.

ASSOCIATION WITH NUTRITIONAL AND METABOLIC FACTORS. Although nutritional factors might be intuitively associated with cataract, their significance is quite difficult to prove. Blood levels of vitamins reflect only current nutritional status and cannot detect previous periods of hypovitaminosis. An association between cataract and diet was observed in the Nepal Blindness Survey, in which vegetarians who never ate meat or fish were found to have twice the cataract prevalence of those who ate fish or meat, even occasionally (Brilliant and others 1988). A caveat in interpreting these data is that vegetarianism was most common in the regions with the highest sunlight exposure and it was impossible to separate these two possibly interacting variables.

In their study of the Punjab, Chatterjee, Milton, and Thyle (1982) reported a relative increase in prevalence of cataract among individuals with lower protein consumption. The authors of the Indian and U.S. case-control study of age-related cataracts (Mohan, Sperduto, Angra, and others 1989) similarly detected an increased risk of posterior subcapsular and nuclear cataract in those individuals who had a history of a diet deficient in protein. Biochemical analysis from the same study

detected an association with lower levels of ascorbic acid. In a case-control study of Americans with and without senile cataract reported by Jacques and co-workers, the risk of cataract was reduced for individuals with higher blood levels of carotenoids, vitamin D, and vitamin E, whereas the risk was increased for those with lower levels of vitamin C (Jacques, Hartz, Chylack, McGandy, and Sadowski 1988).

Carotenoids, along with vitamins C and E, are potent antioxidants and thus quench free radicals. Therefore, if the theory of oxidative stress is valid, it should not be surprising that their levels are associated with cataract risk. Jacques, Chylack, McGandy, and Hartz (1988) reported that higher levels of an "antioxidant index," composed of vitamins C and E and carotenoids, along with antioxidant enzymes found in red blood cells were associated with lower risk of cataract. Corroborating data regarding this antioxidant index were reported from the Indian and U.S. case-control study (Mohan and others 1989).

ASSOCIATION WITH SEVERE DIARRHEA AND DEHYDRATION. Minassian, Mehra, and Jones (1984) have advanced the theory that severe diarrhea and subsequent dehydration might lead to an elevated level of blood urea nitrogen and, thus, to alteration of lens proteins and cataract. This theory, attractive from the biochemical point of view, has not been corroborated in epidemiologic studies. Khan, Khan, and Sheikh (1987) found no correlation between cataract risk and cholera-related diarrhea in a case-control study performed in Bangladesh. Similarly, Bhatnagar and colleagues (1988) found no association between cataract and remembered episodes of severe diarrhea from a study in South India.

Lowering or Postponing Disease Incidence

Currently, there are no proven interventions that prevent cataract or delay its onset. Although cataract surgery is likely to remain the most cost-effective means of treating an existing cataract, strategies that decrease or delay the onset of cataract are of vital importance. Because of the strong association between cataract and aging, a ten-year increase in the average life span in developing countries is likely to double the prevalence of cataract. Similarly, a ten-year delay in the onset of cataract would halve its prevalence in the population. Although this may seem an impossible task, one must remember that eighty-year-old residents of Framingham, Massachusetts, have the same prevalence of cataract as seventy-year-old residents of India and Nepal. Although nutritional and metabolic deficiencies may serve as a risk factor for cataractogenesis, interventions in this area go far beyond the scope of eye disease. Even if improved nutrition does delay the onset of cataract, the interventions required are identical to those required to combat all other malnutrition-associated conditions in developing countries.

If, in fact, exposure to ultraviolet radiation is a risk factor for cataractogenesis, public health interventions that decrease ocular UVR exposure may have a useful role. They are intriguing from the international development point of view in that they may be quite inexpensive. Rosenthal and co-workers (1988) have shown that a brimmed hat reduces ocular UVR exposure by approximately 50 percent, and the addition of UVR-absorbing sunglasses further lowers transmission to 1 percent of ambient UVR. Whereas UVR-absorbing sunglasses are expensive to manufacture and obtain by the standards of developing countries, locally manufactured hats of straw or other ubiquitous materials are practically free. Furthermore, although properly manufactured UVR-absorbing sunglasses may potentially block 86 percent to 99 percent of ambient UVR, a 0.6 centimeter displacement of sunglasses away from the forehead results in a substantial increase in ocular UVR exposure (Rosenthal, Bakalian, and Taylor 1986). Additional studies need to be performed in which individual exposure to UVR is measured during outdoor activities and inexpensive interventions are tested.

Reducing the Burden of Cataract Blindness

The National Eye Institute and its collaborating institutions have embarked on a long-term research effort to develop drugs that may delay the onset of cataract. Although this research has yielded invaluable insight into the biochemistry of the lens and possible metabolic pathways of cataractogenesis, clinical trials are only in the earliest planning stages. A chemotherapeutic strategy that could delay the onset of cataract by ten years in the United States would have the potential to save $500 million or more annually in surgical costs. Because of the low cost of cataract extraction in developing countries and the likely high cost of chronic use of any new drug, it will probably be many years before this can be a cost-effective strategy for the developing world.

Cataract Surgery in Developing Countries

Once cataract has developed, the only known treatment is surgical removal. Helen Keller International has reported that the cost of cataract extraction ranges from $15 in a mass-surgery setting on the Indian subcontinent to $22 in an African mobile surgical facility, to $33 in an urban Latin American public hospital (HKI 1986). Fortunately, cataract extraction is highly successful, even with the limited resources, lower standards of sterility, and older instruments found in developing countries. Substantial improvements in outcome of surgery were achieved during the 1960s and 1970s, when microsurgical techniques and watertight closure of cataract wounds with fine silk or nylon sutures were universally adopted.

There remain two main methods of cataract extraction today: extracapsular cataract extraction (ECCE), which has been adopted by nearly all the industrial world, and intracapsular cataract extraction (ICCE), which is employed in less than 10 percent of cases in the United States and considerably more frequently in the developing world. The latter type of extraction involves removing the entire lens with disruption of the zonular fibers which form the attachment of the lens capsule to surrounding ocular structures. The former entails incising the lens capsule, expressing the lens nucleus and aspirating remaining lens cortex, leaving intact, if all goes well, the lens capsule and its zonular attachments. The ECCE method enables the surgeon to insert an intraocular lens into the remaining lens capsule and is thought to preserve better the anatomy of the eye.

Christy and Lall (1973) reported an infection rate of 0.46 percent for 54,000 ICCEs performed at a mass-surgery program in Pakistan. Although this is higher than the 0.17 percent infection rate following ICCE in the United States (Javitt and others 1991a), it is certainly acceptable by local standards.

In this setting, functional vision is restored to between 85 percent and 92 percent of patients who undergo surgery (Javitt, Venkataswamy, and Sommer 1983; Al Salem and Ismail 1987; Whitfield 1987; Brilliant and others 1988). Suboptimal outcomes are a function of preexisting retinal disorders, as well as complications of surgery. The standard intracapsular cataract extraction commonly performed in developing countries is a mature surgical procedure that requires little in the way of technical improvement.

Because an aphakic eye (one that has undergone cataract extraction) is left with an extreme refractive error, corrective spectacles, contact lenses, or intraocular lens implants (IOLs) are required for visual rehabilitation of the patient. In most developing nations, locally manufactured spectacles in a standard aphakic power are available for $5 to $12. At present, IOLs are considerably more expensive, and contact lenses with their need for frequent replacement and sterile solutions are totally impractical. Davies and colleagues (1986) have shown that IOLs are more cost-effective than contact lenses in the National Health Service of the United Kingdom and may offer considerable advantages in patient comfort and reduction of subsequent complications.

Although conventional wisdom has long held that intracapsular cataract extraction with provision of aphakic spectacles is the appropriate technology for the developing world, this approach needs re-evaluation. Aphakic spectacles are notably thick and uncomfortable to wear. Although straight-ahead vision can be corrected to 20/20, they cause considerable distortion of peripheral vision and complete obscuration of objects between 30° and 45° in the periphery. Moreover, magnification induced by aphakic spectacles makes objects such as steps and curbs appear closer than they are. Ellwein and others (1991) have noticed that as many as half of those who receive aphakic spectacles in cataract surgery programs in the developing world do not wear them and hence, suffer extremely limited postoperative vision.

In recent years, there has been increased interest in converting to extracapsular cataract extraction with intraocular lens implantation, which is currently the dominant procedure in industrial nations. Analysis of 330,000 cases of cataract extraction in the United States reveals that patients who undergo ICCE have a 1.7-fold higher likelihood of infection and retinal detachment than those who undergo ECCE (Javitt and others 1991a and 1991b). Although there is likely to be an improvement in outcome and reduced risk of complication following

ECCE, this procedure requires the use of an operating microscope, more delicate surgical techniques, and sterile irrigating solutions. Approximately three to six months of full-time training is required to teach the newer extracapsular technique to a skilled ophthalmologic surgeon familiar with older methods.

Extracapsular cataract extraction enables the surgeon to place an intraocular lens in the posterior lens capsule (see figure 26-3), where it is least likely to cause ocular discomfort and long-term corneal complications. However, the lens capsule itself is likely to opacify over a period of years in 25 percent of those who undergo the procedure. In the industrial world, this circumstance is routinely managed by using a solid state (Neodymium: YAG) laser to create an opening (capsulotomy) in the opacified lens capsule. An alternative is to incise the lens capsule with a needle-knife, which is easily performed in the physician's office. This latter approach was routinely employed in the United States and Europe until introduction of the solid state laser in the early 1980s. While the capsulotomy procedure is quite simple to perform, opening the lens capsule in this manner increases the risk of subsequent retinal detachment to approximately the same level as that following intracapsular cataract extraction.

An alternative to postoperative capsulotomy in the 25 percent of patients who are likely to develop capsular opacity is to perform a capsulotomy at time of surgery after placement of the intraocular lens. The disadvantage of this approach is that all patients will be subject to higher risk of retinal detachment associated with disruption of the posterior capsule. Conversely, this approach may be the only practical one in settings where long-term follow-up of patients is infeasible.

Current techniques achieve the purpose of restoring functional vision to most of those who are blinded by cataract. Unless an individual is accustomed to reading or performing similarly demanding tasks, the visual outcome of ICCE with spectacle correction may be acceptable. As the price of an intraocular lens continues to decline, however, it may even rival the cost of aphakic spectacles. With improved technology ECCE may become the preferred method of cataract extraction in the developing world, as well.

Economic Return on Cataract Surgery

The economic cost associated with cataract reflects the near-total disability associated with this condition. My colleagues and I performed a pilot study to determine the cost-benefit ratio of restoring sight via cataract surgery in developing countries (Javitt, Venkataswamy, and Sommer 1983). The Aravind Eye Hospital in Madurai, India, is a private charitable institution that currently performs more than 20,000 free cataract extractions annually on indigent patients who are functionally blind at the time of surgery. The cost of surgery is funded by revenues from paying patients and private voluntary organizations. One hundred patients were randomly selected from among those who visited the hospital for follow-up care between six months and two years after surgery. By means of an interview in their native language, the patients were queried as to the effect of losing their sight on their economic and social circumstances. In addition to earning ability before and after surgery, patients were asked about other members of the family who were able to return to work after the patient's surgery or who were forced to leave work when the patient initially became visually incapacitated. The interview data were correlated with the outcome of surgery.

Eighty-five percent of the patients surveyed achieved postoperative visual acuity of 6/36 or better. Eight percent had vision of 6/60, and 7 percent had visual acuity of less than 6/60. Patients were included in the study data regardless of the surgical outcome.

Eighty-five percent of the males and 58 percent of the females who had lost their jobs as a result of blindness regained those jobs. A number of those who did not return to work did free other family members from household duties, thereby enabling them to return to work. Eighty-eight percent of male patients and 93 percent of female patients who reported having lost authority within their family and their community stated that they had regained their social standing.

At the time of the study the marginal cost of performing a cataract extraction was $5 dollars (53 rupees). Economic data were compared with that investment cost. The results showed that the average individual regaining functional vision through cataract extraction in this setting generated 1,500 percent of the cost of surgery in increased economic productivity during the first year following surgery. This benefit was generated both by the patients and by their family members

Figure 26-3. Lense Implant with Subsequent Capsulotomy

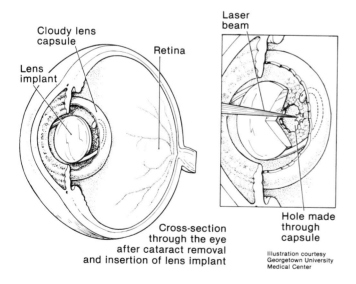

Cloudy lens capsule

Lens implant

Retina

Laser beam

Hole made through capsule

Cross-section through the eye after cataract removal and insertion of lens implant

Illustration courtesy
Georgetown University
Medical Center

Note: Following extracapsular cataract extraction, the lense implant is placed into the remaining capsule of the natural lens (figure left), which may subsequently opacify. The Neodynium: YAG laser can then be used to make an opening (capsulotomy) in the opacified lense capsule without harming the implant (figure right).

who were able to return to work. No data yet exist on the annual return on investment for the long term.

Cost-Effectiveness, or Cost Utility, of Cataract Surgery

Elsewhere in this collection, a year of the life of a functionally blind person has been equated to a loss of 0.5 disability-adjusted life-year (DALY). Torrance (1982) reported empirical data suggesting that individuals associate a utility value of 0.39 (with perfect health represented as 1.0) with a lifetime of being "blind, deaf, or unable to speak." Drummond and co-workers (1987, 1988) employed a utility scale calibrated in disability-adjusted life-years (DALYs) and reported that a year of life for a poorly adjusted (poorly rehabilitated) blind person is valued at 0.35 DALY, whereas a year of life for a well-adjusted (well-rehabilitated) blind person is valued at 0.48 DALY.

For consistency with other chapters, in my comparison of cataract extraction with other potential health care interventions I have employed the DALY model in which healthy years of future life are discounted at a rate of 5 percent. I have assumed a year of life following successful bilateral surgery to equal 1.0 healthy years of life and a year of life following successful unilateral surgery to equal 0.84 healthy years of life. This is consistent with data from a U.S. study of cataract patients in which the improvement in visual function following cataract surgery in the second eye was approximately 50 percent of that associated with improvement following surgery in the first eye (Javitt, Street, Brenner, and others 1993). I have assumed bilateral cataract surgery costs in the developing world to be between $18.00 and $42.50 per eye in 1990 and the cost of spectacles to be $6.00.

In assessing the benefits accruing from any procedure, the survival of the underlying population must be considered. Data from 330,000 U.S. Medicare patients undergoing cataract extraction indicate 75 percent survival at five years after surgery with an absolutely straight survival curve (Street and Javitt 1992). Based on the U.S. data, I have assumed the average patient undergoing cataract surgery in the developing world to have a 5 percent annual mortality risk after surgery. Because cataract patients in the developing world tend to be ten years younger on average than those in the United States, however, survival may be different in that setting.

Surgery in a single eye has an 85 percent chance of restoring vision, for a probable gain of 2.00 DALYs in the patient's expected future lifetime. On the basis of this assumption, bilateral surgery has a 72 percent chance of restoring vision in both eyes, and a 96 percent chance of restoring vision in at least one eye (assuming independence of eyes) for a probable gain of 3.05 DALYs. I further assumed that a new pair of spectacles is required every five years of life.

Table 26-4 is a comparison between the projected cost-utility ratios of unilateral and bilateral cataract surgery and several other health care interventions reported elsewhere in this collection. As can be seen from the table, cataract surgery compares quite favorably with several interventions that are generally accepted without question in the public health arena.

Table 26-4. Cost-Utility of Cataract Surgery and Other Types of Health Interventions

Intervention	Cost per DALY saved (dollars)
Bilateral cataract surgery	
$18.00 per eye	15.70
$26.80 per eye	21.50
$42.50 per eye	31.80
Unilateral cataract surgery	
$18.00 per eye	15.00
$26.80 per eye	19.00
$42.50 per eye	27.00
Noncataract intervention	
Passive case finding and short-term chemotherapy for TB	10.00
DPT and polio immunization	20.00–40.00
Oral hypoglycemic management of NIDDM	330.00

Source: Jamison, chapter 1, this collection.

Increasing Availability of Cataract Surgery

Although shortage of qualified surgeons is commonly invoked as an explanation for the backlog of blinding cataract in developing countries (Wilson 1980; Foster 1987), it bears careful scrutiny. The ratio of ophthalmologists to population in India is 1:100,000, the same as that for Great Britain (Venkataswamy 1987). Yet, in the face of an alarming prevalence of cataract blindness, Indian ophthalmologists remain concentrated in the cities, where many are underemployed, if not unemployed. There remains an undersupply of ophthalmologists in rural areas. The cost of starting a surgical facility is beyond the resources of most individuals, and government jobs that would allow one to practice in a public hospital are scarce. Thus, the Indian subcontinent is faced more with a maldistribution of surgeons than with a true shortage. Africa, to the contrary, truly presents an example of worker shortage, where there is only one ophthalmologist per 1 million people, or one ophthalmologist for every 4,000 blind individuals (Foster 1987; Schwab 1987).

MASS SURGICAL STRATEGY. High-volume surgical facilities have been in place in India and Pakistan for the past twenty years (Christy and Lall 1973; Liu and others 1977; Wilson 1980; Foster 1987; Venkataswamy 1987). They have demonstrated that cataract surgery can be performed inexpensively and safely on an assembly-line basis. Costs have traditionally been borne by a combination of government funding, private voluntary organization support, and patient fees. Not surprisingly, patients recognize the value of sight restoration and will contribute to their own care within their means. Unfortunately, when family resources are stretched thin, even the cost of food during hospitalization may be too large a burden for a family in a subsistence economy.

Fixed surgical facilities may succeed in areas of high population density, but rural areas might best be served by satellite or mobile facilities. A study in Tanzania reported that only 39 percent of patients scheduled for surgery actually appeared if the facility was more than twenty-five miles from home. A decrease in the distance that patients were required to travel meant substantially increased rates of participation (HKI 1985).

Thus far, mass surgery has generally relied upon expatriate ophthalmologists for at least a portion of their surgical workers. This arrangement is necessary if a large volume of surgery is to be performed and the backlog reduced. Because this is clearly not a self-sustaining arrangement, training programs must be devised to provide local ophthalmic surgeons who will remain in the community.

TRAINING OF LOCAL PROVIDERS. An ongoing problem in training local ophthalmologists has been a tendency for those who go to large urban centers for training to remain in those urban centers. The training they receive may not be ideally suited to the problems they will encounter if they do return home. In recent years, Helen Keller International has mounted a highly successful program to train eye surgeons in the Philippine outer islands. General medical officers are selected at the local level and are trained in situ by visiting faculty. Their training focuses on the problems that face their community. Thus far the dropout rate has been minimal and the cost of training far less than would be required if travel and housing were required for training in urban centers.

A pilot program in Kenya has demonstrated that nonphysician ophthalmic clinical officers can be trained to perform cataract surgery with acceptable results (Whitfield 1987). Although the mechanical aspects of surgery can be learned by individuals of good dexterity, there is no evidence yet that surgical judgment and the judgment required to manage complications can be taught without duplicating most of a formal residency in ophthalmology. A second problem in this strategy is that most developing countries have physician licensing laws that are as strict as those of any Western country. Because of the public health menace of semiskilled itinerant cataract surgeons, countries such as Pakistan have laws that mandate jail sentences for nonphysicians who perform eye surgery.

Increasing Participation in Care

Although providing care at an affordable cost (which may mean free of charge in some areas) is an essential step in the eradication of cataract blindness, the simple provision of care is not sufficient to guarantee its acceptance. Only 20 percent of blind individuals in southern India who were offered free cataract extraction appeared for surgery within three years (Venkataswamy and Brilliant 1981). The remaining blind persons declined because of mistrust, lack of access to the facility, inability to pay for food while hospitalized, or other concerns. The result is that community-based facilities may remain underused in the face of an overwhelming backlog of cataract blindness.

Several researchers have studied factors that affect rates of participation in cataract surgery at a community-based pro-

gram in India (Christy and Lall 1973; Venkataswamy and Brilliant 1981). The provision of free transportation to the hospital and food while hospitalized substantially increased the frequency with which patients appeared for cataract surgery (Bhatnagar and others 1988). Since blind individuals are essentially immobile without assistance in that society, the provision of transportation not only relieves the patient of a monetary burden but eliminates the need for another family member to be away from work during the patient's hospitalization. Similar findings have been reported from Nepal by Brilliant and Brilliant (1985).

Research Priorities for Ending Cataract Blindness

In 1986 the National Eye Institute co-sponsored a conference with Helen Keller International in which leading public health ophthalmologists and policymakers articulated long-term research priorities for the eradication of cataract blindness (HKI 1986). Research goals were divided into three focus areas:

Operations research techniques for improving the efficiency and effectiveness of cataract care in developing countries. The aim of specific projects would be the following:

- To compare the effectiveness of various methods of identifying cataract-blind people within a community and, through the reduction of psychosocial and economic barriers, motivate them to seek surgery
- To compare alternatives for improving access to cataract surgery, such as eye camps or the establishment of temporary satellite hospitals
- To evaluate alternative forms of minimum-level ophthalmic surgical facilities in regions that are currently underserved
- To improve operating room efficiency
- To determine ways of reducing the postoperative stay following cataract surgery
- To increase the number of ophthalmic personnel trained to perform cataract surgery in underserved areas

Epidemiologic research designed to measure the magnitude of the cataract blind population in different regions, study the risk factors for cataract, and evaluate methods of delaying the onset of cataract through controlled clinical trials. Following are specific priorities:

- Developing a standard, reproducible system for classifying and documenting the type and severity of cataractous change
- Identifying the risk factors for aging-related cataracts in populations that have widely varying prevalence of disease
- Studying migrant groups who move from high-prevalence areas to low-prevalence areas in order to determine the relative importance of genetic and environmental factors in cataract development

- Developing noninvasive techniques that can be used to measure precisely the progression of human cataract
- Implementing randomized controlled clinical trials to test the potential of strategies intended to delay cataract onset

Biological research designed to elucidate the biochemical and physiologic mechanisms of cataractogenesis. The goal of specific projects would be the following:

- To test the hypothesis that oxidative damage to lens proteins is a significant cause of human aging-related cataract and to develop mechanisms for preventing that damage
- To develop a method to grow human lens cells in tissue culture in order to study the normal and abnormal production of lens proteins
- To study the molecular biology underlying the formation of congenital and hereditary cataracts in the hope of shedding light on the process of age-related cataractogenesis

Conclusions

Cataract is the leading cause of blindness and disability in developing countries. Current surgical methods of treating cataract are highly effective and cost between $15 and $33 per patient. Initial research suggests that the patient who benefits from sight-restoring cataract surgery may generate a 1,500 percent or greater annual return on the cost of surgery.

The elimination of cataract as the main cause of world blindness requires initiatives on multiple levels in order to formulate short-term, intermediate-term, and long-term solutions. The most pressing need is to begin immediately to reduce the backlog of cataract blindness through mass surgery. This requires a commitment of resources along with initiatives in operations research designed to reduce barriers to surgery and increase the effectiveness of public health programs. Economic research is similarly required to study net savings to patients, their families, and society of sight restoration through cataract surgery.

Although the strategy of mass surgery using expatriate ophthalmologists has the potential to reduce the current backlog, only by training local ophthalmologists and ancillary personnel will it be self-sustaining. Additional epidemiologic research is needed in order to elucidate better the relationship between cataract and environmental factors as well as the effects of reducing known risk factors.

The currently used technology for cataract extraction is adequate for the needs of developing countries, but eventually the instrumentation required for extracapsular extraction and lens implantation will become economically feasible in these countries. The new technologies of surgical extraction combined with the long-term hope of affordable pharmacologic intervention may one day make the current burden of cataract blindness a dim vision of the past.

References

Al Salem, M., and L. Ismail. 1987. "Factors Influencing Visual Outcome after Cataract Extraction among Arabs in Kuwait." *British Journal of Ophthalmology* 71:458–61.

Bhatnagar, R., K. P. West, S. Vitale, S. Joshi, G. Venkataswamy, and A. Sommer. 1988. "Risk of Cataract and History of Severe Diarrheal Disease in Southern India." Abstract. *Investigative Ophthalmology* 29:8.

Bochow, T. W., S. K. West, A. Azar, B. Munoz, A. Sommer, and H. R. Taylor. 1989. "Ultraviolet Light Exposure and Risk of Posterior Subcapsular Cataracts." *Archives of Ophthalmology* 107:369–72.

Brilliant, G. E., and L. B. Brilliant. 1985. "Using Social Epidemiology to Understand Who Stays Blind and Who Gets Operated for Cataract in a Rural Setting." *Social Science and Medicine* 21:553–58.

Brilliant, G. E., R. P. Pokhrel, N. C. Grasset, and L. B. Brilliant. 1988. "The Epidemiology of Blindness in Nepal: Report of the 1981 Nepal Blindness Survey." Seva Foundation, Ann Arbor, Mich.

Brilliant, L. B., N. C. Grasset, R. P. Pokhrel, A. Kolstad, J. M. Lepkowski, G. E. Brilliant, W. M. Hawks, and R. Pararajeskgaram. 1983. "Associations among Cataract Prevalence, Sunlight Hours, and Altitude in the Himalayas." *American Journal of Epidemiology* 118:250–64.

Brilliant, G. E., J. M. Lepkowski, B. Zwuta, R. D. Thulasiraj. 1991. "Social Determinants of Cataract Surgery Utilization in South India." *Archives of Ophthalmology* 109(4):584–89.

CDC (Centers for Disease Control). 1983. *Morbidity and Mortality Weekly Report* 32:119.

Chatterjee, A., R. C. Milton, and S. Thyle. 1982. "Prevalence and Aetiology of Cataract in Punjab." *British Journal of Ophthalmology* 66:35–42.

Christy, N. E., and P. Lall. 1973. "Postoperative Endophthalmitis following Cataract Surgery." *Archives of Ophthalmology* 90:361–66.

Davies, L. M., M. F. Drummond, E. G. Woodward, and R. J. Buckley. 1986. "A Cost-Effectiveness Comparison of the Intraocular Lens and the Contact Lens in Aphakia." *Transactions of the Ophthalmologic Society of the UK* 105:304–13.

Dawson, C. R., and I. R. Schwab. 1981. "Epidemiology of Cataract—A Major Cause of Preventable Blindness." *Bulletin of the World Health Organization* 59:493–501.

Drummond, M. F. 1988. "Economic Aspects of Cataract." *Ophthalmology* 95:1147–53.

Drummond, M. R., G. L. Stoddart, and G. W. Torrance. 1987. *Methods for the Economic Evaluation of Health Care Programmes.* Oxford: Oxford University Press.

Ederer, F., R. Hiller, and H. R. Taylor. 1981. "Senile Lens Changes and Diabetes in Two Population Studies." *American Journal of Ophthalmology* 91:381–95.

Ellwein, L. B., J. M. Lepkowski, R. D. Thulasiraj, and G. E. Brilliant. 1991. "The Cost Effectiveness of Strategies to Reduce Barriers to Cataract Surgery." *International Ophthalmology* 15(3):175–83.

Foster, A. 1987. "Cataract Blindness in Africa." *Ophthalmic Surgery* 18:384–88.

HCFA (Health Care Financing Administration). 1986. Summary data on cataract surgery, drawn for Medicare Part-B claims. Distributed by Ms. Michael McMullen, HCFA, Oak Meadows Building, Security Blvd., Baltimore, Md.

HKI (Helen Keller International). 1985. *Kongwa Primary Health Care Report 1984–85.* New York.

———. 1986. *To Restore Sight: The Global Conquest of Cataract Blindness.* New York.

Hiller, R., L. Giacometti, and K. Yuen. 1977. "Sunlight and Cataract: An Epidemiologic Investigation." *American Journal of Epidemiology* 105:450–59.

Hiller, R., R. D. Sperduto, and F. Ederer. 1983. "Epidemiologic Associations with Cataract in the 1971–1972 National Health and Nutrition Examination Survey." *American Journal of Epidemiology* 118:239–49.

Jacques, P. F., L. T. Chylack, Jr., R. B. McGandy, and S. C. Hartz. 1988. "Antioxidant Status in Persons with and without Senile Cataract." *Archives of Ophthalmology* 106:337–40.

Jacques, P. F., S. C. Hartz, L. T. Chylack, Jr., R. B. McGandy, and J. A. Sadowski. 1988. "Nutritional Status in Persons with and without Senile Cataract: Blood Vitamin and Mineral Levels." *American Journal of Clinical Nutrition* 48:152–58.

Javitt, J. C., G. Venkataswamy, and A. Sommer. 1983. "The Economic and Social Aspect of Restoring Sight." In P. Henkind, ed., ACTA: *24th International Congress of Ophthalmology.* New York: J. B. Lippincott.

Javitt, J. C., S. Vitale, J. K. Canner, H. Krakauer, A. M. McBean, and A. Sommer. 1991a. "National Outcomes of Cataract Extraction 2: Endophthalmitis following Inpatient Surgery." *Archives of Ophthalmology,* 109:1085–89.

———. 1991b. "National Outcomes of Cataract Extraction 1: Retinal Detachment following Inpatient Surgery." *Archives of Ophthalmology.*

Javitt, J. C., D. A. Street, H. M. Brenner, and others. 1993. "Improvement in Visual Function following Cataract Surgery in the First and the Second Eye." *Archives of Ophthalmology.*

Khan, M. U., M. R. Khan, and A. K. Sheikh. 1987. "Dehydrating Diarrhoea and Cataract in Rural Bangladesh." *Indian Journal of Medical Research* 85:311–15.

Liu, H. S., W. J. McGannon, F. I. Tolentino, and C. L. Schepens. 1977. "Massive Cataract Relief in Eye Camps." *Annals of Ophthalmology* 1979:503–8.

Minassian, D. C., V. Mehra, and B. R. Jones. 1984. "Dehydrational Crisis from Severe Diarrhoea or Heatstroke and Risk of Cataract." *Lancet* 10: 751–53.

Mohan, M., R. D. Sperduto, S. K. Angra, R. C. Milton, R. L. Mathur, B. A. Underwood, N. Jaffery, C. B. Pandya, Viki Chhabra, R. B. Vajpayee. 1989. "India-U.S. Case-Control Study of Age-Related Cataracts." *Archives of Ophthalmology* 107:670–76.

Rosenthal, F. S., A. E. Bakalian, and H. R. Taylor. 1986. "The Effect of Prescription Eyewear on Ocular Exposure to Ultraviolet Radiation." *American Journal of Public Health* 76:1216–20.

Rosenthal, F. S., C. Phoon, A. E. Bakalian, and H. R. Taylor. 1988. "The Ocular Dose of Ultraviolet Radiation to Outdoor Workers." *Investigative Ophthalmology and Visual Science* 29:649–56.

Schwab, L. 1987. "Cost-Effective Cataract Surgery in Developing Nations." *Ophthalmic Surgery* 18:307–9.

Sperduto, R. D., and R. Hiller. 1984. "The Prevalence of Nuclear, Cortical, and Posterior Subcapsular Lens Opacities in a General Population Sample." *Ophthalmology* 91:815–18.

Street, D. A., and J. C. Javitt. 1992. "National Outcome of Cataract Extraction IV: Increased Mortality following Cataract Extraction in Beneficiaries." *American Journal of Ophthalmology* 113:263–68.

Taylor, H. R. 1980a. "The Environment and the Lens." *British Journal of Ophthalmology* 64:303–10.

———. 1980b. "Prevalence and Causes of Blindness in Australian Aborigines." *Medical Journal of Australia* 1:71–76.

———. 1980c. "The Prevalence of Corneal Disease and Cataracts in Australian Aborigines in Northwestern Australia." *Australian Journal of Ophthalmology* 8:289–301.

Taylor, H. R., S. K. West, F. S. Rosenthal, B. Munoz, H. S. Newland, H. Abbey, E. A. Emmett. 1988. "Effect of Ultraviolet Radiation on Cataract Formation." *New England Journal of Medicine* 319:1429–33.

Torrance G. W., M. H. Boyle, S. P. Horwood. 1982. "Application of Multi-Attribute Utility Theory to Measure Social Preferences for Health States." *Operations Research* 30:1043–69.

Venkataswamy, G. 1987. "Cataract in the Indian Subcontinent." *Ophthalmic Surgery* 18:464–66.

Venkataswamy, G., and G. E. Brilliant. 1981. "Social and Economic Barriers to Cataract Surgery in Rural South India: A Preliminary Report." *Visual Impairment and Blindness* 405–508.

Venkataswamy, G., J. Lepkowski, R. L. Mowery, and the Operations Research Group. 1988. "Operations Research to Reduce Barriers to Cataract Surgery in India." *Investigative Ophthalmology* 29:8a.

Wen-shi, S. 1979. "A Survey of Senile Cataracts among High Altitude Living Tibetans in Changdu District." *Chinese Journal of Ophthalmology* 15: 100–4.

Whitfield, R. 1987. "Dealing with Cataract Blindness Part 3: Paramedical Cataract Surgery in Africa." *Ophthalmic Surgery* 18:765–67.

Whitfield, R., Jr., L. Schwab, N. J. Bakker, G. G. Bisley, and D. Ross Degnan. 1983. "Cataract and Corneal Opacity Are the Main Causes of Blindness in the Samburu Tribe of Kenya." *Ophthalmic Surgery* 14:139–44.

WHO (World Health Organization) Programme for the Prevention of Blindness. 1987. Available data on blindness. 87.14:1-23.34. Geneva.

Wilson, J. 1980. *World Blindness and Its Prevention.* Oxford: Oxford University Press.

27

Oral Health

Douglas Bratthall and David E. Barmes

In contrast to most other diseases, some of the oral diseases are well known and experienced by most people, albeit perhaps only to a mild degree. Those readers, however, who have had toothaches or jaw infections may testify that oral health problems can be so dominant that practically all other problems fade into insignificance until help is received—and, if professional help is not available, removing the aching tooth may be another never-forgotten experience.

A variety of diseases affect the oral cavity. Dental caries, the disease causing cavities in the teeth, is common worldwide. Untreated caries may lead to infection in the pulp, an infection that may spread to the supporting tissues and the jaws, with or without pain to the individual. Other common diseases are the periodontal diseases, including inflammation of the tissues surrounding the teeth and breakdown of bone support and loss of teeth.

Further problems affecting the teeth involve the position of the teeth, varying from simple conditions like too much space between them or overcrowding to serious lip and cleft palate syndromes resulting in chaos for the formation of normal dentition. Traffic accidents, violence, and certain sports and games often involve injuries to the teeth. Disturbances in the formation of normal tooth structures may be caused by inherited diseases or, as in the case of fluorosis, by the intake of too much fluoride through drinking water or food. A number of substances may give disturbing discolorations to the teeth, either when the substances are supplied during the time of formation of the teeth or when they are added to already erupted teeth.

The soft tissues in the oral cavity may be the site of numerous conditions, involving oral cancers, symptoms of infection by the human immunodeficiency virus (HIV), or less harmful but painful conditions. Disturbances in the normal saliva flow are not uncommon and are most prevalent in elderly people; such conditions are usually very uncomfortable for the person affected and may predispose him or her to further dental problems. Unnecessary or poor quality dental care can also be the cause of oral health problems.

From this short introduction, it is clear that the oral cavity is a center for a large variety of possible diseases, some of which can be prevented, some of which can be cured only by compli-cated operations performed by highly skilled personnel, and some of which cannot be treated by any methods known at present. To this should be added the fact that considerable importance is attached to the oral cavity in many cultures in developing countries; this may be illustrated by traditions such as grinding of healthy teeth to certain shapes or knocking out teeth for ceremonial reasons. In industrial countries the increasing number of advertisements for dental materials, and courses, in aesthetic dentistry also reflects this importance. Because the oral cavity is the means of communication, tasting, eating, kissing, and so on, and because it is positioned at a level where it is easily observed, it is understandable that many people regard oral health as very important.

Further information regarding the etiology will be given below for some of the most prevalent oral diseases. This should not be interpreted as an underestimation of the less prevalent diseases. Certainly, such diseases may be most inconvenient or even fatal for those affected. But, from a global point of view, any changes in the prevalence of the common oral diseases will be of such significance, that we, at this stage, can be excused for making such a restriction.

Dental Caries

Dental caries is characterized by the dissolution of the hard tissues of the teeth (enamel, dentin), eventually leading to the destruction of the affected tooth surface, or of the tooth itself. The immediate cause is the organic acids produced by certain microorganisms present on the tooth. The bacteria, together with a matrix made up mainly of extracellular polysaccharides produced from sucrose by the microorganisms, form the so-called dental plaque. The acids are formed when fermentable carbohydrates are added to the plaque. Each time such a process is started, the tooth will be damaged, but if the process does not occur too often, the natural capacity of the body to remineralize the tooth will prevent the formation of a cavity.

From this simple description, some factors that influence the risk of caries disease, and cavities, can be identified:

- The tooth surface may be more or less covered by dental plaque. More plaque, especially if it contains cariogenic microorganisms, includes more bacteria and may result in the formation of more organic acids. All methods aimed at reducing the amount of plaque, such as toothbrushing and use of antiplaque substances, thus are an attempt to reduce the amount of acids to be produced.

• Dental plaque is composed of a variety of oral microorganisms. Some of these microorganisms have a higher cariogenic potential than others. This potential includes factors such as the ability to form acids, to form acids at low pH, to survive at low pH, to adhere to the tooth, and to form extracellular polysaccharides. Among the many microorganisms identified, the so-called mutans streptococci (*Streptococcus mutans, Streptococcus sobrinus*), in particular, have been assigned an important role in the development of caries. Some means are now available for combating the mutans streptococci, although they are not yet in common use.

• Composition of diet, as well as frequency of eating, are further important factors. A diet with a low sucrose content, or less frequent eating, will result in reduced formation of organic acids. This knowledge has resulted in well-known advice regarding the restriction of intake of products that contain sugar and also has led to the development of less cariogenic products, which contain other sweeteners such as xylitol, sorbitol, or aspartame.

• Effective remineralization is another factor that has received increased attention. This factor is dependent on saliva flow and saliva composition, but the presence of fluoride during the active process, in the plaque fluid, has been shown to be of utmost importance. Earlier methods of employing fluorides concentrated mainly on trying to "build in" the fluorides to make the teeth more acid resistant by systemic addition of fluoride during the calcification of the teeth. Although this strategy still has some bearing, the continuous supply of fluorides even in low concentrations now attract most interest. The potential of fluoride to reduce caries has resulted in numerous attempts to use the substance, such as by adding fluoride to drinking water, salt, milk, tablets, fluoride rinses, varnishes, gels, and, of course, toothpaste.

• A number of individual factors may increase, or decrease, the risk of caries. These factors operate mainly through the saliva. Extremely low secretion rates, which, for example, may be an unwanted side effect of certain drugs, often result in high caries scores. Antibodies in the oral fluids are of particular interest because they would be the main mechanism for a caries vaccine.

The factors mentioned above: plaque, specific bacteria, diet, fluoride, and saliva are all involved in the caries process. It is important to understand what happens exactly on the tooth where a caries lesion will, or will not, occur. Once the factors have been identified, further questions will be raised: why do we have this particular combination of factors on this tooth, or in this person, or in this population? We then arrive at points for discussion of why a certain groups of people have a certain type of diet, why they do not clean their teeth, why they do not use fluorides, and so on. The answers to such questions may sometimes be found through research within community dentistry, but often they lie outside the purely odontological field.

Periodontal Diseases

Bacteria are the main cause also of the diseases affecting the supporting tissues of the teeth, and the host's response to the bacteria may result in more or less severe damage. Accumulation of bacteria on the teeth close to the tissues usually results in gingivitis, characterized by a tendency of the gums to bleed, especially when light pressure is applied, as, for example, at toothbrushing. More severe forms involve breakdown of the bone support of the teeth, resulting in more or less mobile teeth, later perhaps in the total loss of the affected teeth.

The processes leading to the more severe forms are the result of presence of bacteria in the gingival pockets and the reaction of the bacteria to the host defense systems. Research during the last fifteen years has pointed out some bacterial species as being particularly associated with periodontal diseases: *Actinobacillus actinomycetemcomitans, Bacteroides gingivalis, Bacteroides intermedius, Peptostreptococcus micros, Veillonella recta*, to name some. But bacteria may be present also in gingival pockets where no periodontal disease appears to follow, illustrating the complex interaction with the host. Periodontal diseases are not considered diseases which unconditionally follow gingivitis, although they may. Individuals at extra risk for periodontal diseases may be persons with immunodeficiencies, malnutrition, or diabetes, and those who smoke. A thorough discussion about the possibilities of identifying individuals at risk for periodontal disease was presented by Johnson (1989).

Prevention of periodontal diseases usually focuses on the dental plaques—the effective removal of the bacterial deposits, including calculus, on the teeth. Treatments of advanced stages usually include surgical methods to get access to the affected parts. Antibiotic therapy is sometimes introduced but can only be looked upon as a support for the local treatment.

Other Oral Diseases

Because dental caries and periodontal disease are or have been so common, less attention has usually been focused on other oral health problems. It would be a great mistake, however, to neglect these diseases and conditions, because they may often result in severe consequences to the person affected. In a survey of the epidemiology of oral diseases other than caries and periodontal disease, roughly one-quarter to one-half of populations examined were affected by conditions like masticatory dysfunction, traumatic dental and maxillofacial injuries, impactions, and oral mucosal disease (Andreasen and others 1986). Some examples of this survey will be mentioned below.

Regarding *dysfunction* of the masticatory apparatus, Andreasen and others reviewed five studies, all dealing with populations in industrial countries. About 25 to 50 percent of the people had subjective symptoms. The authors of the studies pointed out that headache often follows mandibular dysfunction and that headache is a common cause of visits to physicians.

For *traumatic dental injuries*, Andreasen and others reviewed fourteen studies that summarized investigations concerning

Table 27-1. Prevalence of Oral Soft Tissue Lesions in Chiang Mai, Kuala Lumpur, and Sweden

	Prevalence (percent)		
Lesion	Chiang Mai	Kuala Lumpur	Sweden
Infections			
Herpes labialis	0.9	0	3.1
History of herpes labialis	5.6	2.6	14.3
Intraoral herpetiform lesion	0.9	1.3	0.3
Pseudomembranous candidiasis	0	0.4	0.2
Angular cheilitis	0.9	0.9	3.8
Ulcers			
Recurrent aphthae	11.1	5.1	2.0
History of recurrent aphthae	37.2	21.9	15.7
Traumatic ulcer	13.2	12.4	4.3
Whitish lesions			
Leukoplakia	1.3	1.7	3.6
Preleukoplakia	1.7	1.7	6.4
Smoker's palate	3.4	3.4	1.1
Betel chewer's mucosa	0.4	1.3	0
Frictional lesion	3.8	5.2	5.5
Cheek and lip biting	1.7	5.6	5.1
Leukoedema	23.9	29.6	48.9
Lichen planus	3.8	2.1	1.9
Denture-related lesions			
Denture sore mouth	3.4	7.7	16.0
Flabby ridge	0	0.4	8.6
Denture hyperplasia	0.9	0	3.4
Tongue lesions			
Median rhomboid glossitis	1.3	1.3	1.4
Geographic tongue	5.1	6.4	8.5
Plicated tongue	3.4	5.2	6.5
Hairy tongue	0	0.9	0.6
Atrophy of tongue papillae	3.0	1.3	1.1
Pigmentation			
Melanin pigmentation	70.5	88.4	9.9
Amalgam tattoo	0.9	0.4	8.2
Tumors and tumorlike lesions			
Carcinoma	0	0.4	< 0.1
Papilloma	0.9	0	0.1
Hemangioma	2.1	1.7	0.1
Lipoma	0	0.4	0.1
Fibroepithelial polyp	1.7	3.9	3.3
Pyogenic granuloma	1.3	0.9	0.1
Mucocele	0.4	0.4	—

— Not available.
Source: Table based on study of 234 people in Chiang Mai, 233 in Kuala Lumpur (Axéll, Bte Zain, and Siwamogstham 1990), and 20,333 subjects in Sweden (Axéll 1976).

children and adolescents age three to nineteen. The frequency of dental injuries varied from 8 to 35 percent. The authors of a Danish prospective study of children eligible for the preschool dental service pointed out that every third child had experienced trauma of the primary dentition and every fifth child had sustained injury to the permanent dentition before leaving school at age sixteen (Andreasen and Ravn 1972). Data from developing countries were very sparse.

Few reports on *maxillofacial injuries* were available but those reporting data from Scandinavia and England estimated the annual incidence as being 1 to 4 per 10,000 people, traffic accidents and assault being the main cause. A remarkable higher incidence was reported from Greenland, 19 cases per 10,000, usually caused by assault following alcohol abuse.

Tooth impactions and other eruption disturbances were frequent findings in seven studies. About 20 to 30 percent of the populations investigated were affected. The conditions may lead to resorption of teeth, cysts, tumors, and inflammation, in particular, pericoronitis.

Very few studies have presented comprehensive data on the prevalence of the full range of *mucosal lesions*. One such study was performed in Sweden (Axéll 1976), and recently data have become available for most of those lesions from two more areas, Chiang Mai in Thailand and Kuala Lumpur in Malaysia (Axéll, Bte Zain, and Siwamogstham 1990), although based on a much smaller sample and more selected material. The findings are summarized in table 27-1. It should be understood that several of the conditions may be painful or even precancerous. For example, leukoplakia has been recognized as a frequent precursor to oral cancer, and researchers in one study with an average observation period of 7.5 years showed that 17 percent of leukoplakias became malignant.

A chapter in this collection is devoted to cancer, but it should be mentioned here that the prevalence of *oral cancers* differs widely between different areas. In a survey of the literature, the reported incidence rates of oral cancer, including vermilion border of the lip, varied from 5 to 25 cases per 100,000 population in industrial countries and from 2 to 17 in developing countries (Andreasen and others 1986). Smoking tobacco and drinking alcohol are the major etiologic factors. Also, it should be observed that not only the stronger types of alcoholic drinks, like whisky and vodka, are associated with the disease but also wines and other less alcoholic drinks. Chewing tobacco with or without areca (betel) is carcinogenic.

Special oral health problems are associated with HIV infection. Pindborg (1989) proposed a classification for lesions that included a variety of fungal infections, bacterial and viral infections, neoplasms, neurological disturbances, and lesions of unknown cause. The tabulation is preliminary and revisions are foreseen. It is clear, however, that the oral cavity often displays symptoms of HIV infections, and some of the diseases that occur are very serious.

Malocclusions include, for example, crowding or spacing problems, overjet, deep or open bite, crossbite, and scissors bite. Several problems can result from malocclusion, such as

Table 27-2. Changes in Caries Prevalence in Twelve-Year-Olds, by Country

Country	Year	DMFT [a]	Year	DMFT [a]
Asia				
Bangladesh	1979	1.8	1990	3.5
China	1951	0.6	1985	0.7
French Polynesia	1977	10.5	1987	2.5–3.8
Indonesia	1973	0.7	1982	2.3
Myanmar	1977	0.8	1990	1.1
Philippines	1977	2.5	1982	5.5
Singapore	1970	2.9	1984	2.5
Thailand	1977	2.7	1989	1.5
Tonga	1966	0.7	1986	1.0
Industrial countries				
Belgium	1972	3.1	1988	3.1
Canada	1977	6.0	1987	4.3
Finland	1975	7.5	1991	1.2
Japan	1975	5.9	1987	4.9
New Zealand	1973	6.0	1989	2.4
Sweden	1937	7.8	1989	2.2
United Kingdom	1973	4.7	1983	3.1
United States	1965/67	4.0	1986/87	1.8
U.S.S.R.	1972	3.5	1986	3.0
Latin America and the Caribbean				
Argentina	1965	4.5	1987	3.4
Brazil	1976	8.6	1988	6.7
Cuba	1973	5.1	1984	3.9
Mexico	1972	2.7	1984	3.2
Middle East and North Africa				
Algeria	1974	1.9	1987	2.3
Israel	1966	2.4	1989	3.0
Jordan	1962	0.2	1991	1.7
Morocco	1970	2.6	1989	1.8
Syrian Arab Republic	1974	4.4	1989	1.7
Sub-Saharan Africa				
Central African Republic	1974	0.2	1986	4.1
Malawi	1978	0.8	1991	0.7
Sudan	1979	1.1	1984	2.1
Tanzania	1973	0.6	1989	1.0
Togo	1973	1.6	1986	0.3
Zaire	1970	1.0	1985	1.0
Zambia	1971	0.1	1982	2.3

a. DMFT: Number of decayed, missing, and filled teeth.
Source: WHO Global Oral Data Bank.

difficulties in jaw movements and temporomandibular joint disturbances. Speech and swallowing might be affected, and psychosocial problems may occur if aesthetic problems are apparent. In their study from the United States, Kelly and Harvey (1977) indicate that the majority of American children and adolescents have a malocclusion of some type. Actually, they showed that 75 percent of the youths, age twelve to seventeen years, had a deviation from the ideal situation and about 25 to 30 percent had a severe malocclusion. For these conditions, the treatment needs and demands vary among countries. The problem itself is an important factor, and it is compounded by the possibility of requiring specialist treatment, the cost of which is, of course, also an important factor.

Disease Prevalence: Current Levels and Trends

Oral diseases can be measured by various indexes. The indexes may focus on the prevalence of the disease by cross-sectional studies, or the incidence, by longitudinal studies. For dental caries, a cross-sectional study will reveal lifetime caries, or the amount of caries since the first permanent tooth appeared in the mouth. Missing teeth pose special difficulties; a tooth may be missing because advanced caries required its extraction, but it may also be missing for other reasons, such as periodontitis, orthodontic reasons, or aesthetic reasons. It will be appreciated that age is an important factor to be taken into account when evaluating caries data—the older the age, the greater the risk of more damaged teeth. Thus, the caries index always shows higher individual values with age. When caries levels are compared for different populations, the same age groups must therefore be chosen.

Information regarding the prevalence of dental caries is overwhelming. It stretches from ancient times, as recorded by archaeological investigations of skulls, to the present, when, in some areas, all children are subjected to annual checkups, including x-rays, and data are fed continuously into computers so that even minor changes can be seen. To obtain comparable data, it is important that the same recording methods be used, and in this field, the Oral Health Unit at the World Health Organization (WHO) has prepared guidelines for oral health surveys, recommending indicator ages; recording forms are also produced. Since the early 1970s, a powerful instrument to monitor changes in oral health trends has been set up at WHO in Geneva: the Global Oral Data Bank. At present it contains files on more than 1,000 surveys, dating from 1937, with data on caries for 148 countries and on periodontal diseases for 103 countries. Each year global maps regarding caries and periodontal diseases are produced illustrating the latest information using comparable data. In table 27-2 we show examples of caries data from some countries.

Various indexes are also used to estimate the degree of gingival inflammation and periodontal disease. The WHO studies use the Community Periodontal Index of Treatment Needs (CPITN; see Barmes and Leous 1986; Pilot and others 1986). The index is based on three indicators: (a) presence or absence of gingival bleeding; (b) supra- or subgingival calculus; and (c) periodontal pockets, subdivided into shallow (4 to 5 millimeters) and deep pockets (6 millimeters and more). The mouth is divided into sextants and certain index teeth are registered for any of the indicators. The sextant will obtain a score from 0 (healthy) to 4 (≥ 6 millimeter pocket), and the highest score found on the index teeth is chosen for the sextant. The results for some countries are shown in figure 27-1. Johnson (1989) calculated that approximately 5 to 20 percent of most populations that have been adequately surveyed had destructive periodontitis of a "clinically significant" degree.

Figure 27-1. *Observed Periodontal Conditions Measured by* CPITN *at Age 35–44, Selected Countries*

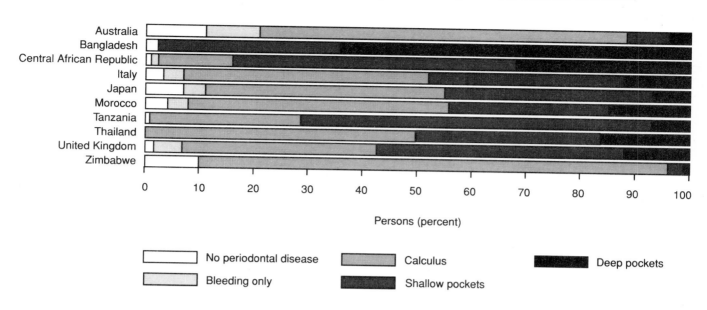

Source: WHO Global Oral Data Bank.

The situation for dental caries has changed during the last decades of this century, as shown in table 27-2. A tremendous decrease in the prevalence of caries has occurred in several industrial countries, at least in younger age groups. Some developing countries, however, show the reverse trend. Some explanations for these facts are listed in table 27-3.

It is clear that a number of factors may have been instrumental in the decrease in caries in industrial countries. It is not possible, as yet, to grade the various factors, because the importance may vary from country to country and the importance of an individual factor is dependent on the original level of caries.

The information available as a whole may illustrate the situation. In historical times, the problem of caries was minor, worldwide. Exceptions can be found in certain populations, and some groups of people showed the presence of root surface caries. An increase was noted in restricted groups of populations when refined sugars were introduced. At the beginning it was mostly people from higher social classes who could afford these products who were affected. In many Western countries, a "caries explosion" started during the period between 1850 and 1900, when industrialization and new dietary habits arrived.

Demand appeared for oral health services, for professional extractions, and for the repair of damaged teeth. Dental schools were built, new instruments were developed, and new filling materials were progressively devised. A golden age for dentists began, brought about by a never-ending demand for oral health services. Eventually, it was realized that fillings, crowns, bridges, and the like did not last very long and that at least one-third of dental treatment involved replacing previous treatment. A growing demand for preventive measures became apparent and a number of methods were devised, resulting in a sudden decrease in caries and periodontitis. The demand for services is now on the decrease in highly industrialized countries. Dental schools face problems because of the reduced need for dentists, some being forced to close and others to reduce the intake of students.

Meanwhile, developing countries are turning to more Western food. Very often these countries have no, or very limited, resources for oral health treatment. Interest in prevention is understandably low, because oral health problems have, until recently, been more or less nonexistent. Caries is increasing, particularly in the cities, resulting in a growing demand for better dental services.

Patterns for the Years 2000 and 2015

The World Health Organization has defined a certain number of goals for oral health for the year 2000.

- Fifty percent of five- to six-year-olds will be caries free.
- The global average will be no more than three decayed, missing, or filled teeth at twelve years of age.
- Eighty-five percent of the population should retain all their teeth at age eighteen.
- A 50 percent reduction in present levels of toothlessness at age thirty-five through forty-four will be achieved.
- A twenty-five percent reduction in present levels of toothlessness at age sixty-five will be achieved.
- A data-based system for monitoring changes in oral health will be established.

Table 27-3. Current Trends in Caries Prevalence

Trend	Intervention	Comments
Decrease in industrial countries	Fluoride in toothpastes	Fluoride has been added since the 1950s; 80–95 percent of toothpastes contain fluoride. It is considered a major reason for the decrease.
	Water fluoridation	Fluoride content of drinking waters may be adjusted to optimal levels. Positive effects may be obtained even with local applications.
	Salt or milk fluoridation	Used in some countries.
	Fluoride tablets, topical application, rinsing, varnishes	Used in various school-based programs, as well as individually.
	Oral hygiene	Information, instruction, and supervised oral hygiene programs may have resulted in improved hygiene.
	Dietary advice	Mainly focused on reduction of sucrose. Total sugar consumption has not dramatically changed. Use of sugar substitutes has increased.
	Oral microflora changes	Temporary suppression through antibiotics. Possible effects on acid production through fluorides and other antimicrobial substances.
Increase in developing countries	Changes in diet	Westernization of diet

Source: Compiled by present authors.

For caries, one important goal is that the mean number of decayed, missing, or filled teeth should not exceed three at the age of twelve. Current trends seem to indicate that many Western countries have a good chance of reaching this goal (Pilot 1988). Other countries, such as Poland, have expressed doubts about the possibilities of reducing caries to that extent (Ja'nczuk 1989). Many developing countries have never exceeded that particular goal, but the crucial question remains: will the increase observed in some countries be halted or not?

The year 2000 is close, and for 2015, no goals have yet been set. Let us therefore present two "scenarios."

THE OPTIMISTIC SCENARIO. The ongoing trend toward a decrease in oral diseases in Western countries continues. New effective prophylactic agents are introduced, special programs for risk groups are designed, and oral diseases in the elderly are kept under control. The profession adjusts itself to the new situation. By agreement, many tasks are transferred from dentists to personnel with less costly education. The number of dentists decreases, but the profession aims at, and succeeds in, distributing the resources according to geographical needs. Although the number of dental schools is reduced, the resources for dental research are not. Politicians are also aware of the fact that oral diseases are not eliminated, just kept in check. Therefore, resources for continuous preventive methods remain intact.

In developing countries, the authorities realize that they have to choose one of two ways—either the expensive one used earlier by the Western countries or the immediate introduction of effective preventive programs. They choose the latter one and are successful in educating the people in the value of prevention before the diseases become prevalent. Traditional foods are retained as far as possible, and if between-meal snacks containing sucrose are introduced, they will come

after the introduction of preventive programs. These programs have been worked out in collaboration with advanced research institutes in industrial countries. Knowledge has thereby been transferred and resources have been allocated to help introduce the programs.

THE PESSIMISTIC SCENARIO. To begin with, the decrease in prevalence of the diseases continues for some time. This is interpreted by the decisionmakers as the elimination of dental diseases. The interest of the individual, the profession, and the politicians in supporting preventive efforts decreases. Preventive programs in schools are reduced; some cities stop adding fluoride to drinking water. Development of new preventive methods are successful, but the research and development costs are high, resulting in high prices for the products; therefore, they are used only by a few.

The elderly population is increasing. They will have more teeth than before. Root surface caries cannot be kept under control. There is a shortage of personnel at homes for the elderly, and the care givers that remain show little interest in taking care of the teeth of their patients, particularly because the task has become increasingly difficult, owing to the fact that the "extra" teeth are situated more posterior than was the case earlier. Many extractions follow, but the elderly demand fixed teeth, and therefore treatments involving extremely expensive implants and bridges increase rapidly. Because the number of dental schools has been reduced, the number of staff (that is, the dental researchers) has also been reduced. At the beginning, endless discussions between the dentists, dental hygienists, nurses, and other supporting groups are held, finally leading to the withdrawal of the possibility for these groups to perform clinical work. All of a sudden, when it is realized that there are too few dentists, it becomes a problem to cover the less popular areas of the countries with professionals.

The consumption of Western type of food, including junk food, is rapidly increasing in developing countries. Starting in the cities, caries is increasing and the demand for restoration, not for prevention, is growing. Dental schools and dental clinics are being established to meet this demand. Preventive programs are launched, but because of the lack of resources, interest, and knowledge, the programs reach only a small proportion of the population. Also, the profession favors the reconstructive approach because it gives higher income and status. Dentists are gathering in and around the big cities, leaving extractions in the underprivileged population to be performed by less-qualified personnel. Advertisements for Western food and other products are flourishing, including cigarettes. In many developing countries, smoking is on the increase, resulting in more and more cases of oral cancer.

In both developing and industrial countries, HIV infections are spreading rapidly, and patients with oral manifestations are frequently seen in clinics. Resources have to be set aside for these patients and, because special, often time-consuming arrangements for infection control have to be made, these patients take more and more time to treat. Due to general environmental problems such as pollution, climatic change, drug abuse, and even war, smaller and smaller proportions of national budgets are being set aside for health purposes, in particular, for oral health.

The coming decades will be extremely important, because the decisions to be taken will influence oral health for many years to come. At the present time, it is possible to have some hope for a positive outcome. The pessimistic scenario, however, was very easy to imagine. Some questions to consider when trying to decide which scenario will come out on top are, for example, is it usual that decisions are made which favor the health of the total population? Is present knowledge about prevention being used properly? How many years does it take to introduce new ideas to an entire population? Will environmental and economic crises be solved? What are the resources for introduction of the negative factors in relation to the health-supporting activities?

All the facts mentioned in the two scenarios will probably happen, somewhere in the world. We will have various combinations of the pessimistic and optimistic scenarios. Some countries will be winners, some losers. The regular monitoring reports from the WHO Oral Data Bank will reflect the net outcome worldwide.

Economic Costs

A patient has a cavity that needs restoration. How much does it cost to get it filled? The directs costs involve time for drilling, filling, and polishing, plus the materials. Further costs include those of office space, dental equipment, salaries for personnel, office supplies, telephone, and so on. If the tooth had been more seriously damaged, perhaps a crown would have been necessary, which would have meant additional costs for impression materials, labor of technicians, gold, x-rays, transportation between dentist and technician, and so on. Other costs cover training personnel, running dental schools, dental supply depots, dental research and dental journals, patient time, traveling costs, and so on, plus administration of the dental programs within the government health divisions and departments. In different countries, the proportion of the total costs varies according to how much is finally charged to the patient and how much is paid through taxes. For this reason, comparisons between fees charged for a filling must be assessed with caution. In addition, trying to get the values in comparable monetary values is almost impossible, but here are some examples.

The fee for one occlusal surface filling in a molar of an adult patient would, in the United Kingdom, be about £5 (corresponding to about US$8), of which the patient would pay directly 75 percent, if the dentist is working within the National Health Service. In Sudan, the patient would have to pay about 12 Sudanese pounds, or about US$1 to $2, and in a Brazilian city, US$25 could be charged. The figures are easily misleading, however, and a WHO/FDI (World Health Organization/Fédération Dentaire Internationale) joint working group, JWG 9, proposed instead a relative value system, in which different treatments were related to a particular item, giving the value 100. The item chosen was a one-surface amalgam filling, in a first molar, including anesthesia and lining.

Data from the following countries are available: Austria, Denmark, Finland, France, Hong Kong, Japan, the Netherlands, and Sweden. The fee index indicates that the price for upper and lower dentures would be about twenty to ninety times more expensive than the filling. One porcelain or metal crown was estimated to cost seven to forty times more than the filling, and a simple extraction was estimated to cost from 33 to 148 percent of the fee for the filling.

Here is another way to illustrate the cost of treatment. In a provincial hospital in a district in Zimbabwe, 48 kilometers from the capital, Harare, a simple filling would cost Z$5.00, equivalent at that moment to about US$2.50. For the same amount of money, 1 to 2 kilograms of meat could be obtained, or two tubes of toothpaste, or 7 kilograms of brown sugar. Or, the patient could have traveled by bus to Harare, enjoying 100 pieces of candy during the trip. At a private clinic in the capital, the patient could be charged four to five times more for the filling.

Total costs for dentistry may be very low at present in some developing countries, where, in some cases, the total budget for health is just a few dollars per person per year. In industrial countries, dental costs may often reach about 10 percent of the health budget. This is the case in Switzerland, for example (6.5 million inhabitants), where total costs have been calculated at about 1.7 billion Swiss francs (SFr), corresponding to about SFr 400,000 per dental surgery (Meier 1988).[1] Ninety-four percent of these costs are paid by the patients, the remainder by the state. In Sweden (about 8.5 million inhabitants), the total cost for dental care was 6,505 million Swedish krona (Skr) in 1985, of which 44 percent was covered by the state, 25 percent by county councils, and 31 percent by patients. These are direct costs only and do not cover such expenses as education of dental personnel or loss of working hours for the patients. Current direct dental costs per inhabitant of Sweden would amount to approximately US$125 per year.

For the purpose of comparison, it is interesting to study the costs for an advanced form of therapy, implants. This treatment is used for patients who do not have teeth in one or both jaws. In 1986, a thorough cost evaluation (Karlsson 1986) of such care, the Brånemark method, was made for ten patients who had received treatment in specialist clinics in a county of Sweden. The treatment involves the following procedures: after detailed examination, titanium fixtures are implanted in the patient's jaws by a surgical operation. After a healing period of three to six months, "distances" are applied, and after a further two weeks, bridges can be inserted, fixed to the distances. This procedure is followed by several checkups. Thus, the result is "fixed" teeth for a patient, for whom the previous alternative was removable dentures.

In the study referred to, Karlsson (1986) calculated direct costs (for treatment time for dental personnel and for equipment) and indirect costs (resources lost because of missing teeth, such as work problems, time, and travel for the patient). Furthermore, the author discussed calculation of costs of a more undefined character, such as the monetary value of the problem of having no teeth. Because of the great difficulties of obtaining such values, these costs were not included in the results. The results showed that the total cost for one jaw was about Skr 40,000 to 60,000 (about US$6,150 to $9,230). This cost is about seven times higher than for removable dentures, under similar conditions.

Certainly, these calculations are relevant only for this particular group of patients, and similar treatment in other countries would give other results because of varying costs for dentists' time, transportation, and so on. Still, the calculations illustrate the enormous costs that could follow if no preventive programs that protect against loss of teeth are implemented and if the population demands fixed teeth.

Elements of Preventive Strategy

The basic elements of a preventive strategy consist of identification of, and action against, the etiological factors for each oral disease. In table 27-4 we illustrate these elements for some diseases. As can be seen, information and motivation are important preventive methods for several conditions. The use of these methods, however, requires that the patient (population) follow certain rules. One definite advantage of a method such as water fluoridation is that people will benefit even if they are unable to follow advice because of sickness, failing interest, lack of education, and the like.

The elements of prevention must be presented within a system, and the industrial countries have developed more or less effective frameworks. In developing countries, this work is still in the beginning stages, and includes a strategy with primary, secondary, and tertiary prevention. One concept for primary oral health care was recently described by Jeboda and Eriksen (1989). They suggested these levels:

- Level 1. Prevention of onset of disease (prepathogenic), including integration of general and oral health; information, advice, control; diet and nutrition; general and oral hygiene; fluorides.
- Level 2. Prevention of further development of disease, including simple fillings; fissure sealing for high-risk patients; professional hygiene.
- Level 3. Relief of pain and debilitating consequences of disease, including emergency treatment, extractions, and medication; referral.

Cost and Effectiveness

An example from Switzerland may illustrate cost and effectiveness in an industrial country. The estimations have been made available by Dr. M. Büttner (personal communication, 1989). In the canton of Basel, 30.4 tooth surfaces per fifteen-year-old child had to be restored in 1961. The cost for these treatments was estimated at SFr 2.8 million per 1,500 children. In 1988, only 3.7 surfaces per child had to be restored, at a cost of SFr 0.3 million, thus a difference of SFr 2.5 million.

In 1962 a water fluoridation program was implemented in Basel, and in 1970 a school-based preventive dentistry program was introduced. During the past two decades, fluoridated toothpaste has become more and more prevalent in the marketplace, and approximately 90 percent of the population now uses such toothpaste. Seventy percent of the population uses fluoridated salt.

The school-based program, which actually starts when the children are three years of age and follows the children throughout secondary school, includes topical fluoride applications and oral hygiene instructions as well as dietary advice. Most tasks are performed by auxiliaries. The cost for this program is estimated at SFr 16 per child per year. Thus, for 1,500 children who participate in the program for ten years, the cost would be SFr 240,000. The cost for the fluoride used for water fluoridation and maintenance in Basel is now estimated to only SFr 0.5 per person per year.

Some further data on the effectiveness of the program can be mentioned: of the fifteen-year-old children leaving school in 1967, 0 percent had no caries. In 1988, 34 percent had no caries. For the same age group, fifteen teeth were affected, as a mean, in 1961, whereas only three teeth were affected in 1988.

It is not possible to estimate exactly how much of the caries reductions are due to the various components in the program. In countries without fluoridated water or salt, substantial reductions in caries have also been observed, if fluoridated toothpaste and school programs are used.

The Future of Prevention Technology

Can we expect new methods that will change, dramatically, the basis for preventive treatment of the oral diseases? Dental research tries to find new ways, in several directions. Intensive studies focus, for example, on plaque-inhibiting substances.

Table 27-4. Preventive Strategies for Oral Health

Condition	Cause	Action needed	Methods
Dental caries	Increased sugar intake	Reduce sugars	Information, recommendations; increase price of sugars, taxes; sugar substitutes
	Plaque present	Reduce plaque	Information and instruction; more effective tooth cleaning; flossing, toothpicks; professional tooth cleaning; less sugars in diet; fissure sealants; antimicrobial products
	High *mutans streptococci* levels	Reduce *mutans streptococci*	More effective tooth cleaning; less sugars in diet; antimicrobial varnish; chlorhexidine gels and rinses; vaccination
	Insufficient fluoride in relation to etiological factors	Increase fluorides	Water fluoridation; daily use of fluoride toothpastes; fluoride-containing drinks and foodstuffs; varnishes, rinsing programs; fluoride tablets, gels
	Reduced saliva secretion	Compensate	Find out reasons and take appropriate actions
Periodontal disease	Plaque present	Reduce plaque	Information and instruction; more effective tooth cleaning; flossing, toothpicks; antimicrobial products; professional tooth cleaning; scaling
	Specific pathogenic bacteria	Reduce bacteria	Antibiotics
Oral cancer and precancer	Increased risk factors, including tobacco, alcohol	Reduce risk factors	Information, motivation
AIDS-related symptoms	Risk behavior	Treatment and prevention	Information, motivation
Lip and palate clefts	Present from birth	Surgical treatment	Care in dental hospital
Fluorosis	High fluoride intake	Reduce intake	Defluoridation of drinking waters; identify other sources; information
Orthodontic problems	Genetic	Treatment	Care by specialized personnel for advanced cases
	Other dental diseases, caries, or periodontal disease	Prevention	Care by specialized personnel for advanced cases
Temporomandibular joint problems	Stress	Treatment and prevention	Individual treatment, information, clinical care
	Other dental diseases, caries, or periodontal disease	Prevention	Individual treatment, information, clinical care
Traumatic injuries	Sports	Treatment and supervision	Individual treatment, mouth guards

Source: Authors' compilation.

Such products could have an effect on the tooth surface, the saliva pellicle covering the teeth, or the oral bacteria. Several products seem to be promising. The products would be administered through mouth rinses, topical application, or tablets. Prices, number of applications, and long-term effects are as yet unknown, and it can be assumed that these products will first be used in industrial countries.

Whereas plaque-inhibiting substances act on most bacterial types forming the dental plaque, other substances try to find means of attacking the pathogenic bacteria. Most studies concern the mutans streptococci. Very promising results have been reported by Sandham and others (1988). They have found that a varnish, containing chlorhexidine, can eliminate the mutans streptococci in many patients. The use of this varnish could be combined with methods which identify persons carrying large amounts of these bacteria. The system seems to be ready for large-scale clinical studies. It is important, however, to evaluate the effects on caries, not only on the bacteria.

Vaccination against dental caries has been discussed for decades, and vaccines that have good protective effects in animals have been produced. Hesitation to test these products on humans stems from concerns for safety. Because caries is not a deadly disease, not one single case of fatal side effect should be accepted. Suspicion of possible unwanted cross-reactions of certain caries vaccine preparations with human tissues has been substantiated, and, therefore, the first generation of these vaccines will probably not come into use. Genetic engineering, however, is making possible the development of new versions, in which antigens of the mutans streptococci are transferred into normal gut microorganisms. It is possible that such a vaccine will reduce the mutans levels on the teeth, with concomitant reduction of caries. Many years of research will still be needed, however, if effective vaccination is to be of use to developing countries.

Although fluorides have been investigated intensively for decades, new products can still be expected. For example, Ögaard and others (1988) have suggested that a hydrogen fluoride solution with low pH, resulting in calcium fluoride-formation on the teeth, could be very effective, and some pilot experiments have supported their hypothesis. More clinical experiments are necessary, however, to prove its usefulness under field conditions.

Dietary modifications through the use of sugar substitutes may be effective, but so far the products are, in general, comparatively expensive and present some side effects if consumed in large amounts. Industrial countries have more opportunity to use the products currently available. It is possible, however, that new products, or modifications of sucrose, will become available which will also be suitable for developing countries.

These few examples serve to illustrate the fact that new strategies may be devised, some within a fairly short time, but those particularly useful for developing countries may yet be years away. Still, that technology will change is now apparent; it will leave drilling and filling for more advanced technology, based on microbiology and chemistry. The examples, however, focus on caries and periodontal diseases. The spectrum of other oral diseases may become affected by the changes exemplified only to a certain degree. Rather, there may be a risk of increase in some conditions in developing countries, such as traumatic injuries from traffic accidents as traffic increases.

Expected Minimum Standards

For a developing country, it is reasonable to expect that the following standards be achieved:

- The population should receive information about the principal oral diseases, thus allowing the individual to avoid

habits and products that increase the risk of disease, such as frequent intake of products that contain sugar. Of course, if sugar-rich products are necessary for survival, that would take precedence.

- If pain is present, possibilities for pain relief must exist.
- If there is any risk of caries occurring, or if caries is already present, a fluoride program should be implemented, and if toothpaste is used, it should contain fluoride. If toothpaste is too expensive, school-based fluoride programs should be started. For cities, water fluoridation can be considered, provided good technical management and safety can be guaranteed.
- Although heavy formation of dental calculus is common in certain populations in developing countries, it might be unrealistic to suggest services like professional removal of calculus for these populations at present. It should be possible, however, to introduce oral hygiene programs among children, which would place the next generation in a better position.
- Oral manifestations of cancers, or precancerous lesions, are common in some populations. These populations should be, or have a chance to be, inspected for early signs of such manifestations at the same time that acceptable services for treatment are built up. If pathogenic processes are diagnosed, it should be possible to obtain surgical or other types of treatment.
- Serious cleft syndromes in newborn babies are not common, but if present, they require advanced treatment. A referral center for these conditions should be available. Such a center should also be able to take care of severe fractures from accidents and other causes.
- If fluorosis is present to a disturbing extent, defluoridation should be performed, if at all possible.

As a basis for all their efforts, the authorities should have an oral health program which includes surveys and other data collection to clarify the distribution of oral diseases within the population and incidence of the diseases. The main "local" etiological factors for the diseases should be known. The effects of preventive programs already implemented should be monitored. Changes in diet should be observed, in particular, any increase in sugar, and sugar-rich snacks, between meals. National authorities should work toward the training of dental personnel and the development of appropriate technology. Those who select personnel should bear in mind geographical distribution. Goals can be formulated: all persons should be able to eat, drink, and talk without discomfort. In addition, the mouth and teeth should have an acceptable appearance.

Oral Health Personnel

Oral health services are expensive, as revealed earlier. Manpower and education account for three-quarters to four-fifths of these costs. Therefore, resource planning should aim at ensuring that both the quantity and type of oral health personnel are adequate. It is certain that savings are possible if less-educated personnel can be used. It is apparent that several functions mentioned above could be performed by personnel other than dentists. It is also clear, however, that certain conditions demand highly skilled personnel. What, then, would be the best strategy for a given situation and the best combination of personnel types?

One should not expect a simple answer to such a question because the basis for decisions differs so widely among countries. But the question has been studied by WHO, and a planning instrument has been drawn up. Using the Lotus computer program, the WHO method for estimating oral health personnel requirements provides a procedure for rapid calculation on the basis of data or estimates for:

- Oral disease levels
- Need for oral care and retreatment frequency
- Demand for care
- Average time per item of care
- Average hours worked

For any single level of disease one can alter the assumptions on the demand for care, on treatment strategies which are more or less interventive, on retreatment frequency, and on time allocations per item for time worked. Thus, one can have widely different estimates of personnel needs for a single oral health status. Also, overall personnel needs can be subdivided on the basis of use of dental professionals only, professionals and auxiliaries, and professionals and auxiliaries and primary health workers. In the latter case, especially, the numbers should read as full-time equivalents rather than simply head counts. Subclassification, on the basis of intervention, allows for an aggressive treatment service, for which a prime example is one in which every tooth recorded as carious would be filled, through a moderate service, to a noninterventive system which uses high-risk assessments to defer filling any tooth as long as some form of prevention, simple surface care, or even "wait and see," can substitute.

In table 27-5 we give an example of this type of exercise for three distinct levels of dental caries, each managed through a range of strategies from interventive to noninterventive and displayed in three main oral health personnel combinations. Clearly, great differences in economic and health consequences are embodied in these comparative figures, for example, from 665 oral health personnel per million for the situation that includes high caries prevalence and an interventive strategy to 95 per million for the situation that embodies low caries prevalence and a noninterventive strategy. Similarly, within one caries prevalence level the differences are considerable; for example, the interventive strategy in the high caries prevalence level calls for 665 dentists per million, whereas the noninterventive strategy for that same prevalence level requires only 175 dentists plus 50 auxiliaries plus 40 primary health workers if the three-level combination of personnel is used.

As large as these differences are, they can be even larger if one varies such items as demand for care, time per item, and hours worked. The figures in table 27-5 are based on a 2,000-hour year. If this is changed to a more likely 1,500-hour year, or even a 1,200-hour year, which is a reality in many countries and not even a minimum, the lowest and highest estimates of personnel needed per million become 130 and 890, respectively, for the 1,500-hour year and 160 and 1,110, respectively, for the 1,200-hour year.

The full versatility of the system extends to extrapolating observed trends in the oral health status and to entering data appropriate to the achievement of stated, measurable goals in the medium to long term. This system is already a powerful planning tool, and the WHO Oral Health Unit hopes to expand it further in the near future with more specific measurement of economic factors. The importance of the system is also reflected when the number of dentists in relation to the number of inhabitants in some countries is considered (table 27-6). Hypothetical cases have been taken from the list in table 27-6 to highlight contrasts based on actual situations for which assumptions which seem most appropriate have been made.

Applying the WHO method and assuming the partially interventive strategy, a 1,500-hour working year, and a stable caries level, we conclude that one dental operator is needed in the following countries for the populations indicated: Brazil,

Table 27-5. Oral Health Personnel Needed per Million Population

Level of caries	Strategy	Dentists only	Dentists plus auxiliaries	Dentists plus auxiliaries plus primary health workers
Low	Interventive	145	75+70	75+30+30
	Partially interventive	105	40+65	40+25+40
	Noninterventive	95	35+60	35+15+45
Moderate	Interventive	255	165+90	165+65+25
	Partially interventive	195	125+70	125+45+25
	Noninterventive	160	95+65	95+35+30
High	Interventive	665	465+200	465+170+30
	Partially interventive	365	245+120	245+85+35
	Noninterventive	265	175+90	175+50+40

Source: Oral Health Unit, WHO, Geneva. Calculations based on 2,000 hours worked per year.

Table 27-6. Dentists per 10,000 Population, by Country

Country	Dentists
Asia	
India	0.1
Indonesia	0.1
Mongolia	0.4
Sri Lanka	0.2
Thailand	0.3
Industrial countries	
Belgium	6.1
Canada	4.9
Denmark	8.8
Finland	9.3
France	7.2
Germany	5.7
Italy	0.6
Netherlands	4.9
Sweden	11.0
United Kingdom	3.1
United States	5.9
Latin America and the Caribbean	
Argentina	2.2
Bolivia	0.6
Brazil	1.3
Colombia	3.6
Costa Rica	3.1
Chile	2.6
Uruguay	7.7
Middle East and North America	
Algeria	1.2
Jordan	2.4
Iran	0.5
Israel	7.1
Oman	0.6
Pakistan	0.1
Saudi Arabia	1.0
Yemen, Rep. of	0.0[a]
Sub-Saharan Africa	
Kenya	0.1
Mali	0.0[b]
Senegal	0.1
Sierra Leone	0.1
Togo	0.0[c]

a. In Democratic Republic of Yemen, only eighteen dentists in country.
b. Only fifteen dentists in country.
c. Only five dentists in country.
Source: World Health Statistics 1988.

2,990; Costa Rica, 5,488; Germany, 2,941; India, 5,696; Jordan, 8,036; Pakistan, 4,036; Sierra Leone, 10,976; Sweden, 2,601; the United Kingdom, 2,616.

Priorities for Resource Allocation

We believe resources in developing countries should be allocated to the following:

- An effective primary oral health organization for prevention and care. If possible, the activities should be combined with other health services or school-based programs.
- Referral centers as mentioned above. Also, developing countries are in need of some highly trained experts in various fields.
- Appropriate technology. It is important that equipment, materials, and methods work under field conditions. There are numerous examples of sophisticated and expensive dental units that are not operating in developing countries.
- Resources for oral health planning, preventive programs, and education. They include surveys, epidemiological studies, and the establishment of national or local registries, with efficient use of informatics and electronics.

We do not think that the present budgets for oral health in most developing countries are sufficient for the addition or enhancement of these items. New resources are necessary, but the many demands already present, as well as those expected in the near future, urgently need to be met.

Priorities for Operational Research

Many important questions and problems for oral health need attention. The list below illustrates some of them as seen from a global standpoint. Another order of priority may very well be chosen locally, which is why the list should not, by all means, be regarded as the universal truth.

- *Prevalence and incidence of oral diseases.* Epidemiological investigations should be performed regularly and records analyzed to monitor the oral health situation. They should, of course, include caries and periodontal disease, but it is important that they be extended to cover also the more common discomforting, premalignant or malignant oral diseases. Children and representative samples of indicator ages among the elderly should be included.
- *Etiological factors.* Concomitant with epidemiological surveys, one should try to identify the main factors causing disease in the population under investigation. Studies should be performed aimed at finding effective means of reducing such factors or risk behaviors.
- *Treatment needs.* Improved methods and tools to evaluate treatment needs and demand for oral care are necessary. The methods should include an attempt to determine the total needs of the population, taking into consideration also the less prevalent diseases.
- *Preventive programs.* A variety of preventive programs should be installed and new strategies should be tested. The possibilities of selecting risk groups should be further investigated, and various combinations of oral health personnel tested. In particular, it is important to establish the effect of primary health care workers during longitudinal studies.

Also, collaboration with nondental personnel within prevention needs further study.

• *Toothpaste and other oral health products*. It is believed that fluoride toothpaste and other fluoride-containing products have been of great importance in decreasing the prevalence of caries in industrial countries. The use of such products in developing countries should be promoted, but the outcome of such activities is also dependent on the price of the products. New products, more afforable than those produced today, must become available.

• *Transfer of knowledge*. The results of various oral health projects must be readily communicated so that good ideas can be picked up quickly by other countries or communities. Research should advise on improved methods to transfer knowledge and skills to developing countries. In particular, the possibilities offered by new technologies should be explored.

Notes

During the preparation of this chapter, we have received valuable comments and suggestions from a number of collegues who have read parts of the manuscript or draft versions. We would like to thank all these persons for their help and for the time they have spent with the issue. In particular, we want to thank A. Adeyinka, J. Ahlgren, T. Axéll, G. Bratthall, J. R. Freed, J. Frencken, D. T. Jamison, J. McCombie, H. Miyazaki, W. H. Mosley, T. Pilot, S. Schweitzer, R. Serinirach, Y. Songpaisan, and W.D. Sithole.

1. A billion is 1,000 million.

References

Andreasen, J. O., J. J. Pindborg, E. Hjörting-Hansen, and T. E. Axéll. 1986. "Oral Health Care: More than Caries and Periodontal Disease. A Survey of Epidemiological Studies on Oral Disease." *International Dental Journal* 36:207–14

Andreasen, J. O., and J. J. Ravn. 1972. "Epidemiology of Traumatic Dental Injuries to Primary and Permanent Teeth in a Danish Population Sample." *International Journal of Oral Surgery* 1:235–39.

Axéll, T. E. 1976. "A Prevalence Study of Oral Mucosal Lesions in an Adult Swedish Population." *Odontologisk Revy* 27(supplement 36):1–103.

Axéll, T. E., R. Bte Zain, and P. Siwamogstham. 1990. "Prevalence of Oral Soft Tissue Lesions in Out-Patients at Two Malaysian and Thai Dental Schools." *Community Dentistry and Oral Epidemiology* 18:95–99.

Barmes, D. E., and P. Leous. 1986. "Assessment of Periodontal Status by CPITN and Its Applicability to the Development of Long-Term Goals on Periodontal Health of the Population." *International Dental Journal* 36:177–81.

Ja'nczuk, Zbigniew. 1989. "Oral Health of Polish Children and WHO/FDI Goals for the Year 2000." *Community Dentistry and Oral Epidemiology* 17:75–78.

Jeboda, S., and Harald Eriksen. 1989. "Primary Oral Health Care: The Concept and Suggestions for Practical Approach." *Odonto-Stomatologie Tropicale* 11:121–26.

Johnson, N. W. 1989. "Detection of High Risk Groups and Individuals for Periodontal Diseases." *International Dental Journal* 39:33–47.

Karlsson, Göran. 1986. "Samhällsekonomisk utvärdering av käkbensförankrade broaren förstudie." Report 8. Center for Medical Technology Assessment, University of Linköping, Sweden 1–78.

Kelly, J., and C. Harvey. 1977. "An Assessment of the Teeth of Youths 12–17 Years." DHEW Publication (HRA) 77-1644. National Center for Health Statistics, U.S. Public Health Service, Washington, D.C.

Meier, C. 1988. "Wieviel ist Prophylaxe wert?" *Schweizerische Monatsschrift für Zahnmedizin* 99:647.

Ögaard, B., Gunnar Rölla, Joop Arends, and J. M. ten Cate. 1988. "Orthodontic Appliances and Enamel Demineralization. 2. Prevention and Treatment of Lesions." *American Journal of Orthodontics and Dentofacial Orthopedics* 94:123–28.

Pilot, Taco. 1988. "Trends in Oral Health: A Global Perspective." *New Zealand Dental Journal* 84:40–45.

Pilot, Taco, D. E. Barmes, M.-H. Leclercq, B. McCombie, and Jennifer Sardo Infirri. 1986. "Periodontal Conditions in Adults, 35–44 Years of Age: An Overview of CPITN Data in the WHO Global Oral Data Bank." *Community Dentistry and Oral Epidemiology* 14:310–12.

Pindborg, J. J. 1989. "Classification of Oral Lesions Associated with HIV Infection." *Oral Surgery, Oral Medicine, Oral Pathology* 67:292–95.

Sandham, J., J. Brown, H. Phillips, and K. Chan. 1988. "A Preliminary Report on Longterm Elimination of Detectable *Mutans streptococci* in Man." *Journal of Dental Research* 67:9–14.

28

Schizophrenia and Manic-Depressive Illness

Peter Cowley and Richard Jed Wyatt

Schizophrenia and manic-depressive illness constitute a tremendous health burden. They affect 2 percent of the world's population during life's most productive years, in turn straining family and other resources (Goodwin and Jamison 1990; Jablensky and others 1992). The diagnoses of schizophrenia and manic-depressive illness rely on objective criteria that can be used by trained health professionals. When broadly defined, schizophrenia can include both brief and chronic forms of the illness. Manic-depressive illness can occur in milder (bipolar II) and severe forms (bipolar I). In both forms of bipolar disorder an individual's mood, energy level, and cognition vary greatly over shorter or longer time periods. In order to limit the scope of this project, manic-depressive illness is used synonymously with bipolar I and II disorders.

Although most epidemiological studies of schizophrenia are from industrial countries, a recent World Health Organization (WHO) study provides epidemiological information from developing communities (Jablensky and others 1992). There is, however, painfully little known about manic-depressive illness in developing countries (Goodwin and Jamison 1990; Robins and Regier 1991).

The treatment of schizophrenia serves as the primary template for the cost-effectiveness calculations of how the program might work for manic-depressive illness. By showing how the cost-effectiveness template can be used for more than one mental illness, we hope that further research can be carried out on the cost-effectiveness of treating other mental illnesses, such as unipolar depression. The treatment protocol presented here has been simplified from what would be expected in the most industrialized parts of the world, making it practical and less costly, if also less exacting. Plans include a referral base (general medical practioners, psychiatrists, families, traditional healers, and herbalists) from which individuals with such symptoms as "odd behavior," nontraditional violent outbursts, and delusional thinking can be sent to a clinic for evaluation and possible medical treatment.

The clinic will be staffed by trained auxiliary health workers and nurses; the client will visit the clinic once a month, and a trained psychiatrist will visit the clinic once a week to attend patient review sessions. Finally, the model assumes a steady-state prevalence; therefore, it includes both old patients and new patients.

Risk Factors

There are few discernible risk factors for schizophrenia and manic-depressive illness; nonetheless, twin and adoption studies indicate that schizophrenia and manic-depressive illness have a genetic component (Gottesman and Shields 1982; Goodwin and Jamison 1990). Schizophrenia and manic-depressive illness have approximately the same incidence and prevalence in males and females (Robins and Regier 1991; Jablensky and others 1992). The peak age for developing schizophrenia and manic-depressive illness is approximately twenty; all but a few cases develop initial symptoms before age thirty-five (Goodwin and Jamison 1990; Jablensky and others 1992).

Socioeconomic class is a possible risk factor for schizophrenia, those living in poor socioeconomic conditions having high incidence and prevalence rates (Robinson and Regier 1991; Jablensky and others 1992). It is not known if the poor socioeconomic conditions in urban areas pose a risk or if persons with schizophrenia, because of their disease, migrate into these socioeconomic conditions. There is less of a "downward" social drift among persons with manic-depressive illness, which may be because manic-depressive individuals often have high energy and enthusiasm, which are correlated with social achievement (Bagley 1973).

Incidence and Prevalence: Schizophrenia

Studies done by WHO indicate that the incidence (derived from the time of the initial provider contact and interviews with family members about a patient's psychiatric history) of "broadly defined" schizophrenic patients who seek treatment is between 15 and 52 per 100,000 people (age fifteen through fifty-four), the developing world reporting the higher figures (Wig 1982; Jablensky and others 1992). "Broadly defined" schizophrenic patients include those with evidence of a psychotic state, such as nuclear schizophrenia, paranoid state, acute paranoid reaction, alcohol- or drug-induced hallucinosis, unspecified psychosis, probable and borderline psychosis (Jablensky and others 1992).

Approximately 30 to 40 percent of individuals in the developing world who have experienced psychotic episodes feel persecuted or neglect daily tasks such as personal cleanliness (Jablensky and others 1992). If only those patients who show nuclear symptoms of schizophrenia (delusions of control, feelings of someone inserting thoughts, or auditory hallucinations) are tabulated, the incidence decreases to between 7 and 14 per 100,000 (age fifteen to fifty-four); such individuals usually show at least intermittent symptoms for the rest of their life (Jablensky and others 1992). Comparison with other annual incidence rates from developing countries is difficult because of differing diagnostic criteria. Nonetheless, other studies from Asia indicate an incidence of between 2 and 11 per 100,000 in those age fifteen and above; Beijing, China, reported an incidence of schizophrenia of 11 per 100,000 in persons age fifteen and above (Yucun and others 1981; Wig 1982).

Incidence and Prevalence: Manic-Depressive Illness

The authors of three studies in northern Europe have found an annual incidence of manic-depressive illness of between 11 and 21 per 100,000 for persons age fifteen and older who seek treatment (reviewed in Goodwin and Jamison 1990). Individuals with manic-depressive illness often present with: inflated self-esteem, distractibility, increased pleasure, decreased sleep patterns or signs of fatigue, feelings of worthlessness, or suicidal ideation. Commonly, the disease course is cyclical in nature, and the threat of a manic or depressive episode continues throughout the rest of the individual's life. It is suspected that manic-depressive illness is not as prevalent in developing countries as it is in industrial ones (Goodwin and Jamison 1990).

Morbidity and Mortality: Schizophrenia

It has been reported that the course of schizophrenia is less severe in developing countries (Jablensky and Sartorius 1988). The differing disease course patterns for suboptimally treated patients from developing and industrial countries are shown in table 28-1. Data in this table indicate that patients from developing countries are more likely to have a brief psychosis.

World Health Organization research indicates that several factors are associated with a good prognosis (being female, married, and having an acute onset); however, these prognostic indicators and the presence or absence of effective treatment do not completely explain the differences in outcome between patients from the developing and industrial worlds (Jablensky and others 1992; Leff and others 1992). The better prognosis for schizophrenic patients from the developing world may be influenced by the use of a broad case definition or differing demands posed by the particular society (Wyatt and Stevens 1987; Jablensky and Sartorius 1988).

*Table 28-1. **Course of Schizophrenic Disease in Developing and Industrial Countries***
(percent)

Location	Acute	Chronic	Intermittent	Total
Developing regions[a]	27.5	37.1	32.7	97.3[b]
Industrial regions[c]	8.5	63.8	25.3	98.6[b]

Note: Acute course: full remission, no further episodes. Chronic course: at least one subsequent psychotic episode, with incomplete remission between episodes, or continuous psychotic episodes. Intermittent: partial remission, no further episodes, or at least one subsequent episode with full remission between episodes.

a. Agra, India; Cali, Colombia; and Ibadan, Nigeria.

b. The course of illness in some patients did not fit the definition of acute, chronic, or intermittent.

c. Aarhus, Denmark; London, England; Moscow, Russia; Prague, Czechoslovakia; and Washington, D.C., United States.

Source: Leff and others 1992.

Morbidity and Mortality: Manic-Depressive Illness

Retrospective studies indicate that 0 to 55 percent of nonprophylactically treated manic-depressive patients had only one episode, whereas 13 to 42 percent had two to three episodes, 8 to 40 percent had four to six episodes, and 2 to 69 percent had more than seven episodes (reviewed in Goodwin and Jamison 1990). It has been estimated that 22 percent of manic-depressive patients (mainly women) have a chronic course with virtually no normal intervals between mania and depression (Tsuang, Woolson, and Fleming 1979).

Burden of Schizophrenia

At fifteen-year follow-up, persons with schizophrenia and other categories of psychosis reported mortality rates 1.8 times greater than the general population, with 5 percent of patients adequately treated (Lin and others 1989). Approximately 8 percent of schizophrenic patients in the United States kill themselves, at an average age of thirty-one; similar rates of suicide are suspected among individuals with schizophrenia from the developing world (Roy 1986; Leff and others 1992).

Psychiatric disorders such as schizophrenia and manic-depressive illness exert a tremendous toll on the emotional and socioeconomic capabilities of both patient and caretaker. It has been reported that between 17 and 50 percent of schizophrenic patients being followed up had severe social impairment (Leff and others 1992). Other research indicates that more than 25 percent of the schizophrenic population in the United States is unable to work or perform homemaker responsibilities and that those capable of working or performing housekeeping have at least a 25 percent disability (ongoing research by Wyatt).

Burden of Manic-Depressive Illness

Untreated manic-depressive illness is reported approximately to double the yearly risk of dying, with suicide causing the majority of the excess mortality (Goodwin and Jamison 1990). It is estimated that one in five manic-depressive patients commits suicide, often within the first five years of the disease onset (Goodwin and Jamison 1990). Suicide is suspected to be less common among manic-depressive patients in the developing world, which may be a result of lower incidence rates, differing cultural manifestations of the disease, or a cultural bias against reporting suicide (Wittkower and Rin 1965). Due to their illness, approximately 20 to 30 percent of individuals with manic-depressive illness in the United States are unable to work (ongoing research by Wyatt).

Therapeutic Strategy for Schizophrenia

Such antipsychotic medications as fluphenazine, haloperidol, and chlorpromazine reduce the length of psychotic episodes in schizophrenic patients and can prevent relapses. Within six weeks after starting treatment with antipsychotic medication, 40 to 50 percent of active and chronic schizophrenic patients experience remission (Rifkin and others 1991). In addition, maintaining patients on antipsychotic medication produces a 50 to 60 percent reduction in relapse rates (Baldessarini, Cohen, and Teicher 1990; Rifkin and others 1991).

Antipsychotic medication has been reported to cause a 50 to 60 percent decrease in the severity of illness for both acute and chronic psychotic patients as rated by standard clinical rating scales (Santos and others 1989; Baldessarini, Cohen, and Teicher 1990). Relapse rates can be further reduced by using long-acting injectable antipsychotic medications (Baldessarini, Cohen, and Teicher 1990). When a schizophrenic patient improves clinically, social outcome also improves. It has been reported that there is a 0.5 correlation between clinical and social improvement as measured by interpersonal relationships, sociability, leisure activity, and work activity (Shepard and others 1989).

Research indicates that once patients have discontinued antipsychotic medication, they tend to have a much poorer social outcome, including a decrease in work productivity and an increase in socially disruptive behavior (Johnson and others 1983). There is an apparent decline in the suicide risk among treated schizophrenic patients, compared with the risk among those who are untreated; one study indicated that 27 percent of schizophrenic patients attempted suicide when neuroleptic medication was discontinued, whereas only 11 percent attempted suicide while on medication (Johnson and others 1983).

Therapeutic Strategy for Manic-Depressive Illness

Roughly 80 to 90 percent of manic-depressive patients on lithium respond favorably, resulting in a 60 to 80 percent reduction in relapses (Goodwin and Jamison 1990). Furthermore, it has been reported that both manic and depressive episodes are 80 percent less frequent in patients treated with lithium (Holinger and Wolpert 1979; Rybakowski and others 1980). Lithium helps to decrease the duration of an episode by reducing the intensity of mania or depression; correspondingly, there is a decreased episode frequency (Goodwin and Jamison 1990). By reducing the intensity of mania or depression, lithium also helps reduce suicide. Research has shown that 1.17 suicide attempts per patient were made before lithium and 0.18 suicide attempts per patient were made after lithium was introduced (Causemann and Muller-Oberlinghausen 1988).

Cost-Effective Schizophrenia Case Management

There is no model available regarding the cost-effectiveness of either a schizophrenia or manic-depressive outpatient medical program in the developing world. The following model is an attempt to provide estimates of the cost and effectiveness of a case management program based on a best-case scenario; it is presented in equation format with results in table 28-2.

The annual cost of a medication treatment program for individuals with schizophrenia per million population age fifteen and above is the sum of:

- *Estimate of treatment costs per acutely psychotic patient treated successfully* ($Cost_{acute}$). The outpatient costs per acutely psychotic patient who responds to medication and will receive antipsychotic medication for one year is equal to: (N_{acute} x V) + C_{acute}, where N_{acute} = number of outpatient visits needed per year by each acutely ill schizophrenic patient; V = cost of one outpatient visit; and C_{acute} = yearly cost of antipsychotic and anticholinergic medication for each acutely ill schizophrenic patient.

- *Estimate of treatment cost per acutely psychotic patient treated unsuccessfully* ($Cost_{acute/unsuccess}$). Because a fraction of the acutely ill psychotic patient pool who will be given antipsychotic medications for a period of up to six months will not respond, the following equation is needed: ($N_{acute/unsuccess}$ x V) + $C_{acute/unsuccess}$, where $N_{acute/unsuccess}$ = the number of visits used by an acutely psychotic patient who is dropped from the program after three months because of nonresponsiveness to medication, and $C_{acute/unsuccess}$ = cost of medication in acutely psychotic patients who are dropped from the program because of nonresponsiveness to medication.

- *Estimate of treatment costs per chronically ill patient served* ($Cost_{chronic}$). The outpatient costs for patients with schizophrenia who will receive long-term antipsychotic therapy is: ($N_{chronic}$ x V) + $C_{chronic}$, where $N_{chronic}$ = number of outpatient visits needed per year by each chronically ill schizophrenic patient, and $C_{chronic}$ = yearly cost of medication for a chronically ill schizophrenic patient.[1]

- *Estimate of treatment costs per intermittently ill patient treated* ($Cost_{intermittent}$). The outpatient costs for patients who will receive intermittent antipsychotic medication is: ($N_{intermittent}$ x V) + $C_{intermittent}$, where $N_{intermittent}$ = number of outpatient visits needed per year for each intermittently ill schizophrenic patient, and $C_{intermittent}$ = yearly cost of medication for an intermittently ill schizophrenic patient.

In order to simplify the equations, the estimated number of treated patients in the treatment groups (number-schizophrenia) is: $(I_{schizophrenia} \times P \times SS) \times (PT \times E)$, where $I_{schizophrenia}$ = incidence of broadly defined schizophrenia per 1 million population age fifteen through fifty-four;[2] P = proportion of broadly defined acutely ill schizophrenic patients of any age ($I_{schizophrenia}$) who will fall into either an acute, a chronic, or an intermittent disease outcome; SS = multiplication factor to account for preexisting patients; PT = proportion of population of each disease outcome who will be correctly diagnosed and appropriately treated at the health center (does not include those who dropped out because of medication side-effects); and E = percentage of each pool of patients that responds to antipsychotic medication.[3]

- *Estimate of disability-adjusted life-years (DALYs) gained per acutely psychotic patient successfully treated (DALY $_{acute}$)*. The number of DALYs gained per acutely ill patient successfully treated can be calculated as follows: $R \times (H_{acute} + CT_{acute} + M_{acute})$, where R = percentage reduction in patient and caretaker's disabilities and patient's excess mortality with medication; H_{acute} = acutely ill patient's quality-of-life disability; CT_{acute} = disability per acutely ill patient from his or her caretaker's reduced quality of life; and M_{acute} = acutely ill patient's yearly increase in the risk of dying.

- *Estimate of DALYs gained per chronically ill patient treated (DALY $_{chronic}$)*. The number of DALYs gained per treated chronically ill patient treated is: $R \times (H_{chronic} + CT_{chronic} + M_{chronic})$, where $H_{chronic}$ = chronically ill patient's disability from his or her reduced quality of life; $CT_{chronic}$ = disability per chronically ill patient from his or her caretaker's reduced quality of life; $M_{chronic}$ = chronically ill patient's yearly increase in the risk of dying.

- *Estimate of DALYs gained per intermittently ill patient treated (DALY $_{intermittent}$)*. The number of DALYs gained per intermittently ill patient treated is: $R \times (H_{intermittent} + CT_{intermittent} + M_{intermittent})$, where $H_{intermittent}$ = intermittently ill patient's disability from his or her reduced quality of life; $CT_{intermittent}$ = disability per intermittently ill patient from his or her caretaker's reduced quality of life; and $M_{intermittent}$ = chronically ill schizophrenic patient's yearly increase in the risk of dying.

In table 28-2 we display the equations used in determining the cost-effectiveness of the model, and in table 28-3 we present inputs used for the schizophrenia medical treatment program.[4] The $223.00 per disability-adjusted life-year gained is less expensive than most of the adult chronic disease interventions, such as coronary artery bypass surgery and cancer treatment programs (Jamison, chapter 1, this collection). The program would cost approximately $0.104 per person (age fifteen or older), not an unreasonable burden for most health care systems. Over 95 percent of the case management benefits are from reductions in the patient and caretaker's quality-of-life disability, with little contribution from averted mortality.

Manic-Depressive Illness Case Management

The cost-effectiveness of a lithium medication program can be calculated using exactly the same equations as those used for the neuroleptic medication program. The input functions for the case management program for lithium treatment of manic-depressive illness are noted in table 28-4. The manic-depressive illness medication intervention program, with total cost figures of $268.00 per disability-adjusted life-year gained and $0.092 per person (age eighteen and above), like the program for schizophrenic patients, is affordable compared with other adult chronic disease interventions, and it has a similar distribution of benefits, as does the schizophrenia treatment program (Jamison, chapter 1, this collection).

Gaps between Good and Actual Practice

Bothersome but nonlethal side effects from antipsychotic medication used to treat schizophrenia are numerous and include dry mouth, constipation, decreased libido, and tremors, all of which often can be treated by lowering the dose; tardive dyskinesia (repetitive involuntary movements) and neuroleptic malignant syndrome (high fever and blood abnormalities), which are potentially more serious, can contribute to the already serious morbidity (Baldessarini, Cohen, and Teicher 1990). Many patients who are given antipsychotic medication, particularly early in their treatment course, are also given anticholinergic and antiparkinsonian medication to prevent acute dystonic reactions (rigidity of muscle groups, especially facial), which, when they occur, are both painful and frightening (McKane and others 1987; Santos and others 1989). Compliance by the patient in taking antipsychotic medication is another important issue, and it has been estimated that as few as 50 percent of schizophrenic patients take their medication as prescribed (Wilcox, Gilian, and Hare 1965). As with all medications, describing potential side effects before they occur and making certain the diagnosis and treatment are appropriate should increase compliance.

Up to 25 percent of patients taking lithium for manic-depressive illness complain of excessive thirst, tremor, or memory problems (Goodwin and Jamison 1990). Lithium may be harmful to fetuses and can also cause decreased thyroid activity (Mannisto 1980). Toxicity due to lithium overdose can cause serious kidney damage and is often fatal (Goodwin and Jamison 1990). Noncompliance of lithium users in taking their medication ranges between 18 and 53 percent and is often thought to be connected to the denial of the disease as well as the side effects (Goodwin and Jamison 1990). Manic-depressive patients need to be monitored for suicidal ideation, particularly during the first few years of the disease, when the risk is the highest.

Ethical and legal issues regarding giving medication to patients who cannot give consent (particularly those in acute psychotic states) need to be considered in relation to local standards, and possible dispositions for aggressive patients also need to be explored. If antipsychotic medication or lithium is

Table 28-2. Derived Variables and Their Most Likely Values

Name or symbol	Variable	Derivation	Most likely value
Number-schizophrenia $_{acute}$	Number of acutely ill patients treated successfully	$(I_{schizophrenia} \times P_{acute} \times PT_{acute}) \times E_{acute}$	18
Number-schizophrenia $_{acute/unsuccess}$	Number of acutely ill patients treated unsuccessfully	$(I_{schizophrenia} \times P_{acute/unsuccess} \times PT_{acute/unsuccess}) \times (1 - E_{acute})$	15
Number-schizophrenia $_{chronic}$	Number of chronically ill patients treated	$(I_{schizophrenia} \times P_{chronic} \times PT_{chronic}) \times E_{chronic}$	696
Number-schizophrenia $_{intermittent}$	Number of intermittently ill patients treated	$(I_{schizophrenia} \times P_{intermittent} \times PT_{intermittent}) \times E_{intermittent}$	141
Cost $_{acute}$	Cost per acutely ill patient treated successfully	$(N_{acute} \times V) + C_{acute}$	$160
Cost $_{acute/unsuccess}$	Cost per acutely ill patient treated unsuccessfully	$(N_{acute/unsuccess} \times V) + C_{acute/unsuccess}$	$63
Cost $_{chronic}$	Cost per chronically ill patient treated	$(N_{chronic} \times V) + C_{chronic}$	$117
Cost $_{intermittent}$	Cost per intermittently ill patient treated	$(N_{intermittent} \times V) + C_{intermittent}$	$140
DALY $_{acute}$	Disability-adjusted life-years gained per acutely ill patient treated successfully	$R \times (H_{acute} + CT_{acute} + M_{acute})$	0.30
DALY $_{chronic}$	Disability-adjusted life-years gained per chronically ill patient treated	$R \times (H_{chronic} + CT_{chronic} + M_{chronic})$	0.60
DALY $_{intermittent}$	Disability-adjusted life-years gained per intermittently ill patient treated	$R \times (H_{intermittent} + CT_{intermittent} + M_{intermittent})$	0.30
U	Total number of disability-adjusted life-years gained from case management program	$(\text{Number-schizophrenia}_{acute} \times \text{DALY}_{acute}) +$ $(\text{Number-schizophrenia}_{chronic} \times \text{DALY}_{chronic}) +$ $(\text{Number-schizophrenia}_{intermittent} \times \text{DALY}_{intermittent})$	465
Z	Total cost of schizophrenia program	$(\text{Number-schizophrenia}_{acute} \times \text{Cost}_{acute}) +$ $(\text{Number-schizophrenia}_{acute/unsuccess} \times \text{Cost}_{acute/unsuccess}) +$ $(\text{Number-schizophrenia}_{chronic} \times \text{Cost}_{chronic}) +$ $(\text{Number-schizophrenia}_{intermittent} \times \text{Cost}_{intermittent})$	$104,999
Q	Cost per disability-adjusted life-year gained	Z/U	$223

Source: Authors.

Table 28-3. Variables for Model of Schizophrenia Case Management

Symbol	Variable	Value Acute	Value Chronic	Value Intermittent
P	Proportion of schizophrenic population	0.28	0.37	0.33
PT	Proportion who will receive correct treatment	0.40	0.60	0.50
SS	Steady-state factor to account for preexisting patients	1.00	17.4	5.8
N	Number of clinic visits needed per year	30[a]	12	21
V	Cost of one outpatient visit	$2.25	$2.25	$2.25
C	Yearly medication costs	$92[b]	$90	$92
E	Percentage of patients responding to medication	0.50	0.60	0.50
H	Patient's decreased quality-of-life disability	0.40	0.80	0.40
CT	Caretaker's decreased quality-of-life disability	0.20	0.40	0.20
M	Patient's yearly increase in risk of dying	0.0035	0.007	0.0035
R	Percentage reduction in patient's/caretaker's disabilities and mortality risk when patient taking medication	50	50	50

Note: Total incidence (*I*) of schizophrenia (broadly defined) is 300 cases per million people age fifteen to fifty-four.
a. Twenty-one visits for acute patient unsuccessfully treated.
b. $16 for acute patient unsuccessfully treated.
Source: Authors.

given by nonpsychiatrists and without serum monitoring, missed opportunities for dosage adjustment and reducing side effects will be increased. Furthermore, the use of antipsychotic medication or lithium in the developing world needs to be investigated, because medication may work better or worse in those areas. The cost-effectiveness of both programs relies heavily on community and family support. If the community does not respond, effectiveness will decrease as the costs increase because patient compliance will not be encouraged and assistance in helping the patient remain in the program (transport, jobs, housing, and so on) will be lacking.

Priorities for Control

Case management with medication is not the only alternative for these patients, but it may be the most cost-effective alternative. Psychotherapy alone has been proven to be of limited benefit compared with medical treatment, but some forms of

psychotherapy aimed at stress reduction and education about the illness together with antipsychotic medication for schizophrenia and lithium for manic-depressive illness appear to make both illnesses more manageable (Baldessarini, Cohen, and Teicher 1990).

Research on the epidemiology of schizophrenia and manic-depressive illness is of importance; of particular importance is a determination of associated disability. There are numerous rating scales which measure social activities, level of anxiety, activity, ability to perform work, self-esteem, and same and opposite gender friendship that could be used with local modification to help determine disability (Weiss and others 1985). A treatment protocol that would enable supervised primary-level health workers to identify and correctly treat psychotic and bipolar disorders needs to be developed. Research also needs to identify contact points (general practitioners, herbalists and traditional healers) that would act as bases for referral of psychiatric patients to

Table 28-4. Variables for Model of Manic-Depressive Illness Case Management

Symbol	Variable	Value Acute	Value Chronic	Value Intermittent
P	Proportion of manic-depressive population	0.22	0.55	0.33
PT	Proportion who will receive correct treatment	0.30	0.50	0.40
SS	Steady-state factor to account for preexisting patients	1.00	16.7	4.2
N	Number of clinic visits needed per year	30[a]	12	21
V	Cost of one outpatient visit	$2.25	$2.25	$2.25
C	Yearly medication costs	$92[b]	$90	$92
E	Percentage of patients responding to medication	70	60	70
H	Patient's decreased quality-of-life disability	0.30	0.60	0.30
CT	Caretaker's decreased quality-of-life disability	0.10	0.20	0.10
M	Patient's yearly increase in risk of dying	0.004	0.008	0.004
R	Percentage reduction in patient's/caretaker's disabilities and mortality risk when patient taking medication	60	60	60

Note: Incidence (*I*) is eighty cases per million people age eighteen and older.
a. Twenty-one visits for acute patient unsuccessfully treated.
b. $16 for acute patient unsuccessfully treated.
Source: Authors.

a clinic-based medicine intervention program and to ensure patient compliance with the program.

Appendix 28A. Sources Used to Obtain Cost-Effectiveness Estimates

This section discusses sources for cost-effective case management of schizophrenia and manic-depressive illness.

Schizophrenia

The yearly incidence rate of broadly defined schizophrenia ($I_{schizophrenia}$) of 300 per 1 million population, age fifteen through fifty-four, is based on published results from the developing world (Jablensky and others 1992). The proportion of individuals with schizophrenia who fall into the three types of disease outcome categories (P) is derived from table 28-1 (developing world data with broad case definition of schizophrenia). P_{acute} patients are projected to need antipsychotics for only one year with no other treatment necessary, whereas $P_{intermittent}$ patients are assumed to need antipsychotics for a year's duration every third year, and $P_{chronic}$ patients will need antipsychotics for the remainder of their lives.

The 17.4 steady-state factor for the chronic ($SS_{chronic}$) patient pool and the 5.8 factor for the intermittent ($SS_{intermittent}$) pool are based on a cohort calculated to remain in the program for thirty-nine years with a 5 percent yearly dropout rate.[5] The steady-state factor of intermittently ill patients is one-third that of chronically ill ones, because they are projected to need medication only every third year. The proportions of each disease pool treated (PT), ranging from 0.40 to 0.60, are clinically based; those in the acute pool are the ones least likely to enter the program, because their illness is of shorter duration.

Thirty outpatient contacts per year (N) are needed to treat an acutely ill schizophrenic patient. This estimate is based on the assumption that the patients will need fourteen consecutive daily visits for initial stabilization, followed by weekly visits for the next six weeks, then monthly visits for the remainder of the year. The acutely ill patient who does not respond to treatment will be treated for two and a half months (twenty-one visits). The intermittently ill schizophrenic patient's course of illness would probably be known to the health center staff, making initial stabilization less time consuming; thus only twenty-one visits will be needed (seven consecutive daily visits, three weekly visits, and eleven monthly visits). The chronic pool of schizophrenic patients was projected to need outpatient visits once a month for antipsychotic medication injections each year. The $2.25 outpatient cost per visit (V) is derived from calculations in table 28A-1 showing a hypothetical summary of capital and annual costs of health clinics and outposts that have a capacity of approximately 30,000 mental health visits per year.

It is projected that all patients diagnosed with schizophrenia are placed on antipsychotic medication, beginning with two weeks of 2 milligrams of generic oral fluphenazine per day, followed by injections once each month of generic long-acting fluphenazine, and that one-half of the patients need 50 milligrams of generic diphenhydramine hydrochloride to prevent dystonic side effects. The medication costs per year for the acutely or intermittently ill schizophrenic patient (C_{acute} or $C_{intermittent}$) is thus $92 (wholesale price from survey of producers). The yearly cost of medication for the acutely ill patient who does not respond to treatment ($C_{acute/nonresp}$) is $16 for the initial two weeks of oral medication plus two months of injectable medication. The cost of the chronically ill patient's medication ($C_{chronic}$) is $90, because these patients do not need the initial stabilizing doses of fluphenazine.

The effectiveness values of antipsychotic medications (E) are derived from data that show that the decrease in relapse rates when using long-acting antipsychotic medications, in patients who show an initial response to antipsychotics, is approximately 60 percent ($E_{chronic}$) and that 50 percent of actively psychotic patients (or relapsing intermittently ill patients; E_{acute} or $E_{intermittent}$) will remit within six weeks after beginning antipsychotic therapy (Johnson and others 1983; Baldessarini, Cohen, and Teicher 1990; Van Putten, Marder, and Mintz 1990).

The reduction of clinical and social impairment, or quality-of-life disabilities (H), for the acute (40 percent), chronic (80 percent), and intermittent patients (40 percent) through medication is based on various clinical rating scales; the caretaker's decreased quality-of-life disability (CT) is projected to be one-half of the patient's quality-of-life disability.[6]

The yearly increase in the risk of dying (M) is from research showing that individuals with schizophrenia in Taiwan (China) had approximately a 200 percent standardized mortality ratio in a fifteen-year follow-up (Lin and others 1989). Survival statistics for Mexican males in 1980 from age twenty to sixty were then used to calculate a 0.007 yearly increase in the risk of dying (M) for the schizophrenic population (United Nations 1982).

The reductions in quality-of-life disabilities for both patient and caretaker and the reduction in excess mortality risk seen for the patient (R) from the patient's taking antipsychotic medication assume that once the patient's life improves, the caretaker's life will improve at the same rate. The reductions also assume a 60 percent clinical improvement by clinical rating scales and a published correlation between clinical and social improvement, resulting in a projected 50 percent reduction figure (Santos and others 1989; Shepard and others 1989; Baldessarini, Cohen, and Teicher 1990). The same reduction input is used for decreasing the patient's excess mortality risk and is based on research indicating a 50 percent reduction in suicide attempts with medication and an assumption that if suicidal behavior is minimized so will other dangerous behavior which causes the high mortality risk (Johnson and others 1983).

The disability associated with decreased quality of life for patient and caretaker and the increase in the risk of dying for the acute and intermittent groups (when relapsed) are projected to be one-half those of the chronic group. The reasoning

Table 28A-1. Annual Costs of Schizophrenia and Manic-Depressive Case Management Programs

Variable	Assumptions	Cost (dollars)
Operating costs		
Salaries: case management officers	Fifteen officers per center; $1,000 per officer per year	45,000
Salaries: nurse practitioners	One per center; $1,500 per nurse per year	4,500
Retirement pensions	5 percent of salaries	2,475
Supplies	$250 per center, not including drugs	750
Utilities	Gas, water, and electric; $150 per center	450
In-service training	$500 per center	1,500
Supervision	One full day each month by psychiatrist at each center; per diem and transportation	2,000
Maintenance and repair: buildings	1.5 percent of construction price per year	900
Maintenance and repair: equipment	15 percent of purchase price per year	112
Transportation between centers and villages	Twelve visits per year by motorcycle to each village; twenty villages per center; fifteen miles round trip; 20 cents per mile for gas	2,160
Public education	None	2,000
Contingencies	None	3,000
Total		64,847
Capital costs		
Buildings	Annualized with thirty-year life span; $20,000 per center original cost	2,000
Equipment	Annualized with ten-year life span; $250 per center	75
Vehicles	One motorcycle per center; annualized with five-year life span; $1,000 per motorcycle	600
Total operating and capital costs		67,522
Cost per clinic visit	30,000 patient visits per year	2.25

Note: Assumes three centers.
Source: Authors; Over 1991.

for this is straightforward: the length of a psychotic episode based on data concerning hospital stays is six months; thus, the disability of these two groups exists for only one-half of the year (Shepard and others 1989).

Manic-Depressive Illness

The incidence of manic-depressive illness ($I_{\text{manic-depressive}}$) in the developing world is projected to be 80 per 1 million people aged eighteen and older, substantially less than the 150 per million reported from the industrial world (Goodwin and Jamison 1990). The proportion of manic-depressive individuals (P) who fall into the acute (only 1 manic-depressive episode), chronic (7 episodes), and intermittent (2–7 episodes) disease categories is a derivative from research with a fifteen-year follow-up period (Goodwin and Jamison 1990).

For chronic manic-depressive patients the steady-state factor is 16.7 (SS_{chronic}) and is formulated much like the program for schizophrenic patients, except the cohort was followed for only thirty-four years (average age of onset: twenty-five) and the yearly dropout rate because of side effects of medication (such as tremors and gastrointestinal effects) was 5 percent. Calculations for the intermittently ill pool of manic-depressive patients use the same data, except this pool of patients will receive lithium for only one out of every four years.

The proportions of the disease category subtype population who will receive care at a health system (PT) are partially based on an assumption that a lower percentage of the manic-depressive population than the schizophrenic population will undergo treatment because the manic-depressive disease can often be "hidden" with greater ease in society. The proportions vary between 0.30 and 0.50, with the chronic patients most likely to enter because of the length of illness.

The number of outpatient visits needed per year (N) and the cost of one outpatient visit (V) are projected to be the same for the course of each subtype of manic-depressive illness as they were for the course of the subtype pools of schizophrenia. The cost of $92 per year for lithium (C) assumes an average daily dose of between 900 and 1,000 milligrams, which is the traditional dose of lithium for the manic-depressive patient (Goodwin and Jamison 1990; wholesale price from survey of producers). This price includes, for the acute and intermittent patient (but not for the chronic patient), a two-week 2-milligram daily dose of oral fluphenazine. As with the schizophrenia case management plan, the acutely ill manic-depressive patient unsuccessfully treated will be in the program for only two and a half months, needing twenty-one clinic visits and medication costing $16.

Lithium has been reported to reduce relapses by 60 to 80 percent in the industrial world and it is projected that lithium will prevent relapses 6 to 60 percent (E_{chronic}) in the developing world (Rybakowski and others 1980). Lithium has also been reported to be 80 to 90 percent effective in lowering the severity of illness in acutely ill patients (E_{acute} or $E_{\text{intermittent}}$), but it is projected to be only 70 percent effective in the developing world (Goodwin and Jamison 1990).

Patient (*H*) and caretaker (*CT*) quality-of-life disabilities are clinical judgments based on clinical and social rating scales. As with the schizophrenia case management model, the acute and intermittently ill manic-depressive patient (30 percent disabled) is projected to suffer from one episode lasting half a year, resulting in both one-half the disability and one-half the mortality increase suffered by the chronically ill patient who is 60 percent disabled the entire year (Goodwin and Jamison 1990). Correspondingly, it is projected that the caretaker's quality-of-life disability is 20 percent when he or she is charged with caring for a chronically ill patient, and 10 percent when an acutely or intermittently ill patient is involved.

Research indicates that mortality rates are 2.2 times greater for manic-depressive individuals than the general population, which, if one uses the previously mentioned survival tables of Mexican males in 1980, translates into a yearly increase in the risk of dying of 0.008 for manic-depressive individuals (*M*) (United Nations 1982; Goodwin and Jamison 1990).

The patient and caretaker's projected 60 percent reduction in quality-of-life disability with lithium usage (*R*) is based on the impressions of clinicians which indicate that the intensity of manic-depressive episodes decreases significantly. The decrease in the excess mortality for the lithium-treated manic-depressive patient (*R*) is derived from published reports showing a 60 percent decrease in suicides in manic-depressive patients who are taking lithium (Goodwin and Jamison 1990). If the suicide rate decreases 60 percent, it is assumed that the generalized excess mortality will also decrease 60 percent.

Notes

An earlier version of this paper was presented at the WHO/World Bank consultation on *Interventions for Nervous System Disorders* held in Washington, D.C. on July 6-7, 1992. We wish to thank Thomas McGuire for his assistance at the consultation and later, when he reviewed this chapter.

1. In contrast to the acutely ill patient pool, there is no need for an adjustment for patients who do not respond to antipsychotics, because the treatment responses of the chronic and intermittently ill groups of patients will be known to the clinic staff.

2. Incidence reported in the WHO study (Jablensky and others 1992) was for a population of 100,000; for the present circumstances we have adjusted that figure to a population of 1 million. Incidence refers to individuals of fifteen through fifty-four years who experienced clearly psychotic symptoms, had never made contact with a helping agency in the past, and were residents of the catchment area. It was also felt that the risk for schizophrenia was negligible after age fifty-four; thus, the incidence rates are for those age fifteen and older.

3. Either of the two pools of acutely ill patients (responders and nonresponders) will not have a steady-state factor by definition. "Incidence$_{schizophrenia}$" is total incidence and will be the same value for each disease outcome. "Effectiveness$_{acute/unsuccess}$" is (1 – Effectiveness$_{acute}$) because it is the pool of acute patients who are treated unsuccessfully (the response of acute patients to medication is unknown because they have never participated in the program).

4. The equations do not include an input for the number of disability-adjusted life-years gained for the acute nonresponding patient pool by definition. In addition, the inputs for this pool are different from the acute responding pool with respect to number of visits needed (number-visits) and the cost of medication (yearly cost-medication$_{acute/nonres}$) and are included at the

bottom of table 28-3. The same rationale applies to the manic-depressive patient treatment program (table 28-4).

5. The contributions to the total for each of the last thirty-nine years were added to this year's patient pool to give an approximate number of patients in treatment in that disease outcome category. This total number of patients treated (in that disease outcome category) divided by this year's contribution to the patient pool (in that disease outcome category) is the steady-state factor.

Because the average age of schizophrenia onset is twenty and the general life expectancy is predicted to be sixty (individuals with schizophrenia generally have a higher standardized mortality rate), a program of thirty-nine years' duration is appropriate.

6. Completely (100 percent) disabled = 1.0 disability quotient; 40 percent disabled = 0.4 disability quotient; and so on.

References

Bagley, C. 1973. "Occupation Status and Symptoms of Depression." *Social Science and Medicine* 7(5):327–39.

Baldessarini, R., B. Cohen, and M. Teicher. 1990. "Pharmacological Treatment." In S. Levy and P. Ninan, eds., *Schizophrenia Treatment*. New York: American Psychiatric Press.

Causemann, B., and B. Müller-Oberlinghausen. 1988. "Does Lithium Prevent Suicides and Suicide Attempts?" In N. J. Birch, ed., *Lithium: Inorganic Pharmacology and Psychiatric Use*. Oxford: IRL Press.

Goodwin, K., and K. Jamison. 1990. *Manic-Depressive Illness*. New York: Oxford University Press.

Gottesman, I., and I. Shields. 1982. *Schizophrenia: The Epigenetic Puzzle*. Cambridge: Cambridge University Press.

Holinger, P., and E. Wolpert. 1979. "A Ten Year Follow-Up of Lithium Use." *IMJ* 156:99–104.

Jablensky, A., and N. Sartorius. 1988. "Is Schizophrenia Universal?" *Acta Psychiatria Scandanavia* 344(supplement):65–70.

Jablensky, A., N. Sartorius, G. Ernberg, M. Anker, A. Korten, J. E. Cooper, R. Day, and A. Bertelsen. 1992. "Schizophrenia: Manifestations, Incidence, and Course in Different Cultures: A World Health Organization Ten-Country Study." *Psychological Medicine* 20(supplement):1–97.

Johnson, D., G. Pasterski, J. Ludlow, K. Street, and R. Taylor. 1983. "The Discontinuance of Maintenance Neuroleptic Therapy in Chronic Schizophrenic Patients: Drug and Social Consequences." *Acta Psychiatria Scandanavia* 67:339–52.

Leff, J., N. Sartorius, A. Jablensky, A. Korten, and G. Ernberg. 1992. "The International Pilot Study of Schizophrenia: Five-Year Follow-Up Findings." *Psychological Medicine* 22:131–45.

Lin, T., H. Chu, H. Rin, C. Hsu, E. Yeh, and C. Chen. 1989. "Effects of Social Change on Mental Disorders in Taiwan: Observations Based on a 15-Year Follow-Up Survey." *Acta Psychiatria Scandanavia* 348(supplement):11–34.

McKane, J., D. Robinson, D. Wiles, R. McCreadie, and G. Stirling. 1987. "Haloperidol Decanoate v. Fluphenazine Deanoate as Maintenance Therapy in Chronic Schizophrenic In-Patients." *British Journal of Psychiatry* 151:333–36.

Mannisto, P. T. 1980. "Endocrine Side-Effects of Lithium." In F. N. Johnson, ed., *Handbook of Lithium Therapy*. Baltimore: University Park Press.

Over, Mead. 1991. *Economics for Health Sector Analysis: Concepts and Cases*. Washington, D.C.: World Bank, Economic Development Institute.

Rifkin, A., S. Doddi, K. Basawaraj, M. Borenstein, and M. Wachspress. 1991. "Dosage of Haloperidol for Schizophrenia." *Archives of General Psychiatry* 48:166–70.

Robins, L., and D. Regier. 1991. *Psychiatric Disorder in America: The Epidemiologic Catchment Area Study*. New York: Free Press.

Roy, Alec. 1986. "Depression, Attempted Suicide, and Suicide in Patients with Chronic Schizophrenia." *Clinics of North America* 2(1):193–205.

Rybakowski, J., M. Chtopocka-Wozniak, Z. Kapelski, and W. Stryzewski. 1980. "The Relative Prophylactic Efficacy of Lithium against Mania and Depressive Recurrences in Bipolar Patients." *International Pharmacopsychiatry* 15:86–90.

Santos, J., J. Cabranes, C. Vazquez, F. Fuentenbro, I. Almoguera, and J. Ramos. 1989. "Clinical Response and Plasma Haloperidol Levels in Chronic and Subchronic Schizophrenia." *Biological Psychiatry* 26:381–88.

Shepard, M., D. Watt, I. Fallon, and N. Smetton. 1989. "The Natural History of Schizophrenia: A Five-Year Follow-Up Study of Outcome and Prediction in a Representative Sample of Schizophrenics." *Psychological Medicine* 15 (supplement):1–46.

Tsuang, M., R. Woolson, and J. Fleming. 1979. "Long-Term Outcome of Major Psychoses: 1. Schizophrenia and Affective Disorders Compared with Psychiatrically Symptom-Free Surgical Conditions." *Archives of General Psychiatry* 36:1295–1301.

United Nations. 1982. *Demographic Yearbook*. New York.

Van Putten, T., S. Marder, and J. Mintz. 1990. "A Controlled Dose Comparison of Haloperidol in Newly Admitted Schizophrenic Patients." *Archives of General Psychiatry* 47:754–58.

Weiss, D., K. DeWitt, N. Kaltreider, and M. Horowitz. 1985. "A Proposed Method for Measuring Change Beyond Symptoms." *Archives of General Psychiatry* 42:703–8.

Wig, N. 1982. "Methodology of Data Collection in Field Surveys." *Acta Psychiatria Scandanavia* 296(supplement):77–86.

Wilcox, D., R. Gilian, and E. Hare. 1965. "Do Psychiatric Outpatients Take Their Drugs?" *British Medical Journal* 2:790–92.

Wittkower, E., and H. Rin. 1965. "Transcultural Psychiatry." *Archives of General Psychiatry* 13:387–94.

Wyatt, R., and J. Stevens. 1987. "Similar Incidence Worldwide of Schizophrenia: Case Not Proven." *British Journal of Psychiatry* 151:131–32.

Yucun, S., A. Weixi, S. Liang, Y. Xiaoling, C. Yuhua, and Z. Dongfeng. 1981. "Investigation of Mental Disorders in Beijing Suburban District." *Chinese Medical Journal* 94(3):153–56.

PART FIVE

Conclusion

29

The Health Transition: Implications for Health Policy in Developing Countries

W. Henry Mosley, José Luis Bobadilla, and Dean T. Jamison

Changing epidemiologic profiles of developing countries are leading—in many countries quite rapidly—to fundamental changes in the volume and composition of demand for health services and needs for health promotion. The purpose of this collection has been to attempt to take stock, in a systematic disease-by-disease manner, of the potential for cost-effective responses to this changing pattern of needs. Although considerations of intervention cost-effectiveness (or value-for-money) were important even before rapid change in epidemiologic profiles, the relatively limited range of key interventions for communicable childhood disease led, through experience, to a reasonable sense of a cost-effective mix of interventions. The situation becomes vastly more complex with the emergence, as quantitatively important, of a broad range of additional conditions; hence the motivation for the systematic analyses reported in this collection.

Chapter 1 described the approach taken in the chapter-specific analyses and summarized the resulting conclusions concerning cost-effectiveness. Our purpose in this chapter is to explore, in a more general way, the implications of the

Figure 29-1. Relationships among Demographic, Epidemiologic, and Health Transitions

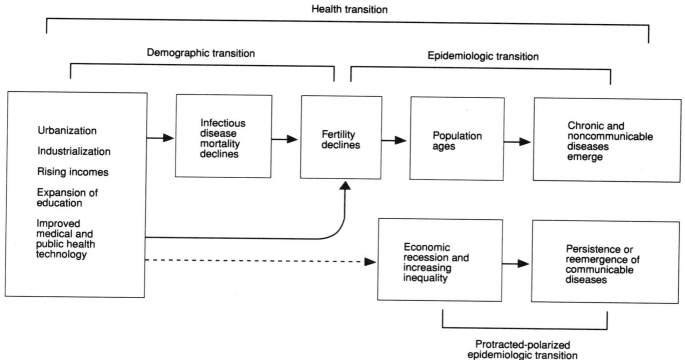

Source: Authors.

epidemiologic and health transition for health policy. We begin by reviewing the global health transition and its constituent demographic and epidemiologic transitions. We then turn to discussion of the implications of these transitions for national governments and, in closing, we explore implications for international aid.

The Health Transition

Essential to an understanding of the evolution of disease control priorities in developing countries is a reasonable projection of probable changes in the pattern of disease. These changes are likely to be profound. Our discussion of these changes divides naturally into four parts—the first deals with the demographic transition, the second deals with the epidemiologic transition, the third deals with the changing risk environment that has been occurring, and the fourth deals with the widening gap in health problems and health needs across social and economic classes. Collectively these changes are coming to be referred to as the "health transition," and figure 29-1 illustrates relations among the demographic, epidemiologic, and health transitions.

The Demographic Transition and Population Aging

Health patterns in the developing world during the next three decades will be profoundly influenced by recent and projected future declines in fertility and mortality as these nations pass through the demographic transition. Figure 29-2, which is drawn from the demographic analyses prepared for this collection, projects declines in the total fertility rates and the gains in life expectancy that might be expected in each of four regions of the developing world during the thirty years 1985 to 2015, assuming reasonable and achievable continuation of established trends. (Table 29-1 provides detail by region on the demographic parameters estimated for 1985–90 and projected for 2000–2005; definitions of the regional groupings that are used may be found in chapter 1, table A-1.) The projected declines in fertility for Sub-Saharan Africa and the Middle East are substantial, averaging 50 percent, whereas the gains projected for life expectancy are more modest, ranging from 10 percent in Latin America to 25 percent in Sub-Saharan Africa.

Long-term projections are inevitably tentative; nonetheless, it should be noted that fertility changes of this magnitude in a thirty-year period are not unprecedented. The total fertility rates in the Latin American and Asian regions ranged from 5.5 to 6.0 births per woman in the late 1950s and declined to their present levels of 3.3 to 3.5 in less than thirty years. Perhaps more problematical are the projected mortality declines. These do not yet take into account the acquired immunodeficiency syndrome (AIDS) epidemic, which has assumed significant proportions in many countries in Sub-Saharan Africa and Latin America. Nonetheless, much of the developing world is now well through a transition from high mortality and fertility rates to low ones; this demographic transition sets the stage for epidemiologic change.

Figure 29-2. Regional Projections of Life Expectancy and Fertility

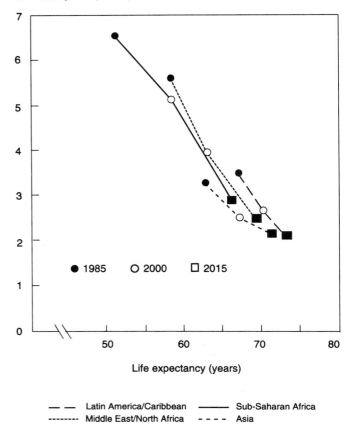

Source: Bulatao and Stephens 1990.

It is commonly assumed that the changing health picture seen in populations undergoing the demographic transition is primarily a function of the declines in mortality. In fact, however, the age structure and, correspondingly, the cause structure of death during the course of the demographic transition is strongly influenced by the rapid decline in fertility. (The role of mortality decline in creating preconditions for fertility decline nonetheless leaves mortality decline as a central *indirect* cause of epidemiologic change. Figure 29-1 illustrates this point.) This occurs because of a phenomenon that is described by demographers as the "momentum" of population growth. To explain simply, with high fertility the age structure of a population is highly skewed toward the young, irrespective of the level of mortality (figure 29-3). With sustained high birth rates and larger numbers of women entering the reproductive ages every year, the base of the population is continually expanding as more births are added every year. With the onset of the fertility transition and rapidly declining birth rates, however, the number of births added each year may remain unchanged or even decline. Consequently the age structure of the population will be progressively transformed

Table 29-1. Demographic Parameters, Globally and by Region, 1985–1990 (Estimates) and 2000–2005 (Projections)

Region[a]	Population (millions)		Crude birth rate (per 1,000 population per year)		Crude death rate (per 1,000 population per year)		Total fertility rate[b]		Life expectancy at birth (years)[c]	
	1985	2000	1985–90	2000–5	1985–90	2000–5	1985–90	2000–5	1985–90	2000–5
Industrialized market economies	760	810	13	12	9	10	1.7	1.8	76	78
Industrialized transition economies	416	453	17	15	11	10	2.3	2.1	70	73
Subtotal, industrialized economies	1,176	1,263	15	13	10	10	1.9	1.9	74	76
Latin American and Carribean	402	529	29	21	7	6	3.6	2.5	67	71
Sub-Saharan Africa	556	720	46	40	15	11	6.4	5.4	52	57
Middle East and North Africa	376	573	40	32	10	8	5.6	4.3	60	65
Asia and the Pacific	2434	3,118	27	21	9	8	3.3	2.6	64	68
Subtotal, developing countries	3,668	4,940	31	25	10	8	3.9	3.1	62	66
World total	4,844	6,203	27	23	10	8	3.4	2.9	65	68

a. Appendix 29A lists countries in each grouping.
b. Number of children a woman would be expected to bear during her reproductive years, based on the age-specific fertility rates prevailing in that period.
c. Average of the male and female life expectancies reported in the source table.
Source: Bulatao and Stephens 1990.

Figure 29-3. Age Distribution of the Population
(figures based on alternative mortality and fertility assumptions)

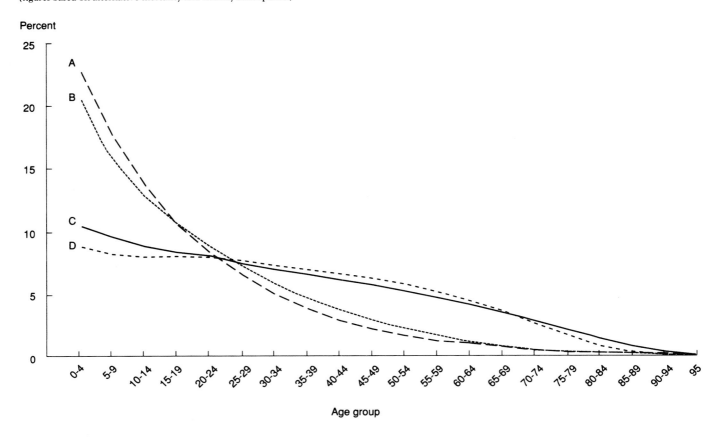

Note: Percent distribution of the female population by age groups in West model life tables. Curves A and B represent a gross reproduction rate of 4.0 (eight births per woman) with life expectancies of seventy five years (curve A) and forty years (curve B). Curves C and D represent a gross reproduction rate of 1.5 (three births per woman) with life expectancies of seventy-five years (curve C) and forty years (curve D).
Source: Coale and Demeny 1983.

from the shape of a broad-based triangle to a rectangular or even trapezoidal shape with a narrowing of the base (figure 29-3). The pace of fertility decline will be directly reflected in an immediate slowing (and even reversal) in the growth of the youngest age groups. The adult population will, however, continue to grow for several decades because of the continuing aging of the larger cohorts of persons already born.

Figure 29-4 illustrates this phenomenon for Latin America. Although the size of the age cohort under five years old changes very little during the thirty-year period, there is a dramatic increase from ages forty-five through sixty-four. In the very long run (more than a century) the numbers of the elderly in the rapidly growing developing countries can increase in size by more than 100 times (Chesnais 1990). Kinsella (1988) examines a broad range of consequences, in addition to the health ones we address here, of population aging in developing countries during the next several decades.

The Epidemiologic Transition

The transformation in the age structure of mortality associated with the demographic transition leads to a transition in its cause structure that has been termed the "epidemiologic transition" by Omran (1971). Omran identifies three phases in this transition: the age of pestilence and famine, the age of receding epidemics, and the age of degenerative and man-made diseases. In table 1-1 (and table 29-7), the "unfinished agenda" and the "emerging problems" illustrate the health conditions that are typically prominent, for children and for adults, in the pre- and postepidemiologic transition environment, respectively. (We consider phase three to be the posttransition phase.)

Olshansky and Ault (1986) proposed a fourth phase in the epidemiologic transition—the age of "delayed degenerative diseases." This phase was proposed because of the progressive decline in the death rates from some chronic diseases associated with steady gains in life expectancy among the aged in the United States and some other industrial countries. Crimmins, Saito, and Ingegneri (1989) have reported for the United States that these gains in survival among the aged have in large measure been in "disabled" years rather than "healthy" life. In this circumstance, improved survival among the aged implies that there will be an increasing, not lessening, demand for health services (Verbrugge 1984, 1989). Fries (1989), however, notes that in the United States in recent years there have

Figure 29-4. *Estimates of Male Population of Latin America, Age Groups 0–4 and 45–64, 1970–2015*

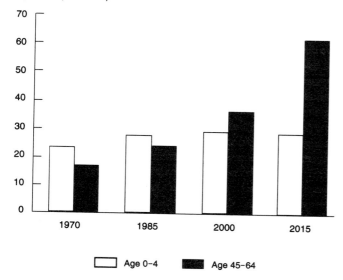

Population (in millions)

☐ Age 0–4   ■ Age 45–64

Source: Bulatao and Stephens 1990.

been substantial declines in the incidence of such conditions as heart disease, lung cancer, and automobile accidents. He observes that "successful aging" with lessened infirmity can be achieved if medical systems pursue vigorously the path of prevention rather than concentrating on developing sophisticated means of treating diseases after they are recognized.

Because of the central role of population dynamics in shaping the profile of illness and the pattern of cause of death, it is worth discussing these matters somewhat further. Preston (1986) has shown that from the time a population comes down to and maintains replacement reproduction levels (total fertility rates approximately 2.1) the entire growth of the population occurs only in the population segment beyond the mean age of childbearing (approximately twenty-eight years). He concludes: "Population momentum turns out to be momentous only for mature adult ages where productivity is typically highest and where concerns regarding the economic effects of rapid growth are probably least" (p. 349). The implications of population momentum in older age groups for the health system are, however, dramatic. Table 29-2, which is derived from World Bank projections, shows the percentage changes in the population size by age group projected to occur in each of the four developing country regions over the thirty-year period 1985 to 2015.[1] This illustrates the marked changes in the age structure of these populations that will result, primarily as a consequence of dramatic declines in fertility. In the cases of Asia and Latin America, where fertility declines have been well under way for the last twenty years, there would be very little change in the size of the populations under age fifteen in the next thirty years; by contrast, the populations over age forty-five would increase by over 130 percent. These increases would represent growth rates of 2.8 to 3.2 percent per year

during the thirty-year period, reflecting the momentum of population growth that follows the historical patterns of high fertility.

At the other extreme, Sub-Saharan Africa, which experienced no significant fertility declines prior to 1985, will continue to show large increases in the population down to age fifteen and then smaller increases in the younger ages, reflecting the much later (probable) onset of a fertility decline. In the Middle East and North Africa, a somewhat earlier onset of fertility decline is projected. Again, the large increases in the older age groups in these regions reflect the momentum of population growth.

It should be clear from table 29-2 that, even if there were no change in age-specific morbidity and mortality rates, projected declines in fertility would have a significant effect on the age structure and, therefore, on the relative frequency of different causes of death simply because the population is aging. For example, in Latin America, all things being equal, we could expect that this change in age structure would be accompanied by more than a doubling of chronic disease among adults in relation to acute diseases among infants and children. In fact, however, mortality rates from these conditions probably will decline. As shown in table 29-2 these projected mortality declines are greatest (decreases of 60 to 70 percent) in the youngest age groups and least (decreases of 7 to 18 percent) in the oldest age groups.

Interactions of changes in mortality with the changes in age structure will result in an even more drastic transformation of the health picture. This is also shown in table 29-2, which gives the percentage changes in numbers of deaths that are projected to occur within each age group by the year 2015. Again taking Latin America as an example, among children under five projections show only a 2 percent increase in the population size but a 62 percent decline in the age-specific mortality rate, resulting in a 61 percent decline in number of deaths. By contrast, in the oldest age group the projections show a 141 percent increase in the population size but only a 12 percent decline in mortality, resulting in more than a doubling of the number of deaths and an even greater increase in chronic disability. This epidemiologic transition will have important consequences for the organization and delivery of health services in the future.

Changing Patterns of Risk

In addition to changes in population age structure, which is the primary determinant of epidemiologic transition, there are global social and economic trends which are transforming the risk factors for different diseases (Kjellstrom and Rosenstock 1990). The most obvious global shift is from rural to urban living. In 1985, only 31 percent of the population of the developing regions of the world resided in urban areas, in comparison with 72 percent in the industrial regions (United Nations 1989). But the urban growth rate in the developing regions is projected at 3.6 percent per year through the end of the century, so its urban population will reach 40 percent by

Table 29-2. Projected Change in Population, Mortality Rates, and Deaths between 1985 and 2015, by Age Group
(percent)

Region	Age group					
	0–4	5–14	15–44	45–64	65+	All ages
Asia						
Population	5	7	53	131	134	51
Mortality rates	–70	–58	–43	–30	–7	–18
Deaths	–68	–55	–13	62	118	23
Latin American and Caribbean						
Population	2	18	57	159	141	63
Mortality rates	–62	–60	–47	–29	–12	–17
Deaths	–61	–53	–21	84	112	35
Middle East and North Africa						
Population	38	70	127	175	150	102
Mortality rates	–64	–65	–57	–36	–18	–43
Deaths	–50	–44	–2	76	105	15
Sub-Saharan Africa						
Population	70	116	163	151	161	132
Mortality rates	–64	–64	–53	–29	–11	–45
Deaths	–40	–22	24	79	132	28

Source: Calculated from Bulatao and Stephens 1990.

the year 2000 and 50 percent by 2015. This rapid shift from a rural subsistence economy to an urban, market-oriented, industrial economy brings with it a range of new health problems (Susser 1981). At the same time, economic growth brings with it the wherewithal and knowledge for populations to acquire the nourishment and sanitation that can reduce the incidence of and fatality rates from communicable disease. Reductions in risk for communicable disease combined with increases in other risks, further discussed below, have the potential to amplify the effects of demographic trends. An important general conclusion from a recent study of adult health in developing countries by Feachem and others (1992), however, is that the *overall* effect of development on age-, sex-, and cause-specific mortality rates for noncommunicable disease is to lower them, despite the often-increasing prevalence of well-established risk factors of modern society.

High rates of injuries related to motor vehicles, industrial accidents, and toxic chemicals (for example, pesticides) are one consequence of rapid urbanization, industrialization, and mechanization of agriculture. Stansfield, Smith, and McGreevey (chapter 25) provide extensive documentation of the dramatic increase of these categories of injuries in developing countries. For example, in Thailand in the age group of one to forty-four years, motor vehicle mortality has been increasing at 30 percent annually, moving from sixth place to first place among all causes of death between 1947 and 1980. In 1978, mortality rates per vehicle were fifty times higher in Ethiopia and Nigeria than in the United States or the United Kingdom. Pesticides in Sri Lanka in 1978 caused almost twice as many deaths as occurred as a consequence of polio, diphtheria, tetanus, and pertussis combined. In India, mechanization of grain mills without appropriate protective shields over

drivebelts resulted in an increased number of serious injuries. Injuries are particularly a problem in many poor countries, which lack the resources and institutions to establish and enforce safety measures. Noteworthy, throughout the world in developing and industrial countries alike, injuries are now the leading cause of death during half the human life span (Stansfield, Smith, and McGreevey, chapter 25).

Chronic conditions such as cardiovascular disease, cancer, and chronic obstructive pulmonary disease are also recognized to be substantially influenced by economic and environmental factors, some of which are amenable to modification by the health system in ways that are reviewed in the chapters in part 4 of this collection. For example, the U.S. Department of Health, Education, and Welfare identified lifestyle and the environment as the primary determinants of mortality for all but one of the ten leading causes of death over age one in the United States in 1975 (USDHEW 1978). A more recent analysis indicated that just three preventable precursors to premature death in the United States—alcohol, tobacco, and injury risks—accounted for 59 percent of all preventable years of life lost before age sixty-five and 54 percent of all preventable days of hospital care (Amler and Eddins 1987).

Smoking provides an excellent illustration of an emerging health problem (Zaridze and Peto 1986; Stanley, appendix A). In the United States it is now well established that tobacco use is currently responsible for more than 30 percent of all cancer deaths, including cancers of the lung, larynx, oral cavity, pharynx, pancreas, kidney, and bladder (Ernster 1988). The most dramatic evidence of this is the tenfold increase in lung cancer mortality in the United States since the turn of this century, with differential trends in males and females reflecting differences in smoking habits (Lopez, chapter 2). Similar dramatic increases in lung cancer mortality associated with cigarette consumption have been observed in Japan since World War II, and rising rates have also been reported from Singapore and Shanghai in recent years (Lee and others 1988; Barnum and Greenberg, chapter 21). In some Latin American and Caribbean cities more than half of the young people smoke; by the mid-1980s it is estimated that at least 100,000 deaths in this region were caused by smoking (USDHHS 1992). The rapid increase in smoking in China has the potential of leading to actual increases in age-specific mortality rates, which would run counter to standard demographic assumptions as reflected, for example, in table 29-1 (Yu and others 1990). Bumgarner and Speizer, chapter 24) have illustrated the plausibility of this outcome with quantitative projection models, and Lopez (chapter 2) summarizes analogous predictions for other parts of the world.

The relation between cigarette smoking and lung cancer illustrates a vitally important feature of chronic noncommunicable diseases—the long latent period between exposure and onset of the disease. Smoking is also one of the strongest risk factors for chronic obstructive pulmonary disease (COPD) and ischemic heart disease (Bumgarner and Speizer, chapter 24, and Pearson, Jamison, and Trejo-Gutierrez, chapter 23); as with cancer, the latency of effect is long for COPD and irreversible; but with ischemic heart disease, cessation confers substantial reduction in risk within a year. These data highlight the importance of taking action to prevent chronic diseases decades before the epidemic appears. Regrettably, a recent review (Masironi and Rothwell 1988) found that the rate of tobacco consumption in developing countries is increasing; consistent with this, Barnum and Greenberg (chapter 21) have found a strong relationship between tobacco consumption and higher levels of national income among developing countries.

Ischemic heart disease and stroke, other major causes of death among adults, are potentially amenable to early preventive interventions. Although all the determinants of ischemic heart disease remain to be defined, and patterns of attributable risk will certainly differ in developing countries from those of the industrial countries, where epidemiologic data are available, several behavioral risk factors are well established. These include smoking, sedentary lifestyle, and high saturated fat diets (Pearson, Jamison, and Trejo-Gutierrez, chapter 23). In general these behaviors are strongly associated with urbanization in low-income countries. For example, Popkin and Bisgrove (1988, p. 9) reported that "urban residents consume increased amounts of processed foods, meats, fats, sugar and dairy products while rural residents consume more coarse grains, roots and tubers and pulses."

China provides a remarkable example of the transition to unhealthy diets. The rapid increase in income and related social and agricultural advances has led to a rapid increase in the proportion of obese Chinese and the proportion of Chinese consuming a very high-fat diet, although a large proportion still have a very low-fat diet and are exceptionally lean. For instance, a nationwide survey found that close to one-fifth (18.3 percent) of the highest tercile of Chinese consumed a diet with over 30 percent energy from fat, whereas close to half (47.8 percent) of the lowest tercile consumed a diet with less than 10 percent of energy from fat (Popkin and others 1992).

An increase in the rate of ischemic heart disease is already being seen in some developing countries as they proceed through the epidemiologic transition. Singapore has experienced a doubling of the heart disease mortality rates during the past two decades in older age groups, although there appears to be a leveling off in the increase among younger males in recent years (Hughes 1986). As shown by the experience of Japan, however, which has a low rate of ischemic heart disease (although not stroke), economic development need not be associated with the disease patterns seen in most Western populations. Developing countries generally have fewer risk factors for some of the diseases associated with Western culture (Rose 1985). The course of these chronic diseases in the future will depend on the choices made by developing countries as they consider alternative health development strategies while proceeding through the epidemiologic transition.

The onset of the global AIDS epidemic has brought sexually transmitted diseases (STDs) to the forefront of the health agenda of many developing countries. The risk factors for STDs are directly related to patterns of sexual behavior. These, in turn, are often related to the development process. For example, in many developing countries, factors contributing to high rates of STDs include increasing urbanization with disruption of traditional social structures, increased mobility for political or economic reasons, poor medical facilities, and high unemployment rates (Piot and Holmes 1989). Over and Piot (chapter 20) present data which show that the high rate of human immunodeficiency virus (HIV) infection in eighteen African cities can be correlated with a low ratio of females to males in urban centers, creating a high demand for prostitutes. An associated factor of significance is the relatively low level of female education, which suggests that where there are fewer alternative economic opportunities for women, prostitution is more frequent. Reducing the risk of HIV in these circumstances will probably require significant social changes relating to the role and status of women (including increasing female education) as well as promoting the use of condoms and treating coexisting STDs.

Epidemiologic Polarization

During the next three decades the most dramatic declines in mortality in the developing regions of the world are projected for the infectious and parasitic diseases that primarily affect infants and young children; relatively modest changes are projected for the death rates for conditions such as cardiovascular disease, cancer, and other chronic diseases.[2] As a result, as tables 29-3 and 29-4 suggest, these chronic, noncommunicable diseases of adults will rapidly emerge as the leading causes of death in developing countries. Table 29-3 shows estimates and projections of mortality by broad category of cause based on model life tables; table 29-4 shows, for 1985 only, the best available empirical estimates, using vital statistics and epide-

Table 29-3. Major Causes of Death in Industrial and Developing Countries, 1985 and 2015
(percent)

Cause of death	Industrial countries		Developing countries	
	1985	2015	1985	2015
Infection	9	7	36	19
Neoplasms	18	18	7	14
Circulatory problems	50	53	19	35
Pregnancy-related deaths	0	0	1	1
Perinatal problems	1	1	8	5
Injuries	6	5	8	7
Other	15	16	21	19
Total number of deaths (millions)	12.0	14.5	37.9	47.8

Note: These estimates (1985) and projections (2015) are based on assumptions about changes in total mortality rates built into the World Bank's demographic projections model and on historically based asuumptions about the relationship between mortality by cause and mortality level. Countries included in the "Industrialized" and "Developing" categories are found in appendix 29A.

Source: Bulatao and Stephens 1990.

miologic data. Both tables, and the preceding discussion, point toward the same conclusion: a health transition of massive proportions is well under way in the developing world, and it will continue for several more decades at least.

A critically important feature of the health transition is the emergence of epidemiologic polarization within and between countries of the developing world. In recent years economic growth in the developing world has not been steady. The worldwide recession, poor economic management, and the excessive accumulation of debt have led to serious setbacks in the economic circumstances of many developing countries. One potential consequence has been the stagnation or even

decay of the health advances that had been achieved in recent decades in some countries, which is often reflected in a rising occurrence of childhood malnutrition (Albanez and others 1989; Cornia, Jolly, and Stewart 1987; and Bell and Reich 1988). These setbacks, combined with a wide disparity in health conditions of different social classes, have been characterized by Bobadilla, Frenk, and their colleagues (Frenk and others 1989; Bobadilla and others, chapter 3) as "epidemiologic polarization."

Available evidence suggests that these setbacks in progress and continuation of polarization rarely result in a reversal in the pace of mortality decline (Hill and Pebley 1990),

Table 29-4. Deaths by Cause, Industrial and Developing Countries, 1985

Cause of death	Industrial countries		Developing countries	
	Number (000)	Percent	Number (000)	Percent
Infectious and parasitic diseases	506	4.6	17,000	45.0
Diarrheal diseases	—	—	5,000	13.0
Tuberculosis	40	0.4	3,000	7.9
Acute respiratory illness	368	3.3	6,300	16.6
Measles, pertusis, diphtheria	—	—	1,500	4.0
Other	—	—	4,800	12.7
Other measles and pertusis	..	..	700	1.8
Malaria	..	..	1,000	2.6
Schistosomiasis	..	..	200	0.5
Other	..	..	800	2.1
Maternal causes	5	0.05	500	1.3
Perinatal causes	100	0.9	3,200	8.4
Cancers	2,293	20.8	2,500	6.6
Chronic obstructive pulmonary disease	385	3.5	2,300	6.1
Circulatory and certain degenerative diseases	5,930	53.7	6,500	17.1
Ischemic heart disease	2,392	21.7	—	—
Cerebrovascular disease	1,504	13.6	—	—
Diabetes	153	1.4	—	—
External causes (injuries)	772	7.0	2,400	6.3
Other and unknown	1,054	9.5	3,500	9.2
Total	11,045	100.0	37,900	100.0

— Not available.
.. Negligible.
Source: Lopez (chapter 2, this collection).

even for Africa (Feachem, Jamison, and Bos 1991). This is best documented in the recent report of the demographic and health surveys (DHS) in twenty-seven countries in Africa, Asia, and Latin America, carried out between 1986 and 1990 (Sullivan 1991).[3] They showed declines in mortality of children under age five in every country; by region the average percentage declines were: North Africa, 46 percent; Latin America, 32 percent; Asia, 28 percent; and Sub-Saharan Africa, 12 percent. Although effective health interventions may have blunted the potential mortality consequences of economic stagnation, evidence is emerging from several countries that low child mortality levels can now be maintained even in the presence of sustained high levels of malnutrition and morbidity (concerning Sri Lanka, see Gunatilleke 1989; concerning Zimbabwe, see Sanders and Davis 1988). It is important that the persistence of these undesirable states, as is emphasized in chapter 3, not be masked by undue focus on (relatively) favorable mortality statistics.

Table 29-5 illustrates the wide disparity in levels of child mortality (under five years) seen among developing countries in every region of the world in the 1980s. Mortality levels range from under 2.5 percent in Costa Rica and Cuba to over 20 percent in Bangladesh and Mali. Within countries as well, significant disparities in health conditions are found among subgroups of the population. Some of the most recent estimates of these conditions are from the recent DHS (Rutstein 1992). Tabulations of the levels and differentials in mortality of children under age five, when grouped according to urban as against rural residence and the mother's level of education, are presented in table 29-6. In general the data indicate child mortality rates 30 percent to 50 percent lower in urban than in rural areas, and a two- to threefold difference between women with no education and those with seven or more years of education.

The relation between maternal education and child survival in developing countries has been observed in multiple studies during the past decade (Caldwell and McDonald, 1981; Cochrane, Leslie, and O'Hara 1982; Hobcraft, McDonald, and Rutstein 1984) and has led some demographers to observe that what counts in child survival is not just the overall health and socioeconomic condition of the country where one resides but the individual's (or family's) social and economic resources. The urban-rural mortality differentials in table 29-6 provide one indicator of the disparity among families in different settings. In this context, because social and economic development usually does not occur uniformly throughout all areas of a country, one will frequently see important differentials in mortality rates in different geographic regions within countries. Examples include Mexico, Brazil, Kenya, Nigeria, India, and Indonesia. Thus, epidemiologic polarization occurs not only across social classes but in regional mortality differentials as well.

The analysis above is limited to infant and childhood mortality primarily because there are relatively few data on mortality differentials by social class among adults in developing countries. Where data are available, the patterns are similar to those well documented in the industrial countries; mortality rates for most chronic diseases among adults are higher among the lower social classes than among the upper classes (Kaplan and others 1987; Feachem and others 1992; World Bank 1989). For example, in a study of mortality in the rich and poor areas of Pôrto Alegre, Brazil, Barcellos and others (1986b, p. 206) found that death rates for men between forty-five and sixty-four were 50 percent higher among the poor, with death rates for cancers, cardiovascular diseases, respiratory diseases, and injuries all higher among men living in poor neighborhoods. The reasons, as in the industrial countries, relate to a high-risk lifestyle that includes alcohol consumption, smoking, lack of exercise, and obesity, as well as poor living and working conditions.

In many countries of the world, particularly across Asia, women experience excess mortality as compared with men because of their marginalized position in society (Das Gupta 1987). These excesses are most evident in the higher rates of infant and childhood mortality among females. Another reflection of the disadvantaged position of women is the extraordinarily high rate of preventable maternal mortality in many developing countries, which is 100 to 500 times higher than in the industrial countries (Walsh and others, chapter 17). Among the surviving women, studies in many parts of the world have documented a higher prevalence of stunting and

Table 29-5. Probability of Dying by Age Five, by Country, 1980–85

Probability of dying by age five (percent)	Latin America	Asia	Africa
25–30	none	none	Mali
20–25	none	Bangladesh	Liberia Senegal
15–20	Haiti	India	Ghana Uganda
10–15	Guatemala Peru	Turkey	Egypt
5–10	Brazil Dominican Republic Ecuador El Salvador Mexico	Philippines Thailand	Botswana
2.5–5	Argentina Chile Colombia Panama Trinidad Uruguay	Kuwait Malaysia Sri Lanka	none
<2.5	Costa Rica Cuba	Hong Kong Singapore	

Source: Hill and Pebley 1990; updated by Hill, personal communication.

Table 29-6. Mortality Rates of Children Younger than Five Years, by Residence and Mother's Education, Selected Countries, 1986–90
(deaths under age 5 per 1,000 births)

Country	Type of residence		Mother's education			
	Rural	Urban	None	1–3 years	4–6 years	7 or more years
Africa						
Egypt	164	88	161	116	108	48
Morocco	137	81	125	76	66	50
Tunisia	88	62	84	71	58	39
Mali	303	203	290	244	214	112
Liberia	239	216	242	*	*	177
Senegal	250	135	226	179	123	75
Uganda	191	164	195	222	173	144
Togo	169	131	170	163	131	89
Ghana	163	131	175	119	169	125
Burundi	186	163	191	167	141	90
Kenya	91	89	109	101	92	70
Zimbabwe	98	55	120	94	83	60
Botswana	56	57	62	52	47	53
Asia						
Indonesia	124	78	144	139	99	48
Thailand	52	35	76	88	47	19
Sri Lanka	43	40	72	47	41	35
Latin America						
Bolivia	168	114	180	166	141	70
Peru	153	74	169	147	113	53
Guatemala	130	99	136	122	84	44
Brazil	121	88[b]	136	137	70	40
Mexico	104	59	112	91	54	29
Ecuador	99[a]	63[a]	159	121	74	49
Dominican Republic	66[a]	69[a]	136	100	96	66
Paraguay	47	43	65[c]	51[c]	41[c]	27[c]
Colombia	32	35	74	—	—	26[d]

— Not available.
* Less than 500 children exposed.
a. Based on last five years.
b. Calculated from urban breakdown.
c. Education categories are 0–2 years, 3–5 years, primary complete, and secondary or higher.
d. Secondary only.
Source: Rutstein 1991.

micronutrient deficiency (Leslie 1991). The enormity of this problem has recently been shown by Coale (1991), who analyzed the estimated deficits in the female population of several Asian countries; the deficits were derived from a comparison of the actual ratio of males to females with the expected ratio if there were no excess female mortality. For China and India, from 5.3 to 5.6 percent of females were "missing," indicative of a deficit of 52 million in these countries.

Although noncommunicable diseases and injury will become more prominent with the epidemiologic transition, the infectious diseases, malnutrition, and excess (unwanted) fertility cannot be ignored. These will, however, become even more concentrated among the poor, leading to the phenomenon of epidemiologic polarization. Tuberculosis is illustrative of a leading disease that remains on the unfinished agenda of developing country health problems. In most developing countries, the annual risk of infection ranges now from 0.5 to

2.5 percent, a level 50 to 200 times greater than in the industrial countries. The estimates of Murray, Styblo, and Rouillon (chapter 11) indicate that this will result in approximately 7.3 million new cases and 2.7 million deaths in 1990. More than two-thirds of these deaths will be among productive adults (ages fifteen through fifty-nine), primarily the poor. Significantly, this disease alone accounts for about 26 percent of an estimated 7 million *avoidable* adult deaths in the developing world. Assuming no change in the present trends of decline and no improvement in case detection and treatments, Murray, Styblo, and Rouillon project as many as 2.9 million tuberculosis deaths still occurring by 2015. Because of the contribution of the HIV epidemic to tuberculosis, coupled with the rate of population growth in Sub-Saharan Africa, the number of deaths projected could increase by more than 100 percent in that region during the next twenty-five years.

Consequences for the Health System

A central consequence of the health transition for health policy is that in most developing countries, pre- and post-epidemiologic transition problems will coexist. Omran (1971) predicted evolution toward this state of epidemiologic diversity in his original essay on the epidemiologic transition; Evans, Hall, and Warford (1981) and Hiroshi Nakajima (World Health Organization, 1988) further described the trend; and the authors of several World Bank country-specific analyses (Jamison and others 1984; World Bank 1989 and 1990a) have attempted to draw appropriate implications for policy. In table 29-7 we attempt to summarize, for each of the age categories we are using, which health problems on the current agenda need continued attention and which neglected or emerging problems are likely to require substantial increases in effort. The latter are considered in the light of the indicated change in the age distribution of mortality. As Foege and Henderson (1986, p. 321) have observed, these countries "will not have the luxury of dealing with two kinds of problems sequentially. For the remainder of this century they will be dealing with both simultaneously." Health systems of developing countries will, then, be facing unprecedented increases in the volume and diversity of problems they must address; the challenge is to respond with maximal effectiveness, given the sharp constraints on their resources. Assessing intervention cost-effectiveness is an essential first step to meeting that challenge.

The composite effect of the demographic transition and the socioeconomic changes on the health system that are foreseeable for the next thirty-five years—mainly urbanization and higher levels of education—will be formidable. Four main effects are highlighted as they apply to most of the developing countries.[4]

First, the total burden of disease, measured by the number of days that people suffer from acute episodes of disease, chronic disabilities, and days lost as a result of premature death, will increase. This is not only because the population will continue to grow but also because the prevalence of disease will increase as more chronic diseases predominate in the health profile. The adult population suffers more diseases simultaneously and these tend to last longer, as compared with child morbidity. In addition the emergence of new health risks as described in the previous section will lead to higher rates of incidence of some conditions, particularly lung and breast cancer, some accidents and violence, and AIDS.

Second, the demand for health services will be greater. Demand is a direct function of three factors that tend to move in the same direction: (a) health needs that were described before; (b) the threshold for converting need into demand, which will decrease as a result of the higher levels of income and education of populations and the accessibility to informa-

Table 29-7. Health Problems Affecting Various Age Groups in Developing Countries

Age group	Population (millions) 1985	Population (millions) 2015	Deaths (millions) 1985	Deaths (millions) 2015	Important health problems — Unfinished agenda	Important health problems — Emerging problems
Young children (0–4 years)	490	626	14.6	7.5	Acute respiratory infection Diarrheal disease Learning disability Malaria Measles, tetanus, polio Micronutrient deficiencies Protein-energy malnutrition	Injury Learning disability
School-age children (5–14 years)	885	1,196	1.6	1.3	Geohelminth infection Micronutrient deficiencies Schistosomiasis	Learning disability
Young adults (15–44 years)	1,667	2,918	5.0	6.0	Excess fertility Malaria Maternal mortality Tuberculosis	AIDS Injury Mental illness Sexually transmitted diseases
Middle-aged (45–64 years)	474	1,131	5.9	10.4	None	Cancers Cardiovascular disease Chronic obstructive pulmonary disease Diabetes
Elderly (65+ years)	153	358	11.0	22.5	None	Cataracts Depression Disability
Total	3,669	6,229	37.9	47.7		

Note: Many conditions for older age groups manifest themselves clinically long after the processes leading to the clinical condition have been initiated; preventive intervention will, therefore, need to be directed to younger populations.
Source: Figures for population and deaths calculated from Bulatao and Stephens 1990.

tion acquired in urban areas through radio and other mass media; (c) finally, the supply of services, particularly those provided by hospitals, that is, the increased proportion of populations living in urban areas will improve the physical access to health facilities and therefore will boost the demand for services.

Third, the emergence of noncommunicable diseases and disabilities due to injury will increase considerably the complexity of the health care services required. In general, health personnel will require higher qualifications and probably some level of specialization. The technology for diagnosis, treatment, and rehabilitation will be more sophisticated, and the organizational arrangements to ensure minimum standards of care will also increase in complexity.

Fourth, all the previously described effects will increase expenditure for health care. The one that has the greatest relevance is probably the higher cost of medical care that will result from the greater complexity of services, particularly the introduction of new health technologies. The greatest effect of the health transition is likely to be seen in hospitals (Barnum and Kutzin 1993). Most developing countries provide hospital services for only a fraction of the population. The demand for services is already greater than the supply. The shortage of hospital beds will, according to the effects described above, be exacerbated. Three primary causes for hospital admission are likely to grow: childbirth, noncommunicable diseases, and injuries.

Policy Implications for National Governments

Chapter 1 assembled the cost-effectiveness findings from each of the disease-oriented chapters. These findings were grouped as population-based interventions and facility-based interventions as described in table 1-2. Notably, this analysis does not weigh preventive as opposed to curative strategies but, rather, considers the cost-effectiveness of the full range of interventions—primary prevention, secondary prevention, curative, rehabilitation, and palliation—on the same scale. Our purpose in this section is to explore the implications for policy. We stress here that conclusions for policy are highly dependent on the local epidemiological, administrative, and financial context; it is within such contexts (at the national or district level) that policy is shaped. All that can be done in a general overview, such as this, is to point to policies that appear approximately valid for a range of countries and that, therefore, are likely to serve as a useful starting point for country- (or district-) specific analysis of policy.

Policy Instruments of Government

When intervention is desirable, governments have available a variety of measures to promote health and prevent disease that include but extend far beyond the usual activities of ministries of health.[5] Governmental interventions may be usefully grouped into five broad categories, the first three of which are associated with modifying the incentives and knowledge of patients and providers. These are listed as the instruments of policy in table 1-2; these instruments are further discussed below.

- *Providing Information.* Fundamental to any improvements in health behavior among the population are information, knowledge, and skills, ideally reinforced with social support. In recent years, governments have begun to use the media and modern communication technologies to reach the public with information to promote good health behaviors through programs of "information, education and communication." Often this is done effectively in partnership with the private sector. Perhaps the most notable examples of this in a number of developing countries are mass mobilization efforts in support of immunization campaigns, as well as communication programs to improve maternal weaning practices and promote the practice of family planning. In the United States, recent publication of selected operative mortality and success rates, by hospital, has allowed more informed consumer choice to stimulate quality assessment and control in hospitals.

- *Regulation/Legislation.* Health ministries generally have considerable regulatory powers, for example, in licensure of practitioners, and in food and drug control and sanitation, though resources for inspection and enforcement are often limited. A central regulatory power of governments lies in the determination of which health services will (can) be privately provided (through market mechanisms or through nongovernmental organizations) and which will be provided by the state. When coupled with effective public education to reach a social consensus, regulatory authority can be an effective tool for health promotion, as evidenced by the ability of some governments to limit pollution levels and to restrict the advertising of cigarettes or the promotion of infant formula and baby bottles.

- *Taxes, Subsidies.* Taxes or price subsidies can be an important tool available to governments to promote or discourage various practices related to health. The judicious application of high taxes can discourage consumption of cigarettes and excess consumption of alcohol, whereas subsidized prices—for example, for contraceptives—can be a tool to promote desirable behaviors. Fuel taxes can reduce motor vehicle use, thereby decreasing pollution and vehicle accidents, to take another example. Similarly, reduction of subsidies of some very high-fat food products can discourage consumption of fat.

- *Direct Investments.* In many circumstances the only (or best) recourse for the government may be direct investments perhaps with policies of partial cost recovery.[6] Immunization programs and vector control are two examples on the prevention side. The complexity and relative infrequency of many case management procedures, combined with the absence of informed consumers, suggest that a prominent role for government in the financing of a basic level of hospital services may be desirable.

• *Research.* Even if research results are protected by patent, it can be difficult for the private sector to recoup the cost of research investment, and, when it is recovered, it is at the expense of fully appropriate use of the research product. (Comanor [1986] reviews an extensive literature on these issues in the context of the pharmaceutical industry.) The economic case is typically strong, then, for heavy contribution by government to finance research. The purpose, of course, is to lengthen the menu for intervention choice.

An Integrated Approach to Policies and Strategies

In this collection we look at diseases or related conditions (for example, cancers, helminthic infections) one at a time. Although this disease-by-disease approach facilitates the technical analyses of costs and effectiveness of specific interventions, in reality, policymakers and health planners must use a more integrated strategy and consider packages of interventions. In this situation, issues of feasibility and sustainability arise (Vilnius and Dandoy 1990).

Feasibility encompasses political, administrative, and logistical considerations. Some policies, such as raising the age of marriage, may not yet be politically acceptable; others, such as establishing environmental monitoring, may not be administratively feasible because of lack of legal authority or trained personnel. Lack of a well-functioning health infrastructure or an efficient distribution system may be a logistical barrier reducing the cost-effectiveness of some strategies in the short run.

Sustainability is a particularly serious concern, since before this decade, few developing countries had seriously attempted to implement a health care program with their own resources, where total population coverage was the objective. Consequently, the international community and national governments are learning that even highly cost-effective interventions like immunization programs may exceed the available resources of some developing countries in the current economic climate. An advantage of the analytical approach taken in this collection is that it identifies a range of health policies and strategies, some of which may require only minimal government resources (for example, regulations) and some that can even generate revenue (for example, taxation on tobacco). This approach does, however, require health ministries to transcend their traditional bounds and look at the entire national development strategy with regard to its consequences for health.

In chapter 1, health interventions are classified as *population-based* or *clinical* (tables 1-5 and 1-8). The population-based interventions encompass five strategies: (a) change of personal behavior; (b) control of environmental hazards; (c) immunization; (d) mass chemoprophylaxis; and (e) screening and referral. Clinical interventions are assumed to occur, for simplicity, at three levels: (a) the clinic; (b) the district hospital; and (c) the referral hospital. The discussion below follows this same framework, elaborating on issues that must be addressed by policymakers in designing cost-effective intervention programs.

BEHAVIORAL CHANGE. Behavioral change includes personal behaviors related to diet, hygiene and sanitation, personal health habits, reproduction, and self-care or self-referral for illnesses. Worldwide experiences with agriculture, nutrition, family planning, and child survival programs have made it clear that effective population-based health care requires active and informed participation by families and communities (Hornik 1988). Programs to prevent deaths from diarrhea and respiratory infections in infants and children require that mothers be motivated and trained to become informed diagnosticians and managers of home therapy (Berman, Kendall, and Bhattacharyya 1989; Mosley 1989). Correspondingly, family and community involvement is essential for appropriate antenatal and childbirth care (Walsh and others, chapter 17), for effective nutrition intervention programs (Pinstrup-Andersen and others, chapter 18), for early diagnosis (Stansfield and Shepard, chapter 4), and for compliance with treatments for chronic conditions such as tuberculosis or hypertension among adults.

Each of the first four of the policy instruments of government noted above may need to be invoked to promote desired behavioral changes. The most direct approach is through mass media. Most governments are using radio and television broadcasts and print mass media to reach the general population with health information and promotional messages. In recent years there have been important developments in mass communication strategies that are greatly enhancing their effectiveness in creating public awareness of health problems and supporting appropriate behavioral changes (Church and Geller 1990; Gilluly and Moore 1986). Key elements of effective communication programs include identifying the target audiences and conducting preliminary research to tailor the message to their specific needs. Also, the media chosen must be able to reach the target group. Most important, implementation of a communication program must be a learning process—all materials must be pretested and modified, and the effect of the program must be carefully monitored and evaluated.

Entertainment for social change is a new concept in health communications that is rapidly gaining worldwide prominence (Coleman 1988; Coleman and Meyer 1990). This method uses the universal appeal of entertainment by bringing together popular entertainers, skilled producers, and health professionals to show people how they can live safer and healthier lives. To date, this strategy has been used most successfully in the field of family planning, with productions ranging from music videos in Latin America and the Philippines to television dramas and soap operas in Nigeria, Egypt, India, and Mexico. Often these productions are of such high quality that they gain top ratings on popularity charts. An advantage of this is that they are often broadcast on commercial channels at no charge, therefore providing a major subsidy to the health education program.

Although the mass media are useful in introducing new ideas and providing information in support of health programs, the production of sustained behavioral changes in the population generally requires a more comprehensive strategy, incorporating the more persuasive instruments of government to consolidate behavioral change. Perhaps the most neglected tool here is taxation: estimated price elasticities of demand for alcohol and tobacco products are substantial.[7] Such integrated strategies are discussed in detail in the chapters on injury (Stansfield, Smith, and McGreevey, chapter 25), protein-energy malnutrition (Pinstrup-Andersen and others, chapter 18), and cancers (Barnum and Greenberg, chapter 21).

ENVIRONMENTAL HAZARDS CONTROL. Environmental health and safety is largely a matter of engineering and regulation to reduce health risks from known environmental hazards, even when occurrences of the hazard may be increasing. For transport-related injuries, although the number of motor vehicles and the distance driven are increasing, it has been shown that the combined effect of seat belts, speed limits, safer roads, better vehicles, drunk driving prevention, and so forth, has been to reduce the health risk (Kjellstrom and Rosenstock 1990). This pattern has been observed in industrial countries and in a few developing countries in which safety programs have been implemented and data are available.

As with motor vehicles, one can project a rapid increase in modern environmental health hazards associated with industrialization and urbanization in developing countries. The problems of environmental control will be compounded in many countries, however, because the low incomes and standards of living mean that the traditional hazards associated with poor sanitation will remain.

The underpinnings of environmental hazards control are: epidemiologic surveillance to detect illnesses or injuries related to environmental risks swiftly; regular monitoring of potentially hazardous environmental conditions; and regulatory or taxation authority to ensure that appropriate risk reduction actions are taken. Traditionally, environmental control programs in ministries of health have been limited to water, food, and sanitation inspection to reduce infectious diseases. Government capabilities and authority in this area must be greatly expanded to monitor and control a much broader range of environmental risks, including air pollution, toxic wastes, traffic hazards, occupational safety, unsafe manufactured goods, and other health risks. Some of the professional and technical capacities required to monitor and regulate environmental hazards may exist in different ministries in government; however, their functions are often limited by insufficient technically trained personnel, limited resources, and, particularly, lack of statutory authority.

Significant government initiatives in environmental hazards control must begin with broad and detailed statutory regulations empowering one or more agencies to take effective actions. Given the scope and magnitude of the tasks to be carried out—which will encompass areas as diverse as law, engineering, medicine, economics, physics, and chemistry—

environmental protection agencies may be set up independently of ministries of health. However the administrative structure is organized, because of the nature of environmental hazards control, the activities must be administered in a way that facilitates maximum coordination and collaboration among diverse government agencies whose operations will directly, or indirectly, impinge on environmental health. Table 29-8 indicates the range of government agencies and programs outside the health sector that may need to be involved in implementing environmental health activities.

Resources are limited in developing countries, but the multisectoral character of environmental control programs means that their cost may be spread across government agencies and, by regulation and taxation, through the private sector. Thus, environmental improvements, although still constrained by overall national resources, are not dependent upon the budget of a single ministry such as the ministry of health. A broad discussion of approaches to environmental improvement is available in the World Bank's *World Development Report* for 1992.

Consider motor vehicle injuries as an example. The health ministry may take the leading role in surveillance and identifying the growing problem. But a policy recommendation limited to establishing emergency care units without involving

Table 29-8. Agencies Responsible for Health-Related Environmental Improvements

Environmental concern	Relevant agencies
Water availability Water quality/fluoridation Waste disposal	Public works Industry Agriculture Forestry Urban development Rural development
Food safety Food fortification	Agriculture Industry Trade
Vector control	Agriculture Urban development
Motor vehicle/road safety	Roads and highways Import control Alcohol control Transportation
Occupational safety	Labor Industry Agriculture Alcohol control Transportation
Air quality	Motor vehicle control Industry Power development
Housing quality	Urban development Rural development Housing Public works

Source: Authors.

other relevant sectors in activities such as initiating measures to upgrade roads, highways, and intersections; improve motor vehicle safety; and reduce drunk driving and pedestrian hazards would rapidly produce diminishing returns. An intersectoral effort toward the prevention of motor vehicle injuries can be expected to have a synergistic effect, thus making the overall strategy more cost-effective. This example can be multiplied with many environmental approaches to health interventions, as table 29-8 indicates. It reinforces the rationale for an environmental protection agency with broad authority to monitor hazards and take legal action.

IMMUNIZATION, MASS CHEMOPROPHYLAXIS, AND SCREENING. The population-based interventions included under the headings immunization, mass chemoprophylaxis, and screening all share certain characteristics: (a) they involve the direct administration of a specific technical intervention to individuals on a one-by-one basis; (b) they are directed to certain target populations; and (c) coverage of the target population is important to producing the desired effect. Technically, each of these intervention strategies is highly effective when correctly applied to a compliant subject, but their actual effectiveness in developing countries is strongly conditioned by the local administrative, managerial, and logistical capabilities, by traditional cultural constraints, and by epidemiologic factors.

It is particularly with the interventions in this category that the decision criteria noted in the section "An Integrated Approach to Policies and Strategies," above, need to be carefully applied by policymakers, because the one-on-one character of these interventions means that they are intrinsically demanding of resources in terms of personnel and logistics. Even if the criteria are satisfied at the planning stage, these interventions require careful monitoring and evaluation for their effect during implementation; any breakdown in the technical requirements of the intervention, any failure to reach the target population, or inadequate compliance with required procedures by the recipients can greatly reduce their cost-effectiveness.

Traditionally child survival interventions which are targeted to the same group (such as immunizations, micronutrient supplementation [particularly vitamin A] and growth monitoring) are combined into an intervention package to make more efficient use of limited resources. This strategy can be very cost-effective if each of the specific interventions is carefully monitored and regularly evaluated to see that it meets the standards required for an effective program and that it produces the desired effect on health in the population. If, however, an activity is simply added to an operating program and no procedures have been properly established to ensure a health effect, efficiency will decline. This has frequently been the case when growth monitoring (a screening tool) has been introduced into child survival programs without any provision to attend to children with faltering growth (Gopalan, cited by Pinstrup-Andersen and others, chapter 18). Conversely, when growth monitoring is used as a tool to manage a population-based nutritional supplementation program, as has been done

in Tamil Nadu State in India, substantial program efficiencies can be achieved (World Bank 1990).

Cost savings to government for these mass interventions may be achieved through the use of mass mobilization campaigns, in which a substantial contribution in kind may be provided by the private sector. This has been the case with polio immunization mass campaigns conducted at intervals of six months in some Latin American countries. Program efficiencies can also be achieved by focusing efforts in places where the target population will be concentrated. Warren and others (chapter 7) propose school-based delivery of "targeted mass chemotherapy" for intermittent (six-month or annual) mass treatment for helminth infections with the objective of reducing worm burdens, and hence morbidity, without necessarily eliminating infections. The rationale is that in heavily infected populations it is not the acute effects of infection that are the major public health concern but the chronic insidious effects of continuous moderate to heavy infection throughout childhood, which reduces the growth and intellectual development of children. Immunizations are among the most cost-effective of interventions discussed in this collection, and school-based anthelmintic chemotherapy also appears highly attractive.

Where provision for treatment and follow-up is available, screening selected populations for infectious diseases is also cost-effective, for example, miners for tuberculosis and commercial sex workers for STDs. The latter strategy has recently gained in significance as an important public health intervention for two reasons. First, there is evidence that some STDs play a role in the transmission of AIDS. Second, theoretical work suggests that reducing the risk of HIV transmission by a small core group of infected carriers with multiple sex partners is a much more effective means of limiting the epidemic than treating a much larger group of people with few sex partners (Over and Piot, chapter 20). Other diseases for which screening and referral are at least moderately cost-effective are breast and cervical cancer (Barnum and Greenberg, chapter 21). Murray, Styblo, and Rouillon, however, the authors of the chapter on tuberculosis (chapter 11), do not recommend active case finding.

CLINICAL INTERVENTIONS. Chapter 1 summarizes the range of health interventions that require medical facilities, the level of facility required, and the estimates of cost-effectiveness. As with population-based interventions, national policymakers should have an informed epidemiologic analysis in the local context, along the lines of the framework given here, to guide the allocation of resources across clinical facilities of varying complexity and cost (Barnum and Kutzin 1993). Operationally, the choices for clinical interventions should actually be for packages of activities, because once certain institutional resources are established (for example, a surgical suite with blood bank), many procedures can be performed at marginal cost. As emphasized in the discussion in chapter 1, however, the factor to consider is not just the marginal cost of the procedure but its cost-effectiveness with regard to disability-adjusted life-years gained. Institutional capacities will be limited, and the time and resources spent on relatively ineffective procedures, such as surgery for lung cancer, will be taken away from resources that could be spent on highly costeffective interventions, such as cesarean section for obstructed labor. From the perspective of developing public policy, the extent to which economies of scale will (or will not) result from a packaging of services or from delivering required volumes of procedures determines the extent to which competitively provided services can be efficient in any given demand environment. There is much anecdotal evidence to suggest that actual economies of scale sharply limit the scope for competition to be efficient, suggesting the importance of government in financing a basic level of care or regulating hospital services.

Barnum and Kutzin (1993) provide a comprehensive analysis of the economic and financial issues surrounding resource allocation to hospitals in the public sector. They note that hospital operating expenses, which commonly absorb from 40 to 80 percent of public sector health resources, are at the core of the gap between required and available health resources in many countries. In addressing this issue, they make several observations that are relevant to this collection. First, they confirm that in low-income economies nonhospital interventions are more efficient in dealing with prevalent health conditions. They point out, however, that in countries with highly successful primary health care programs (China and Sri Lanka) a substantial proportion of health resources (above 60 percent) is spent on hospitals. Still, these are not large, tertiary facilities with sophisticated high-technology equipment, but district-level hospitals.

This leads to Barnum and Kutzin's second point relating to efficiencies within the hospitals. In many low-income countries, a high proportion of hospital expenditure is for personnel. With fiscal constraints, hospitals, particularly lower-level facilities, may be inadequately provided with drugs and other essential supplies, resulting in low admission and turnover rates. This can lead to misuse of tertiary facilities for minor illnesses and can contribute to the inappropriate provision by all hospitals of extended care or convalescence in order to maintain bed occupancy levels. The implication of Barnum and Kutzin's analysis is that hospital efficiency can be improved by more effective allocation of resources to increase the quality of care. This means strengthening both technical and managerial skills, as well as providing for sufficient drugs and supplies to care effectively for a selected group of conditions for which interventions can be cost-effective.

In considering specific activities that may be carried out in different levels of facilities, we briefly discuss certain generic issues related to continuing education for health providers and the assessment, development, and control of technology. We deal with these issues here because they are essential ingredients in the process of selecting and implementing cost-effective interventions in hospitals and other facilities.

CONTINUING EDUCATION FOR HEALTH CARE PROVIDERS. A critical element in developing cost-effective health care systems is the reorienting and retraining of health care providers. The worldwide experience in initiating national programs to provide family planning services and child survival technologies has revealed that the vast majority of doctors, nurses, and other health care providers do not have the necessary training and technical skills to provide even basic contraceptive technologies. Before the introduction of oral rehydration therapy, which rationalized diarrhea management, hospitals in many developing countries were experiencing acute diarrhea case-fatality rates as high as 10 to 30 percent; 99 percent of these ought not to have occurred, given the availability of intravenous fluids. Even now, in countries in which oral rehydration therapy has been introduced and available for five to ten years, many physicians typically administer unnecessary and, at times, dangerous drugs to patients with diarrhea (Mamdani and Walker 1986; Martines, Phillips, and Feachem, chapter 5). Similarly, in cases of acute respiratory illnesses medical practitioners may prescribe as many as three to six drugs, including more than one antibiotic, often in ineffective doses (Quick and others 1988). Furthermore, systematic patient follow-up is rarely carried out in primary health care facilities to see if the treatment has been effective.

Many of the limitations described above are the result of resource constraints; however, it should be apparent that there will be no cost-saving by poorly trained personnel dispensing ineffective treatments (Stansfield 1990). Rather, for health care to be cost-effective, health professionals and their support staff must be trained and motivated to diagnose and treat properly the diseases they see. Much more use of practical diagnostic algorithms, continuing education programs, and careful supervision are essential to achieve this goal. Good records and case follow-up must become an integral part of treatment programs, since most of the benefits of therapeutic regimens are lost without proper patient compliance. With limited resources, gains in cost-effectiveness can be achieved only by limiting the range of conditions to be cared for, and by doing the job well. Although the selective disease-specific strategy of vertical programs is commonly criticized because of the presumed lack of efficiency in the use of medical manpower, it has had the advantage of focusing attention on each critical step necessary to make an intervention effective (Taylor and Jolly 1988; Mosley 1988). At the same time it builds a base of practitioner competence that can later be extended to providing a broader range of services.

An important step in the process of improving the qualifications of health providers is strengthening professional associations. Presently, professional associations in many developing countries are heavily dependent on commercial enterprises (primarily the pharmaceutical industry) for national meetings, publications, and continuing education. With this limited exposure to technical developments, health providers are in no position to judge the merits (much less the cost-effectiveness) of new products for patient care. Continuing education with recertification of competence, which is a requirement in highly developed countries like the United States, where physicians have virtually unlimited access to the medical literature, is essential in developing countries, where resources are severely constrained. National professional associations could play a vitally important role in this area, but government financial support is likely to be required to facilitate provision of unbiased information.

TECHNOLOGY ASSESSMENT, DEVELOPMENT, AND CONTROL. Even in a wealthy nation like the United States, private hospitals are not permitted to introduce expensive high-technology procedures (for example, open-heart surgery) without permission of a government-mandated review board, which assesses the demand for heart surgery and the availability of the procedure in other hospitals in the area. The hospitals themselves are also shortening the duration of inpatient stay and moving many procedures to the outpatient facilities to cut costs. And consumer groups are demanding cost-saving innovations like the availability of less expensive generic drugs instead of the costly proprietary products.

In the financially constrained environment of developing countries, cost containment is even more essential. To move in this direction requires institutional capabilities as described in the section "Policy Implementation and Health System Responses," below. But beyond a control function is the critical need for research to adapt highly effective technologies to developing countries. This was done with oral rehydration therapy for diarrheal diseases, and steps are being taken to simplify the diagnostic requirements for effective treatment of acute respiratory infections (Martines, Phillips, and Feachem, chapter 5; Stansfield and Shepard, chapter 4).

Adaptations of medical technology to developing country settings have not only involved prevention and medical treatments but surgery as well. Female surgical sterilization traditionally had been an inpatient procedure done under general anesthesia. Experience has accumulated over the past twenty years with performance of a mini-laparotomy that can be done under local anesthesia on an outpatient basis (Liskin and Rinehart 1985). Cataract extraction is another procedure adapted to conditions in developing countries. High-volume surgical facilities have been in place in India and Pakistan for the past twenty years. In these settings, cataract surgery can be performed inexpensively and safely on an assembly-line basis. More recently, a pilot program in Kenya has demonstrated that nonphysician ophthalmic clinical officers can be trained to perform cataract surgery with acceptable results (Javitt, chapter 26).

An important case study of the adaptation of technology on a national scale is the "simplified surgery system" developed in Colombia (Velez Gil and others 1983; Yankauer 1983). Controlled trials of selected surgical procedures were conducted, comparing their safety and effectiveness when performed as ambulatory procedures with that when performed as inpatient procedures. The results indicated that 75 percent of surgical interventions did not require hospitalization. The government has now instituted a nationwide program of ambulatory surgery.

Analytic Capacity Building

The fundamental underpinning of any health intervention program is measurement and evaluation. Without measurement of the nature and magnitude of the health problem in a population and its trends and determinants, it is impossible to design intervention strategies that maximize the effectiveness of the health technologies. Correspondingly, in the absence of quantitative indicators of program performance, it is impossible to assess the efficiency of an intervention strategy, much less undertake analyses of the cost-effectiveness ratios of alternative policy options. Managers of the smallpox eradication program stress the central role that outcome measurements played in the success of that program (Fenner and others 1988).

In health intervention programs, measurement problems are complex, but work has begun in developing the survey tools and analytical methods (White 1985; Gray 1987). Feachem, Jamison, and Bos (1991, p. 45) have reviewed experience with (and findings from) a range of analytical advances as applied in Africa and conclude that "several new and powerful approaches—use of indirect demographic methods, case-control epidemiologic techniques, and particularly, expanded use of sentinel districts and facilities—offer highly cost-effective ways for health ministries to meet an important part of their information needs."

The microcomputer is the most important technical advance supporting the development of strengthened information systems (Berge, Ingle, and Hamilton 1986). Microcomputers have now been adapted for a wide range of health care applications in developing countries by the World Health Organization and the U.S. Centers for Disease Control, including managing primary health care programs and drug supply systems, monitoring immunization coverage, and standardizing nutrition surveys (Victora 1986; Wilson and others 1988; Hogerzeil and Manell 1989; Babikir, Dodge, and Pett 1989). Specialized software packages are also available for demographic data analyses, field survey research applications, health and population program planning, and so forth. Wide applicability of epidemiologic and economic analyses will require much more trained manpower in developing countries.

Many governments will need to encourage the creation of new institutions or reconfigure old ones in order to address the issues identified here. Critically needed capacities include:

- *Demographic Analysis*. These capabilities provide the fundamental underpinnings of a population-based health system. There must be accurate measures of the numbers and distribution of the population, its social and economic characteristics, and the trends and determinants of population change. These data will provide the basis for designing intervention strategies as well as for assessing the effect of the disease burden on the population.
- *Epidemiologic Surveillance*. This capacity is essential to assess the magnitude of health problems, define their determinants, and monitor the effect of health program interven-

tions. At the present time in most developing countries, surveillance is limited to measuring the performance of a few infectious disease control programs. Epidemiologic capacities will need to be greatly strengthened as health program strategies move more toward regulation, taxation, subsidies, and information programs in order to reduce acute and chronic disease risks by changing behaviors and improving environmental safety.

- *Economic Analysis.* The demographic and epidemiologic capacities will only measure the burden of disease, its trends, determinants, and the effect of interventions. Economic analysis will be essential to measure the cost-effectiveness of alternative intervention strategies as well as to assess the overall claim of the health sector on scarce development resources (Barnum and Kutzin 1993). Building capacities in this area involve strengthening health service information systems to measure more effectively the resource inputs, the operations of the service delivery system, and its program outputs. Continuing comprehensive analyses of these data will be required to determine the cost-effectiveness of various operational programs. This activity must encompass the private as well as the public health care sector.

- *Health Technology Assessment.* One aspect of cost-effectiveness analysis has become known as health technology assessment; institutional capabilities in this area must include not only the assessment of the effectiveness of new drugs, vaccines, or equipment but also their costs and benefits when introduced into the health system. For example, there may need to be some control of the introduction of expensive high-technology health care interventions such as computerized axial tomography, or CAT, scanners or open-heart surgery in order to control health service delivery costs. More important, because drugs account for 40 to 60 percent of the health budget in many developing countries (not including private expenditure), there is an urgent need to build up the institutional resources to assess these products, not only with regard to safety and effectiveness, but with regard to use and cost (Mamdani and Walker 1986).

Policy Implementation and Health System Responses

The discussion above leads to five central conclusions for policy:

- A comprehensive health policy should move on multiple fronts simultaneously, considering the full range of facility-based and population-based options for any problem being addressed.

- Health strategies should be goal oriented, with specific quantitative intermediate objectives against which program achievements can be measured.

- Planning the appropriate intervention mix should specify as far as possible the quantitative relationships between program inputs (and their costs), outputs, and expected outcomes.

- Information systems must be established that provide timely data on health outcomes, intermediate objectives, and program inputs and costs.

- Regular analyses of input-output-outcome relationships with respect to the instruments of government policy must be carried out to ensure that the instrument mix is, in fact, inducing the desired level of operation of the range of interventions.

Selecting health care priorities in a given setting is only the first step toward improving the allocation of resources in the health sector (Murray 1990). The analysis of the burden of disease would ideally lead to a list of health problems ranked by order of importance. But clearly, the fact that a health problem is high priority does not lead automatically to the decision that the government should invest in prevention or case management. As has been shown in this collection, the role of cost-effectiveness analysis is to inform decisionmakers what interventions are likely to yield more years of healthy life and therefore are preferable. The results from the cost-effectiveness analysis can be used to make decisions at two different levels: first, to set priorities among the alternative interventions available to control a specific disease (for example, measles) or to reduce the exposure of the population to a specific risk factor (for example, tobacco); second, to set priorities within the health sector, selecting the most cost-effective interventions for those health problems that produce the greatest burden of disease.

The identification of these high-priority interventions still is insufficient to justify public investment. For example, it is clear that in many countries, some of the cost-effective interventions are already being delivered by the private sector (including traditional practitioners) or by voluntary organizations and, therefore, intervention by the government is not justified. In family planning, for example, there is strong involvement of the private sector in many countries (Lande and Geller 1991).

High-priority interventions, for which government involvement is justified, deserve a level of investment to achieve the greatest possible coverage and the highest quality standards. But to achieve these goals and the ultimate outcome on health status, the health system needs to have the infrastructure and organization to deliver the services. Table 29-9 shows a framework that integrates three criteria—burden of disease, cost-effectiveness, and health system strength—to set priorities and define more specifically the response from the health system. Strategies are suggested to strengthen the health system, if the system is weak, including development of trained staff and necessary infrastructure. Other possible combinations of these three criteria are also shown, and possible responses from the health system are suggested. Importantly, this framework indicates that an intervention with a very unfavorable

Table 29-9. *Responses of Strong and Weak Health Care Systems to Burden of Disease*

Burden of disease	Intervention cost-effectiveness	Strong health systems	Weak health systems
High	High	Aim for full population coverage Improve quality of services provided	Reorient/train existing staff Develop technical/ management systems Establish infrastructure
	Low	Research to improve interventions Do not expand services Institute cost recovery	Research to improve interventions Restrict or eliminate services
Low	High	Target high-risk groups	Provide services on demand
	Low	Restrict services or provide cost recovery	Eliminate services

Source: Authors' design.

cost-effectiveness ratio that is aimed at controlling a disease with low prevalence and low lethality clearly is a good candidate for rationing or elimination.

Another combination of criteria of interest to developing countries passing through the later phases of the epidemiologic transition is that of available interventions for high-priority diseases that have unfavorable cost-effectiveness ratios. The most obvious example of this situation at present relates to AIDS, where control of transmission in the core population offers the potential for being cost-effective (Over and Piot, chapter 20) but actual application of the interventions is difficult. The proposed response given in table 29-9 is research; operational research aimed at improving the cost-effectiveness of current approaches to patient care and to promoting and supporting behavioral change, and basic research directed to developing new interventions, that is, vaccines or better drugs which will cost less and become more effective. As noted earlier in the discussion of clinical interventions, the control of the emerging noncommunicable diseases, where tertiary hospital care is not now cost-effective, will probably depend on the development of lower-cost interventions that can be provided in district hospitals and health centers or through population-based programs.

Probably one of the earliest attempts to incorporate the analysis of the burden of disease and the cost-effectiveness of interventions into the process of health planning was developed by the Pan-American Health Organization, in collaboration with the Center for Development Studies at Caracas, Venezuela, in 1965. This is, by and large, the most comprehensive planning methodology proposed for developing countries. It provides details of the planning process and the requirements of information. Although the principles proposed were accepted, decisionmakers found them difficult to apply, mainly because the information available was inadequate and the complexity of the estimates demanded expertise not always available. Fortunately, in recent years important developments in informatics, epidemiology, and economic evaluation of health services are making more accessible the advanced methods proposed by the Center for Development Studies planning model (PAHO/WHO 1965).

Despite the importance of using explicit criteria to set health priorities for public investment in developing countries, there is not much experience with country-level applications. An important exercise was undertaken in the late 1970s in Ghana, however, which used the number of healthy days of life lost to assess the effect of diseases on health, and cost-effectiveness analysis to assess the appropriateness of alternative interventions (Ghana Health Assessment Project Team 1981). Five disease conditions were considered, namely, malaria, measles, childhood pneumonia, sickle-cell disease, and severe malnutrition. The results were used in the design of the Ghanian primary health care program, and the methodology proposed has served as a yardstick for subsequent developments in the assessment of the burden of disease.

International Aid

We have shown some of the implications of selecting disease control priorities, from the perspective of national governments, for the process of designing and implementing programs. This section deals with implications for the instruments through which agencies providing development assistance in the health sector can channel their aid. We begin by categorizing these instruments and then turn to the implications of this review's finding—concerning the health transition and intervention cost-effectiveness—for future directions of assistance in the health sector.

Instruments of Aid

One reasonable categorization of aid follows from whether the objective is one of assisting in the provision of services, of helping to improve the policy environment, or of expanding the research base underlying new interventions or improved resource allocation (table 29-10). These instruments of aid relate closely to the instruments of government discussed in the previous section. (See also chapter 1.) Many of the successful experiences with aid in the health sector have had as their objective the *provision of services* where no services, or only inadequate services, were available. The smallpox eradication

Table 29-10. *Instruments of Aid*

	Modality of assistance	
Objective	*Program implementation*	*Capacity strengthening*
Service delivery	Support acquisition of drugs, equipment, and technical assistance for delivery of expanded program of immunization (EPI), vector control programs, hospital services	Invest in institutional development and staff training to improve efficacy of service delivery, for example, through improved logistics and supply systems
Policy improvement	Identify specific areas of policy improvement (such as ban on tobacco advertising or introduction of cost-recovery mechanisms) and include them (usually conditional) as part of an assistance package	Invest in development of policy and planning departments in ministries or universities; invest in staff training and advanced education
Undertaking research (including epidemiologic, evaluational, and economic analyses)	Conduct research or analyses (perhaps with involvement of aid agency or expatriate staff) to strengthen formulation of policy or delivery of service	Invest in national and international capacity for undertaking research relevant to epidemiologic and economic conditions of developing countries, both institutional and human resource development

Source: Authors' design.

effort had this objective, as does its successor, the Expanded Programme on Immunization. Mission hospitals, too, are oriented toward provision of service, as are many other forms of assistance.

The capacity of a country to deliver services will, it is increasingly recognized, depend a great deal on the *policy environment* in which systems for delivering services must function. The policy environment defines a range of key structural conditions: the mandated division of labor among public, private, and nonprofit nongovernmental organization sectors; cost-recovery policy (and financing policy more generally); referral policy; pharmaceutical policy; policy toward prevention; policy toward taxation or subsidization of health-influencing processes or commodities; and policy toward distribution of access to services. Obviously some policy environments will be conducive to inefficiency or inequity; others less so.

The potential importance of aid in assisting with improving policy has been the subject of much attention and debate in the past five to ten years. Policy-oriented aid inevitably has the flavor of exchange of policy reform for financial assistance. The extent to which such exchange is productive depends greatly on the strength of those factions in the country who are intellectually (or otherwise) committed to reform, on the substance and style of the discussions leading to agreement, and on the inherent viability of the measures adopted. Most policy-based aid to date has been concerned with improving macroeconomic policy; more than $1.5 billion of World Bank (and International Development Association) lending in fiscal year 1989, for example, was for "structural adjustment loans" (or SALs) involving fast disbursing resource transfer and macroeconomic conditionality. The World Bank is now also using "sector adjustment lending" instruments; incremental, highly flexible resources are made available to a sector in tranches released on certification of specified progress in policy improvement. Efforts to help improve the policy environment through sector adjustment lending are playing an increasingly

important role in health sector operations at the World Bank, sometimes closely tied to provision of service in so-called hybrid projects.

Some aid to the health sector is channeled to *research and to development of research capacity* in recipient countries (see table 29-11). Among the programs:

• The Programme for Research and Training on Tropical Diseases supports biological and operational research on five major parasitic diseases and one bacterial disease that affect more than 600 million individuals; it is currently expending about $40 million per year.

• The Human Reproduction Program deals with biological and social aspects of fertility and its regulation; it currently operates at a budget of about $23 million per year.

• The International Clinical Epidemiology Program (INCLEN) and blindness-related programs on trachoma and onchocerciasis represent efforts of foundations (the Rockefeller Foundation and the Edna McConnell Clark Foundation, respectively) in two quite different domains.

Other important programs are well established—many of them, like the Programme for Research and Training on Tropical Diseases and the Human Reproduction Program, managed by the World Health Organization and funded by multiple donors. The influential Commission on Health Research for Development has been convened over the past several years and recently completed its work. The commission provided an extraordinarily thorough critical review of current efforts and capacities (Murray and others 1990) and of desirable directions for future effort (Commission on Health Research 1990). The Commission on Health Research has labeled this "essential national health research" and identified support of such research as a high priority. A follow-on secretariat to the commission has been established in Geneva to facilitate research efforts of individual countries.

Much research important for resource allocation is relatively nontransportable—local epidemiologic and operational analyses being important examples. Many research results, however, are transportable; lessons from Senegal and the Gambia about the effectiveness in the field of oral and injectable polio vaccine, for example, are probably almost as relevant in South Asia as they are in West Africa. The transportability of research does vary, of course. Little of use to Zaire in controlling AIDS is likely to emerge from study of sexual practices in San Francisco. Still, it is clear that much in the way of research output is transportable, leading (in economists' jargon) to important informational externalities. Existence of these externalities creates conditions in which any individual country is unlikely to invest fully in (nonpatentable) research because that country reaps only a fraction of a research project's benefits, yet it must pay the full cost. *The existence of these informational externalities, combined with substantial research capacity in donor countries, makes research a particularly viable domain for aid.* In addition, the requirement for a substantial critical mass of highly qualified (and, therefore, highly paid) scientists for much research points toward internationalization of the conduct of that research (as well as of its finances). This suggests the desirability of relatively few (but productive) venues with broad participation on the staff.

Two additional comments are worth making about research. First, despite the existence of programs that were described in the preceding paragraph, the current volume of resources going into research is quite limited. The Commission on Health Research (1990, p. 39) estimated, for example, that perhaps only a few pennies per death per year are going into research on such significant third-world killers as acute respiratory infections and tuberculosis; although relatively more is invested in tropical and parasitic disease research, the overall amount is quite limited. The commission estimates, overall, that only about 5 percent of the $30 billion spent on health research in 1986 was oriented toward developing countries.

Second, vaccine development efforts have the potential both for providing cost-effective prevention for a much broader range of conditions than is now possible and for reducing the cost and logistical complexity of currently available vaccines. In relation to potential, research of this sort currently receives very limited support—although the recent move toward creation of a Children's Vaccine Initiative suggests that solutions to this problem may soon emerge.

In summary the objectives of external assistance involve improving service delivery, improving the policy environment, and supporting the generation of research findings that underpin development of new interventions or more informed choice from among existing ones. Table 29-11 synopsizes these points and divides intervention concerning each objective into two modalities: *program implementation* and *capacity strengthening.* Interventions oriented toward attainment of results in the short term (and, often, this will be important) naturally emphasize the program implementation modality. In the long term, however, strengthening capacity (usually capac-

ity at the national or subnational level) is essential, and, increasingly, assistance programs include substantial resources for capacity strengthening through institutional development. Often this involves direct assistance to an institution—for example, a ministry headquarters or a hospital—designed to improve its overall functioning. Relevant efforts may include staff training, reorganizational advice, or support for development of information systems. Often of particular importance for capacity strengthening is investment in education and training facilities for health professionals, including nursing, medical, and public health faculties. To be effective, such investment may require a long time horizon; but the payoff can be very substantial indeed. The Rockefeller Foundation's more than thirty-year involvement with the Peking Union Medical College, for example, has had an influence on health policy in China, including Taiwan, that extends from the 1920s to the present day (Bullock 1980).

Conclusions

Estimates of the levels and structure of cause of mortality reviewed in this chapter strongly suggest that, not only will the number of deaths rapidly increase in developing countries, but there will also be a substantial (although incomplete) shift in the distribution of causes to the relatively expensive noncommunicable diseases of adults and the elderly. This shift, and the epidemiologic diversity likely to result from a lingering heavy burden of communicable disease, will challenge health systems to mount a broader range of preventive interventions and to develop very low cost protocols for managing cases in increasing numbers. Several general conclusions follow:

- As the increasing burden of noncommunicable disease is initially likely to affect the relatively more affluent and politically vocal older age groups, governments will need to take great care to ensure completion of the unfinished agenda for improving the health of children and the poor in the face of resource demands placed (predominantly) by the relatively better off. Almost certainly this equity objective will be consistent with extending the investments in immunization and other interventions against infectious diseases, which the chapters here have shown to offer the greatest gains in healthy life per dollar invested.[8] A key input to completing the unfinished agenda will be investment in research on vaccines—both to increase the range of conditions to be addressed and, more important, to simplify delivery logistics.

- Many of the risk factors for noncommunicable disease (smoking, sedentariness, increased motor vehicle use) tend, for at least a time, to become more prevalent with increasing affluence; in this they differ from risk factors for most communicable diseases (with the exception of AIDS). The disadvantage of this is obvious; the advantage is that taxation-based preventive policies can actually generate revenue for government while promoting health. More gen-

Table 29-11. Directions for International Aid

	Modality of assistance	
Objective	*Program implementation*	*Capacity strengthening*
Service delivery	Continue strong emphasis on most immunization and family planning programs	Develop drug logistic capacity to support implementation priorities
	Enhance emphasis on: • Measles immunization • Case management of acute respiratory infection • Control of vitamin A deficiency • Tuberculosis chemotherapy • Anthelmintic chemoprophylaxis • Control of sexually transmitted diseases • Control of cancer pain	Offer pre- and in-service training of providers to effectively manage priority procedures Develop capacity to deliver inexpensive rehabilitative services Reduce emphasis on general institutional development in favor of strengthening specific capacities
	Increase selectivity in delivery of ORT (oral rehydration therapy) and BCG (bacille Calmette-Guérin) immunization in low-risk environments	
	Sharply reduce support for hospital facilities	
Policy improvement	Implement full range of policies to limit use of tobacco	Develop instruments for effecting sustainable increases in flow of resources to the health sector
	Implement policies to track and reduce use of procedures of low cost-effectiveness	Develop staff and institutional capacity for formulating and implementing policies involving taxation, regulation, and communication, as well as direct investment
	Implement policies, including control of alcohol use, to reduce occupational and transport injuries	
Undertaking research	Substantially increase aid resources for research	Develop national and international capacity for conduct of essential national health research
	Finance and assist in the conduct of exemplary ENHR programs	Develop and adequately finance international and national capacity for research on cardiovascular diseases in developing countries; also, perhaps, for other noncommunicable diseases and injuries
	Increase epidemiologic operational research on: • Cardiovascular disease • STDs (sexually transmitted diseases) • COPD (chronic obstructive pulmonary disease) • Injury • Mental disorders	Maintain and extend capacity for monitoring epidemiologic trends and efficacy of intervention in well-documented populations (such as Matlab in Bangladesh)
	Assess intervention cost-effectiveness in different environments	

Source: Authors' design.

erally, increasing epidemiologic diversity will require a broader range of preventive measures; increasing use of the full range of government policy instruments (like taxes) can play an important role in implementing them. Of particular importance here is prompt national and international action to control tobacco use. Acquisition of tobacco addiction by today's youth generates the dynamic for lung cancer, COPD, and cardiovascular disease epidemics in fifteen to thirty years. Taxes, prohibition on promotion, and other effective interventions are available, and their prompt implementation is high priority.

• To help preserve resources for the poor and to ensure broad access to reasonable treatment, great effort will need to be devoted to implementing (or developing) low-cost ways of reaching the goals of secondary prevention, cure,

and rehabilitation—and to providing humane palliation for those whose lives could only be marginally extended (if at all) by affordable intervention. Some methods that are reasonably cost-effective have been identified, but significant efforts are required to develop and evaluate a more comprehensive range of low-cost therapeutic interventions.

• Today's allocation of research resources to the health sector in developing countries virtually ignores the problems that will dominate the policy agenda in years to come. This situation may have several roots: a sense that current research priorities should mirror operational ones; a sense that the National Institutes of Health and their sister institutions around the industrial world are doing what needs to be done about chronic disease; and, perhaps, a lack of appreciation for epidemiologic dynamics. Yet, as we have argued, case management of chronic disease will have to proceed in environments drastically more cost-constrained than the ones for which institutions such as the National Institutes of Health are working; relevant research and development efforts must be modified and evaluated for cost-effectiveness in very different environments. Likewise, very little indeed is known, for example, of the descriptive epidemiology of cardiovascular disease in the developing world, and no available risk models are based on developing country data, which might include risk factors not observed in industrial countries. The list of examples could go on; the point is simply that the analytic effort to address the emerging health problems of developing countries in the 1990s and beyond has barely begun.

• Just as manufacturers with older equipment expect higher maintenance costs, older populations will generate, for a variety of reasons, higher health maintenance costs for their country. National economic planners should expect to see, as populations age, expenditure on health steadily rising as a percentage of the gross national product in the coming decades.

Appendix 29A: Regional Groupings of Countries and Territories

The following lists define the countries that are considered in the text.

Industrialized Market Economies

Australia	Japan
Austria	Luxembourg
Belgium	Malta
Canada	Netherlands
Channel Islands	New Zealand
Cyprus	Norway
Denmark	Portugal
Finland	Spain
France	Sweden
Germany, former	Switzerland
Federal Republic of	United Kingdom
Greece	United States of America
Iceland	Other Europe
Ireland	Other North America
Italy	

Industrialized Transition Economies

Albania	Hungary
Bulgaria	Poland
Czechoslovakia	Romania
Former German	Former U.S.S.R.
Democratic Republic	Yugoslavia

Latin America and the Caribbean

Antigua and Barbuda	Jamaica
Argentina	Martinique
Bahamas	Mexico
Barbados	Montserrat
Belize	Netherlands
Bolivia	Antilles
Brazil	Nicaragua
Chile	Panama
Colombia	Paraguay
Costa Rica	Peru
Cuba	Puerto Rico
Dominica	St. Kitts and Nevis
Dominican Republic	St. Lucia
Ecuador	St. Vincent and the
El Salvador	Grenadines
Grenada	Suriname
Guadeloupe	Trinidad and Tobago
Guatemala	Uruguay
Guyana	Venezuela
Haiti	Virgin Islands (US)
Honduras	Other Latin America

Sub-Saharan Africa

Angola	Mali
Benin	Mauritania
Botswana	Mauritius
Burkina Faso	Mozambique
Burundi	Namibia
Cameroon	Niger
Cape Verde	Nigeria
Central African Republic	Réunion
Chad	Rwanda
Comoros	Sâo Tomé and Principe
Congo, People's Rep. of the	Senegal
Côte d'Ivoire	Seychelles
Djibouti	Sierra Leone
Equatorial Guinea	Somalia
Ethiopia	South Africa
Gabon	Sudan
Gambia, The	Swaziland
Ghana	Tanzania
Guinea	Togo
Guinea-Bissau	Uganda
Kenya	Zaire
Lesotho	Zambia
Liberia	Zimbabwe
Madagascar	Other West Africa
Malawi	

Middle East and North Africa

Afghanistan	Bahrain
Algeria	Egypt, Arab Republic of

Middle East and North Africa (continued)

Gaza Strip	Qatar
Iran, Islamic Republic of	Saudi Arabia
Iraq	Syrian Arab Republic
Israel	Tunisia
Jordan	Turkey
Kuwait	United Arab Emirates
Lebanon	West Bank
Libya	Former Yemen, People's
Morocco	Democratic Republic of
Oman	Former Yemen Arab Republic
Pakistan	Other North Africa

Asia and the Pacific

Bangladesh	Malaysia
Bhutan	Maldives
Brunei	Mongolia
Cambodia	Myanmar
China	Nepal
Fiji	New Caledonia
French Polynesia	Pacific Islands
Guam	Papua New Guinea
Hong Kong	Philippines
India	Singapore
Indonesia	Solomon Islands
Kiribati	Sri Lanka
Korea, Democratic	Thailand
People's Republic of	Vanuatu
Korea, Republic of	Viet Nam
Lao People's Democratic	Western Samoa
Republic	Other Micronesia
Macao	Other Polynesia

Notes

We are deeply indebted to a number of our colleagues for comments and discussions concerning earlier drafts of parts of this material; they include Jacques Baudouy, Robert Black, John Briscoe, J. Richard Bumgarner, Donald Bundy, Guy Carrin, Lincoln Chen, E. Chigan, Andrew Creese, Joseph Davis, Nicholas Drager, Davidson Gwatkin, Jean-Pierre Habicht, Ann Hamilton, Alaya Hammad, Jeffrey Hammer, Ralph Henderson, Kenneth Hill, Michel Jancloes, Jeffrey Koplan, Jean-Louis Lamboray, Joanne Leslie, Bernhard Liese, Judith McGuire, Richard Morrow, Mead Over, Thomas Pearson, Richard Peto, Margaret Phillips, Nancy Pielemeier, Barry Popkin, André Prost, William Reinke, Ismail Sirageldin, Robert Steinglass, Eleuther Tarimo, Carl Taylor, Anne Tinker, Kenneth Warren, and David Werner. David Bell and Anthony Measham have provided us particularly extensive and valuable comments. The first section and the first part of the second section of this chapter are based on material we prepared with Donald A. Henderson of Johns Hopkins University (Mosley, Jamison, and Henderson 1990), and we would like to acknowledge both Dr. Henderson's direct contribution and his influence on the chapter as a whole. An early version of those early parts of the chapter was critically reviewed in August 1989 by the Board on International Health of the U.S. Institute of Medicine, and the comments of the chairman of that board, William Foege, as well as of its other members, provided valuable redirection. Likewise, we would like to acknowledge the strong influence on

our thinking of Richard Feachem and the effort he has led for the World Bank to review issues concerning the health of adults in the developing world. Last, we acknowledge those who provided valuable comments on portions of this chapter, which was given by Dean T. Jamison as the Heath Clark Lecture for 1989–90 at the London School of Hygiene and Tropical Medicine.

1. Here and in much of what follows we draw heavily on estimates based on World Bank projections (Bulatao and Stephens 1989), which typically use combinations of model life tables rather than empirical estimates of mortality. Although we are aware of the shortcomings of this method, it provides the only globally complete projection model that is currently available. A more epidemiologically based assessment of the distribution of death by cause in 1985, for the developing and the industrial countries, is presented in the chapter on cause of mortality (Lopez, chapter 2).

2. Uemura (1989) has calculated excess mortality ratios for different countries and age groups at different points in time, using, as a reference, the lowest age- and sex-specific mortality rates so far observed in any country. His conclusions clearly show that the greatest gains to be made in developing countries are in the younger age groups. (Greater gains are also possible, he shows, among females than among males at all ages, even though absolute age-specific mortality rates are typically lower for females.)

3. The Demographic and Health Surveys (DHS) is a nine-year project to assist government and private agencies in developing countries to conduct national sample surveys on population and health. DHS is funded by the U.S. Agency for International Development (USAID) and administered by the Institute for Resource Development. For more information about the DHS program (or copies of individual country reports) write to DHS, IRD/Macro Systems, 8850 Stanford Boulevard, Suite 4000, Columbia, Md. 21045, U.S.A.

4. Most of the implications of the health transition on the health system described here refer to the health care subsystem. The possible effects on the other sectors of the economy are more difficult to anticipate, despite their potential importance. Particularly relevant is the effect of ill-health in the production of goods and services and the policy responses to the potential loss in productivity.

5. For a valuable general discussion of the economic role of government, its limits, and its comparative advantage, see Stiglitz 1989. A somewhat more mathematical treatment of these matters, with an emphasis on project evaluation methods, may be found in Starrett 1988. Birdsall (1989) provides an extended discussion of the role of government in the health sector; she emphasizes its past successes in many developing countries but calls for a redefinition of its role to leave more responsibility in routine areas to private actors and to achieve greater financial and administrative responsiveness in its own operations. Akin, Birdsall, and deFerranti (1987) discuss the financial aspects of these matters at greater length. Behrman (1990) provides a clear overview of the central role of household decisionmaking (in many domains) as determinants of health; this provides a context for assessing the role of government.

6. We define "direct investment" broadly to include not only activities directly administered by government but, also, services contracted for by government or natural monopolies (for example, tertiary facilities) that may be partially privately owned or independently managed but whose policies are closely regulated in the public interest.

7. It is worth stressing, however, that when price elasticities of demand are low, taxation ceases to be effective for changing behavior; for example, raising taxes on salt, even substantially, could be expected to have only a minimal effect on consumption.

8. World Bank (1989) and Feachem and others (1992) have assembled evidence showing, convincingly, that the poor suffer more from chronic diseases than do their well-off counterparts. *Relatively*, though, the poor suffer much more from infectious conditions; hence the desirability, from a distributional perspective, of infectious disease control programs.

References

Akin, John S., Nancy J. Birdsall, and D. de Ferranti. 1987. *Financing Health Services in Developing Countries: An Agenda for Reform.* A World Bank Policy

Study. Policy and Research Division of the Population, Health and Nutrition Department. Washington, D.C.: World Bank.

Albanez, Teresa, Eduardo Bustelo, Giovanni Andrea Cornia, and Eva Jespersen. 1989. "Economic Decline and Child Survival: The Plight of Latin America in the Eighties." Innocenti Occasional Paper 1, UNICEF International Child Development Centre, Florence, Italy,

Amler, Robert W., and H. Bruce Dull, eds. 1987. *Closing the Gap: The Burden of Unnecessary Illness.* New York: Oxford University Press.

Amler, Robert W. and D. L. Eddins. 1987. "Cross-sectional Analysis: Precursors of Premature Death in the United States." In Robert W. Amler and H. Bruce Dull, eds., *Closing the Gap: The Burden of Unnecessary Illness.* New York: Oxford University Press.

Babikir, Adam, Cole P. Dodge, and Ian Pett. 1989. "Monitoring Immunization Coverage in Sudan." *Health Policy and Planning* 4(1):91–95.

Barcellos, T. M., and others. 1986. *Segregacāo urbana e mortalidade em Pôrto Alegre.* Pôrto Alegre: Fundação de Economia e Estatistica.

Barnum, Howard N., and Joseph Kutzin. 1993. *Public Hospitals in Developing Countries: Resource Use, Cost, Financing.* Washington, D.C.: World Bank.

Behrman, J. R. 1990. "A Survey on Socioeconomic Development, Structural Adjustment and Child Health and Mortality in Developing Countries." In Kenneth Hill, ed., *Child Survival Programs: Issues for the 1990s.* Baltimore: Johns Hopkins University School of Hygiene and Public health, Institute for International Programs.

Bell, David E., and M. R. Reich, eds. 1988. *Health, Nutrition, and Economic Crisis.* Dover, Mass.: Auburn House for the Harvard School of Public Health.

Berman, Peter, Carl Kendall, and Karahi Bhattacharyya. 1989. "The Household Production of Health: Putting People at the Center of Health Improvement." In Ismail Sirageldin, W. Henry Mosley, Ruth Levine, Valerie Schwoebel and Kiyomi Horiuchi, eds., *Towards More Efficacy in Child Survival Strategies: Understanding the Social and Private Constraints and Responsibilities.* Baltimore: Johns Hopkins University School of Hygiene and Public Health.

Birdsall, Nancy J. 1989. "Thoughts on Good Health and Good Government." *Daedalus* 118:23.

Bulatao, Rodolfo A., and Patience Stephens. (forthcoming). "Estimates and Projections of Mortality by Cause: A Global Overview, 1970–2015." Policy research working paper. Population Policy and Advisory Service of the Director's Office of the Population and Human Resources Department. World Bank. Washington, D.C.

Bullock, M. B. 1980. *An American Transplant: The Rockefeller Foundation and Peking Union Medical College.* Berkeley: University of California Press.

Caldwell, John C., and Peter F. McDonald. 1981. "Influence of Maternal Education on Infant and Child Mortality: Levels and Causes." In International Union for the Scientific Study of Population, *International Population Conference, Manila, 1981,* vol. 2. Liège, Belgium.

Chesnais, Jean-Claude. 1990. "Demographic Transition Patterns and Their Impact on the Age Structure." *Population and Development Review* 16(2): 327–36.

Church, C. A., and J. S. Geller. 1990. "Lights! Camera! Action!" Population Reports J-38. Johns Hopkins University Population Information Program. Baltimore.

Coale, Ansley J. 1991. "Excess Female Mortality and the Balance of the Sexes in the Population: An Estimate of the Number of 'Missing Females.'" *Population and Development Review* 17(3):517–23.

Coale, Ansley, and Paul R. Dimeny, with Barbara Vaughan. 1983. *Regional Model Life Tables and Stable Populations.* 2nd edition. New York: Academic Press.

Cochrane, Susan, Joanne Leslie, and Donald J. O'Hara. 1982. "Parental Education and Child Health: Intracountry Evidence." *Health Policy and Education* 2(3/4):213–50.

Coleman, Patrick L. 1988. "Enter-Educate: New Word from Johns Hopkins." *JOICFP Review* 15:28–31.

Coleman, Patrick L., and R. C. Meyer. 1990. "The Enter-Educate Conference: Entertainment for Social Change." In *Proceedings.* Baltimore: Johns Hopkins University Center for Communication Programs.

Comanor, William S. 1986. "The Political Economy of the Pharmaceutical Industry." *Journal of Economic Literature* 24(3):1178–1217.

Commission on Health Research for Development. 1990. *Health Research: Essential Link to Equity in Development.* Oxford: Oxford University Press.

Cornia, Giovanni Andrea, Richard Jolly, and Frances Stewart, eds. 1987. *Adjustment with a Human Face.* Oxford: Clarendon Press.

Crimmins, Eileen M., Yasuhiko Saito, and Dominique Ingegneri. 1989. "Changes in Life Expectancy and Disability-Free Life Expectancy in the United States." *Population and Development Review* 15(2):235–67.

Das Gupta, Monica. 1987. "Selective Discrimination against Female Children in Rural Punjab, India." *Population and Development Review* 13(1):77–100.

Ernster, Virginia L. 1988. "Trends in Smoking, Cancer Risk, and Cigarette Promotion." *Cancer* 62(8)Supplement:1702–12.

Evans, John R., Karen Lashman Hall, and Jeremy Warford. 1981 "Health Care in the Developing World: Problems of Scarcity and Choice." *New England Journal of Medicine* 305(19):1117–27.

Feachem, Richard G. A., Dean T. Jamison, and E. R. Bos. 1991. "Changing Patterns of Disease and Mortality in Sub-Saharan Africa." In Richard G. A. Feachem and Dean T. Jamison, eds., *Disease and Mortality in Sub-Saharan Africa.* New York: Oxford University Press.

Feachem, Richard G. A., Tord Kjellstrom, Christopher J. L. Murray, Mead Over, and M. A. Phillips. 1992. *The Health of Adults in the Developing World.* New York: Oxford University Press for the World Bank.

Fenner, Frank, Donald A. Henderson, Isao Arita, Zdenek Jezek, and Ivan D. Ladnyi. 1988. *Smallpox and Its Eradication.* Geneva: World Health Organization.

Foege, William H., and Donald A. Henderson. 1986. "Management Priorities in Primary Health Care." In J. A. Walsh and K. S. Warren, eds., *Strategies for Primary Health Care.* Chicago: University of Chicago Press.

Frenk, Julio, José Luis Bobadilla, Jaime Sepúlveda, and Malaquias Lopez Cervantes. 1989. "Health Transition in Middle-Income Countries: New Challenges for Health Care." *Health Policy and Planning* 4(1):29–39.

Fries, James F. 1989. "The Compression of Morbidity: Near or Far?" *Milbank Quarterly* 67(2):208–31.

Ghana Health Assessment Project Team. 1981. "A Quantitative Method of Assessing the Health Impact of Different Diseases in Less Developed Countries." *International Journal of Epidemiology* 10(1):73–80.

Gilluly, R. H., and S. H. Moore. 1986. "Radio—Spreading the Word on Family Planning." Population Reports J-32. Johns Hopkins University Population Information Program. Baltimore.

Gray, Ronald H. 1987. "A Review of Methodological Approaches to Evaluating Health Problems." IIP Occasional Paper 1. Report of the Workshop on Health Impact Evaluation held at the Johns Hopkins University School of Hygiene and Public Health, Institute for International Programs, October 9–10, 1986, Baltimore.

Gunatilleke, Godfrey 1989. *Government Policies and Nutrition in Sri Lanka: Changes During the Last Ten Years and Lessons Learned.* Ithaca, N.Y.: Cornell Food and Nutrition Policy Program.

Hill, Kenneth, and Anne Pebley. 1990. "Child Mortality in the Developing World." *Population and Development Review* 15(4):657–81.

Hobcraft, J. N., J. W. McDonald, and S. O. Rutstein. 1984. "Socio-economic Factors in Infant and Child Mortality: A Cross-National Comparison." *Population Studies* 38:193–224.

Hogerzeil, Hans V., and Per Manell. 1989. "Computerized Drug Supply Systems for Developing Countries." *Health Policy and Planning* 4(2):177–81.

Hornik, R. C. 1988. *Development Communication: Information, Agriculture, and Nutrition in the Third World.* New York: Longman.

Hughes, Kenneth 1986. "Trends in Mortality from Ischemic Heart Disease in Singapore, 1959 to 1983." *International Journal of Epidemiology* 15(1):44–50.

Ingle, Marcus, Noel Berge, and Marcia Hamilton. 1986. *Microcomputers in Development: A Manager's Guide.* West Hartford, Conn.: Kumarion Press.

Jamison, Dean T., John R. Evans, Timothy King, Ian Porter, Nicholas Prescott, and Andre Prost. 1984. *China: The Health Sector.* A World Bank Country Study. Washington, D.C.: World Bank.

Kaplan, George A., Mary N. Haan, S. Leonard Syme, Meredith Minkler, and Marilyn Winkleby. 1987. "Socioeconomic Status and Health." In Robert W. Amler and H. Bruce Dull, eds., *Closing the Gap: The Burden of Unnecessary Illness.* New York: Oxford University Press.

Kinsella, Kevin. 1988. *Aging in the Third World.* International Population Reports P-95, 79. Washington, D.C.: U.S. Department of Commerce, Bureau of the Census.

Kjellstrom, Tord, and Linda Rosenstock. 1990. "The Role of Environment and Occupational Hazards in the Adult Health Transition." *World Health Statistics Quarterly* 43(3):188–96.

Lande, R. E., and J. S. Geller. 1991. "Paying for Family Planning." Population Reports J-39. Johns Hopkins University Population Information Program. Baltimore.

Last, John M. 1988. *Dictionary of Epidemiology.* 2d ed. New York: Oxford University Press for the International Epidemiological Association.

Lee, H. P., S. W. Duffy, N. E. Day, and K. Shanmugarathnam. 1988. "Recent Trends in Cancer Incidence among Singapore Chinese." *International Journal of Cancer* 42(2):159–66.

Leslie, Joanne. 1991. "Women's Nutrition: The Key to Improving Family Health in Developing Countries?" *Health Policy and Planning* 6(1):1–19.

Liskin, Laurie, and Ward Rinehart. 1985. "Minilaparotomy and Laparoscopy: Safe, Effective, and Widely Used." Population Reports C-9. Johns Hopkins University Population Information Program. Baltimore.

Mamdani, Masuma, and Godfrey Walker. 1986. "Essential Drugs in the Developing World." *Health Policy and Planning* 1(3):187–201.

Masironi, Robert, and Keith Rothwell. 1988. "Tendances et effets du tabagisme dans le monde." *World Health Statistics Quarterly* 41(3/4):228–41.

Mosley, W. Henry. 1988. "Is There a Middle Way? Categorical Programs for PHC." *Social Science and Medicine* 26(9):907–8.

———. 1989. "Interactions of Technology with Household Production of Health." In Ismail Sirageldin, W. Henry Mosley, Ruth Levine, Valerie Schwoebel, Kiyomi Horiuchi, eds., *Towards More Efficacy in Child Survival Strategies: Understanding the Social and Private Constraints and Responsibilities.* Baltimore: Johns Hopkins University School of Hygiene and Public Health.

Murray, Christopher J. 1990. "Rational Approaches to Priority Setting in International Health." *Journal of Tropical Medicine and Hygiene* 93(5):303–11.

Murray, Christopher J. L., David E. Bell, E. de Jonghe, Sarah Zaidi, and Catherine Michaud. 1990. "A Study of Financial Resources Devoted to Research on Health Problems of Developing Countries." *Journal of Tropical Medicine and Hygiene* 93(4):229–55.

Olshansky, S. Jay., and A. Brian Ault. 1986. "The Fourth Stage of the Epidemiologic Transition: The Age of Delayed Degenerative Diseases." *Milbank Quarterly* 64(3):355–91.

Omran, Abdel R. 1971. "The Epidemiological Transition: A Theory of the Epidemiology of Population Change." *The Milbank Memorial Fund Quarterly* 49(4):509–38.

PAHO/WHO (Pan-American Health Organization/World Health Organization). 1965. *Health Planning Problems of Concept and Method.* Prepared at the Center for Development Studies (CENDES) of the Central University of Venezuela, Caracas, in cooperation with the Pan American Sanitary Bureau. Washington, D.C. April.

Piot, Peter, and King K. Holmes. 1989. "Sexually Transmitted Diseases." In K. Warren and A. Mahmoud, eds., *Tropical and Geographical Medicine.* New York: McGraw-Hill.

Popkin, Bury M., and E. Z. Bisgrove. 1988. "Urbanization and Nutrition in Low-Income Countries." *Food and Nutrition Bulletin* 10(1):3–23.

Popkin, Bury M., Ge Keyou, Zhai Fengying, Xuguang Guo, Ma Haijiang, and Namvar Zohoori. 1992. "The Nutrition Transition in China: A Cross-sectional Analysis." Carolina Population Center. University of North Carolina. *European Journal of Clinical Nutrition* (in press).

Preston, Samuel H. 1986. "The Relation between Actual and Intrinsic Growth Rates." *Population Studies* 40(3):343–51.

Quick, Jonathan D., Patricia Foreman, Dennis Ross-Degnan, and others. 1988. "Where Does the Tetracycline Go?: Health Center Prescribing and Child Survival in East Java and West Kalimantan, Indonesia." Unpublished report prepared by Drug Management Program of Management Sciences for Health, Boston, Mass., with the Office of Population and Health, Jakarta, and USAID.

Rose, Geoffrey 1985. "Sick Individuals and Sick Populations." *International Journal of Epidemiology* 14(1):32–38.

Rutstein, S. O. 1991. "Levels, Trends and Differentials in Infant and Child Mortality in the Less Developed Countries." In K. Hill, ed., *Child Health Priorities for the 1990s.* Baltimore: Johns Hopkins University School of Hygiene and Public Health, Institute for International Programs.

Sanders, David, and Rob Davies. 1988. "Economic Adjustment and Current Trends in Child Survival: The Case of Zimbabwe." *Health Policy and Planning* 3(3):195–204.

Stansfield, Sally 1990. "Potential Savings through Reduction of Inappropriate Use of Pharmaceuticals in the Treatment of ARI." In A. Gadomski, ed., *Acute Lower Respiratory Infection and Child Survival in Developing Countries: Understanding the Current Status and Directions for the 1990s.* Proceedings of a workshop held in Washington, D.C., August 2–3, 1989. Johns Hopkins University School of Hygiene and Public Health, Institute for International Programs. Baltimore.

Starrett, D. A. 1988. *Foundation of Public Economics.* Cambridge: Cambridge University Press.

Stiglitz, Joseph E., Mark Perlman, Douglass C. North, Dieter Bös, Chris Freeman, A. H. E. M. Wellink, Ian MacGregor, Jean-Jacques Laffont, and Arnold Heertje (ed.). 1989. *The Economic Role of the State.* Cambridge, Mass.: Basil Blackwell in association with Bank Insinger de Beauford NV.

Sullivan, J. M. 1991. "The Pace of Decline in Under-Five Mortality: Evidence from the DHS Surveys." In IRD/Marco International, Inc., *Proceedings of the Demographic and Health Surveys (DHS) World Conference, Washington, D.C., 1991.* Vol. 1, Columbia, Md.

Susser, Murvyn. 1981. "Industrialization, Urbanization and Health: An Epidemiological View." In International Union for the Scientific Study of Population, *International Population Conference, Manila, 1981,* vol. 2. Liège, Belgium.

Taylor, Carl E., and Richard Jolly. 1988. "The Straw Men of Primary Health Care." *Social Science and Medicine* 26(9):971–77.

Uemura, Kazuo. 1989. "Excess Mortality Ratio with Reference to the Lowest Age-Sex-Specific Death Rates among Countries." *World Health Statistics Quarterly* 42(1):26–41.

United Nations, Department of International Economic and Social Affairs. 1989. *Prospects of World Urbanization, 1988.* Population Studies 112 (ST/ESA/SER.A/112). New York.

USDHEW (U.S. Department of Health, Education, and Welfare), Public Health Service. 1978. *Ten Leading Causes of Death in the United States, 1975.* Atlanta: Centers for Disease Control.

USDHHS (U. S. Department of Health and Human Services). 1992. *Smoking and Health in the Americas.* DHHS Publication (CDC)92–8419. Atlanta: Centers for Disease Control, Office of Smoking and Health.

Velez Gil, Aldolfo, Marco Tulio Galarza, Rodrigo Guerrero, Graciela Pardo de Velez, Osler L. Peterson, and Bernard L. Bloom. 1983. "Surgeons and Operating Rooms: Under-Utilized Resources." *American Journal of Public Health* 73(12):1361–65.

Verbrugge, Lois M. 1984. "Longer Life but Worsening Health?: Trends in Health and Mortality of Middle-aged and Older Persons." *Milbank Memorial Fund Quarterly/Health and Society* 62(3):475–519.

———. 1989. "Recent, Present, and Future Health of American Adults." In Lester Breslow, Jonathan E. Fielding, and Lester B. Lave, eds., *Annual Review of Public Health*, vol. 10. Palo Alto, Calif.: Annual Reviews.

Victora, C. G. 1986. "CDC Anthropometric Software Package (CASP)." PC software review. *Health Policy and Planning* 1(1):84–85.

Vilnius, Douglas, and Suzanne Dandoy. 1990. "A Priority Rating System for Public Health Programs." *Public Health Reports* 105(5):463–70.

White, K. L. 1985. "Health Surveys." *World Health Statistics Quarterly* 38(1):2–14.

WHO (World Health Organization). 1988. *From Alma-Ata to the Year 2000: Reflections at the Midpoint*. Geneva.

Wilson, R. G., B. E. Echols, H. H. Bryant, and A. Abrantes, eds. 1988. *Management Information Systems and Microcomputers in Primary Health Care*. Geneva: Aga Khan Foundation.

World Bank. 1989. "Adult Health in Brazil: Adjusting to New Challenges." Report 7807-BR. Washington, D.C.

———. 1990a. "China: Long-term Issues and Options in the Health Transition." Report 7965-CHA. Environment, Human Resources and Urban Development Division, Asia Country Dept. III. World Bank. Washington, D.C.

———. 1990b. "India–Tamil Nadu Integrated Nutrition Project Completion Report." World Bank. Washington, D.C. Population and Human Resources Division, India Country Department.

———. 1992. *World Development Report 1992*. New York: Oxford University Press.

Yankauer, Alfred. 1983. "Lessons in Surgery for the Third World." *American Journal of Public Health* 73(12):1359–60.

Yu, J. J., M. E. Mattson, G. M. Boyd, M. D. Mueller, D. R. Shopland, T. F. Pechacek, and J. W. Cullen. 1990. "A Comparison of Smoking Patterns in the People's Republic of China with the United States." *Journal of the American Medical Association* 264(12):1575–79.

Zaridze, D. G., and Richard Peto, eds. 1986. *Tobacco: A Major International Health Hazard*. World Health Organization/IARC Scientific Publication 74. New York: Oxford University Press.

Appendixes

Appendix A

Control of Tobacco Production and Use

Kenneth Stanley

Tobacco was cultivated in the Americas more than 3,000 years ago and is believed to have originated there. By the arrival of Columbus in 1492, tobacco was being chewed, smoked, or snuffed in many areas of both North and South America.

Tobacco cultivation was spread, primarily by the Spanish and the Portuguese, to Europe, Africa, India, Turkey, Russia, China, and Japan by the early 1600s. By 1620 the Virginia colony in North America was growing tobacco commercially for export. This lucrative trade helped to develop both the American colonies and the English merchant navy.

In the 1700s and the early 1800s, large quantities of tobacco were being snuffed by the aristocracy of Europe and chewed by the American pioneers as they pushed westward. By the middle of the 1800s, however, the technology for making cigarettes and flue-curing tobacco had been developed, and the chewing of tobacco was beginning to be seen as unhygienic. By World War I the mass production of cigarettes had begun, and smoking rates among men in industrial countries began to rise dramatically. Cigarette smoking became popular among women in industrial countries starting about the time of World War II. At this time, smoking rates also began to rise in men in developing countries. Filtered cigarettes became popular in the 1950s, and in the 1960s low-yield cigarettes entered the marketplace. Today, tobacco is cultivated commercially in more than 120 countries and is consumed in all countries of the world.

Tobacco production and consumption influence various sectors of society in different ways, some negatively and some positively. As a result, it is important to consider the perspectives of these various sectors, including the individual tobacco user, the tobacco grower, the tobacco industry, the health community, and governments. My objective in this chapter is to review the influence of tobacco on each sector, to determine the health and economic effect of tobacco, and to evaluate strategies to control its use.

The Adverse Effects of Tobacco

Although the major diseases associated with tobacco have been known for more than thirty years, only recently have many of the other health problems been firmly established. Similarly, the adverse effects of tobacco on members of the family, coworkers, businesses and the environment have been investigated only in the last few years.

Health Effects

The three leading causes of mortality for the productive age group between fifteen and sixty-five years in both industrial and developing countries are cardiovascular diseases, cancer, and accidents (WHO 1980). Chronic diseases are well recognized as significant health problems in the industrial regions of the world. The prevalence of communicable diseases among children, however, often hides the fact that chronic diseases are also becoming a serious problem in developing countries. Life expectancy in those countries has risen from 41.0 years in 1950–55 to 57.6 years today; it is projected to reach 70.4 years by 2020–25 (United Nations 1989). The correlation between life expectancy and mortality from cardiovascular diseases, cancer, and infection is given in figure A-1.

The association between tobacco use and ill health has been reviewed by many national and international committees and organizations. Consistently, they conclude that tobacco use is a significant cause of disability and premature death (RCP 1983; WHO 1986; USDHHS 1989a). Worldwide, approximately 3 million premature deaths per year are due to tobacco smoking (see table A-1). In Europe alone, there are more than 500,000 such deaths each year; in the United States, the corresponding figure is 434,000, or one-sixth of all deaths. More than a quarter of all regular cigarette smokers die prematurely from smoking-related diseases.

The extent of mortality by disease that can be ascribed to tobacco has been determined for the United States and is presented in table A-2. Lung cancer is the single largest contributor, followed by ischemic heart disease. Lung cancer accounts for 26 percent of the mortality resulting from smoking. In the United States, about 1.2 million years of potential life before the age of sixty-five are lost each year, two-thirds among men and one-third among women (CDC 1991).

The rates of attributable mortality similar to those in table A-2 would be applicable for most industrial countries, in which smoking has been a widespread habit for many years. Smoking

Figure A-1. Relationship between Life Expectancy at Birth and Mortality from Cardiovascular Diseases, Cancer, and Infections

Percentage of all deaths

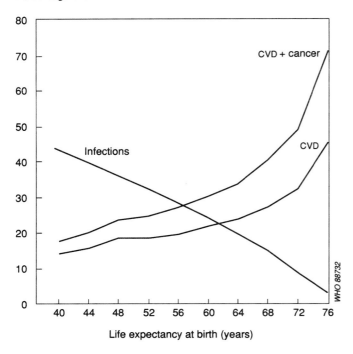

Life expectancy at birth (years)

Source: Based on analysis of United Nations statistics (Omran 1971), modified by Dodu.

has only recently become popular in many developing countries, however, and the delay of twenty to twenty-five years between the time one begins to smoke and the onset of many of the most important associated diseases such as lung cancer means that current attributable rates calculated for developing countries will be somewhat less. Within ten to fifteen years, however, cigarette smoking will have been prevalent in many developing countries for sufficient time to be the cause of a mortality pattern closely approximating that currently seen in industrial countries. The change has already occurred in some regions. For example, in Shanghai County, a rural and urban area near the city of Shanghai, the leading causes of death in

the early 1960s were infectious diseases, accidents, respiratory diseases, digestive diseases, and neonatal deaths. But by the end of the 1970s, the most common causes of mortality in the area were cancer, cerebrovascular diseases, and heart diseases (Gu and Chen 1982). This shift in health problems took place in less than twenty years and is marked by the emergence of diseases caused by tobacco use.

One of the common hindrances of effective action against tobacco is the public's general lack of understanding of the relative importance of the various risks in daily living. Often, the local media provides continuous information about hazards from various factors with considerable sensationalism, in repeated attempts to grab the public's attention. As a result a large portion of the public believes everything causes cancer so why worry only about cigarettes. In reality, however, tobacco is the dominant public health hazard in industrial countries. In the United States and many other industrial countries, smoking is responsible for more deaths than heroin, cocaine, alcohol, acquired immunodeficiency syndrome (AIDS), fires, homicide, suicide, and automobile accidents—combined. In the United Kingdom, a report of the Royal College of Physicians expressed the extent of the problem by stating that among 1,000 young male adults in England and Wales who smoke cigarettes, on average about 1 will be murdered, 6 will be killed on the roads, and 250 will be prematurely killed by tobacco (RCP 1983).

CANCER. In countries in which smoking has been a widespread habit, it is responsible for 80 to 90 percent of lung cancer deaths and 40 percent of bladder cancer deaths. Tobacco is responsible for 30 percent of all cancer deaths, including some cancers of the oral cavity, larynx, esophagus, stomach, and cervix.

An important feature in the relation between cigarette smoking and lung cancer is the strong correlation between the duration of regular cigarette smoking and subsequent lung cancer rates. A doubling of duration of regular tobacco use will result in an increase in lung cancer incidence of approximately twenty-fold. This relationship holds particular relevance for projecting the health problems of countries in which substantial increases in tobacco smoking have occurred in the last decade but the full health effects have not yet been felt.

The concept that atmospheric pollution might be an important cause of lung cancer dates back to the 1930s, when it

Table A-1. Mortality Attributable to Smoking, by Region

Region	Deaths per year	Year	Source
United Kingdom	110,700	1988	Health Education Authority 1991
United States	434,000	1988	CDC 1991
Europe[a]	505,000	1985	WHO Regional Office for Europe 1988
Latin America	98,100	1985	USDHHS 1992
Industrial countries	1.7 million	1985	Peto and Lopez 1992
Worldwide	3.0 million	1990	WHO 1991

a. Exlcuding the former U.S.S.R.
Source: See last column.

Table A-2. Disease-Specific Mortality Attributable to Smoking, United States, 1988

Disease	Males	Females	Total
Neoplasm			
Lip, oral cavity, pharynx	4,942	1,460	6,402
Esophagus	5,478	1,609	7,087
Pancreas	2,775	3,345	6,120
Larynx	2,401	589	2,990
Trachea, lung, bronchus	78,932	33,053	111,985
Cervix	n.a.	1,246	1,246
Urinary bladder	2,951	963	3,914
Kidney, other urinary	2,729	363	3,092
Cardiovascular disease			
Hypertension	3,441	2,254	5,695
Ischemic heart disease			
Age 35–64	29,263	9,105	38,368
Older than 64	41,821	27,990	69,811
Other heart diseases	27,503	14,638	42,141
Cerebrovascular disease			
Age 35–64	5,121	4,504	9,625
Older than 64	11,554	5,134	16,688
Atherosclerosis	4,644	3,612	8,256
Aortic aneurysm	5,798	1,435	7,233
Other arterial disease	1,874	1,111	2,985
Respiratory disease			
Pneumonia, influenza	11,580	8,098	19,678
Bronchitis, emphysema	9,670	5,269	14,939
Chronic airways obstruction	29,838	16,884	46,722
Other respiratory diseases	828	690	1,518
Conditions in infants			
Short gestation, low birth weight	344	261	605
Respiratory distress syndrome	351	233	584
Other respiratory conditions	384	277	661
Sudden infant death syndrome	422	280	702
Burns	850	453	1,303
Passive smoking	1,330	2,495	3,825
Total	286,824	147,351	434,175

n.a. Not applicable.
Source: CDC 1991.

was observed that lung cancer rates were higher in cities than in towns. Subsequent investigations that have considered the effect of smoking habits, however, as well as national and international reviews, have led to the conclusion that no more than 10 cases per 100,000 males each year could be ascribed to atmospheric pollution in the high-risk populations and that the proportion of lung cancer attributable to smoking is of the order of 80 to 90 percent.

Oral cancer is a significant problem in South Asia, where the habit of chewing tobacco in the betel quid is common. Oral cancers almost always occur on the side of the mouth where the tobacco quid is kept, and the risk of cancer rises dramatically for those who keep the tobacco quid in the mouth overnight. Approximately 90 percent of oral cancers in this part of the world can be attributed to tobacco chewing and smoking habits (WHO 1984).

CARDIOVASCULAR DISEASES. Approximately 25 percent of ischemic heart disease deaths are due to smoking in countries in which smoking has been a common habit for many years (WHO 1979). The association with ischemic heart disease depends upon age, with the stronger effect for those at a younger age. As for lung cancer, the risk of death from ischemic heart disease decreases upon cessation of smoking.

Smoking is also associated with atherosclerosis, hypertension, and cerebrovascular disease. In addition to mortality, however, there is also significant morbidity associated with tobacco; for example, amputation due to vascular disease in the legs is common.

CHRONIC BRONCHITIS AND EMPHYSEMA. Soon after beginning to smoke, smokers develop a cough and produce more sputum than nonsmokers; respiratory infections tend to increase, and lung function begins to be impaired. Approximately 75 percent of deaths from chronic bronchitis and emphysema are due to smoking. In pure economic terms, bronchitis is probably the most expensive of the smoking-related diseases because of the associated long-term morbidity. There is benefit in cessation of smoking at any stage of bronchitis.

PREGNANCY, WOMEN, AND CHILDREN. Maternal smoking results in slowing fetal growth because of reduction in the oxygen supply reaching the baby through the placenta, to the extent that children born to smoking mothers weigh an average of 200 grams less than those born to abstaining mothers. Tobacco use causes a twofold increase in the risk of spontaneous abortion and is associated with an increased risk of complications during pregnancy and labor. The perinatal risk is increased by 35 percent for women who smoke more than twenty cigarettes per day. It is estimated that more than 8,000 infant deaths each year in industrial countries are caused by parental smoking. The effects of tobacco use by mothers in developing countries, where birth weights are already low and perinatal risk high, have not yet been determined.

Smoking also increases the risk of cardiovascular disease for women who take contraceptive pills. Tobacco use is associated with increased rates of cervical cancer, and tobacco-related substances such as nicotine have been found in the cervical fluid of smokers. Further, natural menopause occurs about two or three years earlier among smokers than among nonsmokers.

PASSIVE SMOKING. The risk of lung cancer in nonsmokers married to smokers is increased 25 to 35 percent as a result of passive ("enforced") smoking, the breathing of other people's tobacco smoke. Children of parents who smoke have an increased incidence of bronchitis and pneumonia (NRC 1986; USDHHS 1986).

NICOTINE ADDICTION. All tobacco products contain nicotine, a powerful drug that causes addiction, that is, the user's behavior is controlled to a considerable extent by the pharmacologic agent. Mechanisms of this addiction are similar to those of heroin and cocaine (USDHHS 1988).

Effects on the Family

A tobacco habit by one or more family members often drains a significant portion of the family income, typically in the range of 1 to 5 percent of the income of a wage earner in both industrial and developing countries. Tobacco habits are more prevalent among the lower socioeconomic groups, and they tend to be the hardest hit financially. The effect is likely to be greater in the poorest developing countries. It has been calculated for Bangladesh that the smoking of only five cigarettes per day would result in a monthly dietary deficiency of approximately 8,000 calories in a poor household, seriously endangering the survival of a large number of children (Cohen 1981). Of course, smoking-related deaths and morbidity, such as debilitating respiratory diseases, also mean a loss of income to

the family. In addition to the effects on the health of the children of a smoking parent, and on that of nonsmoking adult family members, the children are more likely to grow up to be smokers also, with the resulting health problems for themselves, their spouses, and their children. Tobacco use among children is one of the risk-taking activities which appears to be associated with an increased use of alcohol and other drugs.

Effect on the Workplace

Only within the last few years have the consequences of a smoker in the workplace been realized. Studies in the United States (USDHHS 1985) have revealed the following:

- Smokers take 50 percent more sick leave and are 50 percent more likely to be hospitalized;
- Smokers are more than twice as likely to die during their working years (before age sixty-five);
- Smokers have twice as many on-the-job accidents;
- Smokers waste 2 to 6 percent of their working hours because of the smoking ritual;
- Corporations incur increased cleaning, repair, and maintenance costs because of smokers; and
- Nonsmoking workers suffer significant irritation, discomfort, and health risks caused by smokers.

The increased costs for life insurance (approximately 50 percent) and health insurance (30 percent) have been determined by insurance companies, and programs developed to return this money to the nonsmoking employees have served as inducements to promote some nonsmoking company policies in the United States. A West German branch of a U.S. computer firm recently gave nonsmoking employees an extra six days' vacation to compensate for cigarette breaks given year-round to smokers; as a result, 30 percent of the staff gave up smoking. It was estimated that in 1980 an average smoking employee costs an excess of $400 to $800 each year in 1983 values (Kristein 1983).

Effect on the Environment

Although only 0.3 percent of arable land worldwide is used to grow tobacco, most of this land could also be used to grow food and other crops. The reduction in food production associated with the growing of tobacco is likely to be associated with increased prices for food locally and, hence, lower nutritional status in the general population.

The growing of tobacco requires large quantities of pesticides and herbicides throughout most of its growing season. It also depletes soil nutrients at a higher rate than most other crops and requires either fertile soils or the extensive use of commercial fertilizers. In tropical developing countries, which often have poor soils, the result is that either the farmer consumes considerable fertilizer (at a substantial cost to the farmer or the government) or periodically seeks out new cropland, often by deforestation. A significant problem also arises with the misuse of pesticides (purchased in larger-than-usual quantities because of the increased cash profitability of tobacco as a crop) and possible contamination of village water supplies as a result of poor training and lack of education of the farmers, a problem compounded by lack of health services in the area.

Deforestation has been called the most serious environmental problem now facing developing countries. Approximately one-half of tobacco grown is flue-cured; in poor countries without coal, such as Brazil and most of Africa, this means curing by the burning of wood. Farmers are taught the rule of thumb that one hectare of tobacco will need one hectare of wood for curing. In many developing countries areas of tobacco production are easily located by their lack of trees. The increase in erosion, deforestation, and prices of wood for other uses are among the results associated with the curing of tobacco. In response to this problem in Africa, the British-American Tobacco Company (BAT) has initiated a replanting plan, which, however, as yet has not produced a significant reversal of the trend.

It has been estimated that 7 to 11 percent of fire losses in the United States are associated with tobacco smoking, resulting in an annual cost of approximately one-third of a billion U.S. dollars (Kristein 1983). It is reasonable to suspect proportionally higher tobacco-smoking fire losses in developing countries.

Tobacco Production and Consumption

Tobacco products are among the items manufactured most frequently by mankind. Approximately 5 trillion cigarettes are produced each year, or 1,000 cigarettes for each man, woman, and child on earth.

Tobacco Habits

Worldwide, tobacco is consumed in a wide variety of ways, many in combination with other ingredients. Tobacco consumption can be divided into two broad categories, depending on whether it is smoked or not.

TOBACCO SMOKING. The most common form of tobacco use is the manufactured cigarette. This familiar product is made from a blend of as many as 150 lots of tobacco, wrapped most often in paper. The types of tobacco blended to produce the cigarette vary, depending on the regional taste preference; flue-cured tobaccos are popular in North America and most of Europe, whereas dark air-cured types are preferred in France and parts of North Africa and South America. Tar yields also vary, depending on the blend, lower levels generally being found in the industrial countries. Currently, there are about 280 cigarette brands in the United States alone.

Pipe smoking was probably the earliest form of tobacco use and often has had social or ceremonial significance in the local culture. Water pipes of various types are in common use throughout much of the Middle East, South Asia, China, and parts of Africa (IARC 1986). Often, molasses and other ingre-

dients are added to the tobacco mixture. Cigars are made from air-cured and fermented tobaccos and vary considerably in shape and size. Their smaller cousins, cheroots, are made from heavy-bodied tobaccos.

The most common tobacco product smoked in India and neighboring countries is the bidi, made by rolling a small amount of ground tobacco in a temburni leaf and tying it with a thread. In southeastern India, women practice reverse smoking, in which the smoker turns a cheroot around and keeps the lit end inside the mouth. Cloves are added to the tobacco mixture in Indonesia, to create local cigarettes called *kreteks*. Many other areas of the world also produce local tobacco-smoking products, each with its own special characteristic and name.

SMOKELESS TOBACCO. Smokeless tobacco products, consisting of tobacco leaf and a wide variety of flavoring and other ingredients, are used either orally or nasally. In industrial countries, chewing tobacco is produced by shredding tobacco leaf, pressing the leaf into bricks (plugs), or by drying it out and forming twists. Pieces are bit off and chewed or placed between the cheek (or lip) and gum. Snuff, which may be sniffed or placed in the mouth, has a much finer consistency than chew-

Table A-3. Worldwide Tobacco Leaf Production

Country	Production in 1990 (thousands of metric tons)	Annual change between 1980 and 1990[a] (percent)
China	3,019	10.3
United States	737	(1.0)
India	564	2.1
Brazil	444	1.1
Turkey	288	3.5
Italy	205	4.6
U.S.S.R. (former)	200	(3.5)
Indonesia	150	3.6
Zimbabwe	140	3.0
Greece	125	0
Region		
Africa	378	2.8
North and Central America	940	(1.5)
South America	588	0.5
Asia	4,660	6.0
Europe[b]	667	(0.8)
Oceania	14	(3.0)
Global		
Industrial countries	1,791	(1.7)
Developing countries	5,654	5.1
Developing countries (except China)	2,635	1.3
Worldwide	7,446	3.0
Worldwide (except China)	4,427	0

a. Calculated by author. Baseline values at 1980 are averages of 1979–81. Decreases are given in parentheses.
b. Excluding the former U.S.S.R.
Source: FAO 1991.

ing tobacco and is made from powdered or finely cut tobacco leaves. Moist snuff taken orally (dipped) has been used for many years in Sweden and the United States, and it has recently become popular among adolescent males in those countries. Some tobacco companies have begun marketing it in small paper containers, like tea bags.

For centuries, plant products have been chewed by eastern Mediterranean and South Asian population groups. When tobacco was introduced, it was readily incorporated into many of these chewing habits (WHO 1988b). The most common oral use of tobacco is the betel quid, widely used in South Asia and parts of Oceania. It consists of a leaf from the betel vine wrapped around sliced or shredded areca nut, tobacco, slaked lime, and various flavorings. The large number of variations of oral use of tobacco, especially in South Asia, is remarkable.

TOBACCO PRODUCTION. Tobacco is grown in more than 120 countries worldwide, occupying a small portion (about 0.3 percent) of the world's arable land. This proportion, however, is considerably larger in some countries, such as Malawi (3.8 percent), Greece (3.1 percent), Bulgaria (2.7 percent), and Zimbabwe (2.6 percent). About 5 million hectares are under cultivation currently worldwide, with an average yield of about 1,500 kilograms of tobacco leaf per hectare (FAO 1991).

Global tobacco leaf production is given in table A-3. China is the world's leading producer of tobacco (40 percent), followed by the United States (10 percent) and India (8 percent). The majority of the world's tobacco is grown in Asia; 76 percent is produced in the developing countries worldwide.

The dominant trend in tobacco production is the 10.3 percent annual increase in China. Worldwide production of tobacco is increasing by 3.0 percent each year, but if China is excluded from the calculation, production is virtually stable. Production in the United States is decreasing at an annual rate of 1.0 percent per year.

The majority of tobacco leaf produced today is the flue-cured type because of increasing preference for its use in cigarettes. At the current price of tobacco in most countries of $1.50 to $3.50 per kilogram, the value of the world's annual tobacco leaf production can be estimated at $10 billion to $20 billion.

Approximately 85 percent of tobacco leaf grown worldwide is used for cigarettes. There is considerable variation among countries, however. Whereas virtually all tobacco is used for cigarettes in Japan, in the United States about 80 percent is used for cigarettes, 10 percent for cigars, and 10 percent for other tobacco products. In India, about 30 percent is used for making the bidi, 20 percent for chewing, 15 percent for cigarettes, and the remainder for a wide variety of tobacco products; about seven bidi are produced for each cigarette in India (USDA 1988).

Tobacco Consumption

Cigarette consumption is shown by country and region in table A-4. China is the world's leading consumer of cigarettes (31

Table A-4. Worldwide Cigarette Consumption

	Consumption in 1990 (thousands of millions)	Annual change between 1982 and 1990[a] (percent)
Country		
China	1,641	7.2
United States	547	(1.6)
U.S.S.R. (former)	378	(1.5)
Japan	315	0.1
Brazil	164	2.7
Germany	162	1.5
Indonesia	141	6.3
Poland	104	1.5
Italy	96	(1.3)
France	96	1.1
Region		
Africa	199	1.8
North and Central America	695	(1.6)
South America	270	2.0
Asia	2,734	4.6
Europe[b]	923	0.2
Oceania	43	0.2
Global		
Industrial countries	2,299	(0.6)
Developing countries	2,943	4.5
Developing countries (except China)	1,302	1.9
Worldwide	5,242	2.0
Worldwide (except China)	3,601	0.2

Note: Consumption is defined as output plus imports minus exports.
a. Calculated by author. Decreases are given in parentheses.
b. Excluding the former U.S.S.R.
Source: USDA 1988, 1991.

percent), followed by the United States (10 percent), the Commonwealth of Independent States (former U.S.S.R.; 7 percent), and Japan (6 percent). Fifty-two percent of cigarettes are consumed in Asia. Worldwide, consumption is increasing about 2.0 percent per year, with the greatest rise occurring in the developing countries. Cigarette consumption has been decreasing at an annual rate of about 1.6 percent in the United States and 2.5 percent in the United Kingdom since 1982.

Because of increasing health concerns, the preference worldwide has been moving toward cigarettes with filter tips. In China, the percentage of cigarettes with filter tips was 41 percent in 1990, tripling the percentage of 1986. Filter-tipped cigarettes account for more than 95 percent of the cigarettes in Brazil, Germany, Japan, and the United States but for only 87 percent in Italy, 73 percent in Indonesia, 64 percent in Poland, 60 percent in France, and 28 percent in the former U.S.S.R. (USDA 1988).

Health concerns have also had an effect on the tar and nicotine levels of cigarettes. Median tar levels are less than 20 milligrams per cigarette in Germany, Japan, and the United States, but high levels are found in China (26 milligrams per cigarette) and Indonesia (36 milligrams per cigarette). Tar levels in the United Kingdom and the United States have been falling at an annual rate of about 3 percent during the last twenty years (IARC 1986). Due to advances in technology and the fact that less tobacco is needed in filtered cigarettes, the amount of tobacco per cigarette in the United States has been declining by about 1.5 percent per year during the last thirty years.

The value of cigarette production worldwide is difficult to determine because a large component of the price is taxes. Taking an average price of approximately $1.00 for a pack of twenty cigarettes as a crude benchmark leads to an estimate of the retail value of all manufactured cigarettes of $150 billion to $250 billion—a more than tenfold increase over the price of the tobacco leaf alone.

Few countries have carried out national surveys of smoking prevalence, and rates can vary markedly within a country, especially between the urban and rural areas. Limited surveys have been conducted in nearly all countries, however, and can be used to determine approximate national tobacco-use habits (see table A-5). Worldwide, about half of adult males and 10 percent of adult females smoke. The difference in rates between the sexes is largest in the developing countries, particularly in Asia. In a number of European countries, smoking rates among adolescent girls exceed those of the boys.

Higher education levels tend to be associated with lower smoking rates worldwide (Chasov, Oganov, and Glasunov 1984; Pierce 1989). For example, in China the smoking rate of male peasants was 81 percent, whereas that of white- and blue-collar workers was 42 to 58 percent (Tomson and Coulter 1987).

It is estimated that more than 200 million adults in South Asia use smokeless tobacco. In Indonesia and parts of India, the habit is more common among women than men, who prefer to smoke. Smokeless tobacco habits often begin at very young ages, and prevalence rates of 15 to 25 percent for children ten years of age or younger have been reported (IARC 1985).

More than 10 million people use smokeless tobacco in the United States; annual sales amount to approximately $1 billion. The situation is similar in Sweden, where more than 30 percent of the males age sixteen to thirty-five use snuff. Significant use by children younger than six years of age has been reported in some areas of the United States (Rouse 1989).

Tobacco Industry and Promotion

Approximately 5 million hectares are under cultivation for tobacco, 80 percent of which are in the developing countries. The tobacco manufacturing industry processes tobacco leaf into cigarettes, cigars, chewing tobacco, and a wide variety of other products, thereby increasing the value of the tobacco about tenfold. Few businesses are as profitable and as difficult to enter as this industry.

Tobacco Growers

Whereas an average tobacco farm in the United States has about 2 hectares planted in tobacco, in developing countries tobacco is often cultivated on smaller plots of 0.5 to 1.5 hectares. There are about 4 million tobacco farms worldwide. Each hectare yields an average of 1,500 kilograms of tobacco, resulting in an annual global production of about 7.5 million metric tons of tobacco leaf (FAO 1991). From estimates of labor use per hectare (USDA 1986), it can be determined that the average-size tobacco farm could be managed by a single full-time farmer, who would have substantial time left over, if it were possible to spread the workload evenly over the year. Extra hands are typically used at planting and harvesting time, however. Therefore, although tobacco could provide full-time employment for something less than about 4 million farmers, in reality it provides part-time employment for a larger number of farmers and laborers, very often women in developing countries.

It has been reported that 6 million people in India are employed in tobacco growing, and 35 million people are so employed worldwide (*Tobacco International* 1974; FAO, Committee on Commodity Problems 1989). It is relatively easy to see, however, that these estimates are somewhat excessive, because comparison with the number of hectares under cultivation (FAO 1991) shows that there would be more than fourteen farmers per hectare in India and about seven farmers per hectare of tobacco being grown worldwide.

Nearly always, tobacco is grown in rotation with other crops, such as maize, cotton, wheat, and soybeans. In most areas, tobacco is a competitor with food for the arable land. In parts of Greece, Turkey, Malawi, and Zimbabwe, however, the soil is regarded as unsuitable for other crops, and the issue of competition with food crops does not arise.

*Table A-5. **Smoking Prevalence Rates in Adults, 1985–90***

Most populous countries	Males (percent)	Females (percent)
Country		
China	61	7
India[a]	52	3
U.S.S.R. (former)	65	11
United States	32	27
Indonesia	61	5
Brazil	40	36
Japan	66	14
Pakistan[b]	44	6
Bangladesh	70	20
Nigeria	29	20
Global		
Industrial countries	51	21
Developing countries	54	8
Worldwide	52	10

Note: Regional and global estimates are based on population-weighted results of surveys for the most populous countries in each category.
   a. Includes bidi and other forms of smoking.
   b. Includes chewers.
Source: Author's compilation from World Health Organization surveys.

In many developing countries, either the government or the tobacco industry provides considerable support to the tobacco farmers, often in the form of technical assistance and training, logistical support, and soft loans. Benefits of this support are observed beyond the tobacco crop alone, because the supported tobacco farmers also tend to produce superior yields of other crops grown in rotation or concurrently with the tobacco.

Over the years, improvement in agriculture technology has led to a significant rise in tobacco yield per hectare of land. Tobacco production worldwide would be much greater than the present level if it were not for a network of governmental programs to limit the size of the tobacco harvest each year in order to keep the price high enough to provide a reasonable profit for the farmer. A number of subsidies, incentives, and guaranteed price supports and other mechanisms are provided by governments to keep the tobacco-growing industry healthy. Such mechanisms provide excess income to the farmers, giving them an incentive and the means to band together to exert political influence to retain their preferential treatment. Of course, this phenomenon is not restricted to tobacco farmers.

Crop selection for farmers in a market economy is largely based on the maximization of net profits. For farmers in developing countries, a number of other factors also come into play. Tobacco is a labor-intensive crop, and tobacco provides employment for family and community members. Tobacco farmers can be assured of a relatively stable high price for their crops, often in hard currency. And, they do not face the usual problem of needing rapid transport to avoid spoilage—in areas often bereft of even rudimentary services—that is encountered with most food crops. The record-setting tobacco crop in China in 1985 was largely due to an increase in the relative price for tobacco combined with government policy changes giving the farmers greater freedom in planting decisions.

Tobacco provides the farmers with gross returns per hectare that are significantly higher than for all or most other crops, depending on the soil type. Still, considerable costs are incurred in the growing of tobacco. In the United States, in 1985, the cost of growing flue-cured tobacco amounted to 76 percent of the value of the crop produced; 21 percent was for labor; 19 percent for machinery; 10 percent for curing fuel; 10 percent for the plant bed, fertilizer, and pesticides; and the remainder for marketing and inspection fees and other farm management expenses (Grise and Clauson 1985). This excludes the cost of the land. In the United States, 14 percent of the tobacco farms were operated by tenants. Although the relatively high costs incurred in the growing of tobacco in the United States cannot be extrapolated to the world, the need for labor, fertilizers, pesticides, and transport is virtually certain, and these expenses can be estimated to be approximately half of the value of the crop worldwide.

Nevertheless, net receipts per hectare from tobacco often exceed or are close to the gross receipts from most other crops. For example, in India a hectare of tobacco produced a gross return of approximately 8,000 rupees and a net return of 3,000 rupees, whereas cotton and groundnuts produced gross returns of about 2,500 rupees and net returns of 800 to 900 rupees (FAO 1982). In some developing countries, limits are set by the government on prices for food crops in order to provide low-priced food for urban centers; such limits reduce the incentive for farmers to grow food and increase the incentive to grow tobacco. Nearly all the considerable resources used for growing tobacco could easily be used for producing food instead. The generation of hard currency and the fact that tobacco requires very little arable land notwithstanding, tobacco is grown in a number of areas in developing countries where food is in short supply and could be grown. On the basis of the earlier estimates of approximately $10 billion to $20 billion as the value of world annual tobacco leaf production and approximately 4 million tobacco farmers worldwide (if they were full-time farmers), the average tobacco farmer worldwide would receive a gross return of $2,500 to $5,000 and a net return of about $1,300 to $2,500.

Although there has been considerable interest in determining which crops can be substituted for tobacco that would provide a suitable economic alternative for the farmer, this is a complicated issue. It depends on a number of factors, including soil types, climate, local dietary patterns, available manpower, transportation system, crop-destroying pests, local and external market prices, proximity to urban centers, processing plants, and trade centers; in addition there are the more controllable factors of local government policies on price supports, price limits, subsidies, production quotas and limits, and agricultural extension services for tobacco and other crops. Nevertheless, there appears to be sufficient reason to believe that a multinational effort, including governmental policy modifications, could produce a situation in a number of countries in which it would be financially advantageous for farmers to grow food rather than tobacco.

In the short term, however, the number of individuals addicted to tobacco use worldwide, many of whom would be willing to pay exorbitant prices, would indicate that the considerable industry made up of tobacco growing and tobacco processing will continue to exist for many years. It will exist as either a legal or a black-market activity until society norms change sufficiently to produce a tobacco-free generation.

Tobacco Manufacturing Industry

Approximately 45 percent of world cigarette production is controlled by state industries in centrally planned economies, and 14 percent is controlled by state-level tobacco monopolies; the remaining 41 percent is dominated by a few international conglomerates such as the British-American Tobacco Company and Rothman's International, based in the United Kingdom, and the Philip Morris Companies and the R. J. Reynolds Tobacco Company, based in the United States (USDA 1988). The forces which have led to the situation in which cigarette manufacturing is undertaken by a relatively limited number of large enterprises include the highly automated technology used for cigarette production, the need for sophisticated advertising and promotional techniques (in countries that permit advertising), and the high profitability, which provides funds that can be used to diversify and to deploy for political advantage.

In centrally planned economies, excess income produced by tobacco is often used to offset shortfalls in other areas. There is little, if any, price competition among the conglomerates, primarily because of the high taxes on tobacco products, which minimize the effect of any change in the manufacturer's price. And, although they compete vigorously for market shares through advertising and promotional activities, they cooperate in many other areas, including the sharing of manufacturing facilities.

Over the last few years, the conglomerates have diversified extensively—sometimes into related industries such as transport and fuel, to control their costs, and sometimes into food, clothing, and cosmetics. Although it is often said that this diversification was undertaken because of projected future declines in tobacco consumption, there are significant economic reasons for it, related to the limited size of the tobacco market, surplus cash, and the need for continued growth to be economically competitive.

The U.S. cigarette industry is depicted in figure A-2. Of the retail price of cigarettes, about 30 percent goes for taxes, 25

Figure A-2. Cigarette Business in the United States, 1985
(billions of U.S. dollars)

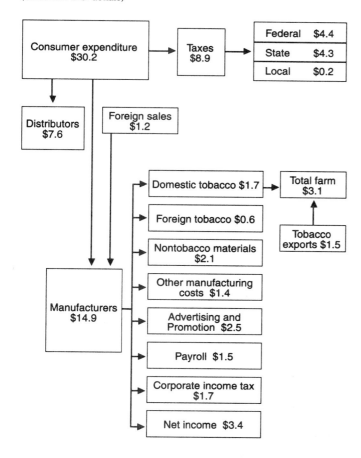

Source: USDHHS 1989b.

percent to the distributors, and the remainder to the manufacturers. A net profit for the manufacturers of approximately 23 percent, after advertising, materials and manufacturing expenses, and taxes are removed, is the source of the considerable pool of funds available for diversification, market expansion, and other activities devised to maintain the position of the tobacco conglomerates.

Tobacco processing and manufacturing is the source of considerable employment—77,000 workers in the United States, 44,000 in Brazil, and 40,000 in Cuba (USDHHS 1992). Ninety-two percent of the cigarettes produced worldwide are consumed domestically (USDA 1988). Many of the tobacco-growing developing countries, however, especially in Africa, supply tobacco leaf but are effectively excluded from participating in the more lucrative industry of manufacturing cigarettes.

The leading exporter of cigarettes in 1990 was the United States, with 27 percent of the world's total, followed by the Netherlands, Hong Kong, Bulgaria, Germany, and the United Kingdom. Hong Kong exports six times more cigarettes than China. In the first half of the 1980s, Bulgaria was the world's leading exporter of cigarettes, mostly to the former U.S.S.R. Since 1989, however, the United States has been exporting more than twice as many cigarettes as any other country (164 billion in 1990). The former U.S.S.R. imports the largest number of cigarettes (65 billion or 15 percent of the total world imports), followed by Japan and France. In 1990, China exported 10.4 billion cigarettes and imported 6.2 billion (USDA 1991).

No large tobacco manufacturing company has yet admitted publicly that tobacco use is harmful to health. The virtual certainty of overwhelming liability suits is probably the primary reason for this position, even though it is indefensible before the battery of extensive evidence that tobacco is clearly the cause of many significant and deadly health problems. The lack of effective public education programs in many developing countries, combined with the efforts of many sectors within some countries which represent vested interests and which therefore do not want to hear about the detrimental effects of tobacco, give rise to the current situation in which tobacco habits are spreading rapidly throughout the developing world.

Advertising and Promotion

Numerous advertising and promotional activities have been undertaken by the tobacco companies. The industry claims that the purpose of advertising is to maintain brand loyalty and to achieve brand switches among smokers, rather than to induce nonsmokers to start, or current smokers to increase consumption. Advertising is viewed by the health sector, however, as one of the strongest inducements to smoking, especially to beginning it, and a ban on advertising is an important milestone in a national tobacco control program. The tobacco industry's arguments are weakened by the fact that they very strongly resist bans on advertising, much more so than other restrictive measures, and that tobacco advertising takes place even in countries where there is only one tobacco company. For example, for many years BAT had a monopoly of the cigarette market in Kenya and still was the country's fourth largest commercial advertiser (Muller 1978). It should be pointed out, however, that advertising is not needed to create a rise in tobacco consumption rates. Smoking increased significantly after World War II in many countries, such as in eastern Europe, where there was no advertising of any products until recently. Often in these countries, tobacco consumption trends were linked to trends in disposable income.

In industrial countries tobacco industry advertising promotes youth, fun, and adventure. In developing countries, it stresses success and a high quality of life. Creation or maintenance of an image is the key strategy in modern advertising. For example, the successful Marlboro cigarette brand advertising has even used a picture of only horses to promote its product—the well-understood image being the free-spirited life of the cowboy. Tobacco advertisements in the industrial countries in the 1960s and 1970s attempted to promote smoking among women by linking it to women's rights, proclaiming in the 1980s, "You've come a long way, baby."

In developing countries, tobacco is often advertised in a manner that would be unacceptable in the industrial countries in which the cigarettes are actually produced. Products have names such as "Long Life," "New Paradise," and "Sportsman," and the advertising is blatant and forceful. In countries in which tobacco's health risks are not widely known, advertising other than that of the tobacco industry's is limited and the general desire to become "Westernized" is extensively promoted in movies, so even a small amount of advertising expenditure can have a dramatic effect (RCP 1983).

A tobacco promotion technique that is becoming increasingly useful to the industry is the sponsorship of sports and cultural events. These activities give the tobacco industry much positive visibility, provide considerable leverage in some sectors, increase contacts with political decisionmakers, and are much more cost-beneficial than direct advertising.

In the United States, about $3.3 billion are spent each year on tobacco advertising and promotion—27 percent for promotional allowances (paid to retailers and others to facilitate tobacco sales), 41 percent for a variety of other promotional activities, 14 percent for newspaper and magazine advertising, 11 percent for outdoor and transit advertising, and 7 percent for point-of-sale advertising (CDC 1990). Tobacco advertising in the United Kingdom amounts to more than 40 million English pounds per year. In Ghana, Malaysia, and Kenya, cigarette advertising accounts for 15 percent , 9 percent, and 5 percent of all advertising, respectively (Wickstrom 1979). The influence exerted on the media industry by this proportion of advertising is, of course, considerable. Eight of twelve American large-circulation women's magazines did not feature a single article on the hazards of smoking for a period of more than twelve years, despite regularly featuring articles on health issues (Whelan and others 1981).

The Role of Governments in Tobacco Promotion

Governments, in virtually all cases, fall short of being homogeneous decisionmaking and implementing bodies. For both market economies and planned economies, they consist of a number of competing factions.

MINISTRY OF HEALTH AND OTHER MINISTRIES. The key governmental factions involved with tobacco are the ministry of agriculture in close alliance with the ministry of finance, and the ministry of health, with, in general, a looser alliance to the ministry of education. The ministry of agriculture and the ministry of finance are nearly always two of the stronger ministries, with the former handling the crucial tasks of keeping the population fed and a large section of the population employed, and the latter handling the allotment of public funds, keeping the economy running, and monitoring the balance of payments. Conversely, although the ministry of health handles an important and politically sensitive function, it is generally thought of as one of the weaker ministries. Further, both the ministry of health and the ministry of education are often viewed by the other ministries as bottomless pits for absorbing public funds.

Ministries are influenced from without by a combination of specific constituencies and broad public opinion. A large group of tobacco farmers with sufficient cash receipts to organize themselves is a political force to be reckoned with. Lucrative taxes from the production, import, export, and sale of tobacco provide a reliable source of government revenues, often providing a significant portion of government income and thereby capturing the alliance of the ministry of finance. In cigarette-producing countries, however, the most important political force to be dealt with is usually the cigarette manufacturing industry, which produces for itself excess revenues that are considerably greater than those available to the farmers.

The specific constituency for the ministry of health largely consists of doctors, who are trained to diagnose and treat disease rather than to deal with disease prevention. Only a small proportion of employees, if any, in a ministry of health is likely to have any training to deal with tobacco control issues, such as legislation, public education, or childhood education. Although it is this ministry which must take the lead in the struggle against tobacco, a considerable portion of its efforts in this regard involve working through other ministries and organizations to achieve the desired results.

Also, rather than disease prevention, the public most often demands more hospitals, clinics, and medicines from the ministry of health. And as always in prevention, the constituency that benefits the most—those who have been prevented from acquiring the diseases and suffering the morbidity and premature death—never know it. Only an epidemiologist can even give an estimate of how many would have been in this group were it not for preventive efforts long ago.

Further, the general public around the world, especially in developing countries, has a difficult time understanding how a tobacco habit today will result in an increased chance (not a certainty) of an internal disease twenty or thirty years later. In some cultures it is not even possible to express this concept in the local language.

TAXES. Governments may tax tobacco in many ways, including taxes on the farmer, based on the amount of tobacco leaf grown; taxes on the tobacco manufacturing companies, based on the numbers of cigarettes or amount of other tobacco products produced; taxes on import of tobacco leaf or manufactured products; and taxes at the time of retail sales. Taxes are a significant factor in the price of tobacco products. For example, they amount to more than 70 percent of the retail price of cigarettes in Brazil, Canada, Denmark, Italy, and the United Kingdom; more than 50 percent in Mexico and Zimbabwe; and about 30 percent of the price in the United States.

Cigarettes provide a considerable portion of government income in many countries—between 1 and 2 percent of total government revenue in Italy, Japan, and the United States; between 2 and 3 percent in Canada and Denmark; and between 3 and 4 percent in Greece and the United Kingdom. In Argentina and Brazil, they provide 22.5 and 7.4 percent of government revenue, respectively (OECD 1985; USDHHS 1992). Tobacco taxes yield more than $1 billion each year for the Indian government.

From a government perspective, taxes on tobacco have a number of advantages. Not only are they a significant source of income for both the central and local governments, they are relatively easy to collect—the tobacco manufacturing companies simply transfer the funds into a government account; a large collection agency is not needed. Further, governments must try to raise tax revenue without too much public resistance. Because tobacco consumption is generally greater in the lower socioeconomic classes, tobacco taxes raise significant revenues from this large public sector voluntarily, with virtually no complaints. Still, tobacco taxes are basically transfers of funds. They do not increase national wealth but are a convenient means of raising government revenue.

SUBSIDIES. As mentioned earlier, governments provide a wide range of direct and indirect supports to promote tobacco, primarily on behalf of the farmers. These include price supports, incentives, production quotas, soft loans, import restrictions, agriculture extension services, foreign-marketing limitations, state trading, and state monopolies. Often a developing country will invest in tobacco cultivation to provide a source of employment and hard currency. In the United States the tobacco price support program cost only $66 million from 1933 to mid-1986; it is estimated that since then, however, it has cost approximately $1 billion (Warner 1988).

EXPORTS AND IMPORTS.. Although significant strides have been taken to control tobacco consumption in the United States, section 301 of the U.S. Trade Act has been used to impose sanctions on countries, such as Japan, South Korea, and Taiwan (China), that have bans on or barriers to imported tobacco products. These countries have subsequently opened their doors to U.S. tobacco to avoid possible trade sanctions. Cigarette advertising jumped from fortieth place to second place in total advertising time in Japan in two years, primarily as a result of American-style advertising campaigns.

In China, producing and marketing are controlled by the government through the China National Tobacco Company, which uses quotas and allocations. China does not export significant numbers of cigarettes, and virtually all imported cigarettes come from Hong Kong. Companies who wish to export cigarettes to China must purchase tobacco leaf grown in China. Foreign tobacco companies were among the first to take advantage of the special economic zones and favored investment conditions recently offered. In 1988, the R. J. Reynolds Tobacco Company opened a $21 million cigarette factory in Xiamen. A German company is building a plant in Hong Kong for the primary purpose of producing cigarettes for China.

Tobacco export and import are a considerable source of currency transfer among countries. Tobacco leaf accounts for 48 percent of the total commodity export earnings for Malawi and 23 percent for Zimbabwe. A comparison of the total value of tobacco imports with that of exports shows that the United States has the most significant positive currency flow (approximately $2 billion per year) from tobacco. Bulgaria, Greece, the Netherlands, Turkey, Zimbabwe, and probably Brazil and Malawi all have a currency flow from tobacco of more than $100 million annually. The former U.S.S.R. incurs the greatest currency loss (approximately $800 million), and China, Egypt, France, Italy, Japan, and Spain have losses of more than $100 million each.

Tobacco Control Strategies

The aim of tobacco control programs is to establish nonuse of tobacco as normal social behavior, and the key to successfully doing so is effective national action. The basic components of a tobacco control program are legislative measures, education and information, and national program organization. These components are described in the following sections and are summarized in table A-6. Focusing on any single component, such as public information alone, however, is unlikely to be successful. The optimal strategy is a comprehensive one in which all important components are integrated; persistent pressure should be maintained across the entire range of activities and greater efforts made in specific areas as priorities dictate and as resources and opportunities make themselves available.

The control of tobacco presents a different problem from most in public health. In this instance, the resistance to action is not an insect vector or a shortage of trained health care workers but rather is often a well-organized international industry with substantial monetary resources and an active media

Table A-6. *Effectiveness, Cost, and Resistance from Tobacco Industry for Components of a National Tobacco Control Program*

Component	Effectiveness	Cost[a]	Resistance from tobacco industry
Legislative measures			
Increased taxation on tobacco products and other economic measures	Very	Inexpensive	Strong
Ban on tobacco advertising	Very	Inexpensive	Strong
Health warnings on tobacco products and advertisements	Marginal	Inexpensive	Moderate
Limiting the amount of harmful substances in tobacco products and specifying the amount on packages	Marginal	Inexpensive	Little
Protecting the rights of nonsmokers[b]	Moderate	Inexpensive	Moderate
Protecting minors	Moderate	Inexpensive	Little
Education and information			
Informing leaders and key social groups	Moderate	Inexpensive	Little
Encouraging medical personnel and public figures to take leadership roles	Very	Inexpensive	Little
Informing the public about health risks	Moderate	Expensive	Little
Encouraging the public, especially children, never to adopt any tobacco habit	Very	Expensive	Little
Encouraging people who use tobacco to stop or decrease use	Marginal	Expensive	Little
Encouraging workers in high-risk industries and pregnant women to stop any tobacco habit	Moderate	Moderate	Little
National program organization			
Establishing a national agency to plan and coordinate the program	Moderate	Moderate	Little

a. For an agency charged with planning and running a national tobacco control program.
b. Such as on public transportation and in restaurants and work sites.
Source: Author.

campaign; in addition the industry provides considerable revenue for governments and the media industry. Therefore, although some national-level strategies have been developed, implementation of these measures often meets with considerable resistance. Continuous evaluation of the strategies of tobacco control and counterstrategies of the tobacco industry form the basis of the modern public health effort in this area.

National tobacco control programs will, of course, differ among countries, depending on a number of factors, including the extent and type of current tobacco use, the extent of current tobacco-associated health problems in relation to other health problems, other pressing social problems, the extent of dependence on the tobacco industry, local cultural attitudes and public perception of the tobacco problem, and the commitment of the national leaders and physicians with respect to disease prevention. In most industrial countries, the diseases associated with tobacco are highly prevalent, and as a result the public is in general agreement with control efforts. In many developing countries, however, cigarette smoking has been common for only a few years, and the resulting health problems are just emerging. The public may therefore not yet see the need for reduction in tobacco consumption.

Legislative Measures

One of the best measures of national commitment to tobacco control is the extent of national legislation. Antitobacco laws vary in rigor and scope: some are stringent, others exert moderate controls, and still others impose only weak restrictions;

some regulate to limit supply and others regulate to limit demand; and some provide a comprehensive range of controls. Further, some laws are enacted on paper but never enforced and hence are only of symbolic importance. The role of legislation in helping to establish nonsmoking as normal social behavior, however, goes beyond its direct effect; legislation expresses public policy and sends a clear message to the population that tobacco use is harmful. The enactment of legislation represents a maturity of public concern about the health effects of tobacco and is a significant milestone in national public health policy. As of 1986, sixty-four countries had enacted legislation, whereas ten years earlier only nineteen had done so (Roemer 1986). Critics say that legislation can be expensive or difficult to enforce. But experience has shown that if the legislation is not leading public opinion by too great a distance and is accompanied by effective education programs, it can be implemented and will serve to change the social environment and hasten the decline of tobacco consumption.

The tobacco industry will vigorously oppose many aspects of legislation, particularly those measures that have been shown to be the most effective—price increases and advertising bans (see table A-6). The industry's opposition is often couched in the form of indirect attacks on the legislation that appeal to people's fears that their right to freedom is being taken away or that "Big Brother" is looking over their shoulder.

Success in achieving the enactment of legislation requires extensive public information efforts and action by citizens to persuade their legislators of the necessity for legislation (Peachment 1984). As the WHO Expert Committee on Smoking Control Strategies in Developing Countries stated in 1983: "It may be tempting to try introducing smoking control programs without a legislative component, in the hope that relatively inoffensive activity of this nature will placate those concerned with public health, while generating no real opposition from cigarette manufacturers. This approach, however, is not likely to succeed. A genuine broadly defined education program aimed at reducing smoking must be complemented by legislation and restrictive measures" (WHO 1983, p. 43).

Admittedly, it is difficult to demonstrate that a single legislative intervention will reduce consumption because so many factors are involved in the use of tobacco. But studies have shown a decline of smoking associated with controls on advertising, introduction of rotating warnings, price increases, and airing of antismoking messages. Multifaceted legislative measures, in conjunction with other tobacco control measures, have resulted in substantial reduction in tobacco consumption, for example in Finland and Norway (Roemer 1987).

Hong Kong, Ireland, Israel, and New Zealand have taken the significant step of banning the importation and sale of smokeless tobacco products. Voluntary agreements between the government and industry, such as those in Denmark and the United Kingdom, have sought to control promotion of tobacco, but problems of interpretation and enforcement of the agreements have led health authorities to call for replacement of those agreements with legislation.

PRICE POLICY. In nearly all countries, the government plays a significant role in setting the price of cigarettes, primarily through taxes, and there is considerable variation in price among countries. For example, in northern and western European countries the retail price of twenty cigarettes varied from $4.17 in Norway and $3.60 in Denmark to $0.80 in France and $1.21 in Italy in 1987. The tax rate on cigarettes in European countries varies from 35 to 87 percent of the retail price, averaging about 53 percent (Roemer 1987). Tax rates are within this range for the majority of countries worldwide.

The most significant reductions in tobacco consumption are apparently produced by a combination of regular price increases of tobacco products and an effective health education program. If either portion is missing, the effect is markedly reduced, and a decrease in tobacco tax rates can easily negate the effect of other components of a tobacco control program.

The effect of raising taxes on tobacco products is measured by the price elasticity of demand, the percentage of change in tobacco consumption associated with a 1 percent increase in price, adjusted for inflation. The price elasticity for cigarettes in North America and western Europe is approximately −0.4; that is, for every 10 percent increase in the price of cigarettes, consumption will fall 4 percent (Townsend and the Advisory Committee 1987; USDHHS 1992). The fall in consumption is greater for teenagers (an elasticity of −1.4 [Lewit 1981]), particularly young males and those in the lower socioeconomic groups. Further, an increase in price will have a greater effect on the decision to start or stop smoking than it will on the

decision to smoke fewer cigarettes; thus it will have an important role in reducing the number starting a tobacco habit.

The strong association between cigarette price and consumption has also been observed in developing countries. For example, in India, cigarette sales declined by 15 percent after the excise tax was more than doubled on the popular manufactured cigarette brands in 1986 (USDA 1987).

An increase in cigarette prices not only affects cigarette consumption; it also results in a switch to lower-priced brands (often unfiltered), to hand-rolled cigarettes, and to other tobacco products, and if excessive it could lead to an increase in bootlegging. Tobacco duties were increased by 39 percent in the Federal Republic of Germany in 1982. By the next year, the sale of name brands had dropped by 17 percent, but the sales of low-priced cigarettes and of tobacco for hand-rolled cigarettes had increased markedly, making up for 60 percent of the decline of sales in name brand cigarettes (Ramstrom 1986). Although increases in cigarette prices are clearly one of the most effective public health tools available to reduce cigarette consumption, only about half of the effect is a real reduction in cigarette consumption, the other half being a restructuring of the market. This problem can largely be solved by market-neutral simultaneous increases in the cost of all tobacco products, with greater proportional increases in the least expensive, such as tobacco for hand-rolled cigarettes, which needs a proportional price increase in relation to cigarettes of more than three to one.

The most frequent arguments against the raising of tobacco prices are that it will lead to a decrease in governmental tobacco tax revenues and that it will increase inflation. In reality, however, an increase in tobacco taxes will cause a rise rather than a fall in tax revenues for a country (Warner 1984; Townsend 1987). The primary reason for this is that although a price increase will result in a decrease in consumption, the decrease in consumption is proportionally smaller than the increase in tax revenues. It has been estimated that a 10 percent increase in the tobacco tax rate will result in a 5 to 8 percent rise in tobacco tax revenues (Godfrey and Maynard 1988; Jones and Posnett 1988). It is obvious that this relationship will not continue to hold if prices are raised to astronomical levels, but they can be raised considerably in all countries before a point of diminishing returns is reached. It must be pointed out also that by price increases, we mean increases above the rate of inflation. If price increases do not keep pace with inflation, consumption will increase and tax revenues will fall.

An increase in tobacco prices could be inflationary, especially if the cost of tobacco items is linked to a cost-of-living index. For this reason, a retail price index excluding the price of tobacco and alcohol products is now calculated by the Commission of European Commodities. An increase in taxes may even be deflationary, however, because taxes take money out of circulation.

BAN ON ADVERTISING. Advertising is the strongest component of the tobacco industry's promotional effort. In the

United States, the tobacco industry puts more than 8 percent of the retail price of the cigarettes directly back into advertising and promotion, an amount in excess of $3 billion annually (FTC 1988; CDC 1990). The magnitude of this financial commitment is perhaps the best evidence that the payoff for the tobacco industry is dramatic. Tobacco advertising has an elasticity of approximately 0.09; that is, for a 10 percent increase in advertising expenditure, the tobacco industry can expect about a 1 percent rise in consumption (Townsend and the Advisory Committee 1987).

As mentioned earlier, the industry claims that the purpose of advertising is only to improve its share of the market, and not to induce nonsmokers to start a tobacco habit. This view has been negated by studies, however, which show, for example, that brand loyalty for cigarettes is higher than for most other consumer products (Tye, Warner, and Glantz 1987) and that the decision of teenagers to start smoking is largely a result of the positive image promoted by the tobacco industry's advertising. Recent advertisements by the R. J. Reynolds Tobacco Company in Europe and the United States have featured the cartoon character "Joe Camel"; targeting of the youth in this campaign was evidenced by a 91 percent name recognition rate in six-year-olds.

The first priority of legislation in this area should be a total ban on tobacco advertising on television, radio, and other mass media. Promotion of tobacco through the industry's sponsorship of sports and cultural events and other indirect advertising should also be restricted. The tobacco industry often evades advertising restrictions by advertising nontobacco products such as clothing, shoes, and lighters, using advertisements that are virtually indistinguishable from earlier tobacco advertisements. A total ban or at least some restriction on tobacco advertising has been enacted in at least fifty-seven countries (Roemer 1987). Of course, it should be mentioned that the former U.S.S.R., China, and some other countries already have complete bans on all commercial advertising; continuing increases of tobacco consumption in those countries is probably related to increases in disposable income and availability of cigarettes.

OTHER TYPES OF LEGISLATION. The placing of health warnings on tobacco product packages is required in at least forty-three countries worldwide (Townsend and the Advisory Committee 1987). The use of strong rotating health warnings has largely solved the problem of the ineffectiveness of a single familiar warning.

Although epidemiological studies indicate that low-tar cigarettes are associated with a reduction in lung cancer rates of approximately 20 percent (Hammond and others 1976), there is no reduction in harmful effect with respect to cardiovascular disease, respiratory function, pregnancy complications, and other diseases. Low-yield cigarettes, however, are used by the industry to promote the erroneous concept that there is such a thing as a safe cigarette. Far from being safe, however, these cigarettes make it easier for youth and women to start smoking. Smokers will change their habits to compensate (such as by inhaling more deeply or smoking more frequently), and the idea itself that these cigarettes may be less harmful leads to the initiation of this habit by large numbers of youth. Further, by giving smokers support for their rationalizing behavior, such cigarettes weaken their will to quit the harmful addictive habit.

Restrictions on tobacco use in public places, such as the banning of smoking or the setting aside of areas for smokers in public places, such as restaurants, public transport, and the workplace, have been enacted in forty-eight countries (Roemer 1987). These restrictions are designed to protect nonsmokers from the effects of passive smoking and to convey the message that smoking is not normal social behavior and can be harmful to nearby nonsmokers. Studies have shown an increase in lung cancer in the nonsmoking wives of smokers that is three and one-half times greater than in the nonsmoking wives of nonsmokers. In fact, some passengers in the nonsmoking sections of airplanes experience nicotine levels comparable to those of individuals in the smoking section. In the United States this has led to the banning of smoking on all internal commercial flights of six or fewer hours.

There has been little resistance from the tobacco industry to legislation enacted to prevent youth from smoking, mostly by sales restrictions and prohibition in schools. The industry is well aware that if one desires to encourage teenagers to do something, just make it illegal until they reach adulthood. Nevertheless, such laws are important because they communicate to the youth that smoking is harmful. When the laws are enforced and supported by strong education programs, the combined effect can be a considerable reduction in the number of young people who start smoking.

In the past, laws concerning sales to minors have been poorly enforced, but recent experience has shown that the imposition of fines in a few well-publicized cases, together with required posting of notices that it is illegal to sell tobacco to minors, can achieve compliance with the laws. Prohibiting or restricting sales of tobacco in vending machines is another measure necessary to prevent sales to minors.

Legislation can also be enacted to eliminate government subsidies of the growing and manufacturing of tobacco. The U.S. and some other governments are against international legislation in the field of tobacco—apparently because of the precedent it would set in further hindering free trade among countries.

Education and Public Information

A common misconception is that people will change their behavior if they are told how dangerous something is. The overwhelming majority of adults worldwide have been informed of the health risks associated with tobacco, but this, by itself, has had little effect in slowing the spread of tobacco habits. Informing populations about the risks is, however, a necessary component of a comprehensive education program; mass media is effective in changing knowledge, attitudes, and beliefs. And although mass media can sometimes influence behavior, individual contact is often necessary to change behavior significantly (Flay 1987).

Some prefer to view the tobacco, alcohol, and drug-control strategy efforts as a situation of supply versus demand, with education leading the effort to reduce demand. The use of this model in the tobacco field, however, is often supported by the tobacco industry, who in general know that their Achilles' heel is legislation and that the industry can easily outspend public education in advertising. Equal resources on both sides of a struggle between advertising and public information to influence the public's perception of tobacco would be theoretically interesting, but the tobacco industry would never agree to a level playing field. The industry strongly resisted the ban on tobacco advertising on television in the United States until the health sector started running television commercials with Brooke Shields showing how socially unattractive smoking was; the industry capitulated shortly thereafter.

KEY GROUPS. The first step in an education program is to inform key groups of the ill effects of tobacco and what should be done (see table A-6). One of the key groups is physicians, who should be persuaded to take leadership roles. If the physicians do not adopt healthy lifestyles, the public will not adopt them either.

THE GENERAL PUBLIC. A cornerstone in a national education program is informing the general public about the risks associated with tobacco. An appeal to fear, however, is ineffective as a long-term information strategy. To be effective, a program must be run for a long time and should be characterized by simple messages on a common theme, affecting society's image of the tobacco user. For an example of highly successful efforts, it is sufficient to observe a few of the tobacco industry's advertising campaigns in industrial countries; these campaigns are well funded, generally involve a variety of medias and extensive visual images, and are of high professional quality. The countering of these images, in the United States, for example, has led to the creation of public information offices which produce similarly high-quality public material, often involving well-known and trusted public figures, that is aimed at establishing nonsmoking as preferable, normal social behavior.

Frequently, the public's perception of risk differs markedly from the epidemiological reality. For example, risk-opinion surveys indicate that the public in the United States views nuclear power, handguns, and motor vehicles as greater risks than smoking (Upton 1982), whereas in reality smoking is far more dangerous: 30 percent of all cases of cancer in the United States are attributable to tobacco use (Doll and Peto 1981). More than one-sixth of all deaths in males over the age of fifteen in India are attributable to tobacco (Gupta 1988). As in Western countries, chronic diseases are the primary cause of adult mortality in India, but whereas tobacco habits are prevalent, other high-risk habits resulting in chronic disease, such as diets high in animal fat and low in fiber, are not common.

One of the few large prospective controlled studies on the primary prevention of cancer was conducted in India. This investigation of more than 36,000 tobacco chewers and smokers showed that a combination of mass media and personal advice led to tobacco habit cessation rates of 4 to 12 percent in three study areas (Gupta and others 1986).

SCHOOLCHILDREN. The most important component in the control of tobacco is childhood education. Health education programs in schools, however, are generally poor worldwide because health is often not a priority and teachers only rarely have training in health education. It is important that schoolchild programs begin at a young age, because by the age of twelve a child's attitudes and skills in health decisionmaking are largely formed. Further, health education should be comprehensive, covering topics from personal hygiene to nutrition, and should not focus only on a single topic such as tobacco.

Over the years, certain strategies in childhood health education have been determined not to work. These include the appeal to fear, in which individuals are told they will get cancer or heart disease if they smoke, and an emphasis on technical information, in which, for example, the aspects of tobacco production and cigarette manufacture are stressed. Often, this latter strategy is counterproductive, leading to experimentation with tobacco. Moreover, the threat of disease and death in far-off years is rarely effective with young people.

A number of comprehensive school-based education programs have been developed, primarily during the last fifteen years. Effective programs consist of two interlinked components—health beliefs and skills development. The beliefs and opinions of the children concerning health should be openly discussed, with small group participation activities whenever possible. The focus should be on susceptibility to problems thought by children to be important; a child is often more concerned about the smell of tobacco smoke or offending others than about the risk of heart disease or cancer. Perceived benefits and barriers to risk-reducing behaviors should also be discussed, with the emphasis on nonuse of tobacco as normal social behavior.

Children also need to develop social resistance skills (to resist peer pressure, poor adult models, advertisements, and mass media), decisionmaking skills, and assertiveness. The setting of lifestyle goals by a child also often forms a basis for resistance of peer pressure in the later childhood years.

Most effective programs use either the existing teachers, older children (peer leaders), or a combination of both, rather than specialized health education teachers. The "child-to-child" program (UNESCO 1988) was designed for use in developing countries and uses older children to teach the younger children, building on a linkage already existing in many of these countries. This UNICEF-sponsored program is used in fifty-eight countries.

Two of the most well known programs in industrial countries are the "Growing Healthy" and "Know Your Body" programs. More than 1 million schoolchildren in the United States are studying "Growing Healthy." Both programs have been shown to reduce the initiation of smoking by more than 50 percent, as well as conferring other health benefits ("Results of the School Health Education Evaluation" 1985; Walter, Vaughan, and Wynder 1989).

SMOKING CESSATION. People continue smoking in the face of overwhelming evidence of its detrimental effects because of the social acceptance of smoking, the addiction, and, where permitted, the constant pressure of advertising. The nicotine in cigarettes is one of the most addictive substances known. There is, however, a wide range in the level of addiction in a smoking population. It has been estimated that about 95 percent of the 37 million Americans who have stopped smoking have stopped on their own with no support groups or other assistance. Still, stopping smoking often requires three, four, or five attempts. Only a small portion of smokers participate in cessation clinics and in the associated research studies.

In the United States, approximately 70 percent of all adults see a physician at least once a year, but only about half of smokers have ever been advised by a physician to stop smoking. Although physicians should play an important role in smoking cessation, the most effective cessation activities involve both physicians and nonphysicians, and frequent contacts with the smokers. Reliance on single methods, such as nicotine chewing gum or counseling, is not as effective as combinations of methods, in which change of the social environment for the smoker is stressed. The average success rate of cessation programs at one year is about 5 to 10 percent (Kottke and others 1988). Routine minimal (30 to 40 seconds) advice to quit smoking, given by physicians and primary health care workers, would produce significant effects worldwide simply as a result of the large number of contacts. Specialized cessation advice for expectant mothers and workers in high-risk industries can easily be incorporated into existing health counseling services.

Tobacco Control Programs

An effective national effort against tobacco normally requires the establishment of a national agency or office to plan and coordinate all aspects of the program. A budget for such a national agency in an industrial country of average size is in the range of $1 million to $10 million. Frequently, the creation of a national group to review the scientific literature and recommend specific national actions to the public is the driving force behind the political will to take the necessary steps. Even though it has been mainly countries in northern Europe and North America that have developed national tobacco control programs, countries such as Chile and India have also taken significant steps in formulating such programs.

In many ways, the war against tobacco is analogous to the war against drugs. Demand-side strategies can help to slow the growth, but supply-side strategies are also necessary in order to reduce consumption dramatically. It should be pointed out, however, that in the United States and most countries, substantially more resources have gone to fighting drugs, which have claimed far fewer lives than tobacco.

The first national-level body to review the evidence against tobacco was the Royal College of Physicians in the United Kingdom, whose first report was published in 1962. This physician-led group drew up recommendations for action and in 1971 established the organization Action on Smoking and Health (ASH) to coordinate voluntary efforts against tobacco

use. In the United Kingdom, smoking among males twenty years and older fell from 52 percent in 1974 to 35 percent in 1986; for females, the corresponding decline was from 41 percent to 31 percent (Pierce 1989). Because of the lack of legislation and poor results from the voluntary agreements with the tobacco industry, the most significant component of the United Kingdom effort against tobacco has been health education.

The comprehensive Tobacco Act was passed in Finland in 1976. This legislation was one of the first and most successful national program actions taken against tobacco; one component of this act obligated the state to set aside 0.5 percent of the tobacco excise tax to combat smoking. In 1975, 40 percent of adult males were daily smokers, and rates had been increasing yearly. But by 1984, there had been a reduction to 33 percent (Leppo and Vertio 1986).

The first report on smoking and health by the U.S. surgeon general in 1964 was an extensive review of the scientific literature, and the key political step against tobacco in the United States. This report was communicated to the public and served as the basis for formulating policy to control tobacco consumption. The series of surgeon general's reports has continued and now numbers twenty-two, and as a set it is the most comprehensive review and analysis of the association between tobacco and health in the world today. In the United States, smoking prevalence among adults fell from 40 percent in 1965 to 29 percent in 1987 (USDHHS 1989a).

Lung cancer mortality (or incidence) rates are perhaps the best marker of significant progress against smoking on the national level. A hard look at the lung cancer mortality trends, however, compels one to conclude that the fight to control this disease worldwide is currently being lost.

In 1985, WHO reported its study of cancer mortality trends covering the period 1960–80 in twenty-eight industrial countries, representing 75 percent of the population of the industrial world. The most dramatic rise in age-adjusted mortality was registered for lung cancer—76 percent for men and 135 percent for women (WHO 1985). Mortality trends for males in selected countries are given in figure A-3. The mortality reductions seen in Finland and the United Kingdom, where comprehensive antismoking campaigns were first implemented, are the strongest evidence of effective national programs.

Economic Analysis and Conclusions

As the debate on the control of tobacco worldwide matures, it is turning more to economic analyses. When the public listens to this debate, it is faced with incomprehensibly large financial amounts on both sides of the issue. In this section the value of the retail market of cigarettes (VRM) is used as a yardstick against which the costs and benefits can be compared.

The Economic Benefits of Tobacco Use

The economic benefits of tobacco can be divided into the following categories:

Figure A-3. **Trends in Age-Specific Lung Cancer Mortality of Males Age 50–54, Selected Countries**

Age-specific death rates per 100,000

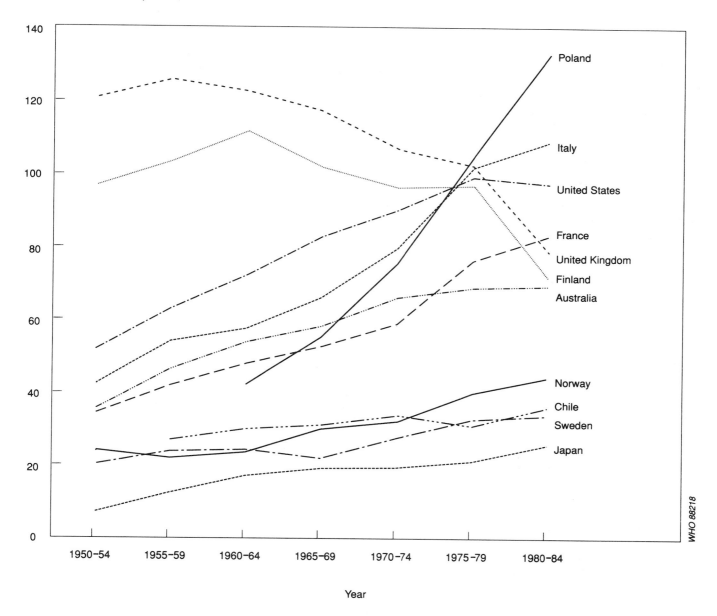

Year

Source: WHO 1987.

- Employment in the tobacco manufacturing industry
- Employment for wholesalers, distributors, and retailers
- Employment in the advertising and media industry
- Income for tobacco farmers
- Taxes raised on tobacco products
- Export of tobacco

For the United States in 1985, about 30 percent of the value of cigarette sales went for taxes, and 25 percent to the distributors. The farmers received about 6 percent of this VRM ($1.7 billion) and a similar amount for tobacco exports. About 5 percent ($1.5 billion) of the VRM was spent by the manufacturing industry for salaries to its workers and 8 percent for advertising and promotion (see figure A-2; USDHHS 1989b). For Canada in 1979, about 50 percent of the VRM went for taxes, 7 percent to the farmers, 17 percent to the retailers and distributors, and 25 percent to the manufacturing industry (Collishaw and Myers 1979). In Northern Ireland in 1984, 74 percent of the VRM was cigarette tax revenue. One-third of the remainder went to retailers and two-thirds to the manufacturing industry as employee earnings (£31.6 million; Nelson

1986). In 1981–82, about 74 percent of the VRM in Egypt was tax revenues; 4 percent went to the retailers and 3 percent to the salary of employees in tobacco manufacturing (£E 21.4 million; Omar 1987).

The export of tobacco leaf is an important source of income for countries such as Brazil, Malawi, Turkey, and Zimbabwe. The majority of cigarettes worldwide are produced with domestic tobacco, however, and the value of the tobacco leaf is typically only 10 percent of the value of the processed tobacco products. The export of tobacco leaf is a source of hard currency transfer from industrial countries to a few developing countries, but on a global scale this is only a small part of the economic picture, less than 1 percent of the value of the worldwide retail cigarette market.

IF TOBACCO WERE ELIMINATED. Consider the changes that would take place if tobacco were eliminated worldwide. As opposed to arguments of the tobacco industry, there would not be an absolute loss equivalent to the total value of all generated salaries and all indirect goods and services associated with the industry and its employees. Rather, the people employed in the tobacco manufacturing industry would move to their "next-best" employment opportunity, with possibly a few being unemployed in the short term and a small number permanently unemployed. Instead of being involved in manufacturing a product that causes harm, they would disseminate to other businesses and the economy would simply adjust. The step down in total income for this group would be no more than a few percent and probably less than 10 percent overall, even when adding in the unemployed. As an example, for Canada, employment in the manufacturing industry has a value of 25 percent of the VRM; the real decrease associated with the elimination of tobacco would be a 2.5 percent drop of the VRM. Similarly, for the people employed in tobacco advertising, distribution, sales, and other businesses related to the tobacco industry, individuals would either have to adjust their businesses or seek "next-best" employment.

For the newspapers and magazines that depend heavily on tobacco advertising, its removal would be, from their perspective, a virtual full loss of tobacco advertising revenues. But again, the resulting staff movement would be to the "next-best" employer. It is conceivable that a small number of newspapers and magazines that depend heavily on tobacco advertising may fail. The cost of those failures, however, is a small price for society to pay for the elimination of tobacco. A rough estimate would be a 10 percent drop from current benefit levels.

If tobacco were eliminated, the farmers would shift to producing the "next-best" crop, often providing considerably less income per hectare. The resources needed for growing a hectare of tobacco, however, such as labor and fertilizer, are considerably greater than those needed for growing the "next-best" crop. If land were not a limiting factor, and it often is not, then the farmer could grow many hectares of another crop with the resources used to grow a single hectare of tobacco. Therefore, although farmers might expect a drop in net return of 50 to 70 percent per hectare from the "next-best" crop, if there were no shortage of arable land the decline in their profits would not be nearly as large.

Tax revenues from tobacco products should not be considered an economic benefit from tobacco because they are merely transfer payments—they do not affect the gross national product or the standard of living. Taxes can be raised in other ways. As mentioned previously, cigarette consumption is greater in the lower socioeconomic groups; perhaps tax revenues could be raised in a more equitable manner.

Thus, if tobacco were eliminated, the real loss in economic benefit to society would be of the order of 5 to 10 percent of the VRM for the industrial countries. In developing countries, even where tobacco-related employment is sometimes considerable, because of the "next-best" employment and crop phenomenon, the economic loss associated with the elimination of tobacco would still be only a small portion of the VRM, probably never nearing 25 percent of the VRM in any country.

It should be noted that the entire VRM came from disposable income paid out by tobacco users. If tobacco were eliminated, nearly all this disposable income of tobacco users and their families would alternatively be used for the purchase of other goods and services—thereby supporting the economic development of those sectors, providing employment and tax revenues, although probably at a lower tax rate. Tobacco is a legal product only because of history. If it were to try to enter the market today, it could not do so because of the built-in safeguards against harmful products that now exist around the world.

The Economic Costs of Tobacco Use

Virtually all analyses of health care expenditure attributable to tobacco have been conducted in industrial countries, and even from a single country the results of those analyses vary considerably. Nevertheless, the broad conclusions are relatively consistent.

The costs of tobacco use are often categorized into one of three groups:

- Direct health care costs—the costs of treating the diseases attributable to tobacco
- Indirect costs of lost productivity—lost income because of illness and premature death attributable to tobacco
- Nonmedical costs—including accidental fires and the loss of wood for the curing of tobacco

For the United States, direct health care costs associated with smoking were estimated in 1982 to be $16 billion (7 percent of the national total health care costs and 73 percent of the VRM) in 1980 (Rice and Hodgson 1983). The corresponding estimate of indirect mortality and morbidity cost was $26 billion (118 percent of the VRM). The Office of Technology Assessment of the U.S. Congress estimated the direct health care costs to be $22 billion (70 percent of the VRM) and indirect costs of lost productivity to be $43 billion (140 percent of the VRM) for 1985, but the office put a wide range on the possible total—from $38 billion to $95 billion (U.S. Congress 1985). In both analyses, the indirect costs alone were greater than the retail value of the cigarettes sold, or the VRM. Economic costs of tobacco have also been calculated separately for six states of the United States and for New York City; for these areas either the total of direct and indirect costs or the indirect costs alone exceeded the VRM (Shultz 1986).

For Canada in 1979, direct health care costs were estimated to be $1.7 billion (Canadian), or 60 percent of the VRM; lost income due to premature mortality was estimated to be $3.3 billion (Canadian), or 110 percent of the VRM; and fire damage was estimated to be $85 million (Canadian), or 3 percent of the VRM (Collishaw and Myers 1979). For Northern Ireland in 1984, the cost to the individual smoker and family was estimated to be $271 million, or 137 percent of the VRM; and the cost to the employer, $135 million, or 68 percent of the VRM (Nelson 1986). For Egypt, direct health care costs associated with tobacco use were estimated in 1982 to be $151 million, or 17 percent of the VRM; and indirect costs of lost productivity, approximately $78 million, or 9 percent of the VRM (Omar 1987). Also, Egypt had to pay an amount equal to 16 percent of the VRM to import foreign cigarettes and the tobacco leaf and other materials to make domestic cigarettes.

Although there is wide variation among countries, it is possible to conclude that in industrial countries in which smoking has been common for many years, the total of the direct health care costs and the indirect costs of lost productivity are significantly greater than the value of the retail cigarette market, and that either the direct cost or the indirect cost, taken alone, is likely to be at least two-thirds of the value of this market. In developing countries, the costs of tobacco use are directly linked to the proportion of disease attributable to tobacco, which in turn is directly associated with the length of time of significant tobacco consumption in the country. The costs in these countries will continue to rise in the next twenty to twenty-five years and will ultimately reach the same levels as in the industrial world.

The previous cost analysis does not take into account that in the absence of tobacco, people will still die and thus incur health costs, although years later. Although tobacco-associated diseases tend to be more expensive to treat than other competing causes of death at the same age, health costs for more elderly individuals would also be more expensive on average. An analysis in Switzerland included a comparison of the health care costs of a smoking population with those of a hypothetical matched nonsmoking population; the costs were virtually identical (Leu and Schaub 1985). It should also be pointed out that direct health care costs are resources that could be directed to other uses and are therefore not real economic losses to society. The indirect costs of lost productivity, however, are real losses to society: contributions of energy and knowledge, often in the years of peak productivity and income, have been wasted.

I conclude that the dominant economic cost of tobacco use in industrial countries is the indirect one of lost productivity, which is approximately two-thirds of the value of the retail cigarette market, or larger. Male smokers are more than twice as likely to die during their working years (before age sixty-five) than nonsmokers (Mattson, Pollack, and Cullen 1987). The cost in developing countries is likely to reach that same level, at a rate which depends on the twenty to twenty-five-year lag time in health problems after the start of considerable tobacco use among the population.

As mentioned previously, a number of governments subsidize tobacco growing or manufacture through a wide variety of measures. Elimination of these subsidies would free these government resources.

There are no reliable estimates of the value of the wood consumed for the curing of tobacco worldwide, but the value is almost certainly in excess of $1 billion. And the price of recovery from desertification is probably also of considerable magnitude—if, indeed, it is possible at all in those areas with insufficient rainfall. Further, if the wood were not used for curing, much of it would probably enter the marketplace and thereby reduce the price of fuel for the general public.

Each year about 3 million premature deaths worldwide are due to tobacco. This tobacco is grown on 5 million hectares of land. Hence, it can be estimated that each seven hectares of tobacco grown will result in approximately four deaths each year: one death from lung cancer, one death from ischemic heart disease, one death from another cancer or cardiovascular disease, and one death from a respiratory or other disease.

Conclusions

When all the economic costs and benefits of tobacco use are summarized and compared, the single element that emerges as determining the conclusion is the simple fact that male smokers are more than twice as likely to die during their working years (before age sixty-five) than nonsmokers. The energy and productivity of these people have been wasted. If tobacco were eliminated worldwide, virtually all other economic concerns related to this event would either be of a much smaller order of magnitude, or the system would simply adjust—individuals would seek employment elsewhere, farmers in developing countries would grow food rather than tobacco, and taxes would be raised by other means.

Of course, the real reason for reducing tobacco consumption is disease and suffering, not economics. It is virtually impossible to put a value on life or suffering. Whatever amount we are willing to pay to keep ourselves alive and healthy is the value of health. On top of the economic loss to society due to tobacco, one must consider the immeasurable suffering and loss deriving from the premature death of millions of individuals.

The control of tobacco is one of the most important public health issues facing mankind, if not the most important. Future generations will look back and wonder why it took so long for us to ban such an obvious hazard.

References

CDC (Centers for Disease Control). 1990. "Cigarette Advertising—United States, 1988." *Morbidity and Mortality Weekly Report* 39(16):261–65.

———. 1991. "Smoking-Attributable Mortality and Years of Potential Life Lost—United States, 1988." *Morbidity and Mortality Weekly Report* 40(4):62–71.

Chasov, E. I., R. G. Oganov, and I. S. Glasunov. 1984. "Prevention of Diseases by Annual Screening of the Population" (in Russian). *Sovietskaja Sdravochranenie* 10:3–6.

Cohen, Nicholas. 1981. "Smoking, Health, and Survival: Prospects in Bangladesh." *Lancet* 1:1090–93.

Collishaw, N. E., and G. Myers. 1984. "Dollar Estimates of the Consequences of Tobacco Use in Canada, 1979." *Canadian Journal of Public Health* 75:192–99.

Doll, Richard, and Richard Peto. 1981. "The Causes of Cancer: Quantitative Estimates of Avoidable Risks of Cancer in the United States Today." *Journal of the National Cancer Institute* 66:1191–1308.

FAO (Food and Agriculture Organization). 1982. "The Economic Significance of Tobacco." ESC: Misc. 82/1. Rome.

———. 1988. *Production Yearbook 1987*. Rome.

———. 1991. FAO *Quarterly Bulletin of Statistics* 3(4), p. 61.

FAO (Food and Agriculture Organization), Committee on Commodity Problems. 1989. "The Economic Significance of Tobacco." CCP:89/17. Rome.

Flay, B. R. 1987. "Mass Media and Smoking Cessation: A Critical Review." *American Journal of Public Health* 77:153–60.

FTC (Federal Trade Commission). 1988. "Report to Congress Pursuant to the Federal Cigarette Labeling and Advertising Act, 1986." Washington, D.C.

Godfrey, C., and A. Maynard. 1988. "Economic Aspects of Tobacco Use and Taxation Policy." *British Medical Journal* 297:339–43.

Grise, V. N., and A. Clauson. 1985. "Costs of Producing and Selling Flue-Cured Tobacco." Tobacco Outlook and Situation Report. U.S. Department of Agriculture, Economic Research, Washington, D.C.

Gu, X. Y., and M. L. Chen. 1982. "Vital Statistics, Health Services in Shanghai County." *American Journal of Public Health* 72:19–23.

Gupta, P. C. 1988. "Health Consequences of Tobacco Use in India." *World Smoking and Health* 13:5–10.

Gupta, P. C., F. S. Mehta, J. J. Pindborg, and others. 1986. "Intervention Study for Primary Prevention of Oral Cancer among 36,000 Indian Tobacco Users." *Lancet* 1:1235–39.

Hammond, E. C., L. Garfinkel, H. Seidman, and E. A. Lew. 1976. "Tar and Nicotine Content of Cigarette Smoke in Relation to Death Rates." *Environmental Research* 12:263–74.

Health Education Authority. 1991. *The Smoking Epidemic—Counting the Cost in England*. London.

IARC (International Agency for Research on Cancer). 1985. *Tobacco Habits Other Than Smoking: Betel-Quid and Areca-Nut Chewing, and Some Related Nitrosamines*. IARC Monographs on the Evaluation of the Carcinogenic Risk of Chemicals to Humans 37. Lyons.

———. 1988. *Tobacco Smoking*. IARC Monographs on the Evaluation of the Carcinogenic Risk of Chemicals to Humans 38. Lyons.

Jones, A., and J. Posnett. 1988. "The Revenue and Welfare Effects of Cigarette Taxes." *Applied Economics* 20:1223–32.

Kottke, T. E., R. N. Battista, G. H. DeFriese, and M. L. Brekke. 1988. "Attributes of Successful Smoking Cessation Interventions in Medical Practice—A Meta-analysis of 39 Controlled Trials." *JAMA* 259:2882–89.

Kristein, M. M. 1983. "How Much Can Business Expect to Profit from Smoking Cessation?" *Preventive Medicine* 12:358–81.

Leppo, K., and H. Vertio. 1986. "Smoking Control in Finland: A Case Study in Policy Formulation and Implementation." *Health Promotion* 1:5–16.

Leu, R. E., and T. Schaub. 1985. *Smoking and Health Care Costs: Plus or Minus?* Proceedings of the 5th World Conference on Smoking and Health, Winnipeg, Canada, 1983. Vol. 1. Canadian Council on Smoking and Health, Ottawa.

Lewit, E. M., D. Coate, and M. Grossman. 1981. "The Effects of Government Regulation on Teenage Smoking." *Journal of Law and Economics* 24:545–69.

Mattson, M. E., E. C. Pollack, and J. W. Cullen. 1987. "What Are the Odds That Smoking Will Kill You?" *American Journal of Public Health* 77:425–31.

Muller, Mike. 1978. *Tobacco and the Third World: Tomorrow's Epidemic?* London: War on Want.

Nelson, Hugh. 1986. *The Economic Consequences of Smoking in Northern Ireland: A Cost-Benefit Analysis of Tobacco Production and Use in the Province*. Belfast: Action on Smoking and Health (Northern Ireland) and Committee of the Ulster Cancer Foundation.

NRC (National Research Council). 1986. *Environmental Tobacco Smoke: Measuring Exposures and Assessing Health Effects*. Washington, D.C.: National Academy Press.

OECD (Organisation for Economic Co-operation and Development). 1985. *Measuring Health Care, 1960–1983*. OECD Social Policy Studies 2. Paris.

Omar, Sherif. 1987. *The Economic Consequences of Smoking in Egypt*. Cancer Institute, Cairo University, Cairo.

Omran, A. R. 1971. "The Epidemiologic Transition: A Theory of the Epidemiology of Population Change." *Milbank Memorial Fund Quarterly* 4:509–38.

Peachment, Allan. 1984. "Learning from Legislative Disasters: The Defeat of the Western Australian Government's Tobacco (Promotion and Sales) Bill." *Medical Journal of Australia* 140(8):482–85.

Peto, Richard, A. D. Lopez, J. Boreham, M. Thun, and C. Heath. 1992. "Mortality from Tobacco in Developed Countries: Indirect Estimation from National Vital Statistics." *Lancet* 339:1268–78.

Pierce, J. P. 1989. "International Comparisons of Trends in Cigarette Smoking Prevalence." *American Journal of Public Health* 79:152–59.

Ramstrom, L. M. 1986. "Worldwide Changes and Tends in Cigarette Brands and Consumption," In D. G. Zaridze and Richard Peto, eds., *Tobacco: A Major International Health Hazard*. IARC Scientific Publications 74. International Agency for Research on Cancer, Lyons.

RCP (Royal College of Physicians). 1983. *Health or Smoking?* London: Pitman.

"Results of the School Health Education Evaluation." 1985. *Journal of School Health* 55:295–355.

Rice, D. P., and T. A. Hodgson. 1983. "Economic Costs of Smoking: An Analysis of Data for the United States." Paper presented at Allied Social Science Association Annual Meetings, San Francisco, December 28.

Roemer, Ruth. 1986. *Recent Developments in Legislation to Combat the World Smoking Epidemic*. World Health Organization, Geneva.

———. 1987. *Legislative Strategies for a Smoke-Free Europe*. Smoke-Free Europe 2. World Health Organization, Copenhagen.

Rouse, B. A. 1989. "Epidemiology of Smokeless Tobacco Use: A National Study." *Journal of the National Cancer Institute* 8:29–33.

Shultz, J. M. 1986. *Smoking-Attributable Mortality, Morbidity, and Economic Costs* (SAMMEC). Center for Nonsmoking and Health, Minnesota Department of Health, Minneapolis.

Tobacco International. 1974. 186(4):717.

Tomson, D., and A. Coulter. 1987. "The Bamboo Smoke Screen: Tobacco Smoking in China." *Health Promotion* 2:95–108.

Townsend, Joy. 1987. "Economic and Health Consequences of Reduced Smoking." In A. Williams, ed., *Health and Economics*. New York: Macmillan.

Townsend, Joy, and the Advisory Committee on Health Education of Finland. 1987. *Tobacco Price and the Smoking Epidemic*. Smoke-Free Europe 9. World Health Organization, Copenhagen.

Tye, J. B., K. E. Warner, and S. A. Glantz. 1987. "Tobacco Advertising and Consumption: Evidence of a Causal Relationship." *Journal of Public Health Policy* 8:492–508.

UNESCO (United Nations Educational, Scientific, and Cultural Organization). 1988. *Child-to-Child: Another Path to Learning*. UNESCO Institute for Education Monograph 13. Hamburg.

United Nations. 1989. *World Population Prospects 1988*. Population Studies 106. New York.

Upton, A. C. 1982. "The Biological Effects of Low-Level Ionizing Radiation." *Scientific American* 246(2):29–37.

USDA (U.S. Department of Agriculture). 1986. *Economic Indicators of the Farm Sector, Production and Efficiency Statistics, 1984*. ECIFS 4-4, ERS. Washington, D.C.

———. 1987. *World Tobacco Situation*. Circular FT-4-87. Foreign Agricultural Service, Washington, D.C.

———. 1988. *World Tobacco Situation*. Circular FT-8-88. Foreign Agricultural Service, Washington, D.C.

———. 1991. *World Tobacco Situation*. Circular FT-8-91. Foreign Agricultural Service, Washington, D.C.

USDHHS (U.S. Department of Health and Human Services). 1985. *A Decision Maker's Guide to Reducing Smoking at the Worksite*. Office of Disease Prevention and Health Promotion, and Office on Smoking and Health, Washington, D.C.

———. 1986. *The Health Consequences of Smoking: Involuntary Smoking*. Report of the Surgeon General. DHHS publication (CDC)87-8398. Office on Smoking and Health, Washington, D.C.

———. 1988. *The Health Consequences of Smoking: Nicotine Addiction*. Report of the Surgeon General. DHHS publication (CDC)88-8406. Office on Smoking and Health, Washington, D.C.

———. 1989a. *Reducing the Health Consequences of Smoking: 25 Years of Progress*. Report of the Surgeon General. DHHS publication (CDC)89-8411, Office on Smoking and Health, Washington, D.C.

———. 1989b. *Smoking, Tobacco, and Health: A Fact Book*. Office on Smoking and Health, Washington, D.C.

———. 1992. *Smoking and Health in the Americas*. A 1992 report of the Surgeon General, in collaboration with the Pan-American Health Organization. DHHS publication (CDC)92-8419. Office on Smoking and Health, Washington, D.C.

U.S. Office of Technology Assessment Health Program, Office of Technology Assessment. 1985. "Smoking-Related Deaths and Financial Costs."

Walter, H. J., R. D. Vaughan, and E. L. Wynder. 1989. "Primary Prevention of Cancer among Children: Changes in Cigarette Smoking and Diet after Six Years of Intervention." *Journal of the National Cancer Institute* 81:995–99.

Warner, Kenneth. 1984. "Cigarette Taxation: Doing Good by Doing Well." *Journal of Public Health Policy* 5:312–19.

———. 1988. "The Tobacco Subsidy: Does It Matter?" *Journal of the National Cancer Institute* 80:81–83.

Whelan, E. M., M. J. Sheridan, K. A. Meister, and B. A. Mosher. 1981. "Analysis of Coverage of Tobacco Hazards in Women's Magazines." *Journal of Public Health Policy* 2:28–35.

WHO (World Health Organization). 1979. *Controlling the Smoking Epidemic*. Technical Report 636. Geneva.

———. 1980. "Sixth Report on the World Health Situation, 1973–1977. Part I: Global Analysis." Geneva.

———. 1983. *Smoking Control Strategies in Developing Countries*. Technical Report 695. Geneva.

———. 1984. "Control of Oral Cancer in Developing Countries." *Bulletin of the World Health Organization* 62:817–30.

———. 1985. "Cancer in Developed Countries: Assessing the Trends." *World Health Organization Chronicle* 39:109–11.

———. 1986. *Tobacco or Health*. EB77/1986/REC/1. Geneva.

———. 1987. *1987 World Health Statistics Annual*. Geneva.

———. 1988a. "A 5 Year Action Plan: Smoke Free Europe." World Health Organization, Regional Office for Europe, Copenhagen.

———. 1988b. *Smokeless Tobacco Control*. Technical Report 733. Geneva.

———. 1991. "Tobacco-Attributable Mortality: Global Estimates and Projections." *Tobacco Alert* 4–5.

Wickstrom, B. O. 1979. *Cigarette Marketing in the Third World: A Study of Four Countries*. University of Gothenburg, Gothenburg, Sweden.

Appendix B

Reducing Mortality in Children under Five: A Continuing Priority

Carl E. Taylor and Vulmiri Ramalingaswami

In recent years, several international agencies have given highest priority to supporting programs for child survival and development in developing countries. This emphasis is justified and should continue at least until the year 2000. Child mortality is still the world's largest public health problem in numbers of individuals dying and years of life lost. The development of children determines the quality of future populations. Another reason children deserve priority is because child health interventions tend to be the most cost-effective health area activities in all parts of the world. In this appendix we will focus on selected issues relevant to the implementation of practical programs.

Some specific justifications for maintaining priority attention on the problems of children are the following:

• Children under five years of age make up about 15 percent of the population in most developing countries, and women in the reproductive age group make up about 20 percent. In poor countries, young children have higher mortality rates than any other age group—30 to 40 percent. Morbidity and malnutrition are also high. Children in unhygienic environments have to cope with the synergistic problems of numerous infections, to which they have to develop immunity at the same time that they are adapting nutritionally to rapid growth on limited diets. The United Nations Children's Fund (UNICEF) annual State of the World's Children reports have clearly demonstrated the many dimensions of the massive need. Estimates and projections of mortality in the present collection provide detailed information on the relative importance of the principal diseases. It is worth noting here that the World Health Organization (WHO) in conjunction with UNICEF has assigned highest priority to immunizable diseases, the pneumonia-diarrhea complex, malnutrition, perinatal problems, and conditions associated with maternal health.

• Both nationally and internationally no appeal for funds and support can match the donor generosity stimulated by children in need. The pathos of a simple picture of a suffering child stirs an eagerness to help. Individual responsive-ness to the basic needs of children is greatly magnified by group response to effective messages in the public media. Communities seem more willing to correct social problems when children are involved than to do so for adults. Political leaders know their image among constituents can be improved by showing concern for the needs of children. In the past ten years, UNICEF's Child Survival and Development Revolution (CSDR) has stimulated unprecedented levels of international support, public awareness, and concern.

• In more rapidly developing countries attention is shifting from straightforward concern about child survival to child development. This includes efforts not only to improve health and nutrition but also to promote intellectual development and learning. Obviously, such child development activities must give intersectoral emphasis to education and strengthening the capacity and role of mothers. The goal is not only that all children should be healthy but that they should be educated.

• Child health interventions have a proven record demonstrating that their implementation is feasible in national programs. It has been repeatedly shown that a cluster of low-cost interventions can dramatically improve survival (UNICEF 1988). The methods can be implemented at home or in peripheral health facilities. They can often be applied best through community participation, and they have greatest long-term sustainability when they become incorporated into local cultural patterns. Education about a definable, locally relevant group of child care practices can produce continuing change in health habits that strengthens a general sense of self-reliance.

• Because of national expectations that international support for CSDR will continue, developing countries have made long-term commitments. If international donors were to reduce support for child health and shift their attention to adult problems, a serious loss of credibility would occur as mortality increased. Many countries have already become skeptical of international donor support because of its "unreliability." Continuity should be maintained until the promised potential has been fulfilled. For instance, very large amounts of international funds are making rapid improvements in child immunization levels. If these funds are reduced after the global targets are achieved, there is no way that costs can be covered by national budgets. It has been calculated that about half of the poor African and Asian countries about whom data were available will not be able to finance present types of immunization programs even using the most optimistic projections of economic growth up to the year 2000 (Rosenthal 1989). Any slackening of international funding will raise the dismaying prospect of future epidemics in unimmunized populations, a situation reminiscent of the collapse of malaria eradication efforts in the 1960s. Alternative and less expensive means of running immunization programs are available as a routine part of primary health care. Instead of expensive campaigns, it has been shown that periodic "pulse" activities are helpful in increasing coverage.

• A global ethic of concern for children seems to be developing. It is fragile, but long-term commitments should follow passage of the United Nations Convention on the Rights of the Child. Promoting equity and disparity reduction are difficult national and international goals, but these concepts are more likely to be implemented in programs for children than in most other activities. All children deserve everything that their society and international resources can provide, because children represent the future in every country of the world.

• Calculations of the cost-effectiveness of child health measures almost automatically look good in comparison with health care for adults. This is usually most apparent when calculations are based on years of life saved.

Some Priority Interventions

Recent experience has demonstrated that the following interventions deserve priority consideration in practical programs.

Immunizations

Rapid progress is being made in worldwide efforts to immunize children against the six diseases covered by WHO's Expanded Programme on Immunization (EPI): measles, poliomyelitis, diphtheria, tetanus, pertussis, and tuberculosis. The best prospects for sustainable control are in situations where good primary health care infrastructure has been built up. Immunizations as part of primary health care should continue to have high priority until herd immunity is acceptably high and immunization services can be integrated into continuing preventive services. As these services are stabilized, other types of immunizations can be added according to local priorities. For instance, as indicated in chapter 15 of this collection, frequent transmission of the hepatitis B virus to babies from mothers who are type B carriers and the availability of an effective hepatitis B vaccine make this immunization a high priority in

some Asian countries. It may be possible to break the cycle of transmission and prevent the long-term sequelae of liver cancer and cirrhosis.

Diarrheal Diseases

The second priority intervention with which considerable progress has been made in the Child Survival and Development Revolution is in the use of oral rehydration therapy (ORT) for watery diarrhea. In the 1980s 4 million deaths of children from diarrhea were estimated to occur each year before current programs were implemented, and that number can probably be halved by the use of ORT. Dehydration can be prevented by early home treatment through the use of simple local adaptations of traditional preparations, particularly those that are cereal-based (Taylor and Greenough 1989). As with immunizations, the most effective ORT programs are where primary health care infrastructure provides backstopping and support. Packets of oral rehydration salts, intravenous fluids, antibiotics, and other appropriate treatment should be used by health facilities for severe cases of dysentery and chronic diarrhea. It is especially necessary to increase efforts to stop the massive overuse of ineffective medicines. A growing priority is recognition of the close linkage between diarrhea and malnutrition. Diarrhea is one of the most important causes of childhood malnutrition, and nutrient loss can be partially compensated for by appropriate feeding during and after illness.

Diarrhea programs are also beginning to pay increasing attention to the promotion of preventive strategies. The World Health Organization's Diarrhoeal Diseases Control Program has sponsored useful analyses comparing the potential effect of more than twenty interventions (Feachem 1986). Measles, which can be prevented by immunization, frequently causes diarrhea. When it becomes available, rotavirus immunization will probably be highly cost-effective. Promotion of breastfeeding during the first four to six months of life, improved personal and domestic hygiene through hand washing and cleanliness, and better preparation and preservation of food are practical and low-cost methods of diarrheal disease prevention. Sanitary disposal of excreta and improving the availability of water are of continuing importance. Particular attention needs to be paid to the safe disposal of stools of children because they have the highest infection rates.

Acute Respiratory Infections

Ranking with diarrhea in importance as a cause of death of children are pneumonia and other infections of the lower respiratory tract. Although little has been done yet in large-scale application of new methods of control, it is possible now to affirm with some assurance that approximately half of the 4 million deaths of children from acute respiratory infection (ARI) each year can be prevented with available methods of case management. Immunizations will prevent of some of these deaths. In addition to the vaccines for measles and pertussis, new pneumococcus and hemophilus vaccines will probably become available in a few years, but they may not be affordable in public programs for some time. Priority attention to the implementation of national programs for improved case management of lower respiratory tract infections in children is overdue (Gadomski 1990). Methods have been developed to train village health workers to make early diagnosis of pneumonia in children with cough by counting respirations and observing difficult breathing. Antibiotic treatment can then be started promptly by the health worker using a simple protocol. As with diarrheal diseases, this strategy requires an effective primary health care infrastructure to provide technical backstopping and professional support. A significant effort is needed to stop the overuse of antibiotics for upper respiratory tract infections. Priorities for prevention have not yet been adequately defined. Improved maternal nutrition will increase resistance in babies of low birth weight who have extremely high neonatal pneumonia mortality rates. The severity of respiratory infections in children seems to be influenced particularly by parents who smoke and by smoke pollution in homes and urban areas. General factors such as crowding and poor housing also seem to be important in transmission. More evidence is needed on practices such as swaddling, which is common in some countries (for example, China and Turkey) and may interfere with respiratory function in newborn babies.

Malaria

Globally, malaria control has long been given high priority because malaria is an important killer of children and a cause of chronic disability and debility at all ages. Despite the collapse of the worldwide program of malaria eradication, control of malaria is one of the great success stories of international health. The massive reduction in mortality and prevalence in Asia and the Americas has saved millions of lives, although control has proved difficult in Africa and parts of Southeast Asia, where resistant strains of mosquitoes and parasites continue to spread. Much of the improvement has resulted from general environmental and socioeconomic change rather than specific health interventions. Malaria remains one of the greatest challenges both for the development of technology and for a delivery system (Breman and Campbell 1988).

Protein-Energy Malnutrition

The high prevalence of protein-energy malnutrition is indicated by the UNICEF estimate that 29 percent (165 million) of the world's children are malnourished according to standard weight-for-age criteria. Of these, 98 million children are in South Asia. The prevalence of maternal malnutrition is most evident in the high proportion of babies with low birth weight. It is estimated that about 16 percent of all babies born each year worldwide, or 20 million, weigh less than 2,500 grams at birth. Control of protein-energy malnutrition continues to deserve high priority because of its effect on child development and because of synergistic two-way interactions with infec-

tions. In many situations it has become evident that simply providing food is not sufficient to reduce malnutrition and that interventions to control infections are also needed. Most studies have focused on single nutritional interventions. Food availability, food affordability, and food use in the family are all key issues that need to be addressed. It is necessary now to develop understanding of how to integrate services adapted to causal patterns in specific situations.

Maternal and Perinatal Health Problems

The fact that 99 percent of pregnancy-related deaths in the world occur in developing countries is clear evidence that many of them could be prevented (World Bank 1987). For both mothers and children, pregnancy and delivery are periods of considerable risk due to the following types of problems: hemorrhage, sepsis, eclampsia, obstructed labor, and complications of abortion. Perinatal mortality among the poor is largely determined by delivery care and the maturity of the fetus, which is indicated best by the birth weight. It is estimated that 2.5 million deaths occur each year from perinatal causes; the long-term developmental defects from conditions such as hypoxia during labor and birth trauma are more difficult to estimate (WHO/UNICEF 1986). Control efforts are concentrated mainly on general preventive measures and improving case management through the use of high-risk monitoring (Backett, Davies, and Petros-Barzovian 1984). Preventive measures are focused mostly on improving maternal health, particular emphasis being given to nutrition of the mother. Deficiencies in specific nutrients, such as iodine, iron, and folate, can seriously interfere with fetal development. Mothers who were themselves malnourished in childhood tend to have small pelvises and stature and are more likely to experience complications at the time of delivery. Sexually transmitted diseases and a variety of organisms in the genital tract can produce serious sequelae when they infect babies (Bang and others 1989).

Improved case management of pregnancy depends on a health care system which can identify high-risk conditions early and arrange for the pregnant mother to be referred for whatever special care is needed. This seems to work best when pregnancy care is part of primary health care and a high-risk surveillance system is adapted to the particular conditions and resources available locally (Lettenmaier and others 1988). Initial screening by personnel who are trusted by mothers should be readily available to foster the goal of achieving complete coverage of all pregnant women. The referral process, then, will depend on local networks of health personnel and facilities and also on communications and transport.

Breastfeeding

Good lactation is the most natural of health interventions. Cessation of breastfeeding is, however, part of modernization trends in many areas of the world. Abundant evidence shows that in the poorest communities the effect of declining breastfeeding rates is disastrous with regard to child mortality and nutrition. Its protective value is shown by the fact that breastfed babies are relatively healthy for the first six months of life and also by the good start they get for subsequent development. Breastfeeding is also the world's most ubiquitous method of family planning.

Birth Spacing

Many studies have shown that family planning is an effective means of improving child health (IPPF 1988). It is usually associated with social and economic conditions in the home associated with being a "wanted child." International programs for family planning, unfortunately, have often been dissociated from health services. For eventual sustainability the two should be naturally linked, especially because this is the way mothers think about their problems. In a two-way interaction, family planning directly contributes to better child health, and child survival increases motivation to practice family planning.

Defining Local Priorities

It has become increasingly evident that only a few interventions, such as immunizations and community environmental control measures, are sufficiently widespread around the world to justify their being given global priority. Once those programs have been introduced, the remaining priority problems will vary greatly, depending on local conditions and available resources. Examples range from infections such as malaria, hemorrhagic dengue, and Japanese B encephalitis to localized prevalence of kwashiorkor and iodine deficiency.

The systematic setting of priorities in health care on the basis of cost-effectiveness criteria will almost automatically give greater emphasis to prevention than to curative care. This is especially true for the communicable diseases which contribute most to childhood mortality, morbidity, and developmental deficit.

Most decisions about priorities require balancing concerns about the technological effectiveness of specific procedures and the feasibility and cost of using them. A health problem that has high priority because of high rates of mortality and morbidity may be given low priority because no effective control measures are available. Our greatest limitations seem to be in community-based delivery systems and in the process of adapting procedures to local conditions.

Decisions about priorities concerning what will actually be done are always influenced more by administrative and political issues than by epidemiological information about diseases. The interventions focused on in this collection are selected mainly because of potential efficacy for particular diseases, but there is also a need for more general types of information. Even though it may be appropriate to start a priority-setting process by considering the cost-effectiveness of disease-specific interventions, it then becomes necessary to consider how those interventions can be integrated in a total health system and what other resources are available within local socioeconomic constraints.

Some people have criticized UNICEF in recent years because its child-survival strategy is said to be based on a "selective" disease-oriented analysis of priorities. The fact is, however, that UNICEF's promotion of the Child Survival and Development Revolution had its origin in the Alma Ata principles of getting complete coverage for equity in primary health care. To this was added focused efforts to accelerate action in the home and community (Taylor and Jolly 1988). An important distinction is that UNICEF's GOBI (growth monitoring, oral rehydration, breastfeeding, immunizations) priorities are interventions and not specific diseases. They were selected largely because they were simple and low cost, had high effectiveness, and were suitable for mass implementation because they used methods which stressed social mobilization and self-reliance. They resulted in high expectations among political leaders who understood that these programs would give them opportunities to be involved in activities which had potential for public recognition at low cost (UNICEF 1988). The expectations UNICEF created in persuading national leaders to support the Child Survival and Development Revolution are now coming due as the people expect to benefit from the significant improvements that were promised. Great effort is being expended in trying to meet deadlines for ambitious targets that were set on the basis of limited analysis. The overall effort will have benefits even if particular interventions do not avert the number of deaths that was originally projected. The point, however, is that without the ambitious targets, much less would have been achieved. In the 1990s there should be more emphasis on building sustainable infrastructures.

Practical programs for control of the main communicable diseases of children require a combination of research and application. A common assumption of research workers has been that all they need to do is to make new findings and technology available, and then implementation will follow spontaneously. This is not necessarily true, as experience with smallpox has shown. Even though an effective vaccine was available, much persuasion and field research had to be done for a very long period of time before countries were willing to make serious efforts to control the disease. The chapters in this collection that are concerned with the high-priority diseases of childhood show the complexity of determinants of effective control even with the simplest interventions. Mass programs have had some clear successes, but the limitations of looking just for simple solutions have also become evident. As initial successes have been achieved, greater effort is needed to identify means of promoting sustainability and cost-effectiveness adapted to the community level. This requires new methods for adapting implementation to the particular cultural, socioeconomic, and administrative traditions of local groups and service sectors in what has been called country-specific health research (Commission on Health Research for Development 1990).

Determinants of Successful Child Survival Programs

The ultimate need is that all special child survival programs should help to build a primary health care infrastructure. If any intervention or technology is introduced as part of a special program, it should eventually be integrated into the local infrastructure except in the rare instances in which eradication seems feasible. The long-standing confrontation between proponents of vertical and horizontal programs should be viewed from the perspective that a balance is needed (Taylor and Jolly 1988). Setting priorities implies giving focused emphasis for a period of time to particular activities. These will not have sustainability, however, unless they are built into continuing services based on community priorities.

To achieve sustainability it is essential from the beginning to have programs that are based on sociocultural appropriateness and sensitivity. Community relationships should be developed in ways that ensure acceptability, accessibility, administrative feasibility, and continuing financing.

Any international initiative should not impose outside priorities but be responsive to continuing dialogue between national and local expressions of effective demand. It is counterproductive to push ahead in global initiatives without adjusting to local perceptions of community priorities.

The most profound and long-term changes in child survival and development will occur as a result of behavioral changes applied in family patterns of child care. Simplified procedures should be established to introduce new home methods in daily routines such as hand washing, oral rehydration, or improving weaning methods. In order for these routines to be accepted as parental behavioral norms, there will need to be strong social support for individual families. For instance, the goal should be for every case of watery diarrhea to be managed by mothers with home-based simple fluids to prevent dehydration.

New strategies are needed to combine interventions into rationalized packages of services as part of primary health care. Such packages should have great cost-effectiveness because of shared costs for programs which have multiple benefits. Little has been done to define entry points at which one type of intervention can facilitate the introduction of other interventions. Problems in measurement methodology need to be resolved to develop means of calculating cost-effectiveness in cases in which input, output, and outcome variables overlap. Sorely needed is quantitative analysis of integrated services seen in the successful national experiences in China and Sri Lanka. It may mean that we should set up new multipurpose studies on integrated services (WHO 1986), which would likely have to be done in relatively small but representative populations exemplified in the district strategy advocated by WHO.

Types of Child Survival Interventions

A simple categorization may contribute to one's understanding of how to focus activities. Three strategic models can help in deciding about how particular child survival interventions can be most effectively implemented.

- *Preventive interventions organized by public or government services (EPI, community water supplies, regulations to control epidemics)*. Some interventions may be considered so important that public health authorities take the initiative to enforce mass implementation using legal or centralized regulatory controls. To make these methods acceptable to the public, the evidence for effectiveness and safety must be so indisputable that the people accept the principle that social good should take precedence over individual choice. Social mobilization can be applied through community pressure to enlist the compliance of individuals and groups.

- *Case management interventions (ORT, ARI, monitoring of high-risk pregnancies and growth)*. In a two-phase process, initiative is taken first by the health system in setting up screening or surveillance procedures to identify specific health problems early, or individuals and groups who are at high risk. The second phase requires an appropriate response by the individual and family to apply preventive or corrective interventions. A strong educational process is necessary to stimulate awareness and motivation to act. Equally important is clear definition of what support is necessary from health services and reliable logistics to make appropriate drugs, equipment, and supplies accessible and available. These responses can range from implementation of interventions that can be readily applied in the home to knowing when to go to a health facility. Examples include knowing the right amount of salt to add to dilute rice porridge for simple home-based ORT, having readily available co-trimoxazole for childhood pneumonia that has been diagnosed by trained community health workers according to the WHO protocol for ARI, having easy access to weighing scales for growth monitoring, and testing blood pressure as part of routine prenatal examination.

- *Primary prevention in the home*. Some of the most positive and lasting changes in promoting better health and nutrition result from basic behavioral changes in routine child care. These depend on family initiative and represent one of the ultimate goals in improving child survival and development. Examples include personal hygiene and home sanitation, preventing the exposure of children to home air pollution and passive smoking, diets for long-term healthy development, and appropriate stimulation for intellectual development of babies.

Competing Concerns

Two competing concerns must be balanced. The first is the need in almost all programs to increase community participation through decentralization. This requires local setting of priorities and dialogue between community leaders and health system workers to ensure technical quality of services, logistics, training, and supervision while taking into account local desires and priorities. Community participation can be a strong force in promoting sustainability.

The second concern is to ensure equity by setting up arrangements so that services reach those in greatest need. By targeting high-risk groups for special attention, a program should be able to reach those who have the highest prevalence of disease. It is only through improving their health that a significant effect on morbidity and mortality can be achieved.

It is, however, especially hard to reach those in greatest need because they tend to be suspicious and poor and they live in places with difficult transport and communication. Their access to care is limited by their own time constraints and well-established social and economic barriers. They are typically bypassed because they do not know where or how to get care. Getting care is not only inconvenient; local arrangements and the arrogance of health workers often violate local cultural patterns.

The conflict between the above two concerns arises because of the ease with which local leaders can manipulate the process of community participation and priority setting. Local leaders responsible for community participation usually make sure that benefits go first to their family and friends. Outside involvement in priority setting may help to ensure equity in coverage. If health service systems set up standard measurement methods as part of community-based surveillance, it should be possible to determine who in the community is in greatest need. Then dialogue between community elite and responsible health workers can allocate resources on the basis of data about relative need. Having to meet clear coverage targets set by national programs requires health workers and local leaders to make sure that special services get to all, especially the population pockets which have the greatest need. Based on systematic monitoring of the priority diseases in an area, the selection of an appropriate mix of priority interventions should become a responsibility shared among the health service workers, the community participants, and representatives of other sectors.

Networks for Health Services Development

As primary health care infrastructure develops, one of the most important skills to be incorporated in local capacity building is the ability in decentralized units to work with communities in setting local priorities. An effective means for developing this capacity is to organize a network of linkages between academic centers and local health services (WHO 1986). This gives institutions with capability in operations research and planning an opportunity to work out practical solutions for local health problems in experimental areas. Solutions that have been adapted to local conditions can then be generally implemented in a systematic extension process. This strategy has the potential of promoting both community participation and equitable distribution. Information systems with rapid feedback to local implementation are a critical component.

Few preventive programs can be completely standardized because they all need to be adapted to local circumstances.

Program development can be greatly facilitated by setting up a learning process to find the best way of organizing locally appropriate services. Problems which arise in day-to-day activities can be brought to the experimental area for study in the field. These field studies should progressively advance knowledge so that there is incremental learning of what works under local circumstances. Regional linkages between such experimental areas and field research teams can be coordinated in a national network to build capacity and to provide mutual support.

References

Backett, E. M., A. M. Davies, and A. Petros-Barzovian. 1984. *The Risk Approach in Health Care, with Special References to Maternal and Child Health including Family Planning.* Public Health Papers 76. WHO, Geneva.

Bang, R. A., M. Baitule, S. Sarmukaddam, A. T. Bang, Y. Choudhary, and O. Tale. 1989. "High Prevalence of Gynaecological Diseases in Rural Indian Women." *Lancet* 1:85–88.

Breman, J. G., and C. C. Campbell. 1988. "Combatting Severe Malaria in African Children." *Bulletin of the World Health Organization* 6:611–20.

Commission on Health Research for Development. 1990. *Health Research: Essential Link to Equity and Development.* Oxford: Oxford University Press.

Feachem, R. G. 1986. "Preventing Diarrhea: What Are the Policy Options?" *Health Policy and Planning* 1:109–17.

Gadomski, Anne, ed. 1990. *Acute Lower Respiratory Infection and Child Survival in Developing Countries.* Baltimore: Johns Hopkins University, Institute for International Programs.

IPPF (International Planned Parenthood Federation). 1988. *Better Health for Women and Children through Family Planning: Report of the International Conference, Nairobi, Kenya, October 1987.* London: IPPF.

Lettenmaier, C., L. Liskin, C. A. Church, and J. A. Harris. 1988. *Mothers' Lives Matter: Maternal Health in the Community.* Population Reports 16(2). Johns Hopkins University, Population Information Program, Baltimore.

Rosenthal, Gerald. 1989. *The Economic Burden of Sustainable EPI: Implications for Donor Policy.* Arlington, Va.: John Snow, REACH (Resources for Child Health).

Taylor, C. E., and W. B. Greenough. 1989. "Control of Diarrheal Diseases." *Annual Review of Public Health* 10:221–46.

Taylor, C. E., and R. Jolly. 1988. "The Straw Men of Primary Health Care." *Social Science and Medicine* 26:971–77.

UNICEF (United Nations Children's Fund). 1988. *The State of the World's Children 1988.* New York: Oxford University Press.

World Bank. 1987. *Preventing the Tragedy of Maternal Deaths.* Report of the International Safe Motherhood Conference, Nairobi, Kenya, February 1987. Washington, D.C.

WHO (World Health Organization). 1986. *National Health Development Networks in Support of Primary Health Care.* Geneva.

WHO/UNICEF (World Health Organization/United Nations Children's Fund). 1986. *Maternal Care for the Reduction of Perinatal and Neonatal Mortality.* Geneva: WHO.

Appendix C

Priority Setting for Health Service Efficiency: The Role of Measurement of Burden of Illness

Gavin Mooney and Andrew Creese

The need to set priorities arises from the fact that not all illness can be eradicated nor all needs met. This failure to be able to meet all needs arises not principally because of the limitations of technology—the technology is currently available to eliminate many of the most important diseases, such as poliomyelitis and measles—but because of the scarcity of resources. Policymakers in the health sector have to manage resources in ways that maximize health outcomes, whether this means redeploying resources, allocating limited new resources, or cutting back on the use of existing resources. They must also get the most out of whatever they have available, which is likely to mean changing the mix of resource allocations.

Priorities are about change. Setting priorities to achieve best possible value for the resources available should be based on considerations of both benefits and costs. Using scarce resources in any way means, by definition, giving up the opportunity to use them in some other way; providing benefits here means forgoing them elsewhere. Priority setting means developing analyses and procedures to ensure that the policies that get priority (that is, those which get a higher call on extra resources) are the ones that provide the greatest benefits per additional dollar spent. If the dollars could have been better spent elsewhere, then they should have been spent elsewhere.

In this appendix we illustrate first how, conceptually, information on the burden of illness can contribute to the process of priority setting. We then identify some of the practical problems entailed in deriving appropriate information on both the costs (briefly) and the outcomes of health interventions. We also consider here the usefulness and limitations of the dollar cost per disability-adjusted life-year (DALY) gained. Finally, using the cost and outcome information summarized for individual chapters, we give examples of how a cost-effectiveness strategy may be used in setting health priorities at sector, project or program, and clinical levels of the health system.

The Burden of Illness and Priority Setting

The notion of illness as a social and economic burden is very old. Quantitative estimates of society's losses from bubonic plague epidemics and natural disasters were made in the seventeenth century by the English physician William Petty (1699). The epidemiological and economic tally of diseases on a national or global basis has been documented more recently in an empirical work by Walsh and Warren (1979). Accounts of the costs of individual health problems, such as road traffic accidents or, more recently, acquired immunodeficiency syndrome (AIDS), are regularly published in journals concerned with health policy. (See, for example, Henke and Behrens 1986; also see the subsequent debate on the cost of illness: Shiell, Gerard, and Donaldson 1987; Behrens and Henke 1988; and Hodgson 1989.) The motivating factors, sometimes implicit, sometimes explicit, behind such analyses appear to be an assessment or reassessment of priorities. Measuring the burden of illness is thus seen as an ingredient in the rational setting of priorities.

The reason for attempting to measure the burden of illness is thus to allow a better (that is, more efficient) use of scarce resources in reducing the effect of illness on a population, a group of individuals, or even single individuals. In some instances, such as when an epidemic or an important new disease manifests itself—and AIDS is a classic case—awareness of the burden of illness in itself forces a reassessment of expenditure priorities. But even in this instance there is a need to assess the benefits and costs of different policy reactions and also to review the priority status of the new problem with the same criteria used to measure illness problems that have been more long standing.

One cannot examine issues of efficiency, however, without looking at both inputs and outputs—costs and benefits. The burden of illness, however measured, is not a particularly useful concept if it is assessed separately from the question of the policies and resources associated with addressing that burden, that is, questions of how effective and how costly different forms of treatment, care, or prevention are in dealing with the illnesses being considered.

Looking solely at the disease or illness side of the equation, and not simultaneously at the resource or input side, does not permit one to say anything conclusive about the assessment or evaluation of priorities. Conceptually, it is necessary to give some consideration to the relationship between the burden of illness and the effect that different treatment, care, or prevention interventions have upon it.

The need to consider the disease and resource sides of the efficiency equation together is not, of course, an argument against measuring the burden of illness; it is only an argument against the belief that the epidemiology of illness in itself is a basis for priority setting and against the idea that, in general (there are exceptions), measuring the total burden of an illness is a valuable thing to do. Thus if, for a particular country the burden of morbidity and premature mortality from childhood infections was greater than the burden of adult respiratory disease, this in itself would tell us nothing about the relative resource allocation priority of these two problems. Assuming for the moment that adult and infant lives are weighted of equal importance, considerations of the cost and effectiveness of available technology for altering the course of the disease must still be introduced before the overall cost-effectiveness of interventions can be ranked. Furthermore, in most instances it will not be the total costs and the total benefits (in the context of the burden of illness, the latter will normally be estimated as a reduction in that burden) that are relevant—or indeed the average costs and benefits.

The prime concern is with assessing change. If resource inputs in one program are increased, to what extent is the burden of illness in that program reduced? If inputs are increased again, how much more is the burden of illness reduced? Conversely, if resource allocations to a program are decreased, to what extent will the burden of illness increase? Economic thinking of this sort has clearly established that what is relevant in the setting of priorities are the marginal benefits and the marginal costs and consequently the marginal effect on the burden of illness of an increase or decrease in the resources deployed in that program.

Thus the prime objective of efforts to estimate the burden of illness is best seen in the context of attempting to estimate the reduction in the burden of illness through the application of some treatment or preventive regime which inevitably involves the use of scarce resources. Such efforts are a means toward allowing the quantification of the effectiveness of a particular policy on a particular disease and help in answering the question, For illness X, does treatment A do more good (reduce more the burden of illness X) than treatment B?

Thereafter the issues of operational efficiency can be addressed: how best, with regard to the cost per unit of output, can the burden of particular illness X be reduced? Here the relevant techniques are cost-effectiveness analysis and cost-utility analysis, the latter having the advantage over the former of being able to consider more than one type of output (for example, both mortality and morbidity reductions). This is discussed in more detail later.

A comparison of the burden of illness across different diseases, if such is possible, leads into still more interesting questions of the relative efficiency of using resources to deal with the effects of different illnesses. The clear implication here is

that if there is a need to choose between spending Y on program C and spending the same amount on program D, then for the sake of efficiency (what is called allocative efficiency) the investment should be in the program in which the benefit is larger. The question then is, where can an increase in resources be deployed to decrease the burden of illness to the greatest extent? It should be noted that the question in the other direction is also relevant: where can a cut in resources be made so that the increase in the burden of illness is minimized? Here the relevant techniques are cost-utility and cost-benefit analyses.

The ideal with cost-benefit analysis is to operate with the three key rules for allocative efficiency:

- If for a particular program costs are greater than benefits, then that program should not be implemented.

- If benefits are greater than costs, proceed with the policy. But further, and ideally, these rules should be applied at the margin.

- In other words, a policy should be pursued up to that point where the marginal benefit equals the marginal cost— but not beyond that point.

Such rules are made in recognition of the scarcity of resources (we cannot do everything) and the importance of efficiency (we accept that society should attempt to provide as much benefit as possible with what resources are available; for good reviews of economic appraisal, see Mills 1985 and Drummond and others 1986).

These issues can be summarized in the following five points:

- Measuring the burden of illness is an important ingredient in rational priority setting.

- Rationally set priorities are obtained by a process of weighing costs and benefits, and benefits are obtained largely through a reduction in the burden of illness.

- Priorities are set on the margin: it is the costs and benefits of change that matter. Accepting this leads to such questions as, if resources are increased, where can they be used to reduce the burden of illness most?

- Priorities are not a function of total costs or total benefits, which means consequently that rational priority setting has no interest in the total burden of an illness unless it is practical both technologically and economically to eliminate that illness—and such instances occur very seldom.

- There are two relevant forms of efficiency in priority setting: operational efficiency when the priority questions relate to how; allocative efficiency when they relate to whether and how much.

Measuring the Effectiveness of Interventions

Our main concerns in this appendix pertain to measurements of the burden of illness. Because of the importance attached to the costs of reducing the burden of illness, however, we briefly look first at some issues of cost measurement.

Information on Costs

Several key principles are associated with all costing. First, what we seek to measure are the so-called opportunity costs, that is, the benefits forgone in the best alternative use of resources. Where markets work well, market prices can often be used in estimating costs. In the health care sector and in developing countries generally, however, the frequent market failures or distortions mean that "shadow pricing" is required.

Second, the relevant cost is always the cost of the change being considered, and this can normally be defined as the marginal cost. If, for example, it is expected that a hospital will have to deal with an extra hundred births next year, the relevant cost relates to the extra use of resources for staff, equipment, and other resources for these births. (It should be noted that this cost may have no similarity to the existing average cost per birth in the hospital.)

Third, the cost should normally include all resource use, no matter on whom it falls. Thus it is not just health service or public sector costs that are relevant but also costs falling on private agencies, the patients themselves, their relatives, and so forth.

Fourth, payments for sickness benefits, pensions, and the like are not costs as such but rather transfers from one group in the community (normally the working population) to another (here, ill people and the elderly). These redistributions of resources are not costs from society's point of view. They are called "transfer payments."

At a more practical level, one of the great difficulties in making estimates of costs according to the above principles is the paucity of existing data. What are often available from accounting data are average costs—and yet it is not these that are required. Because they are available, however, there is a great temptation to use them. We would counsel against this and suggest that crude marginal cost estimates are better than precise average costs.

If the use of average costs is to be rejected and marginal costs calculated, how is this best done? The answer is, quite simply, to ask the appropriate people for their estimates. Thus, in extending care to take account of an extra hundred births next year in a particular hospital (as in the example above), the starting point is to ask the hospital manager or obstetrician what facilities and resources will be needed to cope. An estimate can be made of the extra time of doctors, of nurses, of auxiliary staff, of equipment, of food, and the like—and then each of these resources costed. That then gives the relevant cost figure.

The lack of adequate, readily available, marginal cost data in health care (and not just in developing countries) is perhaps just as big a problem as the lack of good outcome measures. It is normally easier, however, to overcome the problems on the cost side and get a sufficiently accurate estimate of the relevant marginal costs.

Information on the Effectiveness of Health Interventions

It is clear that the measurement of the burden of illness is difficult. This is true for three reasons: first, the effects on health status and illness are multidimensional, involving physical pain, physical impairment, mental disability, mortality, and so on; second, health status is a value-laden concept; and third, the appropriateness of one particular measure is likely to vary, depending on why it is being used. Infant mortality could be a reasonable basis for comparing the effect of child immunization programs across different countries. It would not be a suitable measure for the effectiveness of an antismoking campaign among schoolchildren.

There is also a hierarchy of measurement which has to be noted. If all that is of interest is to answer the question "Is x more effective than y?" then an "ordinal" ranking is all that is required (that is, we can rank the relevant change in the burden of illness as greater or less). If we want to go further and say that a quantified amount more is obtained, then "cardinal" scaling is necessary.

In most contexts, cardinal scaling is necessary in priority-setting exercises because it is not enough to be able to say that x is more effective than y—especially if x is also more expensive than y; we need to know how much more, the issue of cardinality.

HEALTH CARE ACTIVITIES. The most basic methods used in measuring health care outputs are activity measures, such as numbers of cases treated, numbers of consultations, and proportion of population vaccinated, which do not directly measure health at all. Of course, it is reasonable to assume that the more patients who are treated the greater will be the benefit with regard to reduction in the burden of illness. But that assumption requires various other assumptions about the effectiveness of intervention, which it would be preferable to measure more directly. For example, to couch the effectiveness of a family planning campaign in terms of the proportion of women reached in the campaign may be a poor measure of the effect it has on family planning per se or, more explicitly still, on the number of unwanted pregnancies conceived.

HEALTH INDEXES. The simplest methods which incorporate some assessment of health status involve using estimates of mortality or life-years lost. It is clearly the case, however, that these estimates then ignore morbidity and any other aspects of the burden of illness. Of course, there may be some situations in which it is possible to justify such ignoring—for example, in certain instances in which mortality and morbidity are highly correlated. Generally, however, such measures are of rather limited value. In the field of clinical or individual health status measurement, several different types of index exist. Such indexes are important, because the objects of such measurement are those on which population-based health status measures should be based. For assessments of levels of physical and social functioning of individuals, see, for example, the Duke-UNC Health Profile (Parkerson 1981); the Sickness Impact Profile (Bergner and others 1981); the Index of Well-being (Kaplan and Bush 1982). For a general review see Hall and Masters 1986. For population-based measures, the review method of Walsh and Warren (1979) is worth noting. Still, the authors made no attempt to aggregate the morbidity and mortality components of health and simply presented ordinal rankings of the main diseases, first by their morbidity and second by their mortality.

More recent attempts to combine both types of information in a single aggregate have counted both avoided disability and avoided mortality as the number of days of a "normal" life gained. This has provided a common yardstick with which morbidity or spells of temporary incapacity can be arithmetically combined.

The Ghana Health Assessment Project Team's calculations of "healthy days of life" are of particular interest in the context of attempting to use burden-of-illness data in the setting of priorities, particularly with respect to the need to be cautious in using such data. In this study, an index was developed for measuring days of healthy life lost to selected diseases which involves the assumption that days spent being dead, being permanently disabled, and being temporarily disabled are equally valued. That seems a difficult assumption with which to agree, but provided the sensitivity (see the section on uncertainty below) of such assumptions is tested, then such apparently gross assumptions may be defensible. The point is that they ought to be tested—by, for example, determining what difference it makes if the weight attached to being disabled is 0.5 compared to a weight for death of 1.

Certainly such a method is valuable, provided its limitations are recognized and provided it is not used to rank priorities in terms of the total burden of illness. Barnum (1987), for example, makes the very relevant point that weightings should be applied to estimates of lost healthy days, first, to reflect the time dimension (that is, the discounting of losses in the future) and, second, to reflect productivity loss. Even here, however, there are problems because the implication of the productivity loss measure is that anyone older than fifty-seven years has a zero value. (Here we have a variant of the human capital method of estimation without any attempt being made to avoid the problems of zero-weighting retired people.)

Barnum states: "The results [provided by this approach] illustrate that weighting and discounting, and their interaction, potentially ... affect the priorities and strategies that evolve from an epidemiological analysis of the health sector" (1987, p. 838). This interpretation, however, gives the impression that the commentator is assuming that the total burden of different illnesses in itself provides some basis for setting priorities. As we have argued above, it does not, except in some very restricted circumstances. (It may be that such total measures will have more relevance in setting research priorities in situations in which the relative size of a problem is the only basis for setting priorities because we know nothing about either the different costs of research in different areas or the different probabilities of success and therefore have to assume that neither varies with the illness. Such assumptions may be an approximation of reality in setting research priorities; that is unlikely to be true, except infrequently, in the case of health care policy priorities.)

A further problem revealed by the method used by the Ghana Health Assessment Project Team is not only that it deals with totals but also that it deals with averages. We have already considered the need to concentrate on the margin, and in some instances marginal benefits or marginal costs may turn out to be closely approximated by average benefits or average costs, respectively. But they may not.

Thus, and for example, in estimating the value of a death prevented, the relevant formula in the calculations of the Ghana Health Assessment Project Team, when including an allowance for length of survival, considers only the average age at onset and the average age at death. It follows that the value of a death prevented is then always calculated on the basis of the average years of life extended by the program. Yet if there is considerable variability about these averages, then priorities may be wrongly set. Thus, for example, if we consider the priority to be attached to screening women over the age of twenty for breast cancer and use only average figures, the average increase in life expectancy is small. But if we then look at specific age groups or risk groups, the position will be better for some, worse for others. Thus using average figures is likely to lead to a misallocation of scarce resources. We have in this example two lessons to be learned: the danger of using total burden-of-illness data; and the danger of using average burden-of-illness data.

A more recent study, in which program cost information is juxtaposed with an aggregate measure of effectiveness, is that by Prost and Prescott (1984) on onchocerciasis. The authors estimate the cost-effectiveness of prevention measures for onchocerciasis using the alternative measures of effectiveness reproduced in table C-1.

Given the emphasis here on added benefits and on the sensitivity of the results to different measures of effectiveness, this type of empirical work is potentially very useful. As Prost and Prescott themselves state, however, "the relative cost-effectiveness of onchocerciasis control is very sensitive to the choice of effectiveness measure" (1984, p. 801). It is thus clear that there remain problems in improving such measurement of burden of illness to allow relevant measures of effectiveness to be designed.

We accept that this is difficult, but it is what is required for rational priority setting, and no amount of concern about lack of data or about the problems involved in such development will make the basic requirement change. It is, in our judgment, much better to attempt to adopt this methodology in some form or other even if we get no closer than a crude approximation than to adopt what are clearly wrong or inappropriate measures.

A related approach, hitherto used only in industrial countries, entails the adjustment of the quantity of additional days of life by a factor designed to capture (and make comparable) the dimension of quality. In comparing renal dialysis with kidney transplantation, for example, as options for patients with end-stage renal failure, it is clear that a simple comparison of the dollar cost per case would fail to capture the superior quality of outcome of successful transplantation over dialysis. This factor is apparent to all—clinicians, patients and their families, and potential patients, that is, the public. The outcome resulting from transplantation is clearly "better" than

Table C-1. Cost-Effectiveness of Onchocerciasis Control
(U.S. dollars)

Unit of measure	Cost
Per year of healthy life added	20
Per productive year of healthy life added	20
Per disability-adjusted year of healthy life added	150
Per discounted productive year of healthy life added	150

Source: Prost and Prescott 1984.

that from dialysis. Although both options prevent premature death, the difference in the quality of survivors' lives necessitates adjustment to the number of years gained to reflect this, so that the outcomes are comparable.

This approach, it has to be emphasized, tells us only about the relative burden of one disease as compared with others. Its primary use is in attempting to rank for the purposes of priority setting the costs per disability-adjusted life-year (DALY) gained on the margin of different programs. Thus if one program has an extra cost of $10,000 per DALY gained and another program has an extra cost of $100,000, it would be rational, if there were no other considerations, to invest in the first program, because the number of DALYs gained would be greater.

The fundamental problem with DALYs as with all such measures of health status is in getting the appropriate weights for mortality and for all the possible forms of morbidity. Questions here relate to whom to ask to do the valuing; how one life is to be compared with another—normally assumed to be the same; how to allow for uncertainty; and many other issues, including whether the only output of health services is improved health status. Because this last point is a concern with all the methods of measuring the burden of illness in this appendix, it will be considered later in a more general context. (For a critique of DALYs see Loomes and McKenzie 1989).

Two contributions to the field of development of DALYs are particularly noteworthy. We will discuss, first, some of the work of the "father of DALYs," George Torrance, from Canada and, second, the work of Alan Williams, from England (see Torrance 1985; Williams 1985).

One of Torrance's key contributions to the field is with respect to methodology and in various papers he has provided much guidance for researchers in how to measure health states in practice. Thus he gives the main steps in developing health status measures:

- Identify the relevant health states for which preferences are required.
- Describe the health states.
- Select the subjects whose preferences will be measured.
- Determine the type of preferences required (ordinal, cardinal).
- Determine the measurement instrument to be used.

Although we cannot discuss all these steps in detail, it is worth noting, regarding the last, that there are various ways of tackling the question of how to measure burden of illness using health status or DALY measures. All are concerned with attempting to quantify different health states—such as unconsciousness, severe physical impairment, moderate pain—on a scale stretching from perfect health (given a weight, say, of 1) to death (weighted, say, as 0). Thus a year of life with, for example, significant physical impairment and considerable pain might be thought to be only 80 percent as good as a year of perfect life. In such a case, the DALY for this health state would be 0.8.

Various instruments are available to assist in the attempt to measure DALYs. These include the following:

- *The rating scale* normally consists of a line on a page with a scale from, say, 0 at one end to 1 at the other, the end points being defined as death and perfect health, respectively. Other health states are then placed at different points on the line, a point right in the middle being equated with a health state or DALY of 0.5.

- *The standard gamble* involves a choice of the certainty of a health state Y as opposed to the probability of a health state X (where X would normally be preferred to Y). If X were perfect health (weight as 1) and the probability which made the valuer indifferent in this choice were 75 percent, then the DALY for Y would be 0.75.

- The weights of *the time trade-off* are determined by offering choices of different lengths of life in different health states and attempting to get "indifference" across different choices.

The actual use of DALY data linked to costs is provided in table C-2, based on work by Williams (1985). Essentially what this means is that given an additional amount of money, say, £14,000, (approximately $25,000) to spend on the listed programs, spending it on pacemakers would give twenty DALYs, whereas spending it on hospital hemodialysis would give only one DALY.

It is perhaps superfluous to add that the development of DALYs can be difficult. However it is done, attaching weights to different morbidity states in relation to death, so that, ideally, mortality and all forms of morbidity can be placed on a single index, involves value judgments. It is also the case that we know of no "fully fledged" DALY applications in developing countries.

SOME COMMON PROCEDURAL POINTS. Whatever methodology is adopted for assessing the burden of illness, there are five issues that need to be handled with care.

- Determination of the purpose
- Discounting over time
- Other outputs
- Uncertainty
- Equity

Although determining the purpose may seem an obvious point, it is worth stressing that how the burden of illness is best measured or valued is a function of why it is being measured or

Table C-2. Costs and Consequences of Selected Medical Procedures
(pounds sterling)

Procedure	Present value of extra cost per DALY gained
Pacemaker implantation for heart block	700
Hip replacement	750
Valve replacements for aortic stenosis	950
CABG for severe angina with left main disease	1,040
CABG for moderate angina with three-vessel disease	2,400
Kidney transplantation (cadaver)	3,000
Heart transplantation	5,000
Home hemodialysis	11,000
CABG for mild angina with two-vessel disease	12,600
Hospital hemodialysis	14,000

Note: CABG (Coronary artery bypass grafting).
Source: Drummond 1987; Williams 1985.

valued and in what circumstances. Calculations concerning the burden of illness will almost always be used as an estimate of some output measures, and output measures have to be or ought to be related to the purpose or objective of the exercise. It is also clear that if the wrong measure is used it is quite likely that a distorted answer will be obtained. (For example, if breast cancer treatment programs are related solely to percentage of survival over, say, five years, then all aspects of quality of life—pain, dignity, losing a breast, and so on—will be ignored and given a zero weight. Yet it seems clear that women suffering from breast cancer will value more than just survival.)

For calculations of the burden of illness (and also the resource costs of interventions), the value attached at different points in time is not constant. As Barnum states: "Neither the individual nor the community is indifferent as to when the effects of disease occur.... A healthy day of life in the present has a greater intrinsic value to the individual than a day in the future (1987, p. 834)." The way to handle this phenomenon is through "discounting" future benefits and costs at some positive rate of discount; such discounting results in a weighting over time which gives more weight to current effects, less to those of the near future, and still less to those in the distant future. This means, for example, that preventive programs may seem to do rather badly as a result of discounting. This is because they often involve costs now (which are therefore not discounted) and benefits in the future (which are discounted). What rate of discounting to use is problematical, and it is normal procedure to use a range of rates, usually between about 3 and 10 percent.

Although it can generally be agreed that the decrease of the burden of disease on the sufferer is the prime output of any health care system, other outputs are present and relevant for the setting of priorities. For example, if infectious diseases are cured in some people, others who would otherwise have become infected will benefit. Again, nonsufferers may benefit knowing that others' suffering is reduced—what Culyer (1976)

has called the caring "externality." Information is also an output. For example, informing patients about their state of health even if it is not changed or indeed cannot be changed may provide benefit to the patient. Being able to pass difficult decisions to the doctor may also sometimes be of benefit to some patients.

It is difficult to say what weight will be attached to these other outputs. It is clear, however, that their importance is likely to vary both across different diseases and across different patients. Thus, although it is appropriate in assessing priorities to concentrate on the output side on reductions in the burden of disease, these other forms of output may sometimes alter the priority rankings or weightings.

Benefits in the future may be uncertain, and in such cases an adjustment should be made to reflect their expected value. For example, the reduction of infant mortality may lead to greater benefits as a result of a health education campaign concerned with hygiene to reduce childhood diarrhea. Often, however, it will not be possible to state precisely what all the potential effects of an intervention for the treatment or prevention of some disease will be.

Where uncertainty exists, sensitivity analysis should be used in handling it; that is, a range of values should be put in for a particular parameter to see what the effect of the different values is—how sensitive the result is to the change in values. Where the result does change, it may be necessary to devote some effort to trying to reduce that particular uncertainty.

Although we accept that equity is an important goal in most health care systems, we are focusing in this appendix on efficiency. Still, it is important to recognize that equity and efficiency goals can sometimes conflict. Such a conflict may mean that minimizing the burden of illness is not the goal or at least that such a goal is constrained by concerns for equity. For example, although it may in some instances be efficient to concentrate highly specialized facilities in the cities, this is unlikely to provide an equitable system with regard to geographical access.

It is also the case that if equity is concerned with access or use rather than with health per se, then factors other than purely burden of disease have to be taken into account. In other words, if a society values the fact that individuals have equal access to health care irrespective of whether they then use it to obtain effective care, then such a set of values cannot be directly contained within burden-of-illness calculations.

Certainly in many—but admittedly not all—equity measures there will be some need to assess the relative burden of disease across different groups in society. Such cases present the few occasions in which the burden of disease itself, as opposed to its reduction, is the relevant policy measure with which to operate. Whether that is the relevant measure of equity to use is something that cannot be resolved in this appendix (but see for more discussion Mooney 1992). Other factors such as access may become relevant.

METHODS FOR PUTTING MONETARY VALUES ON OUTCOMES. We have seen above that health status measures are more widely usable if they aggregate the relevant components (mortality and morbidity) in a single numeraire, such as healthy days or DALYs. In an analogous fashion, the usefulness of health outcome data for priority setting is substantially increased if an acceptable monetary yardstick can be found, to allow direct comparisons between the value of inputs used in improving health and the value of these improvements. When this is possible, not only can cardinal comparisons be made between competing claims on resources, but the more fundamental cost-benefit questions can be asked and answered.

There are three principal methods for putting monetary values on health outcomes:

- The "human capital" method
- The "willingness-to-pay" (for risk reduction) method
- The "implied values" method

The oldest and simplest of these methods in practice is the human capital one. In this method it is assumed that the objective function that we are trying to maximize through improved health is gross national income in that the measure of value is an individual's output, normally assumed to be equal to the gross labor costs of employment or in some instances simply the earnings of the individual. Thus if a person is unable to work because of illness, we would, using this method, estimate the burden of that illness as being the work output lost, which is equated with the gross labor costs of employing the individual over the relevant time period. If a person dies as a result of illness, the burden is equated with the present value of the gross costs of employment over what would otherwise have been his or her expected working life span.

There are some clear problems with this method. Unless adjustments are made, it means that no weight is attached to retired people, housewives, children (as children), and others not gainfully employed. Also it will give different values to high earners and low earners, which may well be deemed an inequitable basis on which to set health priorities. Further, gross labor costs are at best an approximation of the value of an employee's output. It is also assumed that there is no value to health beyond the capacity it provides to produce output relevant to the gross national product, a somewhat restricted view of the goal of health services.

The willingness-to-pay method, most often applied to the saving of life or, more precisely, the reduction in risk of death, adopts a different value stance. Here the nature of the social welfare function—that is, what it is that is to be maximized from a societal perspective—is based on individuals' values with respect to their willingness to pay for reductions in risk of death (or injury or illness). Thus it is assumed that it is legitimate to ask potential victims or potential sufferers how much they are prepared to pay for a reduction in, say, the risk of death from perhaps 3 in 10,000 to 2 in 10,000. If the response on average to such a question were $5, then the value of a "statistical" life would be $50,000 (that is, 10,000 × $5).

This strategy has some advantage in that the question is put to the potential victim, whose values, it can well be argued, are

the ones that should be allowed to count. Also, the question posed as a probability does seem appropriate. (For example, to ask an individual what he or she is prepared to pay to avoid certain death is almost certainly an unanswerable question.) Whether it is possible to obtain valid answers to such questions, however, remains unclear. It is possible to study the behavior of individuals in risk situations and elicit their implied values (for example, in their willingness to pay for safety devices on their cars), but many of these situations are so far removed from the sorts of choices relevant to health care valuations that the values emerging may not be very useful. Additionally the studies that have been conducted in which this strategy was used yield a very wide range of values—but ones which are normally much higher than those based on the human capital method.

Despite the practical problems of the willingness-to-pay method, it has considerable theoretical advantages in that the valuation basis of individuals' willingness to pay for reductions in the risk of illness and death seems more defensible than that in the human capital method. Of course, if there are equity objections to the method on grounds that priorities in health care should not be based on individuals' ability to pay (on which willingness to pay is inevitably based), then its application has to be handled with care. The use of the method to date has been very restricted and has related more to willingness to pay to reduce the risk of dying than to reduce the risk of having a nonfatal illness and injury.

The third method of evaluating the burden of illness, the implied values method, is somewhat similar to that of willingness of individuals to pay to reduce risk, except that now it is a question of determining what the implied willingness of health care and other health inducing organizations is to pay for various health outputs or reductions in the burden of illness. The basis of the method is simple: if a decision is made, at the margin, to spend $1 million to save a life, then by implication the value of that life must be at least $1 million, otherwise the investment would not be made. If a decision is made not to spend $2 million to save a life, the value of the life is then by implication less than $2 million.

In this process of estimating the implied values of life, ideally one would wish that for similar outputs the willingness of the health care system to pay at the margin of each program would be the same (the condition for an efficient solution). What limited information exists, however, suggests that there is a very wide range of values for like outputs. That does not mean that attempts to make the values explicit should not be pursued. The point is that the aim might first have to be to sort out the inefficiencies implicit in the fact that there is a range of values rather than in the short run to use the values per se in the assessment of the burden of illness. Even then, however, the use of a mean value in the short run would be a possible strategy.

One of the clear advantages of this implied values method is that it does not involve any change in the value system, because the implied values would simply reflect those of the existing system. The method is also relatively easy to apply.

It must be obvious from what has been said that none of the methods outlined is ideal in both principle and practice. The human capital method is simple but tends to treat people like machines, where their only value is as workers. It may be argued, however, that estimates made on this basis can provide at least minimum values of life and sickness avoided. The willingness-to-pay method is, theoretically, to be preferred but has not yet been widely applied even within the mortality field, where it is most frequently found. It also requires substantial investment in data. The implied values method at least provides a basis for improving technical efficiency and is relatively simple to apply. (For a fuller discussion of valuing life, see Mishan 1981 and Linnerooth 1982).

Cost-Effectiveness Comparisons for Priority Setting

At the present stage of development of methods of priority setting it is suggested that a simple, sensible way to proceed is to identify the marginal costs of similar outputs across different programs and adjust the allocation of funds to try to get such marginal costs closer to equality. In other words, if (a) some form of DALY measure can be devised and (b) the cost per DALY gained can be identified on the margin of each existing program, we can then attempt to reallocate resources from programs in which the marginal cost per DALY gained is high to those in which it is low.

The reviews of contemporary empirical experience of cost and outcome relationships contained in chapters of this collection constitutes an important piece of stock taking. Epidemiologic, technologic, and economic characteristics of the main diseases and the principal current interventions are presented in a broadly similar format, which allows estimated average costs per average number of days of healthy life gained to be compared (see figures 1-7 and 1-9).

What conclusions is it possible to draw from these reviews? Of equal importance, what conclusions is it not possible to derive from these data? In the first place, the very existence of such a quantity of information on such a range of interventions is clearly to be welcomed. Too many studies have argued for greater priority in funding for one specific disease or intervention, in the absence of any explicit comparisons. Such studies are the antithesis of an economic way of dealing with the situation, in which the necessity for making trade-offs between activities, in the face of overall resource limitations, is taken as a starting point. A galaxy of alternative patterns of resource use exists, even in the poorest country—in the target groups (for example, adults or children), in the intervention strategy (preventive or case management), and in the type of disease or health problem.

The scope of these reviews, however, is still very modest when compared with the huge quantity of health-related actions coexisting in any country at a given moment, or even in a single small general hospital. The range of available health interventions, differing in input mix, location of treatment, type of patient, type of illness, timing of intervention (primary or secondary preventive, curative, or caring), is so large as to encourage classification, rather than enumeration. The interventions for which cost per DALY gained have been compared are a tiny and nonrepresentative fraction of those available. Indeed, their best use lies more in the illustration of the method of cost-effectiveness in priority setting than for any realistic debate on priorities at a global level. For a full review of priorities, more information is needed and on a more local basis.

Although numerically insignificant, however, the interventions evaluated in the chapters of this collection do have an epidemiologic significance beyond their mere number. They include interventions of known effectiveness against some of the main sources of mortality. Many of these interventions might thus be expected to be prominent among health priorities even if the total number of cost- and outcome-documented additional health interventions were dramatically expanded.

Even for those interventions which are considered, there remains some unevenness in the relevant types of cost and health outcome data presented. In two particular areas this shortage of information may be a critical limitation. First, the sensitivity of the estimated costs per DALY gained is not, in all cases, subject to appraisal. Point estimates, or even "greater than" estimates, are of limited value when there are important margins of uncertainty surrounding them. As indicated above, sensitivity analysis is important in narrowing down the areas in which further information is required and in avoiding overdogmatic priority ranking where the state of available knowledge should indicate caution. Second, the data presented are, in all cases, estimates of the average cost per DALY gained. As emphasized above, such information may lead to inappropriate resource allocation decisions. If studies are conducted to establish the relationship between average costs and marginal costs, then no problem arises. But there are few, if any, such studies for the interventions reviewed in this compilation. By comparing costs and output for health interventions operating at differing scale, we can identify the effects of output variation on total and marginal costs. Once again, in too little of the available empirical work have output variations in relation to costs been assessed.

So, in the absence of empirical information about the relationship between average and marginal cost, what analytical use can be made of the available data? One route to follow is to proceed on the assumption that marginal costs are close to average costs. This is a very special and potentially dangerous assumption. The most casual observation of health care facilities in developing countries suggests that chronic overuse (for example, multiple occupants of hospital beds, "floor patients," long lines at hospital clinics) coexists with equally chronic underuse (for example, less than twenty consultations per month at a health post with a staff of four health workers, and infant immunization rates of under 20 percent). A bold simplifying assumption of equality between marginal and average cost thus seems more sanguine than intuitive.

Without the benefit of either a simplifying assumption or some empirical basis to speculate about the relationship, at current output levels, between marginal and average cost, restraint should be used in applying such data to a review of priorities. This is a disappointing conclusion. If marginal and average costs per DALY were roughly equivalent, if the data incorporated allowances for uncertainty, and if these interventions were taken as in some sense representative of technological options in health care, then the data in figures 1-7 and 1-9 could be interpreted as revealing the following:

- Globally, interventions aimed at children should receive higher priority, whether for case management or prevention, than those aimed at adults.

- Although the average cost per DALY for preventive interventions targeted on children is approximately half of that of case management interventions, the ten most cost-effective activities (at $20 per DALY or less) are a mixture of both preventive and curative actions.

- For adults the overall mean cost for preventive interventions is still lower than for case management, although the differences are now much less.

- The ten most cost-effective interventions for adults entail a mix of preventive and curative actions.

- Some service set providing integrated cure and prevention, rather than discrete vertical programs, would appear to be the most appropriate delivery mechanism.

- The optimal mix of interventions will change as demographic and epidemiologic profiles differ or shift, and thus it needs to be kept under continuous review.

These tempting conclusions are not strictly possible. The data fitted into the cost-effectiveness apparatus are simply not good enough—in quantity and in quality—to warrant such conclusions. This does not mean that the exercise is worthless. If we can reach such conclusions, for a project, country, or region, they are clearly of consequence. That we cannot yet do this—although we may be close—gives urgency to the need to accelerate and improve the collection of relevant data.

Additionally the emphasis on looking at marginal change will normally mean that collecting even crude data on marginal costs at a local level will be better than adopting national or international average cost data. The message is clear. Better to have approximate estimates of local marginal costs than precise, more generalized, average costs.

Concluding Comments

Priority setting is about choice. It is about arranging things in such a way that those policies and programs that are considered most worthwhile stand a better chance of being implemented than others that are considered less worthwhile. In other words, not all needs can be met because resources are scarce. Disease cannot be eliminated; it can only be reduced. So priority should be given to those areas in which the burden of illness can be reduced most per dollar spent. Indeed, we should continue to set priorities according to incremental or decremental changes until it is agreed that no further movement can reduce the burden of disease even more. Clearly, if there are

more or fewer overall resources available, that changes the position—but not the principle. Again if other outputs are deemed relevant (for example, reassurance or information), as we believe they should be, then benefits other than reduced burden of disease must be taken into account.

The link between priority setting and efficiency is crucial in the context not only of the burden of disease per se but of the debate about priority setting more generally. Let us restate clearly what our views are on this matter:

- The need to set priorities arises from the fact that not all illness can be eradicated nor all needs met; this is not just a statement about technology but about the scarcity of resources.

- Priorities are about change. Decisionmakers and policymakers have to try to redeploy resources, allocate some new (but limited) resources, and cut back on the use of existing resources in such a way as to get the most out of whatever resources they have. That means changing deployment.

- Priorities should be based on both benefits and costs. Using scarce resources in one way means, by definition, giving up the opportunity to use them in some other way; providing benefits here means forgoing them there. Priority setting means trying to ensure that those policies that get priority (that is, what gets a higher call on resources) are those providing greatest benefits per dollar spent. If the dollars could have been better spent elsewhere, then they should have been spent elsewhere.

These three statements are central to priority setting. They are very neatly summed up by Shiell, Gerard, and Donaldson (1987) in their critique of studies on the cost of illness: "the total 'costs of illness' can only indicate the benefits of treatment options if an intervention is capable of totally eradicating or entirely preventing the disease in question. This is only likely to be possible in the case of a very few infectious diseases. The most pertinent questions facing policymakers usually relate to scale; that is, by how much should an existing program be expanded or contracted. The answer to this question requires a marginal analysis which compares the expected change in benefits with the costs of the intervention which brings that change about."

From this appendix a number of important conclusions emerge on priority setting in the context of the burden of disease. First, the emphasis of efforts on priority setting ought to be firmly "on the margin": what can be bought with a few dollars more? what shifting of resources from one program to another on the margin can provide the maximum reduction possible of the existing burden of disease? if cuts have to be made, where should this happen to minimize any increase in the burden of disease? Second, developing some common measure of marginal changes in the burden of disease across different diseases is the key to progress in this area. Third, efforts to measure the total burden of any disease ought to be resisted because total burden is not the basis for setting priorities. Fourth, averages are likewise to be resisted except where it can be shown that they are reasonable approximations for marginals. Fifth, care must be exercised to ensure that all relevant factors are accounted for—other nonhealth outputs, equity considerations, uncertainty, discounting. Finally, whatever measures are adopted, sensitivity analysis should be applied to determine how robust the results are to different assumptions.

Notes

Comments from Howard Barnum (World Bank), David Evans (World Health Organization), Karen Gerard (University of Sydney), Richard Morrow (World Health Organization), David Parker (United Nations Children's Fund), Gerald Rosenthal (REACH project), and Carl Stevens (Reed College, Portland, Oregon) were particularly influential in shaping our thinking about this appendix. Remaining errors of fact and interpretation are our own. We are also indebted to Anne Haastrup for her secretarial assistance in preparing and revising the manuscript.

References

Barnum, Howard. 1987. "Evaluating Healthy Days of Life Gained from Health Projects." *Social Science and Medicine* 24(10):833–41.

Behrens, C., and K.-D. Henke. 1988. "Cost of Illness Studies: No Aid to Decision Making? Reply to Shiell et al." *Health Policy* 10:137–41.

Bergner, Marilyn, R. A. Babbitt, W. B. Carter, and B. S. Gilson. 1981. "The Sickness Impact Profile: Development and Final Revision." *Medical Care* 19:787–805.

Culyer, A. J. 1976. *Need and the National Health Service*. London: Martin Robertson.

Drummond, M. F. 1987. "Economic Evaluation and the Rational Diffusion and Use of Health Technology." *Health Policy* 7:309–24.

Drummond, M. F., A. Ludbrook, K. Lowson, and A. Steele. 1986. *Studies in Economic Appraisal in Health Care*. Oxford: Oxford Medical Publications.

Ghana Health Assessment Project Team. 1981. "A Quantitative Method of Assessing the Health Impact of Different Diseases in Less Developed Countries." *International Journal of Epidemiology* 10:73–80.

Hall, J., and G. Masters. 1986. "Measuring Outcomes of Health Services: A Review of Some Available Measures." *Community Health Studies* 10(2):147–55.

Henke, K.-D., and C. S. Behrens. 1986. "The Economic Cost of Illness in the Federal Republic of Germany in the Year 1980." *Health Policy* 6:119–43.

Hodgson, T. A. 1989. "Cost of Illness Studies: No Aid to Decision Making? Comments on the Second Opinion by Shiell et al." *Health Policy* 11:57–60.

Kaplan, R. M., and J. W. Bush. 1982. "Health Related Quality of Life Measurement for Evaluation Research and Policy Analysis." *Health Psychology* 1:61–68.

Linnerooth, Joanne. 1982. "Murdering Statistical Lives . . . ?" In M. W. Jones-Lee, ed., *The Value of Life and Safety*. Amsterdam: North Holland.

Loomes, G., and L. McKenzie. 1989. "The Use of QALYs in Health Care Decision-Making." *Social Science and Medicine* 28(4):299–308.

Mills, Anne. 1985. "Survey and Examples of Economic Evaluation of Health Programs in Developing Countries." *World Health Statistical Quarterly* 38(4):402–31.

Mishan, E. J. 1981. *Cost Benefit Analysis*. London: George Allen and Unwin.

Mooney, G. H. 1992. *Economics, Medicine, and Health Care*. Brighton, Engl.: Wheatsheaf.

Parkerson, G. R., S. H. Gehlback, E. H. Wagner, S. A. James, N. E. Clapp, and L. H. Muhlbaier. 1981. "The Duke-UNC Health Profile: An Adult Health Status Instrument for Primary Care." *Medical Care* 19:806–28.

Petty, Sir W. 1699. *Political Arithmetic or a Discourse Concerning the Extent and Value of Lands, People, Buildings, etc.* London: Robert Clavel.

Prost, A., and N. Prescott. 1984. "Cost-Effectiveness of Blindness Prevention by the Onchocerciasis Control Program in Upper Volta." *Bulletin of the World Health Organization* 62:795–802.

Shiell, A., K. Gerard, and C. Donaldson. 1987. "Cost of Illness Studies: An Aid to Decision-Making?" *Health Policy* 8:317–23.

Torrance, G. W. 1985. "Measurement of Health State Utilities for Economic Appraisal—A Review." *Journal of Health Economics* 5:1–30.

Walsh, J., and K. Warren. 1979. "An Interim Strategy for Disease Control in Developing Countries." *New England Journal of Medicine* 301:967–73.

Williams, Alan. 1985. "Economics of Coronary Artery Bypass Grafting." *British Medical Journal* 291:326–29.

Appendix D

Rationales for Choice in Public Health: The Role of Epidemiology

André Prost and Michel Jancloes

The decisionmaking process in public health has attracted much attention in recent years. The share of the health and social sectors in public and private expenditure has increased to the point that most systems no longer seem to be affordable either in industrial or developing countries. The importance of the economic factor has meant increasing challenge to the rationale for making decisions only on technical grounds, a process which is deeply rooted in a sector managed by a strong technical constituency and which is backed by emotional moves in public opinion expressed as "Health at any cost" or "Nothing is too expensive for the sake of saving life." New processes are introduced, sometimes reluctantly, in the management of the health sector: determination of priorities; advocacy shifting from effectiveness of technology to that of use; preference given to mass benefits over the satisfaction of individual demand; and so on.

Public opinion on health matters makes sectoral choices more than a policy issue: it makes them a political problem. Final decisions result from the combination of technical judgments, economic feasibility (rarely economic consequences), pressure from lobbies, social and psychological implications, and predominantly circumstantial opportunity. Short-term considerations tend to prevail over long-term implications. It is therefore of the utmost importance to identify criteria for decisionmaking which could introduce some rationality in the decisionmaking process and possibly increase the chances of reaching a consensus among all actors: providers, users, payers, and policymakers.

Attempts to use an economic rationale as the main, or even the sole argument, have been opposed by both health providers and users. They cannot accept the imposition, for financial reasons, of any limitation on the degree of sophistication of the technology on one side, or on the benefits they may enjoy on the other. Thus, no consensus can be reached using cost-benefit or cost-effectiveness analyses.

For the last ten years, epidemiology has been promoted as an alternative tool for decisionmaking in health. Epidemiologists aim at describing health and disease phenomena in population groups, their determinants, and changing patterns over certain periods of time. Epidemiology is the instrument of choice for measuring effectiveness. Background data collected before the intervention constitute a resource which must be elaborated into appropriate information in order to document precisely the changes that have occurred and to demonstrate trends. Epidemiological techniques can also be used to assess unforeseen benefits, provided they are accessible through health and demographic indicators.

This role can be extended to the forecasting of the outcome at the planning stage. Usually, several implementation strategies can fit the design of a project and be considered adequate to meet the stated objectives. It is necessary to select the operational strategy that will maximize the outcome in relation to the input. Cost-effectiveness analyses of this type rely heavily on the accuracy of the epidemiological situation and trend analysis.

In addition, epidemiological assessment takes into account the wide range of relationships and interdependencies within health systems and between health and other sectors. The comparative study of the importance of and interactions between health determinants may bring unforeseen side effects to light. It also shows the effect on the health sector of decisions made in other sectors, such as taxation and financial measures, agricultural and industrial reforms, and, more generally, public policies.

Because epidemiology has become the key factor for evaluation and for effectiveness analyses in health, there has been an increasing tendency to use it at earlier stages of the process, namely at the stages of planning, policy setting, and decisionmaking. The technical method used in this discipline together with its ability to rank priorities and to identify selective programs would seem to reflect the concerns of all the actors and make conclusions readily acceptable. Our aim in this appendix is to analyze the advantages and the difficulties of this approach as well as the challenges that epidemiologists face in making a relevant use of their technique. We argue that, although epidemiology is an essential tool for policy setting, it cannot be the ultimate rationale for decisionmaking in health.

Current Methods

The principal conceptual problem lies in the definition of health indicators which represent the variety of diseases, aggregate the differences among population subgroups, and account for changes over a period of time. A single measure of health status has never been unequivocally accepted; it may even never have existed. Because of this difficulty, analyses have usually been limited to the comparison of two diseases, or to the comparative effectiveness of control strategies for a single disease. The lack of a standard measure of health status considerably hampers the use of epidemiology as an instrument for planning and policy setting.

Two methods have been designed in recent years to interpret conceptually the role of epidemiology in public health. One method uses a quantitative compounded indicator—the number of disability-adjusted life-days—to assess the effect of disease.[1] Thus, results are applied to the process of health resource allocation and management (Ghana Health Assessment Project Team 1981; Morrow, Smith, and Nimo 1982; Romeder and McWhinnie 1977). The ranking of diseases is established by using the average estimated number of healthy days lost in a lifetime as a result of disease episodes. The loss attributable to every single disease is the sum of healthy days lost through acute illness episodes (temporary disability), through chronic conditions and sequelae (partial or complete disablement), and through premature death (considered equivalent to complete disablement). The loss to the community is derived by multiplying the average loss attributable to every single disease by the annual incidence of each disease in the community.

Another method is the "measurement iterative loop" developed at McMaster University, Canada (Tugwell and others 1984). It is a framework intended to guide informed decisionmaking in health. The seven successive steps reflect a logical progression from the assessment of the burden of illnesses through hypothesis generation about the causes of disease, and about the efficiency and the effectiveness of prevention and treatment procedures, to evaluating the effect in a community. It is an approach of a programmatic nature, based on a rational scheme of planning, including an in-depth analysis of sector needs and constraints. Epidemiology is used in the determination of priorities for action, which result not only from the assessment of sectoral needs but also from an assessment of effect, and thereof from cost-effectiveness choices.

Both methods are attractive. They represent valuable contributions to the theory of the decisionmaking process in health. Unfortunately, their application to real situations does not meet the high expectations raised at the conceptual stage. We shall attempt to determine reasons for failure.

Validation of the Results

Quantitative epidemiology uses mathematical tools: averages, percentages, ratios, and so on. The resulting figure, which for practical purposes is one single number, tends to express available information with a degree of precision which far from reflects the confidence limits of the assumptions. The development of computerized systems of data collection and information storage increases the illusion of exactness. It can be misleading, especially for nontechnical people who are unfamiliar with the critical assessment of the validity of results.

For example, suppose an estimated incidence of severe gastroenteritis of 130 cases per 1,000 population per year: a critical assessment should consider whether this figure is based on the records of outpatient visits in health clinics or on a survey of a population sample, whether the result has been adjusted to account for differences in the age and sex distribution between the survey population and the whole population of the country, what recall period was used in the survey, what criteria were used in the definition of "severe cases," how the seasonal variations have been taken into account, and so on. The confidence limits represent the range in which the majority of results from different sources will be included. The value of the assumptions and their confidence limits vary between diseases because of varying levels of precision in the data base and because of differences in the complexity of the epidemiological pattern of diseases.

Striking differences in the ranking of diseases by order of importance can occur, depending on the choice of the upper or the lower limit of the range of use in the calculations. Such ranking also depends on the magnitude of the multiplier effect introduced by the various mathematical formula aiming at the calculation of a synthetic indicator (see note 1).

Validity of Indicators

The ranking of diseases for the determination of priorities necessitates the use of a single indicator to allow for comparisons. Thus, ranking of diseases can be established by using, for example, the death toll, or the incidence in the community, or the degree and duration of the resulting disablement. The selection of the indicator represents a value judgment which may reduce the freedom of the decisionmaker and somehow preempt the decision. Using mortality figures could mean, for example, that the social and economic cost of disablement is obliterated. Using national averages does not allow for the identification of population groups especially deprived or particularly at risk.

The use of a compounded indicator is an attempt to reduce these biases. The method of disability-adjusted life-days (DALDs) combines the effects of mortality, morbidity, and disablement; it uses life expectancy as the reference period. There is no significant bias in the analysis when relatively similar health conditions affecting the same age groups are to be compared. For example, the first mention of this indicator in the literature (Dempsey 1947) was applied to a comparison of mortality due to tuberculosis, heart disease, and cancer; all these diseases are chronic and are prevalent mainly in adults.

More recently, the proposal to use the DALDs lost indicator as a general method for assessing the effect of diseases (Ghana

Health Assessment Project Team 1981) has resulted in more complex combinations. It aggregates not only the effects of mortality, morbidity, and disablement, but also it combines the effect of acute and chronic conditions, in all age groups from birth to death. The authors did not discuss the implicit value judgments of this method. For example, the assumption that "the younger the death, the greater the loss to the community" derives directly from computing the difference between the life expectancy and the age at death. It implies that the death of a child is a greater loss than the death of a young adult in the productive period of his or her life simply because life expectancy for a child is much greater than it is for an adult. It implies for the same reason that maternal mortality is of less consequence to the community than the simultaneous death of the newborn. Also, by definition, the measure assumes that one year of complete disability is equivalent to one year of premature death. It could be argued that meeting the needs of a disabled person places a heavier burden on the community. Finally, mixing together the effects of mortality and morbidity results in minimizing the social and economic cost of common though nonfatal diseases, which may represent up to 80 percent of the workload of outpatient clinics and a large share of drug expenditure.

It is obvious that the aggregation of morbidity and mortality into a single measure necessarily involves making value judgments about the relative weights that should be assigned to each component. The assumption that additional years of life are equally valuable, regardless of the age at which they accrue, conflicts with the common notion that adult mortality is more serious than child death. Weighting procedures may alleviate the difficulty. It can be reflected through the assignment of a zero weight to years of life added before age fifteen, and a weight of one to those added beyond age fifteen. Any other weight could be proposed and discussed. This method of weighting for age preference can be combined with the relative weighting of disability and death, and with weighting for time preference (that is, assigning lower weights to benefits which occur in a distant future). Previous studies have shown that assessments of the effect of a disease and of the effectiveness of a health intervention are very sensitive to the choice of different weights (Prost and Prescott 1984; Barnum 1987). Introducing productivity weights (that is, allocating different weights according to the status of the patient as a producer for the community) has even greater policy implications. Thus, there is no straightforward weighting procedure which could lead to noncontroversial measurements. On the contrary, the selection of weights results from value judgments and therefore carries the risk of further distorting the objectivity of the method.

Quality of the Data

Good quality data bases do not exist in most countries. There is no better consensus on the incidence of home accidents in Europe than on the number of diarrheal episodes in African children. When available, data are often limited to specific diseases and they do not cover the broad spectrum of health disorders. In many developing countries, in the absence of any reliable data base, epidemiologists use assumptions derived from scattered surveys, from incomplete reporting systems, or, even worse, from hospital statistics.

To improve the quality of data, health planners direct considerable effort toward the collection of health statistics. An example is given by the comprehensive epidemiological survey conducted by the health services of Mali with support from the World Bank (Duflo and others 1986). The objective of this survey was to help design a regional health development project. The survey was conducted in a random sample of villages during a period of one month. Specific morbidity and mortality rates were determined and were used to estimate the number of days lost as a result of the diseases observed.

This methodologically sound survey provided an accurate picture of the disease situation, with a reasonable degree of precision. It emphasized the relative importance of neglected pathologies, such as eye diseases, cardiovascular disease, and hemoglobinopathy. It did not, however, change the preliminary ranking of the main diseases (malaria, gastroenteritis, measles, malnutrition, pregnancy complications, respiratory infections) which had been established on the basis of poor quality data available from health providers in the area. It can be argued that data collected at a high cost during the survey have not yielded any better information for the project design. The additional precision in the assessment of the burden of diseases made justification of the project more difficult to challenge. More precise data are of a greater value as a baseline for future evaluation of project benefits. They were not used at the planning stage.

Important in the establishment of a data base is that the system be conceived in relation to the needs of the users or potential users. Too often, data which are critically needed are missing, or they are impossible to retrieve from bulk information. Too many epidemiologists, nationally and internationally, perceive their function as that of collecting the greatest possible amount of information in order to combine all possible variables. In fact, the role of epidemiologists is to tailor the collection of data, using a problem-solving approach, in accordance with hypotheses generated at a preliminary stage.

Comprehensive in Contrast to Selective Care

The ranking of diseases, based on whatever epidemiological indicator is selected, singles out a list of diseases or individual health conditions as the target for control, either because they represent a public health scourge, or because of their socioeconomic effect. Six diseases in Ghana (Ghana Health Assessment Project Team 1981) and eight in Mali (Duflo and others 1986) account for 50 percent of the total number of disability-adjusted life-days lost to the community every year. It seems essential, at first glance, to concentrate all efforts on combating these diseases, or the most important of them, because larger benefits will accrue to the community. Thus, the search for maximum efficiency leads to the development of disease-oriented programs, using specially designed control methods (case finding, case management, evaluation), selective logistical support, and targeted retraining of staff.

One application of this concept is the Selective Primary Health Care Strategy proposed by Walsh and Warren (1979). The ranking of priority diseases is based on the assessment of their effect in the community and of the effectiveness of available control methods using the implicit value judgment that reducing infant mortality to improve life expectancy is the objective of efficient health services. Therefore, selective primary health care has focused in most cases on diarrhea and diseases preventable by vaccine, and activities have been almost exclusively concentrated on oral rehydration and immunization campaigns.

This strategy is both conceptually and practically misleading. First, it relates cost figures to disease control effectiveness and not to health benefits. It does not consider that the allocation of resources to one activity can have various types of benefits. For example, in an experiment in Zaire, the villages in which successful treatment for intestinal worms had been carried out have shown improvements in immunization compliance, tuberculosis screening, and health education. There was also a decrease in the average number of patient visits to the health facilities (Jancloes 1989). In such a program, parasite control is used as a catalyst to trigger the compliance of the people with health services, and thus to progress toward the real objective of improving the health of every family member.

Second, on the practical side, it is almost impossible, at the peripheral level, to focus on a limited number of diseases. Health services are multivalent by nature. The definition of tasks results from the people's demand for care and from a comprehensive public health strategy which combines the provision of curative care, prevention, hygiene education, and interaction with other sectors that influence health. Patients have been reluctant to use the facilities available in pilot projects set up to test the feasibility of the selective primary health care strategy, mainly because they realized that these facilities could not cover the broad spectrum of their complaints and that they would have to visit another health post for complementary treatment.

Thus, the determination of "priority diseases" is not only misleading with regard to allocative efficiency but it ignores the multisectorality of the health determinants. It ignores observations that some of the most significant progress in health has derived from nonmedical interventions (for example, decrease in infant mortality with rising education levels, historical decrease in tuberculosis incidence before any efficient control method has been available, and so on).

The Demand for Health Services

The perception of health needs by people differ, often strikingly, from the assessment of needs by epidemiologists. Whereas the latter determine risk groups and priority diseases on the basis of various technical criteria (life expectancy, mortality, and the like), communities use a different value system, which places greater importance on individual conditions and on adult morbidity, for example. Whereas epidemiological surveys might conclude that diarrhea and measles are the priority diseases, a sociological survey might reveal, for example, that hernia, hemorrhoids, blindness, and complications of delivery are the priority concerns of the population.

Moreover, the epidemiological method emphasizes the importance of the determinants of diseases, leading to preventive rather than to curative actions. The failure to appreciate the primacy of prevention is now shared by the general public and by a majority of the health profession (Terris 1980). Policies based on an epidemiological rationale are generally opposed by both providers and users of health services. Especially at times of economic stringency, programs of health promotion and disease prevention are easier targets for short-term savings than is specialized curative care. This attitude coincides with the expectations of the consumers and with the dominant position of the health professionals in the curative technical structures.

In almost all cases, an ethical conflict arises between epidemiological and sociological methods. Should planners ignore it, the community will develop sideline channels to meet the demand (private practice, traditional healers, uncontrolled sale of drugs, and so on). The result is the lack of users' commitment to the successful implementation of the program and the absence of a rational use of resources despite intensive planning efforts.

In the case of the Mali project mentioned above, decisionmakers took the demand aspect into account at the initial stage. They considered that ensuring the effectiveness of the referral level in the treatment of adult diseases was essential to the credibility of the program. In a second phase, they took into account the epidemiologically determined needs, with village interventions aimed at reducing child morbidity and mortality.

The Decisionmaking Process

Decisionmakers act on their own judgment as to whether they themselves or the society at large could derive more benefits from the proposed strategy than from competing health interventions (and sometimes nonhealth interventions). The benefits are both those assessed by project evaluation and those perceived subjectively.

Decisionmaking is a complex process which involves a number of determinants: political, sociological, psychological, cultural, economic, technical, sometimes religious, and so on. Opportunity, feasibility, short-term rather than long-term considerations, legal and administrative settings, financing systems, and institutional framework are also essential. Decisionmakers' approval of programs is often lacking because they do not give indirect benefits the same weight as technicians do. In periods of economic stringency, the practical problem is not to determine sectoral priorities but to find politically realistic ways of moving toward greater economic efficiency in the very short run, considering the role and the power of the actors involved (van der Werff 1986).

Experience has proved that the technical rationale, as provided by, among other things, epidemiological analyses, is relatively low in the hierarchy of factors that influence decisionmaking. The failure of the economic rationality to become the instrument of choice for decisionmaking gives little chance of success to the epidemiological rationality to fulfill this function. Had it been the case, tobacco would have already been banned from the face of the earth.

The comparison of epidemiology with economics as a tool for decisionmaking can be elaborated further in the context of development projects. External assistance sources use efficiency and effectiveness to demonstrate to their constituencies that a high rate of return is obtained. Thus epidemiology is used to quantify health returns and to maximize these returns through appropriate choices at the planning stage. On the other side of the partnership, national authorities and deciders responsible for implementation are sensitive to preferences derived from the value system of the communities. They are in the midst of the ethical conflict described above. Attempts to impose epidemiology as an indisputable tool for decisionmaking, in view of the neutral character of the scientific analysis, are perceived as a limitation to the freedom of judgment, and as a technique to impose targets and objectives which meet the concerns of donors rather than the needs of beneficiaries.

Concluding Remarks

Epidemiological information should be collected as early as possible in public health programs because the quality of any future evaluation depends on the accuracy of baseline data. The lack of such data may hamper the assessment of effectiveness and thus be detrimental to the continuation of activities. There is no alternative to epidemiological methods when evaluating effects on public health.

Epidemiological techniques provide snapshots of the situation as well as indications on trends. They may even allow for a ranking of diseases, using whatever indicator is relevant to the stated objective and provided that associated ethical issues have been properly explored and accounted for. The use of epidemiology for choices in health policy implies a double leap forward: a leap from the ranking of diseases to the setting of priority objectives for action, and a leap from technical priorities to allocating resources on a selective basis.

In both cases, epidemiology alone cannot substantiate the move. The tools used in this discipline are not relevant, and results are often misleading. At the planning stage, objectives are determined on the basis of all the factors involved in the decisionmaking process. The results of epidemiological analyses are to be considered among other factors. The importance of each of these other factors and their interactions should balance the importance of epidemiologically assessed needs. The choice of the epidemiological indicator influences largely the outcome of the results. Thus, these results should not be used to preempt the decision. Epidemiology is not the neutral tool which can lead to unequivocal and unchallengeable choices.

At the beginning of this appendix, we stated that it was of the utmost importance to identify criteria for decisionmaking which could form the basis for a consensus among all actors in the health sector: providers, users, payers, and policymakers. Epidemiology, as a science, is universally praised. Its implications for behavioral changes in users of health services and for the setting of public policies are not readily acceptable unless an intensive educational effort is undertaken. Thus, it is evident that any attempt from the payers and from the deciders to impose policy decisions on the basis of an epidemiological rationality will be rejected. Similar attempts from the health professionals can be opposed by their political and financial partners as a way of preempting the decision for technical reasons. This conflict can be detrimental, because the validity of epidemiology as an analytical tool is at risk to be denied, for reasons of policy implications and not of genuine criticism.

Notes

The authors wish to thank David Parker, Senior Adviser, Health Financing of the United Nations Children's Fund for his extensive review of this chapter.

1. The average number of disability-adjusted life-days lost to the community by each patient with a disease (L) can be calculated as follows (L = Days lost due to [premature death] + [disability before death] + [chronic disability] + [acute illness]):

$$
\begin{aligned}
L = &\ (C/100 \ \times\ [E(A_o) - (A_d - A_o)] \ \times\ 365.25) \\
&+ (C/100 \ \times\ (A_d - A_o) \ \times\ D_{od}/100) \ \times\ 365.25) \\
&+ (Q/100 \ \times\ E(A_o) \ \times\ D/100 \ \times\ 365.25) \\
&+ ([100 - C - Q] / 100 \ \times\ t),
\end{aligned}
$$

in which A_o = average age at onset of the disease; A_d = average age at death attributable to the disease; $E(A_o)$ = life expectancy (in years) at age A_o; C = case-fatality rate (expressed as a percentage); D_{od} = percentage of disablement between onset of the disease and each death attributable to it; Q = percentage of permanently disabled among patients who have recovered; D = percentage of disablement of those permanently disabled; t = average period of temporary disablement during acute episodes; I = annual incidence of the disease (new cases per 1,000 population).

As a result, the total loss to the community attributable to cases of the disease occurring in any single year (R) is the total number of days $R = L \times I$ (per group of 1,000 population) (Ghana Health Assessment Project Team 1981).

References

Barnum, Howard. 1987. "Evaluating Healthy Days of Life Gained from Health Projects." *Social Science and Medicine* 24:833–41.

Dempsey, Michael. 1947. "Decline in Tuberculosis: The Death Rate Fails to Tell the Entire Story." *American Review of Tuberculosis* 56:157–64.

Duflo, Bernard, and others. 1986. "Estimation de l'impact des principales maladies en zone rurale malienne." *Revue d'Epidémiologie et de Santé publique* 34:405–18.

Ghana Health Assessment Project Team. 1981. "A Quantitative Method of Assessing the Health Impact of Different Diseases in Less Developed Countries." *International Journal of Epidemiology* 10:73–80.

Jancloes, Michel. 1989. "The Case for Control: Forging a Partnership with Decision Makers." In D. W. T. Crompton and others, eds., *Ascariasis and Its Prevention and Control.* London: Taylor and Francis.

Morrow, R. H., P. G. Smith, and K. P. Nimo. 1982. "Assessing the Impact of Disease." *World Health Forum* 3:331–35.

Prost, A., and N. Prescott. 1984. "Cost Effectiveness of Blindness Prevention by the Onchocerciasis Control Programme in Upper Volta." *Bulletin of the World Health Organization* 62:795–802.

Romeder, J. M., and J. R. McWhinnie. 1977. "Potential Years of Life Lost between Ages 1 and 70: An Indicator of Premature Mortality for Health Planning." *International Journal of Epidemiology* 6:143–51.

Terris, Milton. 1980. "Epidemiology as a Guide to Health Policy." *Annual Review of Public Health* 1:323–44.

Tugwell, P., K. J. Bennett, D. Sackett, and B. Haynes. 1984. "Relative Risks, Benefits, and Costs of Intervention." In K. S. Warren and A. A. F. Mahmoud, eds., *Tropical and Geographical Medicine.* New York: McGraw-Hill.

van der Werff, Albert. 1986. "Planning and Management for Health in Periods of Economic Stringency and Instability: A Contingency Approach." *International Journal of Health Planning and Management* 1:227–40.

Walsh, J. A., and K. S. Warren. 1979. "Selective Primary Health Care: An Interim Strategy for Disease Control in Developing Countries." *New England Journal of Medicine* 301:967–74.